D0146609

IMMUNOLOGY, IMMUNOPATHOLOGY & IMMUNITY

fifth edition

Stewart Sell, MD
Professor
Department of Pathology and Laboratory Medicine
University of Texas Houston Medical School
Houston, Texas

Contributing authors
Ira Berkower, MD, PhD
Chief, Laboratory of Immunoregulation
Division of Allergenics & Parasitology
Office of Vaccine Research
Center for Biologics, FDA
Bethesda, Maryland

Edward E. Max, MD, PhD
Acting Chief, Laboratory of Cell and Viral Regulation
Food and Drug Administration
Center for Biologics, Evaluation, and Research
Bethesda, Maryland

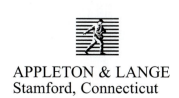

APPLETON & LANGE
Stamford, Connecticut

Notice: The authors and the publisher of this volume have taken care to
make certain that the doses of drugs and schedules of treatment are correct
and compatible with the standards generally accepted at the time of
publication. Nevertheless, as new information becomes available, changes in
treatment and in the use of drugs become necessary. The reader is advised to
carefully consult the instruction and information material included in the
package insert of each drug or therapeutic agent before administration.
This advice is especially important when using new or infrequently used drugs.
The publisher disclaims any liability, loss, injury, or damage incurred as
a consequence, directly or indirectly, or the use and application of any of
the contents of the volume.

Copyright © 1996 by Appleton & Lange
A Simon & Schuster Company

All rights reserved. This book, or any parts thereof, may not be used or
reproduced in any manner without written permission. For information,
address Appleton & Lange, Four Stamford Plaza, PO Box 120041, Stamford, CT 06912-0041

96 97 98 99 / 10 9 8 7 6 5 4 3 2 1

Prentice Hall International (UK) Limited, London
Prentice Hall of Australia Pty. Limited, Sydney
Prentice Hall Canada, Inc., Toronto
Prentice Hall Hispanoamericana, S.A., Mexico
Prentice Hall of India Private Limited, New Delhi
Prentice Hall of Japan, Inc., Tokyo
Simon & Schuster Asia Pte. Ltd., Singapore
Editora Prentice Hall do Brasil Ltda., Rio de Janeiro
Prentice Hall, Upper Saddle River, New Jersey

Library of Congress Cataloging-in-Publication Data

Sell, Stewart, 1935–
    Immunology, immunopathology, and immunity / Stewart Sell;
contributing authors, Ira Berkower, Edward E. Max—5th ed.
        p.   cm.
    ISBN 0-8385-4064-3 (alk. paper)
    1. Immunology. 2. Immunopathology. 3. Immunity.   I. Berkower,
Ira.   II. Max, Edward E.   III. Title.
    [DNLM: 1. Immune System—physiology. 2. Immune System–
–physiopathology. 3. Immunity. 4. Immunologic Diseases.   QW 504
S467i 1996]
QR181.S39   1996
616.07′9—dc20
DNLM/DLC
for library of Congress

ISBN   0-8385-4064-3

9 780838 540640   90000

NB21

Acquisitions Editor: John Dolan
Production Editor: Chris Langan
Designer: Libby Schmitz
Senior Art Coordinator: Maggie Belis Darrow
Illustrator: Alex Teshin Associates

PRINTED IN THE UNITED STATES OF AMERICA

Contents

To: William O. Weigle, Ph.D. and Richard W. Dutton, Ph.D. for their exceptional contributions to the understanding of how cells of the immune system interact to produce tolerance and immunity.

Preface

The goal of this edition of Immunology, Immunopathology and Immunity is to present a systematic accounting of both the beneficial and destructive of the immune system, with emphasis on the effector mechanisms. Since publication of the 1987 edition dramatic advances have occurred in understanding the molecular basis of cell signalling and cellular interactions, as well as some immune mechanisms in immunity and disease, requiring extensive updating and rewriting.

The current availability of many new immunology books begs the question of "Which niche is left unfilled?" This book is unique due to its emphasis on what the immune system DOES. On one hand it protects us from both internal (ie, cancer) and external (ie. infectious diseases) damage, but on the other hand it can be turned against us and cause many diseases: the double-edged-sword. Not only are basic principles of immunology suitable for an introductory course presented, but also there is coverage, in a well organized way, of resource information on immune and infectious diseases normally only found in large reference books. This breadth of material is emphasized in the division of the text into three parts, Immunology, Immunopathology and Immunity.

In the first part, Immunology, the basic structure and function of the immune system is presented with the purpose of providing the essential facts required to understand the second part of the text, Immunopathology. Thus, the immunology section is not intended to present in exhaustive detail all the fine nuances of the induction and control of immunity, but to concentrate on those fundamentals that are believed to be essential for further understanding of immune mechanisms. First the basic structure of the cells and organs is presented. Then, because of the great advances in understanding immune induction and expression, two new authors were sought in order to provide more precise expertise on selected topics in basic immunology. Ira Berkhower provides state of the art understanding of the acquisition of immune recognition and cell interactions in induction and control of immune responses. Similarly, Ed Max condenses an enormous amount of information on the molecular biology and action of immunoglobulins and receptors that should provide the reader with just the right amount of information required for following later chapters. Part one is concluded with chapters on basic aspects of inflammation and wound healing. Understanding basic aspects of inflammation is essential, since immune effector mechanisms responsible for effecting immune diseases and immune protection are essentially variations on the theme of inflammation.

The second part of the book, Immunopathology is, in turn, divided into two parts. The first part, immunopathologic mechanisms, presents the seven immunologic effector mechanisms. Understanding how these mechanisms act individually is essential in unraveling how different mechanisms may interact to produce a particular disease. The effects and characteristics of the way these mechanisms operate are contrasted and compared. In the second part details of specific immune disorders such as drug allergies, skin reactions and auto-immune diseases as examples of the effects of different immune mechanisms are presented, as well as the role of immune mechanisms in transplantation and tolerance. These mechanisms not only cause disease (immunopathology), but also play critical roles in defense against foreign invaders (immune defense mechanisms). Understanding how the immune mechanisms work in producing lesions provides the background for how they work in protecting us against infectious diseases and cancer.

The third part of the book, Immunity, covers how immune mechanisms act in infectious diseases and cancer, as well as what happens when they are unable to function, immune deficiency diseases, and how they may be directed to provide protection, i.e. vaccination. Finally there is a separate new chapter on HIV infection and AIDS that includes up-to-date comprehension of how HIV infection interacts with the immune system to produce AIDS.

Overall this book provides a systematic directed look into how the immune system works that is not available in other immunology books. Most immunology books are designed for basic immunology courses. As such they provide either a brief superficial view of immune induction and a description of immune products for the quick course, or in depth coverage of experimental details and protocols for the more serious student with little space for what is important for students of the medical professions, i.e., how immune effector mechanisms protect us and how they cause disease. Larger multi-authored books on clinical immunology may be excellent reference books to look up a specific subject but because they are multi-authored usually do provide more details and contain overlaps that detract from systematic, organized presentation. Our aim is to present a systematic and readable account of immunology, immunopathology and immunity for those who are interested in how the immune system works in causing and in preventing disease. We hope that this book will fill a niche between the dry basic immunology books and the encyclopedic clinical immunology treatises and be just what the doctor ordered for understanding immunopathology and immunity.

part
I

Immunology

1

Introduction

Immunology

Immunology is the study of the *system* through which we identify infectious agents as different from ourselves and defend or protect ourselves against their damaging effects. From the time of conception, the human organism faces attack from a wide variety of infectious agents and must have ways to identify and react to them. We have many physiologic mechanisms that adjust to environmental variables such as temperature, supply of food and water, and physical injury. The immune system provides us with highly specialized ways to defend ourselves against invasion and colonization by foreign organisms. This defensive ability is called *immunity*.

Immunity

The term *immunity* comes from the Latin word *immunitas*, which means "protection from." In legal terms, immunity means that the protected person is not subject to certain laws (eg, diplomatic immunity) or is exempt from certain duties (eg, not required to serve in the armed forces). In clinical terms, immunity means protection from certain diseases, particularly infectious diseases. For instance, the commonly used statement "She is immune to measles" indicates that the person referred to has had measles once (or has been vaccinated against measles) and will not get measles again. This is a form of **acquired immunity** or **adaptive immunity**.

The protective mechanisms of the body are divided into two major types: innate and adaptive (Table 1–1). Innate resistance is present in all normal individuals, does not require previous exposure to be effective, and operates on different infectious agents in the same way

TABLE 1–1. COMPARISON OF INNATE AND ADAPTIVE (ACQUIRED) IMMUNITY

Characteristic	Innate Immunity	Adaptive Immunity
Specificity	Nonspecific, indiscriminate	Specific, discriminate
Mechanical	Skin, mucous membrane	Immune induced reactive fibrosis (granuloma)
Humoral	pH, lysozyme, serum proteins	Immunoglobulin antibodies
Cellular	White blood cells	Specifically sensitized lymphocytes
Induction	Constitutive, does not require immunization	Requires previous contact (immunization)

every time the individual is exposed. The adaptive, specific immune defense system does not become active until the individual is exposed to the infectious agent; it requires stimulation or **immunization** to become activated. It has the capacity to identify foreign agents and distinguish foreign from self (self and nonself discrimination). It is mediated by products that specifically recognize one agent and do not act on a different agent. In an infectious disease the adaptive immune system is activated during the first infection, so that upon subsequent contact no disease will occur. The immune system has learned to recognize the infectious agent and react specifically to it with an accelerated protective response. This is termed **immune memory**.

INNATE IMMUNITY

Innate defense mechanisms against foreign invaders include mechanical barriers, secreted products, and inflammatory cells (Fig. 1–1). Innate resistance is present at all times in normal individuals. Its effectiveness may be modulated by physiologic conditions (nutrition, age, hormone levels, etc.). It does not distinguish among microorganisms of different species and does not alter in intensity upon reexposure. One of the major nonspecific defense systems is the epithelial surface of the body. Externally, the skin, and internally, the mucous membrane linings of the gastrointestinal tract and the epithelium of the airways of the lungs, provide mechanical barriers to invasion. Secreted products, such as acid in the stomach, lysozyme in tears, sebaceous gland secretions, and certain proteins in the blood, are toxic to potential invaders. White blood cells are attracted to sites of infection by products of infecting organisms or necrotic tissue and attack the invaders.

When the protective epithelial barriers are breached (as by a cut or abrasion of the skin or by penetration of invading organisms past the protective lining of the airways of the lungs), and organisms begin to grow in the tissues of the body, a more specific and more powerful back-up defense system is needed. Since most infectious organisms

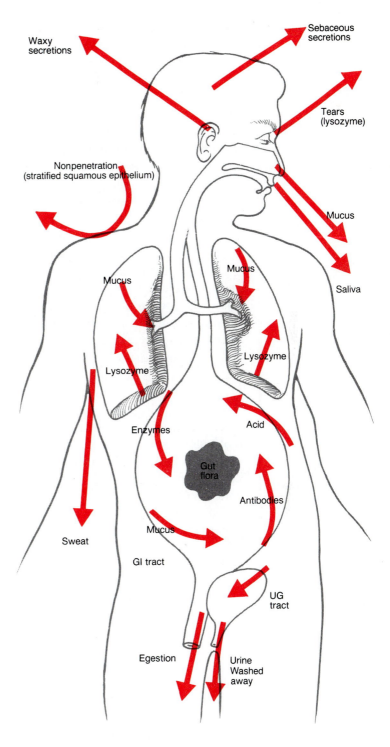

Figure 1–1. Innate immunity. Innate defenses against infectious agents include skin and mucous membrane barriers and secretions that are bacteriostatic or remove foreign agents by washing them away.

**ADAPTIVE
IMMUNITY**

can multiply rapidly and the defensive reaction must be directed specifically to the infection and not to host tissues, this system must be activated quickly, be precisely directed, and be very destructive. These are the characteristics of adaptive immunity.

Immunization (or vaccination) is the process of stimulating adaptive resistance; once induced, a discreet "state of immunity" exists. The adaptive immune system is quiescent until stimulated by a specific infection (**immunizing event**). It is capable of exquisitely distinguishing among microorganisms and significantly alters in its intensity and response time upon reexposure. In normal individuals, the adaptive immune system contains the potential to be activated. This potential is converted to actuality by exposure to substances recognized as foreign by the immune system (**immunogens** or **antigens**).

There are two major arms of the immune response: **humoral** and **cellular**. Humoral immunity is mediated by soluble protein molecules known as **antibodies**; cellular immunity is mediated by specifically sensitized white blood cells known as lymphocytes. **Immunization** or **vaccination** may activate two different classes of lymphocytes. The cells responsible for antibody production are in the **B-lymphocyte** series; those for cellular immunity are in the **T-lymphocyte** series (Table 1–2). Antibodies are made by the B-cells after activation. **Antibodies** belong to a family of molecules found in the blood or external secretions termed **immunoglobulins**. Antibodies are protein molecules that react specifically with structures (**epitopes**) on infecting organisms through specialized receptors (**binding sites** or **paratopes**) on the antibody molecule. **Specifically sensitized T-cells** also have an antibody-like receptor that recognizes antigens. Activated T-cells proliferate and differentiate in specialized organs in the body (**lymphoid organs**) and are released into the blood through specialized vessels known as lymphatics. This allows rapid delivery to other parts of the body, where an infection may be located.

The response of the immune system to immunization has been compared to a motor neuron reflex arc; ie, there is an afferent, efferent, and central limb (Fig. 1–2). *Afferent* refers to delivery of the immunogen to cells of the immune system; *central* refers to the response of the

TABLE 1–2. TWO MAJOR ARMS OF IMMUNITY

	Humoral	Cellular
Cell line	B cells, plasma cells	T cells
Product	Antibody	Sensitized cells
Protection against	Bacteria, viruses	Viruses, mycobacteria, fungi

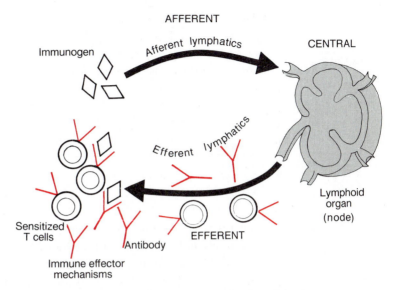

Figure 1–2. Afferent, central, and efferent limbs of the immune response. Afferent—delivery of immunogen to lymphoid organ (lymph node). Central—recognition of antigen by cells of the immune system and production of specifically sensitized cells and humoral antibody. Efferent—delivery of immune products to site of antigen localization and activation of immune effector mechanisms.

reacting lymphoid organs resulting in production of antibody and/or sensitized cells; *efferent* refers to the delivery of these products to the site of antigen deposition. When the antibody or sensitized cells react with antigen (infectious agent) in the tissues, very powerful immune defense mechanisms are activated. Once immunization has occurred, the immunized individual will respond with a more rapid and more intense response upon second exposure to the same immunogen (secondary response or immunological memory).

When an infectious agent begins to grow in our bodies, a "race of life" is started. The race is between the rate of expansion of the infection and the ability of our immune systems to combat the infection. The invaders of our bodies have many ways of evading both innate and the adaptive resistance. These include such properties as the release of "toxins," the formation of protective coatings, the ability to localize in inaccessible sites, and the ability to exist within our own cells or even be incorporated into our DNA, thus evading recognition or destruction (see Chapter 25). Thus, the immune system must be able to react quickly, specifically, and powerfully to an infection. Some of the critical characteristics of the adaptive immune system are listed in Table 1–3.

TABLE 1–3. FUNCTIONAL ABILITIES OF THE ADAPTIVE IMMUNE SYSTEM

1. *Specific recognition* of many different foreign invaders
2. *Rapid synthesis* of immune products upon contact with invaders
3. *Quick delivery* of the immune products to the site of infection.
4. *Variability of effector defensive mechanisms* to combat infectious agents with different properties
5. *Nonself direction* of the defensive mechanisms specifically to foreign invaders rather than one's own tissue
6. *Deactivation* mechanisms to turn off the system when the invader has been cleared

The Inflammatory Response

The response of our bodies to an infection occurs in the form of **inflammation**. The hallmark of an inflammatory response is the passage of proteins, fluid, and cells from the blood into focal areas in tissues. The result is the local delivery of agents that can effectively combat infections. During an inflammatory response, components of the innate and adaptive resistance mechanisms are often both used. These include inflammatory cells, products of inflammatory cells, certain blood proteins (inflammatory mediators), and common pathways of response (see Chapters 8 and 9).

Initiation of an inflammatory response begins by an increase in blood flow to infected tissues and by the separation of the cells lining the blood vessels or capillaries, followed by emigration of cells into the involved tissue (Fig. 1–3). Increased blood flow and vascular permeability allows fluid and/or cells to enter into the tissues. The gross manifestations of acute inflammation were first clearly recognized by Celsus about 25 B.C. as the cardinal signs of inflammation (Table 1–4). The signs of inflammation are manifestations of increased blood flow and infiltration of tissues by inflammatory proteins and cells. Increased blood flow causes redness and increased temperature. The presence of fluid and red blood cells in tissues is grossly recognized by swelling (edema) and redness. White blood cell (inflammatory cell) infiltrations cause a white color. If the site of inflammation is necrotic and filled with white blood cells, the inflammatory site will be recognized as pus. If red blood cells are present, the pus may be yellow or bloody red, depending on the proportion of red cells. The cellular evolution of an inflammatory response eventually results in the healing or scarring of the lesion.

Evolution of Immunity (Phylogeny)

Adaptation to the environment is the driving force in evolution and survival of a species. Organisms must not only accommodate to changes in temperature, pH, nutrients, oxygen, and water, but also

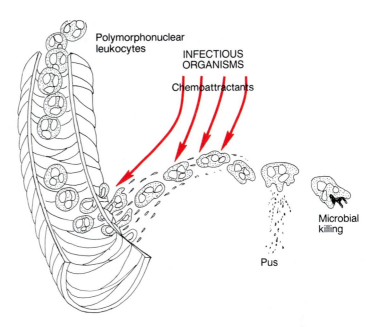

Figure 1–3. Acute inflammatory response to infection. Infectious organisms release chemicals or initiate tissue damage which produces products that are chemotactic (attract) inflammatory cells (polymorphonuclear leukocytes) and cause constriction of vascular endothelial cells. This results in release of fluid into the tissue (edema) and/or infiltration of tissue with inflammatory cells. Polymorphonuclear leukocytes may ingest and kill the infecting organisms or may release proteolytic enzymes into tissue, causing necrosis and formation of pus. Antibody serves to enhance this response and direct the inflammatory cells by reacting with the infecting organisms and activating bloodborne inflammatory mediators brought into the tissue during edema formation. These mediators react with cell surface receptors on the inflammatory cells and enhance the ability of the cells to ingest (phagocytose) and destroy the organisms.

must be able to defend against potentially fatal effects of other organisms (parasites). The most primitive defense system is the ability to recognize that something is foreign (not self). Shared domains in cell

TABLE 1–4. FOUR CARDINAL SIGNS OF ACUTE INFLAMMATION: CELSUS (25 B.C.)

Latin	English
Rubor	Redness
Tumor	Swelling
Calore	Heat
Dolore	Pain

The fifth classic sign of acute inflammation, "functio loosa" (loss of function), was added by Virchow (1821–1902).

recognition molecules, in particular β_2-microglobulin domains of T-cell receptors, and cell adhesion molecules, suggests that the adaptive immune response may have evolved from much older cell–cell interaction mechanisms.

INVERTEBRATES

A simplified phylogenetic tree as related to evolution of immune functions in invertebrates is presented in Figure 1–4.

The ability to identify foreign species and strains is present in each individual species. The defense mechanisms of invertebrates differ from the specific adaptive immunity of vertebrates in three critical features:

1. There is no morphologic development of a lymphoid system or cellular cooperation during defensive reactions.
2. There are no specific antigen recognition molecules such as immunoglobulin antibody or lymphocyte receptors.
3. There is no genetic information for the synthesis of immunoglobulin molecules.

Protozoa are able to recognize other protozoa as different because of different enzymes in different species and can defend themselves by phagocytosis. In this process, they are able to identify foreign (different species) from self (same species). The ability to recognize tissue of different species (self versus nonself) clearly exists in sponges. Identical pairs of sponges will fuse when mixed, whereas foreign pairs show a cytotoxic (necrotic) rejection response at their interface. The strength of rejection depends on the degree of genetic difference. A more rapid and extensive rejection occurs when two allogenic (different) species are put together a second time (secondary rejection response or immune memory). In higher organisms this phenomenon is tested by whether or not an individual will accept a graft of tissue from another individual (graft rejection implies recognition of foreign tissue). In coral the extent of parabiotic incompatibility suggests that each clone of coral is different. This principle of the uniqueness of the individual also applies to humans (*histocompatibility differences*).

White blood cell differentiation appears first in echinoderms and protochordates (for a description of white blood cells, see Chapter 2). In the coelomic cavity of earthworms there are primitive white blood cell types which combine features of polymorphonuclear cells and lymphocytes. These cells appear to be responsible for graft rejection in these species; and some appear to respond to **mitogen** stimulation. A mitogen is a substance that stimulates cell proliferation (mitosis). Protochordates contain nodules of lymphatic cells and circulating lymphocytes which respond to stimulation. Lymphocyte-like cells also infiltrate grafts of sea urchins. Humoral factors also appear in earthworms, and hemolysins (which cause lysis of red blood cells) and

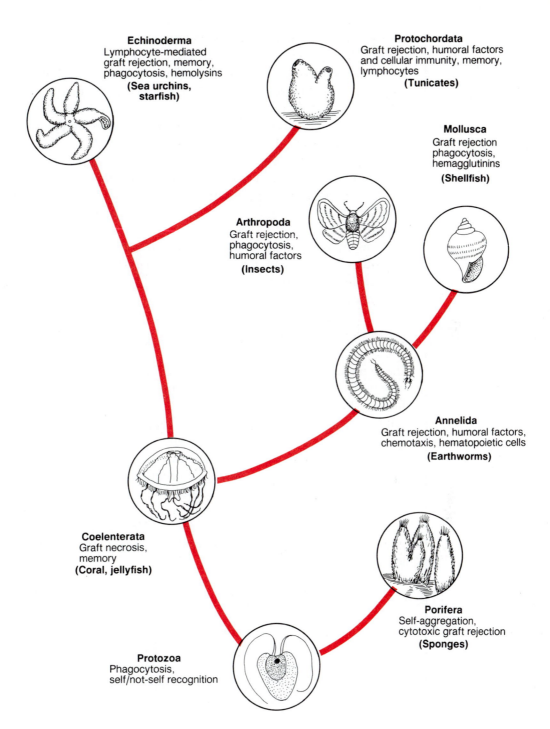

Figure 1–4. Phylogeny of invertebrate immunity.

hemagglutinins (which cause agglutination of red blood cells) are found in starfish and shellfish. However, these are not immunoglobulins and are not antigen specific. Snails have at least four cell types that impede the dissemination of microbes, but the most prominent role in defense is played by mobile **haemocytes** which have phagocytic capacities and granules (phagosomes) with properties similar to vertebrate granulocytes. Tunicates express both cellular and humoral immune factors, including some differentiation of lymphocytes. Some insects (arthropoda), such as cockroaches, have antibody-like proteins that have properties of specificity and memory, as well as cell-mediated ability to reject grafts from other strains of roaches. A major defense mechanism in insects is mechanical isolation (walling off) of parasites by collections (nodules) of blood cells (haemocytes), with deposition of melanin on the surface of the parasites (melanization). In general, cellular immune responses appear to precede the development of humoral responses during evolution.

VERTEBRATES

The phylogeny of immunity in vertebrates is illustrated in Figure 1–5.

T and B Cells

The immune system in vertebrates is characterized by a true two-component (T- and B-cell) system, specific immunoglobulin antibody production, highly developed specific cellular immunity, and specific immune memory. Immunoglobulins first appear at the level of agnatha (jawless fishes), although cyclostomes do not appear to have immunoglobulins. T- and B-like cells exist in teleost fishes but are not clearly defined in agnatha, although a primitive T-cell response can be demonstrated. Table 1–5 lists evolution of lymphoid organs in vertebrates (lymphoid organs of the human are described in Chapter 3). Agnatha demonstrate diffuse lymphoid tissue in the gut but do not have other lymphoid organs. Thymus and spleen appear in fishes, and lymph nodes appear in amphibians.

Clearly defined T and B cells are first seen in amphibians, where thymectomy results in loss of cellular responses such as graft rejection, and T- and B-cell responses can be demonstrated. Reptiles have demonstrable T regulatory cells, cells with surface immunoglobulin, and lymphoid organs that resemble those of mammals. Most amphibians do not have clear-cut graft rejection, but some amphibians have slow chronic graft rejection reactions compared to reptiles, birds, and mammals. The evolutionary trend from slow to fast graft rejection may reflect expression of histocompatibility antigens rather than a weakness in the immune reaction in lower species.

Epithelium and Lymphoid Organs

Associations of epithelial tissue and lymphoid tissue in some lymphoid organs appear to be of critical importance in the development of the mammalian immune system. In order to survive on land, changes in the

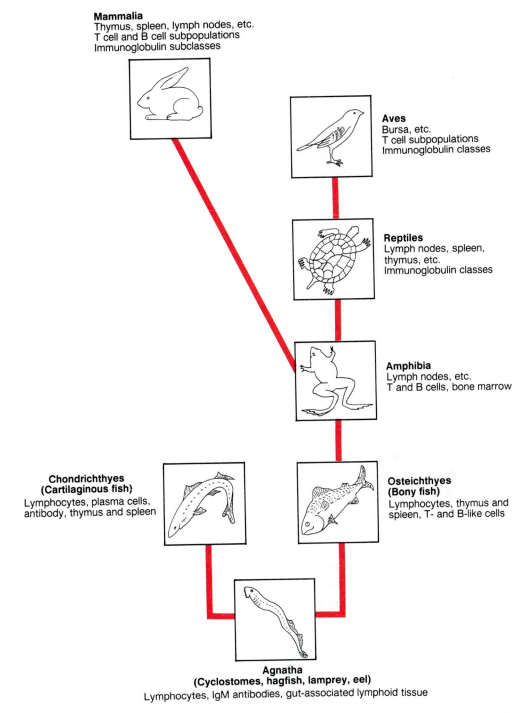

Figure 1–5. Phylogeny of immunity in vertebrates.

gill pouches and cloaca bursa of amphibians had to evolve in birds and mammals. During embryogenesis of higher vertebrates, the five paired gill pouches cease absorbing oxygen and develop to supply epithelium for cervical organs. In primitive coelenterates the coelomic cavity serves not only to absorb nutrients, but also to absorb oxygen. This function evolves into gills in the neck (foregut) of fishes and the hindgut of mollusks and arthropods. The five gill pouches in fish become vestigial in amphibia, but the epithelial tissue of the third pharyngeal pouch provides the stroma of the medulla of the thymus. This epithelial stroma is essential for the maturation of thymocytes (see Chapter 6). The hindgut gills evolve into the cloaca in turtles and further into the cloacal bursa of Fabricius of birds. The bursa of Fabricius is essential for the development of the B-cell system in birds. In mammalia, the gastrointestinal-associated lymphoid tissue (GALT) plays an important role in the development of the B-cell system (see below).

SUMMARY

1. Some form of recognition of self and nonself is present in the simplest animal species.
2. Cellular immunity precedes humoral immunity in evolution.
3. A bifunctional (T- and B-cell) system with developed lymphoid organs is the most recent immunologic development.
4. Epithelium that evolves from the gills of fishes (ie, pharyngeal pouches) plays a major role in the development of the lymphoid organs of mammals (thymus and GALT).

Selective pressures during evolution are believed to have resulted in the development of protective immune mechanisms. Primitive immune mechanisms may have had a number of other functions in lower organisms, such as recognition of cell surface markers required for aggregation of cell types in the early stages of development of multicellular structures (recognition of self and nonself). Immune recognition mechanisms may be variants of the cell–cell interactions that occur during embryologic development. It is likely that the immune system, as we now see it, is expanding and being modified to perform even other new functions such as regulation of neuroendocrine or hormonally expressive cells.

Immuno-pathology (The Double-edged Sword)

The evolution of the immune system did not occur without ambivalence and flaws. This same system which functions so well to protect against foreign invaders may also be turned against us. The term **immunopathology** is an oxymoron (inherently self-contradictory): "immune" means protection or exemption from; "pathology" is the study of disease. Thus, immunopathology literally means the study of the protection from disease, but in usage it actually means the study of how immune mechanisms cause diseases. Immunity is a double-edged

TABLE 1–5. PHYLOGENY OF THE IMMUNE SYSTEM FROM PRIMITIVE FISHES TO MAMMALS[a]

Class or Group	Thymus	Bone Marrow	Lymph Glands or Nodes	Blood Granulocytes and Lymphocytes	Reactions to Primary Tissue Allografts (Cell-mediated Immunity[b])	
					Moderate	Strong
Hagfish and lampreys	0	0	0	+	+	0
Sharks and rays	+	0	0	+	+	0
Bony fishes	+	+	0	+	+	+
Amphibians	+	+	+	+	+	+
Reptiles	+	+	+	+	+	0
Birds	+	+	+	+	+	+
Mammals	+	+	+	+	+	+

[a] + indicates presence of corresponding types of cells or reactivity.

[b] Moderate histocompatibility barriers are found in animals representing all vertebrate classes, but strong barriers are the rule in advanced bony fishes, anuran amphibians, and most birds and mammals.

From Hildemann, WH, in *Frontiers in Immunogenetics*, Elsevier–North Holland Press, New York 1981.

sword: on the one hand, immune responses protect us from infections; on the other hand, immune mechanisms may cause disease. The most compelling evidence that immune reactions are protective is provided by the naturally occurring immune deficiency diseases. Individuals with an inability to mount an effective immune response to infectious agents invariably succumb to infections unless vigorously treated. However, immune reactions may also cause disease. The terms "allergy" and "hypersensitivity" are used to denote deleterious immune reactions. **Allergy** is frequently used for a particular type of rapidly developing explosive immune reaction (anaphylactic), and **hypersensitivity** is used for delayed or cell-mediated immune reactivity. The term "immunity" was once restricted to the protective effects of immune reactions, but by common usage, this is no longer the case. In some diseases, immune mechanisms may actually be directed against our own tissues. This is termed **autoimmunity**.

History of Immunopathology

A listing of the major events in the history of immunopathology is given in Table 1–6. Recognition of adaptive immunity occurred in the ancient societies of China and Egypt. Application of this phenomenon by introduction into lesions scratched on the skin ("variolation") or by

TABLE 1–6. HISTORY OF IMMUNOPATHOLOGY

Fever	Mesopotamia	3000 B.C.
Recognition of adaptive immunity	Egypt, China	2000 B.C.
Anatomic identification of organs	Hippocrates	400 B.C.
Acquired resistance to poisons	Mithridate Eupator, King of Pontus	80 B.C.
Four cardinal signs of inflammation	Celsus	25 A.D.
"Snuff" variolation for smallpox	Sung Dynasty, China	1000
Renaissance of anatomy	Vesalius	1540
Bursa of birds described	Fabricius	1590
Peyer's patch	Peyer	1690
Cowpox vaccination	Jenner	1798
Tuberculous granulomas	Rokitansky	1855
Langhans' giant cell	Langhans	1868
Waldeyer's ring	Waldeyer	1870
Cellular pathology	Virchow	1880
Attenuated vaccines	Pasteur	1880
Phagocytosis	Metchnikoff	1882
Anti-rattlesnake venom	Sewall	1887
Bactericidal antibodies	Nuttall	1888
Neutralization (antitoxin)	Von Behring, Kitasato	1890
Delayed hypersensitivity skin test	Koch	1890

(continued)

TABLE 1–6. HISTORY OF IMMUNOPATHOLOGY (continued)

Bacteriolysis (antibody and complement)	Bordet	1894
Precipitins	Kraus	1887
Blood groups	Landsteiner	1900
Side chain theory, tumor immunity, horror autotoxicus	Ehrlich	1900
Anaphylaxis	Richet, Portier	1902
Arthus phenomenon	Arthus	1903
Osonins	Wright	1903
Serum sickness	Von Pirquet, Schick	1905
Organ transplantation	Correl, Guthrie	1905
Delayed hypersensitivity	Von Pirquet	1906
Immune surveillance of cancer	Ehrlich	1909
Viral cancer immunity	Rous	1910
Passive cutaneous anaphylaxis	Prausnitz, Kustner	1921
Chemical mediators of inflammation	Lewis	1925
Template (Instructional) theory	Breinl, Horowitz	1930
Quantitative precipitin reaction	Heidelberger	1935
Antibody is in gammaglobulin	Tiselius, Kabat	1938
Yellow fever vaccine	Theiler	1938
Rheumatoid factor	Waaler	1940
Hemolytic disease of newborn (Rh)	Levine	1941
Immunofluorescence	Coons	1942
Concept of collagen disease	Klemperer	1942
Immune tolerance	Medawar, Burnet	1944
Passive transfer of cell-mediated immunity	Chase	1945
Chimeras in bovine twins	Owen	1945
Antibodies in plasma cells	Fagraeus	1948
Clonal selection theory	Burnet, Fenner	1949
Agammaglobulinemia	Bruton	1952
Transplantation chimeras in mice	Billingham, Brent, Medawar	1953
Cellular transfer of transplantation immunity	Mitchison	1953
Natural selection theory	Jerne	1955
Mechanism of immune complex disease	Dixon	1956
Autoimmune thyroiditis	Witebsky, Doniach	1957
Histocompatibility antigens	Snell, Dausset	1958
Structure of antibodies	Kabat, Porter, Edelman	1959
Lymphocyte recirculation	Gowans	1959
Mitogenic activation of lymphocytes	Nowell	1961
Function of the thymus	Miller, Good	1961
Classification of immune mechanisms	Gell, Coombs	1962
Migration inhibitory factors	David, Vaughn	1962
Lymphocyte surface immunoglobulin and lymphocyte activation	Sell, Gell	1964
Mixed lymphocyte reaction	Bain, Vas, et al.	1964
Cooperation of T and B cells in antibody response	Claman	1966
In vitro primary immune response	Mishell, Dutton	1967

(continued)

TABLE 1–6. HISTORY OF IMMUNOPATHOLOGY (continued)

IgE as reaginic antibody	Ishizaka	1967
Accessory cell role in immune response	Mosier	1968
Linkage of immune response to MHC	McDevitt, Tyan	1968
Immune response genes	Benacerraf, McDevitt	1969
Tolerance in T and B cells	Weigle, Chiller	1971
T-cell helper factors	Dutton, Schimpl	1972
Idiotype network	Jerne	1974
Hybridoma (monoclonal antibodies)	Kohler and Milstein	1975
Natural killer cells	Kiessling, Herberman	1975
MHC class-restricted T cytotoxicity	Zinkernagel, Doherty	1975
Ig gene rearrangements	Tonegawa	1978
CD4 and CD8 T-cell subsets	Reinherz, Kung, Scholssman	1979
Transgenic mice	Gordon	1980
Antigen-specific T-cell hybridoma	Kappler, Marrack	1981
Antigen-presenting B cells	Chesnut, Grey	1981
Antigen-processing (Class II)	Unanue	1982
(Class I)	Townsend	1985
T-cell receptor	Allison, Haskins, et al.	1982
B-cell antigen presentation	Glimcher, Walker, et al.	1982
Somatic generation of Ig variable regions	Tonegawa	1983
H. influenzae conjugate vaccine	Robbins, Stein, Anderson	1983
Discovery of HIV	Montagnier	1983
T-cell receptor gene	Hedrick, Davis, Mak	1984
Thymic maturation of CD4+CD8+ T-cells	Fowlkes, Mathieson	1984
Cell Adhesion Molecules	Ruoslahti, Springer	1985
Surrogate light chain	Sakaguchi, Melchers	1986
MHC binds antigenic peptides	Buus, Sette, Grey	1986
Antibodies to TCR chains	Kappler, Marrack	1987
Class I MHC antigen-binding site	Bjorkman, Strominger, Wiley	1987
Endogenous superantigens and V-beta chains	Kappler, Marrack, MacDonald	1988
RAG genes	Schatz, Oettinger, Baltimore	1988
Thymic selection of TCR	von Boehmer	1988
Peripheral tolerance	Miller, Schwartz, Lo	1988
Igα, Igβ in membrane Ig	Reth	1990
Peptide transporter proteins (TAP1/2)	Monaco	1990
Immunolopathology of AIDS	Fauci, Levy, others	1992
Molecular diagnosis of immunodeficiencies: Bruton's X-linked agammaglobulinemia-protein kinase deficiency	Bentley	1993
Hyper IgM syndrome–CD40 ligand deficiency	Ochs, Kroczek	1993
X-linked SCID–IL2R γ-chain mutation	Leonard	1993
Autosomal SCID–ZAP70 kinase deficiency	Weiss	1994

inhalation into the nasal cavity of smallpox organisms was practiced by the Chinese about 1000 A.D., and artificial vaccination was introduced in England in 1798. In the late 1800s and early 1900s many immune-mediated phenomena were described. The cellular immune system was emphasized by Metchnikoff and the humoral system by Von Behring. Modern immunology can be said to have begun in the late 1950s with the recognition of histocompatibility antigens, identification of the structure of antibodies, and the study of immune mechanisms that cause disease. More recently, the contributions of molecular biology and genetic engineering have revolutionized our understanding of the molecular mechanisms of antibody diversity and the nature of the T-cell receptor, as well as how immune cells recognize and are activated by antigens. A list of "immunologists" who have been awarded the Nobel Prize is given in Table 1–7.

In the following chapters of this text we shall explore how the specific immune system works (immunology), what happens when it

TABLE 1–7. NOBEL PRIZES AWARDED FOR IMMUNOLOGY

Year	Recipient	Country	Discovery
1901	Emil von Behring	Germany	Antitoxins in serum
1905	Robert Koch	Germany	Cellular immunity (tuberculosis)
1908	Elie Metchnikoff	Russia	Phagocytosis
	Paul Ehrlich	Germany	Antitoxins, side-chain theory
1913	Charles Richet	France	Anaphylaxis
1919	Jules Bordet	Belgium	Complement mediated bacteriolysis
1930	Karl Landsteiner	U.S.A.	Human blood groups
1950	Philip Hench	U.S.A.	Cortisone treatment of rheumatoid diseases
	Edward Kendall	U.S.A.	
	Tadeus Reichstein	Switzerland	
1951	Max Theiler	South Africa	Yellow fever vaccine
1957	Daniel Bovet	Switzerland	Antihistamines
1960	Macfarlane Burnet	Australia	Acquired immunological tolerance
	Peter Medawar	Great Britain	
1972	Gerald Edelman	U.S.A.	Chemical structure of antibodies
	Rodney Porter	Great Britain	
1977	Rosalyn Yalow	U.S.A.	Radioimmunoassay for insulin
1980	George Snell	U.S.A.	Major histocompatibility complex
	Jean Dausset	France	
	Baruj Benacerraf	U.S.A.	
1984	Georges Koehler	Germany	Monoclonal antibody
	Cesar Milstein	Great Britain	
	Neils Jerne	Denmark	Immune regulatory theories
1987	Tonegawa	Japan (U.S.A.)	Immunoglobulin genes
1991	E. Donnall Thomas	U.S.A.	Bone marrow transplantation
	Joseph Murray	U.S.A.	Renal transplantation

goes astray and causes disease (immunopathology), and how these same mechanisms protect us (immunity).

Summary

Higher organisms have evolved effective defense systems to protect themselves against foreign markers. One system is constitutive and consists of mechanical barriers, pH, temperature, phagocytosis, inflammation, etc. (innate resistance). The other is induced and consists of specific products that recognize invaders as foreign (adaptive immunity). After induction (immunization), the adaptive system responds more rapidly and with greater intensity than after first exposure (immune memory). The two major arms of the adaptive immune response are humoral (antibody) and cellular (specifically sensitized cells). Cells of the body known as lymphocytes are responsible for the adaptive immune response (T lymphocytes for cellular immunity and B lymphocytes for humoral immunity). In response to infection, both adaptive and innate inflammatory mechanisms may be activated. During evolution, the adaptive immune response became increasingly complex. Humans have different classes of antibodies and different subsets of T cells that have different functions as immune effectors.

The immune response is not always protective; in many instances, the same immune effector mechanisms that defend against foreign invaders may be turned against us and produce disease (the double-edged sword of immunopathology). In the following chapters, the immune response will be described (Part I—Immunology), the destructive effects of immune mechanisms presented (Part II—Immunopathology), and the role of immune mechanisms in defense analyzed (Part III—Immunity).

Bibliography

PERIODICALS

Advances in Immunology, New York, Academic Press.
Annual Review of Immunology, Palo Alto, CA, Annual Reviews Inc.
Comprehensive Immunology, New York, Plenum.
Progress in Allergy, Basel, Switzerland, S. Karger.
Immunological Reviews, Copenhagen, Munksgarrd.
Immunology Today, New York, Elsevier.
Seminars in Immunology, Philadelphia, PA, WB Saunders.

BASIC IMMUNOLOGY TEXTS

Abbas AK, Lichtman AH, Pober JS: *Cellular and Molecular Immunology.* New York, WB Saunders, 1991.
Eisen H: *Immunology* (2nd ed.). Hagerstown, IN, Harper & Row, 1980.
Golub ES, Green DR: *Immunology: A Synthesis*, 2nd ed. Sunderland, MA, Sinauer, 1991.

Hildemann WH: *Fundamentals of Immunology*, New York, Elsevier, 1984.

Hood L, Weissman IL, Wood WB, Wilson JH: *Immunology*, 2nd ed. Menlo Park, CA, Benjamin Cummings, 1984.

Humphrey SH, White RG: *Immunology for Students of Medicine*, 3rd ed. Oxford, Blackwell, 1970.

Janeway CA, Travers P: Immunology: The immune system in health and disease. New York, Garland, 1994.

Kimball JW: *Introduction to Immunology*, 2nd ed. New York, Macmillan, 1986.

Klein J: *Immunology*. Boston, Blackwell, 1990.

Paul WE: *Fundamental Immunology*, 3rd ed. New York, Raven Press, 1993.

Roitt I: *Essential Immunology*, 7th ed. Oxford, Blackwell, 1991.

Stites DP, Terr AI (eds.): *Basic and Clinical Immunology*, 7th ed. Los Altos, CA, Lange, 1991.

CLINICAL IMMUNOLOGY TEXTS

Brostoff J, Scadding GK, Male D, Roitt IM: *Clinical Immunology*. London, Gower, 1991.

Holborow EJ, Reeves WG: *Immunology in Medicine*. London, Academic Press, 1977.

Lachmann PJ, Peters DK, Rosen FS, Wallport MJ: *Clinical Aspects of Immunology*, 5th ed. Oxford, Blackwell, 1993.

Miescher PA, Muller-Eberhard HJ: *Textbook of Immunopathology*, 2nd ed. New York, Grune and Stratton, 1976.

Sampter M (ed.): *Immunological Diseases*, 4th ed. Boston, Little, Brown, 1988.

INNATE IMMUNITY

Lamont JT: Mucus: The front line of intestinal mucosal defense. *Ann NY Acad Med* 664:190, 1992.

Walker WA, Sanderson IR: Epithelial barrier to antigens. *Ann NY Acad Med* 664:10, 1992.

PHYLOGENY OF IMMUNITY

Brehelin M: Immunity in invertebrates. New York, Springer-Verlag, 1985.

Cohen N: Phylogeny of lymphocyte structure and function. *Am Zool* 15:119–133, 1975.

Cooper EL: *Comparative Immunology*. Englewood Cliffs, NJ, Prentice-Hall, 1976.

Goetz D (ed.): Evolution and function of the major histocompatibility system. Berlin, Springer-Verlag, 1977.

Good RA, Papermaster BW: Ontogeny and phylogeny of adaptive immunity. *Adv Immunol* 4:1, 1964.

Hildemann WH, Clark EA, Raison RL: *Comprehensive Immunogenetics*, New York, Elsevier-Holland, 1981.

Humphries T, Reinherz EL: Invertebrate immune recognition, natural immunity and the evolution of positive selection. *Immunol Today* 15: 316–320, 1994

Karp RD: Cell-mediated immunity in invertebrates: The enigma of the insect. *Bioscience* 40:732, 1990.

Ohno S: The ancestor of the adaptive immune system was the CAM system for organogenesis. *Exp Clin Immunogenetic* 4:181, 1987.

Sima P, Vetvicka V: Evolution of immune reactions. *CRC Critical Rev Immunol* 13:83–114, 1993.

HISTORICAL

Bibel DJ: Milestones in Immunology: A historical exploration. *Science Tech Pub*, Madison, WI, 1988.

Boyd WC: *Fundamentals of Immunology*. New York, Interscience, 1943.

Gell PGH, Coombs RRA: *Clinical Aspects of Immunology*. Philadelphia, PA, FA Davis, 1963.

Haggard HW: *Mystery, Magic and Medicine*. Doubleday, Garden City, NY, Doran, 1933.

Kabat EA: *Structural Concepts in Immunology and Immunochemistry*. New York, Holt, Rinehart, and Winston, 1968.

Landsteiner K: *The Specificity of Serological Reactions*. New York, Dover, 1962.

Long ER: *A History of Pathology*. New York, Dover, 1965.

Majno G: *The Healing Hand*. Cambridge, MA, Harvard University Press, 1975.

Raffel S: *Immunity, Hypersensitivity, Serology*. New York, Appleton-Century-Crofts, 1953.

Silverstein AM: History of Immunology: A History of Theories of Antibody Formation. *Cell Immunol* 91:263–283, 1985.

Silverstein AM: *A History of Immunology*. San Diego, CA, Academic Press, 1989.

2

The Immune System I: Cells

The organs of our bodies that provide the products of immunity (proteins and cells), and the delivery network for these products, comprise the **lymphoid system**. The lymphoid system is a complex network of lymphatic vessels, lymphoid nodules, lymph nodes, spleen, and other organs, distributed throughout the body in places where contact is made with foreign antigens that enter the body through the skin, airways, or gastrointestinal tract. The cells of the body that react to protect us against injury and infection are called white cells (leukocytes). The cells of the immune/inflammatory system are described in this chapter; the lymphoid organs and their development are the subjects of Chapter 3. The major cellular constituents of the immune system are lymphocytes. However, other cells (macrophages) are also involved in induction of an immune response, and other white blood cell types such as macrophages and polymorphonuclear leukocytes take an active part in various effector inflammatory responses associated with immune reactions.

The cells that are present in the blood represent the fully mature products of cell lineages for which the progenitors are found in other organs. There are two major cell types in the blood: red blood cells **(erythrocytes)** and white blood cells **(leukocytes)** (Fig. 2–1).

In smears of peripheral blood stained with a special dye to bring out different cellular structures (Wright's stain), erythrocytes (red blood cells) are small, light pink, and have no nuclei. Erythrocytes are by far the most numerous cells in blood smears. The number of red cells in the blood is indirectly estimated from the **hematocrit** (Fig. 2–2). Red

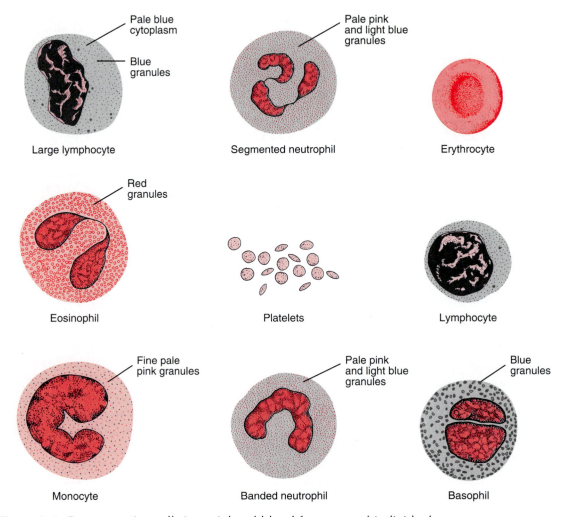

Figure 2–1. Representative cells in peripheral blood from normal individuals.

blood cells do not take part in immune reactions; their major function is to carry oxygen required for metabolism of tissues throughout the body, and remove carbon dioxide produced by cellular metabolism.

WHITE BLOOD CELLS/ LEUKOCYTES

The term "white blood cell" is applied because when anticoagulated blood is lightly centrifuged, white cells sediment in a thin, white layer between the denser erythrocytes (red blood cells) and the plasma. This layer of white cells is called the **buffy coat** (Fig. 2–2). Patients with tumors of the white blood cells often present with a marked increase in this layer and blood that is more white than red—**leukemia** or "white blood." The mature forms of these cells are most easily recognized in peripheral blood smears. The basic structure and function of

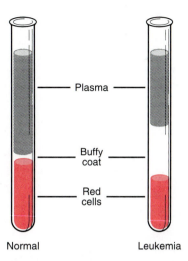

Figure 2–2. Separation of blood components by centrifugation. The red blood cells are the most dense component, sediment most rapidly, and make up approximately 40% of the blood volume. This percentage is known as the *hematocrit*. The hematocrit is used to estimate increases or decreases in the number of circulating red cells in the blood. The plasma component (protein-enriched fluid) makes up the largest percentage (approximately 55% to 60%), and is the least dense. In between the plasma and the red blood cells, the white blood cells form a thin layer called the "buffy coat," which is creamy white in color.

white blood cells is described below; their role in immune responses and inflammation will be presented in more detail in the chapters that follow.

The different white blood cells and their normal representation in the blood are depicted in Figure 2–3.

The terms used by pathologists, immunologists, and hematologists for the different white blood cells reflect different ways of looking at complex cell populations. A simplified classification of blood leukocytes is presented in Figure 2–4.

The large mononuclear cells (macrophages) are phagocytic cells. Macrophages in peripheral blood are termed "monocytes"; in tissues they are called histiocytes. Particular care must be taken in understanding **monocyte** and **mononuclear** cells. Hematologists use the term "monocyte" for the larger, circulating mononuclear white blood cells found in the peripheral blood, which are in the macrophage lineage. Pathologists use the term "mononuclear" or "round cells" for lymphocytes and macrophages seen in tissue to differentiate them from polymorphonuclear cells. These similar terms must be carefully separated to avoid confusion.

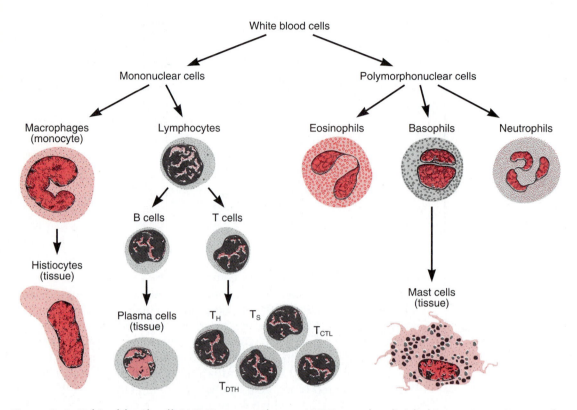

Figure 2–3. White blood cell (WBC) nomenclature. WBC may be divided into two major populations on the basis of the form of their nuclei: single nuclei (*mononuclear* or *"round cells"*) or segmented nuclei (*polymorphonuclear*). Mononuclear cells are further divided into large (*macrophage* or *monocyte*) or small (*lymphocyte*) on the basis of the size of the nucleus. Lymphocytes may be further subdivided into two major populations: *T cells* and *B cells*, on the basis of function and cell surface phenotype (to be described later). B cells are the precursors of the cells that synthesize and secrete humoral antibodies. Subpopulations of T cells are responsible for a number of "cell-mediated" immune activities. T cells and B cells cannot be differentiated on the basis of morphologic appearance, but do have different phenotypic markers. In addition, lymphocytes without distinguishing markers (*null cells*) are present in smaller numbers than T cells or B cells. Some null cells may "kill" certain other cell types in vitro (*natural killer* or *NK cells*) and others may become "armed" by passive absorption of antibody (*antibody-dependent cell-mediated cytotoxicity [ADCC]*), or activated by lymphokines (*lymphokine-activated killer cells [LAKs]*). Polymorphonuclear cells play different roles in inflammation and are defined by different staining characteristics of their prominent cytoplasmic granules as eosinophils (red), basophils (blue), and neutrophils (pink) in standard blood smears.

| Polymorpho-nuclear Leukocytes/ Granulocytes | Polymorphonuclear white blood cells are subdivided into three major populations on the basis of the staining properties of their cytoplasmic granules in standard hematologic blood smears or tissue preparations: neutrophil–pink, eosinophil–red, basophil–blue. Polymorphonuclear cells take part in both immune specific and nonspecific inflammatory |

reactions. Because of the prominence of the granules, cells of these types are also called **granulocytes**.

Neutrophils. Neutrophils are polymorphonuclear leukocytes (PMNs) whose cytoplasmic granules do not take on strong acidophilic (red) or basophilic (blue) staining with the usual dyes used for staining smears of blood, but show only a pale pink coloration. Such cells make up from 50% to 70% of the white blood cells (WBCs) of the peripheral blood and may be found scattered diffusely in many tissues, although they are most frequently found in areas of acute inflammation or acute necrosis. Like other white blood cells, neutrophils are produced from precursor cells in the bone marrow and released into the blood when mature. After entering the circulation, they last only 1 or 2 days, but their exact fate is unknown. Like its relative, the macrophage (large eater), the neutrophil is active in phagocytosis and has been called a microphage (small eater). Neutrophils are rapidly migrating, phagocytic cells that appear in areas of infection or tissue damage. The nucleus of the neutrophil, characteristic of the polymorphonuclear leukocytes, is divided into round or oval lobes connected to one another by thin strands of nuclear material. The other outstanding feature of this type of WBC is the large number of membrane-delineated granules: azurophil granules, specific granules, and short rod-shaped alkaline phosphatase-containing granules (Table 2–1). The role of these granules in inflammation is covered in Chapter 8.

Neutrophils are the first wave of a cellular attack on invading organisms and are the characteristic cells of acute inflammation (see Chapter 8). The appearance of neutrophils in areas of inflammation may be caused by chemicals released from bacteria, factors produced nonspecifically from necrotic tissue, or directed by antibody reacting with antigen (the role of the neutrophil in acute inflammation is taken over by the macrophage in the chronic stage of inflammation).

Eosinophils. Eosinophils are similar in appearance to neutrophils, except that they have prominent eosinophilic (red) granules that may contain rod-like crystalloid inclusions when viewed by electron microscopy. These eosinophilic granules are membrane limited and contain large amounts of hydrolytic enzymes, including peroxidase and catalase, and thus are lysosomes. The granules differ from those of neutrophils by having a high content of peroxidase, which is perhaps related to the crystalloid structure. The chemotactic responses of the eosinophil are similar to those of neutrophils, but eosinophils are found in unusually high numbers around antigen–antibody complexes and parasites in tissues. The eosinophil granule contains major basic proteins and arylsulfatase, which are toxic to parasitic worms and limit the

Cell Type	% of White Blood Cells in Blood	Diameter (μm)	Nucleus	Cytoplasm and Granules	Drawings
Erythrocytes	—	7.5	None	Pink, homogeneous cytoplasm	
LEUKOCYTES					
Polymorphonuclear					
Neutrophils	50–70	10–12	2–5 lobules connected by thin bridges, coarse chromatin	Abundant cytoplasm/ fine pinkish granules	
Eosinophils	1–3	10–12	Usually two oval lobes connected by bridge	Abundant cytoplasm/ coarse reflective granules stained red	
Basophils	< 1	8–10	Bent in S with two or more constrictions; obscured by cytoplasmic granules	Large and irregular granules stained deep blue	
Mononuclear					
Lymphocytes	25–35	6–15	Round to oval; coarse chromatin	Bluish cytoplasm/ about 10% of cells fine azurophilic granules	
Monocytes	3–7	12–18	Kidney shaped, indented; fine chromatin	Bluish cytoplasm/ fine azurophilic granules	

extent of worm infestations. Eosinophils also contain histaminase and may limit or modulate mast-cell-mediated inflammation. The properties of eosinophil granule proteins in inflammation are covered in more detail in Chapter 8. Eosinophils make up from 1% to 3% of the circulating white blood cells.

Basophils/Mast Cells. Basophils have prominent blue-staining cytoplasmic granules. Cells related to basophils but located in solid tissue are called **mast cells**. Cells are found in loose (areolar) connective tissue around small blood vessels. Blood basophils are rounded in appearance, whereas tissue mast cells may be elongated or irregular in cell outline. Blood basophils make up less than 1% of the peripheral WBC. Mast cell and basophil nuclei are round or oval. The outstanding feature of basophils is the abundance of oval basophilic (blue) granules that have a finely granular or reticular ultrastructure. The predominance of granules overshadows other cytoplasmic structures, although mitochondria, endoplasmic reticulum, ribosomes, and a

Golgi apparatus may be seen. Basophil granules contain heparin, histamine, serotonin (5-hydroxytryptamine), membrane-like material that is metabolized to prostaglandins and leukotrienes, and a battery of hydrolytic enzymes. Mast cells also make virtually every other cytokine that has been looked for, including interleukins 1 through 6, tumor necrosis factor, and some inflammatory cytokines that may attract neutrophils and eosinophils to inflammatory sites. In response to a stimulus, mast cells or basophils may spill out the contents of 60% to 70% of their granules. Mast cells have been nicknamed "gate-keeper cells" because they control access of blood proteins and cells to the extracellular space. The release of material from mast cell granules has a marked effect on the smooth muscles of arterioles (dilation) and the permeability of capillaries (contraction of endothelial cells). Release of these pharmacologically active agents by mast cells is the mechanism responsible for early inflammatory changes (see Chapter 8) and for the unleashing of anaphylactic or atopic allergic reactions (see Chapter 14).

Tissue mast cells have different characteristics depending on their location. This is termed **mast cell heterogeneity**. Differences in morphology, mediator content, histochemical staining, responsiveness to cytokines, and sensitivity to drugs have been described. Mast cell heterogeneity is caused by microenvironmental factors. The two major subpopulations of mast cells are identified by those in the mucosa that contain tryptase (MC^T) and those in the connective tissue that contain both tryptase and chymase (MC^{TC}) (Table 2–2). MC^T predominate in lung and mucosa; MC^{TC} predominate in the connective tissue of bowel submucosa and skin. Each is found about equally in nasal mucosa and ocular conjunctiva. The biologic significance of these two mast cell

TABLE 2–2. CHARACTERISTICS OF MAJOR MAST CELL POPULATIONS

Characteristic	MC^T (Mucosal)	MC^{TC} (Connective Tissue)
Neutral protease	Tryptase	Tryptase, chymase
Tissue distribution	Mucosal (lung, bowel mucosa)	Connective tissue (skin, bowel submucosa)
Granule ultrastructure	Scrolls	Gratings/lattices
T-cell dependence	+	−
Compound 48/80 degranulation	−	+
Histamine	+	++
LTC$_4$/PGD$_2$ ratio	25:1	1:40
Cytoplasmic IgE	+	−
Fcε receptors	+++	+
Major proteoglycan	Chrondrotin sulfate	Heparin

Modified from Schwartz LB: Heterogeneity of mast cells in humans. In *Mast Cell Differentiation and Function in Health and Disease*. Galli SJ, Austen KF (eds.). Raven Press, New York, 1989.

populations is not clear, but differences in mediators suggests different functional capacities.

Lymphocytes

"Lymphocyte" is a morphologic term that includes a population of cells of similar appearance, originally identified in lymph fluid, but with different immune functions. The lymphocyte is a small, round cell found in the peripheral blood, lymph nodes, spleen, thymus, tonsils, appendix, and scattered throughout many other tissues. In smears of peripheral blood, lymphocytes appear slightly larger (7 to 8 microns) in diameter than red blood cells (erythrocytes) and make up about 30% of the total white blood cell count (WBC). A typical lymphocyte has very little cytoplasm and is composed mostly of a circular nucleus with prominent nuclear chromatin (Fig. 2–5). The narrow rim of cytoplasm contains scattered ribosomes as well as a few ribosomal aggregates, but in a resting state it is virtually devoid of endoplasmic reticulum or other organelles. Once believed to be a short-lived "end" cell, it is now known that some populations of lymphocytes may survive for months or even years and recirculate from lymph nodes to lymph and blood.

The lymphocyte is responsible for the primary recognition of antigen as well as being an immunologically specific effector cell. Lymphocytes produce cell surface molecules that serve as receptor sites for reaction with antigen. The lymphocyte is the carrier of immunologic specific information. "Immunologically competent cell" and "memory cell" are functional terms for specialized cells found in immunized individuals that are not morphologically distinguishable from other lymphocytes. The lymphocytes that interact during the production of circulating antibody have different functional and antigenic properties but are structurally similar. Two major classes of lymphocytes are T cells and B cells (Table 2–3).

T Cells. The term "T cell" is applied to the **thymus-derived lymphocyte**. T-cell precursors (prothymocytes) are produced in the bone marrow and circulate to the thymus. Thymus-derived cells originate in the thymus from these precursor cells, are re-released into the circulation, and subsequently localize in thymus-dependent areas of the other lymphoid organs (see Chapter 3). Approximately 65% to 85% of lymph node cells and 30% to 50% of spleen cells are T cells.

In the human, T cells were first identified by their capacity to form rosettes with normal sheep erythrocytes (E rosette). A rosette is composed of a central lymphocyte surrounded by a layer of four or more erythrocytes. B cells do not form rosettes with normal sheep erythrocytes but will form rosettes with sheep cells coated with antibody and complement (EAC) because of receptor sites for the third component of complement. In addition, as stated above, human B lym-

TABLE 2–3. SOME PROPERTIES OF T AND B LYMPHOCYTES

Properties	T Cells	B Cells
Site of precursor	Thymus	Fetal liver, GI tract, bone marrow
Surface marker	T antigens	Surface Ig
Rosettes	E	EAC
Tissue distribution	Interfollicular (paracortical)	Follicles (cortical)
Percent of lymphocytes in blood	80%	20%
Radiation inactivation	+	++++
Mitogen response	Con A, PHA	PPD, LPS
Immune functions	Helper Suppressor Killer	Plasma cell precursor
Mixed lymphocyte reaction	Reactive cell	Stimulator cell

E, sheep erythrocytes; EAC, sheep erythrocytes coated with antibody and complement; Con A, concanavalin A; PHA, phytohemagglutinin; PPD, purified protein derivative of *Mycobacterium tuberculosis*; LPS, *Escherichia coli* lipopolysaccharide.

phocytes contain surface immunoglobulin that is detected by immunofluorescence. These techniques have been used to characterize human lymphoid cell populations. Ninety percent to 100% of human thymus cells form rosettes with uncoated (nonsensitized) sheep red blood cells and no rosettes with EAC. Spleen, peripheral blood, and lymph nodes contain approximately 20% to 30% B cells and 60% to 75% T cells by rosetting analysis.

T cells may be further divided into subpopulations on the basis of function and phenotypic markers. Different T-cell subpopulations function to help in antibody formation (T-helper cells, T_H), to kill target cells (T-cytotoxic cells, T_{CTL}), to induce inflammation (T-delayed hypersensitivity cells, T_{DTH}), to inhibit immune responses (T-suppressor cells, T_S). T-helper cells are divided into two major subpopulations: T_{H1} and T_{H2}. T_{H1} cells function primarily as helper cells for induction of B-cell proliferation and differentiation to IgG-producing plasma cells; whereas T_{H2} cells produce factors (interleukins) that induce B cells to differentiate and produce IgE and IgA. The effect of interleukins during induction of immunity is presented in Chapter 7 (see also Appendix A). T_{H1} cells may also differentiate into T_{DTH} cells that are responsible for the inflammatory effects of T cells (ie, delayed hypersensitivity, cytotoxicity) and secrete inflammatory mediators, such as lymphotoxin and interferon-γ. T_{H2} cell products are also believed to stimulate differentiation of other white blood cells, such as eosinophils and basophils (see Chapter 7).

A large number of T-cell subpopulations may now be identified by specific cell-surface markers termed **clusters of differentiation (CD)** (see Appendix C). CD markers are identified by monoclonal antibodies produced to different cell lymphoid cell populations. Thus, T_{Helper} cells in humans are identified as CD4+, and $T_{Cytotoxic}$ cells as CD8+. The expression of these markers during differentiation and in different subpopulations of lymphocytes will be presented in more detail in Chapter 3 and Chapter 7.

T lymphocytes activated by antigens produce effector molecules that activate or deactivate other lymphocytes (interleukins), contribute to immune-mediated inflammation (lymphokines), or interact with other cell types. For instance, interleukins produced by T_{Helper} cells are required to induce activation and differentiation of B cells. A partial listing of some of the functional activities of these factors is given in Table 2–4. Up to 20 different interleukins have now been identified and are numbered from interleukin-1 (IL-1) to interleukin-20 (IL-20) (see Appendix A). T_{H1} cells produce IL-2, γ-interferon and tumor necrosis factor in response to antigen stimulation, whereas T_{H2} cells synthesize IL-4, IL-5, and IL-6. The nature and function of the interleukins will be presented later in this text. In addition, activation and differentiation of T_{CTL} (cytotoxic) cells results in the appearance of cytoplasmic granules (secretory lysosomes). The T_{CTL} granules contain perforin, granzymes, and proteoglycans that act to lyse or kill other cells. The T-

TABLE 2–4. SOME FACTORS PRODUCED BY ACTIVATED LYMPHOCYTES (FOR MORE DETAILS SEE CHAPTERS 7 AND 9 AND APPENDIX A)

Products affecting other lymphocytes (interleukins)
    Helper factors
    Growth-promoting factors
    Differentiating factors
    Suppressor factor
    Transfer factor

Products affecting macrophages (lymphokines)
    Migration-inhibitory factor
    Activation factor
    Chemotactic factor

Products affecting polymorphonuclear leukocytes (lymphokines)
    Chemotactic factors
    Histamine-releasing factor
    Leukocyte-inhibitory factor

Products affecting other cell types (cytokines)
    Cytotoxic factor
    Growth-inhibitory factors
    Osteoclast-activating factor
    Interferon
    Colony-stimulating factor

Many of these factors have now been cloned and characterized by monoclonal antibodies and are included in the larger group of interleukins or lymphokines.

cell population not only contains a variety of effector cells but also is the master regulator of the immune system; the T cell is the director of the immunological orchestra. T cells function to turn off or on other cells in the immune system (T-suppressors, T-helpers, and T-contra-suppressors).

B Cells. B cells are the precursors of the cells that synthesize immunoglobulins (plasma cells). B cells contain readily detectable surface immunoglobulin (sIg), whereas T cells do not have surface immunoglobulin; 10% to 20% of lymph node cells, 20% to 35% of spleen cells, and 0% of thymus cells contain surface immunoglobulin. B cells develop from stem cells that originate in the fetal bone marrow or liver. The site of B-cell differentiation may be in the fetal liver, the gastrointestinal lymphoid tissue, or in peripheral lymph nodes. After antigenic stimulation, B cells differentiate into antibody-secreting plasma cells (see below).

Plasma Cells. The production of immunoglobulins (antibodies) is the primary function of the plasma cell. Plasma cells differentiate from activated B cells. The plasma cell is a small, round or oval cell (9 to 12 μ in diameter) with a small, compact, dense nucleus located at one pole of the cell. Aggregation of the chromatin along the nuclear envelope gives rise to the characteristic "cartwheel" appearance of the plasma cell nucleus under the light microscope. The cytoplasm is dominated by rough endoplasmic reticulum organized in stocked laminae and a prominent Golgi apparatus (Fig. 2–4A). The characteristic lamellar endoplasmic reticulum and the Golgi reflect immunoglobulin synthesis and rapid secretion. They are found in some other cells in which protein secretion is a major function (eg, pancreatic acinar cells). Plasma cells are prominent in the lymph nodes, spleen, and sites of chronic inflammation. Plasma cells increase in number in lymphoid organs, draining the site of antigen injection during the experimental induction of antibody formation. Membrane-bound amorphous densities believed to contain stored immunoglobulins may be observed in more mature plasma cells (Russell bodies).

Null Cells/Natural Killer Cells (Fig. 2–4B). Some lymphocytes do not have detectable surface Ig or T-cell markers; such cells are termed **null cells**. Cells belonging to this general class are active in certain types of lymphocyte-mediated target-cell killing: **natural killer (NK) cells**. The term "natural" is used because NK cells are present without prior immunization and act immediately on target cells; they are part of innate immunity. NK-mediated cytotoxic activity is measured by lysis of selected tumor target cells in vitro. Natural killer cells share some properties of T cells and macrophages, as well as B cells and granulo-

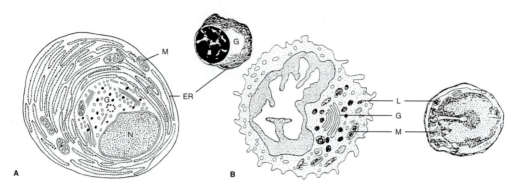

Figure 2–4. **A.** Plasma cell. **B.** Large granular lymphocyte (NK cell). Plasma cell is composed of abundant cytoplasm containing mostly lamellar endoplasmic reticulum and a few other cytoplasmic organelles. In tissue sections, there is polar location of the nucleus and a "cartwheel" appearance of the nucleus produced by condensation of chromatin along the nuclear membrane. The large granular lymphocyte contains mature lysosomes containing cytotoxic enzymes. ER, endoplasmic reticulum; G, Golgi apparatus; M, mitochondria; N, nucleus; L, lysosomes.

cytes (Table 2–5). These cells are believed to arise from a common T-cell–NK-cell progenitor before the migration of prothymocytes to the thymus (see Chapter 3).

NK cells have receptors that recognize plasma membranes of some tumor cells, but the nature of the receptor is not known. Cell adhesion molecules may be important as activation of NK cells by

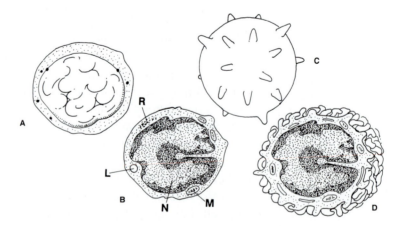

Figure 2–5. Lymphocyte. **A.** Blood smear; **B.** transmission electron micrograph; (c, d) scanning electron micrographs of two functional states of the lymphocyte surface; smooth **C.** and hairy **D.** Cell is composed mainly of a nucleus, with a paucity of cytoplasmic elements. A narrow rim of cytoplasm contains scattered ribosomes, a few membrane-limited bodies (lysosomes), and a few mitochondria. L, lysosome; M, mitochondria; N, nucleus; R, ribosomes.

TABLE 2–5. COMPARISON OF NK CELLS WITH OTHER LYMPHOID CELLS

Characteristic	NK/K cells	Similar to		
		T-1 cells	B cells	Macrophages
Size	16–20 nm	–	–	+
Cytoplasmic/nuclear ratio	High	–	–	+
Nuclear Shape	Lobed	–	–	+
Adherence	Nonadherent	+	+	–
Phagocytosis	Nonphagocytic	+	+	–
Esterase	Absent	+	+	–
Acid phosphatase	Present	+	–	–
FcγRI receptors	Present	–	–	–[a]
Memory	None	–	–	+
ADCC	Strong	–	–	+
Markers				
Asialo-GM1	95%	+	–	–
CD2	80%	+	–	–
CD3	<5%	–	+	+
CR3 and CR4	95%	–	–	+[a]
IL-2 Receptor	<5%	–	–	–[b]
NKH1	95% (NK)	–	–	–
NKH2	5% (K)	+	+	+[c]
TCR	90%	+	–	–[d]

[a]Present on granulocytes.
[b]Present on activated T cells, B cells, and macrophages.
[c]Present on basophils, K cells (ADCC, antibody dependent cell-mediated cytotoxicity).
[d]T-cell receptor gene rearranged.

IL-2 causes an increased expression of several cell adhesion molecules (LFA-1, ICAM-1, and LFA-3) (see Chapter 9). Different NK-cell lines have different specificities and not all tumor cells are susceptible to NK lysis. Because of the presence of large cytoplasmic granules, NK cells are also referred to as **large granule lymphocytes (LGLs)** (Fig. 2–4B). These cytoplasmic granules (lysosomes) contain enzymes and factors that are able to lyse target cells. NK lysis is not restricted by major histocompatibility markers as is T_{CTL}-mediated lysis. Targets for NK lysis include a large variety of tumor cells (leukemias, lymphomas, sarcomas, carcinomas) as well as some normal cell lines. NK activity is increased by infections and is activated by interleukin-2 (IL-2). NK cells activated by IL-2 are called **lymphokine-activated killer cells (LAKs)**. LAKs are now being used in clinical trials to treat cancer patients (see Chapter 30). The role of NK cells in vivo is not clearly established, but they are believed to have an important role in a large number of diverse immunologic functions including defense against microbial, fungal and parasitic infections; regulation of hematopoiesis; natural resistance to foreign grafts; and inhibiting (killing) cancer cells.

NK activity in normal individuals was not recognized for some time because investigators considered the cytolytic activity of control normal cells as background in their assays for T-cell mediated tumor cell killing. For instance, comparisons of killing activity were made using lymphocytes from normal donors to that of lymphocytes from donors that had been cured of cancer (tumor regressor lymphocytes). The lytic effect of the normal NK population, such as determined by inhibition of tumor-cell growth or lysis of tumor cells, was subtracted from the effect of regressor cells, believed to be due to specific T_{CTL} cells. However, it was discovered that lymphocytes from many normal individuals had activity just as high or higher than those from tumor regressors, and that the tumor killing activity was not in the T-cell population, but in null cells, ie, NK cells.

There is marked heterogeneity of natural killer cells in regard to pattern of target-cell specificity, cell surface markers, and response to regulatory factors. In the mouse, for instance, two populations of large granular lymphocytes responsible for MHC nonrestricted killing of target cells are called natural killer (NK) and natural cytotoxic (NC) cells. NK cells express some markers in common with other lymphoid cells and kill a group of tissue culture cell lines called YAC-1-like *within* 4 hours *after* mixing in vitro, whereas NC cells do not have the shared markers and do not kill YAC-1-like target cells, but kill adherent tumor target cells (WEHI-like) *after* 4 hours (16-hour assays). In the human, two classes of large granular NK cells are identified by the cluster of differentiation marked CD3. CD3 is found on T cells and about 5% of NK cells. The CD3+ NK cells also have rearrangement of T-cell receptor genes, whereas the CD3– cells do not. Both classes of NK cells express CD2 and NKH1, a marker associated with NK cells, but not with antibody-dependent cell-mediated cytotoxicity (ADCC) cells. Thus, at least three subpopulations of NK cells may be identified in the human: CD3+NKH1+TCR+, CD3–NKH1+TCR–, and CD3+NKH2 +TCR–(ADCC).

Antibody-Dependent Cell-Mediated Cytotoxicity (ADCC). The cells responsible for ADCC, sometimes called **K cells**, have receptors (FC receptors) for and are able to bind antibodies. Through these antibodies the ADCC cells are directed to lyse target cells to which the antibody is directed. ADCC are believed to be part of the NK-cell population and can be identified by monoclonal antibody-defined surface markers termed NKH1 and NKH2 (see below). NK cells are NKH1+; ADCC cells are NKH2+. ADCC may be an important protective mechanism against certain types of intracellular infections, such as by viruses, or against tumors.

Blast Cells. A well-recognized feature of active immune responses is the presence of large **blast cells**. Blast cells are cells that are activated and are in the process of dividing. These cells have a large nucleus containing finely divided chromatin and prominent nucleoli. The cytoplasm of blast cells is strongly basophilic and contains dense collections of free and aggregated ribosomes. A variety of other subcellular organelles may be found in the cytoplasm, including a Golgi apparatus, varying amounts of endoplasmic reticulum, and mitochondria. Blast cells are found in lymphoid organs draining sites of antigen injection, in active inflammatory lesions (particularly those of delayed hypersensitivity reactions), and may be induced in vitro in pure cultures of lymphocytes by certain mitogenic agents. Antigen-recognizing lymphocytes are stimulated by antigen to undergo transformation into "blast" cells that proliferate, and differentiate into plasma cells or sensitized T cells.

Macrophages

The macrophage (large eater), the primary phagocytic cell, is the largest cell in the lymphoid system, ranging from 12 to 15 microns in diameter when in suspension, but can extend through organs by cytoplasmic extensions (dendritic macrophages). Macrophages in the blood are called monocytes; those in tissue are called histiocytes. The macrophage nucleus usually has a bilobate kidney shape with considerable peripheral condensation of nuclear chromatin. The cytoplasm of the macrophage contains a great variety of organelles, including endoplasmic reticulum, a Golgi complex, mitochondria, free and aggregated ribosomes, and various membrane-limited phagocytic vacuoles (lysosomes, dense bodies, myelin figures, microbodies). The tissue macrophage or histocyte exists in larger size (15 to 18 microns) and may contain many more cytoplasmic vacuoles than blood monocytes. Macrophages invade sites of inflammation after polymorphonuclear cells and serve to clear the site of necrotic debris. The digestive capacity of the macrophage is more effective than that of the polymorphonuclear cell (PMN). It appears that PMNs get in quickly (attack troops) to act on infecting organisms, but macrophages are needed to finish the job (mop-up troops).

Role in the Immune Response. The uptake of antigens by macrophages is the first step in the processing of antigen leading to the production of circulating antibody. In such cases, it appears that antigen is not completely degraded by the macrophage but becomes bound to macrophage RNA or membrane. The macrophage is not the cell that recognizes antigen as foreign, but the macrophage nonspecifically processes the antigen so that it may be recognized by specific antigen reactive cells. Further definitions of the role of the macrophage in the induction of immunity will be discussed in Chapters 5 and 7.

The macrophage also plays a prominent role in the later stages of the inflammatory response and may accumulate in large numbers in sites of inflammation. The migration of macrophages (both blood and tissue) into inflammatory sites is generally believed to be non-antigen specific. Specifically sensitized lymphocytes may, upon reaction with antigen, release substances that attract and affect the migration of macrophages or products that increase the phagocytic or digestive capacity of macrophages (see Table 2–3). The role of macrophages and products of macrophages in inflammation is presented in much more detail in Chapter 9.

Macrophage Subpopulations. Subpopulations of cells in the macrophage family may be recognized by a combination of cell surface markers, morphologic appearance, and location in tissue (Table 2–6). Fixed histiocytes lining the sinusoids of the liver are given the special name of Kupffer cells.

Factors that contribute to induction and expression of immune responses as well as inflammation are also produced by macrophages (see Chapter 9). One macrophage-derived factor, interleukin-1, plays a key role in induction of immune responses, inflammation, and actions of other cells.

Langerhans' Cells. (Fig. 2–6). Langerhans' cells are a population of the macrophage series found within the mammalian epidermis and certain lymph nodes. They are derived from bone marrow macrophage precursors. They are able to present antigen to T cells in vitro and are believed to be important in promoting certain immune-mediated lesions, such as contact dermatitis and skin graft rejection. They are able to pick up antigens encountered in the epidermis and to migrate to the paracortex of the skin-draining lymph nodes, where they transform into interdigitating cells and present antigen to T cells in a class II major histocompatibility complex (MHC)-restricted fashion. A peculiar morphologic term—"veiled cell"—has been applied to cells believed to be Langerhans' cells in the afferent lymphatics and the paracortex of lymph nodes. Veiled cells have multiple long dendritic arms by electron microscopy. Langerhans' cells are not usually visual-

TABLE 2–6. MACROPHAGE SUBPOPULATIONS

Macrophage Subpopulation	Organ	Presumed Function
Stem cell	Bone marrow	Precursor
Monocyte	Blood	Circulating macrophage
Fixed histiocytes	Reticuloendothelial	Phagocytic cells in tissue
Dendritic histiocytes	Lymphoid organs	Process antigen for B cells
Interdigitating reticulum cells	Lymphoid organs	Process antigen for T cells
Langerhans' cells	Skin, lymph nodes	Process antigen for T cells
Kupffer cells	Liver sinusoids	Clear blood of particles

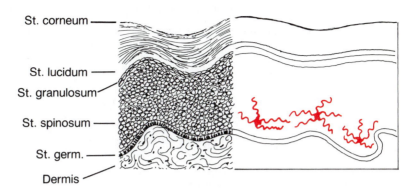

St. corneum

St. lucidum

St. granulosum

St. spinosum

St. germ.

Dermis

Figure 2–6. Langerhans' cells. On the left is a drawing of the layers of the epithelium of the skin. On the right is depicted the location of Langerhans' cells as detected by special markets. Langerhans' cells are not distinguishable from epithelial cells by the usual methods used for staining tissue.

ized in hematoxylin and eosin (H&E) sections but can be distinguished by the presence of class II major histocompatibility markers, by certain CD markers (CD1a, CD1c, CD45), VLA, LFA-1, ICAM-1, C3R, and by the presence of Birbeck granules, which can only be seen by electron microscopy. Birbeck granules are rod-shaped organelles with a central zipperlike striation, occasionally having a vesicular dilation at one end, giving the structure a racketlike appearance. The adhesion molecules LFA-2 and ICAM-1 promote binding to CD2 and LFA-1 on T cells and provide additional activation signals that synergize through the T-cell antigen receptor/CD3 complex (see Chapter 7).

Cellular Interactions in Immune Responses

A simplified diagram of antigen processing and cellular interactions in immune responses is presented in Figure 2–7. Two major types of antigen processing will be presented at this time: exogenous and endogenous. The characteristics and mechanisms of interactions of antigen-presenting cells, T cells, and B cells in induction and expression of immune response will be discussed in more detail in Chapter 7. Exogenous processing can only be accomplished by cells that express class II MHC molecules (macrophages and B cells). During the induction of antibody formation an immunogen is endocytosed by follicular dendritic cells and presented in association with class II MHC molecules on the surface of the antigen-presenting cell to T-helper cells. T-helper cells recognize class II MHC self-markers and antigen and provide proliferation and differentiation signals to the precursors of plasma cells (B cells). The B cell is stimulated to divide and differentiate so that large numbers of specific antibody-producing plasma cells

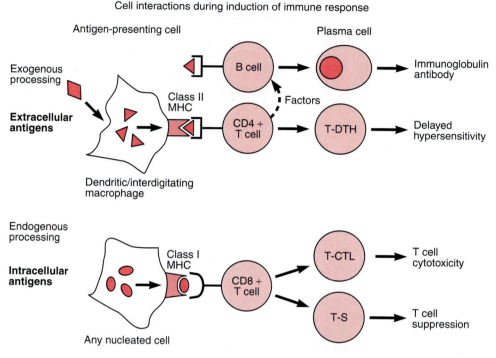

Figure 2–7. Cellular interactions in induction of antibody formation. Exogenous processing results in presentation of antigens in association with class II MHC to CD4+ T-helper cells. During endogenous processing, antigen is presented in association with class I MHC to CD8+ $T_{CTL/S}$ precursors. This subject is only presented here for a preliminary introduction to antigen processing and cell–cell interactions during induction of immunity. For more details see Chapter 7.

are produced. In some instances, B cells can present antigen to T cells and bypass the macrophage requirement or B cells may be stimulated directly (T-independent antibody response). Interdigitating reticulum cells present exogenously processed class II MHC-associated antigen to T-helper cells that proliferate and differentiate into specifically sensitized T_{DTH} cells that mediate delayed hypersensitivity.

Endogenous processing may occur in any nucleated cell that expresses class I MHC molecules. Endogenous antigens are produced by the cell itself or by infectious organisms within the cells. Endogenous processed antigens are presented in association with class I MHC molecules to CD8+ T cells that proliferate and differentiate into T_{CTL} or T_S cells.

HEMATO-POIESIS

Blood cell formation is called hematopoiesis (Greek: *haemia*, blood; *poieses*, production). A general view of hematopoiesis presented in Figure 2–8. The precursors of all blood cells are found normally in the

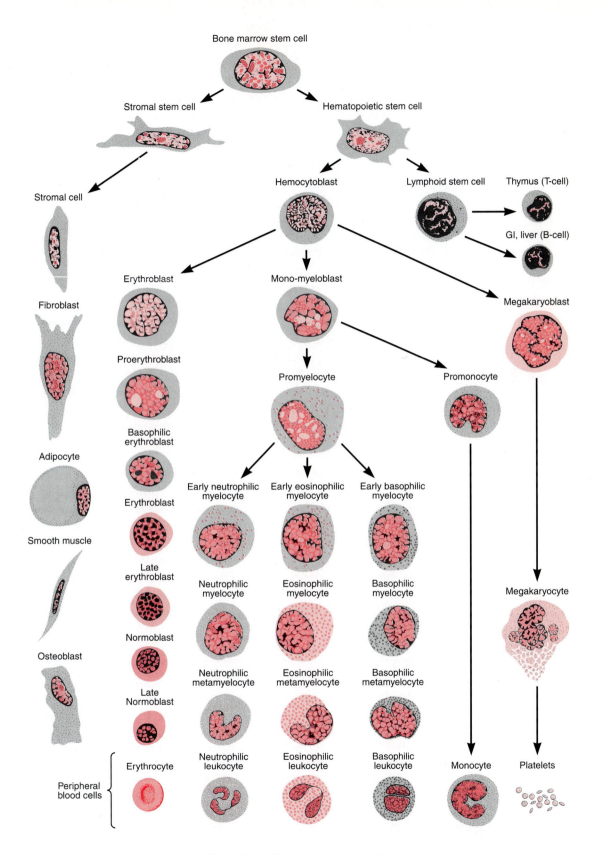

Bone marrow stem cell

Stromal stem cell

Hematopoietic stem cell

Stromal cell

Hemocytoblast

Lymphoid stem cell

Thymus (T-cell)

GI, liver (B-cell)

Fibroblast

Erythroblast

Mono-myeloblast

Megakaryoblast

Proerythroblast

Promyelocyte

Promonocyte

Basophilic erythroblast

Adipocyte

Early neutrophilic myelocyte

Early eosinophilic myelocyte

Early basophilic myelocyte

Erythroblast

Smooth muscle

Neutrophilic myelocyte

Eosinophilic myelocyte

Basophilic myelocyte

Late erythroblast

Megakaryocyte

Normoblast

Neutrophilic metamyelocyte

Eosinophilic metamyelocyte

Basophilic metamyelocyte

Osteoblast

Late Normoblast

Peripheral blood cells

Erythrocyte

Neutrophilic leukocyte

Eosinophilic leukocyte

Basophilic leukocyte

Monocyte

Platelets

Figure 2-8. *Continued on page 42.*

bone marrow. Formation of erythrocytes, monocytes, granulocytes, and platelets is called myelopoiesis. All blood cells arise from a common **bone marrow stem cell**, which represents less than 0.01 percent of bone marrow cells. The putative human hematopoietic stem cell expresses the cell-surface antigen CD34. The primitive mesenchymal stem cell first differentiates into a stromal stem cell that gives rise to bone marrow stroma, as well as fibroblasts, adipocytes, smooth muscle, etc., and the **hematopoietic stem cell** that gives rise to lymphoid and myeloid cell lineages. In the bone marrow the stromal cells interact with the hematopoietic cell to provide a microenvironment which supports continued production and differentiation of blood cells. The myeloid stem cell then differentiates into erythrocyte (normocyte), monogranulocyte (promyelocyte), and platelet (megakaryocyte) lineages. The occurrence of leukemic cells which share markers and properties of monocytes and polymorphonuclear cells (monomyelocytic leukemia) and development of colonies for monocytic and granulocytic cells from a shared precursor in vitro is evidence that there is a common precursor for monocytes and granulocytes. The lymphoid stem cell differentiates into B-cell and T-cell/NK lineages. The ability to induce differentiation of myeloid precursors in vitro has led to a much better understanding of the role of different **colony-stimulating factors** in controlling myeloid differentiation.

Hematopoietic Factors

Three major classes of hematopoietic factors have been identified (Table 2–7). A simplified illustration of the action of these factors is presented in Figure 2–9. The first class is lineage specific and stimulates the final mitotic divisions and terminal differentiation (lineage-restricted colony-stimulating factors). The second class, pluripotent progenitor-stimulating factors, stimulate proliferation of progenitor cells, are not lineage specific, and do not support complete differentiation through mature end cells. The third class acts synergistically with other factors to augment colony development in vitro, but have little or

Figure 2–8. Hematopoiesis. The stroma and blood cells arise from a common bone marrow stem cell which gives rise to a stromal stem cell and a hematopoietic stem cell. The stromal stem cell differentiates into stromal cells, fibroblasts, adipocytes, smooth muscle cells, and osteoblasts that form the supporting structure for the hematopoietic cells. The white blood cell lineages differentiate from a pluripotent hematopoietic stem cell in the bone marrow. The first differentiation step of the hematopoietic stem cell is into lymphoid and myeloid series. Lymphoid cell development takes place in other organs and will be presented in Chapter 3. The hemocytoblast stem cell differentiates into erythroblast, monomyeloblast, and megakaryoblast (platelets) lineages. The monogranulocytic then differentiates into monocytic and granulocytic lineages. A series of maturation stages in each lineage results in the formation of the mature cells of each lineage that leave the bone marrow and circulate in the peripheral blood. The morphologic stages of granulocytic maturation are: promyelocyte, myelocyte, metamyelocyte, band, and segmented.

TABLE 2–7. CLASSES OF HEMATOPOIETIC GROWTH FACTORS

Class	Factor	Cell Lineage
Lineage-restricted colony-stimulating factors	Granulocyte CSF	Granulocytes
	Macrophage CSF	Monocytes
	Erythropoietin	Red blood cells
	Interleukin-5	Eosinophils
Pluripotent colony-stimulating factors	Interleukin-3	Myeloid lineage
	Granulocyte/monocyte CSF	Granulocytes/monocytes
Recruiters	Interleukin-1	Stem cells
	Interleukin-6	Megakaryocytes
	Interleukin-9	Mast cells, erythrocytes

Modified from Mazur EM, Cohen JL: Basic concepts of hematopoiesis and the hematopoietic growth factors. *Clin Pharm Therapeut* 46:250, 1989. Further details on the properties and function of the interleukins during the immune response and in inflammation will be presented later.

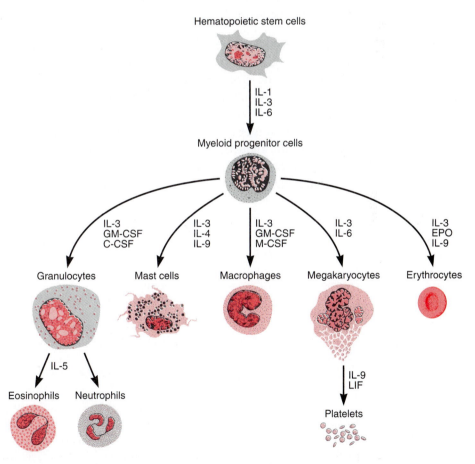

Figure 2–9. Role of Growth Factors in Hematopoiesis. Interleukins, colony stimulating factors and erythropoietin have been shown to induce differentiation during hematopoiesis. Some, such as IL-3, are active on different lineages of cells, whereas others, such as IL-5, M-CSF and G-CSF act on some lineages but not on others (see Table 2-7).

no intrinsic activity. Some of these factors also have critical roles in T- and B-cell differentiation, which will be presented in later chapters.

Hematopoietic Factor Treatment of Human Diseases

The availability of hematopoietic factors produced by recombinant techniques has led to the use of selected factors for the treatment of human diseases in which there is a block in hematopoietic development (Table 2–8). These factors are able to stimulate hematopoiesis in patients with primary hematologic diseases, but so far have had little effect in people with cancer. Erythropoietin has been approved by the FDA for use in anemia secondary to renal failure or azidothymidine (AZT) therapy for acquired immunodeficiency disease (AIDS); granulocyte CSF has been approved for treatment of neutropenia in patients undergoing chemotherapy for cancer, and granulocyte/monocyte CSF for stimulation of patients receiving autologous bone marrow transplants. Other factors are being evaluated by clinical trials but have not yet been approved at the time of this writing.

Summary

A summary of the properties of white blood cells is given in Table 2–9. The cells of the lymphoid system are the white blood cells. This chapter compares the structure and function of leukocytes (white blood cells). Polymorphonuclear cells (neutrophils, eosinophils, and basophils/mast cells) have important parts to play in the inflammatory response, but do not recognize antigen and are not involved in induction of specific induction of immunity. Mononuclear cells (lymphoid cells) include macrophages, lymphocytes (T cells, B cells, and null cells), and plasma cells. These cells are active in inflammation and in

TABLE 2–8. HEMATOPOIETIC GROWTH FACTORS FOR HUMAN DISEASES

Factor	Therapeutic Applications	FDA Status
Erythropoietin	Anemia of renal failure	Approved
	Anemia related to AZT therapy (AIDS)	Approved
Granulocyte CSF	Neutropenia (cancer chemotherapy)	Approved
	Congenital and acquired neutropenia	Not approved
	Myelodysplasia	Not approved
	Aplastic anemia	Not approved
Granulocyte/monocyte CSF	Autologous bone marrow transplant	Approved
	Cancer chemotherapy	Not approved
	AIDS	Not approved
	Myelodysplasia	Not approved
	Aplastic anemia	Not approved
Interleukin-3	Aplastic anemia, myelodysplasia	Not approved
Interleukin-6	Thrombocytopenia	Not approved
Monocyte CSF	Fungal infections, tumor therapy	Not approved

Modified from Groopman JE: Hematopoietic growth factors: Will their promise be fulfilled? *J NIH Res* 3:75, 1991.

TABLE 2–9. SUMMARY OF PROPERTIES OF CELLS OF THE IMMUNE SYSTEM

Cell Type	Function	Markers
B lymphocyte	Precursor of plasma cells, produces antibody, antigen presentation	Surface immunoglobulin, Class II MHC, complement receptors, Fc receptor, CD19, CD20, CD22, CD37, etc.
T lymphocytes		
T_{Helper}	Assists response of other lymphocytes	TCR, CD4, IL-3, IL-4, etc.
T_{DTH}	Initiates delayed hypersensitivity reactions	TCR, CD4, IL-2, IL-3, etc.
T_{CTL}	Kills specific target cells	TCR, CD8, perforin, granzymes
T_S	Suppresses immune responses	TCR, CD8, ? suppressor factor
Null cells	Natural killers, ADCC	FcR, CD16, perforins, granzymes
Macrophages	Antigen presentation, phagocytosis, chronic inflammation	Class II MHC, CD14, CD68, FcR and CR digestive granules (lysozyme, proteases, peroxidases), IL-1
Langerhans' cells	Antigen presentation, epidermis	Class II MHC, CD1, CD45, LFA-3, ICAM-1, VLA, Birbeck granules
Neutrophil	Acute inflammation, phagocytosis, bacteriocidal	CD15, CD67, Fc and C receptors, pink granules (cationic proteins, myeloperoxidase, lysozyme, defensins)
Basophil (mast cell)	Vasodilation, vascular permeability, bronchoconstriction	Fc receptor for IgE, blue granules (heparin, serotonin, arachidonic acid), interleukins 1–6, tumor necrosis factor, etc.
Eosinophil	ADCC to parasites, antiinflammatory	IgG, IgE, C3b receptors, red granules (major basic protein, arylsulfatase, histaminase)

both induction and expression of immune responses. T cells, B cells, and macrophages cooperate in the induction of antibody responses to most antigens. Upon immune induction, T cells differentiate into specifically sensitized lymphocytes responsible for cellular immune reactivity, whereas B cells differentiate into antibody-secreting plasma cells. Null cells are active as killer cells, able to kill (lyse) a variety of target cells. Polymorphonuclear cells (granulocytes) and macrophages are active in the effector states of tissue inflammation in both a specific and nonspecific manner.

Bibliography

This chapter is a general introduction to the cells of the immune system. More recent references on the differentiation, identification of phenotypic markers, genetics, and phenotypic markers of the cells of the immune system are given in later pertinent chapters.

POLYMORPHO-NUCLEAR CELLS

Bainton DF: Developmental biology of neutrophils and eosinophils. In *Inflammation: Basic Principles and Clinical Correlates*, 2nd ed. (Gallin JI, Goldstein IM, Snyderman R, eds.). New York, Raven Press, 1992, 303–324.

de Duve C, Wattiaux R: Function of lysosomes. *Am Rev Physiol* 23:435, 1966.

Galli SJ, Austen KF: Mast cell differentiation and function in health and disease. New York, Raven Press, 1989.

Hallett MB: The neutrophil: Cellular biochemistry and physiology. Boca Raton, FL, CRC Press, 1989.

Kaliner MA, Metcalfe DD: The mast cell in health and disease. New York, Marcel Dekker, 1992.

Kirshenbaum AS, Kessler SW, Goff JP, et al.: Demonstration of the origin of human mast cell from CD34+ bone marrow progenitor cells. *J Immunol* 146:1410, 1991.

Klebanoff SJ, Clark RA: The neutrophil: Function and clinical disorders. Amsterdam, North-Holland, 1978.

Kobayaki TK, Robinson JM: A novel intracellular compartment with unusual secretory properties in human neutrophils. *J Cell Biol* 113:743, 1991.

Lehrer RI, Ganz T, Selsted ME: Defensins: Endogenous antibiotic peptides of animal cells. *Cell* 64:229, 1991.

Oppenheim JJ, Rosenstreich DL, Potter M: *Cellular Functions in Immunity and Inflammation*. New York, Elsevier/North Holland, 1981.

Spitznagel JK: Antibiotic proteins of human neutrophils. *J Clin Invest* 86:1381, 1990.

Spry JF, Kay AB, Gleich GJ: Eosinophils 1992. *Immunol Today* 13:384, 1992.

LYMPHOCYTES

Bianco C, Patrick R, Nuzzenzweig V: A population of lymphocytes bearing a membrane receptor for antigen–antibody complement complexes. *J Exp Med* 132:702–718, 1970.

Gowans JL, McGregor DD: The immunological activities of lymphocytes. *Prog Allergy* 9:1, 1965.

Jondal M, Holm G, Wigzell H: Surface markers on human T and B lymphocytes. I. A large population of lymphocytes forming nonimmune rosettes with sheep red blood cells. *J Exp Med* 136:207–215, 1972.

Katz DH: Lymphocyte differentiation, recognition, and regulation. New York, Academic Press, 1978.

Peters PJ, Borst J, Oorschot V, et al.: Cytotoxic T lymphocyte granules are secretory lysosomes, containing both perforin and granzymes. *J Exp Med* 173:1099–1109, 1991.

Sandor M, Lynch RG: The biology and pathology of Fc receptors. *J Clin Immunol* 13:237–246, 1993.

Sell S, Asofsky R: Lymphocytes and immunoglobulins. *Prog Allergy* 12:86, 1968.

NATURAL KILLER/ADCC

Bykowsky MJ, Stutman O: The cells responsible for a murine natural cytotoxic (NC) activity: A multilineage system. *J Immunol* 137:1120, 1986.

Herberman RB, Reynolds CW, Ortaldo JR: Mechanism of cytotoxicity by natural killer cells. *Annu Rev Immunol* 4:651, 1986.

Lanier LL, Spits H, Phillips JH: The development relationship between NK cells and T cells. *Immunol Today* 13:392–395, 1992.

Moretta L, Ciccone E, Poggi A, et al.: Ontogeny-specific functions and receptors of human natural killer cells. *Immunol Lett* 40:83–88, 1994.

Ortaldo JR: Comparison of natural killer and natural cytotoxic cells: Characteristics, regulation, and mechanism of action. *Pathol Immunopathol Res* 5:203, 1986.

Robertson MJ, Caliguri MA, Manley TJ, Levine H, Ritz J: Human natural killer cell adhesion molecules: Differential expression after activation and participation in cytolysis. *J Immunol* 145:3194, 1990.

Schmidt RE (ed.): Natural killer cells: Biology and clinical application. Farmington CT, S Karger, 1991.

Westermann J, Pabst R: Distribution of lymphocyte subsets and natural killer cells in the human body. *Clin Invest* 70:539, 1992

MACROPHAGES

Axline SG: Functional biochemistry of the macrophage. *Semin Hematol* 7:142, 1970.

Cohn ZA: The structure and functions of monocytes and macrophages. *Adv Immunol* 9:163, 1968.

Holiian A, Scheule RK: Alveolar macrophage biology. *Hosp Pract* 25:49, 1990.

LANGERHANS' CELLS

Knight SC, Stagg A, Holl S, et al.: Development and function of dendritic cells in health and disease. *J Invest Dermatol* 99:33S, 1992.

Schuler G: Epidermal Langerhans' cells. Boca Raton, FL, CRC Press, 1990.

Streilein JW, Bergstresser PR: Ia antigen and epidermal Langerhans' cells. *Transplant* 30:319, 1980.

Teunissen MBM: Dynamic nature and function of epidermal Langerhans' cells in vivo and in vitro: A critical review, with emphasis on human Langerhans' cells. *Histochem J* 24:697, 1992.

CELL INTERACTIONS IN IMMUNE RESPONSE

Braciale TJ, Braciale VL: Antigen presentation: Structural themes and functional variations. *Immunol Today* 12:124, 1991.

Claman HN, Mosier DE: Cell–cell interactions in antibody production. *Prog Allergy* 16:40, 1972.

Miller JFAP, Basten A, Sprent J, Cheers C: Review: Interactions between lymphocytes in immune responses. *Cell Immunol* 2:249, 1971.

Mitchison NA: The carrier effect in the secondary response to hapten–protein conjugates. II. Cellular cooperation. *Eur J Immunol* 1:18, 1971.

Mosmann TR, Coffman RL: Heterogeneity of cytokine secretion patterns and functions of helper T cells. *Adv Immunol* 46:111, 1989.

Rothermel AL, Gilbert KM, Weigle WO: Differential abilities of Th1 and Th2 to induce polyclonal B-cell proliferation. *Cell Immunol* 135:1, 1991.

Yewdell JW, Bennink JR: Cell biology of antigen processing and presentation to major histocompatibility complex class I molecule-restricted T lymphocytes. *Adv Immuno* 52:1, 1992.

HEMATO-POIESIS

Aglieta M: Positive and negative signals in the control of myelopoiesis. *Haematologica* 74:121, 1989.

Buchner T: Hematopoietic growth factors in cancer treatment. *Stem Cells* 12:241–252, 1994.

Champlin RE: Therapeutic use of hematopoietic growth factors for patients receiving high-dose chemotherapy and bone marrow transplantation. *Cancer Bull* 43:197, 1991.

Graber SE, Kranz SB: Erythropoietin: Biology and clinical use. *Hematol Oncol Clin N Am* 3:369, 1989.

Groopman JE: Hematopoietic growth factors: Will their promise be fulfilled? *J NIH Res* 3:75, 1991.

Huang S, Terstappen LWMM: Formation of haematopoietic microenvironment and haematopoietic stem cells from single human bone marrow stem cells. *Nature* 360:745, 1992.

Mazur EM, Cohen JL: Basic concepts of hematopoiesis and the hematopoietic growth factors. *Clin Pharmacol Therapeut* 46:250, 1989.

Mertelsmann R, Hermann F (eds.): Hematopoietic growth factors in clinical applications. New York, Marcel Dekker, 1990.

Till JE, McCulloch EA: Hematopoietic stem cell differentiation. *Biochem Biophys Acta* 605:431, 1980.

The Immune System II: Organs

3

Introduction

Lymphoid organs are compartmentalized collections of specialized lymphocytes, macrophages, and supporting connective tissue that serve as sites for immune responses, producing the antibody and sensitized lymphocytes that provide specific adaptive immunity. Lymphoid organs, which include lymph nodes, spleen, thymus, gastrointestinal-associated lymphoid tissue (GALT), bronchus-associated lymphoid tissue (BALT), and skin-associated lymphoid tissue (SALT), as well as the bone marrow, yolk sac, and liver, have similarities as well as differences in structure and function. Different populations of lymphocytes are selectively located in different domains of a given lymphoid organ forming functional microenvironments with macrophages or epithelial cells of special types.

Lymphatic Vessels

The lymphatic circulation collects interstitial body fluids that pass from blood capillaries and returns the fluid to the systemic circulation, and in doing so delivers foreign antigens to reactive lymphoid organs and products of an immune response to the systemic circulation. The lymphatic circulation is different for each set of organs. Lymph nodes have both afferent and efferent lymphatics (Fig. 3–1). Lymph nodes are located along the course of lymphatic vessels that drain from the skin and are situated in the body in locations where foreign material entering the body will be filtered through the lymph nodes. Specialized antigen-presenting cells in the skin (Langerhans' cells) migrate to the lymph nodes after contact with antigen, thus presenting the antigen to T cells in microenvironments suitable for humoral or cellular immune responses. Gastrointestinal lymphoid organs are located along the

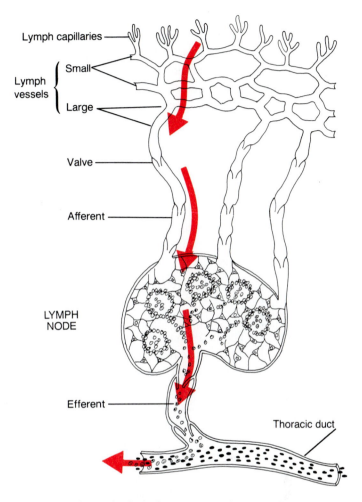

Figure 3–1. Lymph node lymphatics. Lymphatic collecting vessels are similar to veins. Afferent lymphatics deliver lymphatic fluid-containing blood cells that have escaped through capillaries, as well as foreign material that has entered the interstitial spaces of the body. Afferent lymphatics deliver lymph fluid to the lymph node. The lymph nodes act as a filter for the lymphatic fluid, which delivers antigens to the node. Specific antibodies or sensitized cells are produced in the lymph node and delivered to the systemic circulation through the efferent lymphatics.

absorptive areas of the gastrointestinal tract. Lymphatic capillaries of the gastrointestinal tract are called lacteals. Lacteals not only deliver antigens to the lymphoid tissue but also absorb fats in the form of chylomicra. The spleen does not have parenchymal lymphatics and serves as a filter for the circulating blood. The bone marrow and thymus function as sites of production of immature lymphoid cells (central lymphoid organs have no afferent lymphatics). The thymus has efferent lymphatics, whereas the bone marrow delivers maturing cells into the blood through specialized venous capillaries.

In response to the antigens, specific antibodies or specifically sensitized cells are produced in the lymphoid organs and delivered to the systemic circulation by efferent lymphatic vessels. The afferent lymphatic vessels retrieve fluid (lymph) and blood proteins which escape from blood capillaries and venules and return it to the venous system after filtration through the lymph nodes. If this function of the lymphatic circulation is impaired, fluid will collect in the involved tissues (edema). The lymphatic vessels also collect wandering white blood cells in tissues, including lymphocytes that may have contacted antigen in the periphery, and return them to the lymphoid organs. Lymphatic vessels drain every organ of the body except parts of the central nervous system, the eye, the internal ear, cartilage, spleen, and bone marrow (Fig. 3–2).

Lymphoid Organs

CENTRAL LYMPHOID ORGANS

The bone marrow, liver, and thymus are considered **central lymphoid organs** because their function is to provide precursor cells that circulate and take up residence in the **peripheral lymphoid organs**, ie, lymph nodes, spleen, etc. Gastrointestinal-associated lymphoid tissue (GALT) and bronchus-associated lymphoid tissue (BALT) have both central and peripheral functions.

Figure 3–2. A diagram of the human lymphoid system. The system consists of circulating lymphocytes and the lymphoid organs, and includes the network of lymphatic vessels and the lymph nodes stationed along them, the bone marrow (in the long bones, only one of which is illustrated), the thymus, spleen, adenoids, tonsils, Peyer's patches of the small intestine, appendix, lung (BALT), skin (SALT), and mammary gland (MALT). Afferent lymphatic vessels collect the fluid and cells that escape from the blood capillaries and return them via the lymph nodes to the bloodstream. In addition, efferent lymphatics collect lymphocytes and antibody molecules from the lymph nodes and deliver them to the blood. The thoracic duct is the largest lymph vessel in the body and joins the left subclavian vein. The right lymphatic duct joins the right subclavian vein. Seventy-five percent of body tissues are drained by the thoracic duct and 25% are drained by the right lymphatic duct. There is no pump for the lymphatic circulation, such as the heart for the systemic circulation. Lymphatic fluid is propelled by contraction of skeletal muscles or in larger vessels by smooth muscle cells that force the fluid from one level to another past valves that only permit passage of fluid and cells in one direction.

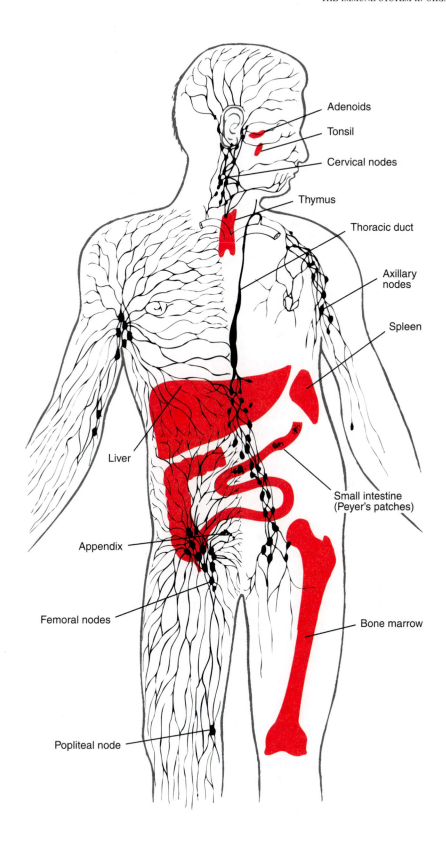

Adenoids

Tonsil

Cervical nodes

Thymus

Thoracic duct

Axillary nodes

Spleen

Liver

Small intestine
(Peyer's patches)

Appendix

Bone marrow

Femoral nodes

Popliteal node

Bone Marrow

The bone marrow is soft tissue found within many bones of the skeleton of the body and is the site of production of new blood cells. It contains fat cells, stromal cells, and the blood forming cells (hematopoietic tissue). The stem cells of all the blood elements, including the precursors of lymphoid cells, are located in the bone marrow. These stem cells (**multipotent hematolymphomyeloid stem cells**) and their progeny are organized into islands of cells within fatty tissue. In the bone marrow, the cell types are admixed so that precursors of red blood cells (erythroblasts), macrophages (monoblasts), platelets (megakaryocytes), polymorphonuclear leukocytes (myeloblasts), and lymphocytes (lymphoblasts) may be seen in one microscopic field. It is impossible to differentiate stem cells for one cell line from those of another cell line by morphologic appearance alone. However, stem cells are usually surrounded by more mature cells of the same cell line so that a given cell may be identified by the company it keeps.

In normal bone marrow, the myelocytic series (polymorphonuclear cells) makes up approximately 60% of the cellular elements, and the erythrocytic series, 20% to 30%. Lymphocytes, monocytes, reticular cells, plasma cells, and megakaryocytes together constitute only 10% to 20%. Lymphocytes make up 5% to 15% of the cells of the normal adult marrow and 20% to 30% of a child's marrow. Normally, lymphocytes are mixed diffusely with the other cellular elements, but focal collections of lymphocytes may be seen in the marrow of elderly individuals. Plasma cells normally constitute fewer than 1% of the marrow cells but increase in percentage with age. Circulating blood enters via arteries that enter through the periosteum and pass through the compact bone in small canals. The marrow is drained by venous sinuses that collect mature blood elements for distribution into the peripheral blood. The mechanism whereby mature cells escape into the bloodstream whereas immature ones are held back is not known.

The bone marrow is not usually a site of reaction with, or response to, antigen. Marrow lymphocytes circulate from the marrow to other lymphoid organs and differentiate into lymphocytes capable of immune function. Cells originating in the marrow populate the thymus where they may differentiate into T cells, whereas other marrow cells differentiate into B cells (see below). Some immunologically reactive cells may be present in the bone marrow but their contribution to the immune response of the whole animal remains unclear. An intriguing observation is that in the human, naturally occurring tumors of plasma cells that produce immunoglobulin (multiple myeloma) are often found in the bone marrow; extramedullary location multiple myeloma is much less frequent. This suggests that the precursors of plasma cells with malignant potential are located in the bone marrow.

Liver

Early in ontogeny, the liver and yolk sac of mammals is the primary site of blood cell formation and, along with the bone marrow, may be the original site of maturation or production of B cells. (For more details, see Development of Lymphoid Organs below.) The yolk sac and liver are closely related embryologically. The fetal liver is made up of immature liver cells (hepatocytes) surrounded by many islands of blood-forming cells containing essentially the same populations of hematopoietic cells as the bone marrow. Attempts to identify a tissue site for maturation of B-cell populations has largely been influenced by the finding that the **bursa of Fabricius**, a gastrointestinal lymphoid organ of birds, is required for normal avian B-cell maturation. A mammalian equivalent for the avian bursa in this regard has not been convincingly demonstrated. The mammalian gastrointestinal lymphoid tissue may also be a site for B-cell development, but studies are inconclusive. Lymphocytes derived from mouse embryo liver develop surface Ig (B cells) when cultured in vitro. From this finding it has been suggested that the fetal liver of mammals is a major tissue site of B-cell maturation. The yolk sac may also serve as a site for production of immature immune cells for the embryo.

Thymus

The thymus is the organ where precursors of T cells develop and mature. T cells are, in fact, **thymus-derived cells**. Cells in the thymus are technically not T cells; T cells are derived from cells that have begun maturation in the thymus and completed it in peripheral lymphoid organs (lymph node, etc). The thymus contains an outside layer of packed lymphoid cells (cortex), an inside layer of less densely packed cells (medulla), a fibrous capsule, prominent trabeculae that divide the organ into lobules, and a hilum with entering arteries and draining veins and lymphatics (Fig. 3–3). The thymus differs from the lymph nodes and the spleen in three important features:

1. Normally, there are no lymphoid follicles and essentially no B cells. The cortex consists of packed small T-cell precursors and many proliferating cells in various stages of differentiation to T cells, as well as many apoptotic cells.
2. The medulla contains remnants of epithelial islands that appear as concentric rings of eosinophilic tissue known as Hassal's corpuscles.
3. The medulla does not contain sinusoids but is a mesenchymal–endothelial reticular network in which are found large numbers of lymphocytes.

The cortex can be differentiated from the medulla because the lymphocytes are much more closely packed in the cortex. There are no afferent lymphatics in the thymus. The drainage of the thymus has not been well characterized; most drainage occurs through the vein, although significant lymphatic drainage has been claimed by some observers. The cortex is an area of active proliferation, with complete

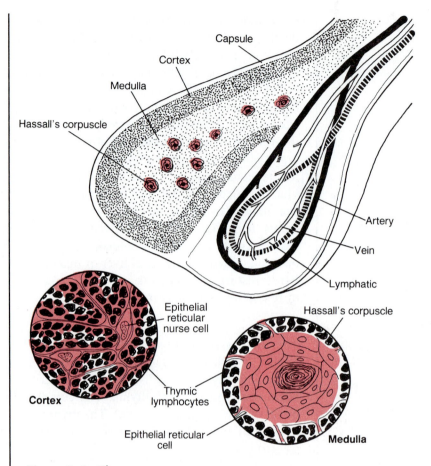

Figure 3–3. Thymus.

turnover of cells believed to occur every 3 or 4 days. The primary function of the normal adult thymus is the production of thymic lymphocytes (thymocytes). However, only about 1% of the lymphocytes produced ever leaves the thymus; the other 99% are destroyed locally
(apoptosis). The thymus is important for the development of immunity
of the cellular type (see Chapter 6) and for normal maturation of the
paracortical areas of the lymph node and of the periarteriolar collection
of lymphocytes in the white pulp of the spleen (see Lymph Node and
Spleen below). Few B cells can be identified in the normal thymus, but
B-cell zones may appear with aging or in certain diseases, such as
myasthenia gravis.

Phenotypic characterization of both the thymocytes and stromal
cells of the thymus reveals a complexity of cell types not apparent by
conventional morphology. The cortical epithelium is derived from
ectodermal branchial cleft cells, whereas the medullary epithelium is

TABLE 3–1. CHARACTERIZATION OF THYMIC STROMA

Location	Tissue Type
Capsule	Mesodermal
Subcapsule	Endocrine epithelium (nurse cells)
Cortex	Nonendocrine epithelium (dendritic endothelium) Dendritic cells/macrophages
Medulla	Endocrine epithelium (Hassal's corpuscles) Dendritic cells/macrophages

derived from the third pharyngeal pouch. The capsule is derived from mesodermal connective tissue (Table 3–1). In addition, both the cortex and the medulla contain macrophages and Langerhans'-type dendritic cells. Maturation of thymocytes requires contact between thymocytes and thymic epithelial cells (see Chapter 6). In the cortex, many thymocytes are located within vacuolar membranes of large epithelial cells known as **thymic nurse cells**. These lymphoepithelial cell complexes provide a close association between intact, actively dividing thymocytes and large cytoplasmic vacuoles of the epithelial nurse cell (Fig. 3–4). It is within the thymic nurse cells that thymocytes may learn to identify self from nonself. Prothymocytes arriving from the bone marrow develop receptors for major histocompatibility complex (MHC) markers. If the cells do not react with these MHC markers during their residence in thymic nurse cells, they are deleted by apoptosis and phagocytosis by macrophages; many macrophages containing dying thymocytes are seen in the cortex. Those that react with class I MHC are destined to become CD8+ T cells, whereas those that react with class II MHC will become CD4+ T cells. High-affinity self-reactive thymocytes that might give rise to autoimmune disease are then removed by negative selection in the medulla after reaction with thymic dendritic cells, which are rich in MHC molecules. The surviving cells are then ready for release into the circulation and for further maturation in the peripheral lymphoid organs. The development of the T-cell receptor and maturation of thymocytes will be presented in more detail in Chapter 6.

The medullary epithelium, represented by Hassal's corpuscles, express different phenotypes as differentiation from medullary endocrine epithelium to mature Hassal's corpuscles occurs. This differentiation parallels that seen in skin keratinocytes (Table 3–2). Thymocytes also show differentiation-related phenotypic changes from cortex to medulla as defined by phenotypic markers identified by monoclonal antibodies (see Fig. 3–17). These markers are called **clusters of differentiation (CD)**. The nature of these markers will be presented in

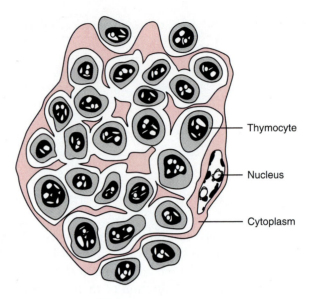

Figure 3–4. Thymic nurse cell. Thymic nurse cells are epithelial-derived cells in the outer cortex that contain from 5 to 20 immature thymocytes within cytoplasmic spaces and are partially enclosed by plasma membranes on the surface of the cell. It is thought that thymic nurse cells play a critical role in the early differentiation of thymocytes. C, cytoplasm of nurse cell; N, nucleus of nurse cell; T, thymocyte.

more detail below and in later chapters. The subcapsular cortex contains the least mature thymocytes. In the deep cortex more differentiated thymocytes are seen and maturation to more mature thymocytes occurs in the medulla. Further differentiation occurs after the cells leave the thymus (postthymic compartment).

The role of the thymus in the development of other endocrine organs is not well known. Thymectomy leads to a reduction of pituitary hormone levels and atrophy of the gonads. Neonatal hypophysectomy results in thymic atrophy and wasting disease; and other evidence sug-

TABLE 3–2. COMPARISON OF DIFFERENTIATION STAGES OF SKIN AND THYMIC MEDULLARY EPITHELIUM

SKIN			
Basal $\longrightarrow$	Spinosum $\longrightarrow$	Granulosum $\longrightarrow$	Corneum
THYMUS			
Medullary	Epithelium	Outer	Inner
Endocrine $\longrightarrow$	around $\longrightarrow$	layer of $\longrightarrow$	layer of
Epithelium	Hassal's	Hassal's	Hassal's
	bodies	bodies	bodies

gests that growth hormone may have an important effect on T-cell maturation.

PERIPHERAL LYMPHOID ORGANS

The functionally mature cells of the immune system are located in the peripheral lymphoid organs, which include lymph nodes, spleen, and other collections of lymphoid cells throughout the body.

Lymph Node

Lymph nodes are located in areas of lymphatic drainage in the body and serve as filters for tissue fluid in lymphatic vessels (Fig. 3–5). Classically, the organ is divided into the inner zone, the **medulla**, surrounded by an outer zone, the **cortex**. The cortex is variable in distribution and content depending on the state of activation (see below). The lymph node cortex contains nodules of lymphocytes (primary follicles), more loosely arranged nodules surrounded by a rim of tightly packed lymphoid cells (secondary follicles or germinal centers), and lymphocytes lying between the follicles (paracortical areas or diffuse cortex) that extend irregularly as bulges into the medulla (deep cortex). Thymectomy of neonatal animals leads to a depletion of lymphoid cells in the paracortical and deep cortical zones; therefore, these zones have become known as **thymus-dependent areas**. On the other hand, depletion of the primary follicles and germinal centers occurs in birds upon removal of a cloacal bursa of Fabricius (bursal-dependent zones); however, in mammals, removal of GALT does not deplete follicular zones. The medulla consists of a network of draining sinusoids formed by a meshwork of phagocytic reticular cells. The follicles are mainly composed of B cells (B-cell domain), and the paracortical zone is mainly composed of T cells (T-cell domain). Specialized dendritic macrophages are also present in each of these domains (see Chapter 2); interdigitating reticulum cells in the T-cell domain (paracortex) and follicular dendritic reticular cells in the B-cell zones (follicles). There are also T cells within the B-cell domains, and these are highly enriched for CD4+ T_{Helper} cells.

Afferent lymphatic vessels drain into a subcortical sinus; lymphatic sinusoids drain through the cortex around follicles and paracortical areas into the extensive sinusoidal network of the medulla. There are also extranodal connections directly between afferent and efferent lymphatics, allowing some lymph flow to bypass the lymph node. Some efferent lymphatics arise at the junction of the paracortex and the medulla. It is here that T lymphocytes produced in the paracortex enter the medullary sinusoids. The medullary sinuses drain into efferent lymphatics, which empty into the main efferent lymphatic vessel and exit through the hilum. The arteries divide into capillaries in the cortex. These capillaries drain into veins in the cortex, so that the cortex

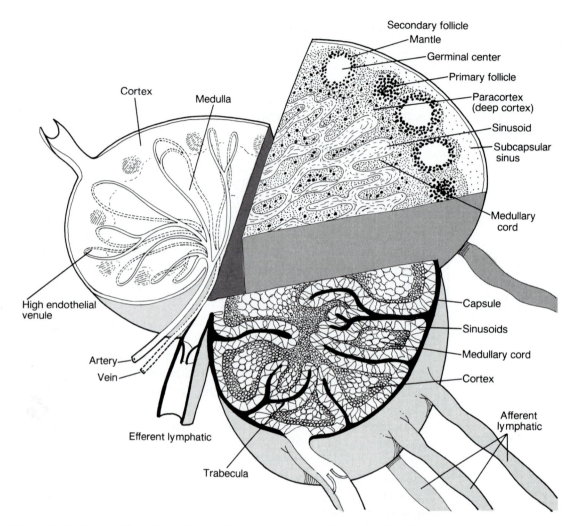

Figure 3–5. Normal lymph node. Nodes are made up of lymphoid cells contained in a meshwork of reticular fibers surrounded by connective tissue capsule. Most lymph nodes are bean-shaped, with an indented area known as the hilus. The cortex (outer layer) contains densely packed lymphoid cells and includes germinal centers responsible for production of antibody-synthesizing plasma cells and paracortical areas where lymphocytes are produced. The medulla (central area) consists of sinusoidal channels maintained by reticular cells. Columns of lymphoid cells are found between sinusoids in areas containing reticular macrophages. Afferent lymphatics drain through cortex around germinal centers into medullary sinusoids. Since the medullary sinusoids contain lymphatic fluid and not blood, there are normally very few red blood cells in the medullary sinusoids. Medullary sinusoids drain into efferent lymphatics and are collected by main efferent lymphatic that drains from hilus. The main artery divides into capillaries supplying the cortex. These capillaries drain into veins that follow the trabeculae and exit at the hilus.

is supplied with circulating blood in a conventional manner, whereas the medulla is mainly supplied with lymph fluid by afferent and efferent lymphatics. Recirculating lymphocytes enter the lymph node via high endothelial postcapillary venules in the paracortex. B cells must pass through the T-cell domain and home to the B-cell domain (follicle). In reactive nodes, B- and T-cell nodular zones are located together in a **composite nodule**, which contains two clearly definable domains. The peripheral, subcapsular zone contains mainly B cells; the deeper paracortical zone contains mainly helper T cells. These composite nodules provide anatomic structures which allow T_{Helper}–B-cell interactions.

Spleen

(Fig. 3–6) The splenic lymphoid tissue is analogous to that of the lymph node, but it is arranged differently. A comparison of the structure and function of the spleen to the lymph node is given in Table 3–3. The lymphoid follicles and surrounding lymphoid tissue are called white pulp, and the sinusoidal area, which usually contains large numbers of red blood cells, is called red pulp because of the color seen on gross examination of the freshly cut organ. The white pulp is not concentrated in an area like the cortex of the lymph node but is organized as a lumpy cylindrical sheath surrounding small arteries (central arterioles) like a bunch of grapes. T cells are located in a tight sheath around the central arteriole called the **periarteriolar lymphoid sheath (PALS)**; the B-cell domain extends as a lumpy eccentric **follicle** of white pulp. These follicles may be primary or secondary (germinal center). There is a tightly packed zone of B cells called the **mantle** surrounding splenic germinal centers. The mantle is composed of cells of the primary follicle pushed aside by formation of the germinal center. The mantle is separated from another lymphoid zone by a venous sinus known as the **marginal sinus**. The **marginal zone** is in turn surrounded by a less dense collection of cells called the **perifollicular zone**, which separates the white pulp from the red pulp. Circulating T and B cells enter the splenic white pulp by transversing the marginal sinus, which is similar to the high endothelial venules in the lymph node. T and B cells may be found mixed in the marginal zone, which may be considered an extension of the outer layer of the PALS around the follicle. The B cells of the marginal zone appear to be in an activated state. It has been claimed that T-independent antibody responses may take place in the marginal zone. There are four types of phagocytic-macrophage cells in the spleen: (1) cells lying free in sinusoids, (2) fixed sinusoid-lining cells, (3) reticular cells lying between sinusoids that form a network of meshwork reticular fibers, and (4) cells found in areas surrounding the white pulp (the perifollicular zone).

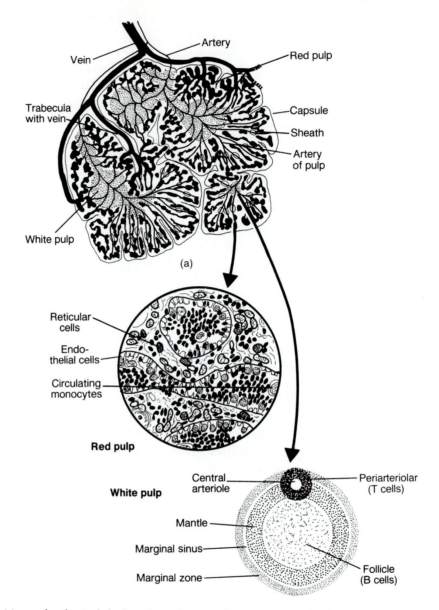

Figure 3–6. Normal splenic lobule. The spleen is composed of a network of sinusoidal channels filled mainly with red blood cells (red pulp). There are no lymphatic vessels. Blood enters through arteries that may empty directly into the splenic sinusoids or into the reticular area between the sinusoids. The sinusoids are drained by veins that exit via trabecular veins to large vein that leaves the spleen at the hilus. A zone of densely packed lymphocytes surrounding the central arteriole contains T cells (thymus-dependent area), while B cells are found surrounding the germinal center. The mantle surrounding germinal centers is composed mainly of B cells, but also T cells, believed to be pushed aside from the B-cell zone by formation of the germinal center. Overlying the mantle is the marginal zone, containing venous capillaries that permit circulating cells to enter the white pulp. Blood flows from the central arteriole through small follicular arterioles into the marginal sinus, which drains into the red pulp. The central arteriole continues through the white pulp. Upon exiting the white pulp, the central arteriole is divided into many small branches—the penicilli arterioles—which drain into the sinusoids or the medullary cords of Billroth.

TABLE 3–3. COMPARISON OF SPLEEN TO LYMPH NODE:
STRUCTURE AND FUNCTION

Structure	Description	Function/Composition	Lymph Node Equivalent
White Pulp			
T-cell zone	Periarteriolar sheath	Predominantly CD4+ T-cells	Paracortex
B-cell zone	Periarteriolar follicles	Production of B cells	Cortical follicle
Mantle	Rim of densely packed small lymphocytes around follicle	Small B cells not taking part in proliferation in follicle	Mantle
Marginal zone	Zone outside mantle inside perifollicular zone	Mixture of T and B cells, large activated B cells	Not known
Perifollicular zone	Zone between white and red pulp, without sinusoids	Place of retarded blood flow with interaction of circulating blood and white pulp	Medulla(?)
Red Pulp			
Sinusoids/ capillaries	Meshwork of sinuses, reticulum cells and capillaries	Clearance of particles from blood, filtering of effete red blood cells	Medullary sinuses, HEV
Nonfiltering zone	Lymphocyte zones in red pulp lacking capillaries	(?) Site of initiation of immune reactions	Primary follicle
Perivascular rim	Thin perivascular zone containing plasma cells	(?) Connected to nonfiltering zone	Medullary cords

The splenic parenchyma contains no lymphatic vessels; there are some in the connective tissue trabeculae. Blood enters through arteries running in trabeculae. The arteries branch and extend into the red pulp. The white pulp is positioned as a sleeve around the smaller arterioles. The arterioles continue out of the white pulp, where they divide into smaller branches, the penicilli arterioles, which supply the red pulp by either direct connection with the medullary sinusoids or drainage into the intersinusoidal reticular tissue, known as the cords of Billroth. The penicilli arterioles resemble the branches of a fine paintbrush (*penicilli*, from the Latin: "hair pencil"). There is not complete agreement as to which arteriolar drainage is predominant, but recent evidence suggests that most penicilli arterioles drain into the cords. Pores in the endothelial lining of the sinusoids permit easy exchange of blood from the cords to the sinusoids. In addition, small arterioles pass through the white pulp (follicular arterioles) and drain into the marginal sinus that surrounds the follicles. The medullary sinusoids have a basic structure similar to that of the lymph node but drain into branches of the splenic vein and not into efferent lymphatics. After injection of antigens, antibody-forming cells are seen in the outer layer of the periarteriolar lymphoid sheath (PALS) from where they migrate to the coaxial sheaths of lymphoid tissue surrounding the terminal arterioles. From here, antibody-producing cells may migrate into the red pulp, where they secrete antibody into the splenic sinusoids.

It was once believed that the spleen was not an important organ for adaptive immunity. However, children who have their spleens removed surgically because of trauma, neoplastic disease, or hematologic disorders are subject to what is termed "the postsplenectomy syndrome." The postsplenectomy syndrome is caused by bacterial sepsis, usually with large numbers (approximately 100/mL blood) of encapsulated bacteria. Thus, the spleen does serve an important function in clearing the blood of infectious organisms!

Mucosal-Associated Lymphoid Tissue (MALT), Gastrointestinal-Associated Lymphoid Tissue (GALT), Bronchus-Associated Lymphoid Tissue (BALT), and Duct-Associated Lymphoid Tissue (DALT)

Local collections of lymphoid tissue underlie the submucosa of many areas of the gastrointestinal tract and airways of the lung. MALT occurs in two forms: organized tissues such as the tonsils (lingual, palatine, pharyngeal, and tubal) (Fig. 3–7), the appendix (Fig. 3–8), and Peyer's patches (Fig. 3–9), and diffuse lymphoid cells in the epithelium and underlying connective tissue that is not organized into recognizable organs. Different domains of lymphoid tissues may be identified in MALT: the dome, the follicle, the thymus-dependent area, and submucosal areas. The tonsils form a ring of lymphoid tissue at the base of the tongue and pharynx, known as Waldeyer's ring, which "guards" the passageway to the esophagus and trachea. The GALT is a major lymphopoietic organ in the adult and may be a source for T and B cells after thymic function declines with age. There is a very high rate of both cell proliferation and cell death (apoptosis) in the follicles of the GALT. Thus, the GALT may take over not only the function of the thymus in producing new T cells but also retain the function of the major B-cell-producing organ. Antigens entering through the gut or lungs may stimulate cells in the GALT or BALT, which can then circulate to other tissues.

The overlying mucosa, listed below, is characteristic of each location: lingual tonsil, stratified squamous; palatine tonsil, stratified squamous; pharyngeal tonsil, pseudostratified columnar; tubal tonsil, pseudostratified columnar; appendix, columnar goblet cells (crypts of Lieberkuhn); and Peyer's patches, specially modified intestinal epithelium (see below). Afferent lymphatics in the form of lacteals deliver material absorbed through the intestine to the lymphatic tissue. Both immunoglobulin (antibody) and lymphoid T cells are produced by the gastrointestinal lymphoid tissue. These are delivered to the systemic circulation by draining lymphatics, but many of the proteins and cells produced are secreted into the gastrointestinal lumen. The gut mucosa contains large numbers of IgA-producing plasma cells, and IgA is

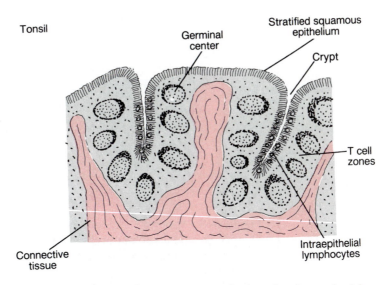

Tonsil

Germinal center

Stratified squamous epithelium

Crypt

T cell zones

Intraepithelial lymphocytes

Connective tissue

Figure 3–7. Tonsil. Tonsils are composed of a closely packed layer of germinal centers underlying epithelium, separated by T-cell zones. There are no afferent lymphatics, but there are prominant efferent lymphatics. Overlying epithelium is characteristic of areas where tonsils are located (see Gastrointestinal Lymphoid Tissue). The epithelium of the crypts of the tonsils has a distinguishing structure of reticulation in contrast to the stratified squamous epithelium of the surface. This reticular structure is a lymphatic labyrinth that contains large numbers of intraepithelial lymphocytes which migrate from the underlying subepithelial lymphoid tissue through a discontinuous basement membrane in the crypt. (Modified from Bloom, W., and Fawcett, D.W.: A Textbook of Histology. ed. 9. Philadelphia, W.B. Saunders, 1969.)

transported across the mucosa in large amounts by specialized processing in mucosal cells by the addition of a transport piece (see below). Lymphocytes found in the mucosal layer of the GI tract appear to be predominantly CD8+ cytotoxic cells. CD4+ helper cells are prominent in the submucosa. The intraepithelial lymphocytes of the GALT contain high numbers of γδ T cells, the type of T cells that appear in the thymic cortex associated with early thymocyte maturation. It is believed that these T cells mature extrathymically and may represent discrete subsets of organ-specific lymphocytes, with unique T-cell receptor repertoires.

The specialized mucosal cells overlying GALT and BALT are known as **M cells** or **follicle-associated epithelium (FAE)**. M stands for microfolds, because of the presence of ridges or folds on the surface of M cells. M cells lack the cilia of bronchial epithelium or the

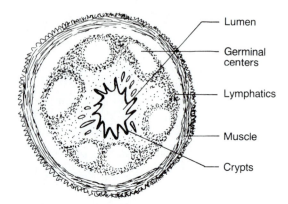

Figure 3–8. Appendix. Appendicular lymphoid tissue is composed of a layer of germinal centers underlying mucosa. Mucosa consists of crypts of goblet cells characteristic of this part of the intestine. Many cells produced in the appendix appear to be discharged into the lumen. Afferent lymphatics drain around germinal centers from origin in crypts; efferent lymphatics drain from germinal centers. (Modified from Bloom W, Fawcett DW: *A Textbook of Histology*, 9th ed. Philadelphia, WB Saunders, 1969.)

microvilli of intestinal mucosal cells. M cells are Class II MHC+; they take up and transport enteric antigens to the underlying lymphoid tissues. Associated with M cells are dendritic macrophages, CD4+ T_{Helper} cells, and clusters of IgM+ B cells. M cells do not contain a transport

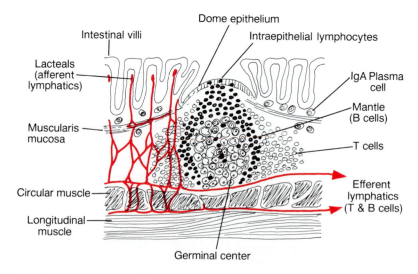

Figure 3–9. Structure of the Peyer's patch (PP).

piece for immunoglobulin found in other mucosal cells. Antigen processing by M cells may be important in immune response to enteric pathogens such as *Vibrio cholera, Salmonella*, and pathogenic *Escherichia coli*. In addition, enteric pathogens, such as poliovirus, may enter the body through M cells. M cells have abundant glycosylated surface proteins that bind to these organisms, as well as human immunodeficiency virus (HIV), through lectin-like receptors.

The mucosal lymphoid tissue produces large amounts of antibody that is secreted into the intestinal lumen. Memory B cells with a high J chain content required for dimeric IgA and pentameric IgM secretion are produced in Peyer's patches and migrate to the lamina propria of the intestine, where they can be activated to produce IgA dimers for secretion by mucosal cells that produce secretory piece (Fig. 3–10). In addition, the lactating breast is a secretory lymphoid organ as are other glands, such as salivary glands (**duct-associated lymphoid tissue [DALT]**). Under the influence of prolactin, antibody-producing cells home to and proliferate in the breast where they produce antibodies that are secreted into the milk. Upon suckling, these antibodies protect the newborn infant against diarrheal pathogens. IgA antibodies are also secreted in salivary glands.

GALT is believed to be a major source of new lymphocytes in the adult animal. Both T and B lymphocytes are delivered from GALT via efferent lymphatics to the thoracic duct and to the systemic circulation. These cells may then localize in any lymphoid organ of the body (except perhaps the thymus) with preferential homing to mucosal lymphoid tissue (eg, GI tract, lacrimal glands, mammary glands, BALT and bladder) (Fig. 3–11).

Mammary Duct-Associated Lymphoid Tissue (DALT)

Local immunization of the mammary gland results in the accumulation of T and B cells around ducts with a histologic appearance similar to BALT. Lymphocytes are seen within the overlying epithelium, and local immunoglobulin production with accumulation of plasma cells follows. A normal lactating breast contains large numbers of IgA-containing plasma cells, believed to be responsible for the high levels of IgA in colostrum and milk that provides early passive immunity to newborns. In addition, transmigration of T cells through the ductal epithelium may provide passive cell-mediated immunity.

Skin-Associated Lymphoid Tissue (SALT)

SALT includes Langerhans' cells in the epidermis, recirculating T cells that pass through the epidermis and dermis, keratinocytes producing epidermal T-cell-activating factors, and local draining lymph

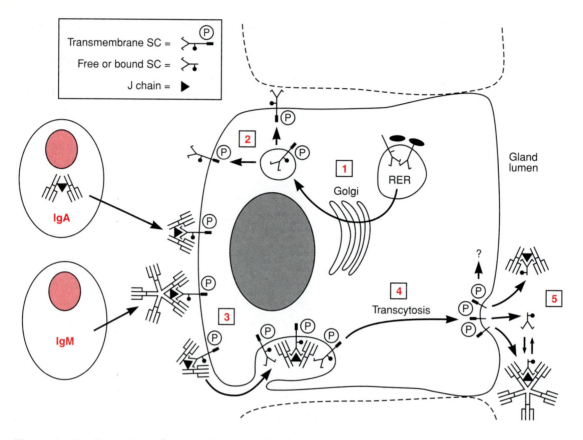

Figure 3–10. Secretion of IgA and IgM antibodies by epithelial cells in the intestine. Secretory component is a protein produced in the rough endoplasmic reticulum and glycosylated by the Golgi apparatus of mucosal epithelial cells (1). The SC is then phosphorylated and processed through vesicles to the cell membrane (2). Dimeric IgA or pentameric IgM containing J-chain complex with the cell surface secretory component and are endocytosed (3). The endocytosed vesicles are transcytosed across the mucosal cell cytoplasm (4). At the intestinal lumen, the tail of the secretory component is cleaved and the IgA or IgM molecules complexed to the head of the secretory component are released into the intestinal lumen (5). (Modified from Brandtzaeg P, Sollid IM, Thrane PS, et al.: Lymphoepithelial interactions in the mucosal immune system. *Gut* 29:1116, 1988.)

nodes. The keratinized layer of the skin provides the first barrier to external organisms (antigens). Antigens that pass through the outer layers of the skin, such as the lipid-soluble antigens eliciting contact dermatitis (ie, poison ivy) will then come into contact with the class MHC II+, FcR+ Langerhans' cells. The Langerhans' cells form an almost closed network of antigen-presenting cells within the spinal cell layer of the epidermis (see Figure 2–7) and in the form of **veiled cells** are found in afferent lymphatic vessels migrating to draining lymph nodes.

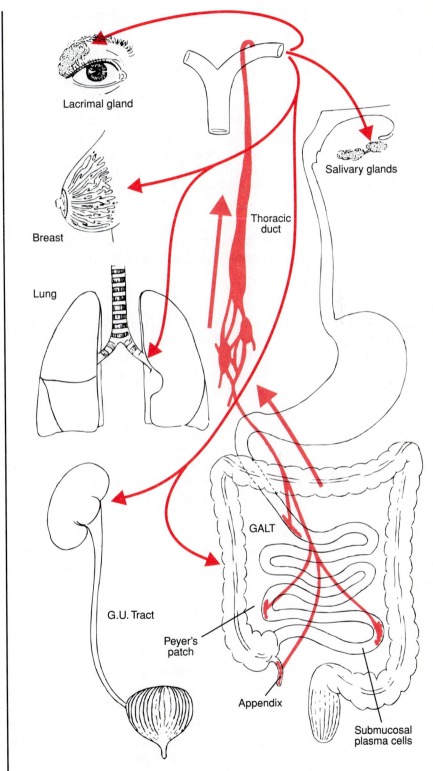

Figure 3–11. Cellular traffic in the secretory system (see text).

Dendritic cells bearing Langerhans' cell phenotypes are found in the lymph nodes draining the skin but not in the mesenteric lymph nodes or spleen. It is believed that Langerhans' cells are in continuous circulation, passing from the skin to the draining nodes, thus delivering processed antigens to the T cells in the paracortex of the lymph node. This system is anatomically ideally organized to react to antigens that are presented in the epidermis, such as contact sensitivity antigens. In addition, there is a subpopulation of lymphocytes that appears to home to the skin **(epidermotropic)**. In the malignant form, these are represented by the cutaneous T-cell lymphomas, in particular, Sezary's cell variant. Sezary's cells have a mature helper T-cell phenotype, indicating a preference for T_{Helper} cells to home to the epidermis. In addition, mice have an epidermal T cell not found in humans. The importance of the skin in immunopathology is recognized in this book by inclusion of a separate chapter on immune reactions in the skin.

Innervation of Lymphoid Organs

The neuroendocrine system is intimately linked and involved in bidirectional communication with the immune system. There are two major linkages: the sympathetic nervous system (ie, epinephrine) and the hypothalamic–pituitary–adrenal axis. Through these connections, one neural, the other endocrine, immune reactivity and inflammation are modulated. The immune system and its products (lymphokines and monokines) can modify neuroendocrine functions, and neuroendocrine hormones can increase or decrease immune reactions. The study of these phenomena has given rise to a variety of terms: **immunoneurology, immunoendocrinology, endocrine immunology, psychoneuroimmunology, psychoimmunology**, etc.

There is innervation of the thymus, spleen, and bone marrow by the autonomic nervous system. The thymus is supplied by nerves derived from the vagus, phrenic, and recurrent laryngeal nerves, as well as from the stellate and other small ganglia on the thoracic sympathetic chain, but most of the innervation of the medulla of the thymus is derived from the vagus nerve, which terminates as a plexus at the corticomedullary boundary, where mid-sized and small thymocytes, believed to be partially differentiated, are located. Undifferentiated T cells occupy the outermost cortex, where nerve fibers from the phrenic and recurrent laryngeal nerve terminate. The possible role of this innervation in the development of thymocytes is poorly understood. The primary innervation of the spleen is sympathetic catecholinergic nerves from the celiac ganglion, which terminate in the central arterioles of the white pulp. It is not clear if these terminals are important for regulating blood flow, since experimental studies have shown that the spleen can contract rhythmically even after ligation of its nerves. However, ligation of the splenic nerves prevents the suppression of immunization caused by intermittent foot shock. In lymph nodes, acetylcholinergic fibers are restricted to the capsule; but catecholinergic fibers form perivascular plexuses, which are believed to regulate blood flow. The nerves that innervate bones arise from the level of the spinal cord that corresponds to the location of the bone. These nerves have medullary branches that enter the bone marrow with the nutrient arteries. The presence of both afferent and efferent nerve fibers in the marrow suggests that an autonomic reflex arc may influence marrow functions, which is the production of blood cells.

Lymphocytes have been shown to have adrenergic receptors, not only for norepinephrine, but also for a variety of neuropeptides, including neurotensin, vasoactive intestinal polypeptide, etc. In addition, activated lymphocytes may be able to secrete neuropeptides. Sympathetic stimulation of lymphoid organs may increase or decrease antibody production, depending on which adrenoceptor type (alpha or beta) is activated: Beta-2 adrenoceptor activation increases early antibody production, but suppresses late responses; the effect of stimulation of alpha adrenoceptors is controversial.

Adrenocorticotropic hormone (ACTH) and cortisone also are active in controlling immune responses. During active immunization, cortisone levels of the blood are elevated and immune responses to a different second antigen given during an active response are depressed (antigenic competition). It has been shown that IL-1 and IL-6 can act to increase ACTH secretion by the pituitary by increasing corticotropic-releasing factor from the hypothalamus. ACTH acts on the adrenal gland to increase corticosteroid production; corticosteroids depress lymphocyte activities. ACTH may also be increased by stress, and a number of studies have shown that immune responses may be depressed during times of psychological stress. Finally, opioids may increase inflammatory effects of neutrophils, macrophages, and mast cells, and NK activity, but decrease antibody production. In conclusion, the role of neurotransmission of specific signals to cells of the immune system and the effect of hormones are not yet understood well enough to provide a clear idea of how they might influence immune responses.

A comparison of the characteristics of lymphoid organs is given in Table 3–4. The structure of each lymphoid organ is related to its functions, the most notable of which are:

1. The thymus, which does not normally respond to antigenic stimulus, has no afferent lymphatics and no apparent structure associated with delivery of antigen to the organ. In addition, the thymus is the site of T-cell development and does not normally contain B-cell domains.

Comparison of the Structure of Lymphoid Organs

2. The spleen, which is a filter for the blood and not the lymphatics, has no lymphatic vessels.
3. The bone marrow, which is the site of formation of blood cells, does not normally contain T- and B-cell domains.

Lymphocyte Circulation

Histologic examination of the lymphoid organs provides a static view that belies the extensive recirculation of lymphoid cells. Lymphocytes, both T and B cells, leave their maturation sites, percolate through the lymphoid tissue, and enter other organs by circulation in the bloodstream. Entrance to the bloodstream occurs either via efferent lymphatics or draining veins. Mature lymphoid cells (memory cells?) as well as naive T and B lymphocytes may reenter lymphoid organs after circulating. Lymphocytes enter the lymph node by transversing specialized cortical capillary venules known as high endothelial venules (HEV), because of the thickness of the endothelial cells. HEVs have specific surface recognition sites for T and B lymphocytes so that these cells transverse HEVs located in different areas of lymphoid organs. At

TABLE 3–4. SOME CHARACTERISTICS OF LYMPHOID ORGANS

	Cortex	Medulla	B-Cell Domains (Follicles)	Afferent Lymphatics	Efferent Lymphatics	Special Features
Thymus	+	+	0	0	+	Hassal's corpuscles, epithelial reticulum, no B cells
Spleen	0	0	+	0	0	White pulp and red pulp, no parenchymal lymphatics
Lymph node	+	+	+	+	+	Subcapsular sinus, prominent follicles, and paracortical zones
GI						
Tonsils	+	0	+	0	+	Zones of T and B cells, no prominent medulla or draining sinusoids, active mitoses
Appendix	+	0	+	±	+	
Peyer's patches	+	0	+	+	+	
Bone marrow	0	0	0	0	0	Hematopoietic cells in fatty tissue, few mature immune cells

Key: +, present; 0, absent

least four functionally distinct lymphocyte–HEV recognition systems control the homing of lymphocytes separately to peripheral lymph nodes, to GALT (Peyer's patches, appendix), and to inflamed synovium. Passively transferred stem cells home specifically to the bone marrow, after bone marrow transplantation, through HEVs. Thus, there is organ selectivity for lymphocyte localization. For instance, lymph node lymphocytes preferentially localize to lymph nodes, whereas GALT lymphocytes preferentially localize to GALT when reinfused into an animal. The nature of the reaction between homing lymphocytes and HEVs has led to identification of specific recognition molecules. The features of the recognition molecules on lymphocytes and endothelial cells through which specific homing is controlled (**cell adhesion molecules [CAMs]**) are detailed in Chapter 9.

T and B cells may enter at the same site but are able to go separately to their respective domains in the lymphoid organ. In the lymph node, B cells must transverse the T-cell domain (paracortical zone) to reach the B-cell domain (follicles). In the spleen, T cells and B cells first localize in the marginal zone. T cells migrate into the periarteriolar lymphatic sheath (PALS) and B cells home to the follicle. In this way, B cells come into contact with T cells and accessory cells on their way to B-cell zones. Recirculating T and B cells enter the medullary or red pulp sinusoids before entering the efferent lymphatics. The lymphocyte fields of the lymph node thus contain slowly percolating masses of T and B cells, most of which are on their way from blood to lymph and back to blood. The ratio of the constitutive population of fixed cells to recirculating lymphocytes is not known.

The Effect of Antigens on Lymphoid Organs

The "normal" structure of the lymphoid organs depends upon antigenic exposure. In germ-free animals that have little antigenic contact, the lymphoid organs contain few primary or secondary follicles, sparse paracortical areas, and serum immunoglobulin levels less than one-tenth that of conventional animals. The medullary areas contain sinusoids relatively depleted of mononuclear cells or lymph fluid. If antigen is introduced, there is a marked increase in cortical follicles and paracortical tissue, and the serum immunoglobulin levels may increase to almost normal levels.

ANTIBODY PRODUCTION

The induction of antibody formation involves the interaction of four major cell types in lymphoid organs leading to formation of germinal centers. The four cell types are B cells, T cells, follicular dendritic cells (FDC), and tingible body macrophages. FDCs, B cells, and T-helper cells interact during the induction process, whereas tingible body macrophages serve to remove B cells that do not survive in the follicle (apoptotic cells). FDCs organize the cellular interactions. In vitro B cells will bind to dendritic cells and form clusters of cells. The B cells in these clusters are protected from apoptosis as compared to B cells not in clusters. Upon contacting a responsive individual, radiolabeled antigens that stimulate the production of both circulating antibody and nonantigens are taken up by the phagocytic cells (macrophages) of the medullary areas of lymph nodes and spleen (Fig. 3–12). After a few days, antigens are found in "dendritic" macrophages in the cortex or white pulp where germinal centers will form. Dendritic macrophages, when activated, develop into elongated spindle-shaped cells with cytoplasmic extensions that envelop differentiating B cells and serve as the site for follicle development. Activated follicular dendritic cells express cell immunoglobulin (Fc) and complement receptors and will take up antibody–antigen complexes. In addition activated dendritic cells have upgraded expression of the cell adhesion molecules, ICAM-1 and VCAM-1, which interact with LFA-1 and VLA-4 on B cells and T-helper cells. (Cell adhesion molecules are presented in more detail in Chapter 9.) The follicular dendritic cell thus provides a cytoplasmic meshwork for cell interactions during development of the immune response. B-cell proliferation around the dendritic macrophages containing the antigen leads to development of a nodule of cells (follicle). Virgin B cells are positive for both IgM and IgD, but on stimulation the proliferating B cells in the germinal center lose their surface IgD. The nonproliferating IgD-positive B lymphocytes are pushed aside to the periphery of the nodule overlying the center of proliferation to form a *mantle* around the follicle.

The stimulated B cells either die within the follicle by apoptosis or mature into plasma cells. The maturing B cells form a light zone of "blast" cells at the base of the follicle where there are few, if any, dendritic cells. Within 5 to 7 days after immunization, plasma cells appear below the germinal center and migrate into the medullary cords, where they produce and secrete immunoglobulin antibody that is released into the medullary sinusoids. Plasma cells may be observed in large numbers in the adjacent medullary cords or red pulp for periods of at least 10 weeks after immunization. Within one to two weeks after primary immunization, memory B cells can be identified in the lymph nodes draining the site of immunization; later, memory B cells are present in distal lymph nodes. After the active phase of antibody production, the germinal center involutes by apoptosis, and tingible body macrophages become more prominent. The residual follicle may form into a collection of lymphocytes in the cortex that is recognized as the primary follicle and may be the location of memory cells. If this is the

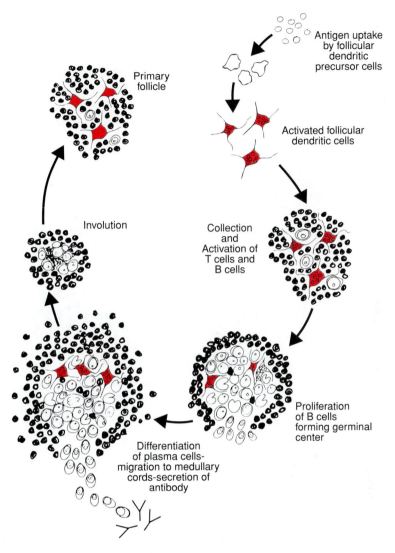

Figure 3–12. Germinal center formation. Localization of labeled antigen in lymph node following immunization demonstrates distribution in both medullary and cortical macrophages. Antigen first appears in the lining cells of the subcortical sinus. On day 2, labeled macrophages are scattered through the cortex. By day 4, the label appears in cells in developing follicles (follicular dendritic cells), and blast cells can be identified underlying the antigen-containing cells. These cells increase in number until a typical germinal center (secondary follicle) is formed, with antigen-containing cells overlying the area of B-cell maturation. By day 7, plasma cells appear deep to the germinal center. These cells then migrate into the medullary cords and secrete antibody into the medullary sinusoids. During involution of the follicle, there are many tingible body macrophages which phagocytose numerous cells, even dividing cells.

case, then the terms "primary" and "secondary" are inappropriate, as a primary follicle may derive from a secondary follicle.

GERMINAL CENTER B CELLS

The morphology of the B cells in an active germinal center is depicted in Figure 3–13. The cell types in an active germinal center serve as prototypes for the changes seen in B cells that occur during proliferation and division. These cell types have been used to classify tumors arising from B cells.

CELL-MEDIATED IMMUNITY

The morphologic changes occurring in a lymph node during the development of specifically sensitized cells (cytotoxic T cells or delayed hypersensitivity, see Chapters 15 and 16) are different from those occurring during the production of circulating antibody (Fig. 3–14).

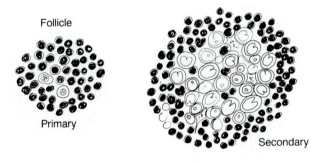

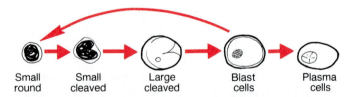

Figure 3–13. Germinal center B cells. The B cells seen in a germinal center range in size and shape from small round cells to large irregular "cleaved" cells on the basis of nuclear appearance. Primary follicles are composed of small round lymphocytes, almost all B cells. Germinal centers contain a mixture of B cells: small round, intermediate round, large round, medium cleaved, and large cleaved. Cleaved cells are believed to represent "activated" B cells; large round cells are "blast" cells that divide to produce two daughter B cells that are small and round. These morphologic cell types have been used to classify tumors arising from B cells (B-cell lymphomas). Small round B-cell tumors have a good prognosis; large round or cleaved cells have a poor prognosis; cell types in between have an intermediate prognosis.

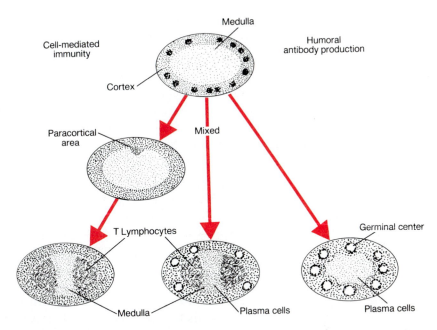

Figure 3–14. Morphologic response of lymph node to antigen stimulus. Induction of pure cell-mediated immunity leads to proliferation of lymphocytes in the paracortical zone. Induction of pure antibody formation results in germinal center formation and appearance of plasma cells in medullary cords. Immunization with most antigens produces both changes with enlargement of paracortical zones and production of germinal centers.

During the induction of cellular immunity, the proliferative changes in the lymph node do not occur in the follicles or germinal centers but in the other areas of the lymph node cortex that contain tightly packed T lymphocytes (the paracortical area). Here, there is a population of macrophages known as interdigitating reticular cells, which process antigens in a manner similar to follicular dendritic macrophages but present the antigens to T cell precursors. A few days after contact with an antigen, large "immature" blast cells and mitotic figures (dividing cells) are seen in the paracortex. A temporary increase in the number of small lymphocytes occurs in this area 2 to 5 days after immunization. It is likely that these are the specifically sensitized cells that are rapidly released into the draining lymph and disseminated throughout the body. It is not precisely clear where antigen is recognized during the development of delayed hypersensitivity. Lymphocytes may be able to recognize antigen at a site distant from the lymph node, where the sensitizing antigen is located, such as in the skin. The reacting lymphocyte may return to the lymph node, lodge in the paracortical area, and undergo rapid replication, resulting in the formation of large numbers of sensitized cells that now may recognize and react with the sensitizing antigen. In addition, the Langerhans' cells of the skin are related to the interdigitating reticular cells of the lymph node paracortex and may carry processed antigen from contact in the skin by migration through lymphatics to the paracortical zone of the lymph node. On the other hand, antigens may be "recognized" first by reactive lymphocytes in the lymph node following delivery of the antigen to the lymph nodes by lymphatics.

Induction of T_{CTL} may take place at sites outside lymphoid organs. Since T_{CTL} precursors recognize endogenous antigen in the context of class I MHC molecules which are present on any nucleated cell, any nucleated cell expressing an immunogen recognized as foreign by a T_{CTL} precursor may serve as an antigen-presenting cell. However, the co-signaling molecules, in particular IL-1, may not be adequate for primary induction of T_{CTL} activation unless macrophages are present. Other cells may be able to function as complete antigen-presenting cells to T_{CTL} precursors. For example, hepatocytes infected with malaria parasites can present antigen in association with class I MHC molecules and may be able to produce and release sufficient co-factors to activate T_{CTL} directly. On the other hand, macrophages in the liver, activated as a result of infection, may produce IL-1 which acts as a co-factor for T_{CTL} precursors engaged with malarial antigens on class I MHC molecules on hepatocytes.

In summary, different immune responses take place in different lymphoid tissue microenvironments (Table 3–5). Specific T-dependent

TABLE 3–5. FUNCTIONAL LYMPHOID ORGAN MICROENVIRONMENTS

Microenvironment	Cells Present	Function
Germinal Center	B cells, blasts, dendritic macrophages, T cells, tingible body macrophages	T-cell dependent B-cell proliferation and differentiation
Paracortex (lymph node) Periarteriolar sheath (spleen)	T cells, interdigitating macrophages	T-cell proliferation and differentiation
Marginal zones	Dendritic macrophages, B cells	T-independent B-cell responses
Medulla (lymph node) Red Pulp (Spleen)	Plasma cells, T cells, Reticular cells	Rapid antibody production and release of sensitive T cells
Primary follicles	B cells, T cells, dendritic macrophages	Storage of memory cells
Mantle of germinal center	B cells	B-memory cell differentiation

B-cell proliferation occurs in germinal centers, T-cell proliferation in the paracortex or periarteriolar sheath, T-independent B-cell proliferation in marginal zones, and antibody secretion in medullary cords. Memory B cells may differentiate in the mantle of germinal centers and be stored in primary follicles.

Development of Lymphoid Organs (Ontogeny)

The first identifiable hematopoietic cells from which lymphoid stem cells arise appear in the yolk sac, then in the bone marrow, spleen, and liver of the developing fetus. It is not clear from where the progenitor hematopoietic cells that precede those in the yolk sac arise, but embryologists have evidence that these cells migrate from the primitive neural crest (Fig. 3–15). The first major determination stage in the differentiation of blood-forming cell lineages is the formation of oligopotent stem cells for the formation of lymphoid cells and those for the formation of myeloid cells. The morphologic development of T and B

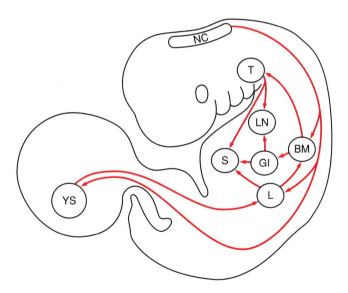

Figure 3–15. Postulated migration of hematopoietic stem cells from neural crest precursors during fetal development. Neural crest precursor cells migrate to the fetal yolk sac or liver. From the yolk sac or primitive liver, hematopoietic stem cells migrate to fetal bone marrow, spleen, and liver. Prothymocytes arising in the bone marrow migrate to the thymus (T-cell development); pro-B cells in the bone marrow migrate to the gastrointestinal tract or mature in the liver to functional B cells. Maturing T and B cells migrate to the spleen or lymph nodes, where final differentiation steps occur. BM, bone marrow; GI, gastrointestinal tract; L, liver; N, neural crest; S, spleen; T, thymus; YS, yolk sac.

cells will be presented first, followed by a brief description of the production of the myeloid series of cells.

ONTOGENY OF LYMPHOID ORGANS

A model for the cellular development of lymphoid organs was proposed by Robert Good in the 1960s. According to this model, the precursor stem cells for all lymphoid cells arise in the bone marrow. During fetal development, the stroma for the peripheral lymphoid organs appears first in the absence of lymphoid cells and consists of epithelial or mesenchymal supportive tissue. T and B cells are derived from bone marrow precursors and acquire immune competence by maturation in inductive microenvironments (Fig. 3–16).

T-cell Differentiation

The critical role of the thymus in the development of T cells was recognized by Jacques Miller in the early 1960s when he noted that surgical removal of the thymus **(thymectomy)** led to an absence of T-cell function and a depletion of T cells in the thymus-dependent zones of the peripheral lymphoid organs. T-cell maturation involves **prothymocyte** "stem" or "progenitor" cells produced in the bone marrow that circulate to and mature in the thymus (see Fig. 3–3). Until a few years ago prothymocyte referred to a putative functional cell population that had not been identified by any markers.

CD Markers of T-cell and B-cell Differentiation. Human T-cell and B-cell differentiation markers are recognized by monoclonal antibodies (clusters of differentiation [CD]) (see Appendix B). Only a few of these markers will be introduced here in order to present a simplistic view of T- and B-cell maturation. Some representative CD markers are listed in Table 3–6.

The expression of CD markers during differentiation of thymocytes is shown in Table 3–7. CDs 34, 7, and 45 identify prothymocytes as well as cells in the thymus. Early in the cortex thymocytes acquire CD2 and CD5 and then lose CD34. CD34 is also found on hepatopoietic stem cells. In the thymic cortex, cells that recognize class II MHC molecules and survive acquire CD4 (helper phenotype) and cells that recognize class I MHC molecules acquire CD8 (T_{CTL} phenotype). Further selection for nonself in the medulla is associated with production of the T-cell receptor complex, identified by CD3.

CD45, otherwise known as the leukocyte common antigen, exists in isoforms of molecular weight 180, 190, 205, and 220 that identify cells that die or develop further in the thymus. Thymocytes that express CD45 p180 are designated CD45RA and are destined to die in the thymus; those with CD45 205/220 are called CD45RO and are in the lin-

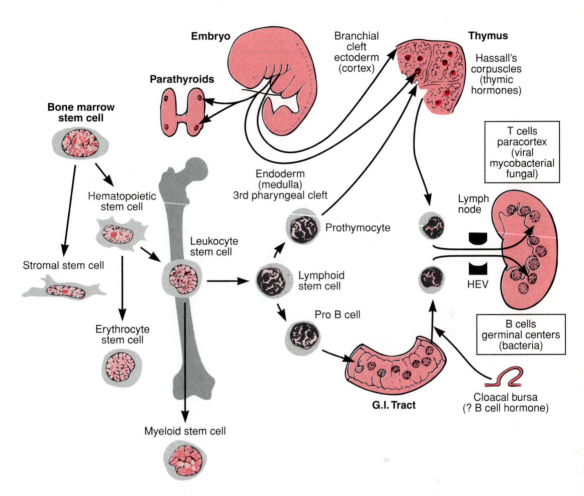

Figure 3–16. Scheme of hematopoiesis and differentiation of T and B cells. Precursors of all blood cells, as well as T cells and B cells, arise from a common stem cell in the bone marrow. The first step in determination is between lymphoid stem cells and myeloid stem cells. Cells determined to become T cells (prothymocytes) migrate to the thymus. Interaction of these cells with thymic epithelium and thymus factors produced by thymic epithelial cells induce maturation of thymocytes to T cells. T cells are "thymus-derived cells," which leave the thymus and migrate to thymus-dependent zones of the spleen and lymph nodes, where they undergo further maturation. B-cell maturation occurs in the bone marrow, liver, or gastrointestinal tract (cloacal bursa in fowl) and migrate to the "bursa"-dependent zones of peripheral lymphoid organs. Myeloid differentiation occurs in the bone marrow (see below).

eage that will become functional T cells. In the periphery, 60% of T cells are CD45RA and 40% CD45RO. On peripheral T cells, CD45 p180 (RA) identifies resting memory T cells. Activation of these cells in the periphery is associated with conversion to re-expression of CD45 p205/220 (RO). It is concluded that inappropriate rearrangement

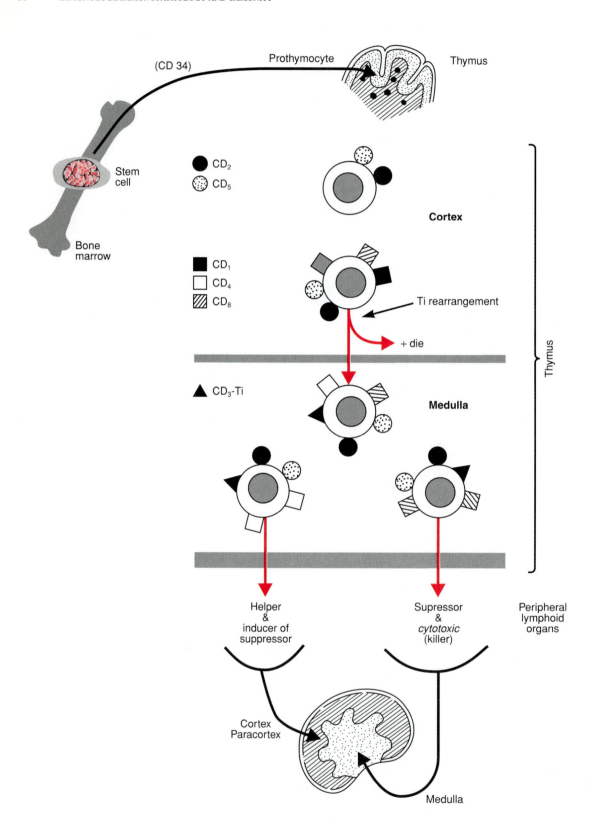

TABLE 3–6. A BEGINNER'S CD SUBCLASSIFICATION OF LYMPHOID CELLS

Marker	Property	Tissue Distribution
CD1	Cell surface glycoprotein	Cortical thymocytes, Langerhans' cells, interdigitation cells, Reed–Sternberg cells
CD2	Sheep RBC receptor	All T cells and thymocytes, T-cell leukemias and lymphomas
CD3	T-cell receptor chain	Medullary thymocytes, peripheral T cells, T-cell leukemias and lymphomas
CD4	Receptor for HIV	T-helper cells, T_{DTH} cells
CD7	Glycoprotein	T-cells and bone marrow prothymocytes
CD8	Glycoprotein	T-cytotoxic cells (suppressor cells)
CD5	Glycoprotein	All T cells, some B-cell tumors (chronic lymphocytic leukemia [CLL])
CD10	Glycoprotein	B cells early in differentiation (acute lymphocytic leukemias [ALL])
CD19	Glycoprotein	All B cells (ALL, CLL, and large-cell lymphoma [LCL])
CD22	Glycoprotein	All B-cells except late in differentiation (ALL and CLL, not LCL)
CD34	Glycoprotein	Precursors of T and B cells (stem cells)
CD45	Membrane protein tyrosine phosphatase	Most white blood cells; differentiates lymphomas from other small cell tumors

Cluster of differentiation (CD) markers define different stages of T-cell development as thymocytes pass through maturation stages in the thymus (Table 3–7). A simplistic presentation of this maturation is presented in Figure 3–17. It is now known that bone marrow precursor cells for both T and B cells may be identified by CD7, CD34, and CD45. A common prothymocyte/NK cell progenitor has cytoplasmic CD3 (cyCD3+, mCD3−). In the thymus, CD5 and CD2 are expressed in cortical thymocytes, in the absence of other markers of T-cell differentiation. CD7+CD34+CD45+ cells may be seen in the yolk sac, fetal liver, neck, and upper thorax of the human fetus as early as 7 to 8 weeks' gestation associated with fetal mesenchyme, and in the fetal thymus by 9 to 10 weeks. In addition, in experimental systems, prothymocyte cell clones have been derived from cultures of bone marrow cells.

Figure 3–17. T-cell differentiation and acquisition of CD markers in the human thymus. Prothymocytes, bearing CD7, CD34, and CD45 markers arise in the bone marrow and migrate to the thymus, where they mature into T cells and CD8. "Thymocytes" refers to cells in the thymus, and T cells to thymus-derived cells that have matured in the thymus and have migrated to peripheral lymphoid markers. The first identifiable markers in the thymic cortex are CD2 and CD5; CD1, CD4, and CD5 are acquired as the cortical thymocytes mature. In the thymic medulla, CD1 is lost, and CD3, part of the T-cell receptor, is acquired. As a final differentiation step CD4+ cells and CD8+ cells segregate into two separate populations. CD4 designates the $T_{helper/delayed\ hypersensitivity}$ population; CD8 designates the $T_{suppressor/cytotoxic}$ population. After leaving the thymus, $T_{H/DTH}$ cells locate preferentially in the cortex of lymph nodes; $T_{S/CTL}$ localize in the medulla, although there is considerable overlap (for details see Chapter 6).

TABLE 3–7. CD Markers of T-cell Differentiation in the Thymus

Marker	Prothymocyte	Cortex		Medulla		Post-Thymic
		Early	Late	Early	Late	
CD34	XXXXXXXXXXXXXXXXXXXXXXXXXX					
CD7	XXXXXXXXXXXXXXXXXXXXXXXXXXXXXXXXXXXXXXXXXXXXXXXXXXXXXXXXXXXXX					
CD45	XXXXXXXXXXXXXXXXXXXXXXXXXXXXXXXXXXXXXXXXXXXXXXXXXXXXXXXXXXXXX					
CD2		XXXXXXXXXXXXXXXXXXXXXXXXXXXXXXXXXXXXXXXXXXXXXXXX				
CD5		XXXXXXXXXXXXXXXXXXXXXXXXXXXXXXXXXXXXXXXXXXXXXXXX				
CD1			XXXXX			
CD4			XXXXXXXXXXXXXXXXXXXXXXXXXXXXXXXXXXXXXXXXXX			
CD8			XXXXXXXXXXXXXXXXXXXXXXXXXXXXXXXXXXXXXXXXXX			
CD3					XXXXXXXXXXXXXXXXXXXXXXXXX	

or specificity of the T-cell receptor in the thymus activates expression of CD45 p180 and cell death.

Selection of Recognition. In the thymus, developing cells not only acquire T-cell surface markers, but also the T-cell receptor for antigen, and the ability to identify self and nonself (see Chapter 6). There is an enormous amount of proliferation, as well as cell death in the thymus, related to selection of cells that will recognize foreign antigens in association with self antigens, but not react to and be activated to self-antigens (ie, not cause autoimmunity). On the other hand, some T cells must be able to recognize the self-markers of the major histocompatibility system in order to function in helping B cells to respond to antigen. This type of self-recognition is imprinted and maintained during the maturation of thymocytes. The antigen receptor of T cells is fixed in the thymus by rearrangement of the T-cell receptor genes. During development of T cells, the thymus "selects the useful, neglects the useless, and destroys the harmless." Two pairs of rearranging T-cell receptor genes have been identified: γδ and αβ. γδ T cells appear early in development, preceding αβ T cells and rapidly disappearing so that they represent only a minor fraction of the T lymphocytes in the adult immune system. Understanding the process of T-cell development of recognition specificity has been one of the major advances in immunology to occur within the last 10 years and is presented in detail in Chapter 6. After proliferation and maturation in the thymus, some of the **thymocytes** leave the thymus to become **thymus-derived cells (T cells)**, and lodge in the **thymus-dependent zones** in the spleen, lymph nodes, and other peripheral lymphoid organs.

Thymic Hormones. Thymic endocrine epithelial cells produce factors known as **thymic hormones** that induce phenotypic maturation of thymocytes in vitro. Over 20 different factors have been described; the four most important of these are listed in Table 3–8. Each of these factors added in vitro to thymus cells has the property of inducing the appearance of T-cell differentiation markers, activating adenosine monophosphate (cAMP), and inducing mature T-cell functions. However, the role of these thymic hormones in normal T-cell development in vivo is questionable. Most studies indicate that maturation of thymocytes requires direct contact between thymic epithelial cells and thymocytes.

B-cell Differentiation

Bone marrow stem cells are influenced by the microenvironment of the bone marrow, liver, and gastrointestinal tract to differentiate into B cells, the precursors of plasma cells. B cells differentiate into plasma cells after induction of specific antibody responses by antigen. Thus, the early stages of B-cell differentiation are antigen-dependent, whereas the later stages of differentiation into plasma cells is antigen-dependent.

Stages of B-cell Differentiation. Pro-B, pre-pre-B, pre-B, and B cells are defined by the configuration of their immunoglobulin genes and the expression of immunoglobulins (see Chapter 4). Progenitors for B cells (pro-B cells) have immunoglobulin genes in germline configuration. Rearrangement of these genes to allow immunoglobulin expression is the essential feature of B-cell differentiation. Ig gene rearrangement occurs in pre-pre-B cells, but no Ig is expressed. Pre-B cells express cytoplasmic IgM and surface μ-chains associated with omega and iota light chains, which are products of nonrearranged light-chain genes. The function of this pre-B-cell receptor is not known. Immature B cells

TABLE 3–8. A SUMMARY OF THYMIC HUMORAL FACTOR EFFECTS

	T-cell Induction	B-cell Induction	Mitogenic	cGMP or cAMP	MLR[a]	Helper[b]	Suppressor[b]
Thymosin	+	0	+	cGMP	+	+	+
Thymopoietin	+	+	+	cGMP	+	+	+
Thymic humoral factor	+	+	+	cAMP	+	+	
Facteur thymique serique (thymulin)	+	+	0	cAMP	0	+	+

[a] MLR—induce ability to respond to mixed lymphocyte reaction.
[b] Helper, suppressor—induce these functions in thymocytes.

and memory B cells express surface IgM but not IgD. Mature and activated B cells express heavy-chain molecules with rearranged light-chain gene products. They may coexpress IgM and IgD, or express another surface Ig class. The details of immunoglobulin gene rearrangements and expression of cytoplasmic and cell surface immunoglobulins associated with B-cell development and current concepts of generation of antibody diversity in B cells will be presented in Chapter 4.

CD Markers of B-cell Differentiation. The expression of CD markers during B-cell differentiation is presented in Table 3–9. These markers have been used to aid in defining the stage of differentiation of B-cell lymphomas (see Chapter 24).

Site of B-cell Differentiation. In mammals, the actual site of B-cell differentiation remains uncertain. In birds, a special lymphoid organ, the bursa of Fabricius, located near the anus, is clearly responsible for B-cell maturation. In the 1950s it was reported that hormonal or surgical removal of the bursa at hatching leads to a loss of development of B cells and a deficiency of immunoglobulin production. Later it was found that bursaless birds could produce immunoglobulins, and a role for extrabursal homing of prebursal cells had to be considered. There appears to be an association between follicle–epithelium in the gastrointestinal tract and bursal mesenchymal dendritic cells to form a

TABLE 3–9. EXPRESSION OF SOME CD MARKERS DURING B DIFFERENTIATION

Antigen	Antigen Independent				Antigen Dependent			
	Pro-B	Pre-pre-B	Pre-B	Immature B	Mature B	Activated B	Memory B	Plasma Cell
CD10	XXXXX	XXXXX	XXXXX					
CD19	XXXXX	XXXXX	XXXXX	XXXXX	XXXXX	XXXXX	XXXXX	
CD22/24		XXXXX	XXXXX	XXXXX	XXXXX	XXXXX	XXXXX	
CD21			XXXXX	XXXXX	XXXXX	XXXXX		
CD23					XXXXX	XXXXX	XXXXX	
CD38		XXX	XXXX					XXXXXXXX
CD39				XXXXX	XXXXX	XXXXX	XXXXX	XXXXXXXX
PAC1								XXXXXXXX

IL, interleukins (see Chapter 7); H-BCGF, high MW B-cell growth factor; L-BCGF, low MW growth factor.

Modified from Uckun FM: Regulation of B-cell ontogeny. *Blood* 76:1908, 1990.

microenvironment for B-cell development. However, a clear role for the gastrointestinal-associated lymphoid tissue (GALT) in B-cell differentiation of mammals has not been demonstrated. Mammalian B cells may arise from determined stem cells in the yolk sac, fetal liver, or bone marrow and mature in the liver, bone marrow, or GALT.

After B cells develop, they migrate through the lymphatics to the B-cell zones of other lymphoid organs. B cells are concentrated in the lymphoid follicles of the lymph node, spleen, and GALT. B-cell maturation depends on interaction with and humoral factors produced by epithelial tissue in the inductive microenvironment of the liver or GALT, similar to the effect of epithelial-produced thymic factors on maturation of T cells. A factor extracted from the bursa of Fabricius of chickens, **bursapoietin**, apparently induces differentiation bone marrow B-cell precursors. Another factor, ubiquitin, may be extracted from the thymus as well as other tissues. Ubiquitin induces differentiation of both T cells and B cells in vitro and functions as a receptor for homing of circulating lymphocytes to lymphoid organs. Again, the in vivo significance of these factors remains unclear. Attempts to restore immune competence in patients with immune deficiencies using such factors have not yet provided convincing beneficial effects.

Interleukins and B-cell Development. More recently, the role of interleukins in B-cell development has been studied extensively in bone marrow cell culture systems. The appearance of interleukin receptors on B cells at different stages of differentiation indicate when, during differentiation, various interleukins act. The role of growth factors and interleukins in B-cell activation after exposure to antigens will be presented in more detail in Chapter 7.

Summary

The lymphoid cells responsible for specific immune responses are distributed in blood, lymphatics, and a number of tissues known as lymphoid organs. The morphologic characteristics and functional properties of lymphoid organs are different. The bone marrow serves as the major source for lymphoid stem cells. T cells develop from stem cells that migrate to the thymus and subsequently recirculate to home in thymus-dependent areas of other lymphoid organs—the spleen, lymph nodes, and gastrointestinal tract. B cells mature in the bone marrow, liver, or gastrointestinal lymphoid tissue and migrate to B-cell areas (follicles) of the other lymphoid organs. Induction of antibody formation is associated with a hyperplasia of follicles and plasma cell production, whereas cellular sensitivity is associated with hyperplasia of thymus-dependent areas.

Hematopoiesis is the process of blood cell formation. The cells of the blood and the lymphocytes of lymphoid organs arise from bone marrow precursors. There is a common bone marrow stem cell that undergoes progressive determination, ie, commitment to different cell lines, under the influence of maturation factors produced in different microenvironments. A variety of colony-stimulating factors in the bone marrow drives the maturation of erythrocytes, granulocytes, monocytes, and platelets. T cells develop from prothymocytes that leave the bone marrow and mature under the influence of interactions with epithelial-derived stromal cells and factors produced in the thymus. The site of B-cell development is not clear. Antigen-independent maturation of B cells is believed to be driven by factors produced in the liver or gastrointestinal tract; antigen-dependent B-cell maturation is driven by factors secreted by activated T cells (interleukins).

Bibliography

LYMPHATICS

Grey H: *Anatomy of the Human Body*, 29th ed. Goss C.M. ed. Chapter 10, The Lymphatic System. Philadelphia, Lea & Febiger, 1973.

Job TT: The adult anatomy of the lymphatic system of the common rat (*Epimys norvegicus*). *Anat Rec* 9:447, 1915.

Yoffey JM, Courtice FC: *Lymphatics, Lymph and the Lymphomyeloid Complex*. New York, Academic Press, 1970.

CENTRAL LYMPHOID ORGANS

Bone Marrow

Becker RP, DBruyn PPH: The transmural passage of blood cells into myeloid sinusoids and the entry of platelets into the sinusoidal circulation: A scanning electron microscopic investigation. *Am J Anat* 145:183, 1976.

Lemischka IR, Roulet DH, Mulligan RC: Development potential and dynamic behavior of hematopoietic stem cells. *Cell* 45:917, 1986.

McGregor DD: Bone marrow origin of immunologically competent lymphocytes in the rat. *J Exp Med* 127:953, 1968.

Wu AM, Till JE, Siminovitch L, McCulloch EA: Cytological evidence for a relationship between normal hematopoietic colony-forming cells and cells of the lymphoid system. *J Exp Med* 127:455, 1968.

Thymus

Aguilar LK, Aguilar-Cordova E, Cartwright J, Belmont JW: Thymic nurse cells are sites of thymocyte apoptosis. *J Immunol* 152:2645–2651, 1994.

Boyd RL, Tucek SL, Godfrey DI, et al.: The thymic microenvironment. *Immunol Today* 14:445–459, 1993.

Cooper MC, Peterson RDA, South MA, Good RA: The functions of the thymus system and the bursa system in the chicken. *J Exp Med* 133:75, 1966.

Defresne MP, Goffinet G, Boniver J: In situ characterization in freeze-fractured mouse thymuses of lymphoepithelial complexes ultrastructurally similar to isolated thymic nurse cells. *Tissue Cell* 18:321, 1986.

Good RA, Gabrielsen AE (eds.): *The Thymus in Immunobiology*. New York, Harper & Row, 1965.

Gregoire C: Thymus and immunity. I. Early thymus research. *Eur J Cancer Clin Oncol* 24:1249, 1988.

Malefijt R de Wall, Leene W, Roholl PJM, Wormmeester J, Hoeben KA: T-cell differentiation within thymic nurse cells. *Lab Invest* 55:25, 1986.

Miller JFAP, Marshall AHE, White RG: The immunological significance of the thymus. *Adv Immunol* 2:111, 1965.

Miller JFAP: The role of the thymus in immunity: Thirty years of progress. *Immunologist* 1:1, 1993.

Ritter MA, Sauvage CA, Cotmore SF: The human thymus microenvironment: In vivo identification of thymic nurse cells and other antigenically distinct subpopulations of epithelial cells. *Immunol* 44:439, 1981.

Singer KH, Haynes BF: Epithelial–thymocyte interaction in human thymus. *Human Immunol* 20:127, 1987.

von Boehmer H: Thymic selection: A matter of life and death. *Immunol Today* 13:454, 1992.

Waksman BH, Arnason BG, Jankovic BD: Role of the thymus in immune reactions in rats. III. Changes in the lymphoid organs of thymectomized rats. *J Exp Med* 116:187, 1962.

Liver

Melchers F: B-lymphocyte development in the liver. II. Frequencies of precursor B cells during gestation. *Eur J Immunol* 7:482, 1977.

Owen JJT, Cooper MD, Raff MC: In vitro generation of B lymphocytes in mouse fetal liver, a mammalian "bursa equivalent." *Nature* 249:361–363, 1974.

PERIPHERAL LYMPHOID ORGANS

Goldschneider I, McGregor DD: Anatomical distribution of T and B lymphocytes in the rat: Development of lymphocyte specific antisera. *J Exp Med* 138:1433, 1973.

Makinodan T, Allbright JF: Proliferative and differentiative manifestations of cellular immune potential. *Prog Allergy* 10:1, 1967.

Rocha B, Freitas AA, Coutinho AA: Population dynamics of T lymphocytes: Renewal rate and expansion in the peripheral lymphoid organs. *J Immunol* 131:2158,1983.

Weiss L: The cells and tissues of the immune system: Structure, functions and interactions. In *Foundations of Immunology Series*, Englewood Cliffs, NJ, Prentice-Hall, 1972.

Lymph Node

Bowen MB, Butch AW, Parvin CA, Levine A, Nahm MH: Germinal center T cells are distinct helper–inducer T cells. *Human Immunol* 31:67, 1991.

Cottier H, Turk J, Sobin L: A proposal for a standardized system of reporting human lymph node morphology in relation to immunological function. *Bull WHO* 47:375, 1972.

Fossum S, Ford WL: The origin of cell population within lymph nodes: Their origin, life history, and functional relationship. *Histopathol* 9:469, 1985.

Kowala MC, Schoefl GI: The popliteal lymph node of the mouse: Internal architecture, vascular distribution, and lymphatic supply. *J Anat* 148:25, 1986.

Van den Oord JJ, Wolf-Peters CD, Desmet VJ: The composite nodule: A structural and functional unit of the reactive human lymph node. *Am J Pathol* 122:83, 1986.

Spleen

Claasen E, Kors H, Dijkstra CD, et al.: Marginal zone of the spleen and the development and localization of specific antibody-forming cells against thymus-dependent and thymus-independent type-2 antigens. *Immunol* 57:399, 1986.

Liaunigg A, Kastberger C, Leitner W, et al.: Regeneration of autotransplanted splenic tissue at different implantation sites. *Cell Tissue Res* 269:1, 1992.

Pabst R, Westermann J, Rothkotter HJ: Immunoarchitecture of regenerated splenic and lymph node transplants. *Int Rev Cytol* 128:215, 1991.

Van Krieken JHJM, Te Veld J: Normal histology of the human spleen. *Am J Surg Pathol* 12:777, 1988.

GALT

Brandtzaeg P, Sollid LM, Thrane PS, et al.: Lymphoepithelial interactions in the mucosal immune system. *Gut* 29:1116, 1988.

Erhak TH, Owen RL: Differential distribution of lymphocytes and accessory cells in mouse Peyer's patches. *Anat Rec* 215:144, 1985.

Kraehenbuhl J-P, Neutra MR: Molecular and cellular basis of immune protection of mucosal surfaces. *Physiol Rev* 72:853–877, 1992.

Lefrancois L: Extrathymic differentiation of intraepithelial lymphocytes: Generation of a separate and unequal T-cell repertoire? *Immunol Today* 12:436, 1991.

Miller K, Nicklin S (eds.): *Immunology of the Gastrointestinal Tract*. CRC Press, Boca Raton, FL, 1987.

Owen RL, Jones AL: Epithelial cell specialization within human Peyer's patches: An ultrastructural study of intestinal lymphoid follicles. *Gastroenterol* 66:189, 1972.

Pabst R, Reynolds JD: Evidence of extensive lymphocyte death in sheep Peyer's patches. I. The number and fate of newly formed lymphocytes that emigrate from Peyer's patches. *J Immunol* 136:2011, 1985.

Pavli P, Hume D, Van De Pol E, et al.: Dendritic cells, the major antigen-presenting cells of the human colonic lamina propria. *Immunol* 78:132–141, 1993.

Press C, McClure S, Landsverk T: Computer-assisted morphometric analysis of absorptive and follicle-associated epithelia of Peyer's patches in sheep foetuses and lambs indicate the presence of distinct T- and B-cell components. *Immunol* 72:386, 1991.

Quiding-Jarbrink M, Granstrom G, Nordstrom I, et al.: Induction of compartmentalized B-cell responses in human tonsils. *Infect Immunity* 63:853–857, 1995.

Sato Y, Wake K: Lymphocyte traffic between the crypt epithelium and the subepithelial lymphoid tissue in human palatine tonsils. *Biomedical Res* 11:365, 1990.

Sicinski P, Rowinski J, Warchok JB, et al.: Poliovirus type-1 enters the human host through intestinal M cells. *Gastroenterol* 98:56, 1990.

Waksman BH: The homing pattern of thymus-derived lymphocytes in calf and neonatal mouse Peyer's patches. *J Immunol* 111:878, 1973.

Waksman BH, Ozer H: Specialized amplification elements in the immune system: The role of nodular lymphoid organs in the mucous membranes. *Prog Allergy* 21:1, 1976.

BALT

Bienenstock J: Bronchus-associated lymphoid tissue. *Int Arch Allergy Appl Immunol* 76(Suppl 1):62, 1985.

Pankow W, von Wichert P: M cell in the immune system of the lung. *Respir* 54:209, 1988.

Reynolds HY: Immunologic system in the respiratory tract. *Physiol Rev* 71:1117, 1991.

DALT

Lee CS, Meeusen E, Brandon MR: Local immunity in the mammary gland. *Vet Immunol Immunopathol* 31:1, 1992.

Nair PNR, Schroeder HE: Duct-associated lymphoid tissue (DALT) of minor salivary glands and mucosal immunity. *Immunol* 57:171, 1986.

SALT

Bergstresser PR, Tigelaar RE, Dees JH, et al.: Thy-1 antigen-bearing dendritic cells populate murine epidermis. *J Invest Dermatol* 81:286, 1983.

Bos JD, Kapsenberg ML: The skin immune system: Its cellular constituents and their interactions. *Immunol Today* 7:235, 1986.

Fichtelius KE, Groth O, Liden S: The skin, a first-level lymphoid organ? *Int Arch Allergy Appl Immunol* 37:607, 1970.

Schuler G: *Epidermal Langerhans' Cells*. CRC Press, Boca Raton, FL, 1990.

Shamoto M, Shinzato M, Hosokawa S, et al.: Langerhans' cells in the lymph node: Mirror section and immunoelectron microscopic studies. *Virchows Archiv B Cell Pathol* 61:337, 1992.

Streilein JW: Skin-associated lymphoid tissues (SALT): Origins and functions. *J Invest Dermatol* 80(Suppl):12, 1983.

Innervation

Ader H. Cohen N: Conditioned immunopharmacologic effects on cell-mediated immunity. *Int J Immunopharmac* 14:323, 1992.

Bateman A, Singh A, Kral T, et al.: The immune–hypothalamic–pituitary–adrenal axis. *Endocrine Rev* 10:92, 1989.

Bellinger DL, Lorton D, Felten SY, et al.: Innervation of lymphoid organs and implications in development, aging, and autoimmunity. *Int J Immunopharmac* 14:329, 1992.

Bulloch K: Neuroanatomy of lymphoid tissue: A review. In *Neural Modulation of Immunity*. Guillemin R et al., eds. New York, Raven Press, 1985, 111–141.

Dunn AJ: Psychoneuroimmunology for the psychoneuroendocrinologist: A review of animal studies of nervous system–immune system interactions. *Psychoneuro-endocrinol* 14:251, 1989.

Jankovic BD: Neuroimmunology: Facts and dilemmas. *Immunol Let* 21:101, 1989.

Sanders VM, Munson AE: Norepinephrine and the antibody response. *Pharmacol Rev* 37:229, 1985.

Sibinga NES, Goldstein A: Opioid peptides and opioid receptors in cells of the immune system. *Annu Rev Immunol* 6:219, 1988.

Wan W, Vriend CY, Wetmore L, et al.: The effects of stress on splenic immune function are mediated by the splenic nerve. *Brain Res Bull* 30:101–105, 1993.

LYMPHOCYTE CIRCULATION

Brahim F, Osmond DG: Migration of bone marrow lymphocytes demonstrated by selective bone marrow labeling with thymidine-H^3. *Anat Rec* 168:139, 1970.

Butcher EC: The regulation of lymphocyte traffic. *Curr Top Microbiol Immunol* 128:85, 1986.

Ford WL: Lymphocyte migration and immune responses. *Prog Allergy* 19:1, 1975.

Goldschneider I, McGregor DD: Migration of lymphocytes and thymocytes in the rat. I. The route of migration from blood to spleen and lymph nodes. *J Exp Med* 127:155, 1968.

Gowans JL, McGregor DD: The immunological activities of lymphocytes. *Prog Allergy* 9:1, 1965.

Husband A: Migration and Homing of Lymphoid Cells. Boca Raton, FL, CRC Press, 1988.

Picker LJ, Nakache M, Butcher EC: Monoclonal antibodies to human lymphocyte homing receptors define a novel class of adhesion molecules on diverse cell types. *J Cell Biol* 109, 927, 1989.

Marchesi VT, Gowans JL: The migration of lymphocytes through the endothelium of venules in lymph nodes: An electron microscopic study. *Proc R Soc Biol* 159:283, 1964.

Stamper HB, Woodruff JJ: An in vitro model of lymphocyte homing is characteristic of the interaction between thoracic duct lymphocytes and specialized high-endothelial venules of lymph nodes. *J Immunol* 119:772, 1977.

Stevens SK, Weissman IL, Butcher EC: Differences in the migration of B and T lymphocytes: Organ-selective localization in vivo and the role of lymphocyte–endothelial cell recognition. *J Immunol* 128:844, 1982.

EFFECT OF ANTIGEN

Heinen E, Cormann N, Kinet-Denoel C: The lymph follicle: A hard nut to crack. Immunol Today 9:240, 1988.

Heinen E, Kinet-Denoel C, Bosseloir A, et al.: B-cell microenvironments during antigen stimulation. In *Cytokines*. Sorg C, ed. Basel, Switzerland, S Karger, 1990, 24–60.

Imhof BA, Berrih-Akinin S, Ezine S: Lymphatic Tissues and in vivo Immune Responses. New York, Marcel Dekker, 1991, 1040.

Koopman G, Parmentier HK, Schuurman H-J, et al.: Adhesion of human B cells to follicular dendritic cells involves both the lymphocyte function-associated antigen 1/intercellular adhesion molecule 1 and very late antigen 4/vascular cell adhesion molecule 1 pathways. *J Exp Med* 173:1297, 1991.

Lindhout E, Mevissen MLCM, Kwekkeboon J, et al.: Direct evidence that human follicular dendritic cells (FDCs) rescue germinal center B cells from death by apoptosis. *Clin Exp Immunol* 91:330–336, 1993.

Miller C, Steda J, Kelsoe G, Cerny J: Faculative role of germinal centers and T cells in the somatic diversification of IgV_H genes. *J Exp Med* 181:1319–1331, 1985.

Nossal GJV, Ada GL, Austin CM: Antigens in immunity. IV. Cellular localization of 125-I and 131-I labelled flagella in lymph nodes. *Aust J Exp Biol Med Sci* 42:311, 1964.

Thorbecke GJ, Amin AR, Tsiagbe VK: Biology of germinal centers in lymphoid tissue. *Federation of American Societies of Experimental Biology Journal (FASEB J)* 8:832–840, 1994.

Turk JL, Oort J: Germinal center activity in relation to delayed hypersensitivity. In *Germinal Centers in Immune Responses*, Cottier H, Odortchenko N, Schindler R, Congdon CC (eds.). New York, Springer, 1967.

Van Rooijen N: The "in situ" immune response in lymph nodes: A Review. *Anat Rec* 218:359, 1987.

ONTOGENY OF IMMUNITY

T-cell Development

Auerbach R: Experimental analysis of the origin of cell types in the developing thymus. *Dev Biol* 3:336, 1961.

Clement LT: Isoforms of the CD45 common leukocyte leukocyte antigen family: Markers for human T-cell differentiation. *J Clin Immunol* 12:1, 1992.

Egerton M, Pruski E, Pilarski: Cell generation with human thymic subsets defined by selective expression of CD45 (T200) isoforms. *Human Immunol* 27:33, 1990.

Fesus L: Apoptosis fashions T and B cell repertoire. *Immunol Let* 30:277, 1991.

Good RA, Gabrielsen AE (eds.): *The Thymus in Immunobiology.* New York, Harper & Row, 1985.

Hale ML, Greiner DL, McCarthy KF: Characterization of rat prothymocyte with monoclonal antibodies recognizing rat lymphocyte membrane antigenic determinants. *Cell Immunol* 107:188, 1987.

Haynes BF: Phenotypic characterization and ontogeny of components of the human thymic microenvironment. *Clin Res* 32:500, 1984.

Haynes BF, Martin ME, Kay HH, et al.: Early events in human T-cell ontogeny: Phenotypic characterization and immunohistologic localization of T-cell precursors in early human fetal tissues. *J Exp Med* 168:1061, 1988.

Komuro K. Boyse EA: Induction of T lymphocytes from precursor cells in vitro by a product of the thymus. *J Exp Med* 138:479, 1973.

Miller JFAP, Osoba D: Current concepts of the immunological function of the thymus. *Physiol Rev* 74, 1967.

Owen JJT, Jenkenson EJ: Early events in T-lymphocyte genesis in the fetal thymus. *Am J Anat* 170:301, 1984.

Palacios R, Pelkonen J: Prethymic and intrathymic mouse T-cell progenitors: Growth requirement and analysis of expression of genes encoding TCR/T3 components and other T-cell-specific molecules. *Immunol Rev* 104:5, 1988.

Rothenberg E, Lugo JP: Differentiation and cell division in the mammalian thymus. *Develop Biol* 112:1, 1985.

Safieh-Garabedian B, Kendall MD, Khamashta MA, et al.: Thymulin and its role in immunomodulation. *J Autoimmunity* 5:547, 1992.

Strominger JL: Developmental biology of T-cell receptors. *Science* 244:943, 1989.

Stutman O, Good RA: Thymus hormones. *Contemp Top Immunol* 2:229, 1973.

Tranin N, Small M: Thymic humoral factors. *Contemp Top Immunol* 2:321, 1973.

Turpen JB, Cohen N: Localization of thymocyte stem cell precursors in the pharyngeal endoderm of early amphibian embryos. *Cell Immunol* 24:109, 1976.

Van Ewjk W: Immunohistology of lymphoid and nonlymphoid cells in the thymus in relation to T-cell differentiation. *Am J Anat* 170:311, 1984.

Von Boehmer H, Teh HS, Kisielow P: The thymus selects the useful, neglects the useless, and destroys the harmful. *Immunol Today* 10:57, 1989.

B-cell Development

Archer OK, Sutherland DER, Good RA: Appendix of the rabbit: A homologue of the bursa in the chicken. *Nature* 200:337, 1963.

Brand A, Gilmour D, Goldstein G: Lymphocyte-differentiating hormone of bursa of Fabricius. *Science* 193:319, 1976.

Burrows PD, Cooper MD: B-cell development in man. *Current Biol* 5:201–206, 1993.

Cambier JC: B-lymphocyte Differentiation. Boca Raton, FL, CRC Press, 1986.

Cooper MD: Current concepts: B lymphocytes: Normal development and functions. *N Eng J Med* 317:1452, 1987.

Cooper MD, Peterson RDA, South MA, et al.: The functions of the thymus system and the bursa system in the chicken. *J Exp Med* 133:75, 1966.

Glick B: Historical perspective: The bursa of Fabricius and its influence on B-cell development, past and present. *Vet Immunol Immunopathol* 30:3, 1991.

Hamaoka T, Ono S: Regulation of B-cell differentiation. *Annu Rev Immunol* 4:167, 1986.

Kishimoto T, Hirano T: Molecular regulation of B-lymphocyte response. *Annu Rev Immunol* 6:485, 1988.

Sharp JG, Crouse DA, Purtillo DT: Ontogeny and regulation of the immune system. *Arch Pathol Lab Med* 111:1106, 1987.

Shields JW: Bursal dissections and gill pouch hormones. *Nature*: 259:373, 1976.

Uckun F: Regulation of human B-cell ontogeny. *Blood* 76:1908, 1990.

Warner NL, Szenberg A: The immunologic function of the bursa of Fabricius in the chicken. *Am Rev Microbiol* 18:253, 1964.

4

Antibodies, Immunoglobulins, and B-Cell Receptors

Edward E. Max

One of the two arms of specific immunity is immunoglobulin or antibody—produced by plasma cells. Plasma cells are the differentiated progeny of B cells. An individual must be able to make thousands of different antibody molecules in order to identify and react with many potential infectious agents. Yet each plasma cell makes only one type of antibody. Antibody diversity resides in the vast number of different B cells in any individual that have immunoglobulin receptors for different specific antigens. After antigen binding and stimulation of a specific B cell via receptors for its antigen, the specific B cell is activated. Activation leads to proliferation; and the progeny of the specifically activated B cell differentiate into plasma cells that synthesize and secrete the specific antibody. In this way large numbers of antibodies that react with different infectious agents are produced in a very short period of time. The subjects of this chapter are the nature of antibodies, their reaction with antigens, and how they are produced.

Antibodies

Antibodies were the first components of immune specificity to be recognized. The key experiments providing evidence for immune proteins in blood were performed about a century ago by pioneering immunologists trying to understand how an initial exposure to a specific pathogen could confer immunity to a second attack. It was shown, for instance, that after an animal was exposed to the bacterium *Vibrio cholerae*, protein components of serum from that animal—but not from a "naive animal"—were capable of killing live Cholera organisms. Other early experiments documented other manifestations of antibodies, including their ability to neutralize and precipitate toxins and other bacterial proteins, to agglutinate bacteria, and to confer immunity when injected into a "naive" animal challenged with the specific organism. All of these manifestations have been shown to result from tight and specific binding between an antibody and a microbial component (antigen). Although all antibodies are proteins (also known as immunoglobulins), a variety of macromolecules act as antigens, including proteins, polysaccharides, nucleic acids and proteolipids.

At this point in the history of immunology, it could have been assumed that vertebrates are endowed through evolution with a repertoire of antibodies designed to interact with the microbial molecules to which they are commonly exposed; however, a vastly larger repertoire was indicated by subsequent experiments. Landsteiner and others showed that antibodies could be induced against many nonbiological chemicals if these were injected into experimental animals after being coupled to proteins, eg dinitrophenol coupled to serum albumin. The resulting antibodies could bind with specificity to small molecules like dinitrophenol, known as **haptens**, yet the administration of haptens alone failed to elicit antibodies (ie the haptens were not **immunogenic**) unless they were attached to a macromolecule (a **carrier**). The ability of the immune system to generate specific antibodies against a variety of nonbiological haptenic chemicals that were presumably never encountered in the evolutionary history of vertebrates suggested that antibody repertoire was not limited to any particular set of commonly encountered antigens but could potentially include specificities against a much larger universe of antigens. This raised the question of how such vast diversity might be encoded in the organism's genome; the answer could not be clarified until the development of the techniques of molecular genetics, as discussed below. A related mystery was the mechanism by which a molecule could act as an **immunogen**, ie induce an organism to produce a set of highly specific antibodies directed against the administered antigen, while not inducing antibodies against other antigens.

ANTIGEN BINDING

Antibodies vary considerably in function and structure. One parameter that bears importantly on the function of an antibody is its affinity for antigen, ie how tightly it binds the antigen molecule. As a simple paradigm for measuring affinity consider the binding reaction between a hapten H and antibody molecule A, a reversible reaction:

$$H + A \underset{kd}{\overset{kb}{\rightleftharpoons}} HA$$

where kb is the rate constant for binding and kd is the rate constant for dissociation. If antigen is introduced into an antibody-containing solution, the above reaction will proceed to the right until at equilibrium the rate of binding equals the rate of dissociation: [H] [A]kb = [AH]kd or K = kb/kd = [HA]/[H] [A], where K is known as the association constant, a measure of affinity.

This association constant can be measured by equilibrium dialysis. For this determination, a known amount of antibody is placed inside a dialysis bag and variable amounts of radioactively labeled hapten are added to the solution outside the bag. The large size of the antibody molecule prevents efflux across the dialysis membrane, but the hapten can readily diffuse through the membrane into the bag and then bind to the antibody. At equilibrium the concentration of hapten outside the bag must equal the concentration of free (unbound) hapten inside the bag, so any excess of radioactivity/volume measured inside the dialysis bag is due to hapten bound to antibody. For a pure antibody that binds monovalently to antigen and shows no cooperativity effects, the same association constant will be calculated from the experimental data determined at every concentration of hapten. If similar experiments are performed with an antiserum containing a mixture of many antibodies with a range of affinities, the calculated association constant at low hapten concentration will reflect the antibodies of highest affinity, while at higher concentrations of hapten the calculated association constant will be lower. In this situation, an average association constant can be estimated from the K measured when the antibody is 50% saturated with hapten. When such average association constants are measured in serum samples collected at various times after immunization, it is generally observed that this average association constant increases during the course of an experimentally induced immune reaction (**affinity maturation**). The mechanism of affinity maturation is addressed later in this chapter.

CLONAL SELECTION

Early in the study of antibodies it was recognized that an understanding of how these molecules recognize antigens would require knowledge of their primary structure, ie amino acid sequence. However, attempts to determine the amino acid sequences of antibodies were hampered by the fact that any antibody response in an experimental animal includes a large number of different antigen-specific antibodies with heterogeneous structure; little useful sequence information could be obtained from such mixtures. A logical solution to this technical problem derives from an understanding of the answer to a question posed above: how does a particular antigen elicit a narrow antibody response specifically targeted against that antigen?

The **clonal selection** hypothesis championed by Burnett in the 1950s, and subsequently proven correct, suggested that any one B lymphocyte can make only a single species of antibody. Early in the development of an antibody-producing cell, at the B-cell stage, very little of this antibody is secreted; instead the antibody is expressed on the outside surface of the cell membrane. This form of membrane immunoglobulin serves as an antigen-specific receptor that, on binding antigen, can trigger the B cell to proliferate and mature to an antibody secreting stage. Many millions of resting B cells circulate in the normal animal, each displaying on its surface an antibody of a different structure and binding specificity. When a foreign antigen is administered, only the small population of B cells expressing a membrane antibody capable of binding the antigen will be triggered. These antigen-specific B cells then proliferate and subsequently mature into cells capable of secreting antibody of the same specificity originally displayed on the surface of the clonal progenitors. This hypothesis provided a satisfactory explanation for the selective elicitation of antibodies specific for an injected antigen, though it raised several additional questions addressed later in this chapter: (1) What is the difference in antibody structure between that expressed on the surface and the secreted form? (2) What mechanism explains the shift between these two forms? and (3) Why does each B cell express only a single antibody, given the fact that it should have many genes for antibodies in each antibody gene locus and, as a diploid cell, two copies of each gene locus?

The clonal selection hypothesis provides a theoretical solution to the technical problem of obtaining a pure homogeneous antibody preparation for amino acid sequence analysis: homogeneous immunoglobulin can be obtained from a clonal population of lymphocytes derived from a single progenitor cell. Initially such **monoclonal antibodies** were derived from **myelomas**, which represent clonal expansions of a single malignantly transformed B-lymphoid cell; myelomas occur in humans and can be induced experimentally at high frequency in several inbred mouse strains. Generally such myelomas are not targeted against a known antigen. To generate monoclonal antibodies against specific antigens, **hybridoma** technology was developed, originally by Milstein and Kohler. In this technique, a mouse is immunized with antigen and, after variable lengths of time, individual mice are sacrificed to obtain splenic B cells. These B cells are fused to a nonsecreting myeloma to yield hybrid cells: hybridomas. The antigen-specific splenic B cells contribute the antigen specificity of antibody production, while the myeloma contributes the transformed phenotype, allowing sustained proliferation. Cells secreting antibodies of desired properties can then be cloned from the fusion population and propagated, providing an immortal source of homogeneous antibody suitable for amino acid sequence determination.

Immuno-globulin Structure

ISOTYPES

A comparison of amino acid sequences of various myeloma proteins yielded several important generalizations. Human antibodies can be classified into nine classes or **isotypes**, which are defined by "effector" properties that are independent of antigen specificity. The most abundant isotype in normal human serum is IgG, which exists in four subclasses designated IgG1 to IgG4, in decreasing order of abundance in normal serum (Table 4–1). All IgG antibodies have about the same molecular weight (about 150 kD) and are composed of four disulfide-linked chains which can be separated by reduction in mercaptoethanol to yield two identical heavy (H) chains (about 50 kD) and two identical light (L) chains (about 25kD); the antibody thus has a chain structure designated H_2L_2. The isotype of an antibody is defined by that of its heavy chain, which confers the effector properties. The same two light chain classes—κ or λ—can occur with any of the nine heavy chain isotypes. The heavy chain contributing to IgG is known as γ, whereas the H chains of the other isotype classes—IgA, IgD, IgM, and IgE—are known by the corresponding Greek letters α, δ, μ, and ϵ, respectively. Each heavy chain isotype has a characteristic component of carbohydrate covalently bound at specific amino acid residues.

PROTOTYPE MOLECULE

Because of the high abundance of IgG (about 14 mg/ml in normal human serum) and its frequent representation in myelomas, it was the first isotype whose structure was determined and it remains a conceptual prototype for antibodies. The analysis of IgG structure was facilitated by the observation that the proteases papain and pepsin could clip the H_2L_2 IgG molecule in two different ways, defined by the position of the cleavage sites relative to the disulfide bonds linking the heavy chains (Fig. 4–1). Papain cleaves on the N-terminal side of these disul-

TABLE 4–1. BIOLOGICAL PROPERTIES OF IGG SUBCLASSES

Property	IgG_1	IgG_2	IgG_3	IgG_4
Percentage of total IgG in serum	65	23	8	4
Complement fixation	++	+	+++	0
Placental transfer	+++	++	+++	+++
Passive cutaneous anaphylaxis[a]	+++	0	+++	+++
Receptor for macrophage	+++	0	+++	0
Reaction with staph protein A	+++	+++	0	+++
Prominent antibody activity	Anti-Rh	Anti-levan, anti-dextran	Anti-Rh	Anti-factor VIII

[a]Heterocytophilic antibody (see Chapter 18).

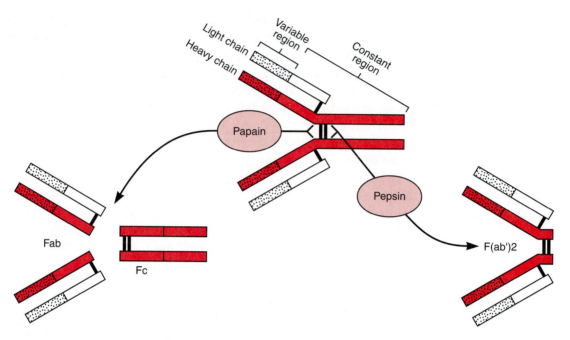

Figure 4–1. Proteases cleave IgG to generate characteristic fragments. In the intact IgG molecule (center) the heavy chain is indicated as a red bar and the light chain as a shorter white bar; in each case the N-terminal variable domain is stippled and the constant domains are not. The thin black bars represent the disulfide bonds that link the heavy and light chains. The figure shows the positions of cleavage by the proteases papain and pepsin and illustrates the useful fragments that are generated.

fide bonds producing three fragments. Two identical fragments are known as Fab because they are capable of monovalent antigen binding. The third fragment is known as Fc because (in rare instances) it can be crystallized even when obtained from polyvalent antiserum (because Fc pieces lack the diversity of the antigen-binding fragments). In contrast to papain, pepsin cleaves on the C-terminal side of the disulfide linkages, yielding a fragment—F(ab')$_2$—that is divalent but lacks the effector properties characteristic of intact antibody. Apart from the significance of these protease fragments in the early protein structural analysis of IgG, they have also become important laboratory tools because of their distinct functional properties.

Amino acid sequence analysis of purified fragments of heavy and light chains from IgG revealed repeated internal sequence similarities which reflect a domain structure of these polypeptide chains. Each domain contains 100 to 110 amino acids (representing about 12 kD) containing an internal disulfide loop and certain other characteristic amino acids. Similar "immunoglobulin domains" have been found in a large number of surface proteins, probably reflecting a primitive and very ancient gene that underwent extensive duplication and diversification during evolution. These related proteins form a group known as the immunoglobulin superfamily which includes T cell receptors (the closest relatives of the immunoglobulins), major histocompatibility antigens, numerous cell adhesion molecules, and a number of other surface proteins with important function in the immune system (including CD4 and CD8).

VARIABLE AND CONSTANT DOMAINS

Sequence comparison between monoclonal antibody chains revealed a remarkable dichotomy between the N-terminal domain, which is highly variable, and all the remaining domains, which show essentially identical sequence when the corresponding domains are compared between different monoclonal chains of the same class. The diversity of the variable (V) domain reflects the function of this part of the molecule in binding diverse antigens, whereas the constant (C) domains confer the isotype-specific properties or effector functions of the immunoglobulin. The number of constant region domains in heavy chains (CH domains) depends on the isotype: μ and ϵ heavy chains have four CH domains, while δ-, γ-, and α- heavy chains each have 3 CH domains, plus a "hinge" region between CH1 and CH2 that may be the evolutionary remnant of a primordial fourth domain. Three-dimensional structure analyses by X-ray crystallography have defined a common general structure in all immunoglobulin domains, which is conserved even in the nonimmunoglobulin members of the immunoglobulin superfamily. In this structure the polypeptide backbone is folded into 7 more or less parallel strands in the configuration known as β-pleated sheet (see Fig. 4–2). In the intact H_2L_2 molecule, the VH and VL domains contact each other, as do the CL and CH1 domain; each remaining CH domain contacts the corresponding domain of the other heavy chain partner. These interactions lead to an H_2L_2 structure whose "Y" shape has been visualized by electron microscopy and, in greater detail, by X-ray crystallography (Fig. 4–3).

EFFECTOR FUNCTIONS

The structural differences between the various heavy chain isotypes are responsible for some differences in "effector" functions of antibodies, ie their ability to act in certain locations or engage secondary protective mechanisms. These effector functions include the following:

1. **Opsonization** is the ability of an antibody to bind to a microorganism or particle to facilitate its phagocytosis or killing by cellular phagocytes (neutrophils, macrophages, etc.).
2. **Complement fixation** involves the activation of a complex

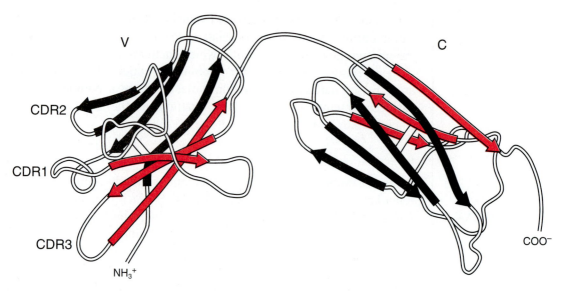

Figure 4–2. Ribbon diagram of a light chain. This 3-dimensional view of the folding of the α carbon chain backbone is a visualization based on X-ray diffraction of immunoglobulin crystals. The V and C domains are rotated 160° with respect to each other. The broad arrows ("ribbons") show the seven segments of β-pleated sheet structure in each domain, with one face of three strands (colored) roughly parallel to another face of four strands. The loops projecting out at left represent the three complementarity determining regions (CDR1, CDR2, and CDR3) which, together with three similar loops from the heavy chain variable region, form the antigen combining site.

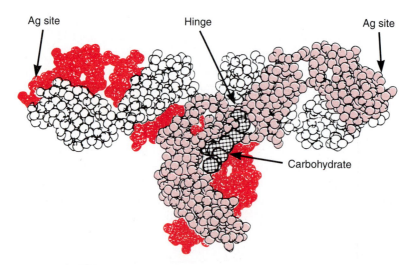

Figure 4–3. This 3-dimensional view shows the structure of an IgG molecule in a space-filling model derived from X-ray crystallographic results. One complete heavy chain is pink and the other is red; each light chain is white, and carbohydrate is crosshatched. The positions of the heavy chain hinge and the two antigen (Ag) binding sites are shown.

cascade of serum proteins—known collectively as **complement**—which can lyse bacteria by chemically punching holes in them. Other functions of complement include **chemotaxis** (the attraction of phagocytes to an inflammatory site), enhancement of opsonization, and increasing the permeability of blood vessels (see Chapter 8). Complement can be activated as a result of binding of antibody to antigen (the "classical" pathway) or directly by certain bacterial products (the "alternative," probably more primitive, pathway).

3. Neutralization (inactivation) of viruses or toxins may result from binding of appropriate antibodies. An antibody that neutralizes a toxin is known as an **antitoxin**.

4. Antigen clearance refers to the ability of the reticuloendothelial system to remove antigen from the serum; the presence of antigen-specific antibody can speed up antigen clearance (see Chapter 10).

5. The release of chemical mediators can be induced by binding of antigen to "cytophilic" antibody, ie antibody noncovalently bound to cell surface immunoglobulin receptors that bind via the Fc portion of the immunoglobulin molecule (Fc receptors); the classic example is IgE, discussed below.

6. Isotypes can be distinguished by their time of appearance after antigen administration or their ability to appear in certain locations, eg to cross the placenta or to appear in secretions.

HEAVY-CHAIN ISOTYPES

A simplified comparison of the structure of the five major immunoglobulin classes is shown in Figure 4–4. Many of their different effector functions are discussed in the brief description of the human immunoglobulin isotypes below and are listed in Table 4–2.

IgM, at about 1.2 mg/ml in normal serum, contributes about 10% of serum immunoglobulin and is present mostly as a pentamer with five H_2L_2 units covalently linked by disulfide bonds. IgM pentamers can be visualized by electron microscopy and appear to be joined at their C-terminal tips. Pentamer formation is facilitated by the presence of a 15 kD protein known as J chain, one molecule of which is linked by disulfide bonds to the $(IgM)_5$ creating a complex of about 950,000 kD (with a sedimentation constant of 19S). This immunoglobulin was designated IgM because it is larger than the other immunoglobulins (macroglobulin). IgM is the first isotype expressed during fetal development and is also the first expressed during the development of each B lymphocyte. As a lymphocyte matures it generally switches to expression of other isotypes, but, remarkably, the heavy chain V region is not altered during this process so the antigen-binding specificity does not change; the mechanism of the switch at the genetic level is discussed later in this chapter. The multivalency of serum IgM allows

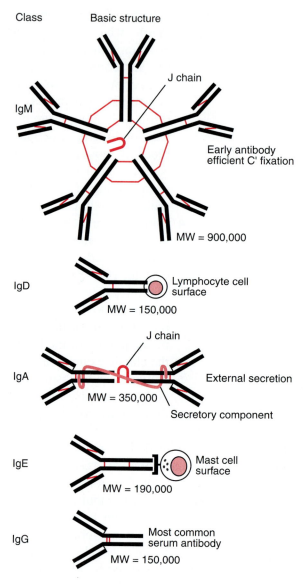

Figure 4–4. Human immunoglobulin classes in human. The five isotype classes (IgM, IgD, IgA, IgE, IgG) each contain similar basic subunits composed of two identical heavy chains (known as μ, δ, α, ϵ, and γ, respectively) and two identical light chains (either κ or λ). There are four human γ subtypes. Disulfide bonds link heavy and light chains as shown (red lines), and also link IgA into dimers and IgM into pentamers; the latter two polymeric forms also include the 15 kD J chain polypeptide. Two isotypes exert their major function bound to cells: IgD is shown bound to the lymphocyte that synthesized it, while IgE is shown bound to a mast cell via the Fcϵ receptor.

TABLE 4–2. SOME PROPERTIES OF HUMAN IMMUNOGLOBULINS

Property	Immunoglobulin Class				
	IgG	IgA	IgM	IgD	IgE
Serum concentration (g/100 ml)	1.2	0.4	0.12	0.003	<0.00005
Sedimentation coefficient (S)	7	7 (9,11,13)*	19 (24,32)*	7	8
Molecular weight	140,000	160,000$^\Delta$	900,000	180,000	200,000
Electrophoretic mobility	γ	Slow β	Between γ and β	Between γ and β	Slow β
H-chains	γ	α	μ	δ	ε
L-chains	λ or κ	λ or κ	λ or κ	λ or κ	λ or κ
Complement fixation	Yes	No	Yes	No	No
Placental transfer	Yes	No	No	No	No
Percent intravascular	40	40	70	—	—
Half-life (days)	23	6	5	3	2.5
Percent carbohydrate	3	10	10	13	10
Antibody activity	Most Ab to infections; major part of secondary response; Rh isoagglutinins; LE factor	Present in external secretions	First Ab formed; ABO isoag-glutinins; rheumatoid factor	Antibody activity rarely demonstrated, found on lymphocyte surface	Reagin sensitizes mast cells for anaphylaxis

* Figures in parentheses indicates the existence of other molecular forms, such as polymers.

Δ Serum IgA 160,000 MW; secretory IgA 350,000 MW, may activate alternate pathway (see Chap. 10) (Modified from Fahey, J.L.: J.A.M.A. 194:183, 1966).

this isotype to bind efficiently to polyvalent antigen particles (such as microbes) even when the intrinsic affinity of each monomeric VH-VL pair for antigen may be relatively low. This isotype thus plays a particularly important role early in infections before affinity maturation has occurred. Because of its large size, IgM does not cross the placenta; thus the presence in cord blood of IgM antibodies against a particular virus is presumptive evidence for fetal infection.

IgD is present in only low amounts in serum (about 0.04 mg/ml) where it has no known function. It is present, along with IgM of the same antigen specificity, on the surface of immature B-cells where it is capable of triggering cell activation in response to antigen exposure. It is possible that IgD has its primary function in this membrane form, though extensive investigation has not fully clarified its role. Mice from a strain genetically engineered to lack IgD are competent to generate an antibody response to antigen challenge but take longer than normal mice to develop high affinity antibodies through affinity maturation.

IgA contributes only about 10% to 15% of serum immunoglobulin (normal range about 2 to 3 mg/ml). However, since it is the predominant isotype in secretions (saliva, milk, tears, and secretions of lung, nasal, and intestinal mucosa), it is actually the predominant immunoglobulin in terms of daily production by the whole animal, playing a key role in defense against environmental pathogens. In secretions, it is generally present as a dimer of H_2L_2 units linked by a molecule of J-chain protein and covalently associated with a protein known as secretory component (SC). The latter protein is not made by B lymphocytes but represents a fragment of the poly-Ig receptor on the surface of epithelial cells, a protein that mediates transepithelial transport of the IgA dimer into lumenal secretions. In humans, there are two IgA subclasses: IgA1, which predominates in serum, and IgA2, which is the (slightly) more abundant form in secretions.

IgE is by far the least abundant isotype in the serum of normal individuals (normal concentration below 0.5 μg/ml) but it is the isotype whose manifestations are perhaps most apparent to the lay observer in that it accounts for all allergic reactions. IgE binds extremely tightly to receptors on the surface of mast cells and basophils. These receptors are known as FcεRI to distinguish them from lower affinity FcεRII receptors found on some lymphocytes. When contact between antigen and surface-bound IgE causes cross-linking of the associated FcεRI molecules, the latter can trigger the release of granules containing allergic mediators such as histamine, causing swelling, itching, rhinitis, bronchoconstriction, etc. (see Chapter 14). This isotype is thought to play a beneficial role in defense against parasites, since helminth infestations are associated with striking increases in IgE concentrations.

IgG is by far the most abundant isotype in serum, contributing about 75% to 85% to total immunoglobulin. The four human IgG subclasses all have a similar monomeric H_2L_2 structure as described above, although the γ3 subclass is distinguished by a very long hinge region containing 15 disulfide cross-links. All four subclasses cross the placenta, consistent with a major role for maternal IgG in fetal and neonatal immunity, but the subclasses do appear to have distinct functional roles. For example, IgG1 and IgG3 are able to fix complement well (Chapter 8), whereas IgG2 is much weaker in this regard and IgG4 does not fix complement at all. IgG2 is the major subtype of anti-carbohydrate antibodies, for reasons unknown. Several forms of Fcγ receptor exist on macrophages, granulocytes and natural killer cells. Cross-linking of these receptors by interaction of bound antibody with polyvalent antigen particles leads to activation of cellular attack mechanisms (phagocytosis or antibody-dependent cell-mediated cytotoxicity or [ADCC]). This mechanism explains the role of antibodies in promoting the killing of bacteria (opsonization), one of the earliest effects of antibodies to be described.

LIGHT-CHAIN ISOTYPES

The two light-chain classes in mammals, κ and λ, are present in human serum in a ratio of about 60% to 40%, respectively (in mice the ratio is about 95% to 5%). Although one or the other light-chain class may predominate in certain immune responses, this ratio is thought to result from chance differences in the V region repertoire for these two classes; and no important functional distinction between κ and λ is known.

DIVERSITY OF ANTIBODY SPECIFICITY

The most remarkable feature of immunoglobulins is the striking diversity of the variable regions. With few exceptions, all myelomas have distinct variable regions, and even hybridoma antibodies specific for a particular antigen are generally distinct. When this immense diversity was discovered, it was unprecedented in biology, and even now it is unmatched except for the related diversity of T-cell receptors. The puzzle of how such diversity might be encoded in the genome of an organism was complicated by the fact that the variability ended precisely at the boundary between the V and C regions of the protein. The molecular explanation for immunoglobulin diversity will be discussed later. A plot of the amount of sequence variability at each of the approximately 110 positions in the V region (a "variability plot"; Fig. 4–5) shows that the variability is not evenly distributed but rather is clustered into three "hypervariable" regions. These three hypervariable clusters were hypothesized to represent the "complementarity-determining regions" (CDRs), ie, the amino acid residues that actually contact the diverse world of foreign antigens. This hypothesis was substantiated by the three-dimensional structures of antibody molecules determined by x-ray crystallography. The three hypervariable regions of the VL and VH domains form six loops that together constitute a surface capable of interacting with antigen (Fig. 4–2). The remaining residues of the V region domain create a framework (FR) that holds the CDR loops in proper position to contact antigen. Crystallographic analysis of several antigen–antibody complexes have characterized features of the interface between these two molecules, which generally conform to early models of a lock-and-key fit. For example, in the complex of lysozyme with antilysozyme, a "bump" projecting from the antigen surface fits into a cavity on the antibody and vice versa. The forces that bind protein antigens to antibodies are essentially the same as those that hold together the subunits of multimeric proteins: van der Waals forces, hydrophobic interactions, hydrogen bonds and salt bridges (ie electrostatic forces between a positive charge on one surface and a negative charge on the other).

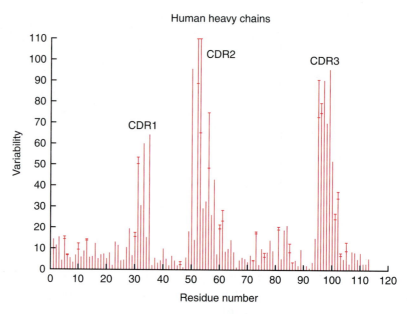

Figure 4–5. A variability plot. A parameter reflecting sequence variability at each codon position in the heavy chain V region shows three clusters of hypervariability at the regions of the protein that contact antigen, known as the complementarity determining regions (CDR1, CDR2, and CDR3).

ANTIGEN DETERMINANT (EPITOPE)

The specific region on a macromolecular antigen that contacts the antibody is known as an **epitope** or **antigenic determinant** (see Fig. 4–6). Most protein antigens have several epitopes. An epitope may be a linear sequence of amino acids or a protein surface composed of several loops that are not contiguous on the linear amino acid sequence of the antigen (**conformational epitopes**). Because antibodies themselves are proteins, they can serve as antigens in some circumstances (see below). The antibodies produced in a given animal are part of that individual's "self" and thus not usually recognized as foreign by the immune system. The mechanism of this crucial discrimination, known as **tolerance**, is not fully understood, but there is evidence that during the fetal and early neonatal development of the immune system, lymphocytes making antibodies that are capable of recognizing "self" antigens are either eliminated or disabled from producing antibody. Failures of development of self-tolerance are responsible for autoimmune diseases, as discussed in Chapter 21.

IDIOTYPES

In contrast to the tolerizing effects of potential antigens during the neonatal period, when a new foreign antigen is encountered later in life, it generally provokes an antibody response. Some V regions—either

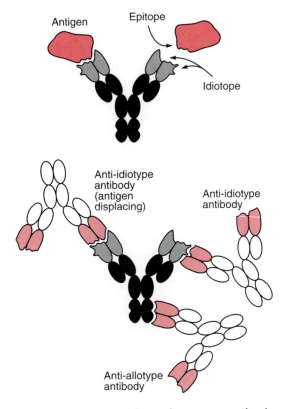

Figure 4–6. The two contact surfaces between antibody and antigen (upper panel) are known as idiotope (on the antibody) and epitope (on the antigen). An antibody may be recognized as an antigen by other antibodies (lower panel), and depending on the part recognized, these are known as anti-idiotype or anti-allotype antibodies.

from antibodies newly synthesized in vivo or from antibodies injected into syngeneic animals—may look sufficiently foreign to the immune system that these antibody V regions induce their own second level of immune response. The resulting antibodies are known as **anti-idiotypic** and are said to recognize an **idiotype** in the V region of the injected antibody. An anti-idiotypic antibody may interfere with the binding of the injected antibody to its antigen if it is directed against an epitope in the complementary determining region (paratope), but anti-idiotype antibodies may also recognize FR residues in the V region and thus fail to interfere with antigen binding (Fig. 4–6). Considerable theoretical discussion has been devoted to mechanisms whereby the immune response might be regulated by an idiotype/anti-idiotype network of interactions, but there is little solid evidence for a significant physiological role of such regulation. For a discussion of the role that idiotypic determinant may have in producing autoimmune diseases see Chapter 11.

XENOTYPES AND ALLOTYPES

Another way an antibody may act as an antigen is if it is injected into a recipient whose own antibodies differ in structure from the injected antibody. This may occur if the injected antibody derives from a different species (a **xenogeneic** antibody). Even within the same species, genetic polymorphisms between individuals—allelic genes—can create differences in immunoglobulin structure sufficient to induce an antibody response in a recipient. Such differences within a species are known as **allotypic** (see Fig. 4–6), and the resulting anti-allotypic antibodies can be useful laboratory reagents. For example, if B cells from a mouse of allotype 1 are injected into a recipient mouse of allotype 2, the production of antibody by the donor cells can be monitored by measuring the production of allotype 1 antibody. The allotypic variations most commonly studied are in the constant regions, but V region allotypes are also known. In human immunoglobulins, about 30 different allotypic specificities are known.

Antibody–Antigen Reactions (Immunotechnology)

The laboratory techniques used to detect and measure antigen–antibody reactions have been critical tools in the development of immunological knowledge; because of the extreme specificity and sensitivity of antibodies, these techniques have also been widely used in other fields, including protein chemistry, molecular biology, forensics, and clinical medicine. The laboratory methods developed first employed natural (unmarked) antigens and antibodies; in these methods, detection of antigen–antibody complex formation depends on a resulting visible change (precipitation, agglutination) or a physiological consequence of such formation (complement fixation).

PRECIPITIN REACTION

Many techniques for detecting antigen–antibody complexes using unlabeled antibodies depend on formation of insoluble particles (precipitation). The insolubility of antigen–antibody complexes results from the fact that each H_2L_2 antibody molecule is divalent (has two antigen-combining sites) while most natural antigens are also multivalent. Thus, under appropriate conditions, a complex lattice containing large numbers of antibodies and antigens forms, leading to an insoluble particle (Fig. 4–7); such particles accumulate as a visible precipitate (precipitin reaction). Precipitates do not form if either antigen or antibody is present in too high a concentration. The sensitivity of the precipitin reaction to both antigen and antibody concentrations means that if the antibody concentration is held constant, a measure of the antigen concentration can be obtained by determining the dilution of antigen that produces optimal precipitation, ie the "equivalence" concentration; conversely, if antigen concentration is held constant the precipitin reaction can be used to estimate antibody concentrations.

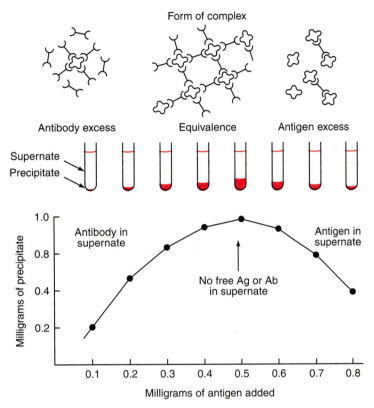

Figure 4–7. The quantitative precipitin reaction. If increasing amounts of antigen are added in separate tubes to constant amounts of antiserum, the amount of precipitate increases to a maximum point and then decreases. This phenomenon results from the nature of the precipitate: a large network in which multivalent antigen and antibody form a lattice structure that becomes insoluble. When either antibody or antigen is in excess, the amount of crosslinking is insufficient to form an insoluble lattice. The concentration ratio yielding maximum precipitation defines the "equivalence point." Determination of the equivalence point by this type of titration can be used to measure antibody if antigen concentration is known or antigen if the antibody concentration is known.

IMMUNO-DIFFUSION

Several laboratory techniques are based on the fact that precipitin reactions can occur in aqueous gels like agar, which can support a concentration gradient because convection is prevented. In a simple **radial diffusion** assay (Fig. 4–8), antibody is incorporated into a flat gel matrix at a uniform concentration. Cylindrical holes, or wells, are cut in the gel. Then a solution of antigen, whose concentration is to be determined, is pipetted into one well, while a series of known concentrations of antigen is distributed into the other wells. A diffusion gradient of antigen concentration forms around each well, and a precipitin

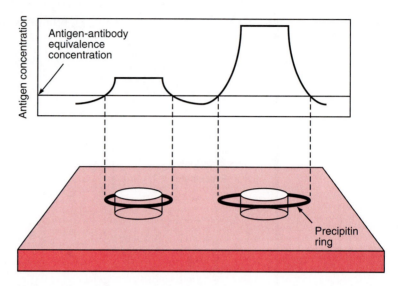

Figure 4–8. A simple method for quantitation using the principle of the equivalence point between antibody and antigen is the radial diffusion assay. Antibody (at a known constant concentration in the agar gel) confronts antigen, which is added to the wells cut into the agar. Forming at the equivalence point, the precipitin ring will be larger for higher antigen concentrations.

ring forms at a position where the diffusing antigen and the constant concentration of antibody reach the equivalence point. This will occur far from a well containing abundant antigen, producing a large ring, while a smaller ring will form around a well containing less antigen. The concentration of the unknown can be determined from the diameter of the precipitin ring it produces, based on the diameters of the rings formed by the standards. The assay can be reversed to measure antibody concentration against a standard of antibody dilutions in a gel containing a constant concentration of antigen.

An elegant variation of the radial diffusion assay is the **double diffusion** or **Ouchterlony** technique. Antigen and antibody solutions are placed separately in two nearby wells cut in a gel. As both molecules diffuse out from the wells, they form a precipitin line at a position reflecting the equivalence point. If one well containing an antiserum is placed near two wells containing two antigen preparations (Fig. 4–9), the pattern of precipitin lines can indicate whether more than one different antigen, or epitopes on the same antigen, are recognized by the antiserum.

IMMUNO-ELECTRO-PHORESIS

If an antiserum recognizes many different antigens, precipitin lines in Ouchterlony plates may be too complex to be interpreted. In that case, **immunoelectrophoresis** may be useful (Fig. 4–10). In this method,

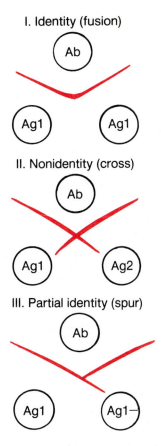

I. Identity (fusion)

II. Nonidentity (cross)

III. Partial identity (spur)

Figure 4–9. If two identical antigen solutions (Ag1) are placed in adjacent wells and an apropriate antiserum (Ab) is placed in an equidistant well, two precipitin lines will form, which will fuse (reaction of identity). If different antigens (Ag1 and Ag2) are placed in adjacent wells and an antiserum containing antibodies to both antigens is placed in the equidistant well, the two precipitin lines cross since the two antigen-antibody precipitations occur independently (reaction of non-identity). If an antigen with multiple epitopes is placed in one well (Ag1) and a related antigen sharing some but not all epitopes is placed in the second well (Ag1⁻), the antibodies directed against the shared epitopes will form a fused precipitin pattern; but antibodies against epitopes of Ag1 missing in Ag1⁻ will not interact with that molecule and will form a "spur," extending the precipitin line between Ab and Ag1.

the antigen mixture, typically serum proteins, is placed in a well and subjected to a voltage gradient which partially separates the proteins from one another electrophoretically. Antiserum is then placed in a linear well parallel to the row of separated antigens and allowed to diffuse towards the antigens, creating curved precipitin lines that allow visualization of many different antigens.

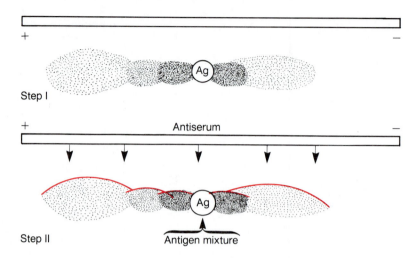

Figure 4–10. To visualize the precipitin lines formed between multiple protein antigens and a mixture of antibodies, the antigens are placed in a well cut into an agar gel (Ag) and subjected to a voltage gradient, which causes the proteins to move by electrophoresis (Step 1); the final position of each protein (shaded areas) depends on its charge and size. After electrophoresis, the antibody mixture is placed in a linear well and allowed to diffuse towards the separated protein antigens (Step II). An arc-shaped precipitin line is formed at the equivalence point between each antibody-antigen combination.

AGGLUTI-NATION

Antibodies may be detected by **hemagglutination** when present in concentrations too low to form a visible precipitate. This method depends on the formation of a link between two red blood cells (or bacteria or antigen-coated latex particles) by a single divalent antibody recognizing an antigen on the surface of the particles (Fig. 4–11). The complexed particles form a diffuse mat, coating the round-bottomed well of a microtiter plate, whereas in the absence of agglutinating antibody, the free particles roll to the bottom in a tight pile. The highest antibody dilution showing agglutination can be used as a measure of antibody concentration. Soluble antigen can inhibit agglutination by competing for antibody molecules, providing a sensitive assay for soluble antigen.

COMPLEMENT FIXATION

Antibodies that fix complement can be detected by the consumption of complement activity. In such a **complement fixation assay**, a test antiserum is mixed with antigen, and then a small amount of complement is added. After incubation to allow for immune complexes to consume complement, red blood cells (RBC) and an anti-RBC anti-

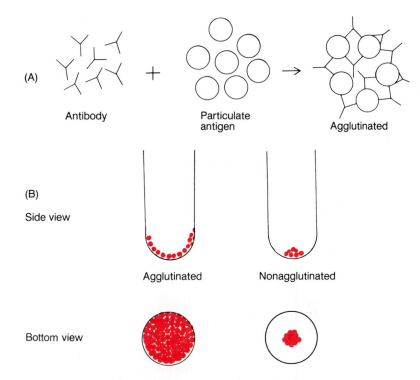

Figure 4–11. Agglutination of particulate antigens. *(A)* Divalent antibody forms a lattice with multivalent particulate antigen. *(B)* Agglutinated particles settle to the bottom of a round-bottomed tube in a diffuse mat, whereas nonagglutinated particles roll down the sides of the container to form a tight heap at the bottom. The difference between these outcomes is easily apparent in a view from below.

body are added. The amounts of reagents are adjusted so that the complement added should be just enough to lyse the RBCs; then the persistence of intact RBCs can be used as a measure of complement consumed by the initial antigen–antibody reaction. Some antisera may contain preexisting complement-consuming immune complexes, and some sera or antigen preparations contain complement inhibitors; these possibilities require careful controls for complement fixation assays (see Chapter 8).

RADIO-IMMUNOASSAY

The detection of binding between antigen and antibody has in recent years benefitted from a variety of technologies that allow one or the other reactant to be bound to solid supports or to be tagged with dyes, enzymes, or radioactive markers. A diverse repertoire of assay techniques has resulted.

In the **radioimmunoassay (RIA)**, antibodies have been used to assay for the presence of a specific antigen. A standard amount of radioactively labeled antigen is incubated with an antigen-specific antibody in amounts that bind to about 60% to 70% of the antibody. The antibody is removed from solution by ammonium sulfate precipitation or adsorption to a solid support, taking with it any bound radioactive antigen, which can be measured by measuring the radioactivity. If unlabeled antigen is added in the initial incubation, some radioactive antigen will be displaced from the antibody. By measuring the displacement caused by standard amounts of unlabeled antigen, a standard curve can be prepared that allows one to deduce the amount of antigen in an unknown sample by the amount of radioactivity it displaces.

IMMUNO-LABELING

Antibodies can be tagged with fluorescent dyes or enzymes using chemical techniques that leave the antigen-binding function intact. With antibodies specific for cell components or surface markers, *tagged* antibodies can be used to stain tissue sections or live cells. An indirect staining strategy relieves investigators of the necessity to individually tag multiple antibodies: nontagged murine monoclonal antibodies against various cell components can be reacted with tissue sections, and then the location of bound antibodies determined by staining with a single fluorescently tagged xenogeneic antibody directed against murine immunoglobulin. In these techniques, it is important to control for natural fluorescence of the cells and for nonspecific binding of the fluorescence-tagged antibody. One variation of fluorescent antibody staining with clinical importance is a test used to detect antibodies against *Treponema pallidum*, the infectious agent of syphilis. A patient's serum is incubated with a slide on which *T. pallidum* bacteria have been fixed and the slide is treated with fluorescence tagged antihuman antibody; the presence of fluorescently stained bacteria indicates that the patient was exposed to this agent.

Fluorescent antibody tagging has been extensively exploited in a technique widely used in immunology to characterize different cell populations in the immune system by the surface markers exposed on their cell membranes. In **flow cytometry**, a population of cells is stained with a fluorescent antibody against a specific membrane antigen. The solution with suspended cells is then passed in a thin stream through a laser fluorometer that measures the fluorescence of each cell as it passes the detector, and stores the information on a computer. Antibodies with different colored fluorescent dyes can be used to stain simultaneously for more than one antigen. In a powerful preparative variation of this technique known as **fluorescence-activated cell sorting (FACS)**, cells with particular staining characteristics can be sorted into separate tubes; this is done by converting the stream into droplets containing single cells, giving each droplet a measured charge according to its staining characteristics, and then deflecting the charged droplets into the appropriate tube by a controlled electric field (Fig. 4–12).

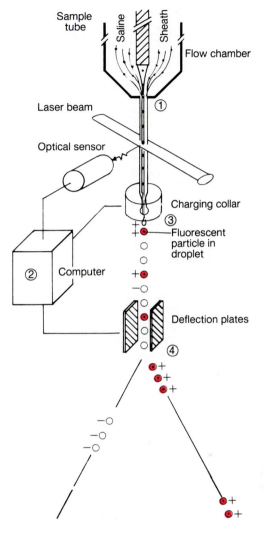

Figure 4–12. Fluorescence activated cell sorting. *(1)* Fluorescently stained cells are forced out of a small nozzle forming a stream in which they pass through a laser beam one cell at a time. *(2)* An optical sensor linked to a computer detects fluorescent characteristics and classifies each cell according to conditions set by the investigator. *(3)* As the stream forms droplets—containing no more than one cell—the computer imparts a positive, negative, or zero charge to each droplet based on the fluorescence class of the cell in the droplet. *(4)* The charged droplets pass between charged plates, which deflect the droplets into appropriate collection tubes.

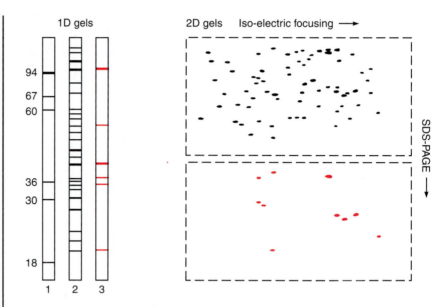

Figure 4–13. Immunodetection of proteins on 1D and 2D gels. The left panel shows three lanes from a "Western blot." The first 2 lanes show protein bands as detected by a non-specific protein stain. Lane 3 shows the result of transferring the same set of proteins in lane 2 onto a filter, and then immunostaining with a labelled antibody; a subset of the total proteins are detected (red bands). The right panel shows a similar comparison between proteins detected by non-specific protein stain after 2D gel electrophoresis (upper panel) and the subset detected after blotting and immunostaining (red spots in lower panel).

An alternative to fluorescence, antibodies can be labeled with enzymes, whose catalytic activity can be used to amplify the signal of an antigen–antibody complex by causing the deposition of an insoluble product or the release of a colored or fluorescent product. Such labeled antibodies can be used to stain tissue sections (**immunohisto-chemistry**) or proteins that have been separated by electrophoresis and then blotted onto a membrane support (**Western blotting**, Fig. 4–13). One of the most versatile and widely used techniques involving enzyme tagging is the **enzyme-linked immunoabsorbance assay (ELISA)**. In a simple ELISA method for assaying antigen, varying amounts of the antigen—a standard curve and unknowns to be assayed—are adsorbed to the wells of a 96-well plastic microtiter plate; after "blocking" nonspecific protein absorption by treatment with a protein mixture and washing steps, an enzyme-linked antibody is pipetted into the wells and allowed to react with the antigen. Unbound antibody is then washed out and a chromogenic substrate of the enzyme is pipetted into the wells. The amount of colored dye

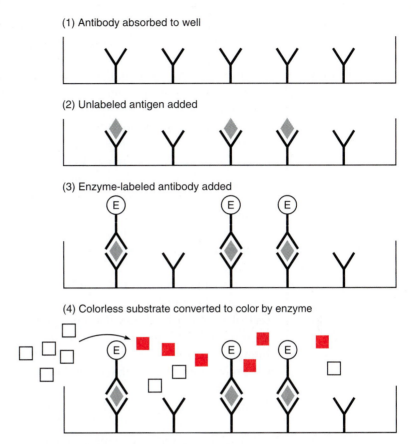

(1) Antibody absorbed to well

(2) Unlabeled antigen added

(3) Enzyme-labeled antibody added

(4) Colorless substrate converted to color by enzyme

Figure 4–14. This figure illustrates a variation of ELISA technology often referred to as a "sandwich" assay because the antigen is detected sandwiched between two antibody molecules–an unlabeled molecule bound to the plate and an enzyme-linked antibody. After the wells of a microtiter plate are coated with a constant amount of antibody and then "blocked" by non-specific protein absorption, varying known amounts of antigen are added to different wells and allowed to bind to antibody on the plate. An enzyme-linked antibody against the antigen is then added in excess, and unbound antibody removed by washing. Finally a solution containing chromagenic substrate is added, and the rate of color production is measured in an automated plate reader; fluorogenic substrates may also be used with fluorescence detecting plate readers.

released by the bound enzyme can then be determined by an automated plate reader and used to measure antigen based on the standard curve of known antigen concentrations. Numerous variations of this technique have been devised to take advantage of the convenience of a solid support that can be used to process multiple samples in automated machines.(eg, see Fig. 4–14).

ANTIBODY-AFFINITY CHROMATOGRAPHY

Many of the methods discussed above require purified antibody for their operation. An antibody may be purified by column chromatography through a support on which antigen is displayed. The antigen-specific antibody is bound tightly while contaminating proteins are washed away; then the antibody can be released by altering the salt concentration or pH. Conversely, columns made with purified antibodies bound to a solid support have been widely used to purify the corresponding antigen. Recent genetic technologies have made it easier to clone genes than it is to purify low-abundance proteins. In many cases it has been possible to generate antisera reactive against a protein whose structure is known only from its gene; such antisera can be obtained by immunizing with peptides synthesized according to the amino acid translation of the cloned gene. C-terminal peptides are frequently useful for this strategy.

Cell Membrane Immunoglobulin

As briefly mentioned before, the structure of antibody expressed on the surface membrane of a B lymphocyte differs on the C terminus from that of secreted antibody. The membrane form is longer, including a 25 amino acid lipophilic transmembrane segment that anchors the immunoglobulin to the membrane lipids, and several additional C-terminal amino acids that extend into the cytoplasm of the cell forming a cytoplasmic "tail." The cytoplasmic tail varies in length between 3 amino acids (μ and δ) and 28 amino acids (ϵ and γ).

ANTIGEN PRESENTATION BY B CELLS

The membrane form of immunoglobulin plays a critical role in B-cell function—signaling the detection of antigen and thereby triggering proliferation and maturation of the B cell to the secretory stage. Two general mechanisms for this triggering have been suggested. In the **T-cell-dependent** mechanism, the binding of a protein antigen to membrane antibody facilitates ingestion of the antigen by the B lymphocyte. The B lymphocyte then acts as an **antigen-presenting cell**, degrading the ingested antigen and displaying some of the resulting peptides on its surface in the binding groove of the specialized peptide-display proteins known as **class II MHC proteins**. The displayed peptides are recognized by T cells, which then become activated and in consequence return activation signals—collectively known as **T-cell help**—to the B cell, triggering proliferation and antibody secretion. Antigen presentation and T-cell activation are discussed in more detail in Chapters 5 and 7. The unique property of B cells as antigen presenting cells (APCs) is that they can efficiently present an antigen at more than 1000-fold lower concentrations than other APCs, as long as the antigen is specifically recognized by membrane immunoglobulin. The mediators of B-cell help include T-cell-derived lymphokines such as IL-2, IL-4, IL-5, and IL-10, as well as signals generated by B-cell–T cell-contact (see Chapter 7). One example of a contact signal that mediates B-cell activation is the interaction between the B-cell protein CD40 and its ligand on the T cell; this signal is required for isotype switching, as discussed later in this chapter.

SIGNAL TRANSDUCTION MEDIATED THROUGH MEMBRANE IMMUNO-GLOBULIN

In addition to the T-cell-dependent mechanism, there is clear evidence that antigen-recognition by B cells can lead to activation signals independent of T cells. Signal transduction mechanisms triggered by various receptor–ligand interactions in nonlymphoid cells are known to depend on enzymatic reactions carried out by cytoplasmic domains of receptor proteins, and it initially seemed puzzling that the cytoplasmic tails of membrane immunoglobulin were too small to support such reactions. This suggested that membrane immunoglobulin might be associated with other components mediating signal transduction. Recent work has indeed identified such components, a disulfide-linked heterodimer known as Igα-Igβ, products of the mb-1 and B29 genes, respectively. Igα and Igβ each have a single extracellular immunoglobulin domain, a transmembrane segment and a cytoplasmic domain large enough to mediate enzymatic reactions typical of signal transducers. The heterodimer binds noncovalently to membrane immunoglobulin and is required for the appearance of immunoglobulin on the cell surface. The mb-1 and B29 genes encode proteins of 21–23 kD predicted molecular weight; but both proteins are heavily glycosylated, leading to molecular weights of about 47 kD (Igα) and 37 kD (Igβ) for the complex associated with human IgM (differing glycosylation and resulting molecular weights of the subunits are found associated with different heavy chain isotypes). A hypothetical model for the B-cell antigen receptor of IgM class is shown in Figure 4–15. The mechanism by which the antigen-binding signal is transduced to activate B cells is an area of active investigation. It is known that the cytoplasmic domains of Igα and Igβ become rapidly phosphorylated on tyrosine residues after membrane immunoglobulin is engaged and cross-linked. At least one member of the *src*-like tyrosine kinase family appear to be involved. Phospholipase C activation leads to the appearance of second messengers inositol triphosphate (IP_3) and diacylglycerol, which induce a rise in intracellular Ca^{++} concentration. The complete signaling pathway leading to proliferation and secretion remains to be elucidated.

Immunoglobulin Genes

Many of the questions raised in the preceding sections concerning the genes encoding immunoglobulins required the techniques of recombinant DNA analysis for their elucidation. These techniques allow specific genes to be isolated ("cloned") and the sequence of nucleotides encoding the genes to be determined. By cloning multiple overlapping segments of DNA, large stretches of the genome can be examined and the sequence of genes on the chromosome determined.

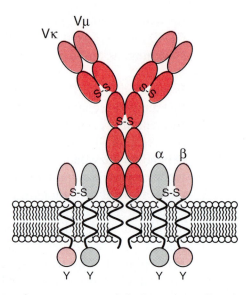

Figure 4–15. Membrane immunoglobulin on B cells. The B cell antigen receptor is composed of an immunoglobulin molecule (L_2H_2) associated with a disulfide linked heterodimer of two smaller proteins known as Igα and Igβ. These proteins each have an extracellular portion composed of a single immunoglobulin-like domain and a cytoplasmic domain containing a phosphorylatable tyrosine residue (Y in the figure).

GENERATION OF DIVERSITY

The most profound puzzle of immunoglobulin gene structure was to understand the generation of the vast diversity of antigen binding specificities, which, as discussed above, was found to lie in the diversity of N-terminal V regions of light and heavy chains. The explanation for this diversity lies in genetic mechanisms unique to the immune system. These mechanisms were discovered when the genes encoding myeloma proteins were compared to the corresponding DNA in germline DNA. In brief, it was found that nucleotide sequences encoding variable regions of immunoglobulins are not present in the germline DNA as contiguous segments as they are in myelomas but must be assembled during the development of each individual B lymphocyte. Each lymphocyte assembles one functional heavy-chain gene and one functional light-chain gene; and variability in the way these genes can be assembled means that the two functional immunoglobulin V genes in a B lymphocyte are almost never assembled in exactly the same way in another lymphocyte. Therefore, the collective pool of circulating lymphocytes develops a repertoire of antibody sequences so huge that when antigen is administered, there will be available some B cells with a membrane antibody capable of binding to that antigen. These antigen-binding B cells are triggered to proliferate and mature into secreting plasma cells, as discussed above, leading to the synthesis of antigen-specific antibodies. An additional process accounts for affinity maturation (the progressive increase in average affinity of antibodies observed during the course of an immune response). A unique somatic mutation mechanism recognizes the functional immunoglobulin V region genes in antigen-activated B lymphocytes and somehow targets these DNA segments for random mutations. Although most mutations in antibody structure probably impair antigen binding or leave it unchanged, rare mutations that increase binding affinity are selected by their improved capacity to bind antigen and thereby receive the antigen-dependent signal for proliferation and secretion. Successive rounds of mutation and selection lead to the progressive increases in antibody affinity observed. The processes of gene assembly and somatic mutation will now be examined in more detail.

V-GENE ASSEMBLY

The human genome contains three independent immunoglobulin gene loci capable of assembling functional immunoglobulin genes: The κ locus on chromosome 2, the λ locus on chromosome 22 and the heavy chain locus on chromosome 14. In the development of a B-lymphocyte, heavy chain gene assembly occurs first, followed by light-chain assembly. However, because the light-chain genes are simpler, they will be considered first.

κ locus

The V regions of functional κ light-chain genes isolated from human B cells or B-cell lymphoid malignancies encode about 108 amino acids in a contiguous DNA segment. In the DNA lying 5′ of the gene—corresponding to the N-terminal direction—additional codons specify the sequence of a "signal peptide." Signal peptides, found in all nascent proteins destined for secretion or membrane expression, are typically the first amino acid residues to be translated by the ribosome and serve as tags to attach the ribosome to the endoplasmic reticulum. As the ribosome continues the translation process, the signal peptide is cleaved by a peptidase and the remainder of the protein is formed inside the endoplasmic reticulum, en route to ultimate secretion or membrane expression. In immunoglobulin genes, the DNA encoding the signal peptide is generally interrupted by an intron within codon -4, that is, the fourth codon counting backwards from the N-terminal amino acid of the mature secreted protein. (Introns are nontranslated sequences that interrupt the coding sequences of a gene; they appear in the primary RNA transcript, but are removed by RNA "splicing" before the RNA is translated into protein.) If the V gene from a B cell is compared to the corresponding DNA in a nonlymphoid cell (loosely described as "germline" DNA), it is found that the germline V gene lacks the C-terminal 13 or so codons found in the assembled V region gene cloned from lymphocytes. These 13 residues have become known as J-region residues since they "join" the V region to the C region. The

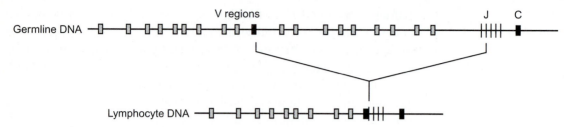

Figure 4–16. V-J rearrangements. In non-lymphoid ("germline") DNA, there are no functional, complete immunoglobulin genes. The two segments that can form a complete κ gene lie in two clusters: the V gene segments and the much smaller cluster of J region segments. A complete functional κ gene is expressed in a lymphocyte after one of the V segments (shown in black in the figure) recombines with one of the J regions.

J-region amino acids in the human κ locus are encoded in five Jκ-region gene segments which lie 5′ of the single Cκ region gene. A particular B cell assembles an intact Vκ gene by a DNA rearrangement that joins one of the Jκ region gene segments to one of approximately 80 germline Vκ sequences which lie 5′ of the J-C cluster (Fig. 4–16). A germline complement of 80 Vκ sequences and five J-gene segments could theoretically lead to 4000 different Vκ-Jκ pairings. However, the number of potentially functional VκJκ genes is different from the number of theoretical Vκ-Jκ pairs for two reasons. First, of the 80 Vκ sequences only about 50 are functional; the remainder are "pseudogenes," that is, these sequences contain mutations that introduce termination codons or other alterations that would preclude their translation to functional κ light-chain proteins. On the other hand, a particular pair of functional Vκ-Jκ gene segments can actually give rise to several different κ light-chain sequences. This is because the DNA recombination mechanism that joins these two segments by deleting the intervening DNA is somewhat imprecise, so the position of the crossover between V and J is somewhat flexible (Fig. 4–17). This flexibility causes additional diversity at the Vκ-Jκ junction. This extra diversity is functionally important for antigen binding since the VκJκ junction forms part of CDR3 generally at, or at least near, the antigen-binding site. After the assembly of a complete κ variable-region gene, the entire κ gene is transcribed into RNA, and the two introns—one within the signal peptide coding region and the other between J and C—are spliced out before the RNA is translated.

DNA Signals for V-gene Assembly

A single common DNA recombination mechanism is thought to assemble V genes of κ, λ, and heavy-chain loci, as well as those of the four T-cell-receptor gene loci (see Chapter 6). Although little is known about the enzymatic mechanism of the recombination, sequences in the

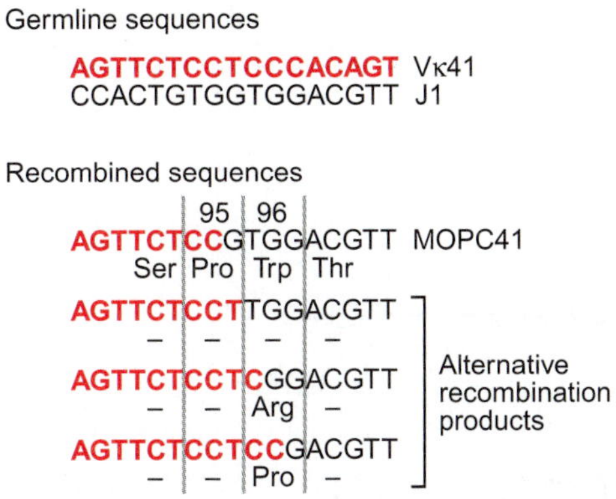

Germline sequences

AGTTCTCCTCCCACAGT Vκ41
CCACTGTGGTGGACGTT J1

Recombined sequences

```
                   95 | 96
      AGTTCTCCGTGGACGTT  MOPC41
      Ser|Pro|Trp|Thr

      AGTTCTCCTTGGACGTT  ⎤
       – | – | – | –      |
                          |
      AGTTCTCCTCGGACGTT    ⎬ Alternative
       – | – |Arg| –      |  recombination
                          |  products
      AGTTCTCCTCCGACGTT  ⎦
       – | – |Pro| –
```

Figure 4–17. Junctional diversity in V gene assembly. The figure shows the DNA sequence of two germline murine κ elements in the region involved in recombination during V gene assembly: the germline Vκ41 segment (highlighted in color) and Jκ1. The next four lines show possible recombination junctions. The first, which was found in the myeloma MOPC41, includes Vκ41 sequence up to the second nucleotide of codon 95 and then switches to Jκ1 sequence. The next shows the consequences of a recombination junction one nucleotide further downstream; the G→T change in the last nucleotide of codon 95 does not change any encoded amino acids. The last two lines, illustrating two other possible recombination products, are associated with amino acid changes that have been observed in actual murine κ chains. The examples shown maintain the triplet reading frame between V and J, which is required for a functional gene but occurs in only about one third of recombination events.

DNA that serve as signals to target the recombination machinery (recombination signal sequences [RSS]) have been identified. These are composed of a 7-mer and a 9-mer sequence (Fig. 4–18) that are separated by a spacer of about 12 bp or about 23 bp of DNA. Recombination occurs between one DNA segment flanked by a RSS with a 12 bp spacer and another with a 23 bp spacer (12 + 23 rule). For example, in the κ system the signal sequences flanking the V region genes have 12 bp spacers, whereas those 5′ of the J-region segments have 23 bp spacers. The conserved 7-mer and 9-mer sequences appear to be targets for the binding of specific protein components of the recombination machinery; although several such proteins have been identified, their precise roles in the recombination machinery remain obscure at present. The expression of two *recombination activating genes* (RAG-1 and RAG-2) is required for V assembly recombination to occur. The function of the encoded proteins has not been definitively determined, but current evidence indicates that they represent components of the recombinase machinery. Mice engineered to lack func-

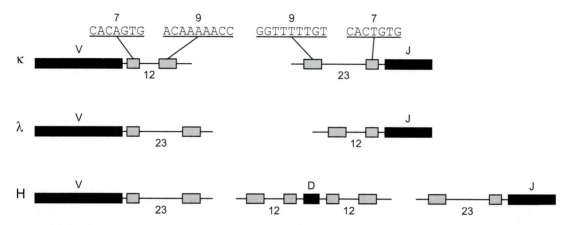

Figure 4–18. Recombination signal sequences (RSSs). The conserved 7-mer and 9-mer sequences that target V assembly recombination are shown flanking the elements involved in these rearrangements. The V, J, and D coding regions are depicted as black rectangles. The spacing between the 7-mer and 9-mer is either about 12 bp or about 23 bp as indicated. Recombination occurs almost exclusively between pairs of elements with different RSS spacing.

tional copies of either RAG-1 or RAG-2 lack B- and T-lymphocytes because they cannot assemble any immunoglobulin or T-cell receptor V genes. According to current working model for the mechanism of recombination, the initial step is a DNA cleavage that occurs exactly at the end of the 7-mer sequence near the V and J segments; this produces two "7-mer signal ends" and two "coding ends" (V and J). The two resulting 7-mer ends are thought to become joined directly, since "signal joints" containing directly apposed 7-mers from V and J can be recovered from B-cells in the process of V assembly recombinations. Before the coding ends are joined, a variable amount of exonuclease nibbling of the DNA ends occurs, accounting for the variable number of V and J nucleotides that ultimately appear in the assembled VJ coding joint (the "flexibility" of VJ assembly). One consequence of the variable trimming of coding ends is that in most VJ recombinations the reading frame of the V region is not maintained through the J region; this leads to a recombination product that is non-functional because it does not encode a Cκ region. On average an in-frame joint would be expected to be generated in about one third of VJ recombinations, approximately what has been observed.

λ locus

The assembly of a human Vλ gene occurs between V and J gene segments similar to those of the κ system. However, the germline organization of the λ constant region locus is significantly different from that of the κ locus. There are four nonallelic functional Cλ genes, whose

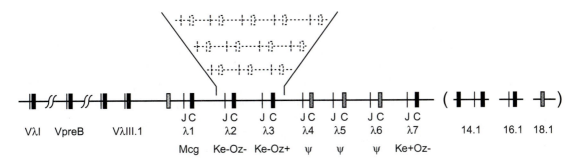

Figure 4–19. Structure of the human λ light chain gene locus. Four of the seven Jλ-Cλ regions in the most frequent haplotype are functional (black rectangles), while three (regions 4, 5, and 6) are pseudogenes (grey retangles) in almost all individuals. Variant loci containing extra duplications between the second and third λ genes are indicated by dashed lines. Flanking regions containing λ-related sequences are shown.

protein products were identified by specific antibodies long before the genes were cloned. These are known by their serological designations Kern⁻Oz⁻, Kern⁻Oz⁺, Kern⁺Oz⁻, and Mcg. The amino acid sequences of these four constant regions differ from each other in only 5 positions. In the human Cλ locus, the genes for these four forms are present in a cluster that also contains three pseudogenes. Each Cλ sequence is associated with a single Jλ gene segment located 5′ to the C sequence. Further upstream in the λ locus lie the V sequences, which are less well characterized than those of the κ system. The overall organization of the locus is shown in Figure 4–19. The λ genes also differ from κ in having the opposite distribution of RSS spacer lengths; that is, Vλ genes are flanked by signal sequences with 23 bp spacers, while those upstream of Jλ have 12 bp spacers (see Fig. 4–18).

Expression of the heavy-chain locus is more complex than κ or λ owing to (1) additional mechanisms for diversity generation in V-H gene assembly, (2) alternative RNA splicing pathways accounting for production of a membrane-bound versus secreted protein from the same gene; and (3) the heavy chain isotype switch. The additional complexity of VH-gene assembly is revealed by comparing the sequence of an assembled gene (isolated from a B cell or myeloma) to that of its germline precursors. Between the DNA derived from a germline VH-region gene and that derived from a JH-region gene segment, one typically finds a variable length of sequence derived from neither. Part of this DNA derives from an additional germline element known as the D ("diversity") segment. In human germline DNA, the heavy-chain locus has about 30 D-region genes located between six JH regions and about 120 V regions. These D elements contain coding sequences of between 11 and 31 bp in length which are flanked by 7-mer and 9-mer signal sequences generally having 12 bp spacers (complementing 23 bp spacing of RSSs associated with both VH and JH regions). In the course of B-cell development, an initial recombination event joins one D region to one of the JH regions. A second V-assembly recombination then joins a VH region to the already assembled DJH segment.

As in the case of light-chain genes, considerable diversity can occur even within V regions assembled from a particular set of germline elements (that is, a particular V, D, and J segment) because of variations at the VD and DJ junctions. The exonuclease trimming of coding ends in the heavy-chain locus is apparently considerably more extensive than that in light-chain genes. Furthermore, assembled heavy-chain V-region genes have variable numbers of "extra" bases between V and D and between D and J. Most of these extra bases, known as "N" regions, appear not to be specified by any germline DNA sequence but instead are added to coding ends of DNA by the enzyme terminal deoxynucleotide transferase (or a similar enzymatic activity) without a template. For a productive VDJ recombination, the V and J region must be in the same reading frame, but the D-region sequence can be read in all three reading frames. Thus, several mechanisms contribute to enormous heavy-chain CDR3 diversity of expressed antibodies: the combinatorial joining of three separate classes of sequence elements (V, D, and J); the extensive variation in trimming of these elements before joining; the three reading frames of the D regions; and the addition of untemplated "N" nucleotides.

Membrane and Secreted Immunoglobulin

The mechanism by which a single heavy chain gene can encode either the membrane or secreted form of immunoglobulin has been explained through the analysis of the C genes and their expressed transcripts. A typical example is the $C\mu$ gene, which lies about 3 kb (kilo base pairs) downstream of the human JH regions. Each of the four domains of internal sequence similarity observed at the amino acid sequence level of $C\mu$ is encoded in a separate exon. The exon encoding the fourth constant domain, CH4, includes the C-terminal codons of the μ-heavy chain form found in secreted antibody. The alternative C-terminal amino acid residues of μ chain expressed on the membrane of B lymphocytes are encoded in two "membrane exons" lying downstream of CH4 (Fig. 4–20). Investigations of RNA transcripts of the μ gene have demonstrated that the primary transcription product of the μ gene can be spliced to encode the last residues of CH4 characteristic of the secreted form, or may be alternatively spliced so as to exclude these residues and join the remainder of the $C\mu$ transcript to the membrane exons encoding the hydropho-

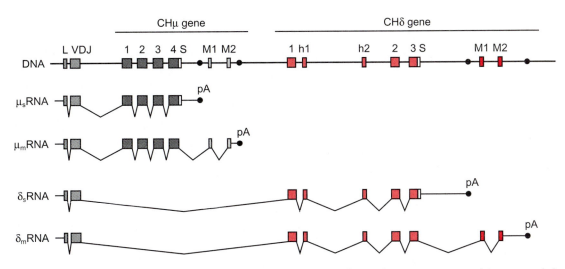

Figure 4–20. Splicing of heavy chain exons in formation of membrane vs secreted immunoglobulin and μ vs δ heavy chain. The exons of a rearranged heavy chain gene are shown, including both μ and δ loci. Sequences that are spliced out at the RNA level are shown as V shaped lines. In the case of μ heavy chain, all mature mRNAs show removal of the intron separating most of the signal peptide sequence from the V region, the JH-Cμ intron, and the three intra-Cμ domain introns. In μs mRNA the transcript includes the last two codons of the secreted heavy chain and terminates at a poly(A) addition site (black dot) close downstream.

bic transmembrane region and cytoplasmic tail characteristic of surface IgM. Analogous splice patterns account for the membrane and secreted forms of the other isotype-heavy chains.

Isotype Switching

The isotype initially expressed in the development of all B lymphocytes is IgM. Most B cells also express surface IgD along with IgM. The simultaneous expression of μ and δ heavy chains appears to result from a long RNA transcript that begins at VDJ, reads through Cμ and continues through the Cδ gene, which lies several kb downstream of Cμ (Fig. 4–20). Such a transcript can be alternatively spliced to yield mature transcripts including either VDJCμ (encoding the μ-heavy chain) or VDJCδ (encoding δ); both RNAs are produced in most early B cells. After a B cell is triggered for activation by an encounter with antigen, the cell may mature to express another isotype such as IgE, IgA or one of the IgG subtypes. This isotype switch is the result of a unique class of DNA rearrangements in which the C region gene of the new isotype moves to lie downstream of VDJ in the position formerly occupied by the Cμ gene. The nature of this rearrangement has been clarified by cloning of the complete set of CH regions and the compilation of a map that orients them with respect to each other. In germline DNA, the constant region genes encoding the γ, ε, and α chains are

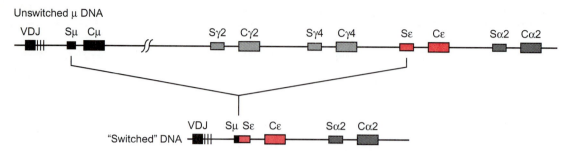

Figure 4–21. Isotype switch recombination. The human heavy chain gene locus is spread out over roughly 300 kb and includes two duplication units of γ-γ-ε-α genes, of which only the more downstream γ2-γ4-ε-α2 unit is shown here. Isotype switching involves DNA deletion events whose endpoints usually fall within the repetitive Switch (S) regions that lie 5′ of each constant region. In the isotype switch deletion illustrated here a composite Sμ-Sε region is formed by the recombination; as a consequence, the Cε gene is moved downstream of VDJ to the position formerly occupied by Cμ. The resulting DNA is a template for transcription of VDJ-Cε mRNA that encodes the ε heavy chain.

arrayed downstream of Cμ and Cδ as shown in Figure 4–21. Thus, in the example illustrated in this figure, the isotype switch to ε is associated with a DNA deletion that removes all the C regions from Cμ through Cγ4, leaving VDJ near the Cε gene. The recombination junctions typically occur within internally repetitive segments of DNA known as "switch regions," which lie on the 5′ side of all the constant region genes (except Cδ, which is rarely involved in a switch rearrangement). In the example of μ to ε switching, the 5′ part of the μ switch region (Sμ) becomes joined to the 3′ part of Sε, forming a composite Sμ-Sε switch region. The exact position of the switch is irrelevant to the final structure of the expressed protein since the recombination occurs within intron sequence that is spliced out of the RNA transcript before it is translated into protein.

Certain types of antigen exposure are known to promote responses dominated by specific isotypes. For example, IgE is most prominent after the exposure of respiratory mucosa to inhaled allergens and in helminth infestations, whereas the B cells of Peyer's patches in the intestinal mucosa respond predominantly with IgA. The detailed mechanism of isotype selection by specific immunogen exposure is not known, but both T cells and the cytokine milieu of the B cell appear to play important roles in the isotype switch. The role of T cells was indicated by investigations of a rare genetic immunodeficiency in which serum IgM is elevated and all other isotypes are essentially absent (hyper-IgM immunodeficiency). Incubation of B cells from affected patients with T cells from normal individuals was found to restore isotype switching by the B cells, whereas the patients' T cells were inactive. The specific B-T interaction implied by these results has been

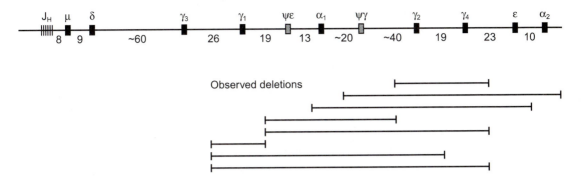

Figure 4–22. The human immunoglobulin heavy chain locus. This map shows the JH regions and the entire constant region gene locus. Black rectangles represent constant region genes for the 9 expressed isotypes; grey rectangles represent two pseudogenes in the locus. The numbers represent the approximate distances between the constant region genes in kilobases. This map order has been deduced from overlapping clones and Southern blotting of large fragments, and is confirmed by analysis of natural germline deletion mutations in humans (represented by the lines at bottom).

traced to the binding of a B-cell membrane protein known as CD40 to a T-cell membrane protein known as the CD40 ligand (CD40L); it is the gene for the latter protein that is abnormal in hyper-IgM immunodeficiency (see Chapter 27). One result of the interaction between these two proteins is B-cell proliferation, which seems to be required for isotype switching. The importance of cytokines is exemplified by the example of switching to IgE. For this switch, it is clear that IL-4 is necessary, while interferon-γ is inhibitory. Since these cytokines are characteristic of two different classes of CD4+ helper cells—Th2 and Th1, respectively (see Chapter 7)—it is apparent that selective isotype switching can depend on T cells in several different ways.

Despite the observation that specific isotypes play unique roles in specific immune responses, several human pedigrees are known with patients who are homozygous for extensive deletions in the CH locus (see Fig. 4–22). These patients generally do not present with serious clinical immunodeficiency, suggesting that there is considerable potential for functional compensation by the remaining available isotypes.

Allelic Exclusion and the Regulation of V Assembly

Most autosomal genes are expressed in roughly equal amounts from the two homologous loci on the maternal and paternal chromosomes. In contrast, each B lymphocyte expresses only a single light-chain gene and a single heavy-chain gene; the allelic light-chain and heavy-chain locus in each cell is excluded from expression ("allelic exclusion"). If both alleles were expressed, each cell might be capable of producing four different VHVL pairs, some of which might react with self-antigens; and individual H_2L_2 molecules with two different VHVL pairs might be produced. Allelic exclusion is apparently important for efficient clonal selection of immunoglobulin targeted against a specific foreign antigen and not against extraneous molecules. But how is allelic exclusion maintained?

The answer appears to lie in the tight developmental regulation of the DNA rearrangements of V-gene assembly. The initial recombination in the B lymphocyte is D-JH joining, which commonly occurs on both heavy-chain alleles before germline VH-region genes become activated for recombination and before any recombinations have occurred in the light-chain genes. When VH genes do become activated and a VDJ rearrangement first occurs in a cell, a μ heavy chain can be produced only if the VDJ recombination is "in-frame" (or "productive"), which happens in roughly one third of recombinations as discussed above. If the initial VDJ recombination is "productive," a μ-heavy chain is made, a step defining the developmental stage known as a pre-B cell. The heavy chain appears on the surface of the cell and transmits a signal that shuts off further heavy chain recombination, thus preventing expression of the allelic heavy-chain locus. (Because heavy chains apparently cannot be expressed on the cell membrane in isolation from a light chain, and at this stage no light chain gene has yet been assembled, the μ protein of the pre-B cell is expressed on the membrane with a "surrogate" light chain composed of a V-like protein and a C-like protein known as ι and ω respectively. These proteins are encoded near the λ locus and show sequence similarity to that chain.) If the initial VDJH recombination is out-of-frame ("nonproductive"), then no μ protein is made to generate a shut-off signal, so recombination can proceed on the other allelic locus. Some cells undoubtedly recombine both alleles nonproductively; these cells may be lost to the immune system as functional participants.

In addition to shutting off VDJH recombination, the production of a μ-heavy chain in the pre-B cell has a second regulatory effect: it activates the κ locus for rearrangement. A feedback mechanism similar to that described for heavy chains prevents the production of two different κ chains; in this case, the signal that shuts off further κ rearrangement is the appearance of functional IgM antibody ($H_2\kappa_2$) on the surface of the cell, an event which defines the cell as developmentally at the B-cell stage.

The λ locus is apparently not activated for recombination in human lymphocytes unless κ recombination is nonproductive on both chromosomal κ loci. The evidence for this is that B-cell leukemias and lymphomas expressing κ chains almost always have their λ-chain genes in germline (ie unrecombined) organization. Surprisingly, if B-cell malignancies expressing λ-light chain are examined, not only are their λ genes in recombined organization (as expected), but their Cκ genes are generally deleted from both allelic κ loci. This deletion represents a programmed step in B-lymphocyte maturation and occurs at specific sites in the DNA.

Exactly how the feedback mechanisms described above activate or shut off recombination at specific loci is not known in detail. According to the current model, the enzymatic machinery for each V-assembly recombination (referred to as "recombinase") is essentially identical for κ, λ, and heavy-chain genes, but the recombination reactions can occur at a particular locus only after that locus becomes "accessible" to the recombinase. Accessibility appears to be associated with gene transcription, since a cell capable of recombination at a particular immunoglobulin locus generally transcribes the germline elements that are targets for the recombination. The resulting transcripts of isolated V regions and C regions are known as germline or "sterile" transcripts, because they cannot encode a functional immunoglobulin chain. The regulation of recombinational accessibility may thus be achieved by transcriptional regulatory mechanisms, which are actively being investigated.

GENE REARRANGEMENTS IN LYMPHOMAS AND LEUKEMIAS

Because the V-assembly recombinations that occur in any one B lymphocyte are generally unique, these recombinations provide genetic markers that are clinically useful in diagnosis and management of B-cell malignancies (see Chapter 24). A V(D)J recombination can be readily detected in DNA from a clonal source by Southern blotting (Fig. 4–23). In a nonclonal population such as peripheral blood lymphocytes, rearranged immunoglobulin genes resulting from diverse recombination events produce a faint smear on a Southern blot rather than specific bands. In the context of such a smear, DNA from a clonal population constituting as few as 5% of the lymphocytes can generate discernible Southern blot bands. Thus, the intensity of a rearranged band in DNA from a blood sample or bone marrow biopsy of a leukemia patient can be used to assess the extent of clonal cells representing residual disease after treatment. An even more sensitive method for detecting clonal rearrangements is the polymerase chain reaction (PCR), which can detect an immunoglobulin rearrangement characteristic of a leukemic cell when such cells are as rare as one leukemic cell in ten thousand normal cells.

SOMATIC MUTATION

The mechanism responsible for affinity maturation of antibodies during the course of an immune response is somatic mutation plus selection. This process can lead to increases of over 100-fold in affinity for antigen. The process has been most fruitfully investigated in mice, where the availability of inbred strains—with identical complements of germline V-region genes—facilitates recognition of individual mutations. Thus, the extensive published sequence data on germline V-region genes cloned from the BALB/c mouse generally means that if the VH and VL gene sequences of any BALB/c myeloma or

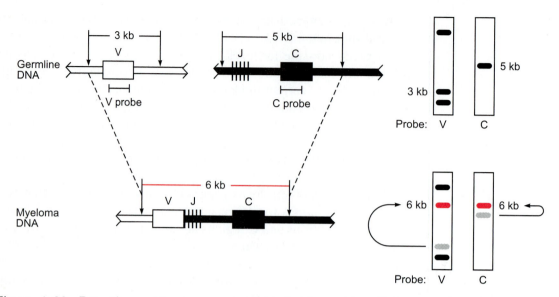

Figure 4–23. Detecting a VJ rearrangement by Southern blot. The upper figures show non-lymphoid ("germline") DNA (left) and resulting Southern blots (right); the lower figures show the corresponding features of DNA from myeloma containing a Vκ–Jκ rearrangement. When germline DNA is digested with a restriction endonuclease (having sites indicated by the arrows in the figure), and Southern blots are probed with a V and C probe, the resulting blot images will in general show bands of different sizes for V and C probes. After VJ recombination, both V and J may lie on a single restriction fragment, here illustrated as 6 kb. With appropriate choice of endonuclease, a given myeloma should always show at least one rearranged band representing the rearranged gene expressed by the myeloma. If the κ allele on the other homologous chromosome has not rearranged a germline band may be visible (grey band); alternatively, a second rearranged band may be seen, or no second band at all if the other allele has been deleted.

hybridoma protein are known, the germline V-region precursors can be identified; therefore, any V-region sequence differences between the expressed gene and its germline precursor can be attributed to somatic mutation. (By contrast, the potential for genetic polymorphisms of germline V genes in humans complicates the identification of somatic mutations.)

The time course of somatic mutation during an immune response has been studied by immunizing mice and analyzing the V-region sequences of hybridomas made at various times after immunization. In the first week after immunization, antigen-specific antibodies are generally not mutated. After this time, mutations begin to appear and increase over the next week or so. Late booster immunizations can induce additional mutations. The mutations are clustered around the rearranged V_HDJ_H or V_LJ_L gene, but extend beyond these coding sequences into flanking DNA in both 5′ and 3′ directions; the homologous sequences on the other chromosome remain essentially not mutated. Apparently a specific "hypermutation" mechanism is able to recognize an assembled immunoglobulin V region as a target for mutation. The mutations are not specifically targeted to CDRs to create higher affinity antibodies, but occur in FR codons as well as CDRs and indeed in intron and flanking regions as mentioned above. In accordance with the evolution-like model discussed earlier in this chapter, mutated V regions may encode an antibody with an affinity for antigen that is higher, lower, or unchanged in comparison to the non-mutated antibody. However, cells making high-affinity antibody have a proliferative advantage as antigen concentration falls, since they are better able to receive antigen-dependent activation signals than are lower affinity cells which bind antigen less efficiently. This proliferative advantage—which acts like evolutionary selection pressure—has been demonstrated by experiments in which antigen concentration was maintained at a high level by repeated injections; this protocol abolished the development of affinity maturation, as would be expected from the reduced selection pressure for efficient antigen binding.

The anatomic location of B cells undergoing somatic mutation has been identified as the germinal center by experiments in which PCR was used to clone immunoglobulin genes from selected regions of thin sections of lymphoid tissue. Each germinal center is apparently colonized by very few B cells before the onset of somatic mutation, since the cells in a particular germinal center appear to be clonal progeny derived from very few founder cells. In several cases it has been possible to analyze multiple mutated sequences from a single germinal center and to derive a genealogic tree which traces how early mutations were retained in later progeny sequences that have additional mutations. Some evidence suggests that the germinal center B cells undergoing somatic mutation represent a separate B-cell lineage, different from the population that responds in the first few days after antigen administration. The population susceptible to mutation appears to require T-cell help to initiate the hypermutation process; the antibody response to T-cell independent antigens like polysaccharides does not show affinity maturation.

The combination of the diversity resulting from joining of multiple gene elements (VL, JL, VH, D, and JH) plus the amplification of that diversity by somatic mutation together provide powerful and flexible mechanisms capable of creating antigen-combining sites of extremely high affinity, exquisitely tailored to the specific foreign antigen under immunologic attack.

Biotechnology Applications of Antibody Genes

The recognition that immunity to a disease could be conferred by administration of serum fractions to experimental animals (**passive immunity**) led to numerous applications in clinical medicine, including the use of animal antibodies (now largely abandoned because of the risks of serum sickness), immunoglobulin-containing human serum fractions (**gamma globulins**) from normal donors and immunoglobulins from humans known to have recovered from a specific disease (see Chapter 26). More recently monoclonal antibodies have been proposed for the diagnosis and treatment of cancer. In diagnostic applications, antibodies against tumor antigens have been tagged with radioactive elements and administered to patients so that cancers, including metastases, can be visualized by nuclear medicine imaging. Therapeutic approaches involve both antibodies tagged with radioactivity to provide localized radiotherapy and antibodies tagged with various toxins (see Chapter 30).

The antibodies that have been used to target these poisons specifically to tumor cells have frequently been murine monoclonal antibodies, since in comparison with human hybridomas, murine hybridomas are easier to make, more productive of antibody, and more stable. Some murine antibodies have shown some promise in clinical situations in humans, but a major drawback is that the murine proteins are frequently recognized as foreign by the patient's immune system, leading to the development of a **human antimouse antibody (HAMA)** response. Such a response diminishes the effectiveness of the murine antibody and carries the risk of serum sickness (see Chapter 13).

The availability of immunoglobulin genes of mouse and human has led to several strategies aimed at avoiding the HAMA response. An initial idea was to fuse murine V genes carrying the specificity for the tumor antigen to human C genes, and to express the encoded chimeric antibody by transfecting the genes into a nonexpressing myeloma; the resulting **transfectoma** expresses an antibody that carries murine determinants only on the VH and VL regions. An even more elegant approach has exploited our understanding of the three-dimensional structure of immunoglobulin V-region protein domains. As discussed earlier, it is the three CDR loops of each chain that contact antigen, while the remaining framework residues serve primarily to hold the CDR loops in the correct position. Therefore, it was reasoned that it should be possible to use genetic engineering to graft the CDR sequences from a murine antitumor antibody onto human V-region framework codons to produce an antibody that is human except for murine sequences at the antigen-binding site. Such "humanized" antibodies have in fact been found to carry the antigen specificity of the original murine monoclonal, but to evoke almost no HAMA response. Antibody genes have been altered in various ways to construct novel proteins with the desired properties of immunoglobulins. One interesting engineered structure is the **Fv chain**, which contains a VH domain directly linked to a VL domain through a spacer polypeptide of about 15 residues.

Several other strategies may also prove useful for generating human monoclonal antibodies. Large segments of the human germline immunoglobulin locus can be introduced into murine strains creating **transgenic mice** that can synthesize human antibodies. Alternatively, immunodeficient mice engrafted with human B-cell precursors may be immunized and then used to generate human hybridomas (though it is not clear whether the murine advantages of stability and high antibody production would be achieved by this approach).

A completely different strategy avoids hybridoma technology completely. A "library" of human V_H and V_L genes is constructed so that Fv proteins are expressed on the surface of bacteriophages; the resulting **phage display library** is then selected for the desired antigen specificity by affinity chromatography on a column support containing antigen. The bound bacteriophages are then eluted, and the resulting V_H-V_L gene pair can be used for further constructions.

These approaches illustrate the potential of biotechnology for providing new therapeutic strategies for passive immunization targeted against specific molecules on tumor cells or microbial invaders, all based on immunoglobulin gene structure.

Summary

Antibodies are proteins that show vast diversity in the antigens that they can bind, yet fall into subclasses showing common effector functions. The basic structure of an antibody is the L_2H_2 unit composed of two identical heavy chains and two identical light chains. The vast diversity of antibodies resides in the N-terminal "variable" regions of both light and heavy chain, whereas the common effector functions are determined by the heavy chain constant regions structure. Antibodies are important clinically (eg their roles in virus neutralization, bacterial opsonization, autoimmunity, allergy, etc.), and an impressive technology has developed for analyzing their presence in body fluids. Specific antibodies developed against antigens of interest can also be used in the laboratory to purify or assay those antigens. One great mystery of antibodies was how their binding diversity could be encoded in the genome; this has been explained by the finding that unique antibody variable region genes are assembled in each B lymphocyte from a common germline endowment of V_H, D, J_H, V_L, and J_L genes. In addition to this combinatorial diversity, the precise junctions between any two germline gene elements may vary depending on how many nucleotides are "nibbled" from the coding sequence ends and the nature of the "N" nucleotides added before the elements are joined. A final measure of diversity results from V gene somatic mutation, which occurs within cells residing in germinal centers of lymphoid tissues; rare mutations that increase antibody affinity are selected for expression by a signalling mechanism acting through the form of antibody that is displayed on the cell membrane of B lymphocytes. After a B lymphocyte has been committed to a particular antigen specificity, the effector functions of the expressed antibody may be altered by isotype switch recombination, a process regulated by the immunologic milieu, including the mix of locally expressed cytokines. The potential importance of specific antibodies as reagents for diagnosis and therapy has motivated scientists to engineer new genes encoding immunoglobulin segments in novel contexts, a technology offering exciting prospects for the future.

Bibliography

ANTIBODIES

Benjamin DC, Berzofsky JA, East IJ, et al: The antigenic structure of proteins: a reappraisal. Ann Rev Immunol 2:67, 1984.

Burnet FM: *The Clonal Selection Theory of Acquired Immunity.* Vanderbilt U. Press. Nashville, TN, 1959.

Burnet FM, Fenner F: *The Production of Antibodies.* MacMillan, Melborne, 1949.

Dick GF, Dick GH: Results with the skin test for susceptibility to scarlet fever. Preventive immunization with scarlet fever toxin. JAMA 84:1477, 1925.

Farr RS: A quantative immunochemical measure of the primary interaction between I*BSA and antibody. J Infect Dis 103:239, 1958.

Heidelberger M: *Lectures in Immunochemistry.* Academic Press, New York, NY, 1956.

Jerne NK: The natural selection theory of antibody formation. Proc Natl Acad Sci USA 41:849, 1955.

Kabat EA, Mayer MM: *Experimental Immunochemistry,* Charles C Thomas, Springfield, Ill, 1958.

Kennett RH, M'Kearn TJ, Bechtol KB: *Monoclonal Antibodies: Hybridomas: A New Dimension in Biological Analysis.* Plenum Press, New York, NY, 1980.

Kitagawa M, Yagi Y, Pressman D: The heterogeneity of combining sites of antibodies as determined by specific immunoabsorbents. J Immunol 95:446, 1965.

Kohler G, Milstein C: Continuous cultures of fused cells secreting antibody of predefined specificity. Nature 256:495, 1975.

Landsteiner K: *The Specificity of Serological Reactions.* Dover Pub Inc., New York, NY, 1962.

Raffel S: *Immunity, Hypersensitivity, Serology.* Appleton-Century-Crofts, Inc. New York, NY, 1953.

Romer PH: Veber Den Nachwis Sehr Kleiner Mengen des Kiphtheriegiftes. Z Immunitaetsforsch 3:208, 1909.

Schick B: Die Diphtherietoxin-Hautreaktion des Menschen Als Vorprobe Der Prophylaktischen Diphtherieheilserum Injection. Munch Med Wochenschr 60:2608, 1913.

Schultz W, Charlton W: Serologische Beobactungen Am Scharlachexanthum. Z Kinderheikd 17:328, 1917.

Talmadge DW, Dixon FJ, Bukantz SC, Dammin GJ: Antigen elimination from the blood as an early manifestation of the immune response. J Immunol. 67:243, 1951.

Weigle, WO, Dixon FJ: The elimination of heterologous serum proteins and associated antibody response to guinea pigs and rats. J Immunol 79:24, 1957.

IMMUNOGLOB- ULIN STRUCTURE

Bernier GM: Structure of human immunoglobulins: myeloma proteins as analogues of antibody. Prog Allergy 14:1, 1970.

Capra JD, Edmundson AB: The antibody combining site. Sci Am, 236:50, 1977.

Cohen S, Milstein C: Structure and biologic properties of immunoglobulins. Adv Immunol 7:1, 1967.

Edelman GM, Cunningham BA, Gall WE, Gottlieb PD, Rutishauser U, Waxdal MD: The covalent structure of an entire G-immunoglobulin molecule. Biochemistry 63:78, 1969.

Fahey JL: Antibodies and immunoglobulins. JAMA 194:141, 183, 1966.

Franklin EC: Immune globulins: their structure and function and some techniques for their isolation. Prog. Allergy 8:58, 1964.

Green NM: Electron microscopy of the immunoglobulins. Adv Immunol 11:1, 1969.

Halpern MS, Koshland ME: The stoichiometry of J chain in human secretory IgA. J Immunol 111:1563–1660, 1973.

Kabat EA: The nature of an antigenic determinant. J Immunol 97: 1, 1966.

Kabat EA: Origins of antibody complementarity and specificity—Hypervariable regions and the minigene hypothesis. J Immunol 125:96, 1980.

Kabat EA: General features of antibody molecules. In Pressman D, Tomasi TB Jr, Grossberg AL, Rose NR (eds.): Specific Receptors of Antibodies, Antigens and Cells. Basel, Karger, 1973.

Karush, F: Immunological specificity and molecular structure. Adv Immunol 2:1, 1962.

Kindt TS, Capra JD: The Antibody Enigma. Plenum Press, New York, 1984.

Marquart M, Deisenhofer J, Huber, R, Palm W: Crystallographic refinement and atomic models of the intact immunoglobulin molecule Ko1 and its antigen binding fragment at 3.0 A and 1.9 A resolution. J Mol Biol 141:369, 1980.

Novotony J, et al.: Molecular anatomy of the antibody binding site. J Biol Chem 258:14433, 1983.

Ohno S, Mori N, Matsunaga T: Antigen binding specificities of antibodies are primarily determined by seven residues of V_H. Proc Natl Acad Sci 82:2945, 1985.

Padlan EA: Structural basis for the specificity of antibody-antigen reactions and structural mechanisms for the diversification of antigen-binding specificities. Rev Biophys 10:35, 1977.

Painter, RH: The C1q receptor site on human immunoglobulin G. Canad J Biochem Cell Biol 62:418, 1984.

Pressman D, Grossberg AL: The Structural Basis of Antibody Specificity. New York, Benjamin, 1968.

Richards FF, Konigsberg WH, Rosenstein RW, et al.: On the specificity of antibodies. Biochemical and biophysical evidence indicates the existence of polyfunction antibody combining regions. Science 187:130, 1975.

Rowe DS, Hug K, Forni L, Pernis B: Immunoglobulin D as a lymphocyte receptor. J Exp Med 138:965, 1973.

Scharff MD, Laskov R: Synthesis and assembly of immunoglobulin polypeptide chains. Prog Allergy 14:37, 1970.

Silverton EW, Navia MA, Davies DR: Three dimensional structure of an intact human immunoglobulin. Proc Natl Acad Sci USA 74:5140, 1977.

Spiegelberg HL: Biological activities of immunoglobulins of different classes and subclasses. Adv Immunol 19:259, 1974.

Svehag SE, Bloth B: Ultrastructure of secretory and high-polymer serum immunoglobulin A of human and rabbit origin. Science 168:847, 1970.

Thorebecke GJ, Leslie GA (eds.): Immunoglobulin D: Structure and Function. New York, Acad Sci, 1982.

Tomasi TB, Bienenstock J: Secretory immunoglobulins. Adv Immunol 9:1, 1968.

Wilkelhake JL: Immunoglobulin structure and effector functions. Immunochem 15:695, 1978.

ANTIBODY-ANTIGEN REACTIONS

Avrameas S, Ternynck T: The cross-linking of proteins with glutaraldehyde and its use for the preparation of immunoadsorbents. Immunochemistry 6:53–66, 1969.

Avrameas S: Indirect microenzyme techniques for intracellular detection of antigens. Immunochemistry 6:825, 1969.

Bullock G (ed.): Techniques in immunochemistry. Academic Press, Orlando, Fla. Vol 1, 1982; Vol 2, 1983.

Campbell DH, Luescher E, Lerman LS: Immunologic absorbents. I. Isolation of antibody by means of cellulose protein antigen. Proc Natl Acad Sci USA 37:575, 1951.

Coons AH: Histochemistry with labelled antibody. Int Rev Cytol 5:1, 1956.

Crowle AJ: Immunodiffusion. New York, Academic Press, 1961.

Engvall E, Perlmann P: Enzyme linked immunoabsorbant assay (ELISA). Quantitative assay of immunoglobulin G. Immunochem 8:871, 1971.

Gill TJ III: Methods for detecting antibody. Immunochemistry 7:997–1000, 1970.

Hapke M, Patil K: The establishment of normal limits for serum proteins measured by the rate nephelometer. Human Path 12:1011, 1981.

Heidelberger M: Lectures in Immunochemistry. New York, Academic Press, 1956.

Hsu SM, Cossmann J, Jaffe ES: A comparison of ABC, unlabeled antibody and conjugated immunochemical methods with monoclonal and polyclonal antibodies. An examination of the germinal centers of tonsils. Am J Clin Path 80:429, 1983.

Kabat EA, Mayer MM: Experimental Immunochemistry, 2d ed. Springfield, IL, Thomas, 1961.

Lefkowits I, Pernis B: Immunological Methods. Academic Press, Orlando Fla. Vol 1, 1979; Vol 2, 1980.

Linthicum DS, Sell S: Topography of lymphocyte surface immunoglobulin using scanning immunoelectron microscopy. J Ultrastruct Res 51:55, 1975.

Loken MR, Stall AM: Flow cytometry as an analytical and preparative tool in immunology. J Immunol Meth 50:85, 1982.

Mancini G, Carbonara AO, Heremans JF: Immunochemical quantitation of antigens by single radial immunodiffusion. Immunochemistry 2:235, 1965.

Merrill D, Hartley TF, Claman HN: Electroimmunodiffusion (EID): A simple, rapid method for quantitation by immunoglobulins in dilute biological fluids. J Lab Clin Med, 69:151, 1967.

Minden P, Reid RT, Farr RS: A comparison of some commonly used methods for detecting antibodies to bovine albumin in human serum. J Immunol 96:180, 1966.

Nakane PK, Pierce GB Jr: Enzyme labeled antibodies for the light and electron microscopic localization of tissue antigens. J Cell Biol 33:307, 1967.

Ouchterlony O: Diffusion-in-gel methods for immunological analysis. Prog Allergy 6:30, 1962.

Oudin J: Method of immunochemic analysis by specific precipitation in gel medium. C R Acad Sci (D) (Paris) 222:115, 1946.

Rodbard D, Weiss GH: Mathematical theory of immunoradiometric (labeled antibody) assays. Anal Biochem 52:10–44, 1973.

Rodbard D, Catt KJ: Mathematical theory of radioligand assays: the kinetics of separation of bound from free. J Steroid Biochem 3:255–273, 1972.

Schuurs AHWM, Van Weemen BK: Enzyme-Immunoassay. Clin Chim Acta 81:1, 1977.

Shnitka TK, Seligman AM: Ultrastructural localization of enzymes. Ann Rev Biochem 40:375, 1971.

Skelley DS, Brown LP, Besch PK: Radioimmunoassay. Clin Chem 19:146–186, 1973.

Stein H, Gatter K, Asbahr H, Mason DY: Use of freeze-dried paraffin-embedded sections for immunohistologic staining with monoclonal antibodies. Lab Investig 51:676, 1985.

Towbin H, Gordon J: Immunoblotting and dot immunoblotting—current statis and outlook, J Immunol Meth 72:313, 1984.

Weetall HH: Preparation and characterization of antigen and antibody adsorbents covalently coupled to an inorganic carrier. J Biochem 117:257–261, 1970.

Weir DM: Antigen-Antibody reactions. In Cruickshank R (ed.): Modern Trends in Immunology. London, Whitefriar, 1963.

Wilchek M, Bocchini V, Becker M, Givol D: A general method for the specific isolation of peptide containing modified residues, using insoluble antibody columns. Biochemistry 10:2828–2834, 1971.

Yalow RS: Radioimmunoassay: A probe for the fine structure of biologic systems. Science 200:1236, 1978.

CELL MEMBRANE IMMUNOGLOBU-LIN

Davidson HW, Reid PA, Lanzavecchia A, Watts C: Processed antigen binds to newly synthesized MHC class II molecules in antigen-specific B lymphocytes. Cell 67: 105, 1991.

Gold MR, Chan VW, Turck CW, DeFranco AL: Membrane Ig cross-linking regulates phosphatidylinositol 3-kinase in B lymphocytes. J Immunol 148:2012, 1992.

Gold MR, DeFranco AL: Biochemistry of B lymphocyte activation. Adv Immunol 55: 221, 1994.

Hombach J, Tsubata T, Leclercq L, Stappert H, Reth M: Molecular components of the B-cell antigen receptor complex of the IgM class. Nature 343:760, 1990.

Rogers J, Early P, Carter C, Calame K, Bond M, Hood L, Wall R: Two mRNAs with different 3′ ends encode membrane-bound and secreted forms of immunoglobulin μ chain. Cell 20:303, 1980.

IMMUNOGLOBU-LIN GENES

Bernard O, Gough NM: Nucleotide sequence of immunoglobulin heavy chain joining segments between translocated VH and μ constant regions genes. Proc Natl Acad Sci USA 77:3630, 1980.

Brack C, Hirama M, Lenhard SR, Tonegawa S: A complete immunoglobulin gene is created by somatic recombination. Cell 15:1, 1978.

Calame K, Rogers J, Early P, Davis M, Livant D, Wall R, Hood L: Mouse Cμ heavy chain immunoglobulin gene segment contains three intervening sequences separating domains. Nature 284:452, 1980.

Durdik J, Moore MW, Selsing E: Novel κ light-chain gene rearrangements in mouse λ light chain-producing B lymphocytes. Nature 307:749, 1984.

Early P, Huang H, Davis M, Calame K, Hood L: An immunoglobulin heavy chain variable region gene is generated from three segments of DNA: VH, D and JH. Cell 19: 981, 1980.

Hesse JE, Lieber MR, Mizuuchi K, Gellert M: V(D) recombination: a functional definition of the joining signals. Genes Dev 3:1053, 1989.

Hieter PA, Korsmeyer SJ, Waldmann TA, Leder P: Human immunoglobulin kappa light-chain genes are deleted or rearranged in lambda-producing B cells. Nature 290:368, 1981.

Hofker MH, Walter MA, Cox DW: Complete physical map of the human immunoglobulin heavy chain constant region gene complex. Proc Natl Acad Sci USA 86: 5567, 1989.

Jacob J, Kelsoe G: In situ studies of the primary immune response to (4-hydroxy-3-nitrophenyl)acetyl. II. A common clonal origin for periarteriolar lymphoid sheath-associated foci and germinal centers. J Exp Med 176: 679, 1992.

Jacob J, Przylepa J, Miller C, Kelsoe G. In situ studies of the primary immune response to (4-hydroxy-3-nitrophenyl)acetyl. III. The kinetics of V region mutation and selection in germinal center B cells. J Exp Med 178:1293, 1993.

Kataoka T, Kawakami T, Takahashi N, Honjo T: Rearrangement of immunoglobulin γ 1 chain gene and mechanism for heavy-chain class switch. Proc Natl Acad Sci USA 77:919, 1980.

Kim S, David M, Sinn E, Patten P, Hood L: Antibody diversity: Somatic hypermutation of rearranged VH genes. Cell 27:573, 1981.

Kurosawa Y, Tonegawa S: Organization, structure, and assembly of immunoglobulin heavy chain diversity DNA segments. J Exp Med 155: 201, 1982.

Matsumura R, Matsuda F, Nagaoka H, Fujikura J, Shin EK, Fukita Y, Haino M, Honjo T: Structural analysis of the human VH locus using nonrepetitive intergenic probes and repetitive sequence probes. Evidence for recent reshuffling. J Immunol 152:660, 1994.

Max EE, Seidman JG, Leder P: Sequences of five potential recombination sites encoded close to an immunoglobulin kappa constant region gene. Proc Natl Acad Sci USA 76: 3450, 1979.

Oettinger MA, Schatz DG, Gorka C, Baltimore D: RAG-1 and RAG-2, adjacent genes that synergistically activate V(D)J recombination. Science 248:1517, 1990.

Roth DB, Menetski JP, Nakajima PB, Bosma MJ, Gellert M: V(D)J recombination: broken DNA molecules with covalently sealed (hairpin) coding ends in scid mouse thymocytes. Cell 70:983, 1992.

Sakaguchi N, Melchers F: Lambda 5, a new light-chain-related locus selectively expressed in pre-B lymphocytes. Nature 324: 579, 1986.

Sakano H, Hüppi K, Heinrich G, Tonegawa S: Sequences at the somatic recombination sites of immunoglobulin light-chain genes. Nature 280: 288, 1979.

Sakano H, Maki R, Kurosawa Y, Roeder W, Tonegawa S: Two types of somatic recombination are necessary for the generation of complete immunoglobulin heavy-chain genes. Nature 286: 676, 1980.

Schiff C, Milili M, Bossy D, Fougereau M: Organization and expression of the pseudolight chain genes in human B-cell ontogeny. Int Rev Immunol 8:135, 1992.

Seidman JG, Max EE, Leder P: A κ-immunoglobulin gene is formed by site-specific recombination without further somatic mutation. Nature 280:370, 1979.

Shimizu A, Takahashi N, Yaoita Y, Honjo T: Organization of the constant-region gene family of the mouse immunoglobulin heavy chain. Cell 28:499, 1982.

Tomlinson IM, Walter G, Marks JD, Llewelyn MB, Winter G: The repertoire of human germline VH sequences reveals about fifty groups of VH segments with different hypervariable loops. J Mol Biol 227:776, 1992.

Tsubata T, Reth M: The products of pre-B cell-specific genes (lambda 5 and VpreB) and the immunoglobulin μ chain form a complex that is transported onto the cell. J Exp Med 172:973, 1990.

van Gent DC, McBlane JF, Ramsden DA, Sadofsky MJ, Hesse HE, Gellert M: Initiation of V(D)J recombination in a cell-free system. Cell 81:925, 1995.

Vasicek TJ, Leder P: Structure and expression of the human immunoglobulin lambda genes. J Exp Med 172:609, 1990.

Waldmann TA: The arrangement of immunoglobulin and T cell receptor genes in human lymphoproliferative disorders. Adv Immunol 40:247, 1987.

BIOTECH-NOLOGY APPLICATION OF ANTIBODY GENES

Boulianne GL, Hozumi N, Shulman MJ: Production of functional chimaeric mouse/human antibody. Nature 312:643, 1984.

Clackson T, Hoogenboom HR, Griffiths AD, Winter G:Making antibody fragments using phage display libraries. Nature 352:624, 1991.

Morrison SL: Transfectomas provide novel chimeric antibodies. Science 229:1202, 1985.

Taylor LD, Carmack CE, Schramm SR, Mashayekh R, Higgins KM, Kuo CC, Woodhouse C, Kay RM, Lonberg N: A transgenic mouse that expresses a diversity of human sequence heavy and light chain immunoglobulins. Nucleic Acids Res 20: 6287, 1992.

5

T-cell Recognition of Proteins and the Major Histocompatibility Complex

Ira Berkower

The immune system is organized to solve the problems of rapid and specific recognition of an enormous number of potential antigens by cell-to-cell collaboration and by clonal expansion of cells specific for the antigen. The immune response depends on T cells acting at each step. The first collaboration, between antigen presenting cells (macrophages) and T cells, will be discussed in this chapter, and the second collaboration, between helper-T cells and antibody-producing B cells, will be discussed in a later chapter. In both steps, the ability of T cells to respond in an antigen-specific manner is central to the strategy of the immune system.

Besides recognizing foreign proteins, T cells also retain a functional memory of virtually all self-proteins, which enables them to distinguish between self and nonself antigens. T cells are born in the bone marrow and mature in the thymus, where they learn tolerance for self antigens. T-cell tolerance will be discussed in the next chapter.

Although potential invaders contain a variety of proteins, nucleic acid, carbohydrates, and, quite often, lipids, T cells respond almost exclusively to proteins of the pathogen. In the case of viruses, this focuses the immune response on structural and nonstructural proteins encoded by viral genes. To recognize these protein antigens, T cells depend on the function of accessory cells, called antigen-presenting cells (APCs), and on the major histocompatibility complex (MHC) molecules of the APC. They utilize their own T-cell receptor (TCR) for antigen, as well as additional accessory molecules expressed on the T-cell surface, including CD4 and CD8.

T cells respond to antigen by cell activation and proliferation with release of factors called cytokines, or interleukins. Activated T cells can then act as helper-T cells by providing essential signals needed for the clonal expansion of other antigen-specific cells, including B cells and cytolytic T cells (CTLs). The B cells make antibodies, including some capable of inactivating viruses before they invade cells. CTLs recognize infected cells during viral replication and destroy them before they can release new virus and infect other cells (see Chapter 15). Considering their central role in a variety of plays making up the immune response, T cells can be compared to the quarterback of the immune system. The coordinated response of different cellular players follows prearranged patterns, or plays, and these are controlled and directed via signals from the T cell. In addition, progeny of the helper-T cells provide specific recognition for T-cell-mediated activation of macrophages, leading to a type of inflammatory reaction known as delayed hypersensitivity (see Chapter 16).

The immune response starts when foreign proteins are ingested by macrophages (Fig. 5–1). These antigen-presenting cells (APCs) are not antigen specific, but they are capable of processing the antigen into fragments and presenting the antigenic fragments to helper-T cells in a form that is highly immunogenic. APCs take up the antigen by endocytosis (upper left in the figure), and the early endosomes become acidified, which activates proteases. Partial enzymatic degradation of proteins occurs, yielding peptides. The most antigenic peptides bind to MHC molecules, which transport them to the cell surface of the APC for T-cell stimulation (lower right). Antigen presentation gets the immune response going, by triggering the response of antigen-specific helper-T cells.

T Cell Clones

A good way to measure the T-cell response to antigen is to mimic clonal expansion in culture. T cells are cultured with antigen plus antigen-presenting cells. As the responding T cells start to grow, they actively synthesize new DNA. By adding radiolabeled thymidine, a building block of DNA, to the culture, the T-cell response can be measured as the incorporation of radioactive counts into newly synthesized DNA. This assay, which has revealed many properties of antigen recognition by T cells, exploits the basic strategy of the immune system, namely, clonal selection by exponential growth of antigen-specific T cells. Through several lines of evidence, the proliferation assay revealed that T cells cannot respond directly to protein antigens, but can only respond to antigen after processing. First, most proteins can be replaced by synthetic peptides corresponding to the appropriate site. Second, although the T cell cannot normally distinguish between these two forms of the same antigenic sequence, the two become quite different when processing is turned off. Thus, if a protease inhibitor such as leupeptin is added to the culture (Fig. 5–2), the two forms of antigen are no

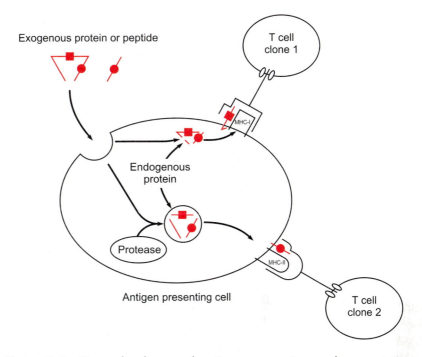

Figure 5–1. General scheme of antigen processing and presentation. Exogenous antigen is taken up in endosomes (lower pathway), where it is partially degraded to peptide fragments. Those peptides that bind MHC class II will be transported to the cell surface for presentation to T cells. Alternatively, endogenously expressed antigen is processed by cytoplasmic proteases, and the peptide fragments that bind MHC class I are transported to the cell surface.

longer equivalent. The response to native protein is blocked completely by leupeptin, but the response to peptide, which is "preprocessed," is unaffected, since it needs no further processing. In a sense, peptides are the natural currency of T-cell recognition. This result also demonstrates that leupeptin inhibition is not due to a toxic effect, since it does not inhibit the peptide response. Third, early studies of T cells showed that they are unable to distinguish between native and denatured proteins. Rather than a sign of nonspecificity, this indicates processing, since the native conformation is destroyed before the T cell sees the antigen.

A further extension of the T-cell proliferation assay was to use repeated cycles of antigen stimulation to derive a line of antigen specific T cells. Consecutive rounds of antigen stimulation must be separated by a resting culture in the absence of antigen. This is necessary because antigen stimulation leads to temporary nonresponsiveness, but the cells can recover during a rest without antigen. A second useful trick is to add T-cell growth factor, now called interleukin-2 (IL-2), to the

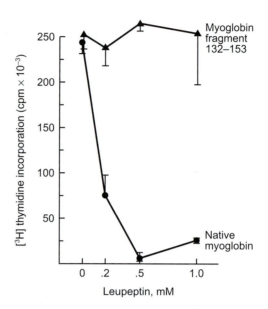

Figure 5–2. In the absence of protease inhibitors, native myoglobin or a peptide fragment are processed and presented equally well to a myoglobin-specific T-cell line. But leupeptin inhibits processing and blocks presentation of the protein completely. It has no effect on presentation of the peptide, since the peptide requires no further processing.

cultures. This cytokine, found in the culture medium of stimulated T cells, is able to keep T-cell lines growing even in the absence of other signals and is particularly useful in maintaining T cells in resting cultures. Viability and expansion of antigen specific T cells is enhanced by IL-2 because antigen stimulation induces expression of the receptor for IL-2 on the responding cells. As shown in Figure 5–3, during the early rounds of antigen stimulation, the total number of cells in culture (mostly not antigen-specific) falls rapidly, while the number of antigen-specific cells increases from nearly undetectable to the point where they exceed the number of nonspecific cells. By the third or fourth round of stimulation and rest, nearly all the cells of the line are antigen-specific, as shown by exponential growth of the total cell number with subsequent rounds of antigen stimulation.

At this point, T-cell "lines" may be "cloned" by limiting dilution. In this method, the cells are spread among hundreds of microtiter wells at a low cell density so that, on average, there is less than one cell per well. In the presence of IL-2 and feeder cells, a line of T cells can be grown from a single cell. After two or three weeks in culture, some of the wells contain clumps of growing T cells. After further expansion, many of these growing colonies are found to be antigen-specific T cells. Since the original cloning was done, on average, at less than one

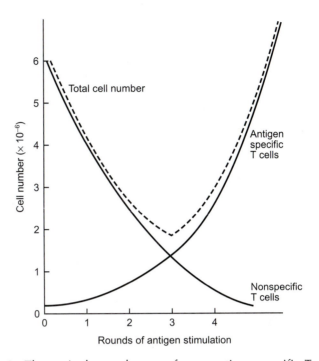

Figure 5–3. Theoretical growth curve for an antigen-specific T cell line. Initially rare, these cells increase exponentially through successive rounds of antigen stimulation. In contrast, the nonspecific cells decline over time, due to lack of stimulation. The total cell number declines initially, then increases as antigen-specific T cells become the majority of the population. At this point, cloning by limiting dilution will give a good yield of antigen-specific T cells.

cell per well, each of the cells in a well should be derived from the same parental cell, and they all should have the same specificity for antigen and MHC. Cloned T cells have been very useful in defining antigenic determinants (epitopes) recognized by T cells, as well as the MHC restriction and antigen processing pathways, as described below.

Another highly successful technique is to fuse the antigen-specific T cells, after a single step of antigen stimulation, with a drug-sensitive T-cell tumor. The normal cells provide antigen specificity and the ability to survive drug selection, whereas the tumor cells confer unlimited growth potential on the product of cell fusion. After a few days in culture, the selecting drug is added to the culture, so only the fused cells can grow out. Thanks to the insight of John Kappler, the antigen-specific cells are detected by their production of IL-2 in response to antigen in combination with antigen-presenting cells, providing a way to measure the response to antigen, independent of T-cell growth. These T-cell hybridomas have become the best way to establish long term T-cell lines in sufficient quantity to study the T-cell receptor (TCR) for antigen.

An example of a proliferative T-cell line is shown in Figure 5–4. A human donor, who had never been infected with hepatitis B virus, was immunized with hepatitis B surface antigen (HBsAg), and peripheral blood lymphocytes were expanded by antigen stimulation. After three rounds of stimulation and rest, the cells were cloned by limiting dilution, at one cell per well, and expanded in the presence of IL-2. As shown, a T-cell line obtained by this procedure gave a dose-dependent proliferative response to HBsAg. However, the response also depended on the MHC antigens (HLA in humans) of the antigen-presenting cell, since maximal proliferation was obtained with presenting cells from donor JL, who matched for HLA type, but there was no response with presenting cells from donor GY, who did not match. This experiment illustrates the dual specificity of T cells for antigen and MHC; the cloned lines make it possible to analyze each requirement independently.

Epitope Mapping

Because they are cloned, with a single antigen specificity, we presume that the T-cell line responds to the same antigenic site, regardless of whether it occurs in a protein, polypeptide, or short peptide. If true, then the precise antigenic determinant can be mapped by replacing the

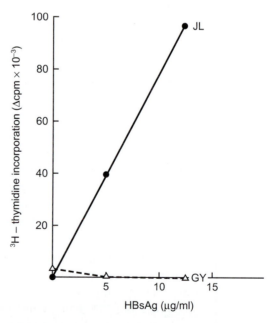

Figure 5–4. Proliferative response of a T-cell line specific for HBsAg. The response is antigen-specific and MHC-restricted, since donor JL, who matches for MHC, presents antigen to the T-cell line, while donor GY, differing at MHC, does not.

native protein with large fragments or short peptides and measuring the T-cell proliferative response to each. This strategy allows us to map precisely the antigenic determinants (epitopes) on protein antigens that are recognized by T cells.

For the HBsAg specific T-cell line, the epitope was mapped starting with large polypeptide fragments of the antigen and proceeding to a set of overlapping peptides (Fig. 5–5). Since native HBsAg protein exists in two forms, "Pre-S + S" and "S," the first step was to determine which form stimulated the T-cell line. As shown at the bottom of the figure, the T-cell line responded to "Pre-S + S" but not to "S" alone, indicating that it was specific for a site contained in the Pre-S sequence.

T-Cell Response to Synthetic Peptides of HBsAg

Antigen	Site	^{3}H – TdR Incorporation (Δcpm)	
		Expt I	Expt II
Pre S$_1$	1 ———— 120	31,521	54,321
Pre S$_2$	121 —— 174	– 1401	ND
1 – 21	⊢—⊣	4937	ND
1 – 28	⊢——⊣	29,866	65,432
12 – 32	⊢—⊣	23,601	ND
21 – 47	⊢——⊣	25,475	39,921
32 – 53	⊢—⊣	1567	ND
53 – 73	⊢—⊣	–197	ND
94 – 117	⊢—⊣	1801	1715
120 – 145	⊢—⊣	1336	ND
Pre S + S Antigen		ND	62,944
S Antigen		ND	174
Medium Control		5374	1,731

Figure 5–5. Mapping the epitope specificity of a human T-cell line. The response to large recombinant fragments of HBsAg showed specificity for the Pre-S1 region. A series of synthetic peptides were tested, and three overlapping peptides stimulated the line, mapping the epitope to the 8 amino acid sequence shared by all three peptides.

Similarly, large fragments of Pre-S, called Pre-S1 and Pre-S2, were tested (top of the figure), and the response mapped to Pre-S1. Then a series of synthetic peptides corresponding to the Pre-S1 sequence were tested, and three peptides, corresponding to amino acids 1 to 28 and 21 to 40, as well as amino acids 12 to 32, were found to stimulate the line. Since these three peptides overlap at just eight residues, the results map the site to amino acids 21 to 28 of the Pre-S region. They clearly show that peptides, large or small, can replace a native protein for stimulation of T cells, provided that they contain the antigenic sequence. By repeating this process for a number of T-cell clones, the predominant epitopes of HBsAg can be identified.

An alternative approach to mapping the epitopes recognized by T cells is to synthesize a series of overlapping peptides covering the entire protein sequence. These peptides should be 20 to 25 amino acids in length (based on peptides eluted from major histocompatibility complex (MHC) class II, see below), and they should overlap with their neighbors, so that epitopes are not missed between them. Each peptide is tested individually, to identify the most important sites for T-cell recognition.

A similar approach has been used to find the epitopes recognized by cytolytic T lymphocytes (CTLs). These cells are capable of recognizing virally infected cells at an early stage in the viral life cycle, before infectious virus has assembled. By lysing the cells at this time, it is possible to kill the infected cell without releasing hundreds of infectious virions (Fig. 5–6A).

The lytic activity of these CTLs against infected cells can be measured by release of Cr51 from labeled target cells. The infected target cells are first allowed to take up Cr51, which binds covalently to intracellular proteins. The labeled target cells are then mixed with CTLs at various ratios of CTL effectors to infected targets (E:T ratio). As the target cells are broken open, or lysed, by the action of CTLs, Cr51 labeled proteins will be released. These can be detected by measuring Cr51 radioactivity released into the culture supernatant.

Using this assay, the ability of CTLs to destroy infected target cells was shown to depend on the MHC class I antigens of the host, as well as the viral proteins synthesized inside the target cell. Even uninfected cells could be made into targets of CTLs by uptake of viral peptides, suggesting that antigen processing was occurring within target cells. Since newly synthesized viral proteins were processed inside the cell (endogenous processing), CTL specificity was not limited to proteins naturally expressed on the cell surface. Rather, viral proteins localized inside the target cell were also good target antigens for CTLs.

For example (Fig. 5–6B), when a CTL line specific for influenza virus-infected cells was tested on target cells expressing individual viral proteins, lysis was specific for influenza nucleoprotein. Although

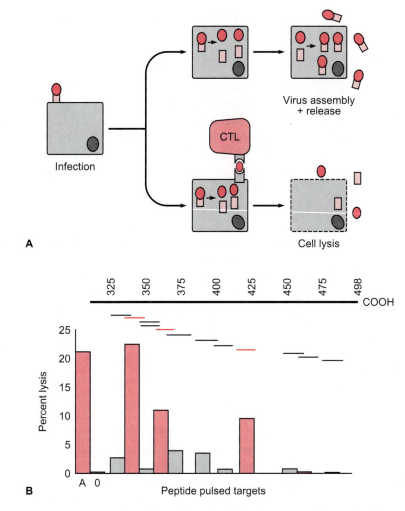

Figure 5–6. **A.** CTLs lyse the infected cell before assembly and release of new infectious virus, terminating the infection. **B.** Epitope mapping with a series of peptides from influenza nucleoprotein. Target cells were labeled with Cr51 and either infected (A), uninfected (0), or pulsed with nucleoprotein peptides as indicated. They were then incubated with influenza-specific CTLs from the same donor. Cell lysis was detected as the release of Cr51 from the target cells. (Modified from Townsend, et al.)

this protein does not normally localize to the cell surface, it is a good target for CTLs, because it can be processed to antigenic fragments and presented on the cell surface during infection. Using a series of synthetic peptides of the nucleoprotein sequence, the major antigenic epitopes recognized by CTLs were localized to just a few sites on nucleoprotein. Thus, epitope mapping for antigens presented with both MHC class I and II indicates that antigen processing is required for presentation with both types of MHC antigens.

Genetic Control
of the Immune
Response

For certain protein antigens, the immune response to the entire protein is under genetic control, and the high response phenotype is inherited as a Mendelian dominant trait. Typically, these antigens are small proteins, such as whale myoglobin, beef insulin, or pigeon cytochrome-c or simple synthetic polymers, such as poly-L-lysine. To demonstrate the genetic relationship, the response is compared between congenic strains of mice, which have the same background genes, but differ only at the MHC locus. At first, whale myoglobin, with 153 amino acids, appears to be a complex antigen. But since mice are presumably tolerant of their own myoglobin, the shared sequences between whale and mouse myoglobin may be subtracted, leaving only the amino acid differences between whale and mouse as potential targets for the immune response. In this view, whale myoglobin represents a collection of nonimmunogenic shared sequences, studded with a few foreign epitopes, corresponding to the evolutionary differences between whale and mouse myoglobin. Murine T cells could respond to some or all of these differences, depending on MHC type. Certain strains of mice would recognize no differences, resulting in nonresponsiveness to the entire protein.

MHC

The genes coding for the immune response to these proteins map to a genetic locus that also controls tissue type, known as the major histocompatibility complex (MHC). In the mouse, this is called H-2 and is located on chromosome 17. In humans, it is called HLA and is located on chromosome 6. The organization of MHC genes in mouse and man is shown in Figures 5–7 and 5–8. The MHC genes code for two classes of proteins, class I and II, which share many similarities between mouse and man. MHC class I proteins in the mouse are called H2-K, -D, and -L and in man are called HLA-A, -B, and -C and have two subunits, of 45 kD and 12 kD. The class I antigens are found on virtually every nucleated cell in the body, but are not found on red blood cells. This is why blood transfusions must match for the blood group antigens A, B, and O, but not for tissue type, whereas organ transplants must match for both or be rejected. Only the larger subunit is coded in the MHC locus, and it is highly polymorphic, differing among individuals of the same species. The smaller MHC class I subunit is 12 kD and does not vary with MHC type. It is found in two places: bound to the MHC heavy chain to form class I molecules on the cell surface or free in the serum, where it is called beta-2 microglobulin. Since each person inherits two copies of HLA-A, -B, and -C, his or her tissue type may include up to six different class I alleles.

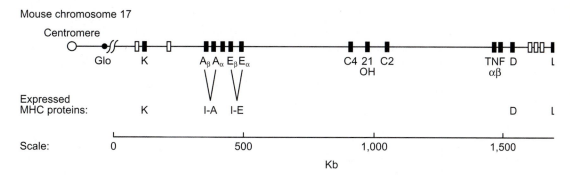

Figure 5–7. Mouse MHC genes on chromosome 17. Class I genes for H-2K, D, and L are separated by the class II genes coding for I-A and I-E. Complement components (C2 and C4), enzymes (21-hydroxylase, 21-OH and glyoxalase, GLO) and cytokines (tumor necrosis factor, TNF) are also located in this genetic region. Filled boxes indicate expressed genes, while empty boxes indicate defective pseudogenes.

A. Complete MHC locus

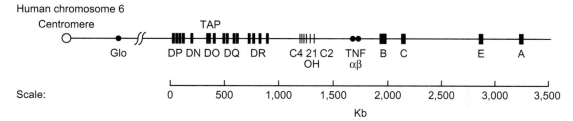

B. Expanded view of MHC class II

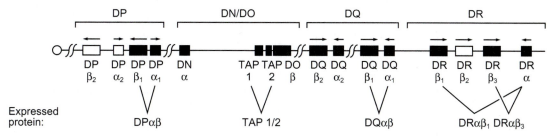

Figure 5–8 **A.** Human MHC genes on chromosome 6. Class I genes for HLA-A, -B, and -C are located on the right side of the figure, while class II genes coding for HLA-DP, -DQ, and -DR are on the left. Once again, C2, C4, 21-hydroxylase, and TNF are located in between, as they were in mouse, and the gene for glyoxalase (GLO) is located between the MHC locus and the centromere. **B.** Expanded view of the HLA-D region. Expressed genes are shown as solid boxes, while defective pseudogenes are empty boxes. Note the TAP 1 and 2 genes located near DO.

The large number of variants of the human HLA class I genes are illustrated in Table 5–1A. Within the human population, the number of possible combinations would be the product of 24 HLA-A alleles times 52 HLA-B alleles times 11 HLA-C alleles, or about 13,700 combinations. This number is increased further, since each person has two

TABLE 5–1A. HLA CLASS I ANTIGENS

HLA-A		HLA-B		HLA-C	
Allele	Frequency (%)	Allele	Frequency (%)	Allele	Frequency (%)
A1	17.4	B7	12.2	Cw1	2.2
A2	27.1	B8	11.9	Cw2	2.2
A3	15.5	B13	2.2	Cw3	15.1
A11	3.0	B18	6.1	Cw4	7.5
A23	4.1	B27	2.8	Cw5	7.3
A24	10.5	B35	8	Cw6	7.9
A25	2.2	B37	1.1	Cw7	30.4
A26	2.8	B38	3.3	Cw8	5.5
A28	5.5	B39	2.8	BLANK	21.8
A29	2.8	Bw31	0.8		
A30	3	Bw42	0.8		
A31	3.9	B44	13.3		
A32	2.8	B45	0.3		
Aw33	1.1	B49	0.8		
BLANK	0.3	Bw50	0.6		
		B51	4.2		
		Bw52	1.4		
		Bw53	0.3		
		Bw54	0.3		
		Bw55	0.6		
		Bw57	3.3		
		Bw58	1.4		
		Bw60	5.5		
		Bw61	1.1		
		Bw62	7.8		
		Bw63	1.1		
		Bw64	1.4		
		Bw65	4.2		
		BLANK	0.6		

Table 5–1A. HLA class I antigens. Note the many alleles of each gene and their relative frequency in a Caucasian population. This distribution will differ in different population groups. (Reprinted from Baur, et al., *Histocompatibility Testing 1984*, Albert ED, Baur MP, Mayr WR, eds. New York, Springer-Verlag, 1984.)

copies of chromosome 6, but reduced somewhat by the fact that certain alleles tend to occur together (linkage disequilibrium). As indicated in the figure, some HLA types, such as HLA-A2, are relatively common, whereas others, such as HLA-Aw33 are very rare. Thus, the likelihood of finding a matched organ donor may be reduced further in those individuals with a rare HLA type.

The MHC class II proteins also have two subunits, an alpha chain of 34 kD and a beta chain of 29 kD. As shown in Figure 5–7, class II proteins in the mouse are called I-A and I-E. The human class II genes (see Fig. 5–8B) code for three proteins, called DP, DQ, and DR, and both subunits are polymorphic. Each locus has one alpha chain; DP and DQ have one beta chain, while DR has two functional beta-chain genes. The expression of these class II proteins is generally limited to specialized antigen-presenting cells of the immune system, including B cells, macrophages, tissue resident macrophages, and dendritic cells of skin and lymph nodes. However, they also can be induced on activated T cells and in other tissues when stimulated by inflammatory cytokines such as interferon.

Each person has two copies of the three class II genes, giving up to six MHC class II tissue types. As shown in Table 5–1B, the 20 alleles at DR times 9 at DQ times 6 at DP gives 1,080 possible combinations, assuming just one copy of each. These provoke a strong T-cell response when lymphocytes from mismatched individuals are mixed in cell culture, and the ensuing mixed lymphocyte reaction was the earliest way to detect MHC class II differences in humans. The large number of possible combinations of class I and II tissue types produces the marked HLA diversity observed in human populations and accounts

TABLE 5–1B. HLA CLASS II ANTIGENS

Allele	Frequency (%)	Allele	Frequency (%)	Allele	Frequency %
DR1	9.5	DQw1	32.3	DPw1	4.3
DR2	15.8	DQw2	18.1	DPw2	11.5
DR3	12	DQw3	23.3	DPw3	4
DR4	12.7	BLANK	26.3	DPw4	41.8
DR7	12			DPw5	4.4
DRw8	3			DPw6	0
DRw9	0.8			BLANK	40
DRw10	0.8				
DRw11	12.3				
DRw12	2				
DRw13	5.4				
DRw14	5.8				
BLANK	7.9				

Frequencies are approximate gene frequencies in Causcasian populations.

for the low probability of finding a perfect HLA match between unrelated organ donors and those in need of a transplant.

Within a family, however, all of the HLA alleles on each parental chromosome 6 are inherited together in a block, called a haplotype. The pedigree of a typical family, with parental haplotypes AB and CD, is shown in Figure 5–9A. According to Mendelian genetics, the children will inherit one haplotype from each parent, giving just four possible combinations: AC, AD, BC, and BD. For each child, the likelihood of matching another sibling for HLA is 25% for a perfect match at both haplotypes, and 50% for matching at just one haplotype. Neither parent will match perfectly, since the children must inherit one haplotype from the other parent. For transplantation purposes, it makes an enormous difference whether both haplotypes are shared between

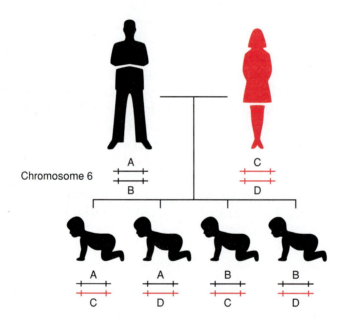

A

	Donor	Recipient	Skin graft (mean survival) days	Kidney graft (1-year graft survival), %	Bone marrow graft
Siblings	a/c →	a/c	20.0	90	Often successful
	a/d →	a/c	13.8	70	Failure
	b/d →	a/c	12.5	60	Failure
Unrelated	x/y →	a/c	12.1	50	Failure

B

Figure 5–9. **A.** HLA inheritance within a family, where the probability of a perfect match between two siblings is 0.25. **B.** Effect of HLA mismatches on the survival or graft rejection of a transplanted organ.

donor and recipient, in which case most transplanted organs will be accepted. This is reflected in the 90% one-year survival of renal allografts from a perfectly matched sibling donor (Fig. 5–9 bottom). In contrast, haplotype mismatched organs are frequently rejected, and renal graft survival decreases in proportion to the number of HLA mismatches.

In the special case of transplanted bone marrow, the donor lymphocytes may recognize the tissues of the recipient as foreign. The ensuing rejection episode can be severe, involving the skin, GI tract, and liver of the recipient in a process known as graft versus host disease. At the present time, graft versus host disease is the major impediment to the use of bone marrow transplantation in a variety of conditions, and only perfectly HLA matched donors are used.

Returning to the human T-cell line against HBsAg shown in Figure 5–4, MHC specificity is a very important part of the T-cell response. Antigen-presenting cells sharing one MHC haplotype (from JL) with the T-cell donor elicited a maximal response, whereas mismatched antigen-presenting cells from GY elicited no response at any dose of antigen. Further studies with this T-cell line revealed that it was specific for the class I antigen HLA-A11 of the donor. Antigen-presenting cells from unrelated subjects, who matched only for HLA-A11, were able to present HBsAg to this T-cell line, even though they differed at other HLA alleles. This is typical of the results with many protein antigens, which must be presented to T cells in association with MHC.

PEPTIDE–MHC BINDING

The basis for T-cell recognition of antigen in association with MHC is that antigenic peptides bind directly to MHC molecules. To demonstrate this binding, an antigenic peptide fragment of ovalbumin (egg albumin) corresponding to amino acids 323 to 339 was radiolabeled and incubated with MHC class II molecules purified from mouse antigen-presenting cells (I-A^d). Bound peptides were separated from free peptides by passing the mixture over a sephadex column, which separates molecules by size (Fig. 5–10). Since the complex of peptide + MHC is quite large, it comes through the column first, while unbound peptide comes through later. The extent of peptide binding can be estimated by comparing the area under the two peaks.

These experiments demonstrated several important properties of peptide binding to MHC class II. First, the binding sites on MHC are saturable, since excess unlabeled peptide could compete off the radiolabeled peptide. Second, two different peptides can bind the same site on MHC, since they also compete for binding. Third, those peptides capable of binding a particular MHC type correspond closely to those known to be immunogenic in mice of the same MHC type. Thus, if a peptide was immunogenic in H-2^d mice, it also showed good binding to the murine class II molecules I-A^d or I-E^d.

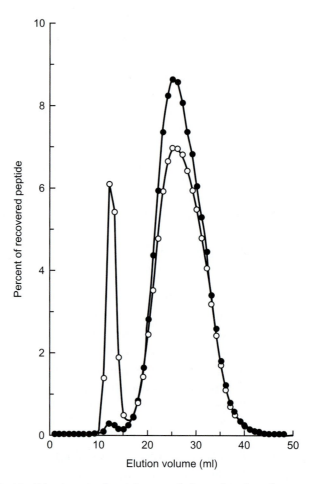

Figure 5–10. Biochemical evidence of direct binding between antigentic peptide and MHC class II. Radiolabeled peptide was mixed with purified I-A protein and passed through a Sephadex sizing column (open circles). By binding I-A, the labeled peptide would elute in the early fractions. Unbound peptide came out in the later fractions (closed circles). (Modified from Buus, et al, 1986.)

Peptide-binding Groove of MHC

These results suggested that MHC should have a peptide-binding site. The three dimensional structure of MHC (Fig. 5–11), solved for HLA-A2 by Bjorkman et al., showed that MHC class I molecules have a lower part anchored in the cell membrane and an upper part with a binding groove large enough to bind antigenic peptides. The sides of the groove consist of alpha helical structures of the HLA heavy chain, and the floor consists of beta pleated sheet. The walls and floor provide numerous contact sites for bound peptides. Those peptides which form noncovalent bonds to the amino acid sidechains of the binding groove will bind stably. Other peptides, lacking "goodness of fit," will come

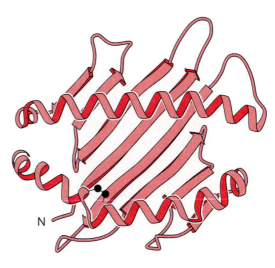

Figure 5–11. Structure of the peptide-binding groove of HLA-A2. Peptide interactions with the floor and walls of the groove determine immunogenicity. (Modified from Bjorkman, et al.)

out of the groove as fast as they go in and will not survive long enough for antigen presentation to T cells.

Since the walls and floor of the peptide-binding groove are lined with residues that vary from one MHC type to another, this structure explains why different peptides will bind to different MHC types. Since a given peptide could bind stably to the MHC of one type and not another, different peptides will be immunogenic in different people, depending on their MHC types. This could present a major obstacle to developing a vaccine based on synthetic peptides, since a number of different peptides might be needed to immunize a population of diverse MHC types.

Peptides Eluted from the MHC Groove

Since the MHC binding groove is accessible to intracellular peptides as well as foreign peptides, how can the foreign peptides compete successfully for MHC binding sites? To answer this question, an ingenious method was developed for detecting natural peptides occupying the MHC binding site, even in uninfected cells. MHC molecules were purified in their native state, with peptide still bound, by affinity chromatography on a monoclonal antibody column. The purified MHC molecules were then denatured with acid, releasing their bound peptides. This method has been used to study both the endogenous peptides that normally occupy the groove and new peptides that appear after viral infection.

The peptides were analyzed in several ways. First, they were separated by high-performance liquid chromatography (HPLC) into discrete peaks (Fig. 5–12), some of which contained more than one peptide. Each MHC molecule gave a distinct pattern, indicating that different peptides were bound. Second, comparing the peptide peaks before and after infection showed new peaks, which were peptide fragments of viral proteins. Third, the eluted peptides were sequenced, to identify shared "anchor residues" corresponding to MHC binding motifs. A fourth method was to pool the eluted peptides and sequence the mixture. Assuming that peptides binding the same MHC groove share a binding motif, amino acid analysis of the non-binding positions might be mixed, but those involved in binding should give a unique amino acid at that position. Such shared anchor residues were indeed found for MHC class I molecules and correspond to the binding motif for the MHC groove.

For example, peptides eluted from the mouse class I molecule H-2 K^d gave more than ten well-resolved peaks, plus many additional minor peaks. The peptides were pooled and sequenced (Fig. 5–13). The resulting sequence showed that most peptides were 9-mers, with variable sequences at seven positions, but fairly strict conservation of amino acids Tyr (or Phe) at position 2 and Ile or Leu at position 9. This motif was also found among peptide epitopes from viruses, tumors, and parasites that were previously known to be presented by H-2 K^d.

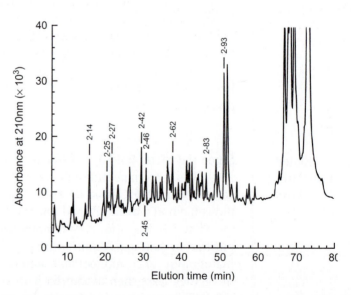

Figure 5–12. Peptides eluted from the binding groove of purified HLA-B27 were separated by high-performance liquid chromatography, and the peak fractions were ready for sequencing (see Fig. 5-14, below). (Modified from Jardetzky, et al.)

	1	2	3	4	5	6	7	8	9	Position / Protein source
Dominant anchor residues		Y							I L	
Strong				N I L	P	M	K F	T N		
Weak	K A R S V T	F	A H V R S F E Q K M T	A E S D H N	V N D I L S T G	H I M Y V R L	P H D E Q S	H E K V V F R		
Known epitopes, aligned	T	Y	Q	R	T	R	A	L	V	Influenza PR8 NP 147–154
	S	Y	F	P	E	I	T	H	I	Self-peptide of P815
	I	Y	A	T	V	A	G	S	L	Influenza JAP HA 523–549
	I	Y	S	T	V	A	S	S	L	Influenza PR8 HA 518–528
	L	Y	Q	N	V	G	T	Y	V	Influenza JAP HA 202–221
	K	Y	Q	A	V	T	T	T	L	P815 tumour antigen
	S	Y	I	P	S	A	E	K	I	*Plasmodium berghei* CSP 249–260
	S	Y	V	P	S	A	E	Q	I	*Plasmodium yoelii* CSP 276–288

Figure 5–13. Peptides eluted from the binding groove of mouse H-2K^d were sequenced without separation. Virtually all the peptides shared sequences at positions 2 and 9, indicating that these residues were important for binding H-2K^d, as anchor residues. The same amino acids were also found on viral peptides recognized by CTLs in association with H-2K^d, as determined by the epitope mapping method shown in Figure 5–6. The single letter amino acid code is used, in which Y= Tyr, I = Ile, L = Leu, N = Asn, P = Pro, M = Met, K = Lys, T = Threo, F = Phe, and A = Ala. (Modified from Falk, et al, 1991.)

Using this method, the shared anchor residues have been determined for other MHC class I binding molecules as well, including H2-, -K^b, and -D^b in the mouse and HLA-A2.1 and -B27 in man. In general, all peptides binding MHC class I are 8 or 9 amino acids long. The second or fifth and the eighth or ninth positions are shared by all the peptides binding a given MHC molecule, but they are unique for each MHC type. Although the anchor residues are conserved, the rest of the peptide sequence can vary widely, allowing many different peptides to bind the same MHC groove, provided they conform to the binding motif. Once an MHC binding motif is known, it can be used to search for as yet unidentified antigenic sites on foreign proteins.

Another example is based on sequencing peptides eluted from HLA-B27 and purified by HPLC (Fig. 5–14). The anchor residues are

Peptides eluted from HLA-B27				Peptide sequence										Source of peptide
	1	2	3	4	5	6	7	8	9					
2–27	R	R	Y	Q	K	S	T	E	L					Human histone H3, H3.3
	R	R	I	K	E	I	V	K	K					Human Hsp89α
2–14	R	R	V	K	E	V	I	K	k					Human Hsp89β
2–83	R	R	W	L	P	A	G	d	a					Human elongation factor 2
2–25a	R	R	S	K	E	I	T	V	R					Human ATP-dependent RNA helicase
2–42	G	R	I	D	K	P	I	L	K					Ribosomal protein (yeast/slime mould
2–62b	F	R	Y	N	G	L	i	H	r					Rat 60S ribosomal protein L28
1–14	K	R	F	E	G	L	T	Q	R					—
2–45	R	R	F	T	R	P	E	H	—					—
2–46	R	R	I	S	G	V	D	R	Y					—
2–62a	A	R	L	F	G	I	R	A	K					—
Viral Peptides														
	S	R	Y	W	A	I	R	T	R					Influenza A nucleoprotein 383–391
	K	R	W	I	I	L	G	L	N	K	I	V		HIV GAG p24 protein 265–276
	G	R	A	F	V	T	I	G	K					HIV gp120 314–322

Figure 5–14. Peptides eluted from HLA-B27 and separated as in Figure 5–12 were sequenced. The same anchor residue (arginine at position 2) was also found on viral peptides discovered by epitope mapping. Many of the self peptides come from indentifiable cellular proteins. In the single letter amino acid code, R = Arg, Y = Tyr, F = Phe, Q = Gln, K = Lys, S = Ser, T = Threo, E = Glu, L = Leu, A = Ala, G = Gly, N = Asn, H = His, and C = Cys. (Modified from Jardetzky, et al.)

Arg at position 2 and Lys or Arg at position 9. These anchor residues, spaced seven amino acids apart, can be used to scan amino acid sequences in search of new antigenic sites likely to bind HLA-B27. Some of these were found on foreign proteins, such as HIV-1 envelope glycoprotein gp120 and influenza virus nucleoprotein, while others derived from cellular proteins (last column of Figure 5–14).

Continuous presentation of self peptides by normal cells may be important for maintaining tolerance to self antigens. But during an infection, processing and presentation of viral proteins activates the immune response. In the case of HLA-B27, something may go wrong with the process of distinguishing self from foreign peptide antigens. This MHC type is closely associated with certain autoimmune diseases, including ankylosing spondylitis (arthritis of the spine) and Reiter's syndrome (arthritis and urethritis with uveitis of the eye). The relative risk of these two syndromes is increased 87- and 37-fold, respectively, for people with HLA-B27, as compared to those lacking HLA-B27. Perhaps the disease could be triggered when foreign peptides bind to HLA-B27 and initiate a T-cell response. Then it may be perpetuated by self peptides, which could direct the response to target organs. According to this hypothesis, the cause and pathogenesis of these diseases may be found among the self and foreign peptides that bind HLA-B27.

MHC molecule	Source of peptide	Peptide sequence	Position	Length
I–A^b	MuLV env protein	H N E G F Y V C P G P H R P	145–158	14
		– – – – – – – – – – – – –	145–157	13
	I–E α chain	A S F E A Q G A L A N I A V D K A	56–73	17
	I–A γ chain	K P V S Q M R M A T P L L M R	39–53	15
	Undefined	X Y N A Y N A T P A T L A V D		15
		– – – D – F – D F – – P T – L		(15)
I–E^b	MuLV env protein	S P S Y V Y H Q F E R R A K Y K	454–469	16
		– – – – – – – – – – – – – – –	454–468	15
		– – – – – – – – – – – – – –	454–467	14
	Bovine serum albumin	G K Y L Y E I A R R H P Y (F)	141–153 (4)	13 (14)
	Undefined	X P Q S Y L I H E X X X I S		14

Figure 5–15. Peptides were eluted from mouse class II molecules (I-A or I-E). Sequences did not reveal shared anchor residues, although in many cases, the protein of origin could be determined. Note that some peptides came from the same site on MuLv envelope protein but were different lengths, suggesting trimming at the carboxyl end. (Modified from Rudensky, et al.)

Applying similar techniques to MHC class II molecules gave a quite different set of eluted peptides (Fig. 5–15). These peptides ranged from 13 to 17 amino acids, longer than peptides bound to class I. The sequences varied more, and anchor residues were not readily apparent. The variability in peptide length suggested that the class II binding site may be groove-shaped, binding peptides from the side and allowing part of the sequence to hang out at either end. In contrast, the class I binding site interacts with peptide at both ends, which forces it to conform to a specific length (8 or 9 amino acids) and fixes the anchor residues at a specified distance from each end. Sequence variability is supported by the crystal structure, which shows class II molecules binding the peptide backbone rather than the ends. This may allow each class II type to bind a greater diversity of peptide antigens, but makes it difficult to assign anchor residues or to predict peptides which will bind a given class II molecule.

By matching the sequences of eluted peptides with known proteins, the protein of origin has been identified for many of the peptides eluted from MHC class II. Although some came from outside the cell, as expected, many others were derived from known intracellular proteins. Based on the protein sequence flanking the peptides, it was anticipated that preferred antigen processing sites could be identified, but, in fact, no consistent processing site was found.

TWO ANTIGEN-PROCESSING PATHWAYS

T cells cannot respond to protein antigens unless they have been processed and presented in the MHC groove of an antigen-presenting cell (APC). Two processing pathways have been distinguished, based on their sensitivity to protease inhibitors or mutations of transport proteins. The two processing pathways, called endosomal and nonendosomal or cytoplasmic, show economy of design, since the immune system has adapted well-established pathways of intracellular protein trafficking in order to process antigens for immune recognition.

Endosomal Processing of Exogenous Proteins

In the endosomal pathway, extracellular proteins, called exogenous antigens, are taken up by endocytosis into early endosomes (Fig. 5–16). Acidification of endosomes activates resident proteases, such as cathepsin D, which partially degrade the foreign proteins into antigenic fragments. As the proteins are cut to smaller fragments, they are also unfolded, exposing the anchor residues for MHC binding.

Meanwhile, MHC class II proteins, following their synthesis on polyribosomes and assembly in the endoplasmic reticulum, travel through the Golgi and enter endosomes. When first assembled, they consist of three chains, called alpha, beta, and invariant chain. The invariant chain apparently binds the other chains and blocks the peptide-binding groove. Invariant chain is removed in the endosomes, and the peptide binding groove is exposed for peptide binding. At this point, MHC can acquire any available peptides and, if the peptide binds stably, the peptide–MHC complex will be transported to the cell surface for presentation to T cells. Thus, producion within endosomes, plus binding affinity for MHC class II determine which peptides will be immunogenic and which will not.

Since endosomal proteases are activated by the acid pH of endosomes, they can be inhibited by weak bases that prevent acidification, such as chloroquine and ammonium chloride. They are also sensitive to the protease inhibitors leupeptin and E-64. Inhibition by these agents is evidence that the protein was processed via the endosomal pathway. In contrast, the nonendosomal pathway uses a different protease and is not sensitive to any of these inhibitors.

Nonendosomal Processing of Endogenous Proteins

Nonendosomal or endogenous processing usually begins when a virus takes over the cell and directs the cell's transcription and translation machinery to synthesize viral proteins. A small percentage of these "endogenously" synthesized proteins are diverted from the cytoplasm for processing by a proteolytic particle, called the proteasome. Proteasomes are assembled from 15 to 20 low-molecular-weight proteins, and they normally function to remove defective or senescent proteins from the cell. During infection, they also degrade a sample of viral proteins that have reached the cytoplasm, producing viral peptides for MHC binding and presentation to T cells (Figure 5–17, lower left).

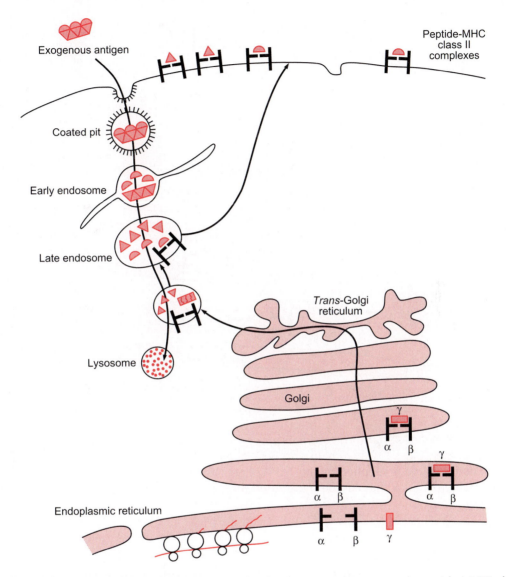

Figure 5–16. Endosomal processing pathway leading to antigen presentation with MHC class II. Class II alpha and beta chains assemble with invariant chain (γ chain) in the endoplasmic reticulum. They are transported to endosomes, where the invariant chain comes off so peptide can bind. They are then transported to the surface with peptide in the binding groove.

However, before they can bind MHC, the peptides must get into the same intracellular compartment as MHC. Newly synthesized MHC class I molecules are held in the endoplasmic reticulum (ER) and wait there until they either bind peptides or are degraded. Thus, it is essential for peptides to be transported from the proteasome to the ER, which requires the activity of a peptide transporter called TAP.

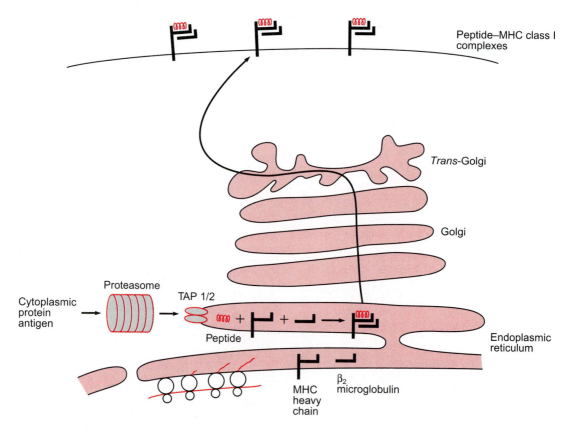

Figure 5–17. Nonendosomal (proteasomal) processing pathway leading to antigen presentation with MHC class I. Class I heavy-chain and beta-2 microglobulin must wait in the endoplasmic reticulum until peptide is supplied by the TAP-1/2 peptide transporter. MHC class I needs peptide to form a stable complex that can be transported through the Golgi apparatus and on to the cell surface.

Most of our information about the transporter comes from two mutant cell lines, called RMA-S and CEM.174, which have a deletion in the MHC class II region that includes the TAP-1 and 2 genes (see Fig. 5–8B) coding for the transporter. The mutants have low expression of MHC class I on the cell surface and fail to present endogenous antigens to T cells. Thus, deletion of the transporter can block MHC class I assembly and transport in uninfected cells, as well as the ability to process and present antigens during infection.

Studying the region of the deletion, Monaco and coworkers found at least four genes that are implicated in the supply of peptides for antigen presentation. Two of these, TAP-1 and -2, closely resemble peptide transport proteins found in other species. Together, they form a heterodimer that transports peptides from the proteasome to the endoplasmic reticulum for MHC class I binding. In normal cells, the supply of self peptides maintains the normal level of MHC class I expression. But mutant cells, which lack the peptide supply factor, fail to transport MHC class I to the cell surface.

The RMA-S and CEM.174 mutants have also deleted two proteins associated with the proteasome. These two proteins, called LMP-2 and -7 (for low-molecular-weight proteins), may play some role in the specificity of proteasomal degradation. During infection, the MHC-encoded proteins function as an elaborate protein processing and peptide transport system, starting with the proteasome (LMP-2 and -7), followed by peptide transport into the ER (TAP-1 and -2) and out to the cell surface (MHC class I heavy and light chains) for presentation to T cells.

The difference between the two processing pathways may be blurred in certain cases. What distinguishes them is the intracellular compartment in which peptide binds to MHC. Exogenous proteins are usually degraded to peptides in the endosomal compartment, where they are taken up by MHC class II molecules. Endogenous proteins are usually degraded in cytoplasmic proteasomes and transported into the ER by TAP-1 and -2 for MHC class I binding. However, exceptions to this simple rule are accumulating, particularly for endogenous proteins presented with MHC class II. This could occur if some endogenous proteins were processed endosomally or if proteasomal peptides could escape the TAP-1 and -2 transporter and reach endosomes instead.

Due to the large number of self peptides, it might be difficult for viral peptides to compete for the available binding sites on MHC class I molecules. Recent studies have shown that viral peptides need to bind only a small fraction of MHC class I molecules, as few as 200 per cell, in order to trigger a T-cell response. This suggests that the immune system may be tuned to respond to virus-sized aggregates of foreign proteins, while ignoring smaller units. This may be important for vaccine design, since particulate antigens such as HBsAg, which contain about 200 copies of HBsAg protein per particle, have 100 times greater vaccine potency than the same amount of HBsAg monomers.

Summary

T cells do not respond to protein antigens directly. Instead, they require partial proteolytic degradation to antigenic peptides. Two processing pathways have been identified: endosomal for exogenous proteins and nonendosomal for endogenous proteins. The endosomal pathway produces peptides for association with MHC class II in endosomes. The proteasomal pathway produces peptides for association with MHC class I in the endoplasmic reticulum, and this requires the function of the TAP-1 and -2 transporter. The peptide–MHC complex is transported to the cell surface for presentation to T cells. Immunogenicity reflects high-affinity binding between a peptide and the peptide binding groove of MHC.

Bibliography

GENETIC CONTROL OF THE IMMUNE RESPONSE

Benacerraf, B. 1978. A hypothesis to relate the specificity of T lymphocytes and the activity of I region-specific Ir genes in macrophages and B lymphocytes. *J. Immunol.* 120:1809.

Rosenthal AS, Shevach EM: Function of macrophages in antigen recognition by guinea pig T lymphocytes. I. Requirement for histocompatible macrophages and lymphocytes. J Exp Med 138:1194, 1973.

Zinkernagel RM, Doherty PC: Activity of sensitized thymus-derived lymphocytes in lymphocytic choriomeningitis reflects immunologic surveillance against altered self components. Nature 251:547, 1974.

T-CELL CLONES

Kappler JW, Skidmore B, White J, Marrack P: Antigen-inducible H-2-restricted, interleukin-2-producing T-cell hybridomas. Lack of independent antigen and H-2 recognition. *J Exp Med* 153:1198–1214, 1981.

Kimoto M, Fathman CG: Antigen-reactive T-cell clones. I. Transcomplementing hybrid I-A-region gene products function effectively in antigen presentation. *J Exp Med* 152:759–770, 1980.

MHC

Baur MP, Neugebauer M, Peppe H, et al.: Population analysis on the basis of deduced haplotypes from random families. In *Histocompatibility Testing 1984,* Albert ED, Baur MP, and Mayr WR (eds.), Springer-Verlag, Berlin, 1984, Berlin 333.

ANTIGENIC PEPTIDES AND EPITOPE MAPPING

Berkower IJ, Kawamura H, Matis LA, et al.: T-cell clones to two major T-cell epitopes of myoglobin: Effect of I-A/I-E restriction on epitope dominance. *J Immunol* 135:2628-2634, 1985.

Lamb JR, Eckels DD, Lake P, et al.: Human T-cell clones recognize chemically synthesized peptides of influenza hemagglutinin. *Nature* 300:66–69, 1982.

Matis LA, Longo DL, Hedrick SM, et al: Clonal analysis of the major histocompatibility complex restriction and the fine specificity of antigen recognition in the T-cell proliferative response to cytochrome c. *J Immunol* 130:1527–1535, 1983.

Streicher H, Berkower IJ, Busch M, et al.: Antigen conformation determines processing requirements for T-cell activation. *Proc Natl Acad Sci USA* 81:6831–6835, 1984.

Unanue ER: Antigen-presenting function of the macrophage. *Annu Rev Immunol* 2:395–428, 1984.

Schwartz RH: T-lymphocyte recognition of antigen in association with gene products of the major histocompatibility complex. *Annu Rev Immunol* 3:237–260, 1985.

Townsend ARM, Rothbard J, Gotch FM, et al.: The epitopes of influenza nucleoprotein recognized by cytotoxic T lymphocytes can be defined with short synthetic peptides. *Cell* 44:959–968, 1986.

PEPTIDE–MHC BINDING

Bjorkman PJ, Saper MA, Samraoui B, et al.: Structure of the human class I histocompatibility antigen, HLA-A2. *Nature* 329:506, 1987.

Buus S, Sette A, Colon SM, et al.: Isolation and characterization of antigen-Ia complexes involved in T-cell recognition. *Cell* 47:1071, 1986.

Buus S, Sette A, Colon SM, et al.: The relation between major histocompatibility complex (MHC) restriction and the capacity of Ia to bind immunogenic peptides. *Science* 235:1353–1358, 1987.

Brown JH, Jardetzky T, Saper MA, et al.: A hypothetical model of the foreign antigen-binding site of class II histocompatibility molecules. *Nature* 332:845–850, 1988.

PEPTIDES ELUTED FROM MHC

Falk K, Rotzschke O, Rammensee HG: Cellular peptide composition governed by major histocompatibility complex class I molecules. *Nature* 348:248, 1990.

Falk K, Rotzschke O, Stevanovic S, Jung G, Rammensee H-G: Allele-specific motifs revealed by sequencing of self peptides eluted from MHC molecules. *Nature* 351:290–296, 1991.

Jardetzky TS, Lane WS, Robinson RA, et al.: Identification of self peptides bound to purified HLA-B27. *Nature* 353:326, 1991.

Rudensky AY, Preston-Hurlburt P, Hong S-C, et al.: Sequence analysis of peptides bound to MHC class II molecules. *Nature* 353:622–627, 1991.

ANTIGEN PROCESSING PATHWAYS

Endosomal Pathway

Germain RN: The ins and outs of antigen processing and presentation. *Nature* 322:687, 1986.

Jin Y, Shih JWK, Berkower I: Human T-cell response to the surface antigen of hepatitis B virus (HBsAg). Endosomal and nonendosomal processing pathways are accessible to both endogenous and exogenous antigen. *J Exp Med* 168:293, 1988.

Morrison LA, Lukacher AE, Braciale VL, et al.: Differences in antigen presentation to MHC class I- and class II-restricted influenza virus-specific cytolytic T-lymphocyte clones. *J Exp Med* 163:903, 1986.

Nonendosomal Pathway

Townsend ARM, Bastin J, Gould K, et al.: Cytotoxic T lymphocytes recognize influenza hemagglutinin that lacks a signal sequence. *Nature* 324:575, 1986.

Townsend ARM, Rothbard J, Gotch FM, et al.: The epitopes of influenza nucleoprotein recognized by cytotoxic T lymphocytes can be defined with short synthetic peptides. *Cell* 44:959–968, 1986.

Transport Proteins TAP-1 and -2

Deverson EV, Gow IR, Coadwell WJ, et al.: MHC class II-region encoding proteins related to the multidrug-resistant family of transmembrane transporters. *Nature* 348:738–741, 1990.

Kelly A, Powis SH, Kerr LA, et al.: Assembly and function of the two ABC transporter proteins encoded in the human major histocompatibility complex. *Nature* 355:641–644, 1992.

Monaco JJ, Cho S, Attaya M: Transport protein genes in the murine MHC: Possible implications for antigen processing. *Science* 250:1723–1726, 1990.

6

The T Cell, Maestro of the Immune System: Receptor Acquisition, MHC Recognition, Thymic Selection and Tolerance

Ira Berkower

T cells acquire the ability to recognize specific epitopes associated with major histocompatibility complex (MHC) molecules through a series of maturation steps in the thymus. Thymocyte precursors originate in the bone marrow and migrate to the thymus, where they develop into mature T cells. The term "T cell" was originally derived from the observation that the T cells disseminated throughout the body came from the thymus and thus were "thymus-derived" or "thymus-dependent" cells. T cells failed to appear if the thymus of certain strains of mice was removed at birth (neonatal thymectomy). When T cells come out of the thymus, they undergo a final maturation step in peripheral lymphoid organs and play a crucial role in immunity, both as T cells functioning to help B cells make antibodies (helper-T cells) and as cytotoxic T cells (CTL) capable of destroying cells infected by a virus. In certain pathological conditions, which render the thymus nonfunctional (see Chapter 27), the absence of mature T cells results in profound cellular immunodeficiency, manifested by increased frequency and severity of infections, particularly those due to intracellular parasites such as viruses, mycobacteria, and certain parasites, as well as inability to reject a foreign skin graft.

T cells may be indentified by characteristic marker proteins on their cell surface (Table 6–1). These cell surface markers include the T-cell antigen receptor (CD3) and the cell phenotype markers CD4 or CD8 defined by monoclonal antibodies specific for these marker proteins. Among mature T cells, CD4 and CD8 are mutually exclusive. Normally, about two-thirds of mature T cells in the blood, lymph

TABLE 6–1. SURFACE STRUCTURES INVOLVED IN ANTIGEN RECOGNITION BY HUMAN T LYMPHOCYTES

Chains		Molecular Weight		Function
		Nonreduced	Reduced	
A. T-cell receptor complex				
α and β		90,000	41,000–43,000 (two chains)	Dual recognition of antigen and MHC
"CD3 complex"	- δ	25,000	25,000	Phosphorylated during cell activation
	- γ	26,000	26,000	Unknown
	- ε	21,000	21,000	Phosphorylated during cell activation
	- ζ	32,000	16,000	" " "
B. CD4		51,000	51,000	MHC class II recognition
C. CD8		76,000	31,000+33,000	MHC class I recognition
D. Protein tyrosine kinases				
Lck		56,000		CD4 and CD8-associated signal transduction
ZAP-70		70,000		TCR-associated signal transduction

nodes, and spleen express surface CD4 (CD4+), whereas the remaining one-third express CD8 on their surface (CD8+) (see Chapter 2).

These two T-cell subsets perform different cellular functions and react with different antigen-presenting MHC molecules. CD4+ T cells respond to antigen presented with MHC class II molecules, whereas CD8+ T cells respond to antigen associated with MHC class I. Generally, CD4+ T cells tend to have a helper function, assisting B cells to make antibodies, whereas CD8+ T cells are cytolytic T cells (CTL), capable of killing infected cells expressing viral antigens in association with MHC class I.

T-cell specificity for antigen and MHC is determined by the T-cell receptor (TCR). As described in the previous chapter, the T-cell receptor is specific for antigen in the form of peptide bound to an MHC protein. Only when presented in this form by an antigen-presenting cell does an antigen elicit a T-cell response. The T-cell antigen receptor forms a complex of six proteins (Fig. 6–1), two of which (TCR α and β chains) have variable regions coding for the antigen plus MHC

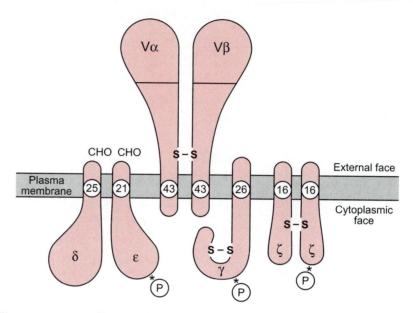

Figure 6–1. T-cell receptor proteins. α and β chains have variable regions that bind antigen plus MHC. γ, δ, and ε chains hold the complex together. The phosphorylated form of ζ binds a tyrosine kinase, which generates the internal signal for T-cell activation.

specificity. To demonstrate this, transfer of transcriptionally active DNA coding for the α and β chains from one T-cell line was able to transfer antigen plus MHC specificity to another T-cell line. The TCR γ, δ, and ε chains, known as the CD3 complex, assemble first, and then add on the α and β chains to form the complete receptor complex. The transmembrane and nearby segments of the CD3 proteins hold the complex together, while the cytoplasmic tails of CD3 and ζ (zeta) are important for receptor signaling. Once the T-cell receptor binds antigen in association with the appropriate MHC structure, the intracellular segments of the CD3 and ζ chains become phosphorylated (see Fig. 6–1) as an important early step in T-cell activation (discussed below).

The TCR α and β chains are like surface immunoglobulin on B cells and must recognize each foreign antigen with a high degree of specificity, despite the tremendous diversity of potential antigens. As with surface immunoglobulin, the TCR is preformed on the T-cell surface before antigen enters the system, and antigen recognition leads to rapid clonal expansion of antigen-specific T cells. The general scheme for generating diversity of the TCR α and β chains is remarkably similar to heavy and light chains of antibodies. Like the immunoglobulin isotypes, there are two types of receptors on the T-cell surface. About

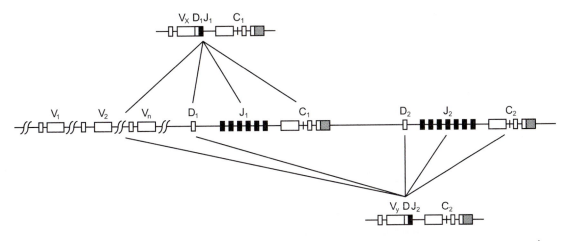

Figure 6–2. Combinatorial joining of V, D, J, and C gene segments to form an active TCR β chain. Two possible gene rearrangements are shown, one above and the other below the germline genes for the β chain.

95% of mature T cells express T-cell receptors with an α and a β chain ($T_{\alpha\beta}$ cells), whereas 5% bear γ- and δ-chain receptors ($T_{\gamma\delta}$ cells). These two groups of T cells are derived from distinct T-cell lineages. The $T_{\gamma\delta}$ cells are found more often in specialized locations, such as the gastrointestinal tract and skin, and are thought to play a role in early immunosurveillance of infections.

As shown in Figure 6–2, the considerable diversity of T-cell receptor V_{β} chains can be generated by recombination between separate variable, diversity, joining, and constant regions. The germline V regions are arranged in tandem, and one of them must recombine with a diversity region, which then recombines with one of the J_{β} regions, to form a transcriptionally active unit. In general, besides forming a contiguous gene, recombination also brings a promoter upstream of the V region into proximity of an enhancer region located near the constant region, causing active transcription of the rearranged gene. Given the seventy variable regions times two D regions times six joining regions for each C region, recombination can generate over a thousand distinct T-cell receptor α and β chains with different specificities (Table 6–2A). This is further greatly increased by junctional diversity, in which new sequences are filled in at the junctions between the V, D, and J regions, in just the right location to produce new contact residues for antigen binding. Altogether, over 10^5 α and β chains can be constructed, and the product of these (10^{10}) gives an upper estimate of the number of different receptor specificities that could be made.

Unlike the surface immunoglobulin on β cells, once the TCR genes have recombined, there is no further somatic mutation. While this may prevent affinity maturation (stronger antigen binding), it may have the important advantage of preventing changes in receptor speci-

TABLE 6–2A. ESTIMATE OF HUMAN TcR REPERTOIRE

	α	β
V	50	70
D	?	2
J	50	13
C	1	2
Combinations	2.5×10^3	3.6×10^3
N sequences added	2.5×10^5	3.6×10^5
$\alpha\beta$ Combinations	Approximately 10^{10}	

TABLE 6–2B. CHROMOSOMAL LOCATIONS OF TCR GENES IN THE HUMAN AND MOUSE

Gene	Human	Mouse
TcR-α	14q11	14C-D
TcR-β	7q32-35	6B
TcR-γ	7p15	13A2-3
TcR-δ	14q11	14C-D

ficity that could lead to autoimmunity after thymic selection has occurred. Similar to immunoglobulins expressed by B cells, T cells show allelic exclusion of V_β chains, so each T cell can express only one V_β chain and has a single antigen specificity. Of the 70 germline V_β genes, each is expressed on between 1% and 10% of all T cells. An extreme example of allelic exclusion occurs in transgenic mice, which have had transcriptionally active T-cell receptor $V\alpha$ and V_β genes inserted into their germ line. Since these mice express the TCR transgenes early in T-cell development, other $V\alpha$ and V_β genes are not expressed, due to allelic exclusion. Thus, virtually every T cell in these mice expresses the $V\alpha$ and V_β chains of the transgene.

The chromosomal location of genes coding for all four variable and constant regions (α or β chains) of the TCR are indicated in Table 6–2 B. Interestingly, the δ-chain locus is contained completely within the variable and constant genes coding for the α chain. One might imagine that prior rearrangement of δ could occur in a precursor T cell, followed by rearrangement of α, with deletion of δ. However, there is no evidence for gene switching between these two subsets. Instead, they appear to represent distinct T-cell lineages, starting in the thymus.

T-cell receptor V_β chains can be stimulated by a special type of antigen called a superantigen. To trigger T cells, these superantigens must first bind to MHC class II of the antigen-presenting cell, but they do not require antigen processing. Then they bind the TCR V_β chain, regardless of the antigen specificity of the V_β chain. By binding all T cells bearing a particular V_β chain, superantigens can activate an entire T-cell subset at once. Certain bacterial toxins, such as staphylococcal enterotoxin A, act by stimulating all murine T cells bearing V_β1, 3, 10, 11, and 17 (Table 6–3). Others, such as toxic shock syndrome toxin TSST-1, induce massive release of cytokines by stimulating all T cells with V_β2, resulting in the toxic shock syndrome. The hallmarks of superantigen-induced T-cell stimulation are (1) lack of antigen processing; (2) flexible MHC requirements; (3) stimulation of all mature T cells with a particular V_β chain, regardless of antigen specificity; and (4) ability to delete all immature thymocytes of the same V_β type.

Thymic Maturation

When they first migrate from the bone marrow to the thymus, precursor cells do not express the major CD markers and have the surface phenotype CD3⁻, CD4⁻, CD8⁻. Over the next five days, as they traverse the thymus from the outer cortical layers to the inner medulla, they become immature thymocytes and then mature T cells ready to leave the thymus. Technically, the term "T cell" means **thymus-derived cell** and should be used only for cells that have left the thymus as mature T cells. Thymic maturation of T-cell precursors is reflected in changes in their cell surface markers. First, the cells acquire both CD4 and CD8, becoming CD4⁺, CD8⁺ (called double-positive) thymocytes. These changes can be measured by staining the cells with two fluorescent antibodies, such as a green fluorescent monoclonal antibody against CD4 and a red fluorescent monoclonal antibody specific for CD8. The cells are then analyzed for red or green fluorescence (or both) in a fluorescence-activated cell sorter. As each cell passes through a beam of laser light, its fluorescence is analyzed for the two colors corresponding to antibodies against CD4 and CD8.

As shown in Figure 6–3, by plotting CD4 fluorescence on the Y axis and CD8 fluorescence on the X axis, each cell can be placed in one

TABLE 6–3. TcR-V_β SPECIFICITIES OF BACTERIAL SUPERANTIGENS

Toxin	V_β specificity	
	Mouse	Human
Staph enterotoxin A	1, 3, 10, 11, 17	1.1, 5, 6, 7.3-7.4, 9.1
Staph enterotoxin B	7, 8.1–8.3	3, 12, 14, 15, 17, 20
Staph enterotoxin C1	3, 8.2, 8.3, 11	3, 6.4, 6.9, 12, 15
Toxic Shock Toxin1	15, 16	2

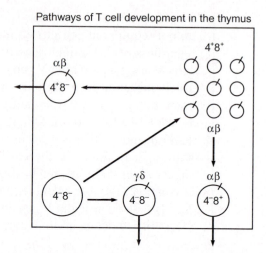

Pathways of T cell development in the thymus

Figure 6–3. Pathways of T-cell development as measured by double immunofluorescence analysis of immature T cells. Each cell is stained with a red-colored monoclonal antibody to CD4 and a green-colored monoclonal antibody to CD8, and its fluorescence measured in both channels simultaneously. The green CD8 signal is plotted on the X axis versus the red CD4 signal plotted on the Y axis. The four quadrants in the figure, representing the four possible combinations of red and green fluorescence, correspond to the stages of T cell maturation. Immature thymocytes (lower left) start as CD4$^-$CD8$^-$ and become CD4$^+$CD8$^+$ and express TCR. These "double-positive" cells are selected for receptor specificity, and the survivors become CD4$^+$CD8$^-$ or CD4$^-$CD8$^+$ mature T cells, which are ready for release from the thymus. (Modified from von Boehmer, 1988).

of four quadrants, depending on its surface phenotype. In this way, thymic maturation can be followed as a progression from one quadrant to another. Immature double-negative thymocytes begin in the left lower quadrant (CD4$^-$, CD8$^-$). In the first maturation step, these cells progress from the lower left quadrant to the upper right quadrant, as they become double-positive (CD4$^+$, CD8$^+$) immature thymocytes. In the second maturation step, thymocytes develop a mature single-positive phenotype, either (CD4$^+$, CD8$^-$) or (CD4$^-$, CD8$^+$). Graphically, they move from the upper right quadrant into either the upper left quadrant (CD4$^+$, CD8$^-$) or the lower right quadrant (CD4$^-$, CD8$^+$). Most thymocytes (80%) are immature double positives, whereas only 15% are mature single positives, ready to leave the thymus, and the remainder are double negative.

In thymic organ culture, double-positive cells appear first, and single positives come later. In addition, pretreatment with antibodies to CD8 can reduce the number of single positives of both phenotypes (CD4$^+$ CD8$^-$ as well as CD4$^-$ CD8$^+$), suggesting that even CD4$^+$ CD8$^-$ mature T cells derive from double-positive thymocytes.

At the double-positive step, thymocytes begin to express the antigen receptor CD3, first at a lower level and later at the same level as mature T cells. Since this is the T cell receptor for antigen plus MHC, its specificity is important in determining whether the maturing thymocytes will retain CD4$^+$ and respond to antigen with MHC class II or retain CD8$^+$ and respond to antigen plus MHC class I. In addition, now that their antigen receptor is expressed, the maturing thymocytes can be rigorously selected according to their antigen specificity, so only those maturing thymocytes with acceptable specificity will be released to the periphery as mature T cells.

Thymic Selection

To ensure that T cells will be able to distinguish between foreign and self-protein antigens, maturing thymocytes are subjected to both positive and negative selection (Fig. 6–4). Positive selection allows thymocytes specific for foreign antigen plus self-MHC to proliferate and mature. In contrast, negative selection deletes any thymocytes that respond to self-antigen plus MHC; in this way, self-reactive T cells are eliminated before they can initiate autoimmune reactions.

Positive selection expands clones of thymocytes capable of recognizing foreign peptides bound to MHC. How the thymus can anticipate foreign antigens for positive selection is unclear. Perhaps it may synthesize a specialized set of generic peptides capable of binding the MHC groove and stimulating a variety of thymocytes with diverse TCRs, which are actually specific for foreign antigens. As mimics of foreign peptides, these thymic peptides could bind MHC tightly but the T-cell receptor weakly. Alternatively, thymic MHC could be modified to bind the TCR, regardless of peptide specificity, as occurs with superantigens. Unfortunately, neither generic peptides nor superantigens have yet been detected in the thymus.

Once released to the periphery, these positively selected T cells must recognize foreign peptides plus self-MHC with considerable specificity. Somehow, positive selection must generate T cells with sufficient diversity to respond to the enormous variety of foreign peptide antigens. Lacking positive selection, T cells that don't respond to antigen plus self-MHC will die in the thymus, perhaps due to lack of essential trophic factors.

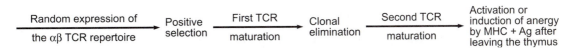

Figure 6–4. Thymic selection. Each thymocyte must be positively selected, usually at the double-positive stage, in order to mature further. If self-reactive, it will be eliminated by negative selection.

In some respects, positive selection resembles the proliferative response of mature T cells to antigen plus MHC, as described in the previous chapter. During thymic maturation, blocking MHC class II with monoclonal antibodies will prevent positive selection of thymocytes specific for this MHC, just as it blocks proliferation of mature T cells. But, unlike the recognition of antigens by mature T cells, thymocytes may rely more on MHC binding and less on the peptide in the groove. Alternatively, positive selection by a thymic superantigen would have to stimulate only those V_β receptors that bind self MHC, which is not the case with peripheral T cells. And, unlike the known superantigens, it would have to expand, rather than delete, immature thymocytes.

Negative selection occurs by clonal deletion and results in the death of T-cell precursors with undesirable specificity. About 50 million immature cells are produced each day in the thymus cortex, but only two million (4%) become mature T cells for release to the periphery; most of the loss is believed to be caused by negative selection. Though inefficient, the combination of T-cell precursor generation and destruction may be necessary, in order to generate the required diversity of antigen receptors, while avoiding self-reactivity.

Negative selection of self-reactive thymocytes may be a logical necessity, but the exact mechanism is unclear. For those thymocytes reacting to self-antigens, antigens expressed on thymic epithelium or macrophages may simply trigger cell death. However, this model contains the implicit assumption that antigen presentation to the same T-cell receptor that normally triggers activation in mature T cells will instead cause death of immature T cells. It is unclear how the same T-cell receptor could deliver different signals at each stage in maturation.

Clearly, for both positive and negative selection to work together, most of the cells positively selected at one step must not be negatively selected at the other. One way to avoid this would be if the two selection steps were based on different affinities for self-MHC. Thus, if high-affinity binding to self-antigens caused negative selection, whereas positive selection would accept either high- or low-affinity binding, then only those cells with relatively low affinity for self-MHC would survive both processes. Alternatively, if positive and negative selection occurred simultaneously, rather than sequentially, positive selection would guarantee survival. Two illustrative examples follow, the first involving negative selection of T cells expressing $V_\beta 17$ by an endogenous superantigen, and the second involving positive selection in females of thymocytes specific for the male H-Y antigen plus H-2^b.

NEGATIVE SELECTION

One type of negative selection of thymocytes involves clonal deletion by endogenous superantigens. Superantigens are proteins capable of V_β-specific T-cell stimulation in the periphery or V_β-specific clonal deletion (negative selection) in the thymus. They were originally found among the bacterial toxins, such as the toxic shock syndrome toxin TSST-1 produced by certain staphylococci. These toxins bind to and activate all peripheral T cells with a particular V_β gene, regardless of their antigen specificity (see Table 6–3). In many ways, this specificity is analogous to staphylococcal protein A, which binds all immunoglobulins of the IgG1, 2, and 4 subclasses, regardless of antibody specificity. In contrast to peripheral T cells, immature thymocytes bearing the same V_β are killed by exposure to a superantigen. Thus, the absence of a given V_β among peripheral T cells suggests negative selection in the thymus.

Similarly, endogenous superantigens can cause deletion of all T cells expressing a particular V_β chain. For example, a superantigen that binds the mouse MHC class II antigen I-E was found to delete all T cells expressing the $V_\beta 17a$ chain. As shown in the top panel of Figure 6–5, BALB/c mice, which express I-E, have undetectable levels of T cells expressing $V_\beta 17a$. In contrast, strain SJA mice, which lack I-E,

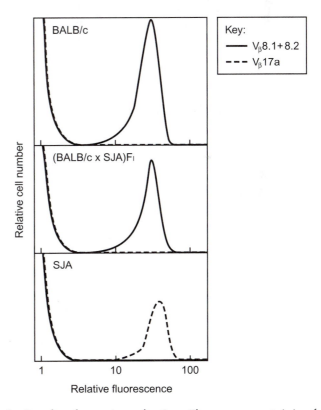

Figure 6–5. Results of negative selection. Fluorescence staining for $V_\beta 17a$ (dotted line) or $V_\beta 8.1$ & 8.2 (solid line) shows that $V_\beta 17a$ T cells are eliminated by negative selection in BALB/c mice (top panel). But in SJA mice, which lack the I-E needed by the superantigen, they survive thymic selection and appear in the peripheral circulation (bottom panel). In the (BALB/c X SJA) F1 hybrid, negative selection is dominant (middle panel). (Modified from Kappler, et al).

express a much higher level of $V_\beta 17a$ (Fig. 6–5, bottom panel). The middle panel of Figure 6–5 illustrates that when BALB/c animals are mated with strain SJA, the (BALB/c X SJA) F1 progeny, which are I-E$^+$, have virtually no T cells expressing $V_\beta 17a$. Thus, deletion of $V_\beta 17a$ T cells recognizing I-E and the superantigen was inherited in F1 animals as a dominant trait.

To determine which developmental stage is affected by negative selection, immature cells in the thymus of these animals were analyzed for CD4, CD8, and $V_\beta 17a$ expression. Among immature double-positive thymocytes, surface expression of $V_\beta 17a$ was the same for two strains, despite differences in I-E expression. But among the single-positive (CD4$^+$, CD8$^-$) mature thymocytes, expression was normal in the I-E negative strain but low in the strain expressing I-E. Thus, negative selection by the superantigen plus I-E must occur after the double-positive stage, since double-positive thymocytes are allowed to express the undesirable V_β gene. They are not, however, allowed to mature into single-positive thymocytes. Negative selection may either block maturation, or it may eliminate cells with undesirable specificity as soon as they reach maturity.

What kinds of self antigens act as superantigens, capable of clonal deletion in the thymus? Several endogenous superantigens have been identified as protein products of retroviruses inherited in the mouse germline. As shown in Table 6–4, endogenous mouse mammary tumor viruses 1 and 6 (mmtv-1 and -6) are inherited on chromosomes 7 and 16, respectively. Mouse strains inheriting these viruses delete their T cells expressing $V_\beta 3$, 5, and 17. Because these superantigens must bind I-E for T-cell activation, clonal deletion also depends on I-E expression. Thus, deletion of $V_\beta 17$ cells, described above, was at first thought to be due to I-E itself, but in fact is due to an I-E-dependent virally coded superantigen.

Besides deleting their own immature T cells with certain V_β chains, lymphocytes from animals expressing endogenous superanti-

TABLE 6–4. MOUSE V_β SELECTION BY ENDOGENOUS SUPERANTIGENS DUE TO MOUSE MAMMARY TUMOR VIRUS

Superantigen	Mouse V_β selection	Mammary tumor virus	Chromosome
Mls-1[a]	6, 7, 8.1, 9	7	1
Mls-2[a]	3, 17	1	7
Mls-3[a]	3, 5, 17	6	16
Mls-2[a]-like	3	13	4
vSAG-3	3	3	11
Etc-1, DVβ11-2	5.1, 5.2, 11, 12, 17	9	12
DVβ11-1	11, 12, 17	8	6
DVβ11-3	11, 12	11	14

gens can also stimulate proliferation of mature T cells from other mouse strains, which lack the superantigen and fail to delete T cells with this reactivity. When first discovered, this phenomenon was described as minor lymphocyte-stimulating antigens: Mls-a, -b, and -c. All three Mls antigens were subsequently shown to be superantigens produced by endogenous mmtv's inherited in the mouse germ line (see Table 6–4). If similar agents exist in man, they could limit TCR expression by thymic deletion in some individuals and contribute to the observed differences in immune responses to infection and vaccination. Alternatively, lack of thymic expression of superantigens in other individuals could produce partial self-tolerance, resulting in autoimmunity in those cases where incomplete clonal deletion permitted survival of self-reactive T cells.

POSITIVE SELECTION

One successful approach for studying positive selection is to make a transgenic mouse by inserting the α and β chain genes for a functional T-cell receptor into the germline of an immunodeficient mouse, such as the severe combined immune deficient (SCID) mouse. These mice are incapable of forming their own T-cell receptors, due to a genetic defect in rearranging either the TCR α and β genes or the immunoglobulin genes. This defect is manifested by a severe immunodeficiency affecting both T cells and B cells. By inserting the rearranged TCR genes for both Vα and V_β chains, T cells will reappear in these animals, and every T cell will have the specificity of the inserted TCR genes. In this way, von Boehmer was able to study mice that expressed a TCR of known specificity for antigen and MHC. The TCR gene came from a female T-cell line responding to the male H-Y antigen. This TCR was also specific for the MHC type (H-2^b) of the female donor. Since the TCR genes were already rearranged, they could be expressed in spite of the SCID defect. Also, since SCID mice have no T-cells of their own, the transgenic mice became, in effect, monoclonal T cell producers. Thus, thymic selection in these mice operates on T cells sharing the same TCR specificity.

By breeding the TCR transgenic mice with other strains, thymic selection could be studied under a variety of conditions. Positive selection should occur in female mice of the H-2^b type, whereas negative selection should occur in male mice of the same H-2 type. T-cell development without positive or negative selection could be examined in female mice of a different H-2 type (H-2^d). As before, the CD4 and CD8 markers were followed through maturation in each thymic environment. In Figure 6–6, the Y axis shows surface CD4; the X axis shows CD8 expressed on the same cells. Immature double-positive thymocytes are found in the upper right quadrant. Mature T cells should appear in the lower right quadrant (CD4$^-$, CD8$^+$), since the TCR genes came from a mature T cell of this phenotype.

As shown in Figure 6–6A, female H-2^b mice gave a normal distribution of T cells bearing the TCR specific for H-Y. Immature double-positive thymocytes appeared first, and these matured into single-positive CD4$^-$CD8$^+$ T cells (lower right). Thus, given a functionally rearranged TCR gene, SCID mice had the ability to mature and select normal T cells. In contrast, in female mice of the wrong H-2 type (H-2^d), positive selection did not occur, as shown by the lack of mature T cells bearing the receptor (Fig. 6–6C lower right). Although immature double-positive T cells formed, they never matured further, and single-positive T cells were not produced. Thus, positive selection is not needed to reach the double-positive stage, but is required for double-positive thymocytes to progress to single-positive mature T cells. Clearly, the TCR participates in this step, since selection depends on thecorrect H-2 (MHC) type. But the selecting antigen remains unknown, since H-2^b females would not be expected to have a surrogate H-Y peptide.

Figure 6–6B, shows negative selection of the H-Y specific TCR in male H-2^b mice. Since in these mice H-Y is a self-antigen, these self-reactive T cells must be clonally deleted to prevent an autoimmune reaction. As shown by the lack of cells in the upper right quadrant, not even immature double-positive T cells of this specificity are detected. This result indicates that negative selection occurs at the double-positive step, probably as soon as the T-cell receptor is expressed. If any T cells reach the double-positive stage, they are eliminated as quickly as they appear. Alternatively, they may never reach this stage. In contrast to these results, clonal deletion due to endogenous superantigens allows double positives to appear, but blocks them from becoming mature T cells (compare Fig. 6–5). This difference may represent stronger negative selection by a cellular antigen as compared to a superantigen.

Negative selection produces self tolerance through clonal deletion. Since it occurs in the thymus, it is called "central" tolerance. Because the undesirable T cells are eliminated, the tolerance is irreversible. Negative selection is more than the lack of positive selection, as shown by the difference between Figures 6–6B and 6–6C. In the absence of positive selection, lack of necessary trophic factors may result in T-cell death after the double-positive step (6C). But negative selection appears to be an active process, blocking the appearance of double-positive thymocytes or removing them as fast as they form (6B). Although clonal deletion is a durable form of tolerance, it is not the only mechanism to prevent a T-cell response to self-antigens.

Peripheral Tolerance

Even if self-reactive T cells manage to escape thymic selection, there is a second mechanism to tolerize these cells in the periphery and to prevent a serious autoimmune reaction. When self-reactive T cells contact self-antigens in the periphery, they often become anergic, ie, unre-

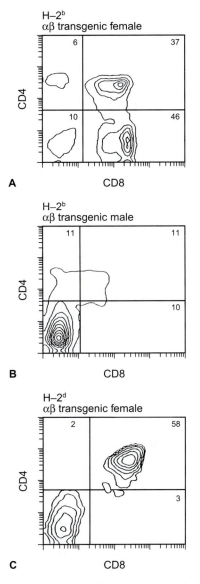

Figure 6–6. Thymic selection of T cells specific for the male H-Y antigen. TCR α and β genes specific for H-Y antigen plus H-2^b were introduced into a transgenic mouse. Thymocytes were analyzed for maturation and selection in a variety of environments, which would favor positive or negative selection. **A.** Positive selection in an H-2^b female. The T cells mature all the way to CD4$^-$CD8$^+$ T cells. Numbers in each quadrant indicate the percentage of cells in that quadrant. **B.** Negative selection in an H-2^b male. In this case, H- Y is a self-antigen, and T cells bearing the transgenic TCR would be self-reactive. Therefore, they are deleted, and no double-positive thymocytes appear. **C.** Lack of positive selection in a female of a different H-2 type, H-2^d. In this animal, H-Y- specific T cells reach the double-positive stage but fail to mature further. (Modified from von Boehmer, 1990).

sponsive to antigen. The anergic state appears to result when self antigen plus MHC are presented by cells lacking additional features of the "professional" antigen-presenting cells. Once anergized, the T cell may remain unresponsive for up to two months. But, unlike central tolerance, the T cell survives, so peripheral tolerance is not permanent and may be reversed over time if the T cell is not continuously exposed to the tolerizing antigen.

An example of peripheral tolerance is provided by an experimental model designed to induce autoimmune diabetes. SJL mice, which do not express the MHC class II molecule I-E, are given I-E as a transgene expressed under the transcriptional control of the insulin promoter. Because insulin is normally expressed only in the islet cells of the pancreas, these mice express I-E in this tissue only. Since I-E is not expressed in the thymus, central tolerance to I-E cannot be acquired, and the negative selection of certain V_β chains by I-E dependent superantigens (as described above) would not occur. This absence of thymic selection would allow I-E-reactive T cells to mature and leave the thymus as single-positive T cells. Then, on reaching the pancreas, they would be expected to reject I-E as a foreign antigen, and cause inflammation and islet cell destruction leading to diabetes. Despite the potential for autoimmune diabetes, however, pancreatic inflammation did not occur.

Instead of being stimulated, these self-reactive T cells were anergized. Their inability to reject I-E$^+$ islet cells was not due to thymic deletion of I-E-reactive T cells. In fact, the V_β17a T cells, which would be deleted by an I-E$^+$ thymus (see strain 107-1 in Table 6–5), were present in normal numbers in the Ins-I-E transgenic mice, comparable to the I-E$^-$ SJL controls (Table 6–5). These T cells would be expected to reject the I-E$^+$ pancreatic cells, but instead, they are anergized. Anergy to I-E antigen was further demonstrated by grafting the I-E transgenic animals with skin from I-E$^+$ animals. The skin grafts were not rejected. However, over time, as expression of the I-E transgene reached toxic levels, the pancreatic cells expressing I-E died off, leaving the animals without I-E. About 30 days later, tolerance was broken, and the skin grafts were rejected. The results indicated that V_β17a T cells were there all along but remained anergized as long as I-E was expressed. Unlike thymic tolerance, peripheral tolerance can be lost when T cells recover from the anergic state.

Induced anergy has been proposed as a treatment for chronic autoimmune conditions, in which tissue damage appears to be caused by self-reactive T cells, possibly reflecting a lack of self-tolerance. Viral infections may trigger an autoimmune response, arising from a temporary loss of self-tolerance. For example, in juvenile onset diabetes, viral infection is suspected of triggering a T-cell response to pan-

TABLE 6–5. T CELLS BEARING I-E-SPECIFIC RECEPTORS ARE NOT DELETED IN INS-I-E TRANSGENIC MICE

Mouse	I-E expression	Percent $V_\beta 17a^+$ T cells
SJL	None	9.7
Ins-I-E Transgenic	Pancreatic β cells, kidney	8.3
107-1	Normal	2.2

creatic islet beta cells, leading to insulitis and permanent loss of islet cells. In theory, if these T cells could be anergized to the appropriate self-antigens, the disease process might be halted and further tissue damage prevented, until normal anergy could be restored by continuous exposure to self-antigens.

T-cell Activation

The T-cell antigen receptor (TCR) consists of six different proteins. The α and β chains have both variable and constant regions, and, like antibodies, the variable regions determine specificity. But the α and β chains have short cytoplasmic tails, so they are not capable, by themselves, of triggering the cellular response to antigen. Instead, they rely on the CD3 chains (γ, δ, and ε) and the ζ chains to transmit a signal across the plasma membrane (Fig. 6–7A). These chains interact with enzymatic machinery on the cytoplasmic side of the membrane to generate intracellular activation signals. During T cell activation, the cytoplasmic tails become phosphorylated at specific sites suggesting the activity of a receptor-associated protein tyrosine kinase. In each of these chains, activation motifs have been identified, consisting of a pair of Tyr-X-X-Lys sequences, and the ζ chain has three of these motifs in tandem (indicated as boxes in Fig. 6–7A). Two tyrosine kinases, p56^{lck} and ZAP-70, appear to be directly involved in CD3 and ζ-chain phosphorylation and the generation of the intracellular activation signal.

p56^{lck} is a member of the src family of protein tyrosine kinases. Typically, the amino half of the protein sequence contains src homology sequences, called SH2 and SH3, while the carboxyl half contains the catalytic site. Other sequences near the amino terminus form the binding site for CD4 and CD8. Up to 90% of the p56^{lck} molecules are bound to CD4 in a CD4$^+$ T cell. Together, CD4 plus p56^{lck} form a combined receptor for MHC class II, with CD4 providing the ligand-binding function, and p56^{lck} generating the signal once ligand has bound (Fig. 6–7B). Similarly, CD8 and p56^{lck} form a combined receptor for MHC class I in CD8$^+$ T cells. When other proteins are brought near to CD4 or CD8 during antigen recognition, they can be phospho-

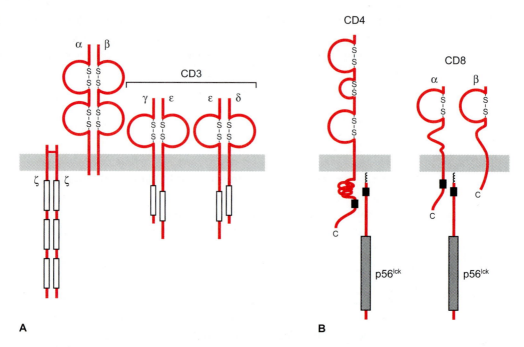

Figure 6–7 **A.** Structure of the TCR proteins, showing activation motifs on the cytoplasmic tails of the γ, δ, ε, and ζ chains. **B.** Structures of CD4 and CD8, showing binding sites for association with the tyrosine kinase p56^{lck} to link MHC binding with signal generation. (Modified from Weiss and Rudd).

rylated by p56^{lck}. The importance of p56^{lck} in signal transduction is shown in mutant cell lines, which are unable to be activated via the TCR, and in genetic knockout mice lacking the p56^{lck} gene, which show a failure of thymic maturation to double positive thymocytes.

A second src kinase, ZAP-70, is also critical for TCR-mediated cell activation. This protein tyrosine kinase also has two src homology-2 domains and a catalytic domain, and it binds ζ chains as well as the CD3 chains. Binding increases in activated T cells, apparently because ZAP-70 has greater affinity for the phosphorylated ζ chains. Together, these two protein kinases may work together in an integrated model of T-cell receptor-mediated cell activation.

As the antigen presenting cell approaches the T-cell surface (Fig. 6–8, left), peptide plus MHC are bound both by the TCR α and β chains and by CD4. Binding brings the CD4-p56^{lck} receptor close to the CD3 plus ζ complex, providing a substrate for the p56^{lck} protein kinase. In the second step, the phosphorylated CD3 and ζ chains induce binding of ZAP-70 kinase (Fig. 6–8, right), which is then activated by p56^{lck}. ZAP-70 then phosporylates downstream effectors, which activate the entire cell. Presumably, this process would occur each time a T cell encounters antigen plus MHC throughout its life, starting with primary immunization, and including the activation of B cells by helper T cells, as described in Chapter 7. It may also occur during thymic maturation, although negative selection suggests the possibility that a different internal signal may be generated, producing clonal deletion.

A genetic defect in ZAP-70 has recently been described in humans by Weiss, et al. Homozygous patients have a form of severe combined immunodeficiency, causing a defect in T cells, as well as antibody formation. In these patients, the mutated ZAP-70 was unstable, depriving T cells of detectable ZAP-70 protein or function. As expected, peripheral T cells lacked the ability to signal via the TCR, measured as loss of response to either mitogens or antibodies that crosslink the TCR. In contrast, receptor-independent cell activation, via phorbol ester and calcium ionophore, was normal. Thymic maturation of CD8+ T cells was blocked. Surprisingly, however, normal numbers of mature CD4+ T cells were produced, suggesting the possibility that other protein kinases, such as syk or fyn, may supply this function during thymic development of CD4+ cells. However, once they

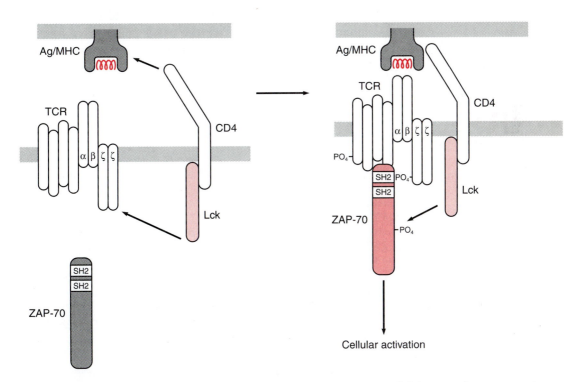

Figure 6–8. Antigen plus MHC binding brings CD4- associated p56lck kinase close to its substrate in the activation motifs of CD3 and ζ chains. These phosphorylated proteins then bind ZAP-70 kinase and trigger cellular activation. (Modified from Weiss).

matured, these T cells were unable to function without ZAP-70, and the result was a profound T-cell deficiency syndrome, despite normal numbers of CD4[+] T cells.

The complexities of TCR signaling may allow the response of activated T cells to fit the stimulus. In addition, certain signals may be responsible for a specific step in T-cell maturation, such as thymic selection or peripheral tolerance, while others may be used for a variety of responses by differentiated mature T cells.

Summary

T-cell specificity for antigen plus MHC resides in the T-cell receptor and is augmented by CD4 affinity for MHC class II or CD8 affinity for MHC class I of the antigen-presenting cell. During thymic development, immature T cells progress from CD4[−]CD8[−] (double-negative) to CD4[+]CD8[+] (double-positive) thymocytes and then become single-positive (CD4[+]CD8[−] or CD4[−]CD8[+]) mature T cells before leaving the thymus. Positive selection in the thymus, based on receptor specificity, is required for cells to progress through these steps. Negative selection operates on self-reactive cells at the double-positive thymocyte stage and eliminates them or prevents further maturation. In addition, any self-reactive T cells that manage to leave the thymus may become unreactive (anergic), through a process of peripheral tolerance. After binding antigen plus MHC, the T cell receptor generates a signal for T-cell activation, through the combined functions of two protein tyrosine kinases, p56^{lck} and ZAP-70.

Bibliography

THYMIC TOLERANCE

Blackman M, Kappler J, Marrack P: The role of the T-cell receptor in positive and negative selection of developing T cells. *Science* 248:1335, 1990.

Fowlkes BJ, Schwartz RH, Pardoll DM: Deletion of self-reactive thymocytes occurs at a CD4[+]8[+] precursor stage. *Nature* 334:620–623, 1988.

Kappler JW, Roehm N, Marrack P: T-cell tolerance by clonal elimination in the thymus. *Cell* 49:273–280, 1987.

Kisielow P, Bluthmann H, Staerz UD, et al.: Tolerance of T-cell receptor transgenic mice involves deletion of nonmature CD4[+]8[−] thymocytes. *Nature* 333:742, 1988.

von Boehmer H: The developmental biology of T lymphocytes. *Ann Rev Immunol* 6:309–326, 1988.

von Boehmer H: Developmental biology of T cells in T-cell receptor transgenic mice. *Ann Rev Immunol* 8:531–556, 1990.

PERIPHERAL TOLERANCE

Lo D, Burkly LC, Flavell RA, et al.: Tolerance in transgenic mice expressing class II major histocompatibility complex on pancreatic acinar cells. *J Exp Med* 170: 87–104, 1989.

Miller JFAP, Morahan G, Allison J: Extrathymic acquisition of tolerance by T lymphocytes. *Cold Spring Harbor Symp* 54:807, 1989.

SUPER-ANTIGENS

Abe R, Hodes RJ: T-cell recognition of minor lymphocyte stimulating (Mls) gene products. *Ann Rev Immunol* 7:683–708, 1989.

Choi Y, Kappler JW, Marrack P: A superantigen encoded in the open reading frame of the 3′ long terminal repeat of mouse mammary tumor virus. *Nature* 350:203, 1991.

Dyson PJ, Knight AM, Fairchild S, et al., Genes encoding ligands for deletion of Vβ11 T cells cosegregate with mammary tumor virus genomes. *Nature* 349:531–532, 1991.

Frankel WN, Rudy C, Coffin JM, Huber BT: Linkage of Mls genes to endogenous mammary tumor viruses of inbred mice. *Nature* 349:526–528, 1991.

Kotzin BL, Leung DYM, Kappler J, et al., Superantigens and their potential role in human disease. *Adv Immunol* 54:99, 1993.

Marrack P, Kushnir E, Kappler J: A maternally inherited superantigen encoded by a mammary tumor virus. *Nature* 349:524–526, 1991.

White J, Herman A, Pullen AM, et al.: The Vβ-specific superantigen staphylococcal enterotoxin B: Stimulation of mature T cells and clonal deletion in neonatal mice. *Cell* 56:27–35, 1989.

T-CELL ACTIVATION

Elder ME, Lin D, Clever J, Chan AC, Hope TJ, Weiss A, Parslow TG: Human Severe Combined Immunodeficiency Due to a Defect in ZAP-70, a T Cell Tyrosine Kinase. *Science* 264:1596–1599, 1994.

Rudd CE: CD4, CD8 and the TCR-CD3 complex, A novel class of protein–tyrosine kinase receptor. *Immunology Today* 11:400–406, 1990.

Weiss A: T-cell antigen receptor signal transduction: A tale of tails and cytoplasmic protein–tyrosine kinases. *Cell* 73:209–212, 1993.

7

How T Cells Help B Cells Make Antibodies

Ira Berkower

Processing of antigens by antigen-presenting cells (APC) and interactive signaling between T cells and B cells are required for antibody responses to T-dependent antigens. The antibody-producing cell is a B cell derived from bone marrow precursors. As B cells mature, they express surface immunoglobulin (sIg), which can be detected by staining the cells with fluorescent antibodies to immunoglobulin. This membrane-bound form of Ig serves as the antigen receptor of the B cell, which will ultimately synthesize and secrete antibodies of the same specificity. As described in the immunoglobulin chapter, due to gene rearrangement, each B cell is committed to a single antibody specificity well before it encounters the antigen. Once antigen appears, antigen-specific B cells undergo rapid and selective clonal expansion, in order to produce antibodies of suffcent quality and quantity to fight infection. Thus, control of B-cell activation is a central strategy of the immune response to foreign antigens.

Adoptive Transfer of T cells and B cells

Antigen-driven B-cell activation depends on help provided by T cells. This requirement was first observed in adoptive transfer experiments, in which cells from immune donor animals were transferred to a non-immune recipient. As shown in Figure 7–1, if T cells were from a donor immunized with bovine gamma globulin (BGG), and B cells were from a second donor immunized with dinitrophenol (DNP) bound to a different protein, then both cell types were required for the recipient animal to produce anti-DNP antibodies in response to the combined antigen DNP-BGG. Without BGG-immune T cells, the transferred B cells could not respond by themselves, and no anti-DNP antibodies were made.

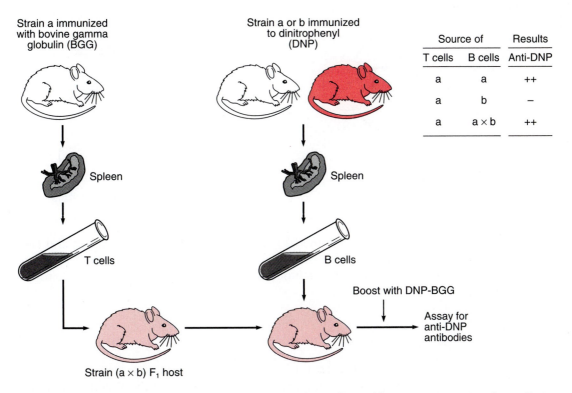

Source of		Results
T cells	B cells	Anti-DNP
a	a	++
a	b	–
a	a × b	++

Figure 7–1. Adoptive transfer of carrier BGG-primed T cells and hapten DNP-primed B cells into an MHC–compatible host. Subsequent immunization with the conjugate DNP–BGG results in antibodies due to T-cell–B-cell collaboration. However, T-cell help requires MHC matching with the B cell (insert).

Although the T cells and B cells recognized different parts of the antigen, they could still cooperate to produce antibodies. The part of the combined antigen recognized by B cells is called the hapten (DNP), and the part recognized by T cells is the carrier protein (BGG). Both parts must be covalently attached, not simply mixed together, in order to elicit a response. The first plausible interpretation of these results was that the combined antigen held together the T and B cells by forming an "antigen bridge" (Fig. 7–2A), so that "helper" factors secreted by the T cell could migrate across and activate the B-cell response.

Besides demonstrating the antigen specificity of each cell type, adoptive transfer also allowed the testing of T and B cells from strains of mice with different MHC types. As shown in the insert of Figure 7–1, the B cells only made antibodies when they matched the MHC type of the helper-T cells. This indicates direct contact between the two cells and could be explained as dual recognition of both antigen and MHC by T cells. As we now know, the T-cell receptor can respond to

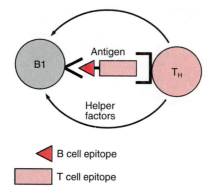

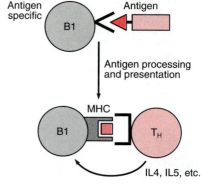

A. 'Traditional' antigen bridge model of T cell help   B. Antigen presentation model of T cell help

Figure 7–2. **A.** Traditional antigen bridge model of T-cell help. Explains why hapten and carrier must be covalently attached. **B.** Antigen presentation model of T-cell help. B cell takes up the antigen via hapten-specific surface Ig. B cell then processes and presents peptide fragments plus MHC to the T cell.

antigen only after it is processed to antigenic fragments and presented by the MHC of the presenting cell, which is the B cell. The need for MHC compatibility is explained by the T-cell receptor's specificity for self MHC.

The results can be explained by the antigen presentation model of T-cell/B-cell help (Fig. 7–2B). In this model, surface immunoglobulin serves as a high-affinity receptor for antigen binding to specific B cells. Antigen is internalized by endocytosis, followed by partial degradation to peptide fragments in endosomes. Those peptides which bind MHC class II are transported to the B-cell surface for presentation to helper-T cells. When the T-cell receptor binds this antigen plus MHC complex, the T cell is triggered to produce a variety of cytokines needed for B-cell activation and differentiation. This model is supported by the observation that B cells function as efficient antigen-presenting cells and can stimulate T-cell proliferation and cytokine secretion, even at low antigen concentrations. Only those B cells with antigen-specific surface immunoglobulin would take up sufficient amounts of antigen to elicit T-cell help.

According to the model, covalent linkage between hapten and carrier is not needed to hold the two cells together via an antigen bridge (Fig. 7–2A), but simply allows both hapten and carrier determinants to enter the B cell together (Fig. 7–2B). In the experiment shown in Figure 7–1, DNP-BGG is taken up by a DNP-specific B cell via its surface anti-DNP immunoglobulin. Partial degradation produces BGG peptides for presentation on the surface of the B cell. Helper-T cells specific for these BGG peptides then respond by releasing helper factors as well as providing contact-mediated help. Since antigen recognition by the two cells is sequential, the B cell can respond to native antigen prior to processing, while the T cell responds to denatured fragments after processing. In this way, the antigen receptors of both cells contribute to the specificity of the response. The more they stimulate T cells, the greater the help B cells will receive.

ACTIVATION SIGNALS

B cell activation signals can be divided into three types. Signal 1 is generated when surface Ig binds the antigen. This signal is particularly important for T-independent antigens, such as bacterial polysaccharides. These antigens can activate B cells directly by crosslinking surface Ig, without antigen processing or presentation to T cells. Antigen valency is important for crosslinking, so polymers are more likely to activate B cells this way.

For protein antigens, however, B cells rely on T cell help. Signal 2 is contact-mediated help, whereas signal 3 is mediated over a short distance by soluble cytokines, such as interleukin-2 and interleukin-4 secreted by helper-T cells.

CONTACT-MEDIATED HELP

Direct contact between the helper-T cell and B cell permits bimolecular interactions to occur at the cell surface (Fig. 7–3). Some of these simply hold the two cells together, whereas others confer antigen specificity or transmit activation signals. As described earlier, each cell contributes to specificity via its antigen receptor. The B cell internalizes and processes antigen based on specific binding to surface Ig. Then, the processed peptides must bind MHC for antigen presentation. Finally, T cell receptor binding of peptide plus MHC leads to activation of T cell help.

Cell adhesion molecules (see Chapter 8), such as LFA-1 on the T-cell surface and ICAM-1 on the B cell, hold the two cells together without contributing to antigen specificity. Similarly, CD2 on the T cell binds LFA-3 on the B cell and stabilizes the pair. But the interaction between CD40 on the B cell and a T cell surface molecule called CD40 ligand (CD40L) provides an essential activation signal for resting B cells (Table 7–1 and Fig. 7–3). CD40 ligand is a 39-KD molecule that is induced on activated T cells but absent from resting T cells. Once expressed, CD40L is quite stable, surviving cell fixation with paraformaldehyde or even cell fractionation, when membrane fractions are prepared from activated T cells. The CD40L sequence shares homology with other cytokines, such as tumor necrosis factor-alpha (TNF-alpha). Thus, CD40L functions as a T-cell membrane-bound cytokine with potent B-cell activating properties.

The B-cell receptor for this signal is CD40. It has a molecular weight of 45 to 50 KD and resembles the receptor for tumor necrosis

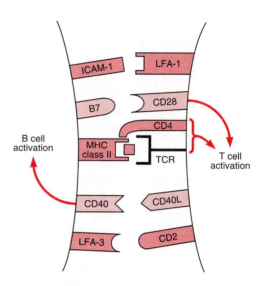

Figure 7–3. Interactions at the T-cell–B-cell interface. Some are antigen specific, such as TCR binding MHC plus peptide. Others are MHC-specific, such as CD4 binding MHC class II. Other interactions are stimulatory, such as CD40L binding CD40 and B7 binding CD28. Finally, some simply help hold the two cells together, such as ICAM-1 and LFA-1 or LFA-3 and CD2.

factor. When CD40L binds its receptor on B cells, and in cooperation with IL-4 (see below), it activates B cells for clonal expansion and stimulates immunoglobulin class switching. In this process, the B cell switches from producing surface IgM to secreted IgG, A, or E by rearranging its immunoglobulin variable gene with a different constant region. However, it retains its original antigen specificity by keeping the same variable region.

In the X-linked inherited immunodeficiency known as hyper-IgM syndrome, the B cells begin to make IgM antibodies but fail to progress through class switching, so they make increased amounts of IgM but no IgG or IgA. Recently, the mutation has been mapped to the gene for CD40L. This defect in T-cell help can be corrected by culturing a patient's B cells in the presence of normal T cells. Thus, CD40L provides an essential signal for B cells to switch from IgM to the other Ig classes.

In the normal lymph node (Fig. 7–4B), antigen specific B cells respond to antigen by forming germinal centers. Within these germinal centers, under nearly continuous T-cell help, B cells proliferate rapidly and switch classes from IgM to IgG, IgA or IgE. They also show affinity maturation, in which they accumulate point mutations in the immunoglobulin variable region genes, allowing the production of

TABLE 7–1. B-CELL ACTIVATION SIGNALS

Signal 1: Antigen bound to surface Ig

Signal 2: Contact Mediated Help

Surface Protein	MW	Found on	Function
B7	44–54 KD	B cells	Binds CD28
CD28	44 KD	T cells	Activates T cell
CD40	45–50 KD	B cells	Activates B cell
CD40L	39 KD	T cells	Binds CD40

Signal 3: Cytokines

Soluble Factor	MW	Produced by	Receptor	Effect
IL-2	15 KD	Th1 cell	55, 70, 64 KD	Growth factor
IL-4	20 KD	Th2 cell	140, 64 KD	Growth factor Ig class switch
IL-5	30 KD	Th2 cell	140, 70 KD	IgA production

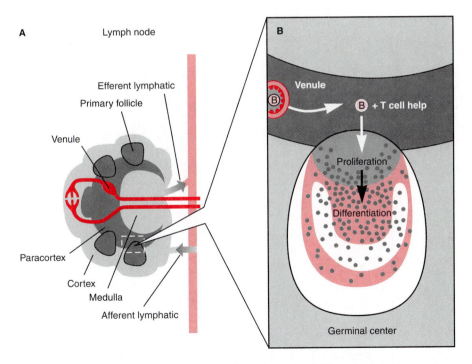

Figure 7–4. Germinal centers form in lymph nodes when dendritic cells bearing antigen meet antigen-specific T cells and B cells. Activated helper T cells express CD40L and stimulate proliferation of antigen-specific B cells. As they progress through the germinal center, these cells mature through class switching and affinity maturation (modified from Clark, et al).

antibodies with progressively higher affinities. But in the hyper-IgM syndrome the normal architecture is lost. Without CD40 ligand, germinal centers do not form, and class switching and affinity maturation cannot occur.

A second activation signal results when CD28 protein on the T-cell surface (a 44-KD homodimer) binds B7 protein on the surface of activated B cells. But in this case, the direction of activation is reversed, as the B cell activates the helper T cell to proliferate and release cytokines needed for further B-cell development. This stimulatory effect (Fig. 7–5) sets up a potential feedback loop in each helper T-cell/B-cell pair. Activation signals flow in both directions, causing the T cells to proliferate and release more cytokines, as the B cells also proliferate and undergo class switching.

Besides T-cell help, the germinal center has two types of resident antigen-presenting cells that provide continuing antigen stimula-

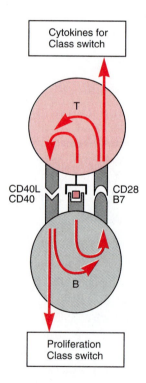

Figure 7–5. Feedback stimulation between activated helper-T cell expressing CD40L and activated B cells expressing B7. Stimulatory signals flow in both directions, resulting in T cell production of cytokines. The B cell responds to CD40L plus cytokines by proliferating and by activating class switching (modified from Clark, et al).

tion throughout the immune response. When antigen first appears, it can be taken up by specialized phagocytic cells in the skin, called Langerhans' cells. Besides processing the antigen, these cells are mobile and transport antigen to the lymph node. Once they arrive in the lymph node, where they are called dendritic cells, these cells present antigen to T cells. The activated helper-T cells express CD40L and stimulate antigen-specific B cells through contact-mediated help and through cytokine production. The collaboration between T cell and B cell results in germinal center formation and provides essential stimuli for B cells to undergo class switching and affinity maturation.

Germinal centers also provide prolonged antigen stimulation of B cells over time. The lymph node follicles contain follicular dendritic cells, which bind antigen in the form of antigen–antibody complexes and may trap and retain antigen for weeks to several months. These cells remain in close association with B cells throughout their stay in germinal centers and provide a continuous supply of antigen. This antigen may stimulate B cells directly, by crosslinking surface immunoglobulin, or indirectly, by supplying antigen for presentation to helper-T cells. The ongoing helper effects may be essential for establishing long-term B-cell memory.

SOLUBLE HELPER FACTORS

Activated T cells release cytokines that play a crucial role in B-cell proliferation and differentiation to antibody-secreting cells (see Table 7–1). The first to be discovered was called B-cell stimulatory factor 1, now known as interleukin-4 (IL-4). This 20-KD protein diffuses from helper-T cells to the IL-4 receptor found on resting and activated B cells.

IL-4 has multiple effects on B cells, including increased expression of MHC class II and co-stimulation of B-cell proliferation. But the most striking effect of IL-4 is to induce class switching. In this process, the variable region of surface immunoglobulin is retained, while the constant region is changed from IgM to the other immunoglobulin classes. This preserves the antigen specificity, while changing from membrane-bound IgM to secreted antibodies with a variety of biologic activities. Class switching can be demonstrated in cell culture, where B cells stimulated by the mitogen lipopolysaccharide (LPS) can be switched from making IgM exclusively to IgG1 or IgE by adding IL-4. Under these conditions, the IL-4 effect can be directly antagonized by interferon. In turn, interferon elicits its own signal for class switching, but directs the B cells to produce IgG2a instead. The physiological importance of IL-4 in class switching can be demonstrated in vivo, since mice pretreated with monoclonal anti-IL-4 fail to make an IgE antibody response to parasites.

Several important lessons can be learned from IL-4. Each T cell can secrete more than one cytokine, usually in a pattern, and one cytokine may have multiple effects on the same cell. Thus, IL-4 may act on a B cell to induce MHC class II expression, enhance B-cell proliferation, and trigger Ig class switching. Once resting B cells have been activated by antigen, the multiple effects of IL-4 may combine to move them along the scheme shown in Fig. 7–6 to become antibody secreting cells producing IgG and IgE. Alternatively, IL-5 can switch these cells to IgA production. Because it has early and late effects on B cells, IL-4 affects switching to all the other Ig classes, besides IgE. Thus, cytokines such as IL-4 and IL-5 have the potential to control the production of IgG antibodies to viral and bacterial pathogens, IgE antibodies to allergens, and IgA antibodies for mucosal immunity.

Any cell that expresses the IL-4 receptor can respond to it, and different cells may respond in different ways. Thus, in addition to B cells, a subset of T cells depend on IL-4 as a growth factor. The pattern of cytokines produced, including IL-4, serves as an important marker distinguishing two types of helper-T cells.

The first type, called Th1, secretes interleukin-2 (IL-2) and interferon γ (IFN), but not IL-4. In contrast, the second type (Th2) secretes

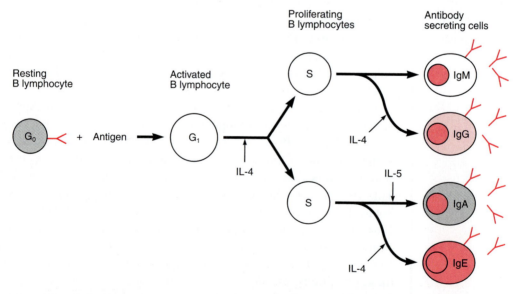

Figure 7–6. Cytokines released by the T cell activate resting B cells (with surface Ig) and lead them through the scheme of proliferation and differentiation to become antibody secreting cells, producing each class of immunoglobulins.

IL-4 and IL-5, but not IL-2 or IFN. Both types secrete IL-3 and granulocyte–monocyte colony-stimulating factor (GM-CSF). Originally used to characterize mouse T-cell lines, these T-cell phenotypes are considered important in regulating the B-cell response to antigens as manifested by the different Ig classes produced.

For example, if some people have increased numbers of IL-4 producing Th2 helpers, they may be more likely to develop allergies: excess IL-4 could increase class switching to produce more IgE in response to allergens. Alternatively, a relative lack of interferon producing Th1 cells could also account for this, since the direct antagonist effect of IFN against IL-4 would be reduced. Finally, since Ig class switching depends on the combined signals from CD40L and IL-4, and both are inducible on activated T cells, it is also possible that increased IgE may simply reflect increased T-cell activation in allergy prone individuals. Further delineation of how different T-helper cell subsets affect the type of immune response is given in the introduction to Part II, immunopathology (see II-5).

How a Vaccine Works

For most successful vaccines, collaboration between the helper-T cell and B cell is a crucial step in generating protective levels of antibodies in virtually all vaccine recipients. To induce high antibody levels, it is often necessary to prime and boost one or more times with vaccine antigen. A typical response to primary immunization and boosting is shown in Figure 7–7. Primary immunization elicits antibodies after a lag time of 10 to 14 days. These are mostly of the IgM class and have low titer and affinity.

After a rest period of four or more weeks, secondary immunization gives a more rapid "memory" antibody response within 7 to 10 days, and the antibody titer generally increases greatly, by two logs or more. These antibodies differ qualitatively as well as quantitatively from the primary response. They are of the IgG class and have greater affinity for the antigen than in the primary response. Subsequently, an infectious challenge will elicit a rapid increase in antibodies resembling the secondary response in titer, immunoglobulin class, and affinity.

These observed serologic phenomena of immunization can be explained in terms of the underlying cellular responses to antigen. During the primary immunization, the few antigen-specific T cells and B cells must quickly expand their numbers through clonal selection. Since antigen-specific helper-T cells are scarce at this time, helper-T function is limiting. Without contact help or IL-4, B cells fail to form germinal centers, so little class switching or affinity maturation occurs. Thus, primary immunization elicits mainly IgM antibodies of low-to-moderate affinity.

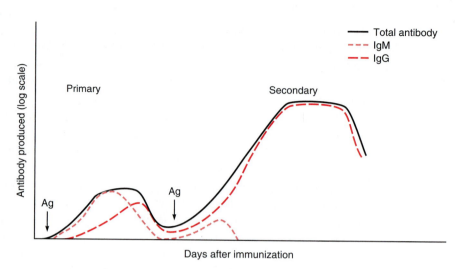

Figure 7–7. Antibody class switching during primary and secondary immunizations. Priming elicits IgM antibodies of low affinity. During the secondary immunization, B-cells receive abundant T-cell help under optimal conditions for class switching from IgM to IgG production and maturation to high affinity antibodies.

But primary immunization greatly expands the number of antigen specific helper-T cells. By the secondary immunization, primed B cells respond to antigen in the presence of excess T-cell help. These B cells increase rapidly and produce a corresponding rise in the level of specific antibodies. Under the influence of T-cell help, both contact mediated help and cytokines such as IL-4, antigen-specific B cells mature in germinal centers, where they switch from IgM to IgG or IgA. Somatic mutation of V-region genes, followed by selective growth, yields B cells producing antibodies with progressively greater affinity for the antigen. While some B cells are actively dividing, others enter a resting phase that can last for decades. Upon subsequent infection, these "memory" B cells can be quickly activated to produce high titers of IgG antibodies with high affinity for the antigen.

VACCINE DESIGN

For many pathogens, the first infection elicits durable immunity against subsequent infections. In such cases, it should be possible for vaccines to elicit protective immunity by eliciting neutralizing antibodies comparable to those found after infection. In designing such a vaccine, the two most important issues are (1) identifying the major neutralizing sites (the target of neutralizing antibodies) and (2) achieving sufficient vaccine potency to elicit protective levels of neutralizing antibodies in virtually all vaccine recipients. While the first issue depends primarily on the virus or pathogen, the second depends on the ability of vaccine antigens to mobilize T cells and B cells to collaborate in producing a vigorous immune response.

NEUTRALIZING SITES

Most antibodies to viral proteins are ineffective for neutralizing the virus. Relatively few sites on the virus are neutralizing sites, which perform essential viral functions that are susceptible to antibodies binding nearby. For example, the neutralizing sites on a viral envelope protein may perform an essential envelope function, such as binding to a host cell receptor, fusing with the cell membrane to allow viral entry, or uncoating inside the cell. By binding these sites, antibodies can neutralize the virus either by blocking an essential function or by triggering a change in the virus. For example, neutralizing antibodies against poliovirus trigger a conformational change that closely parallels inactivation.

A variety of approaches have been used to locate and characterize the major neutralizing sites of a virus. In the case of influenza virus, these sites were found by combining epidemiologic data with data from the research laboratory. Influenza is highly mutable. Its hemagglutinin protein, a predominant target of neutralizing antibodies, accumulates mutations from one year to the next in a process called antigenic drift. Some years, this random process yields a virus variant that escapes from the antibodies that neutralized earlier influenza strains. This results in a new influenza epidemic among previously infected populations, whose antibodies no longer protect them. Epidemiologic studies of these variants indicate that a limited number of point mutations can account for the epidemics, due to escape from neutralizing antibodies directed at these sites.

As shown in Figure 7–8, the accumulated mutations accounting for the decade 1977 to 1986 can be mapped to a few nearby sites on the three-dimensional structure of hemagglutinin. As shown, the sites are generally close to the receptor-binding site of hemagglutinin, at the top of the figure. Quite often, these sites consist of residues that are far apart in the primary sequence, but are brought together by the three-dimensional folding of the protein, and these are called "conformational sites." For a vaccine antigen to elicit neutralizing antibodies to these sites, the correct protein folding is just as important as the correct sequence.

A second approach was to generate "escape mutants" in the laboratory, using a panel of neutralizing monoclonal antibodies specific for hemagglutinin. Virus was grown in the presence of a lethal amount of antibody. Since each antibody binds a single neutralizing site, it applies enormous selective pressure on the virus to escape neutralization by mutating at this site. When surviving viruses were detected, they were analyzed for mutations in the hemagglutinin gene. The neutraliz-

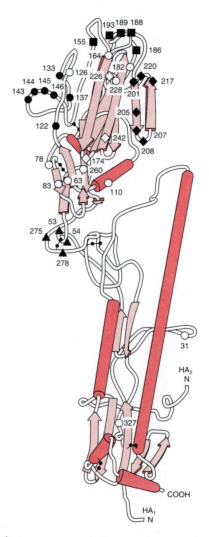

Figure 7–8. Neutralizing sites on influenza hemagglutinin are indicated by solid symbols. Residues forming each conformational site share the same symbol. Hemagglutinin structure based on X-ray crystallography (modified from Wiley, et al).

ing sites identified by "artificial selection" agreed with those observed among the naturally selected strains causing influenza epidemics. These sites are important to vaccine design, because just as the virus changes from year to year, so must the vaccine. Changes affecting neutralizing sites may herald a new epidemic of influenza.

Some viruses, such as human immunodeficiency virus-1 (HIV-1), mutate even more quickly than influenza, varying from one subject's isolate to another. However, variation per se is not proof of selection by neutralizing antibodies. As appreciated by Darwin, random variation is necessary, but not sufficient for evolution. The second step is selection of variants, in this case for escape from neutralizing antibodies. This could occur if virus reinfected a previously immune person. Otherwise, it is premature to conclude that variation in HIV-1 is anything more than random variation produced by a promiscuous reverse transcriptase. This hypothesis could be tested, if an effective vaccine can be found, as the vaccinees become exposed to live virus.

In contrast to variants generated by escape mutation or random variation, stable differences may be found among different isolates of the same virus. For example, the many strains of poliovirus fall within three serotypes. Within a serotype, antibodies to one strain will neutralize all members of the same serotype. But these antibodies do not neutralize members of another serotype. To be effective, a vaccine must contain at least one representative of each serotype, and each serotype should be given on more than one occasion.

IMMUNOGE-NICITY

The second major issue is immunogenicity or vaccine potency. This can be particularly important when the group at risk of serious infection is unable to respond to the neutralizing determinant in its native form. For example (Fig. 7–9A), meningitis due to *Hemophilus influenzae* occurs most often in children between two months and two years of age. Younger babies are protected by maternal antibodies, and older children develop natural immunity. As with many other bacteria, neutralizing antibodies are directed at the polysaccharide capsule surrounding the bacteria. But young children are unable to respond directly to the polysaccharide. Because the antigen is multivalent, B cells should respond without T-cell help. But the T-independent response is weak in young children, so another way had to be found to elicit antibodies to the bacterial polysaccharide.

CONJUGATE VACCINES

The solution was to enlist T-cell help to increase the response to polysaccharides in young children. Although the capsular polysaccharide was T-independent by itself, it was converted to a T-dependent antigen by covalent coupling to a protein carrier. As explained above (Fig. 7–2B), during immunization, the conjugate is taken up by B cells specific for the polysaccharide. The B cells process and present the antigen to helper-T cells specific for the carrier protein. These T cells then provide contact help and cytokines needed by B cells to make antibodies to the polysaccharide. Thus, a conjugate vaccine allows collaboration between T cells and B cells, even though each cell responds to a different antigenic component of the conjugate.

The advantages of conjugate vaccines include flexibility in choosing a highly immunogenic carrier protein. Babies as young as two to six months could respond to the polysaccharide in the conjugate, although they were unable to respond to the polysaccharide by itself (Fig. 7–9B). A theoretical disadvantage of conjugate vaccines is that

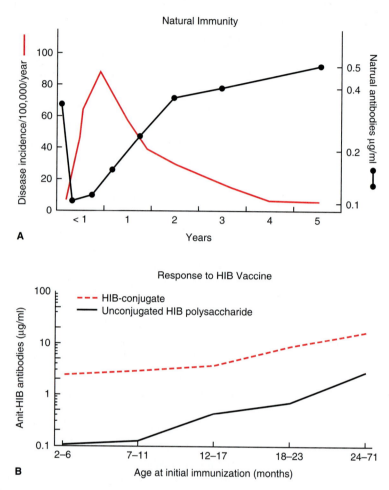

Figure 7–9. **A.** Incidence of *H. influenzae* meningitis (in red) during the first five years of life and the corresponding level of anticapsular antibodies (in black). Most disease occurs in the first two years of life, after maternal antibodies have waned, but before natural exposure has elicited antibodies in the baby. **B.** Response to Hib conjugate vaccine. Unlike the free polysaccharide, the conjugate elicits high-titered anticapsular antibodies at an early age, when protection is needed (modified from Peltola, et al and Ahonkhai, et al).

natural exposure may not boost immunity, since the carrier protein is missing from the pathogen. This is not a problem for Hemophilus influenza b vaccine however, since older children can respond to the polysaccharide alone.

MULTIMERIC ANTIGENS

A second way to enhance immunogenicity is to assemble a virus-sized particles consisting of multiple copies of the antigen. Examples include killed virions, such as inactivated poliovirus, or self-assembling proteins, such as hepatitis B virus surface antigen or hepatitis B core protein. The surface antigen particles contain about 200 proteins each and are up to 1,000 times more immunogenic than the same weight of monomers. Recently, a possible explanation for this phenomenon has appeared. Demotz and Sette found that the minimum number of peptide–MHC complexes on an antigen-presenting B cell or macrophage needed to trigger a T-cell response was around 100 to 300 complexes per cell. This suggests that the immune system may be tuned to respond to "virus-sized" particles, and that particulate antigens may be more immunogenic because they exceed the threshold for T-cell stimulation. These findings suggest that the immunogenicity of recombinant protein monomers could be enhanced by polymerization to form 100-mers.

Other novel vaccines under development include synthetic peptides corresponding to the neutralizing sites on viral proteins. Advantages include ease of synthesis, purity and safety. However, peptides lack the native conformation, so they could not elicit antibodies to conformational neutralizing sites. In addition, a single peptide vaccine may fail to immunize an entire population, since it is unlikely to bind all MHC types, and MHC binding is an essential step in eliciting T-cell help.

Summary

T-cell/B-cell collaboration is a sequential process, starting with antigen recognition on the B cell surface, followed by antigen-presentation to the helper T cell. The T cell provides help via direct contact and also secretes diffusible cytokines. Under the influence of T-cell help, the B cell proliferates and activates class switching, and affinity maturation within the germinal centers of lymph nodes. In order to achieve protection, a vaccine must elicit significant levels of antibodies to the neutralizing determinants of the pathogen. Vaccine potency depends on cooperation between T cells and B cells to elicit a high level response in virtually all vaccine recipients.

Bibliography

B-CELL PRESENTATION MODEL OF T-CELL/B-CELL HELP

Chesnut RW, Colon SM, Grey HM: Requirements for the processing of antigen by antigen-presenting cells. I. Functional comparison of B-cell tumors and macrophages. *J Immunol* 129:2382–2388, 1982.

Chesnut RW, Grey HM: Studies on the capacity of B cells to serve as antigen-presenting cells. *J Immunol* 126:1075–1079, 1981.

Gershon RK: T-cell control of antibody production. *Contemp Top Immunobiol* 3:1, 1974.

Michison NA: The carrier effect in the secondary response to hapten-protein conjugates. II. Cellular cooperation. *Eur J Immunol* 1:18, 1971.

CONTACT-MEDIATED HELP

Allen RC, Armitage RJ, Conley ME, et al.: CD40 ligand gene defects responsible for X-linked hyper-IgM syndrome. *Science* 259:990, 1993.

Aruffo A, Farrington M, Hollenbaugh D, et al.: The CD40 ligand, gp39, is defective in activated T cells from patients with X-linked hyper-IgM syndrome. *Cell* 72:291–300, 1993.

Clark, EA, Ledbetter JA: How B and T cells talk to each other. *Nature* 367:425–428, 1994.

June CH, Ledbetter JA, Linsley PS, et al.: Role of the CD28 receptor in T-cell activation. *Immunology Today* 11:211, 1990.

Korthauer U, Graf D, Mages HW, et al.: Defective expression of T-cell CD40 ligand causes X-linked immunodeficiency with hyper-IgM. *Nature* 361:539, 1993.

Mayer L, Kwan S-P, Thompson C, et al.: Evidence for a defect in "switch" T cells in patients with immunodeficiency and hyperimmunoglobulinemia M. *New Engl J Med* 314:409–413, 1986.

SOLUBLE HELPER FACTORS

Mosmann TR, Coffman RL: TH1 and TH2 cells: Different patterns of lymphokine secretion lead to different functional properties. *Ann Rev Immunol* 7:145–173, 1989.

Paul WE: Pleiotropy and redundancy: T-cell derived lymphokines in the immune response. *Cell* 57:521–524, 1989.

VACCINE DESIGN

Ahonkhai VI, Lukacs LJ, Jonas LC, et al.: *Haemophilus influenzae* type b conjugate vaccine (meningococcal protein conjugate) (Pedvax-HIB™): clinical evaluation. *Pediatrics* 85:676–681, 1990.

Cabral GA, Marciano-Cabral F, Funk GA, et al.: Cellular and humoral immunity in guinea pigs to two major polypeptides derived from hepatitis B surface antigen. *J Gen Virol* 38:339–350, 1978.

Demotz S, Grey HM, Sette A: The minimal number of class II MHC antigen complexes needed for T-cell activation. *Science* 249:1028–1030, 1990.

Harding CV, Unanue ER: Quantitation of antigen-presenting cell MHC class II/peptide complexes necessary for T-cell stimulation. *Nature* 346:574–576, 1990.

Mandel, B. (1979): Interaction of viruses with neutralizing antibodies. In: *Comprehensive Virology 15: Viral–Host Interactions*, edited by H. Fraenkel-Conrat and R.R. Wagner, Chap. 2. Plenum, New York.

Milich DR, McLachlan A, Thornton GB, et al.: Antibody production to the nucleocapsid and envelope of the hepatitis B virus primed by a single synthetic T-cell site. *Nature* 329:547, 1987.

Peltola H, Kayhty H, Sivonen A, et al.: *Haemophilus influenzae* type b capsular polysaccharide vaccine in children: A double-blind field study of 100,000 vaccinees 3 months to 5 years of age in Finland. *Pediatrics* 60:730–737, 1977.

Wiley, D.C., Wilson, I.A., and Skehel, J.J. (1981): Structural identification of the antibody-binding sites of Hong Kong influenza haemagglutinin and their involvement in antigenic variation. *Nature*, 289:373–378.

Wilson, I.A., Cox NJ: Structural basis of immune recognition of influenza virus hemagglutinin. *Ann Rev Immunol* 8:737–771, 1990.

8

Acute Inflammation

Inflammation is the primary process through which the body repairs tissue damage and defends itself against infection. Inflammation may be initiated by either immune or nonimmune pathways, but both pathways employ similar effector mechanisms. Nonimmune inflammation is initiated by injury, or by release of bacterial products or components of dying tissue cells. Immune inflammation is initiated by a specific reaction of immunoglobulin antibody or sensitized T lymphocytes with antigen. The *in vivo* effects of immune inflammation are determined by amplification mechanisms that are also components of nonimmune inflammatory processes. These amplification mechanisms, rather than the specific immune reaction alone, are largely responsible for the tissue lesions actually observed.

ACUTE INFLAMMATION

The function of acute inflammation is to deliver plasma and cellular components of the blood to extravascular tissues. The extravasation of plasma fluid into tissue (edema) causes dilution of toxic materials and increases lymphatic flow. Phagocytic blood cells infiltrate inflamed tissue, destroy infectious agents, clear the tissue of necrotic debris and release cytokines that activate healing.

CHRONIC INFLAMMATION

The function of chronic inflammation is to "heal" the lesion produced by the acute inflammation by clearing the site of the products of acute inflammation and replacing damaged tissue. At later stages, fibrosis may occur, which serves to wall off foci of dead tissue or infection. As a physiologic response to injury, inflammation clears and restores damaged tissue; as a pathologic process, inflammation produces tissue damage (lesions). General inflammatory mechanisms will now be

TABLE 8–1. PHASES OF INFLAMMATION

Stimulus	Response			Healing and Repair
Initiating event ------->	Acute vascular ------------> Response (minutes)	Acute cellular ------------> Response (hours)	Chronic cellular ------------> Response (days)	Scarring (Granulation tissue) Resolution (weeks)
Trauma, ---------------> necrosis, infection	Vasodilation, ---------> increased vasopermeability (hyperemia, edema)	Neutrophil ------------> infiltrate (pus)	Mononuclear ---------> cell infiltrate*	Fibrosis or clearing

* Lymphocytes, macrophages, and plasma cells.

described in this and the next chapter; their pathogenic effects in mediating immune-activated lesions will be presented under the different immunopathologic mechanisms discussed in the chapters that follow.

The phases of tissue inflammation are given in Table 8–1. The following sequence of events occurs during an inflammatory response: (1) Increased blood flow (vasodilation) preceded by transient vasoconstriction, (2) increased vascular permeability leading to edema (vasopermeability), (3) infiltration by polymorphonuclear neutrophils, (4) infiltration by lymphocytes and macrophages (chronic inflammation), leading to (5) resolution (restoration of normal structure) or (6) scarring (filling in of areas of tissue destruction by fibroblasts and collagen) (see Fig. 8–1). The first three events are considered acute inflammation; the latter three stages, chronic inflammation.

INITIATION OF INFLAMMATION

Inflammation is initiated by trauma, tissue necrosis (death), infection, or immune reactions. The immediate response is a temporary vasoconstriction. The mechanism for this is not well understood but is believed to be mediated by the sympathetic nervous system. This is followed within seconds by the acute vascular response resulting in increased blood flow (hyperemia) and edema. If there has been only mild injury, such as caused by stroking the skin, the inflammatory process may be limited to this phase only. However, if there is sufficient cell death or infection the acute cellular phase will follow. Changes in blood flow lead to **margination** of neutrophils next to endothelial cells, followed by **emigration** of neutrophils into the adjacent tissue. Margination is recognized by the lining up of neutrophils along the endothelium of vessels. Emigration occurs by passage of inflammatory cells between endothelial cells. Contraction of endothelial cells also causes leakage (diapedesis) of red blood cells, which may progress to hemorrhage if there is necrosis of endothelial cells.

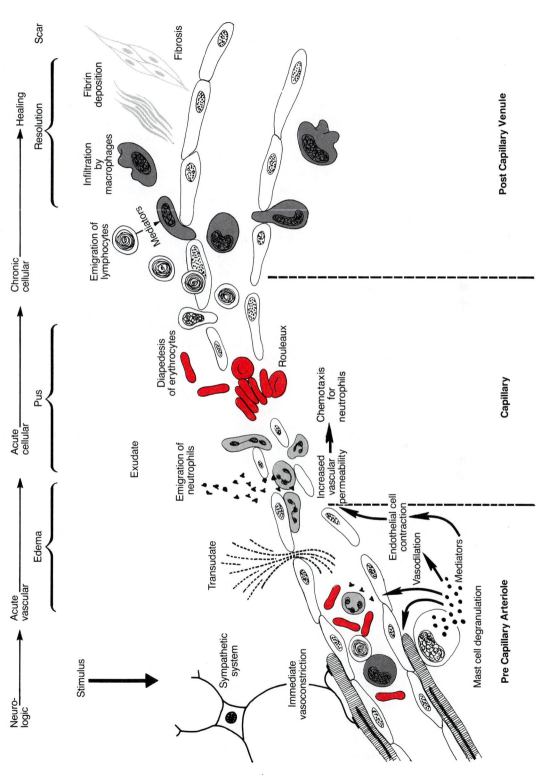

Figure 8–1. The sequence of events in the process of inflammation.

Exposure of fibrinogen and fibronectin in tissues provides sites for platelet aggregation and activation. Alterations in the viscosity of the blood and the charge of plasma may cause red cells to aggregate into stacks like pancakes (rouleaux formation) as the normal negative repelling charge of the erythrocytes is lost. Depending on the degree of injury or infection, the acute cellular phase may be sufficient to clear the tissue. However, it is often necessary for the chronic cellular infiltrate of lymphocytes and macrophages to effect removal of tissue debris or dead bacteria. The macrophage is the major player in this process. If there is damage sufficient to result in loss of normal tissue that must be replaced, fibroblastic proliferation and scarring will occur.

CHEMICAL MEDIATORS

Chemical mediators are signaling molecules that act on smooth muscle cells, endothelial cells, or white blood cells to induce, maintain, or limit inflammation. The agents that act first in the sequence primarily affect smooth muscle cells of precapillary arterioles to produce dilation and increased blood flow. Increased vascular permeability occurs in two phases: early (within minutes) and late (6 to 12 hours). The early phase is mediated by histamine and serotonin, whereas several other mediators contribute to the later phase. Late-phase mediators of acute inflammation are derived from a variety of sources, including arachidonic acid metabolites, breakdown products of the coagulation system (fibrin split products) or peptides formed from blood or tissue proteins (bradykinin), activated complement components (C3a, C5a), as well as factors released from bacteria (f-Met-tripeptides), necrotic tissue, neutrophils (inflammatory peptides), lymphocytes (lymphokines), and monocytes (monokines). The generation of these factors and their effects will be presented in more detail below.

ADHESION MOLECULES

Adhesion molecules are responsible for cell–cell interactions and cell–matrix interactions that take place during inflammation. A more complete characterization of these molecules is included in Chapter 9 (see Table 9–8). Of critical importance in acute inflammation is the interaction of granulocytes with endothelial cells. In the process of inflammation, polymorphonuclear neutrophils (PMNs) circulating in the blood bind to adherence molecules on endothelial cells (ECs) activated by inflammatory mediators. The strength of this initial reaction may not be sufficient to overcome the shear force of the flowing blood, resulting in the characteristic "rolling" seen as PMNs rotate along the EC surface. The adhesion of PMNs to ECs is strengthened by upregulation of other surface molecules (tethering molecules). Further reaction of PMNs and ECs stops the rolling and is followed by transmigration of PMNs through the vascular wall.

TABLE 8–2. ENDOTHELIAL SIGNALING AND TETHERING MOLECULES FOR NEUTROPHILS

Molecule	Structure	Expression Mechanism	Agonists	PMN receptor
Signaling Molecules:				
PAF	Phospholipid	Rapid synthesis	Histamine, thrombin, LTC_4	G-protein
IL-8	Polypeptide	Transcription	TNF-α, IL-1, LPS	G-protein
Tethering Molecules:				
P-selectin (GMP-140)	Glycoprotein	Translocation synthesis	Histamine, thrombin, others	Sialyated Lewis x
E-selectin (ELAM-1)	Glycoprotein	Transcription	IL-1, TNFα, LPS	Sialyated glycoprotein

Modified from Zimmerman GA, Prescott SM, McIntyre TM: Endothelial cell interactions with granulocytes: Tethering and signaling molecules. *Immunol Today* 13:93, 1992.

PMN–EC interactions during acute inflammation involve an overlapping sequence of expression of signaling and binding molecules on both the EC and the granulocyte. Activated ECs produce signaling (platelet activating factor [PAF] and interleukin-8 [IL- 8]) and tethering (binding) molecules (P- and E-selectins) for polymorphonuclear neutrophils (PMNs) (Table 8–2). The selectin family of adhesion molecules consists of three related glycoproteins that extend from the cell surface: L- (leukocyte), E- (endothelial), and P- (platelet) selectin. Selectins contain a lectin, epidermal growth factor-like and a series of complement binding-like domains. P- and E-selectin are expressed on activated ECs.

There appear to be four stages resulting in increasing binding affinity of molecules on PMNs (Table 8–3) to molecules on activated ECs: (1) Reversible "rolling" mediated by L-selectin on PMNs and P-

TABLE 8–3. ENDOTHELIAL ADHESION MOLECULES ON NEUTROPHILS

Molecule	CD Designation	Other Names	Endothelial Receptor
β_2-integrins	CD11a–CD18 LFA-1		ICAM-1, ICAM-2
	CD11b–CD18 Mac-1, Mo1		ICAM-1, IC3b, others
	CD11c–CD18 p150-95		ICAM-1, others
L-selectin	MEL-14, LAM-1		P-selectin (GMP-140)
	LEU-8, etc.		E-selectin (ELAM-1)

Modified from Zimmerman GA, Prescott SM, McIntyre TM: Endothelial cell interactions with granulocytes: Tethering and signaling molecules. *Immunol Today* 13:93, 1992.

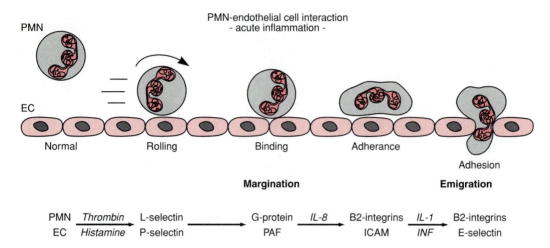

Figure 8–2. PMN-endothelial cell interactions during acute inflammation. Receptors on PMN interact with a series of cell adhesion molecules that are upregulated during the inflammatory process by mediators such as thrombin, histamine, IL-8, IL-1, and interferon. The cell adhesion molecules are P-selectin, platelet-activating factor (PAF), intercellular adhesion molecules (ICAMs), and E-selectin.

selectin on ECs, (2) enhanced binding by G-proteins on PMNs to PAF on ECs, (3) stronger adherence mediated by β_2- integrins on PMNs and P-selectin on ECs, followed by (4) stable binding (adhesion) and migration mediated by β_2-integrins on PMNs and E-selectin on ECs (Fig. 8–2). Immediate low-affinity binding occurs when L-selectin, which is constitutively present on PMNs, binds to the C-terminal lectin domains of P-selectin expressed on ECs within seconds after activation by thrombin, histamine, or leukotriene C_4. This is followed within minutes by synthesis and expression of platelet-activating factor (PAF) on the EC surface, which binds to a G-protein on neutrophils. This reaction produces immediate nontranslational upregulation of expression of CD11 to CD18 heterodimers (β_2-integrin) on the neutrophil, which binds to intracellular adhesion molecules (ICAMs) (ICAM-1 and ICAM-2) (see Chapter 9) on ECs. β_2-integrin is formed by rapid translocation of CD18 from subcellular granules to the PMN cell surface and formation of CD11 to CD18 heterodimers. This is referred to as functional upregulation of the cell surface molecules and may be rapidly reversed. β_2-integrin is also functionally upregulated after activation of PMNs by chemotactic factors or ionophores. Finally, stronger adhesion of PMNs occurs after E-selectin expression on and interleukin-8 (IL-8) secretion by ECs, and is stimulated by TNF-α, IL-1, or lipopolysaccharides (LPS). IL-8 (NAF, NAP-1) is released into the fluid phase and is a potent chemotactic factor for PMNs. IL-8 binds to

G-proteins on the neutrophils, stimulates longer-lasting translational upregulation of β_2-integrins, and enhances adhesion to ECs and to the subendothelial matrix, facilitating transendothelial migration. CD designations and other names for these molecules reflect their origin from monoclonal antibody identification.

Understanding of the role of these adhesion molecules in acute inflammation has been a major advance, but there are still many unknown aspects of acute inflammation. This is most likely due to other combinations and interactions of recognition molecules that take place during the course of acute inflammation.

Activation of ECs by cytokines, such as IL-1 and tumor necrosis factor (TNF) induces adherence of all granulocytic cell types, but there are also specific recognition molecules for eosinophils and basophils. The adherence of eosinophils and basophils to endothelium involves the expression of vascular cell adhesion molecule-1 (VCAM-1) an ECS after activation of ECs by IL-4, and binding of VCAM-1 to very late activation antigen-4 (VLA-4) on eosinophils or basophils to VCAM-1. VLA-4 is a β_1-integrin; neutrophils do not adhere to ECs under these conditions.

GROSS MANIFESTATIONS

The gross manifestations of the acute vascular response may be evoked by scratching the skin (the triple response). The triple response proceeds as follows:

1. 3 to 50 sec, thin red line (vasodilation of capillaries).
2. 30 to 60 sec, flush (vasodilation of arterioles).
3. 1 to 5 min, wheal (increased vascular permeability, edema).

The term "wheal" refers to pale, soft, swollen areas on the skin caused by leakage of fluid from capillaries. Some individuals react to skin stroking by marked wheal formation. The areas of skin will stand out after stroking so that words may actually be written on the skin by whealing (dermatographism).

The ancient Greeks considered inflammation to be a disease. Shortly after the birth of Christ, Galen grossly recognized the four classic cardinal signs of inflammation (Fig. 8–3). Later, the fifth sign (loss of function) was added by the great German pathologist Rudolf Virchow. Increased blood flow is manifested grossly by redness (rubor) and increased local temperature (calor). The increased blood flow delivers serum factors and blood cells to the tissue, causing an increase in tissue mass (tumor). The increase in vascular permeability permits exudation of plasma from the capillaries or postcapillary venules into the tissue, causing edema. Tissue swelling and chemical mediators act on nerve endings to produce pain (dolor). Swelling and pain lead to loss of function (functio loesa).

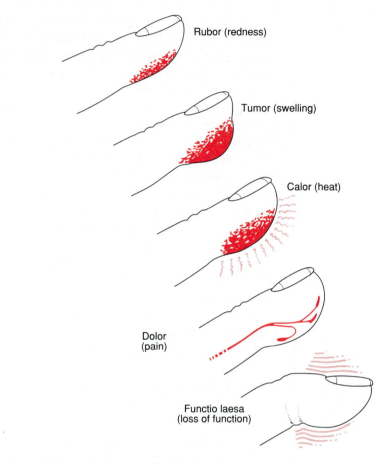

Rubor (redness)

Tumor (swelling)

Calor (heat)

Dolor
(pain)

Functio laesa
(loss of function)

Figure 8–3. The five cardinal signs of inflammation.

HISTOLOGIC FEATURES OF ACUTE INFLAMMATION

The essential pathological feature of acute inflammation is infiltration of the tissue by neutrophils. Neutrophils pass through gaps in capillary endothelium and are attracted to sites of inflammation by chemotactic factors. Tissue necrosis is caused by release of proteolytic enzymes into the tissue from the lysosomes of the neutrophils. Neutrophil infiltration is followed by infiltration by mononuclear (round) cells, ie, lymphocytes and macrophages. Macrophages are also attracted by chemotactic mediators and are activated to phagocytize and digest necrotic tissue or inflammatory products, including effete neutrophils that have become damaged in the inflammatory process. If tissue damage is not extensive, the inflammation will be limited by controlling factors such as enzyme inhibitors and oxygen scavengers. Macrophages will then be able to clear the inflamed area, and the tissue will return to normal (resolution). However, if tissue damage is extensive or the initiating stimulus persists, then mediators of chronic inflammation are activated. If tissue damage is significant or the organ has limited ability to regenerate, resolution cannot be achieved, and the damaged tissue will be replaced by fibroblast proliferation and collagen deposition (fibrous scar). If extensive, fibrous scarring may lead to a compromise of normal function. The fibrotic process may include proliferation of both fibroblasts and endothelial cells (capillaries) which form a highly vascular reaction known as granulation tissue because grossly it has the appearance of small granules like sand. If the inflamed tissue contains material that is difficult for macrophages to digest (such as silica or complex lipids), a particular form of chronic inflammation, granulomatous (like granulation tissue), may be seen (see Chapter 17). The process of inflammation is modified by infection, immune products, tissue death (necrosis), and foreign bodies. Examples of the lesions of different stages of inflammation in different tissue will be given later in the next chapter.

CLASSIFICATION OF INFLAMMATION

Some terms used to describe various manifestations of the inflammatory process are listed in Table 8–4. The manifestations of inflammation depend upon the severity and location of the reaction as well as the nature of the inflammatory stimulus. Systemic effects of inflammation

TABLE 8–4. DEFINITION OF TERMS USED TO DESCRIBE MANIFESTATIONS OF INFLAMMATION

Hyperemia: Increased blood in tissue; caused by vasodilation.

Edema: Excess fluid in tissues; caused by increased vascular permeability.

Transudate: Physiologic, low-protein concentration edema fluid, containing albumin; specific gravity below 1.012; cleared by lymphatics.

Exudate: Pathologic, high-protein edema fluid containing Igs and macroglobulin; specific gravity above 1.02.

Pus: Exudate rich in white cells and necrotic debris; caused by emigration of neutrophils and release of enzymes.

Fibrinoid necrosis: Enzymatic digestion of tissue that looks like fibrin, such as fibrinoid necrosis of vessels in vasculitis.

Types of Exudate:

Serous: Thin fluid (like transudate).
Fibrinous: Stringy, fibrin-containing.
Suppurative: Pus (Neutrophils and necrotic debris).
Hemorrhagic: Bloody (vascular necrosis).
Fibrous: Healed exudate, scar, adhesions.

Types of Lesions:

Ulcer: Surface erosion.
Abscess: Cavity filled with pus.
Cellulitis: Diffuse inflammatory infiltrate in tissue.
Pseudomembrane: Fibrous or necrotic layer on epithelial surface.
Catarrhal: Excess mucous production.

include fever and increased numbers of white blood cells (leukocytosis). Fever is caused by an increase in the metabolic rate in muscular tissue secondary to effects of "pyrogens" released from damaged tissue that act on the hypothalamus. Leukocytosis is caused by increased production and release of white cells from the bone marrow.

The Cells of Acute Inflammation

The cellular players in the process of acute inflammation include mast cells (basophils), platelets, eosinophils, and neutrophils. These granulocytic cells are activated by a variety of chemical processes and in turn produce and release a number of chemical mediators. Most of the manifestations of the acute vascular response are the result of chemical mediators released from mast cells.

MAST CELLS

Mast cells contain granules with a variety of biologically active agents (Table 8–5), which, when released extracellularly (degranulation), cause dilation of the smooth muscle of arterioles (vasodilation), increased blood flow, and contraction of endothelial cells, opening up vessel walls to permit egress of antibodies, complement, or inflammatory cells into tissue spaces. Mast cells were observed by early histologists to be filled with cellular material (granules). The term "mast cell" was applied to indicate that these cells appeared to be stuffed as if by overeating (mastication). However, the cellular granules are now known to contain biologically active agents produced by the mast cell that are released upon activation of the cells. Mast cells are usually located adjacent to small arterioles and in submucosal membranes where released vasoactive mediators would be expected to be most active in causing dilation of smooth muscle cells of arterioles. In classic anaphylactic reactions, mast cells are degranulated by reaction of antigen with IgE antibody that adheres to the surface of mast cells because of a specific configuration of the Fc part of the antibody molecules.

$F_{c\epsilon}$ Receptors

There are two F_cRs for IgE: high-affinity receptors on mast cells ($F_{c\epsilon}RI$) and low-affinity receptors on lymphocytes, monocytes, eosinophils, and platelets ($F_{c\epsilon}RII$) (Fig. 8–4A). Upon reaction of antigen with IgE antibody on the surface of the mast cells, a complex cellular activation mechanism causes the mast cells to release the pharmacologically active agents contained in cytoplasmic granules (Fig. 8–4B). The low-affinity $F_{c\epsilon}RII$ receptors may act to direct effector eosinophils and monocytes to parasites. The role of the $F_{c\epsilon}RII$ on T cells is not known, although the number of T cells with this receptor increases in asthmatics during pollen season.

Pharamacologically active agents of mast cells are the chemical mediators of atopic or anaphylactic hypersensitivity. The effects of

TABLE 8–5. MAST CELL MEDIATORS

Mediator	Structure/Chemistry	Source	Effects
Histamine	β-Imidazolylethylamine	Mast cells, basophils	Vasodilation; increase vascular permeability (venules), mucus production
Serotonin	5-Hydroxytryptamine	Mast cells (rodent), platelets, cells of enterochromaffin system	Vasodilation; increase vascular permeability (venules)
Neutrophil chemotactic factor	MW > 750,000	Mast cells	Chemotaxis of neutrophils
Eosinophil chemotactic factor A	Tetrapeptide	Mast cells	Chemotaxis of eosinophils
Vasoactive intestinal peptide	28-Amino-acid peptide	Mast cells, neutrophils, cutaneous nerves	Vasodilation; potentiate edema produced by bradykinin and C5a des-Arg
Thromboxane A_2	(structure: bicyclic oxygenated ring with COOH side chain; labels O, O, COOH, 12, OH)	Arachidonic acid (cylooxygenase pathway)	Vasoconstriction, broncho-constriction, platelet aggregation
Prostaglandin E_2 (or D_2)	(structure: cyclopentane ring with COOH side chain; labels O, COOH, 15, HO, OH)	Arachidonic acid (cylooxygenase pathway)	Vasodilation; potentiate permeability effects of histamine and bradykinin; increase permeability when acting with leukotactic agent; potentiate leukotriene effect; hyperalgesia
Leukotriene B_4	(structure: fatty acid chain with COOH; labels H OH, H OH)	Arachidonic acid (lipoxygenase pathway)	Chemotaxis of neutrophils; increase vascular permeability in the presence of PGE_2
Leukotriene D_4	(structure: fatty acid chain with COOH and cysteinylglycine; labels C_5H_{11}, H OH, COOH, HS—CH_2, $CHCONHCH_2COOH$, NH_2)	Arachidonic acid (lipoxygenase pathway)	Increase vascular permeability
Platelet-activating factor	Acetylated glycerol ether phosphocholine	Basophils, neutrophils, monocytes, macrophages	Release of mediators from platelets, neutrophil aggregation, neutrophil secretion, superoxide production by neutrophils; increase vascular permeability

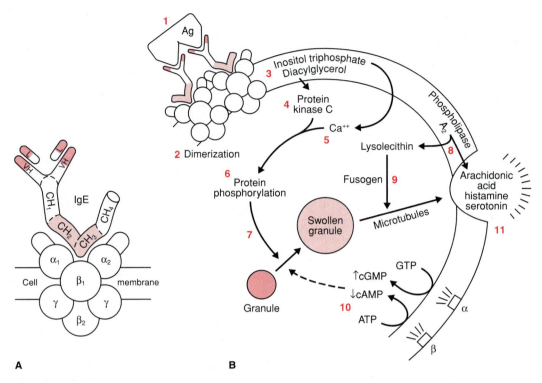

Figure 8–4. **A.** Diagram of the high-affinity $F^{c\varepsilon}R$ on mast cells. The high-affinity $F_{c\varepsilon}R$ on mast cells ($F^{c\varepsilon}I$) is composed of 6 subunits ($\alpha 1$, $\alpha 2$, $\beta 1$, $\beta 2$, $\gamma 1$, $\gamma 2$). The α subunits and $\beta 1$ extend from the cell surface and bind to the CH2 and CH3 domains of the IgE molecule; the γ subunits (connected by a single disulfide bond) and the $\beta 2$ subunit project through the cell membrane into the cytoplasm. **B.** Postulated steps in mast cell degranulation: (1) Binding of antigen (allergen), crosslinking two IgE molecules on mast cell surface. (2) Dimerization of IgE receptors. (3) Alteration of methyltransferases. (4) Conversion of membrane phospholipids to phosphotidylcholine. (5) Opening of Ca++ channel and influx of Ca++ into cells. (6) Activation of Ca++ dependent protein phosphorylation. (7) Enlargement of granules by protein kinases. (8) Activation of phospholipase A_2 with formation of lysolecithin and arachidonic acid. (9) Lysolecithin acts as "fusogen" causing granules to fuse with cell membranes with release of contents. (10) Activation of granules is dependent on levels of cAMP and cGMP, which in turn are regulated by α and β adrenergic receptors.

their release are described in more detail in Chapter 14. The mediators and their effects of mast cell mediators are listed in Figure 8–5. The major early events in inflammation, vasodilation, and increased vascular permeability (which occur within the first 30 minutes) are mediated by the immediate degranulation of mast cells and the release of histamine and serotonin. The second phase (between 1 and 2.5 hours) is believed due to bradykinin (see The Kinin System, later in this chapter). The third phase of persistent edema (occurring 6 to 12 hours after

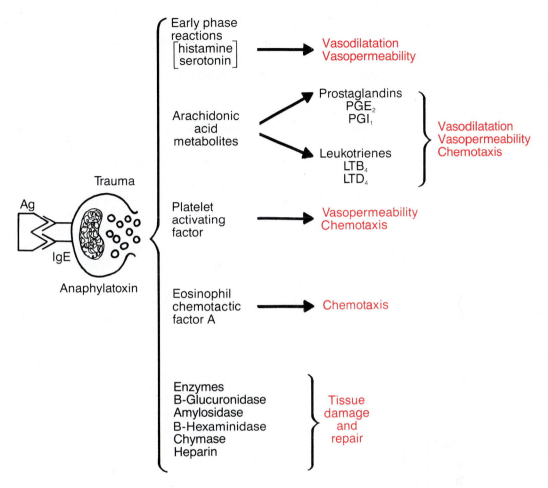

Figure 8–5. Mast cell mediators and inflammation. (Modified from Wasserman SI, Solter NA. *Advances in Allergy and Applied Immunology.* Pergaman Press, 1980, 192.)

initiation of inflammation) are mediated by prostaglandins and leukotrienes produced as a result of metabolism of phospholipids from membranelike material released from mast cell granules (see below). Chemotaxis of neutrophils and eosinophils is affected by leukotrienes as well as by platelet-activating factor. Enzymes activated by solubilization of granular material may also contribute to tissue damage and/or repair.

Cytokines

Mast cells also produce cytokines in a pattern similar to T-helper-2 cells and are believed to play a role in regulation of IgE synthesis. These cytokines include, but are not limited to: IL-2, IL-3, IL-4, IL-5, IL-6, GM-CSF, TNFα, and IFNγ. In particular IL-4 drives CD4+ T-helper cells to express the Th2 phenotype and IL-4, IL-5, and IL-6 drive differentiating B cells to IgE and IgA production. The cytokine profile of mast cells helps explain the longstanding observation of a relationship between mast cell numbers and IgE levels.

Histamine

Histamine is the major preformed mast cell mediator. Injection of histamine into the skin produces the typical wheal and flare reaction of the immediate acute vascular response. Histamine causes endothelial cell contraction and vasodilation leading to edema (wheal) and redness (flare). Histamine is formed from the amino acid L-histidine by the action of an enzyme called L-histidine decarboxylase found in the cytoplasm of mast cells and basophils. The biologic effects of histamine are mediated by two distinct sets of receptors H_1 and H_2 (Table 8–6). Effects mediated through H_1 receptors are the classic acute vascular inflammatory events. Antiinflammatory effects, as well as vasodilation, are mediated through H_2 receptors. Thus, histamine may activate acute vascular effects, yet inhibit acute cellular inflammation. Acute cellular inflammation is mediated by products of arachidonic acid.

Arachidonic Acid Metabolites

Major mediators of inflammation are the metabolic derivatives of arachidonic acid. Arachidonic acid is derived from membrane phospholipids that are broken down by phospholipases. In the human, membrane phospholipids are released from mast cells during the early

TABLE 8–6. H_1 AND H_2-DEPENDENT ACTIONS OF HISTAMINE

H_1-Receptor Mediated	H_2-Receptor Mediated
Increased cGMP	Increased cAMP
Smooth muscle constriction (bronchi)	Smooth muscle dilation (vascular)
Increased vascular permeability	Gastric acid secretion
Pruritus	Mucous secretion
Prostaglandin generation	Inhibition of basophil histamine release
	Inhibition of lymphokine release
	Inhibition of neutrophil enzyme release
	Inhibition of eosinophil migration
	Inhibition of T-lymphocyte-mediated cytotoxicity
Antagonized by "classical" antihistamines	Antagonized by Cimetidine

H_1 and H_2
Vasodilation (hypotension)
Flush
Headache

Modified from Metcalfe DD, Kaliner M. *Mast Cells and Basophils in Cellular Functions in Immunity and Inflammation*. Oppenhiem, Rosenstriech, and Potter, eds. New York, Elsevier, 1981.

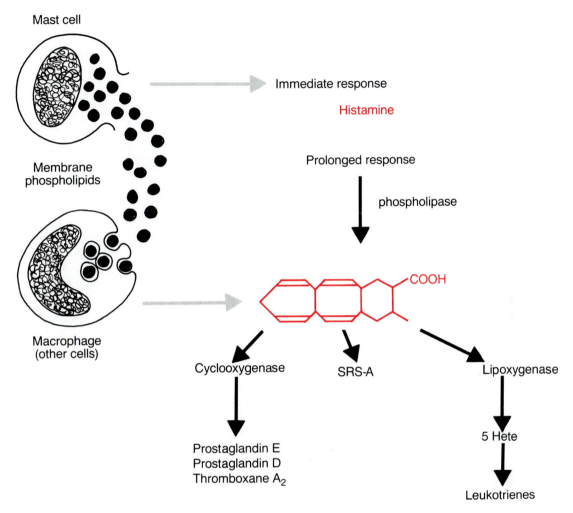

Figure 8–6. Arachidonic acid metabolism. (Modified from Metcalfe DD, Kaliner M. *Cellular Functions in Immunity and Inflammation.* New York, Elsevier, 1981, 353.)

phase of acute inflammation but may also be derived from other cell membranes. The metabolism of arachidonic acid is believed to occur mainly in macrophages but metabolites may also be synthesized by most, if not all, cells that take part in an inflammatory response including the mast cell. Metabolism of arachidonic acid occurs via two major pathways: the cyclooxygenase pathway and the lipoxygenase pathway (Fig. 8–6). The cyclooxygenase pathway gives rise to prostaglandins, and the lipoxygenase pathway to leukotrienes.

Prostaglandins. The prostaglandins are derived by oxidation of prostanoic acid (cyclooxygenation). The numerical subscript in each

Prostanoic Acid

prostaglandin (PG) refers to the number of unsaturated bonds. PGE_1 has one unsaturated bond at the 13–14 position; PGE_2 has 2 unsaturated bonds—one at the 5–6 and one at the 13–14 position. The letter designations refer to the position of bonds in the ring structure.

Prostaglandins were originally identified in seminal fluid and were believed to be produced by the prostate. It is now known that other tissue cells are the major source of prostaglandins, particularly mast cells. Prostaglandins are prominent in anaphylactic reactions (see Chapter 14). The most active components are PGE_2 and PGD_2, which produce vasodilation, increase vascular premeability, and cause hyperalgesia (increased sensitivity to pain). The primary source for thromboxane A_2 is the platelet. Thromboxane A_2 is also produced by the cyclooxygenase pathway and is active in vasoconstriction, bronchoconstriction, and platelet aggregation. These metabolites are rapidly metabolized to inactive forms (PGE_1, PGD_1, and thromboxane B_2) by further oxygenation. Prostaglandin E (PGE) and prostacyclin (PGI_2) also act to suppress a variety of inflammatory cells, including mast cells, PMNs, monocytes, and macrophages, as well as natural killer (NK) cells by increasing intracellular cyclic adenosine monophosphate (cyclic AMP). PGE_1 also inhibits production of leukotriene B_4, suppresses lymphokine production, and inhibits increased vascular permeability and tissue injury during acute inflammation. The nonsteroidal antiinflammatory drugs (NSAIDs), such as aspirin, act to inhibit cyclooxygenase and block formation of these inflammatory mediators.

Leukotrienes. The products of the lipoxygenase pathway are called leukotrienes. They are generated by leukocytes and mast cells. Again, the subscript denotes the number of double bonds. The activity of leukotrienes C_4, D_4, and E_4 is believed to be responsible for a factor previously called slow-reacting substance of anaphylaxis (SRSA), whereas that of leukotriene B_4 is chemotactic for eosinophils (eosinophilic chemotactic factor of anaphylaxis [ECFA]) and neutrophils. Although prostaglandins are responsible for some of the late vascular effects of anaphylaxis, they may also serve to modulate anaphylaxis by increasing cyclic nucleotide levels of mast cells and inhibiting histamine release. Leukotriene B_4 enhances adherence of PMNs to endothelial cells, a process blocked by PGE and PGI_2. In addition, LTB_4 activates PMNS to migrate, degranulate, and generate superoxide anions.

PLATELETS

The role of platelets in inflammation is complex. Platelets contain heparin and serotonin, so that release of these mediators may contribute to the acute vascular phase of inflammation. Platelets also produce oxygen radicals that may cause tissue damage. However, the major role of platelets is to block damaged vessel walls and prevent hemorrhage. Platelets react with ligands in damaged vessel through a family of receptor proteins, the glycoprotein (GP) system.

Platelets react differently at sites of arterial (high pressure, high flow) damage than in veins (low pressure, low flow). Because of the high-flow rate in arteries, platelets must first slow and stop before they can attach to the subendothelium. In arteries, platelets initially react via a single receptor on the platelet surface (glycoprotein Ib [GPIb]), which binds specifically to von Willebrand factor (vWf) on the vessel surface. In the absence of shear forces created by high flow, these ligands will not bind to each other. Shear forces sufficient to initiate platelet–vessel binding occur when arterial blood flows over the static subendothelial surface. After initial binding, platelets are "activated" and the platelet GPIIb surface receptor undergoes a conformational change that permits it to bind to peptide, arginine-glycine-asparagine (Arg-gly-asp), present in fibrin, fibronectin, and vitronectin. At sites of vascular damage the extracellular matrix proteins fibronectin and vitronectin are exposed, and fibrin is formed through activation of the coagulation system (see below). Platelets bind to these molecules forming clumps of platelets that plug up leaks in the vascular system. The platelet and coagulation system (see below) complement each other since platelet aggregation accelerates thrombin formation and fibrin deposits strengthen platelet aggregates. Once activation and spreading of platelets are underway, the platelet becomes a nidus for binding of other platelets and for deposition of fibrin, which strengthens the platelet aggregate by providing links between individual platelets. In the venous system, fibrin forms in the presence of red cells, and platelet deposition is less prominent.

EOSINOPHILS

Acute
Inflammation

Polymorphonuclear eosinophils, discovered by Paul Ehrlich in 1879, are distinguished from other granulocytes by the affinity of their cytoplasmic granules for acidic dyes such as eosin, resulting in an intense red staining. This staining is primarily due to the presence of a major basic protein (MBP), which binds acid dyes. Eosinophils are found predominantly in two types of inflammation: allergy and parasitic worm infections. Some chemotactic factors for eosinophils are listed in Table 8–7. These factors are derived from inflammatory cells, complement, or worm extracts. On the one hand, there is evidence that enzymes in eosinophils may serve to limit the extent of inflammation by neutralizing mediators of anaphylaxis, such as LTC4, histamine, and platelet-activating factor. On the other hand, there is increasing evidence that the cationic proteins in eosinophil granules are mediators of acute inflammation. Eosinophil activation is associated with acute tissue injury. Activated eosinophils cause an initial intense vasoconstriction in lung microvasculature, followed by increased pulmonary vascular permeability and pulmonary edema. The cationic proteins that are active in this process are eosinophil peroxidase (EPO), major basic protein (MBP), and eosinophil-derived neurotoxin (EDN), which make up about 90% of the granule proteins. In addition, these proteins can directly injure endodermal cells, increasing the transudation of fluids into alveolar spaces as well as type II epithelial cells, leading to a decreased secretion of surfactant. This may contribute greatly to the respiratory distress syndromes (see below). Charcot–Leyden crystal protein is also found in some eosinophil granules. This protein belongs to the "S-type" lectin family and may neutralize natural lung surfactants, causing collapse of air spaces (atelectasis).

The distribution and localization of eosinophils involves a family of adhesion molecules on endothelial cells and eosinophils similar to those for neutrophil margination and emigration. Weak binding occurs between eosinophil membrane sialyl Lewis X Carbohydrate to L-selectins on endothelial cells, followed by upregulation of E-selectin

TABLE 8–7. CHEMOTACTIC FACTORS FOR EOSINOPHILS

Factor	Origin
Histamine	Mast cells
Eosinophilic chemotactic factor A	Mast cells
Neutrophil peptides	Neutrophils
Eosinophil stimulator promoter	Lymphocytes
C_5a	Complement
Worm extracts	Ascaris

and PAF on the endothelial cell and binding to β_2-integrins on eosinophils. High-affinity binding specific for eosinophils occurs after activation by IL-4 of expression of VCAM-1 on endothelial cells, which binds to integrin $\alpha4\beta1$ (VLA-4) on eosinophils. Expression of β_2-selectins on eosinophils is required for them to emigrate into tissues.

Eosinophils are "activated" by phosphorylation of signal-transducing proteins to release granular proteins by exocytosis. Activated eosinophils produce platelet-activating factor (PAF), which acts as an autocrine to increase the activated state of the eosinophil, but endothelial cells are the major source of PAF for eosinophil activation. Some eosinophils have receptors for IgA and can be activated by crosslinking of these receptors by antigen.

Parasitic Diseases

Eosinophils play a major role in the killing of parasites. The components of eosinophilic granules active against parasites and against some human tumor cells are listed in Table 8–8. Eosinophils are cytotoxic to schistosome larvae through an antibody-dependent cell-mediated mechanism. Eosinophil cationic proteins (ECPs) are highly toxic for schistosomes and are responsible for binding of eosinophils to worms in a way not possible for neutrophils. ECPs cause fragmentation of worms and are ten times more toxic than the major basic proteins (MBPs), although MBPs make up over 50% of the eosinophilic

TABLE 8–8. PROPERTIES OF EOSINOPHIL GRANULE PROTEINS

Name	Molecular Weight (x 10^3)	pI	Site	Activities
Major basic protein (MBP)	14	10.9	Core	Toxic to parasites, tumor cells: causes histamine release, neutralizes heparin
Eosinophil cationic proteins (ECP)	21	10.8	Matrix	Toxic to parasites, neurons; histamine release, alters fibrinolysis and coagulation, inhibits lymphocytes
Eosinophil-derived neurotoxin (EDN)	18	8.9	Matrix	Potent neurotoxin, RNase activity
Eosinophil peroxidase (EPO)	71–77	>11	Matrix	Forms H_2O_2, inactivates leukotrienes, causes histamine release, kills microorganisms and tumor cells

granule and form the characteristic granule core seen in electron microscopy. Eosinophilic peroxidase is active in generation of H_2O_2, which is active in killing bacteria and in degranulation of mast cells. Finally, eosinophils contain collagenase, which may function to aid remolding connective tissue during healing.

POLYMORPHO–NUCLEAR NEUTROPHILS (PMNs)

Neutrophilic polymorphonuclear leukocytes are the major cellular component of the acute inflammatory reaction. Neutrophils are characterized by numerous cytoplasmic granules that contain highly destructive hydrolytic enzymes that must be kept isolated from the cytoplasm (Table 8–9). These granules contain a number of oxygen-independent enzymes, as well as oxygen-dependent mechanisms for killing. Upon attraction to sites of inflammation, neutrophils attempt to engulf and digest bacteria coated with antibody and complement. However, phagocytosis by neutrophils is usually accompanied by release of the lysosomal enzymes from these cells into the tissue spaces, particularly if the organisms is difficult for the polymorphonuclear neutrophil to ingest. The lysosomal acid hydrolyses cause local tissue digestion at the site of the reactions. The characteristic lesion is fibrinoid necrosis—areas of acellular digested tissue that look like fibrin but lack any fibrillar appearance.

Oxygen-independent Killing

At least three cytoplasmic granules are identifiable: specific granules (lactoferrin, etc.), azurophilic granules (lysosomes in PMNs containing acid hydrolases and other enzymes), and a third granule compartment containing gelatinase. Specific granules contain a specific β cytochrome, the complement receptor CR3 and β_2-integrin, which binds to the endothelial cells during acute inflammation. These protiens are translocated to the cell surface by certain stimuli and are important for cell activation and adhesion. The azurophil granules contain **anionic granule proteins** and include myeloperoxidase, defensins, cathepsin G, azurocidin and "lysosomal enzymes." These proteins bind to microbial cells and disrupt complex membrane functions or are released into tissues where they may destroy host structures as well as microorganisms. For instance, defensins of humans include four 29–34

TABLE 8–9. ANTIMICROBIAL SYSTEMS IN NEUTROPHILS

Oxygen-dependent	Oxygen-independent
Myeloperoxidase	Lysozyme
Superoxide anion (O_2-)	Lactoferrin
Hydroxyl radical (OH-)	Cationic proteins
Singlet oxygen ($^1O_2$)	Neutral proteases
Hydrogen peroxide	Acid hydrolases

amino acid peptides (human neutrophil proteins, [HNPs]) designated HNP-1, HNP-2, HNP-3, and HNP-4, which make up 30% to 50% of the azurophil granules. Defensins kill a wide variety of bacteria, fungi, and viruses by changing the permeability of outer membranes of these organisms. Alkaline phosphatase activity is also upregulated during neutrophil activation; this activity is located in the separate rod-shaped granule compartment, which also contains gelatinase. These enzymes may assist in migration of PMNs into tissue spaces.

Oxygen-dependent Killing

Reactive oxygen metabolites (see Table 8–9), primarily involved in bacterial killing, may also damage endothelial cells and adjacent tissues, resulting in the formation of pus. Reduction of molecular oxygen (O_2) by addition of a single electron results in formation of superoxide (O_2^-) anion from which are formed products such as hydrogen peroxide (H_2O_2), hypochlorous acid (HOC1), hydroxyl radicals (HO^-), and singlet oxygen species ($^1O_2$). The formation of these metabolites results from the action of enzymes such as superoxide dismutase, nicotinamide adenine dinucleotide (phosphate) oxidase, and myeloperoxidase, which are present in inflammatory cells and are activated during inflammation. Cellular injury is mediated by formation of lipid peroxidases within cellular membranes and organelles, protein polymerization, or activation of arachidonic acid metabolites. Oxygen radicals are also formed during ischemic injury (loss of blood supply) due to proteolytic conversion of xanthine dehydrogenase to xanthine oxidase, which, in the presence of O_2, catabolizes the conversion of hypoxanthine and xanthine to uric acid with the generation of O_{2-} and H_2O_2. This subsequently results in generation of chemotactic mediators, neutrophil recruitment, and further tissue injury. Studies employing specific antioxidants suggest that products of O_{2-} and H_2O_2 reactions and the myeloperoxidase-H_2O_2-halide systems are the most toxic mediators of acute tissue damage. In addition, O_{2-} may stimulate fibroblast proliferation, and H_2O_2 activates transcription factors, such as NFkB.

Chemotactic Factors

Neutrophils may be attracted to sites of inflammation by a number of chemotactic factors (see Table 8–10). Neutrophils have cell surface receptors for some of these factors, such as activated fragments of complement (see below) and formyl-methionyl tripeptides. The adherence of neutrophils to cells and surfaces is mediated by cell adhesion molecules known as integrins (see above). Acute inflammatory reactions need not be initiated by immune mechanisms and are frequently associated with bacterial infections (such as staphylococcal and streptococcal infections) or traumatic tissue injury. In these situations, neutrophils are attracted into sites of inflammation by chemotactic factors released

TABLE 8–10. CHEMOTACTIC FACTORS FOR NEUTROPHILS

Complement
 C_5a
 C_5a-desarg
Kallikrein
Fibrinopeptide B
f-met tripeptides
Collagen peptides
Transfer factor (lymphokine)
Neutrophil chemotactic factors of:
 Fibroblasts
 Macrophages (interleukin-1)
 Lymphocytes
Platelet-activating factor
Leukotriene B_4

by the infecting organism (f-met peptides) or by products of damaged tissue, such as fibronectin, fibrin or collagen degradation products, or factors produced by other inflammatory cells. In immune complex reactions, neutrophils are attracted by formation of activated complement components (see below) following antibody–antigen reaction in tissues.

Acute-Phase Reactants

Acute-phase reactants are a heterogeneous group of serum proteins that have in common a rapid increase in concentration in the serum following acute tissue injury. They have a varied function in inflammation, but in general serve to increase or limit the damage caused by inflammatory mediators such as IL-1, TNF, INF- γ, and INFβ-2. The role of these cytokines in inflammation will be presented in more detail in the next chapter, but one of their actions is to stimulate production of acute-phase reactants by the liver. In fact, IFNβ-2 has recently been shown to be identical to hepatocyte-stimulating factor (HSF), which stimulates liver cell release of acute-phase reactants, as well as proliferation of liver cells. A listing of the functions of some acute-phase proteins is given in Table 8–11.

C-REACTIVE PROTEIN (CRP)

CRP is the most widely used indicator of an acute-phase response in man for the early indication of infections, inflammation, or other disease associated with tissue injury. Normally, the serum concentration of CRP is 0.1 mg/dL or less. After injury, rapid production in the liver results in concentrations as high as 100 mg/dL. CRP is synthesized only in the liver, and synthesis is stimulated by IL-6 and IL-1. It is composed of five identical subunits forming a unique ring-shaped molecule known

TABLE 8–11. FUNCTIONS OF SOME ACUTE-PHASE PROTEINS OF HUMANS

Class of Function	Protein	Specific Function
Mediators:	C-reactive protein	Ligand binding, complement activation
	Complement components:	
	C2, C3, C4, C5, C9	Opsonization, mast cell
	Factor B	degranulation
	Coagulation factors:	
	Factor VIII	Clotting, formation of fibrin matrix
	Fibrinogen	for repair
Inhibitors:	C1-inactivator	Control of mediator pathways
	α_1-Antitrypsin	Elastase, collagenase
	α_1-Antichymotrypsin	Cathepsin G
	α_2-Macroglobulin	Proteinase
Scavengers:	C-reactive protein	Ligand binding (clearance of toxins)
	Serum amyloid A protein	?Cholesterol binding
	Haptoglobin	Hemoglobin binding
	Ceruloplasmin	$[O_2^-]$ inactivation
Immune regulation:	C-reactive protein	Interaction with T and B cells
	α_1-Acid glycoprotein	T-cell inhibitor
Repair and resolution:	C-reactive protein	Opsonization, chemotaxis
	α_1-antitrypsin	
	α_1-Antichymotrypsin > Binds to surface of new elastic fibers	
	C1-inactivator	
	α_1-Acid glycoprotein	Promotes fibroblast growth, interacts with collagen

From Whicher JT, Dieppe PA: Acute phase proteins. *Clin Immunol Allergy* 5:425, 1985.

as a pentraxin. A pentraxin is made up of five monomers covalently joined to form a pentamer which has cyclic pentameric symmetry. Serum amyloid P component is also a pentraxin but does not increase in serum after injury. CRP got its name because it was first identified in the serum of patients with pneumonia because it precipitated with the C-polysaccharide on the pneumococcal cell wall. Cleavage of CRP by enzymes from neutrophils produces fragments that promote chemotaxis and contain the tetrapeptide thr-lys-pro-arg, known as tufsin, that is also present in the CH_2 domain of the immunoglobulin heavy chain. Thus, the biological effects of CRP are like those of immunoglobulins, including the ability to precipitate, to function as a primitive opsonin through binding to macrophages, and to fix complement. It also reacts with low affinity to other immune and inflammatory effector cells, but immunomodifying effects are controversial.

SERUM AMYLOID A PROTEIN (SAA)

SAA and CRP are the major human acute phase proteins. In its denatured form, SAA is related to the amyloid A protein found in the tissues of patients with secondary amyloidosis. There are at least three closely related proteins in the SAA family: SAA1, SAA2, and SAA3. The function of SAA in inflammation is not clear.

α1-PROTEINASE INHIBITOR

API, also known as α1-antitrypsin, inhibits the activity of proteases. It acts to limit the effect of neutrophil-derived proteases, thus preventing systemic effects of these enzymes, as well as limiting the damage at the site of inflammation, so that repair can be initiated. API is produced not only in the liver, but also in macrophages. It is a single-chain glycosylated polypeptide of 394 amino acids.

α1-ACID GLYCOPROTEIN

AGP, also known as orosomucoid, is a heterogeneous protein with at least seven polymorphic forms that have up to 40% carbohydrate. Its serum concentration increases up to 5-fold within 24 hours after acute injury. Its function is not clear.

FIBRINOGEN

Fibrinogen is a central player in coagulation, and the fibrinopeptides produced during clotting are chemotactic for neutrophils (see below).

α_2-MACROGLOBULIN

α_2-Macroglobulin inhibits the proteolytic activity of a wide variety of proteinases, including all classes of endopeptidases, serine, cysteinyl, aspartyl, and metallo. Most α-macroglobulins are tetramers formed from paired 180-kDa subunits. Because of its high molecular weight (720 kDa), α_2-macroglobulin does not normally pass from the blood into other tissues. Thus, it is believed to function as an acceptor of proteinases released into the blood, preventing systemic effects of proteinase release. Although much more prominent in rats than in humans, it once was suspected that α_2-M might be defective in patients with cystic fibrosis, but this idea is not supported by more recent data.

COMPLEMENT

In humans, the serum concentration of C_3, the highest of any complement component, more than doubles during the acute phase response (normal concentration is 150 to 300 mg/dL). Other complement components, which also increase during inflammation, play key roles for activation of complement-mediated inflammation (see below).

Serum Protein Systems

A number of different serum proteins are included in systems of activation and control of inflammatory reactions. These include the complement, coagulation, and kinin systems.

THE COMPLEMENT SYSTEM

The complement system consists of a set of up to twenty serum proteins that form a controlled sequence for production of activated molecules (Table 8–12). The complete activation sequence occurs on the surface of cells and involves a series of molecular interactions during which fragments, as well as new multimolecular complexes with biologic activity, are formed. Complement fragments ("split products")

TABLE 8–12. COMPLEMENT COMPONENTS

Component	Function	Molecular Weight	Number of Polypeptide Chains	Serum Concentration μg /mL	Site of Synthesis
Classical pathway					
Cl_q	Recognition	400,000	18	200	Small
$_r$	Enzyme	160,000	2	—	Intestine
$_s$	Enzyme	80,000	1	120	Epithelium
C2	Activation	115,000	1	30	Macrophages
C3	Activation	180,000	2	1,200	Macrophages
C4	Activation	210,000	3	400	Liver epithelium
C5	Attack	180,000	2	75	Macrophages
C6	Attack	128,000	1	60	Liver
C7	Attack	150,000	3	60	—
C8	Attack	150,000	3	15	—
C9	Attack	75,000	1	trace	Liver
Alternate pathway					
Properdin		190,000	4	20	Macrophages
Factor B	C3 Activator	100,000	1	225	Macrophages
Factor D	C3 Co-activator	25,000	4	trace	Macrophages
C3	Activation	210,000	3	400	Macrophages

are released into the fluid phase, where they serve as inflammatory mediators. The multimolecular cell-bound components serve as receptors for phagocytic cells (opsonize) or produce "lesions" in the cell membrane that lead to lysis of the cell. Activation of the complement system may occur via two pathways: the "classical" and the "alternate" pathways. Activation via the classical sequence is initiated by antibody–antigen reactions, whereas the alternate pathway may be activated by certain bacterial products. In addition to cell lysis, activated components mediate a variety of tissue responses, including chemotaxis of neutrophils and monocytes, enhancement of phagocytosis, and increased vascular permeability. These activated components also interact with other accessory systems, including the coagulation and fibrinolytic systems, to amplify and/or limit the acute inflammatory reaction. The major inflammatory functions of activated complement fragments are to open blood vessels, and to attract and activate PMNs.

Classical Pathway

A simplified diagrammatic representation of the classical pathway for complement activation is shown in Figure 8–7 and the sequence described in detail in Table 8–13. The first component of complement, C_1, has the capacity to bind and be activated by antibody molecules that have been altered in their Fc region by reaction with antigen. The Ig classes that are active in fixing complement are IgG and IgM. One molecule of IgM is capable of activating C_1, whereas two molecules of IgG reacting close together are required. Activation of C_1 may take

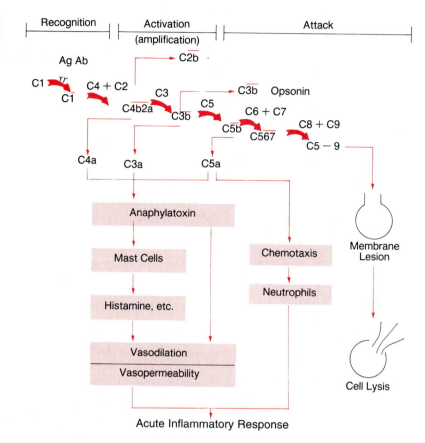

Figure 8–7. Classical pathway of complement activation. Following reaction of antibody with antigen, a cascade reaction of complement components is activated. C1 functions as a recognition unit for the altered Fc regions of two IgG or one IgM molecule(s): C2 and C4, as an activation unit leading to cleavage of C3. C3 fragments have a number of biological activities: C3a anaphylatoxin, and C3b, recognized by receptors on macrophages (opsonin). C3b also joins with fragments of C4 and C2 to form C3 convertase, which cleaves C5. C5 then reacts with C6 through C9 to form a membrane attack unit that produces a lesion in cell membranes, through which intracellular components may escape (lysis).

place in a fluid phase, such as when antibody reacts with soluble antigens in the bloodstream, or activation may occur on the surface of cells, as is the case when anti-erythrocyte antibody reacts with a red cell. In order for two IgG molecules to achieve close enough apposition on a red cell to activate C_1, approximately 600 to 1,000 molecules must bind to the cell, whereas only one IgM molecule is required.

Upon reaction of antibody with antigen, and formation of aggregated Fc regions, a cascade of complement components is activated.

TABLE 8–13. SEQUENCE AND MECHANISM OF IMMUNE HEMOLYSIS

Reaction	Biochemical Event
$E + A \rightarrow EA$	Reaction of erythrocyte and antierythrocyte antibody.
$EA + C1 \rightarrow EAC1q^*$	C1q attaches to antibody at a site on Fc portion of Ig antibody bound to the cell.
$C1r \rightarrow \overline{C1r}$	Bound $C1q^*$ converts C1r to active form by cleavage of C1r.
$C1s \rightarrow \overline{C1s}$	$\overline{C1r}$ activates C1s by cleavage of C1s.
$C4 \rightarrow \overline{C4a} + C4b^*$ $C2 \rightarrow C2a^* + \overline{C2b}$	$\overline{C1s}$ cleaves C4 into $\overline{C4a}$ and $C4b^*$ and C2 into $C2a^*$ and $\overline{C2b}$; plasmin acts on C_2b to produce C_2b kinin; $\overline{C4a}$ has weak anaphylatoxin activity.
$C4b^* + C2a^* \rightarrow \overline{C4b2a}$ $C3 \rightarrow \overline{C3a} + C3b^*$	$C4b^*$ and $C2a^*$ combine to form C3 convertase. $\overline{C4b2a}$ cleaves C3 into $\overline{C3a}$ and $C3b^*$; $\overline{C3a}$ (anaphylatoxin) causes smooth muscle contraction and degranulation of mast cells.
$C3b^* + C4b2a \rightarrow \overline{C4b2a3b}$	$C3b^*$ binds to activated bimolecular complex of $\overline{C4b2a}$ to form a trimolecular complex, C5 convertase, that is a specific enzyme for C5. Macrophages have receptors for C3b, so that C3b acts as opsonin.
$C5 \rightarrow \overline{C5a} + C5b^*$	C5 is cleaved into $\overline{C5a}$ and $C5b^*$ by C5 convertase; $\overline{C5a}$ has anaphylactic and strong chemotactic activity for polymorphonuclear neutrophils.
$\overline{C5b}^* + C6789 \rightarrow \overline{C5b.9}$	$C5b^*$ reacts with other complement components to produce a macromolecular complex that has the ability to alter cell membrane permeability. $\overline{C8}$ is most likely the active component, with $\overline{C9}$ increasing efficiency of $\overline{C8}$ and producing maximal cell lysis.

E, erythrocyte; A, antibody to erythrocyte.

$\overline{C1}$, $\overline{C4}$, etc.: a line above the C number indicates the activated form of the component.

C4a, C4b, etc.: the lower-case letters indicate cleavage products of the parent complement molecule.

$C4b^*$, $C2a^*$: the asterisk indicates a cleavage product that contains an active binding site for other complement components.

C_1 functions as a recognition unit for the altered Fc regions of two IgG molecules or one IgM molecule; C_2 and C_4 act as an activation unit leading to cleavage of C_3. C_3 fragments have a number of biologic activities: C_3a is anaphylatoxin, and C_3b is recognized by receptors on macrophages (opsonin). C_3b also joins with fragments of C_4 and C_2 to form C_3 convertase, which cleaves C_5. C_5 then reacts with C_6 through C_9 to form a membrane attack unit that produces a lesion in cell membranes through which intracellular components may escape (lysis).

The components of the classical pathway leading to cell lysis are C_1 through C_9. In the activation sequence occurring at the cell surface, C_1 functions as a recognition unit, C_2–C_4 as an activation unit, and C_5–C_9 as a membrane attack unit. When C_1 attaches to antibody, it becomes activated as an enzyme (C_1 esterase), which cleaves C_4 and C_2 each into two fragments (C_4a and C_4b, C_2a and C_2b). One of the fragments of C_4 (C_4b) and one of the C_2 fragments (C_2a) join together and bind to new sites on the cell surface. Other fragments, C_4a and C_2b, are released into the fluid phase. C_4a has weak anaphylatoxic activity, whereas C_2b is converted by plasmin into a C_2b kininlike molecule believed to be responsible for the lesions of hereditary angioedema (see below). The complex of C_4b_2a forms an enzyme, C_3 convertase, which binds and cleaves C_3 into C_3a and C_3b. C_3b binds to new sites on the cell surface. Since activated C_1 can cleave many molecules of C_4 and C_2 and the C_4b_2a complex can cleave many molecules of C_3, these serve as amplification steps. C_3a is released into the fluid phase where it functions as anaphylatoxin. Phagocytic cells have receptors for C_3b; C_3b serves as an opsonin (receptor for phagocytes). In addition, C_3b forms a trimolecular complex with C_4b_2a ($C_4b_2a_3b$) that is able to cleave C_5 into C_5a and C_5b (C_5 convertase). C_5a is released into the fluid phase, and C_5b binds to the cell surface. C_5a is a 15,000-MW polypeptide with the most potent chemotactic and anaphylatoxic activity of any chemical mediator. C_4a and C_3a do not have chemotactic activity. In tissues, C_5a is rapidly broken down to C_5a-des-arg by cleavage of the N- terminal arginine. C_5-des-arg is inactive as anaphylatoxin but retains potent chemotactic activity for neutrophils in the presence of whole serum. Anaphylatoxins C_5a or C_3a (and weakly C_4a) produce direct contraction of smooth muscle (see the Schultz–Dale test in Chapter 14). Addition of these complement fragments will produce contraction of intestinal, uterine, tracheal, or other smooth muscle in vitro, followed by a refractory period termed tachyphylaxis, that is specific for C_3a or C_5a, ie, C_3a desensitizes the muscle to further stimulation by C_3a, but not to C_5a. This suggests separate distinct receptors for C_3a and C_5a on smooth muscle. In addition, anaphylactoxic complement fragments induce the release of histamine from mast cells via receptors for C_3a and C_5a. C_5a induces acute inflammation if activated in tissue by soluble antibody–antigen complexes (toxic complex reactions). C_5b binds to the cell surface, where it reacts with the remaining complement components, C6–C9, to produce a multimolecular complex that is capable of inserting itself into the cell membrane, forming a channel that permits release of the cytoplasm (lysis).

Alternate Pathway

The complement cascade may be activated by another set of proteins similar to C_4, C_2, C_1, and C_3; this is called the alternate pathway. A more detailed schematic representation of both the classical and alternate pathways of complement activation is shown in Figure 8–8. The alternate pathway is activated by materials such as bacterial lipopolysaccharide (endotoxin), yeasts (zymosan), or IgA antibody. Three factors—initiating factor, factor B, and factor D—interact in a manner similar to that of the first three complement components of the classical pathway, producing a complex of activated B (Bb) and D that

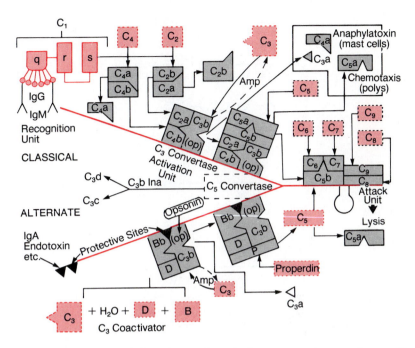

Figure 8–8. Details of the classical and alternate pathway of complement activation. For description, see text.

functions as a C_3 convertase. A trimolecular complex of Bb, D, and C_3b is then formed that is stabilized by the addition of another component, properdin. This complex functions as C_5 convertase in activation of C_5 and the remaining components of the membrane attack unit.

C_3 plays a central role in both the classical and alternative pathways of complement activation. Concealed within the C_3 molecule are at least 10 binding sites for different kinds of interactions that underlie the biologic activities of C_3. As the C_3 molecule is processed by C_3 convertase and then by I and its cofactors, sites appear and disappear. Some of these binding sites are to the cell membrane, to H-factor, to properdin and conglutinin, and to CR2, the C_3d and Epstein–Barr virus receptor on human B lymphocytes. Cleavage of C_3 to form active fragments is illustrated in Figure 8–9. Human C_3 is a 195-kDa glycoprotein containing two polypeptide chains ($\alpha = 120,000$ kDa; $\beta = 75,000$ kDa). The α-chain contains an unstable thioester bond between a cysteinyl residue and a glutamic acid residue that provides a site for covalent bonding reactions. Hydrolysis of the α-chain thioester bond causes "dead end" inactivation. During activation, the first cleavage produces a small fragment, C_3a, which has anaphylactic properties (see below). The larger fragment, C_3b, has a molecular weight of 185,000 Da and undergoes a complex arrangement of its tertiary structure, which

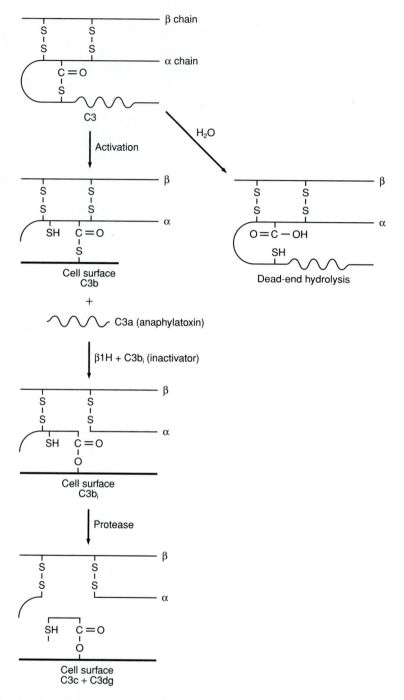

Figure 8–9. The binding and decay of C_3.

exposes the internal thioester bond in the α-chain. This bond can be broken by aldehydes, carboxyl groups, nitrogen nucleophiles, or water, forming a new covalent bond. An ester bond between C_3b and erythrocytes or bacteria is formed, whereas amide, as well as ester, bonds are formed with proteinaceous immune complexes. Since water is usually present in vast molar excess and can hydrolyze the thioester, most activated C_3b does not bind to cell surfaces or immune complexes. Thus, the presence of water serves to neutralize the activated C_3b, and to concentrate the activity of the activated fragments to the protected sites on the cell membrane where complement activation was initiated.

C_3 Receptors

There are four cellular receptors for the activated fragments of C_3: CR1, CR2, CR3, and CR4. C_3 receptors are instrumental in the localization of fragments of C_3 that enhance phagocytosis (opsonize) bacteria, yeast, and other complement-coated particles. Foreign organisms, such as bacteria, become coated with C_3 upon reaction with antibody. Such coated bacteria will become attached to normal red blood cells because of receptors of RBCs for the C_3 fragments. This phenomenon is called "immune adherence." All primate erythrocytes have such C_3 receptors. C_3 receptors are also found on lymphocytes, polymorphonuclear leukocytes, monocytes, and podocytes of the renal glomerulus. A listing of the properties of some C_3 receptors is given in Table 8–14.

Regulation and Amplification Mechanisms

Regulation of the complement system is accomplished by a set of inactivators. Complement activation occurs at low levels normally at all times as well as at high levels during inflammation. If left uncontrolled, the cascade of activation could result in serious damage to normal tissue. A number of inactivators of complement have been identified that act on different stages of complement activation (Table 8–15). Included are C_{1q} inhibitor, C_1 esterase inhibitor, the C_3 esterase inhibitor system, a membrane activation complex (MAC) inhibitor that competes with cell membrane sites for C_{5-9}, and serum carboxypeptidase N, which inactivates anaphylatoxin (C_5a). A deficiency of the C_1

TABLE 8–14. COMPLEMENT RECEPTORS

Receptor	Fragment	Cell Location	Function
CR1	C_3b	Leukocytes, erythrocytes	Cofactor for C3 inactivator
CR2	C_3dg	Lymphocytes, epithelium	C_3dg recognized by phagocytic cells through CR3 and CR4
CR3 (MHc1)	iC_3b	Polymorphs, lymphocytes	Binding of ADCC and NK cells to targets
CR4 (p150–95)	iC_3b	Polymorphs, lymphocytes	May bind to activated endothelium, causes margination of PMNs

TABLE 8–15. REGULATORY COMPONENTS OF THE COMPLEMENT SYSTEM

C_1q Inhibitor	Inactivates C_1q binding
C_1 esterase inhibitor	Inactivates esterase activity
C_3 convertase inhibitor system	Inactivates C_3 convertase
MAC inhibitor	Competes with cell surface for C_{5-9}
Serum carboxypeptidase N	Inactivates anaphylatoxin

esterase inhibitor is found in hereditary angioedema (see Chapter 14). These patients exhibit massive acute transient swelling of areas of the skin, the bronchi, or the gastrointestinal tract associated with depressed serum levels of C_4 and C_2 because of an inability to inactivate C_1 esterase. This reaction results in the continued formation of C_4 and C_2 fragments, particularly C_2b. C_2b is converted by plasmin to a molecule with kininlike activity. The C_2b kinin causes contraction of endothelial cells and edema. The reaction continues for approximately 24 hours, which is essentially the biological life of C_1 esterase in the absence of C_1 esterase inhibitor.

C_3 Convertase System (C_3b/C_4b). C_3 convertase plays a critical role in both the classical and alternative pathways of complement activation. The activity of C_3 convertase is dependent upon the association of C_4b and C_2a in the classical pathway and C_3b and Bb in the alternative pathway. C_3 convertase activity is regulated by a family of proteins, termed regulators of complement activation (RCA), the members of which react with C_3b or C_4b (Table 8–16). This family includes C_2, which reacts with C_4b during classical activation and factor b, which reacts with C_3b during alternative pathway activation, as well as at least six other proteins that serve to regulate the activity of C_4b/C_2a and C_3b/Bb (see Table 8–15). The genes for these proteins are closely linked on the long arm of human chromosome one, and each protein contains from eight to over thirty short, homologous, repeating units approximately sixty amino acids in length. The CR1, CR2, C_4, Bb, and decay activating factor (DAF) genes are very closely spaced and also show a high degree of homology, suggesting origin from a common ancestral gene.

Two RCA proteins, DAF and membrane cofactor protein, protect cells from the action of C_3b and C_4b by inactivating these fragments on the surface of cells. DAF is a 70-kDa glycolipid protein anchored in cellular membranes. MCP is composed of two distinct but highly homologous proteins (MCP-1 and MCP-2) with molecular weights of 68 and 63 kDa. Both of these are present on a wide variety of normal cells and provide protection from autologous tissue destruction by

TABLE 8–16. REGULATORY PROTEINS OF C3 CONVERTASE INHIBITOR SYSTEM

Regulator	Binds to:	Properties	Function	Deficiency State
Factor I inactivator	(C3b, C4b)	MW 90,000 Serine protease endopepidase	Inactivates C3b or C4b by cleavage of α chain; requires cofactors	Low C3, recurrent infections, angioedema
CR1	(C3b/C4b)	MW 160,000–250,000 Cell membrane of neutrophils, macrophages, and erythrocytes	Promotes phagocytosis and degranulation; cofactor for C3b inactivator; increases decay of C4b2a and C3bBb (C3 convertases)	Hemolytic anemias, chronic granulotous disease
CR2	(C3d,g)	MW 145,000 B cell membrane	Membrane activator for B cells	Receptor for Epstein-Barr virus
Factor H	(C3b)	MW 150,000–160,000 Serum glycoprotein	Cofactor for C3b INH; binds C3b, increases decay of C3bBb in the alternative pathway	Low C3, recurrent infections, C3 detectable on erythrocytes
C4-binding protein	(C4)	MW 540,000–590,000 Serum protein	Cofactor for C3b INH; increases decay of C4b2a	
Decay-activating factor (DAF)	(C3b, C4b)	MW 70,000 Cell membrane glycoprotein	Binds C3bBb or C4b2a; increases decay of C3 convertase of both classical and alternative pathway	Paroxysmal nocturnal hemoglobulinuria (lysis of RBC)
JP45-70 (MCP)	(C3b, C4b)	MW 45,000–70,000 membrane	Inactivates C3 convertase (preferential for classical pathway)	

inactivating complement-mediated destruction. Another restriction factor, homologous restriction factor (HRF20) is present on the surface of blood and endothelial cells and inhibits the terminal stage of the formation of membrane attack complexes by interfering with the binding of C_8 to C_{5b67}.

Factor H is an abundant plasma protein of 150 kDa that binds to C_3b, preventing the formation of the alternate pathway convertase (C_3bBb) and causing dissociation of the C_3bBb complex. C_4bp is a 550-kDa plasma protein formed from seven identical 70 kDa subunits. It serves as a cofactor for the proteolytic digestion of C_4b.

CR1 is a polymorphic 190 to 200-kDa receptor which primarily binds C_3b and C_4b. It is found mainly on mature blood cells. It binds C_3bC_4b complexes and processes them for clearance. Immune complexes in the circulation coated with C_3bC_4b bind to erythrocytes and are delivered to the reticuloendothelial system. The C_3bC_4 complexes are stripped from the cells and degraded.

CR2 is a 145-kDa receptor for the 40-kDa degradation fragment of C_3b (C_3dg) as well as for Epstein–Barr virus. CR2 is linked to surface IgM of mature B cells and plays an accessory role in activation of B cells.

Role of Complement in Immune Reactions

Activation of complement components is an essential feature of cytotoxic and immune complex reactions and may play a role in initiating some cellular reactions. The fixation of complement to a cell surface by action of antibody or via the alternate pathway is responsible for cytolytic reactions. Opsonization is activated because of coating by C_3b (or C_4b), and lysis of cells by formation of the membrane attack complex C_{5-9}. The chemotactic effect of C_5a attracts polymorphonuclear leukocytes and is largely responsible for the participation of these cells in immune complex reactions. The anaphylatoxic effects of C_3a and C_5a cause separation of endothelial cells. This serves to open vascular barriers to inflammatory cells so that neutrophils, lymphocytes, and macrophages may emigrate from the blood and induce inflammation in tissues.

THE COAGULATION SYSTEM

Any significant inflammation will result in activation of the coagulation system; several components of this system may serve as inflammatory mediators (Fig. 8–10). The coagulation system responds to various stimuli by the formation of platelet plugs and insoluble protein aggregates (fibrin) formed from soluble precursors. Fibrin forms clots that stop bleeding following injury to blood vessels. The fibrinolytic system is activated soon after clot formation in order to limit the extent of fibrin deposition and to initiate dissolution of fibrin so that circulation can be restored to injured tissues. Fibrin may also act as a scaffold for the ingrowth of fibroblasts and capillaries to initiate repair. If fibrin formed intravascularly is not cleared, multiple areas of tissue necrosis (infarcts) may occur; this is known as disseminated

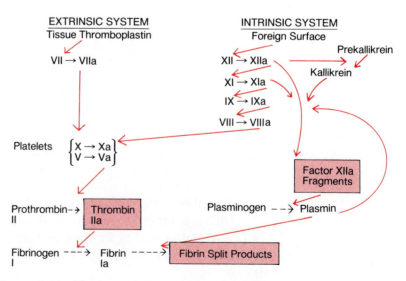

Figure 8–10. The coagulation system and inflammation.

intravascular coagulation (see Shwartzman reaction, Chapter 10). The kinin system increases vascular permeability in areas of inflammation and may be activated by intermediate products of the coagulation cascade.

The major components of the coagulation system are designated by roman numerals; a roman numeral followed by the letter "a" indicates an active fragment of that factor. Coagulation is basically a cascading sequence of enzyme-driven activations. Coagulation products active in inflammation are fragments of Hageman factor (XIIa), thrombin (IIa), and fibrin split products. The coagulation system consists of three major parts: the extrinsic system, the intrinsic system, and the common thrombin–fibrin pathway. The extrinsic system is activated by the action of tissue thromboplastin on factor VII. The intrinsic system involves activation of a series of components beginning with factor XII (Hageman factor). The common pathway is the activation of factors X and V on platelets with the subsequent formation of thrombin and fibrin. Kallikrein, activated factor XI, and plasmin can all act to cleave activated factor XII to produce fragments that initiate fibrinolysis and kinin release and generate a plasma factor that enhances vascular permeability. Activated factor XII converts prekallikrein to kallikrein (see The Kinin System, below) so that activation of the intrinsic coagulation system also generates inflammatory mediators.

The Kinin System

Peptides that are active as mediators of inflammation may be generated from a number of cells and tissue products. Of these, the most active is the kinin system. The components of this system are generated by the cleavage of plasma proteins into active peptides by proteolytic enzymes of the kallikrein system or by trypsin. Kallikreins are small, proteolytic enzymes found in tissues (particularly glandular organs) and in plasma that act on larger molecules such as kininogens to produce active peptides. Kallikreins are activated from prekallikreins by the action of activated factor XII (Hageman factor) of the intrinsic coagulation system. Prekallikrein in plasma exists as a single polypeptide chain with an intrachain disulfide bond. There is also a tissue form that is slightly different. Activated factor XII (XIIa) cleaves the polypeptide chain to form an active two-chain disulfide-linked kallikrein molecule.

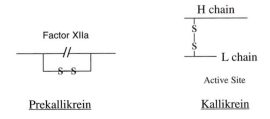

Kallikrein, factor XIIa, factor XI, or trypsin further cleaves high-molecular-weight kininogen to liberate vasoactive peptides. Kallikrein in turn acts on kininogens to produce biologically active fragments (Fig. 8–11). The active peptides are kallidin and bradykinin. Kallidin is a decapeptide and bradykinin is a nanopeptide formed by cleavage of the N-terminal lysine from kallidin. These mediators, particularly bradykinin, are highly active in stimulating vasodilation and increased vascular permeability but are rapidly catabolized by kininases into inactive peptides.

Adult Respiratory Distress Syndrome

The adult respiratory distress syndrome (ARDS) is a disorder in the regulation of acute inflammation. It is the result of diffuse damage to the alveolar epithelium and capillary endothelium of the lung (alveolar wall). This causes increased capillary permeability, interstitial and intraalveolar edema, fibrin exudation, and hyaline membrane formation. ARDS is an increasingly frequent cause of death of patients with diffuse respiratory infections, burns, oxygen toxicity, narcotic overdose, and open cardiac surgery.

The etiology of ARDS is not well defined but is thought to be due to shock, oxygen toxicity, complement activation, bacterial products, or a combination of these. In oxygen toxicity associated with artificial assisted respirators, free radicals injure both endothelium and epithelium, causing increased permeability and inducing alveolar edema. Complement activation generates C_5a, which causes leukocyte aggregation and activation in the lung. Eosinophils release cationic proteins, which injure endothelial cells and alveolar type II pneumocytes. Alveolar cell injury leads to loss of surfactant and collapse of air spaces. Surfactant is a complex mixture of lipids, proteins, and carbohydrates that lowers alveolar surface tension and greatly reduces the work of breathing. A deficiency of surfactant is responsible for neonatal respiratory distress syndrome (NRDS). Surfactant is produced by type II alveolar epithelial cells that are sensitive to different toxic agents. A loss of surfactant is believed to play a major role in both

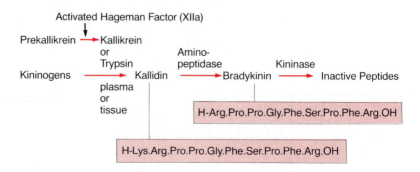

Figure 8–11. The Kinin System.

NRDS and ARDS. The role of the different acute inflammatory mechanisms in ARDS is not clear at this time but most likely involves multiple mediators and may be potentiated by a failure of inactivation mechanisms.

Interrelationships of Inflammatory Cells and Protein Systems in Acute Inflammation

A composite of inflammatory mechanisms and interrelationships is illustrated in Figure 8–12. The complement, kinin, coagulation, and mast cell systems, as well as bacterial products, contribute to vasodilation, increased vascular permeability, and chemotaxis of the neutrophil, the primary cellular mediator of acute inflammation. The anaphylactic peptides C_3a and C_5a are the major inflammatory mediators derived from complement. Cells destroyed by the activation of complement may contribute indirectly through release of intracellular contents that

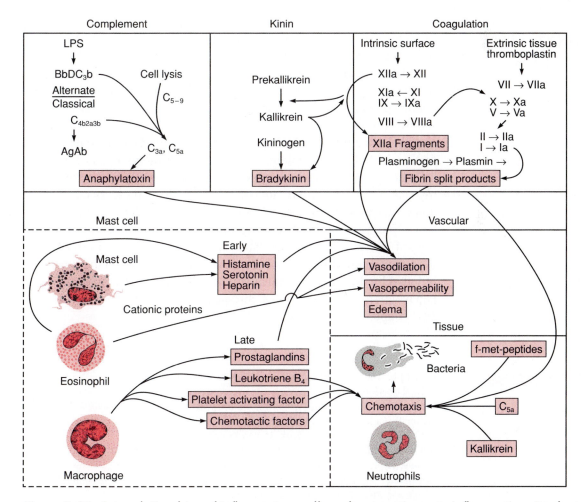

Figure 8–12. Interrelationships of inflammatory cells and systems in acute inflammation. Products of the complement, kinin, coagulation, and mast cell systems produce vasoactive and chemotactic mediators of acute inflammation. The major mediators are highlighted by boxes.

may cause further tissue destruction (enzymes) or activate the extrinsic coagulation system. Activation of the intrinsic coagulation system produces a series of active fragments. Activated factor XII (Hageman factor) contributes to generation of three inflammatory mediators—bradykinin, Hageman factor fragments, and fibrin split products. Mast cells contribute directly by release of mediators such as histamine and serotonin and indirectly by providing arachidonic acid precursors for generation of leukotrienes, prostaglandins, and other factors. These systems act to increase blood flow and vascular permeability leading to edema as well as attracting polymorphonuclear neutrophils and eosinophils to sites of inflammation. Neutrophils destroy infecting organisms by phagocytosis and digestion but also release lysosomal enzymes that may produce tissue damage. Eosinophils are believed to modulate inflammatory reactions by deactivating mast cell mediators, but also contain toxic cationic proteins.

Summary

Inflammation is the process of delivery of proteins and cells to sites of tissue damage or infection and their activation at these sites. The process moves from acute to subacute and chronic stages, and to resolution or scarring. The extent of tissue lesions produced by the inflammatory process are determined by mechanisms mediated by activated serum protein or blood cells, as well as by extracellular matrix and endothelial cells. The serum protein systems involved in acute inflammation include complement, coagulation, fibrinolysis, and kinin; the cellular systems include polymorphonuclear neutrophils, eosinophils, mast cells (or basophils), and platelets. Each of these systems has a homeostatic function and is controlled by interrelated feedback systems. Excessive or prolonged activation, as well as inadequate activation of these systems may have serious effects. Manifestations of inflammation in different tissues are similar even though the process is initiated by different events (infections, tissue necrosis, antibody–antigen reactions). The process of chronic inflammation is presented in the next chapter.

Bibliography

General

Bray MA, Anderson WH: *Mediators of Pulmonary Inflammation.* New York, Marcel Dekker, 1991.

Florey HW (ed.): *General Pathology,* 4th ed. Philadelphia, Saunders, 1970.

Gallin JI, Goldstein IM, Snyderman R: *Inflammation: Basic Principles and Clinical Correlates,* 2nd ed. New York, Raven Press, 1992.

Movat HZ (ed.): *Inflammation, Immunity, and Hypersensitivity.* New York, Harper & Row, 1971.

Oppenheim JJ, Rosenstreich DL, Potter M: *Cellular Functions in Immunity and Inflammation.* New York, Elsevier, 1981.

Spector WG, Willoughby DA: The inflammatory response. *Bacteriol Rev* 27:117, 1963.

Zweifach BW, Grant L, McClusky RT (eds.): *The Inflammatory Response,* vol 3. New York, Academic Press, 1974.

Adhesion Molecules

Butcher EC: Leukocyte–endothelial cell recognition: Three (or more) steps to specificity and diversity. *Cell* 67:1033, 1991.

Godin C, Caprani A, DuFaux J, Flaud P: Interactions between neutrophils and endothelial cells. *J Cell Sci* 106:441–452, 1993.

Granger DN, Kubes P: The microcirculation and inflammation: Modulation of leukocyte-endothelial cell adhesion. *J Leukocyte Biol* 55:662–675, 1994.

Lasky LA: Selectin: Interpreters of cell-specific carbohydrate information during inflammation. *Science* 258:964, 1992.

Piker LJ, Warnock RA, Burns AR, et al.: The neutrophil selectin LECAM-1 presents carbohydrate ligands to the vascular selectins ELAM-1 and GMP-140. *Cell* 66:921, 1991.

Schleimer RP, Stervinsky SA, Kaiser J, et al.: IL-4 induces adherence of human eosinophils and basophils but not neutrophils to endothelium: Association with expression of VCAM-1. *J Immunol* 148:1086, 1992.

Zimmerman GA, Prescott SM, McIntyre TM: Endothelial cell interactions with granulocytes: Tethering and signaling molecules. *Immnuol Today* 13:93, 1992.

Mast Cells

Anderson P, Slorach SA, Uvnas B: Sequential exocytosis of storage granules during antigen-induced histamine release from sensitized rat mast cells in vitro: An electron microscopic study. *Acta Physiol Scand* 88:359, 1973.

Bach MK: Mediators of anaphylaxis and inflammation. *Annu Rev Microbiol* 36:371, 1982.

Chakrin L, Bailey D: Leukotrienes. Orlando, FL, Academic Press, 1984.

Davis P, Bailey PJ, Goldenberg MM, et al.: The role of arachidonic acid oxygenation products in pain and inflammation. *Annu Rev Immunol* 2:335, 1983.

Dvorak HF, Dvorak AM: Basophils, mast cells, and cellular immunity in animals and man. *Hum Pathol* 3:454, 1972.

Feuerstein G, Hallenbeck JM: Leukotrienes in Health and Disease. *Federation of American Societies of Experimental Biology Cell.*

Metcalf DD, Kaliner M, Donlon MA: The mast cell. *CRC Crit Rev Immunol* 3:24, 1981.

Plaut M, Pierce JH, Watson CJ, et al.: Mast cell lines produce lymphokines in response to crosslinkage of Fc epsilon RI or calcium ionophores. *Nature* 339:64, 1989.

Uvnas B: Mechanism of histamine release in mast cells. *Ann NY Acad Sci* 103:278, 1963.

Wodnar-Filipowicz A, Heusser CH, Moroni C: Production of the hemopoietic growth factors GM-CSF and interleukin-3 by mast cells in response to IgE receptor-mediated activation. *Nature* 339:150, 1989.

Zurier RB: Inflammatory Diseases. In *Prostaglandins in Clinical Practice.* Watkins D, et al., eds. New York, Raven Press, 1989, 79–96.

Platelets

Roth GJ: Platelets and blood vessels: The adhesion event. *Immunol Today* 13:100, 1992.

Eosinophils

Beeson PB, Bass DA: *The Eosinophil.* Philadelphia, Saunders, 1977.

Gleich GJ, Adolphson CR: The eosinophilic leukocyte: Structure and function. *Adv Immunol* 39:177, 1986.

Gleich GJ: The eosinophil and bronchial asthma: Current understanding. *J Allergy Clin Immunol* 85:422, 1990.

Harmann KJ, Barker RL, Ten RM, et al.: The molecular biology of eosinophil granule proteins. *Int Arch Allergy Appl Immunol* 94:202, 1991.

Rowen JL, Hyde DM, McDonald RJ: Eosinophils cause acute edematous injury in isolated perfused rat lungs. *Am Rev Respir Dis* 142:215, 1990.

Spry CJF, Kay AB, Gleich GJ: Eosinophils 1992. *Immunol Today* 13:384, 1992.

Neutrophils

Becker EL: Enzyme activation and the mechanism of neutrophil chemotaxis. *Antibiot Chemother* 19:409, 1974.

Boyden S: The chemotactic effect of mixtures of antibody and antigen on polymorphonuclear leucocytes. *J Exp Med* 115:453, 1962.

Cochrane CG: Immunologic tissue injury mediated by neutrophilic leukocytes. *Adv Immunol* 9:97, 1968.

Goldstein IM: Polymorphonuclear leukocyte lysosomes and immune tissue injury. *Prog Allergy* 20:301, 1976.

Halliwell B (ed.): Oxygen Radicals and Tissue Injury. A symposium published by FASEB. Bethesda, MD, 1988.

Morel F, Doussiere J, Vignais V: The superoxide-generating oxidase of phagocytic cells: Physiological, molecular, and pathological aspects. *Eur J Biochem* 210:523, 1991.

Naccache PH, Shaafi RI: Granulocyte activation: Biochemical events associated with the mobilization of calcium. *Surv Immuno Res* 3:288, 1984.

Schiffmann E, Corcoran BA, Wahl SA: N-formylmethyl peptides as chemoattractants for leukocytes. *Proc Nat Acad Sci USA,* 72:1059, 1975.

Spicer SS, Harkin JH: Ultrastructure, cytochemistry, and function of neutrophil leukocyte granules. *Lab Invest* 20:488, 1969.

Thomas EL, Lehrer RI, Rest RF: Human neutrophil antimicrobial activity. *Rev Infect Dis 10 (Suppl.)*2:450–456, 1990.

Varani J, Ward PA: Mechanisms of endothelial cell injury in acute inflammation. *Shock* 2:311–319, 1994.

Winrow VR, Winyard PG, Morris CJ, et al.: Free radicals in inflammation: Second messengers and mediators of tissue destruction. *Brit Med Bull* 49:506–522, 1993.

Acute-Phase Proteins

Baumann H, Gauldie J: The acute phase response. *Immunol Today* 76:74–80, 1994.

Dowton SB, Colten HR: Acute-phase reactants in inflammation and infection. *Sem Hematol* 25:84–90, 1988.

Kolb-Bachofen V: A review of the biological properties of C-reactive protein. *Immunobiol* 183:133, 1991.

Kushner I: Regulation of the acute phase response by cytokines. *Persp Biol Med* 36:611–622, 1993.

McCarty M: Historical perspective on C-reactive protein. *Ann NY Acad Med* 77:1, 1982.

Roberts RC, Nelles LP, Hall PK, et al.: Comparison of the structure and aspects of the proteinase-binding properties of cystic fibrotic α_2-macroglobulin with normal α_2-macroglobulin. *Pediatr Res* 16:416, 1982.

Schwick HG, Haupt H: Properties of acute phase proteins of human plasma. *Behring Inst Mitt* 80:1, 1986.

Sottrup-Jensen L, Sand O, Kristensen L, et al.: The α-macroglobulin bait region: Sequence diversity and localization of cleavage sites for proteinases in five mammalian α-macroglobulins. *J Biol Chem* 264:15781, 1989.

Complement

Cohen S: The requirement for the association of two adjacent rabbit γ-G antibody molecules in the fixation of complement by immune complexes. *J Immunol* 100:407, 1968.

Frank M: Complement: Current Concepts. Kalamazoo, MI, Upjohn, 1985.

Hourcade D, Holers VM, Atkinson JP: The regulators of complement activation (RCA) gene cluster. *Adv Immunol* 45:381–416, 1989.

Hugli TE: Structure and functions of the anaphylatoxins. *Springer Semin Immunopathol* 7:93, 1984.

Humphrey JH, Dourmaskin RR: The lesions in cell membranes caused by complement. *Adv Immunol* 11:75, 1969.

Mayer MA: Membrane damage by complement. *Johns Hopkins Med J* 148:243, 1981.

Muller-Eberhard HJ: Complement: Chemistry and pathways. In *Inflammation: Basic Principles and Clinical Correlates,* 2nd ed. Gallin JI, Goldstein IM, Snyderman R (eds.). New York, Raven Press, 1992, 33–61.

Nose M, Katoh M, Okada N, et al.: Tissue distribution of HRF20, a novel factor preventing the membrane attack of homologous complement, and its predominant expression on endothelial cells in vivo. *Immunol* 70:145, 1990.

Pangburn MK, Muller-Eberhard HJ: The alternative pathway of complement activation. *Springer Semin Immunopathol* 7:163, 1984.

Wilson JG, Andriopoulos NA, Fearon DT: CD1 and the cell membrane proteins that bind C3 and C4: A basic and clinical review. *Immunol Res* 6:192–209, 1987.

Coagulation

Ratnoff O: The interrelationship of clotting factors and immunologic mechanisms. In *Immunology.* Good RA, Fisher DW (eds.). Stanford, CA, Sinauer, 1971, 35.

Roberts HR, Lozier JN: New perspectives on the coagulation cascade. *Hosp Pract* 27:73, 1992.

Sundsmo JS, Fair DS: Relationship among the complement, kinin, coagulation, and fibrinolytic systems in the inflammatory reaction. *Clin Physiol Biochem* 1:225, 1983.

Kinin

Kaplan AP, Ghebrehiwet B, Silverberg M, et al.: The intrinsic coagulation–kinin pathway, complement cascades, plasma kinin–angiotensin system, and their interrelationship. *CRC Crit Rev Immunol* 3:75, 1981.

Schachter M: Kallikreins and kinins. *Physiol Rev* 49, 1969.

Sharma JN: The role of kallikrein–kinin system in joint inflammatory disease. *Pharmacol Res* 23:105, 1991.

Spragg J: Complement, coagulation, and kinin generation. In *Immunopharmacology.* Sirois P, Rola-Pleszcynski M (eds.). New York, Elsevier, 1982.

Webster ME: Kinin system. In *Cellular and Humoral Mechanisms in Anaphylaxis and Allergy.* Movat HZ (ed.). New York, Karger, 1969.

ARDS

Caminiti SP, Young SL: The pulmonary surfactant system. *Hosp Pract* 27:57, 1991.

Hallgren R, Samuelson R, Venge P, et al.: Eosinophil activation in the lung is related to lung damage in adult respiratory distress syndrome. *Am Rev Respir Dis* 135:639, 1987.

Perry TL, Ashbaugh DG: The adult respiratory distress syndrome. *Chest* 60:233, 1971.

Welbourne CRB, Young Y: Endotoxin, septic shock, and acute lung injury: Neutrophils, macrophages, and inflammatory mediators. *Br J Surg* 79:988–1003, 1992.

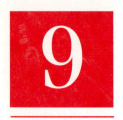

Chronic Inflammation and Wound Healing

Chronic inflammation follows acute inflammation if there is tissue damage or if the acute response is not adequate to clear the tissue. The function of chronic inflammation is to clear the tissue of necrotic debris produced from acute necrosis, provide more powerful defensive weapons against persistent infections, and complete the process of wound healing. If the tissue can be cleared with little or no damage, the structure will be returned to normal (**resolution**); if some of the normal tissue architecture is destroyed, it may be necessary to fill in the zones of destruction with connective tissue (**scarring**).

The Cells of Chronic Inflammation

The cells of chronic inflammation are lymphocytes, macrophages, and plasma cells (see also Chapter 2). To contrast these to the "polymorphonuclear cells" that are the hallmark of acute inflammation, the cells of chronic inflammation collectively are termed "mononuclear cells." Plasma cells are present in many forms of chronic inflammation and represent antibody-producing cells resulting from stimulation of B cells by antigens that migrate from lymph nodes to inflammatory sites.

LYMPHOCYTES

Lymphocytes are prominent in chronic inflammation and are the immune-specific effector cells of T-cytotoxicity (CD8+ T_{CTL}) and of delayed hypersensitivity (CD4+ T_{DTH}). The immune-specific effects of T_{CTL} and T_{DTH} lymphocytes in cell-mediated immunity will be presented in detail in Chapters 15 and 16. In nonimmune chronic inflammation, cytokines produced during acute inflammation and adhesion molecules (see below) attract and activate lymphocytes. In addition to the interleukins that act on other cells during induction of immunity, activated lymphocytes secrete a number of biologically active inflammatory mediators (Table 9–1). The major inflammatory function of these mediators (lymphokines) appears to be the attraction and activation of macrophages, but other functions such as increasing vascular permeability, killing target cells, and controlling lymphocyte proliferation have been attributed to lymphokines.

MACROPHAGES

Macrophages play an important role in chronic inflammation, in general, and in delayed hypersensitivity reactions, in particular. Macrophages usually infiltrate sites of inflammation several hours after lymphocytes. The main function of macrophages is to phagocytize

TABLE 9–1. CLASSIC INFLAMMATORY LYMPHOKINES

Factor	MW	Produced by	Effect
Migration inhibitory factor	15,000–70,000	Activated T_{DTH} cells	Inhibits migration of macrophages
Macrophage activating factor (INF-γ)	35,000—55,000	Activated T_{DTH} cells	Increases lysosomes in macrophages; increases phagocytic activity
Macrophage chemotactic factor	12,500	1. Activated T_{DTH} cells 2. Lysates of PMNs 3. Ag-Ab complexes (complement)	Attracts macrophages; gradient chemotaxis
Lymphotoxin (cachexin)	Multiple (10,000–200,000)	Activated TK or NK cells	Causes lysis of target cells
Lymphocyte stimulating factor	85,000	Activated T_{DTH} cells	Stimulates proliferation of lymphocytes
Proliferation inhibitory factor	70,000	Activated T_{DTH} cells	Inhibits proliferation of lymphocytes
Aggregation factor		Activated T_{DTH} cells	Causes lymphocytes and macrophages to adhere together
Interferon	20,000–25,000	Activated T_{DTH} cells	Inhibits growth of viruses; activates NK cells
Lymphocyte-permeability factor	12,000	Lymph node cells	Increases vascular permeability
Transfer factor	10,000	Activated T_{DTH} cells	Induces antigen-specific delayed hypersensitivity after passive transfer
Skin reactive factor	10,000	Activated T_{DTH} cells	Induces inflammation upon injection into skin
Cytophilic antibody	160,000	Plasma cells	Binds to macrophages; stimulates phagocytosis of specific antigen
Leukocyte inhibitory factor	68,000	Activated T cells	Inhibits neutrophil mobility
Osteoclast activating factor	17,000	T and B cells	Stimulates osteoclasts to absorb bone

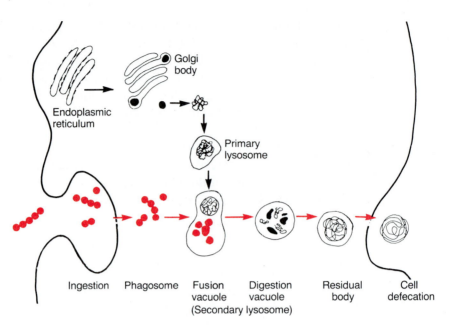

Figure 9–1. Phagocytosis. Foreign material is ingested into a phagosome. Phagosome fuses with primary lysosome (formed by Golgi body), which contains enzymes to digest ingested material. Resulting fusion vacuole is termed a secondary lysosome. When digestion is ended, some material may remain in residual body, or be eliminated from cell by cell defecation. (Modified from de Duve C: *Sci Am* 208:64, 1963. Copyright 1963 by Scientific American, Inc. All rights reserved.)

damaged tissue components, microorganisms, or other cells (Fig. 9–1). In this manner, by the action of potent macrophage lysosomal enzymes, macrophages clear the tissue of the products of inflammation and set the stage for resolution of the inflammatory process. In delayed hypersensitivity reactions, macrophages are attracted and activated by lymphokines produced by reaction of antigen with specifically sensitized lymphocytes (T_{DTH} cells) (see Table 9–3 and Chapter 16). Activated macrophages also secrete cytokines (monokines) that are largely responsible for later events in wound healing (see below).

Phagocytosis

The stages of phagocytosis are illustrated in Figure 9–2. Coating of bacteria by complement or antibody enhances phagocytosis, although phagocytosis may occur in the absence of antibody and complement. Cell surface aggregation of receptors precedes invagination of the cell membrane. Ingestion of material is accompanied by ion fluxes (positive ions entering cell), and superoxide formation. After formation of a phagocytic vacuole, fusion with enzyme containing lysosomes (phagolysosome) and digestion of phagocytosed material occurs.

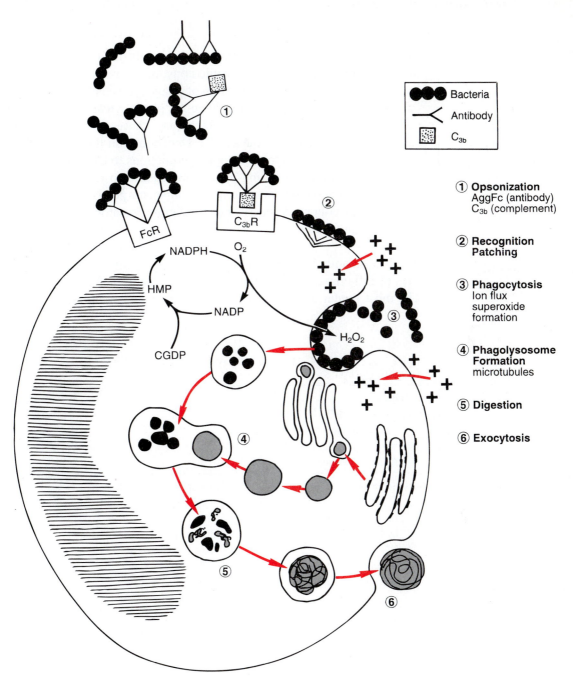

Figure 9–2. Schematic drawing of steps in phagocytosis:

1. Opsonization—aggregated Fc of antibody, activation of C_3b.
2. Recognition through receptors and patching of receptors.
3. Ingestion—cation influx stimulates transduction of hexosemonophosphate shunt and conversion of O_2 to H_2O_2.
4. Fusion of lysosome and phagosome to form phagolysosome involving microtubules.
5. Digestion of bacteria in phagolysosome.
6. Exocytosis of remnants.

Products of Macrophages

The products of macrophages that are important for consideration in inflammation are (1) the cytoplasmic constituents responsible for cellular metabolism and the degradation of phagocytosed material; (2) the cell surface receptors that contribute to phagocytosis; and (3) the secreted products (monokines), which may cause tissue damage or stimulate wound healing (Table 9–2). Depending on the nature of the inflammatory stimulus, the macrophage functions to clear necrotic tissue and to eradicate invading organisms leading to resolution of the acute inflammatory response or, if the organism persists, to initiate a chronic or prolonged defensive reaction, granulomatous inflammation (discussed in Chapter 17).

The importance of macrophages in inflammation was emphasized by Eli Metchnikoff over 100 years ago. Macrophages are attracted to sites of inflammation by a number of chemotactic factors (Table 9–3). The most potent are those derived from activated lymphocytes (lym-

TABLE 9–2. CELLULAR, CELL SURFACE, AND SECRETED PRODUCTS OF MACROPHAGES

I. Cellular
    Peroxidase (RER)
    5′nucleotidase
    Aminopeptidase
    Alkaline phosphatase

II. Cell Surface Receptors	
Fc receptor I (IgG_2a)	High-density lipoprotein
Fc receptor II (IgG_2b)	Lactoferrin
IgM	Insulin
C_3b	Fibrinogen
Lymphokines	Asialoglycoprotein
Protein aggregates (nonspecific)	f-met-leu-phe
Fibronectin	

III. Secreted Biologically Active Products of Macrophages	
Hydrolytic Enzymes	Cell Stimulatory Proteins
Lysosomal hydrolases	Colony-stimulating factor
Neutral proteases	Interleukin-1
Collagenase	Interferon
Plasminogen activator	Tumor necrosis factor
Elastase	Osteoclast activating factor
Lysozyme	Others
Arginase	Complement components (C_2, C_3, C_4, C_5, factor B)
	Oxygen Intermediates
	α_2 Macroglobulin
	Prostaglandins

TABLE 9–3. GROWTH-STIMULATING, CHEMOTACTIC, AND ACTIVATION FACTORS ACTING ON MACROPHAGES

Substance	Physicochemical Characteristics (MW)	Source	Functional Properties
Macrophage colony-stimulating factor (CSF)	70,000	Fibroblasts	Macrophage colony formation from bone marrow cells. Also induces macrophage secretion
Macrophage growth factor (MGF)	Same as CSF	Fibroblasts, activated T lymphocytes	Acts on promonocytes
Factor inducing monocytosis (FIM)	18,000–23,000	Unknown	Increases macrophages in blood
Leukocyte-derived chemotactic (LDCF)	12,000	Activated T lymphocytes	Chemotactic for macrophages
Plasminogen activator inducer (IPA)		Activated T lymphocytes	Stimulates plasminogen activator secretion
Macrophage stimulatory protein (MSP)	100,000	Unknown	Increases spreading and phagocytosis
Factor Bb	65,000	Alternate complement pathway	Increases spreading and phagocytosis; inhibits migration
Macrophage activating factor (INF-γ)	50,000–60,000	Activated T lymphocytes	Increases macrophage tumoricidal and microbicidal function
Migration inhibitory factor (MIF)	25,000–60,000	Activated T lymphocytes	Inhibits migration
Soluble immune response suppressor (SIRS)	Similar to MIF	Activated T lymphocytes	
Interferon	Several MW species	Fibroblasts, activated T lymphocytes	Both types I and II activate macrophages
Macrophage aggregating factor	> 100,000	Activated T lymphocytes	Distinct from MIF. Causes clumping of macrophages in vivo and in vitro; may be fibronectin
IL-8	CXC chemadain	T-cell	Chemotactic
Monocyte Chemotactic Proteins (MCPs)	3 doses cxc chemotein	Osteosarcoma cells	Chemotactic
C5a	15,000	Complement activation	Chemotactic
f-Met peptides	Tripeptides	Bacteria	Chemotactic
Phorbol esters (PMA)		Tumor promotors	Activate macrophage secretion
LPS (endotoxin)		Bacteria	Activates macrophages

Modified from Rosenstreich DL: The macrophage, in Oppenheim JJ, Rosenstreich DL, Potter M (eds.) *Cellular Functions in Immunity and Inflammation.* New York, Elsevier, 1981, 140.

phokines), but factors may also be derived from other cell types. In addition, macrophages are attracted by C_5a and to f-met peptides. Thus, macrophages are attracted to sites of acute inflammation both by products of immune specific activation of lymphocytes and by products of nonimmune cells. In addition, lymphocytes activated by non-immune-specific mitogens, such as endotoxin (lipopolysaccharide [LPS]) or other bacterial products will stimulate production of lymphokines active on macrophages.

Activated macrophages have an increased capacity for phagocytosis, an increased capacity to digest phagocytosed objects and, in addition, secrete factors (monokines) active in inflammation and immune reactions (see Table 9–2). Activated macrophages have changes in lysosomal enzyme content—a decrease in 5′ nucleotidase and increase in aminopeptidase and alkaline phosphatase, as well as an increase in adenosine triphosphate and production of superoxide anion and hydrogen peroxide. There is also an increase in activity of cell surface receptors on macrophages, in particular for Fc regions of immunoglobulin and for C_3b.

Phagocytic Deficiencies

In some cases, because of either the nature or amount of the phagocytized material or because of an insufficiency in lysosomal hydrolases, ingested particles or organisms are not killed and digested. Some organisms (eg, *Histoplasma capsulatum*) have the ability to survive phagocytosis and reproduce within phagocytes. Infection with such an agent may result in the presence of large numbers of viable organisms in the cytoplasm of phagocytic cells. Some inorganic particles (silica) cannot be digested, remain in phagocytic cells, and eventually cause destruction of the phagocyte (phagocytic suicide), tissue damage and fibrosis, and increased susceptibility to certain infections. Certain human diseases are characterized by abnormalities in phagocytosis (phagocytic dysfunction). Such phagocytic deficiencies are usually associated with susceptibility to infections. These diseases are presented in more detail in Chapter 27. In addition, macrophages may not be able to clear tissues of some proteins that are produced in excess or abnormal proteins that are difficult to catabolize. Accumulation of these proteins in tissues leads to a condition known as amyloidosis (see Chapter 10).

Activated Macrophages

An acquired cellular resistance to microbial infection may be observed in an infected host whose mononuclear phagocytes have an increased capacity for destroying infected organisms (ie, has activated macrophages). Macrophage activation may occur by increasing the number of lysosomes per cell, by increasing the amount of hydrolytic enzymes in each lysosome, or by increasing the number of phagocytes available. Once such an increased capacity has been established, it is active against infections caused by unrelated organisms. A number of agents have been found that cause activation of macrophages. These include Bacillus Calmette–Guerin (BCG), *Listeria monocytogenes*, toxoplasma, endotoxin, levamisole, and polynucleotides (Fig. 9–3). Activation may occur by release of macrophage-activating factors from lymphocytes (see Table 9–3) or through an "autocrine" production of interferon-α, -β, or monocyte/macrophage colony-stimulating factor. A considerable interest in the role of this phenomenon in enhancing tumor immunity has developed because of the possibility

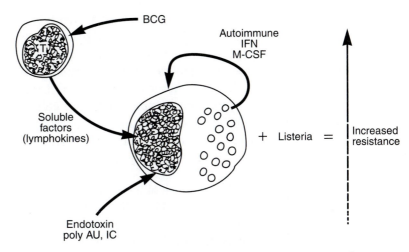

Figure 9–3. Nonspecific macrophage activation. Macrophages may acquire an increased capacity to destroy infective organisms or target cells after treatment with a variety of agents. BCG acts upon a T$_{DTH}$ cell, which produces soluble factors that affect macrophages. Endotoxins and polynucleotides act directly on macrophages. The mechanism of action of these agents is not understood, but as a result of macrophage activation, an experimental animal will resist a normally infectious challenge dose of an infectious agent. The chart (*bottom*) indicates that the dose of *Listeria monocytogenes*, which is required to kill an experimental animal, is significantly higher after treatment of the animals with BCG.

of limiting tumor growth with activated macrophages (see Chapter 30). This type of cellular immunity has been termed **immune phagocytosis**, even though this "immunity" is nonspecific.

In addition, macrophages are activated by a number of factors produced by other cells (**cytokines**). These factors (see Table 9–3) produce a variety of effects on macrophages that may be critical in inflammation.

Cytokines in Chronic Inflammation

Cytokine is a term used for a large group of proteins that are produced by a variety of cells in the body and act to stimulate or inhibit the functions of cells in an autocrine or paracrine fashion. Lymphokines are a subgroup of cytokines produced by lymphocytes; monokines are produced by macrophages. Cytokines are heterogeneous but have the following characteristics in common:

1. They have a low molecular weight (<80 kDa).
2. They are secreted from cells, often glycosylated.
3. They regulate immunity and inflammation.

4. They are produced transiently and act locally.
5. They react with high-affinity receptors on target cells.
6. After reaction, they activate cytoplasmic tyrosine kinases through the stepwise formation of a receptor complex.
7. They alter metabolism and behavior of the responding cell through phosphorylation of cellular kinases.
8. They have multiple and overlapping functions.
9. They act in a network, either inducing or inhibiting the effect of other cytokines.

The response of a cell to a cytokine depends on the local concentration of the cytokine, the simultaneous presence of other cytokines or regulators present, and the state of activation of the cell. In earlier chapters, the role of cytokines (interleukins) in the induction of immunity and in control of hematopoiesis was presented. One cytokine may have many actions (pleiotropy), and different cytokines may produce very similar effects (redundancy). The overlapping and varied effects of the cytokines may seem inefficient, but because there are different ways to accomplish the same thing, inflammation or other processes dependent on cytokine action may be effected successfully under many different circumstances. Thus the cytokines provide a network of back-up systems for vital functions. In this chapter, the cytokines that are active in the chronic inflammatory response will be discussed (Table 9–4). These include interleukin-1 (IL-1), interferon gamma (INF-γ), tumor necrosis factor-beta (TNF-β), tumor growth factor-beta (TGF-β), and interleukin-2 (IL-2).

INTERLEUKIN-1 (IL-1)

IL-1 is the epitome of a **pleotypic** cytokine with many different sources and actions. It is produced by macrophages, dendritic cells, T cells, B cells, and endothelial cells. It was originally called lymphocyte activation factor because of its ability to stimulate proliferation of lymphocytes (T cells). IL-1 production is stimulated by a variety of activation signals. Not only is it critical for activation of T cells and B cells during induction of a specific immune response, but IL-1 also serves as a cofactor for stimulation of proliferation of hematopoietic cells by colony-stimulating factors. The precise effect of IL-1 in inflammation is not easily explained since it has so many different direct and indirect functions. It stimulates production of other lymphokines, such as IL-2, IL-3, IL-4, INF-γ, and TGF-β. It promotes generation of cytotoxic effector cells. It stimulates production of colony-stimulating factors and synergizes with them to increase production of inflammatory cells in the bone marrow. It induces fever, lethargy, and shock; stimulates the release of prostaglandins; and is found in high levels in the joint fluid of patients with rheumatoid arthritis. Thus, IL-1 affects different

TABLE 9–4. MAJOR CYTOKINES INVOLVED IN CHRONIC INFLAMMATION AND WOUND HEALING

Name	Source	Action
IL-1	Activated macrophages, T and B cells, endothelial cells, and other cell types	Activates T and B cells; stimulates production of IL-2, IFN-γ, IL-3, IL-4 and TGF-β; many other effects
IL-2	Activated T cells	Stimulates proliferation of T and B cells; increases IL-1 and IFN-γ production, arguments NK activity and cytotoxicity at macrophages
INF-γ	Activated T cells, LGL, and LAK cells	Upgrades class I and II MHC expression; enhances T$_{CTL}$, NK, and macrophage activity; margination of lymphocytes; increases TNF and IL-1 production
TNF-α (cachectin) TNF-β	Activated macrophages, lymphocytes T$_{DTH}$, NK, LAK	Increases class I MHC expression on fibroblasts and endothelial cells; enhances class II MHC expression; activates macrophages; promotes angiogenesis; induces tumor necrosis, fever, cachexia
TGF-β	Platelets, macrophages, lymphocytes	Stimulates wound healing; controls inflammation; inhibits IL-2, IL-4, INF-γ, and TNF

stages of induction of the specific immune response, as well as acting at many stages of the process of inflammation and healing.

INTERLEUKIN-2 (IL-2)

IL-2 acts primarily during induction of immunity but also has effects in inflammation. It is produced mainly by activated T cells but also in smaller amounts by activated B cells. Its main action is as an autocrine or paracrine stimulator of proliferation of T or B cells. It also enhances the expression of other lymphokines by activated lymphocytes, especially IFN-γ and IL-1, and it synergizes with other interleukins to induce differentiation of B cells to become immunoglobulin-secreting cells. It augments natural killer (NK) cell activity and increases the cytotoxicity of macrophages. The major effect of IL-2 in inflammation appears to be indirect, through stimulation of production of IFN-γ and IL-1. IL-2 has been reported to have some beneficial effect on patients with solid tumor metastases, perhaps through increasing cytotoxicity of NK cells or macrophages.

INTERFERON-GAMMA (IFN-Γ)

IFN-γ (type II interferon) is a major mediator of inflammation. It is produced by activated T cells, large granular lymphocytes, and lymphokine-activated killer (LAK) cells. It upgrades expression of HLA class I markers on most cell types and class II markers on immune cells and vascular endothelium. The action on endothelial cells may be critical in the attraction of inflammatory cells to vessel walls during inflammation (margination). It also markedly increases the expression of integrin receptors on endothelial cells. It directly enhances the cytotoxic effect of cytotoxic T lymphocytes (CTLs), NK cells, and macrophages. (One of the earlier names for INF-γ was macrophage-activation factor.) It also affects the expression of a number of other cytokines. It enhances the transcription of TNF and IL-1 but inhibits production of GM-CSF. It synergizes with other cytokines in a variety of different effects. It has been used effectively in treatment of leprosy and chronic granulomatous disease, but is contraindicated in patients with rheumatoid arthritis, where it appears to increase inflammation.

TUMOR NECROSIS FACTOR (TNF)

TNF was discovered by its ability to cause necrosis of tumors in experimental animals and was originally called **lymphotoxin** because of its ability to kill certain tumor target cells in vitro. It was also shown to have many other effects (pleiotropy). TNF was independently identified by the occurrence of wasting in animals by a substance called **cachexin**, which was later found to be identical to TNF. It is produced mainly by activated macrophages but also by LAK cells and some T-cell lines. It enhances class I MHC expression by fibroblasts and vascular endothelium, synergizes with IFN-γ to enhance class II MHC expression on most cell types, and facilitates macrophage activation and IL-1 release. It promotes angiogenesis during wound healing (see below). In addition to producing hemorrhagic necrosis of tumors, it causes fever, hypotension, and profound weight loss (cachexia). TNF may produce dramatic regression of some tumors, but its effects are not consistent (depending on the immunocompetence of the patient) and are limited by severe systemic toxicity. TNF-β is produced by activated T_{DTH} and NK cells and acts to kill target cells.

TRANSFORMING GROWTH FACTOR-BETA (TGF-B)

TGF-β is named for the original function described for TGF-β—the ability to stimulate growth of some cultured cells in vitro—but actually it has much broader and more significant effects. TGF-β is a multifunctional cytokine playing an important role in embryonal development, as well as in regulating repair and regeneration following tissue injury. Platelets contain high concentrations of TGF-β and upon degranulation release TGF-β at sites of tissue injury. TGF-β is chemoattractive for white blood cells, induces angiogenesis, controls cytokine production, and causes increased deposition of extracellular matrix as well as decreased matrix degradation by lowering the synthesis of proteases and increasing the levels of protease inhibitors. Thus, TCF-β plays a key role as the "chief executive officer" of wound healing. However, like many CEOs, TGF-β sometimes has a vested interest in increasing its influence at the expense of the organization. In chronic progressive inflammatory diseases, TGF-β may act as an autocrine to increase TGF-β production, autoactivating overproduction of extracellular matrix and producing scarring and fibrosis. This has been termed the "dark side" of tissue repair. Controlling TGF-β production may be the key to preventing scarring and fibrosis in diseases such as glomerulonephritis or progressive pulmonary fibrosis.

Wound Healing

The process of wound healing begins during the earliest phase of injury or inflammation. Wound healing involves complex interactions among different cell types, as well as extracellular matrix, inflammatory mediators, and growth factors. The time of onset of healing depends on the extent of damage and whether or not the inflammatory process has been enhanced by infection, immune mechanisms, or chronic injury. Growth factors present in the area of injury promote cell migration and proliferation. The cell types involved in healing include platelets, lymphocytes, endothelial cells, macrophages, and fibroblasts. In uncomplicated sterile wounds, platelets serve to limit hemorrhage and as a source for platelet-derived growth factor (PDGF), which is most likely the first growth factor to take part in the healing process. Polymorphonuclear cells and macrophages clear necrotic tissue by phagocytosis. Once lymphocytes and macrophages enter the wound, the healing process is controlled not only by cytokines but also by various growth factors, as well as by cell matrix interactions mediated by integrins and cell adhesion molecules.

GROWTH FACTORS

Various growth factors originally recognized for their effects on tissue culture cells have been found to be critical pharmacologic agents for wound healing, and some are being successfully used to treat previously incurable wounds. Growth factor therapy is being tested on burns, ulcers, surgical incisions, dental extractions, skin grafts, and others. The most important growth factors for wound healing are listed in Table 9–5. The names of the growth factors are based on the original studies that identified the factor and do not necessarily reflect what is now known about them. For instance, PDGF is also produced by macrophages, endothelial cells, and smooth muscle cells. Transforming growth factors, originally isolated from tumor cells, are also produced by normal cells and mediate many normal functions. TGF-β, originally described as a growth factor, is a potent stimulator of extracellular matrix formation and serves to limit proliferation and stimulate differentiation of many cell types.

TABLE 9–5. GROWTH FACTORS ACTIVE IN WOUND HEALING

Factor	Source	Responding Cells	Receptor
Platelet-derived growth factor (PDGF) (MRI:30 kDa)	Platelets, endothelium, macrophages	Fibroblasts, smooth muscle, glial cells	Tyrosine kinase 185,000
Acidic fibroblast growth factor (aFGF, ECGF) (MRI:15.6 kDa)	Brain, retina, fibroblasts, chondrocytes	Endothelium	150,000
Basic fibroblast growth factor (bFGF) (MRI:16.4 kDa)	Pituitary, brain	Endothelium	150,000
Epidermal growth factor (EGF) (MRI:5.7 kDa)	Salivary gland, epithelium	Mesenchyme, epithelium	Tyrosine kinase 170,000
Transforming growth factor-alpha (TGF-α) (MRI:5.7 kDa)	Tumor cells, epithelium	Mesenchyme, epithelium	Tyrosine kinase 170,000
Transforming growth factor-beta (TGF-β) (MRI:25 kDa)	Platelets, bone, many	Many	500,000
Insulinlike growth factor-1 (IGF-1) (MRI:7.5 kDa)	Liver	Mesenchyme, epithelium	Tyrosine kinase 450,000
Insulinlike growth factor-2 (IGF-2)	Liver	Mesenchyme, epithelium	Tyrosine kinase 200,000, 400,000

Modified from Blitstein-Willinger E: The role of growth factors in wound healing. *Skin Pharmacol* 4:175, 1991.

The precise role of these and other growth factors in wound healing is not yet well understood. The sequence of release of various factors and activation at the site of injury controls cell proliferation, chemotaxis, and cell adhesion and interactions, as well as differentiation and extracellular matrix formation. Thrombin, formed during clotting, stimulates the release of alpha granules from aggregated platelets. The alpha granules contain growth factors such as TGF-β, PDGF, and fibroblast growth factor (FGF). Thus, platelet-derived factors initiate wound healing very early after injury. The influx of macrophages into the wound sets the stage for tissue repair. Macrophages release a variety of biologically active substances, including at least seven "growth factors": IL-1, TNF-α (cachexin), IL-6, FGF, TGF-β, and PDGF, which alter fibroblast growth and metabolism (Table 9–6). Two of these factors—TGF-β and PDGF—stimulate the production of connective tissue. TFG-β stimulates the expression of collagen and fibronectin genes, as well as protein production by fibroblasts. It increases the rate of healing, enhances angiogenesis, and stimulates the release of other growth factors.

TABLE 9–6. EFFECT OF MACROPHAGE-DERIVED CYTOKINES ON FIBROBLAST GROWTH AND METABOLISM

Cytokine	Source	Fibroblast Proliferation	Connective Tissue Production
IL-1	Monocytes, alveolar and peritoneal macrophages	+	+
IL-6	Alveolar macrophages	+	+
TNF-α	Monocytes, alveolar macrophages	±	±
FGF	Peritoneal macrophages	+	ND
TGF-β	Monocytes	−	++
PDGF	Monocytes alveolar and peritoneal macrophages	+	+

Macrophages play a central role in wound healing. Macrophages serve to clear the wound of necrotic tissue and initiate granulation tissue formation. TGF-β may also inactivate macrophages and prevent continuing damage to normal tissue by deactivating superoxide production. Fibroblast growth factors stimulate proliferation of endothelial cells, cells surrounding nerves (Schwann cells), and chondrocytes, as well as fibroblasts, so it is likely to be very important for initiating the proliferative phase of healing and the formation of granulation tissue. Acidic FGF stimulates endothelial cells and thus could be critical for the proliferation of capillaries during healing. TGF-β and PDGF most likely act later in healing to stimulate connective tissue differentiation and extracellular matrix formation. Epidermal growth factor (EGF) is chemotactic and mitogenic for epithelial cells and thus may stimulate reepithelization of a damaged surface. TGF-β and PDGF may act to remodel connective tissue by stimulating collagen production by fibroblasts, as well as proteinase inhibitors and collagenases. The final outcome of matrix formation and collagen remodeling is scarring or resolution.

ADHESION MOLECULES

The interaction of inflammatory cells with the extracellular matrix involves cell receptors and matrix components. The role of selectins and integrins in acute inflammation was covered in Chapter 8. The deposition of fibrin, fibrinogen, and fibronectin from the serum during acute inflammation provides a temporary matrix into which white blood cells, fibroblasts, and endothelial cells migrate. This migration is mediated by specific cell adhesion molecules, the expression of which are upregulated during wound healing. This interaction is still under active investigation, and a number of molecules involved have been identified and characterized. These include **integrins, cell adhesion molecules (CAMS), selectins, vascular agressins,** and **lymphocyte homing receptors** (Table 9–7).

TABLE 9–7. A SIMPLIFIED FAMILY TREE OF ADHESION MOLECULES

Family	Subfamily	Examples
Integrins	β1	VLAs 1-6:
		Collagen receptor
		Fibronectin receptor
		Laminin receptor
	β2	LFA-1 (CD11a/CD18)
		MAC-1 (CD11b/CD18)
		p150.95 (CD11c/CD18)
		ICAM-1, ICAM-2 Receptors
		iC3r, Fibrinogen Receptors
	β3	Platelet protein gpIIb/IIIa
		Vitronectin receptor
Ig Supergene Family		ICAM-1
		ICAM-2
		VCAM-1
Selectins		
	L-selectin	LAM-1
	E-selectin	ELAM-1
	P-selectin	GMP-140
Vascular Addressins		Peripheral lymph node addressins
		Mucosal addressins
Intercrines/chemokines		IL-8, MCP, MIP-1β
Lymphocyte homing receptors	Peripheral lymph node	LAM-1
		LEU-8
	Mucosal	HCAM
		VLA-4, LFA-1

Modified from Montefort S, Holgate ST: Adhesion molecules and their role in inflammation. *Respir Med* 85:91, 1991.

Integrins

Integrins are cell surface molecules found on the surface of almost all cell types, which provide recognition structures for binding to other cells or to extracellular matrix (Fig. 9–4). Integrins belong to a family of heterodimeric receptors made up of α and β subunits. Each subfamily has a common β subunit, with the individual members of the subfamily each having a different α subunit. The three subfamilies are named after the common β chain—β1, β2, and β3. So far eleven α polypeptides and six β polypeptides have been identified in humans (Table 9–8). The β1 subfamily consists of β1 joined to one of the eight α subunits; the β2 subfamily has αL, αM, or αx joined with β2; the β3 has αIIb or αV joined with β3.

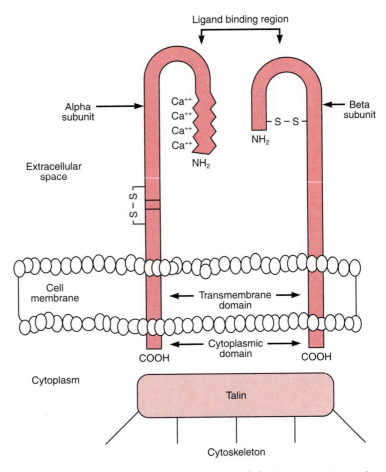

Figure 9–4. General polypeptide structure of the integrins. Integrins are composed of two similar polypeptide chains (α and β) with an extracellular receptor for matrix proteins, a membrane domain and a cytoplasmic "tail." There is about 40% to 50% homology in amino acid sequence among the various α chains and among the three β chains but no homology between the α and β chains. The α chains subunit of each integrin has a matrix-binding domain, and binding to their respective ligands requires a divalent cation such as Ca^{2+} or Mg^{2+}. About one-quarter of the β subunit consists of a repeating unit with a high cysteine content. Both subunits span the cell membrane and have a cytoplasmic COOH terminal that may provide a link between the extracellular matrix and the cytoskeleton. Phosphorylation of the cytoplasmic domain may regulate the binding functions of the receptors. The integrin phenotype expressed by a particular cell imparts specificity for binding to ligands on other cells or to different extracellular matrix components. (Modified from Ruoslahti E: Integrins. *J Clin Invest* 87:1–5, 1991.)

TABLE 9–8. HUMAN INTEGRINS

α-subunits	CD	β-subunits	CD	Molecules	Designation	Receptor
α1	49a	β1	29	$\alpha_1\beta_1$	VLA-1	Coll
α2	49b	β2	18	$\alpha_2\beta_1$	VLA-2, pla, Ia/IIa	Coll, laminin
α3	49c	β3	61	$\alpha3\beta1$	VLA-3	Coll, laminin, fibronectin
α4	49d	β4	-	$\alpha_4\beta_1$	VLA-4	Fibronectin, VCAM-1
α5	49e	β5	-	$\alpha_5\beta_1$	VLA-5, Pla Ic/IIa	Fibronectin
α6	49f	β6	-	$\alpha_6\beta_1$	VLA-6	Laminin
α7				$\alpha_7\beta_1$		Laminin
α8				$\alpha_8\beta_1$		Laminin
αL	11a			$\alpha_L\beta_2$	LFA-1	ICAM-1, ICAM-2
αM	11b			$\alpha_M\beta_2$	iC3bR, Mac-1	iC3b, fibrinogen, LPS, ICAM-1
αx	11c			$\alpha_x\beta_2$	p150, 95	ic3b
αV	51			$\alpha_V\beta_3$	Vitronectin receptor	Vitronectin, etc
α11b	41			$\alpha_{II}\beta_3$	Platelet IIb/IIIa	Fibrinogen, Vitro, fibronectin
				$\alpha_V\beta_1,$		Vitronectin, etc.
				$\alpha\beta_5,$		
				$\alpha_V\beta_6$		

CD, cluster designation identified by monoclonal antibodies; coll, collagen; laminin; lympho, lymphocytes.

Leukocyte Integrins. The leukocyte integrins (β2-integrins) have been identified by a number of monoclonal antibodies (see Table 8–3), including lymphocyte function associated antigen-1 (LFA-1), macrophage antigen-1 (Mac-1), and p150, 95 (molecular weight [MW] designation) (see Table 9–8). The MW of the α subunits of LFA-1, Mac-1, and p150,95 are 180,000, 170,000, and 150,000 Da respectively, while the β chain MW is 95,000. Thus, p150,95 is a heterodimer of a 150,000 and a 95,000 KDa chain. Monoclonal antibodies recognize the different α chains but do not distinguish among the β chains (see Table 9–8). LFA-1 binds to a molecule called intracellular adhesion molecule-1 (ICAM- 1), which is located on endothelial cells. The expression of ICAM-1 is upgraded during inflammation under the influence of cytokines TNF, lipopolysaccharide, IFN-γ, and IL-1 (see below). β_2-integrin (LFA-1) plays an important role in the localization of lymphocytes to tissues during inflammation, as well as in conjugation of CTL and NK cells to target cells and lymphocyte–lymphocyte interactions during primary induction of T-cell responses to antigens. Mac-1 is a receptor for C3bi (CR3), and p150,95 is also a receptor for C3bi (CR4). Mac-1 and p150,95 are active in phagocytosis of objects coated with C3bi (erythrocytes or organisms coated with complement), in chemotaxis of monocytes, and for adherence of monocytes to endothelial cells.

Understanding of the role of the leukocyte integrins in inflammation has been enhanced by the study of leukocyte adhesion deficiency (LAD), a naturally occurring disease of humans. Patients with LAD have recurrent necrotic, indolent infections of soft tissues caused by a variety of different fungi and bacteria. A feature of the lesions is the relative absence of granulocytes, normally a predominant feature of such lesions, in the face of elevated peripheral blood leukocyte counts (five to twenty times normal). In vitro, neutrophils and monocytes from LAD patients show marked defects in adhesion-related functions and deficiency in cell granule and cell surface expression of integrin molecules. Chemoattractants fail to cause upgrading of integrins on the cell surface. Neutrophils and monocytes from LAD patients fail to adhere or spread on glass and do not react to C3bi coated particles.

Other Integrins. In addition to the leukocyte integrins, there are the very late antigens of activation (VLA), the vitronectin receptor (VNR), and the platelet aggregation molecule IIbIIIa. The nonleukocyte integrins bind to extracellular matrix components such as fibronectin, collagen, and laminin. The interaction of different integrins with connective tissue molecules (see Table 9–8) mediates migration of different cell types during wound healing. One of the major binding sites is the tripeptide recognition sequence Arg-Gly-Asp (RGD). Although this tripeptide will inhibit binding of VLA5 (fibronectin receptor), VNR, and IIbIIIa to their respective matrix structures, each is specific, indicating that amino acid substitutions adjacent to the RGD sequence determine specificity of binding. Other receptors, such as those that bind to collagen, also require the RGD sequence but have a separate specificity related to the conformation conferred on the RGD-binding tripeptide by adjacent amino acids.

Ig Supergene Family/Cell Adhesion Molecules

This group of cell adhesion molecules includes a pair of homologous molecules called intercellular adhesion molecules-1 and -2 (ICAM-1 and ICAM-2) as well as vascular cell adhesion molecule-1 (VCAM-1). ICAM-1 and ICAM-2 are ligands for the β_2-integrin lymphocyte function antigen-1 (LFA-1), on all activated leukocytes. ICAM-1, but not ICAM-2, is also a ligand for the β_2-integrin Mac-1. VCAM-1 reacts with the β_1-integrin VLA-4. ICAM-1 and VCAM-1 expression on endothelial cells is increased by inflammatory cytokines, such as IL-1, TNF, IFN-γ, and IL-4. When produced during inflammation, these cytokines will selectively increase expression of different adhesion molecules, so that induction of specific adhesion molecules can provide a means of selective recruitment of inflammatory cells.

Selectins

Binding of leukocytes to endothelial cells is not only important in normal cell circulation between blood and tissues but is also the initial step in infiltration of lymphocytes during inflammation. During normal recirculation of lymphocytes, the circulating cells bind to specialized high-endothelial venules in lymphoid organs. The endothelial cell receptor belongs to another family of vascular cell adhesion molecules. These include **lymphocyte adhesion molecule-1 (LAM-1)** on lymphocytes, **endothelial leukocyte adhesion molecule (ELAM-1)** on endothelial cells, and **granule membrane protein of 140 kDa (GMP-140)** on platelets (Table 9–9).

L-selectin (LAM-1) was originally identified by the monoclonal antibody Mel-14 in mice and by Leu-8 in humans. It functions as the homing receptor for lymphocytes. E-selectin mediates the interaction of cytokine-activated endothelial cells with neutrophils early in inflammation, and P-selectin serves as a site for the binding of monocytes and neutrophils to activated platelets. These proteins share a similar domain structure, including a lectin domain, an EGF-like domain, a series of consensus repeats homologous to regulatory proteins, a transmembrane domain, and a small cytoplasmic domain (Figure 9–5). P-selectin is located within membrane-bound granules in cells that can exocytose rapidly upon induction and appear on the cell surface. This provides a rapid mechanism of expression not requiring new protein synthesis. Expression of P-selectin may play a role in the assembly of cellular components necessary for clot formation by attachment of platelets to granulocytes and monocytes, or a mechanism of clearance of activated platelets from the circulation by attachment of platelets to reticuloendothelial cells.

During the inflammatory process, cytokines may initially cause increased expression of E-selectin (ELAM-1) on endothelial cells, which favors the adhesion of neutrophils during acute inflammation. Over a period of 6 to 12 hours, E-selectin expression declines, while VCAM-1 expression increases, perhaps under the influence of IL-4. Now neutrophils will adhere less well but adhesion of lymphocytes will be increased. Later, strong adhesion is mediated by binding of β_2-integrin (LFA-1) upregulated on activated lymphocytes to ICAM-1 and

TABLE 9–9. PROPERTIES OF SELECTINS*

Selectin	MW (kDa)	Cells Expressing	Cells Binding
L-selectin (LAM-1)	100	Granulocytes, monos, lymphs	Activated ECs
E-selectin (ELAM-1)	115	Activated ECs	HEVs of lymph nodes
P-selectin (GMP-140)	140	Activated ECs, platelets	Granulocytes, monos

*See also Tables 8–2 and 8–3. ECs, endothelial cells; monos, monocytes; lymphs, lymphocytes; HEVs, high endothelial veins.

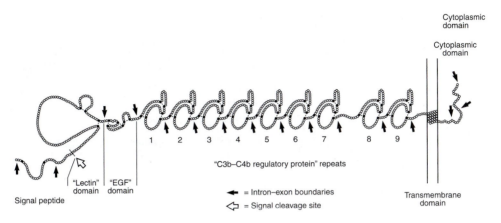

Figure 9–5. Structure of selectin. Selectins have a similar overall structure: a cytoplasmic domain, a series of C3b-C4b-like domains, an ECF domain, and a lectin domain, and a signal peptide. L-selectin has only two C3b-C4b regulatory protein repeats; E-selectin has six, and P-selectin has nine. (Modified from Johnston BI, Bliss GA, Newman PJ, et al.: Structure of the human gene encoding GMP-140, a member of the selectin family of adhesion receptors for leukocytes. *J Biol Chem* 265:21381, 1990.)

ICAM-2 upregulated on endothelial cells. Continued stimulation may result in the appearance of high endothelial venulelike postcapillary venules seen at sites of chronic inflammation, which appear to be the major site for extravasation of lymphocytes into the lesion. A schematic drawing of the sequence of events leading to lymphocyte adhesion and emigration during chronic inflammation is presented in Figure 9–6.

In addition, binding of the cell surface integrins with extracellular matrix structures initiates differentiation of the cells and apparently is vital for the process of wound healing. Binding of fibroblasts to extracellular matrix fibers initiates organization and eventual reepithelization of wound surfaces. This process depends on reaction of basic amino acid sequences on epithelial cells with matrix components and eventual formation of basement membranes. Exactly how this process takes place and the role of different cellular adhesion reactions remain to be elucidated.

Vascular Addressins/ Lymphocyte Homing Molecules

The final group of adhesion molecules aid lymphocytes in homing to a specific type of vascular endothelium. Endothelial cells express addressins which are either mucosal (MAd) or peripheral lymph node in type (NAd); expression is associated with selective homing of lymphocytes to high-endothelial venules (HEV) of the mucosa or lymph node. In animal studies IgE and IgA expressing B cells home selectively to mucosa, whereas IgG-expressing B cells home to lymph nodes.

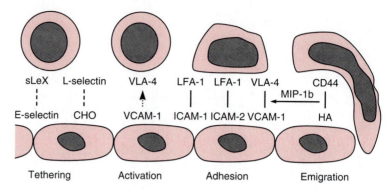

Figure 9–6. Proposed adhesion and emigration cascade of lymphocytes and endothelial cells during the early stages of chronic inflammation. The sequence includes four stages: (1) Weak binding through selectin molecules, (2) an activation signal to upregulate integrin expression, (3) strong integrin-mediated adhesion, and (4) migration through the vessel wall. MIP-1β, a member of the intercrine family increases the adhesiveness of the $\alpha_4\beta_1$-integrin VLA-4 on CD8+ T$_{CTL}$ to VCAM-1. HA = hyaluronate. (Modified from Shimizu Y, Newman W, Tanaka Y, et al.: Lymphocyte interactions with endothelial cells. *Immunol Today* 13:106, 1992.)

At least four major lymphocyte surface molecules are involved in reaction with HEVs (Table 9–10). These include: **L-selectin (lymphocyte adhesion molecule-1 [LAM-1]), homing-associated cell adhesion molecule (H-CAM), β_2 integrin (lymphocyte function antigen-1 [LFA-1]), and a$_4\beta_1$-integrin (very late antigen-4 [VLA-4]).** L-selectin is a peripheral lymph node homing receptor. H-CAM is a homing receptor for all lymphocytes, but is primarily reactive with a 58–66-kDa protein on HEVs identified as **mucosal vascular addressin (MAd)**. Two integrins, VLA-4 and LFA-1, are implicated in lymphocyte homing. The ligand for VLA-4 is VCAM-1; that for LFA-1 is ICAM-1. VLA-4 directs lymphocytes to mucosal tissue; LFA-1 to

TABLE 9–10. LYMPHOCYTE SURFACE MOLECULES REACTING WITH HEVs

Surface Marker	Monoclonal Antibodies	MW (kD)	Species	HEV ligand
L-selectin	LAM-1, MEL-14, Leu-8	75–100	Mouse	Mannose-6-phosphate
H-CAM	CD44, Hermes Pgp-1	90	Human	MAd
B$_2$-integrin	LFA-1, CD11a/CD18	95/150	Human/mouse	ICAM-I
$\alpha_4\beta_1$- integrin (VLA-4)	CD49d/CD29	130/1150	Human/mouse	VCAM-I

both mucosa and lymph node HEVs. LFA-1 is also involved in the interaction of cytotoxic T cells with their target cells.

Proteoglycans

Proteoglycans are macromolecules composed of a protein backbone and one or more glycosaminoglycan side chains. There are four major types of glycosaminoglycans: Heparan/heparan sulfate, chondroitin sulfate/dermatan sulfate, keratan sulfate, and hyaluronic acid. Many different kinds of proteins have sites for noncovalent binding of sulfated glycosaminoglycans. These binding sites are characterized by sequences of basic amino acids such as BBXB and BBBXXB. The capacity of glycosaminoglycans for many different interactions confers on them the function to serve as the "glue" to bind together extracellular matrix components, to bind cells to the matrix and to concentrate soluble biologically active proteins such as growth factors. In addition to the glycosaminoglycan binding, many of these macromolecules can bind through domains in the core protein, such as the lectin-like domain found in the large cartilage proteoglycan. A model of adhesion molecules in a cell membrane binding to extracellular matrix is shown in Figure 9–7.

The role of cell–proteoglycan and growth factor–proteoglycan interactions during inflammation and healing is becoming increasingly clear. Each of the glycosaminoglycans has a strong negative charge, making it possible for them to bind many substances, including some growth factors. Binding of fibroblast growth factors (FGFs) to heparan or heparan sulfate protects the FGF from degradation. FGF and other factors are normally tightly bound to collagens, fibronectin, and heparin sulfate in the extracellular matrix. After wounding, active FGF-glycosamine complexes can then be generated by proteolysis of the proteoglycans, such as occurs during inflammation. Other growth factors, such as GM-CSF and IL-3, as well as platelet factor-4, the prototype of a number of growth factors and cytokines, also bind to heparan and heparan sulfate. In addition, TGF-β binds to proteoglycan through the core protein. The inflammatory mediators of neutrophil granules are able to break down the extracellular matrix leading to the formation of pus, thus destroying the normal tissue organization.

Reestablishment of tissue during the healing process involves the reorganization of the extracellular matrix and reepithelialization of the surface of the wound. Reformation of the extracellular matrix requires synthesis of connective tissue fibers (mainly type I collagen) by fibroblasts and reattachment of extracellular matrix structures to cell surface receptors and proteoglycans. Fibroblasts responding to growth factors released from the damaged matrix, such as FGF, migrate to the wound area, proliferate, and lay down extracellular matrix. During reepithelialization, keratinocytes break free and migrate to the site of

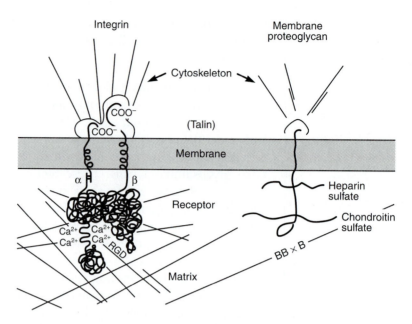

Figure 9–7. Schematic model of binding of a cellular integrin and cell surface proteoglycan to the extracellular matrix. Both the α and β chains of the cell adhesion molecule integrin bind to the cytoskeleton and extend through the cell membrane to attach to proteoglycans in the extracellular matrix, involving Ca++ and the RDG sequence. Cell surface proteoglycans, such as heparan sulfate/chrondroitin sulfate proteoglycan, bind to basic amino acid sequences in fibronectin through the heparan sulfate side chains. (Modified from Ruoslathi E: Proteoglycans in cell regulation. *J Biol Chem* 264:13369, 1989.)

injury, attracted by a variety of chemical signals. The activated keratinocytes also display increased expression of integrins, influenced by TGF-β, that enable them to recognize and attach to matrix molecules.

Review of Mediators in Inflammation

A summary of the role of different mediators at different stages of the inflammatory process is given in Figure 9–8. The early vascular stages are largely caused by mast cell mediators. In some instances, products of the coagulation, kinin, and complement systems may be active. The acute cellular stage is mediated by complement, leukotrienes, or bacterial or tissue products. The chronic cellular stage is influenced mainly by cytokines. The outcome of the inflammatory process depends on the degree of injury and is affected mainly by macrophages which either clear the inflamed tissue or set the stage for fibroblast proliferation and scarring. Because of the difficulty in studying this complex process, which can really only be duplicated in vivo, the precise action of the various mediators is not well understood.

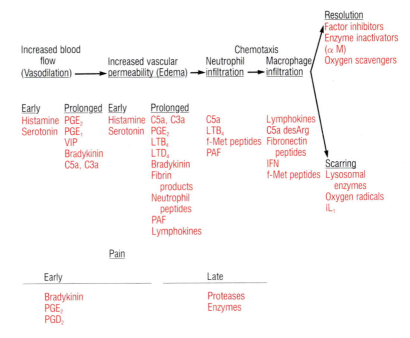

| Increased blood flow (Vasodilation) | Increased vascular permeability (Edema) | Chemotaxis Neutrophil infiltration | Macrophage infiltration | Resolution
Factor inhibitors
Enzyme inactivators
(α M)
Oxygen scavengers |

Early	Prolonged	Early	Prolonged			
Histamine	PGE$_2$	Histamine	C5a, C3a	C5a	Lymphokines	
Serotonin	PGE$_1$	Serotonin	PGE$_2$	LTB$_4$	C5a desArg	
	VIP		LTB$_4$	f-Met peptides	Fibronectin	
	Bradykinin		LTD$_4$	PAF	peptides	
	C5a, C3a		Bradykinin		IFN	Scarring
			Fibrin		f-Met peptides	Lysosomal
			products			enzymes
			Neutrophil			Oxygen radicals
			peptides			IL$_1$
			PAF			
			Lymphokines			

Pain

Early	Late
Bradykinin	Proteases
PGE$_2$	Enzymes
PGD$_2$	

Figure 9–8. Summary of the role of mediators in the process of inflammation. PGE, prostaglandin E; PGD, prostaglandin D; CC, complement components; VIP, vasoactive intestinal polypeptide; LTB, leukotriene B; LTD, leukotriene D; PAF, platelet-activating factor; IFN, interferon; IL-1, interleukin-1; TGF, transforming growth factor.

Manifestations of Inflammation in Tissues

Examples of the morphologic manifestations of different stages of inflammation in four different organs in which inflammation is initiated differently is given in Table 9–11:

1. Vessels: Vasculitis induced by antigen–antibody reaction or inflammatory mediators.
2. Lung: Pneumonia induced by infection.
3. Heart: Myocardial infarction induced by blockage of blood flow (coronary thrombus).
4. Kidney: Glomerulonephritis induced by antibody–antigen reaction and activation of complement.

The initiating event is different, but the subsequent sequence of events is similar. Acute inflammation is first manifested in vessels by increased blood flow (congestion) and increased vascular permeability (edema). Chemotactic factors attract and activate polymorphonuclear neutrophils. If enzyme release occurs in the vessel walls, fibrinoid (looks like fibrin) necrosis is seen. This will be followed by

TABLE 9–11. MANIFESTATIONS OF INFLAMMATION IN TISSUE

Organ	Etiology	Inciting Event	Stages of Inflammation		
			Acute	Subacute	Chronic
Vessel (vasculitis)	Multiple	Multiple; cell injury, infection	Increased blood flow and vasopermeability (edema) Poly infiltrate (pus) — Mononuclear cells Necrosis — Hemorrhage		Resolution Scarring
Lung (pneumonia)	Infection	Release of bacterial products	Edema, congestion Poly infiltrate —Macrophages Hemorrhage — Necrosis — Fibroblast proliferation		Resolution Scarring
Heart (infarct)	Disturbance of flow	Necrosis of myocardial cells	Edema, congestion Poly infiltrate — Macrophage — Fibroblast proliferation		Scarring
Kidney (glomerulonephritis)	Immune inflammation	Deposition of Ag-Ab complexes, activation of complement	Increased glomerular permeability (proteinuria) Poly infiltrate — mononuclear infiltrate Necrosis — Hematuria Epithelial proliferation		Resolution Scarring (uremia)

lymphocyte and macrophage infiltration. If resolution does not occur, subendothelial fibroblastic proliferation leads to narrowing of the vessel wall (endarteritis) and eventually to infarction of tissue. In the lung, congestion and edema due to increased blood flow and vascular permeability are followed by polymorphonuclear infiltration and then macrophage infiltration, fibroblast proliferation, and scarring (organizing pneumonia). In myocardial infarction, necrosis of myocardial cells is seen first. Release of cytoplasm from necrotic cells produces vasodilation and endothelial cell contraction (increased vascular permeability—edema), and chemotaxis for polymorphonuclear cells. This is followed by macrophage infiltration, fibroblast and capillary proliferation (granulation tissue), and scarring. In the renal glomerulus, the sequence of events is initiated by activation of complement following deposition of antibody–antigen complexes in the basement membrane. This produces changes in the endothelial cells and basement membrane that results in leakage of protein in the urine (proteinuria—the equivalent of edema in other organs) and chemotaxis of polymorphonuclear neutrophils. Enzymes released by polymorphonuclear cells cause destruction of the basement membrane, and red cells pass into the urine (hematuria—the equivalent of hemorrhage in other tissues). Subacute glomerular inflammation is manifested by proliferation of epithelial cells and continued thickening of the basement membrane (membranoproliferative glomerulonephritis). The major consequence of the inflammatory process changes from increased glomerular permeability (proteinuria, hematuria) to decreased filtration as the basement membrane becomes thickened (uremia). As in other organs, chronic inflammation is manifested by fibrosis and scarring. Thus, in each organ, even though the initiating event is different, the process of inflammation is essentially the same, leading to resolution or scarring through similar stages.

Cytokines, Adhesion Molecules, and Growth Factors in Atherosclerosis

The cytokines, adhesion molecules, and growth factors of chronic inflammation are critical to the development of atherosclerotic plaques in blood vessels. The endothelial cells of blood vessels constitute a critical interface with the blood and the underlying tissues, particularly the smooth muscle cells of the vascular media. In hyperplastic arterial disease, such as atherosclerosis, the endothelial cells lose their anticoagulant properties and become "sticky" due to increased expression of adhesion molecules. Smooth muscle cells begin to produce increased extracellular matrix. Mononuclear cells from the blood penetrate the arterial wall and infiltrate the smooth muscle cells and begin to accumulate oxidized low-density lipoproteins (LDLs). The proliferation of smooth muscle cells and accumulation of lipid-laden macrophages leads to the formation of "fatty streaks" in the subendothelium and, eventually, atherosclerotic plaques.

This progressive tissue lesion is mediated by an hypothesized series of changes in growth factors, cell adhesion molecules, and cytokines. First, hypercholesteremia promotes lipid uptake by vascular walls. These lipids initiate a cycle of local cytokine production and lipid modification (oxidation of low density lipoproteins [LDLs]). Adhesion of blood monocytes (macrophages) to vascular endothelial cells is mediated by ICAM-1 and VCAM-1 on endothelial cells binding to LFA-1 and VLA-4 on the monocytes. Emigration and activation of monocytes (macrophages) is enhanced by production of MCP-1, an adhesion molecule for monocytes, by endothelial cells. Activated macrophages in the vessel wall produce monocyte/macrophage colony-stimulating factor (M-CSF), a ubiquitous growth factor that auto-upregulates production of the cytokines IL-1, TNF, and INF-γ. As activators of endothelial cells, both IL-1 and TNF induce syntheses of specific glycoproteins that further increase leukocyte adherence and induce rearrangements of the endothelial wall cytoskeleton, as well as augment synthesis of PAF and prostacyclin, which serve to increase vascular permeability and cause vasodilation. IL-1 and TNF also stimulate production of IL-8, which activates neutrophils. In addition to mediating permeability and emigration, IL-1 and TNF induce endothelium to produce platelet-derived growth factor, which serves to recruit smooth muscle cells to the subendothelium and stimulate their proliferation. Within the intima, the accumulating macrophages express an acetyl-LDL receptor for oxidized low-density lipoproteins and the macrophages take up and accumulate modified LDL, thus becoming lipid-laden "foam" cells in fatty streaks. Fatty streaks along the endothelium are the first grossly recognizable changes in atherosclerosis and progress by smooth muscle proliferation, lipid and matrix accumulation, remodeling, calcification, ulceration, hemorrhage, and thrombosis to lesions characteristic of atherosclerotic arterial disease.

Summary

Inflammation is the process of delivery to and activation of proteins and cells at sites of tissue damage or infection. The process proceeds from acute, subacute, and chronic stages to resolution or scarring. Tissue lesions and extent of reaction are substantially determined by accessory inflammatory mechanisms mediated by serum protein or cellular systems. The serum protein systems include complement, coagulation, fibrinolysis, and kinin; the cellular systems include polymorphonuclear leukocytes, mast cells (or basophils), platelets, eosinophils, lymphocytes, macrophages, and the reticuloendothelial system. Each of these systems has a homeostatic function and is controlled by interrelated feedback mechanisms. Excessive or inadequate activation of these systems may have serious effects. Manifestations of the stages of inflammation in different tissues are similar, even though the inflammatory process is initiated by different events (infections, tissue necrosis, antibody–antigen reaction).

Bibliography

LYMPHOCYTES

Cohen S: The role of cell-mediated immunity in the induction of inflammatory responses. *Am J Pathol* 88:502, 1977.

Ford WL, Gowans JL: The traffic of lymphocytes. *Semin Hematol* 6:67, 1969.

Oppenheim JJ, Jacobs D (eds.): *Leukocytes and Host Defense: Progress in Leukocyte Biology,* vol 5. New York, Liss, 1986.

MACROPHAGES

Cohn ZA: The structure and function of monocytes and macrophages. *Adv Immunol* 9:163, 1968.

DeDuve C, Wattiauk R: Functions of lysosomes. *Annu Rev Physiol* 28:435, 1966.

Mackaness GB, Blanden RV: Cellular immunity. *Prog Allergy* 11:89, 1967.

Nelson DS: *Immunobiology of the Macrophage.* New York, Academic Press, 1976.

Schulta RM: Autocrine versus lymphocyte-dependent mechanisms for macrophage activation. *Cell Signal* 3:515, 1991.

WOUND HEALING (GROWTH FACTORS, CYTOKINES, AND ADHESION MOLECULES)

Albelda SM: Endothelial and epithelial cell adhesion molecules. *Am J Respir Cell Mol Biol* 4:195, 1991.

Anderson DC: Leukocyte adhesion deficiency: An inherited defect in the MAC-1, LFA-1, and P150,95 glycoproteins. In *Gene Transfer and Therapy*. Liss, 1989, 315–323.

Beutler B, Cerami A: The history, properties, and biological effects of cachectin. *Biochem* 27:7575–7582, 1988.

Bevilacqua MP, Stengalin S, Gimbrone MA Jr, et al.: Endothelial leukocyte adhesion molecule-1: An inducible receptor for neutrophils related to complement regulatory proteins and lectins. *Science* 243:1160–1165, 1989.

Border WA, Ruoslahti E: Transforming growth factor-β in disease: The dark side of tissue repair. *J Clin Invest* 90:1, 1992.

Cochrane CG, Gimbrone MA (eds.): *Cellular and Molecular Mechanisms of Inflammation: Vascular Adhesion Molecules*. Orlando, FL, Academic Press, 1992.

Dijke P, Iwata KK: Growth factors for wound healing. *Bio/Technology* 7:793–798, 1989.

Dustin ML, Springer TA: Role of lymphocyte adhesion receptors in transient interactions and cell locomotion. *Annu Rev Immunol* 9:27, 1991.

Holzmann B, Weissman IL: Integrin molecules involved in lymphocyte homing to Peyer's patches. *Immunol Rev* 108:45, 1989.

Kishimoto TK, Larson RS, Corbi AL, et al.: The leukocyte integrins. *Adv Immunol* 46:149–182, 1989.

Kovacs EJ, DiPietro LA: Fibrogenic cytokines and connective tissue production. *FASEB J* 8:854–861, 1994.

McEver RP: Selectins: Novel receptors that mediate leukocyte adhesion during inflammation. *Thrombos Haemostas* 65:223, 1991.

McIntyre BW, Bednarczyak JL, Passini CA, et al.: Integrins: Cell adhesion receptors in health and disease. *Cancer Bull* 43:51, 1991.

Montefort S, Holgate ST: Adhesion molecules and their role in inflammation. *Resp Med* 85:91, 1991.

Poole AR: Proteoglycans in health and disease: Structures and functions. *Biochem J* 236:1–14, 1986.

Raghow R: The role of extracellular matrix in postinflammation wound healing and fibrosis. *FASEB J* 8:823–831, 1994.

Ruoslahti E: Proteoglycans in cell regulation. *J Biol Chem* 264:13369, 1989.

Ruoslahti E, Pierschbacher MD: New perspectives in cell adhesion RGD and integrins. *Science* 238:491, 1987.

Ruoslathi E, Yamaguchi Y: Proteoglycans as modulators of growth factor activities. *Cell* 64:867, 1991.

Shimizu Y, Shaw S: Lymphocyte interactions with extracellular matrix. *FASEB J* 5:2292, 1991.

Stahl N, Yancopoulos GD: The alphas, betas, and kinases of cytokine receptor complexes. *Cell* 74:587–590, 1993.

Tanake Y, Adams DH, Hubscher S, et al.: T-cell adhesion induced by proteoglycan-immobilized cytokine MIP-1β. *Nature* 361:79, 1993.

Tavassoli M, Hardy CL: Molecular basis of homing of intravenously transplanted stem cells to the marrow. *Blood* 76:1059, 1990.

Wawryk SO, Novotny JR, Wicks IP, et al.: The role of the LFA-1/ICAM-1 interaction in human leukocyte homing and adhesion. *Immunol Rev* 108:135, 1989.

CHRONIC INFLAMMATION AND ATHEROSCLE-ROSIS

Brody JL, Pickering NJ, Capuzzi DM, et al.: Interleukin 1α as a factor in occlusive vascular disease. *Am J Clin Pathol* 97:8, 1992.

Libby P: Do vascular wall cytokines promote atherogenesis? *Hosp Pract* 27:47, 1992.

Ross R: The pathogenesis of atherosclerosis: A perspective for the 1990s. *Nature* 362:801–809, 1993.

The Reticuloendothelial System/ Blood and Tissue Clearance

Clearance of the products of coagulation, immune complexes, effete blood cells, and products of tissue breakdown from the blood stream, as well as removal of products of inflammation and tissue damage or metabolism from organs, is the function primarily of phagocytic cells belonging to the reticuloendothelial system. Degradation of proteins may be enhanced by enzyme-mediated ligation to heat shock proteins (ubiquitin). Failure of this system to cleanse the blood can lead to a condition known as disseminated intravascular coagulation (Shwartzman reaction). Accumulation of poorly degradable protein deposits that are resistant to phagocytosis and digestion leads to extracellular deposits known as amyloid, or to similar intracellular accumulations responsible for conditions such as Alzheimer's disease. These conditions represent diseases caused by an inability of the body to "turn over" or catabolize products of inflammation, metabolism, or mutated protein molecules.

The Reticuloendothelial System (RES)

The reticuloendothelial system is a multiorgan collection of cells whose primary common functional capacity is phagocytosis. This includes monocytes, macrophages, and endothelial cells. Two general functional types of mononuclear phagocytes are recognized–wandering and fixed macrophages (histiocytes).

WANDERING MACROPHAGES

The wandering cells are the monocytes of the peripheral blood. These cells may be found in other organs, such as the sinusoids of lymphoid organs or the connective tissue stroma of many organs where they may be only temporary residents. The wandering phagocytes are largely responsible for clearing debris from tissue.

HISTIOCYTES

The fixed phagocytes (histiocytes) are more permanent residents in tissue. Histiocytes may be found in liver (Kupffer cells or sinusoid-lining cells), spleen (sinusoid-lining cells, reticular cells, dendritic macrophages), lymph nodes, connective tissue, brain (microglia), bone marrow, adrenals, thymus, and lungs (alveolar macrophages). If particles, such as carbon or vital dyes, are injected into the blood, the Kupffer cells of the liver and the phagocytic cells of the spleen ingest most of them; if the particles are inhaled, the pulmonary alveolar macrophages ingest them; if they are injected into connective tissue, the local phagocytes ingest them; if the particles are injected into the brain, the microglia destroy them. All these cells have in common the ability to ingest foreign materials.

PHAGOCYTIC INDEX

Measurement of the phagocytic capacity of an animal may be accomplished by determining the rate of disappearance of stable, inert, uniform particles such as gelatin-stabilized carbon particles. Upon intravenous injection of such particles, about 90% are taken up by the liver; most of the remainder are taken up by the spleen. Carbon clearance is measured after saturation of the clearing mechanism, because a dose of particles lower than the saturation dose is cleared during the first few passages of the blood through the liver. Determination of carbon clearance under these conditions primarily measures liver blood flow. If a dose large enough to saturate the reticuloendothelial system is given, a two-stage elimination occurs: (1) A rapid clearance as the particle-laden blood first passes through the liver and spleen, and (2) a slower clearance, which occurs upon recirculation through the previously saturated reticuloendothelial system. The slope of this second curve is the phagocytic index. It measures regeneration of phagocytic capacity after saturation.

The clearance of particles from the blood by the reticuloendothelial system follows first-order reaction kinetics:

Reactant —> product
or
particles in blood —> ingestion by RES

The change in concentration of the particles in the blood over a given time is related to the concentration at the start of the experiment, as follows:

$$dC/dt + KC_o$$

This becomes:

$$Ct = C_o \, 10^{-kt}$$

where Ct   = concentration at time t
C_o = initial concentration
t   = time
K   = constant (phagocytic index)

solving for K:

$$K = \frac{\log C_1 - \log C_2}{t_2 - t_1}$$

After injection of a dose of carbon particles sufficient to saturate the reticuloendothelial system, the concentration of carbon in the blood at a given time is determined (C_1, t_1). After a period of several hours, the animal is bled and the concentration of carbon again determined (C_2, t_2). K, the phagocytic index, can then be determined from the formula given above.

STIMULATION OF THE RES

A number of agents may affect the phagocytic index. Products of microorganisms, such as the cell wall of yeast (zymosan), bacterial endotoxins, extracts of *Mycobacterium tuberculosis,* living and killed organisms, simple lipids such as triglycerides, and hormones such as estrogen, have all been shown to increase carbon clearance. The ability of some organisms, such as *Salmonella typhimurium* or *Cornybacterium parvum,* to increase phagocytic activity results in increased resistance of the host to other infecting microorganisms (immune phagocytosis). Antibody to a given organism or particle may increase the capacity of the host to phagocytize antibody-coated particles (opsonin).

IMMUNE ELIMINATION

The presence of antibody in the circulation leads to rapid clearance of antigens injected into the blood. Reaction of antibody with antigen results in formation of aggregated Fc regions of Ig as well as activation of complement, which opsonizes the complexes. The complexes then bind to phagocytic cells and are removed from the circulation by the reticuloendothelial system (Fig. 10–1).

BLOCKADE OF THE RES

Phagocytic clearance may be depressed by overloading the RES. Thus, a saturating dose of carbon may decrease the clearance of a second dose of carbon. Blockade of the RES with fibrin results in a decreased clearance of fibrin formed after the blockade (see Shwartzman reaction below). Agents that blockade the system have similar properties. Injection of colloidal carbon blockades the system for clearance of a second dose of carbon or for similar agents but does not affect the clearance of chromic phosphate. This suggests that there are different phagocytic receptors for different particles.

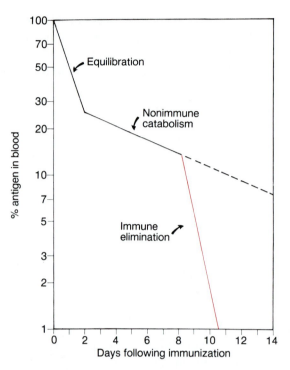

Figure 10–1. Immune elimination. If antibody is present in vivo, antigen is rapidly cleared from the blood stream. There is a three-stage elimination of diffusible antigen from the blood stream of a previously nonimmunized animal. Immediately after intravascular injection, the blood level of the antigen drops rapidly because of diffusion from the capillaries into the extravascular space until approximately 40% of the injected antigen remains in the blood. Following this rapid equilibration phase, antigen is slowly removed by nonimmune catabolism of the injected protein, which lasts for about 7 to 10 days, when the onset of antibody formation results in rapid clearance of the remaining antigen by the reticuloendothelial system. During the phase of immune elimination, soluble antibody–antigen complexes in antigen excess may be demonstrated in the blood. At this time, lesions of serum sickness may occur (see Chapter 13). After antigen is cleared, free antibody appears in the blood. If antigen is injected into an animal that already has circulating antibody, the antigen is removed in one rapid immune elimination phase.

Shwartzman Reaction

The Shwartzman reaction is not an immune reaction but an alteration in factors affecting intravascular coagulation and reticuloendothelial clearance.

LOCAL SHWARTZMAN REACTION

The local Shwartzman reaction is a lesion confined to a prepared tissue site (usually skin) and is a two-stage reaction (preparation and provocation). The tissue site is prepared by local injection of an agent (gram-negative endotoxin) that causes accumulation of polymorphonuclear leukocytes. It is believed that the granulocytes condition the site by releasing lysosomal acid hydrolases that damage small vessels, setting up the site for reaction to a provoking agent. A relatively mild inflammatory reaction may serve as a preparative event. Provocation is accomplished by injection into the prepared site agents that initiate intravascular coagulation (gram-negative endotoxins, antigen–antibody complexes, serum, starch, etc.). The lesion is caused by intravascular clotting with localization of platelets, granulocytes, and fibrin at the site of preparation-forming thrombi that lead to necrosis of vessel walls and hemorrhage. The administration of nitrogen mustard (decreased granulocytes) or vasodilators inhibits the reaction, while agents that block the RES (carbon) increase the intensity of the reaction. Specific immunization is not necessary. Although immune reactions may serve as either a preparatory or provocative event, nonimmune reactions are also effective.

GENERALIZED SHWARTZMAN REACTION (DISSEMINATED INTRAVASCULAR COAGULATION)

The classic generalized Shwartzman reaction is elicited by giving a young rabbit two intravascular injections of endotoxin 24 hours apart (Fig. 10–2). The first injection serves as the preparative step, and the second, the provocation step. After the first injection, a few fibrin thrombi are found in vessels of liver, lungs, kidney, and spleen capillaries. Following the second injection, many more thrombi are found. Bilateral renal cortical necrosis and splenic hemorrhage and necrosis are characteristic. The fibrin thrombi do not contain clumps of platelets or leukocytes. In human disease, the generalized Shwartzman reaction may develop as an acute and frequently fatal complication of an underlying disease, such as an infection, and is known as disseminated intravascular coagulation. It is triggered by one or more episodes of intravascular clotting leading to the formation of multiple fibrin or fibrinlike thrombi that lodge in small vessels. Such thrombi are prominent in the kidney or adrenal glands and cause necrosis and/or hemorrhage. Three steps appear to be necessary:

1. Intravascular clotting with fibrin formation.
2. Deposition of fibrin in small vessels. In order for this to happen, at least one (and usually all) of the following conditions must apply: Depression of reticuloendothelial clearance of altered fibrinogen, decrease in blood flow through affected organs, or liberation of enzymes by granulocytes, which helps precipitate fibrin.
3. Once deposited, the fibrin is not removed by fibrinolysis.

Administration of agents that cause blockade of reticuloendothelial clearance (thorotrast, carbon, endotoxin, cortisone) serve as preparative agents, and agents that activate intravascular clotting (endotoxin, antigen–antibody complexes, synthetic acid polysaccharides) serve as provoking agents.

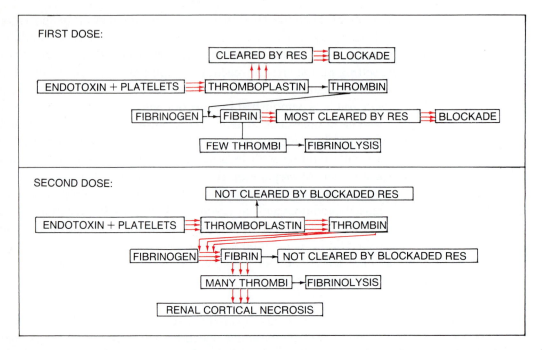

Figure 10–2. Mechanism of generalized Shwartzman reaction induced by endotoxin. Classic generalized Shwartzman reaction is elicited by giving rabbits two doses of endotoxin 24 hours apart. The primary effect of the first (preparatory) dose of endotoxin is to cause release of platelet thromboplastin. Most of this thromboplastin is cleared by the reticuloendothelial system (RES). Some thrombin triggers conversion of fibrinogen to fibrin, but again most of this fibrin is cleared by the RES. If an animal is examined after one dose of endotoxin (preparative dose), a few fibrin thrombi are found in vessels of the liver, lungs, and spleen. These thrombi appear to be quickly removed by fibrinolysis, with no damage to the treated rabbit. However, because of the action of the RES in clearing thromboplastin and fibrin, blockade of the reticuloendothelial system occurs. This blockade permits a second dose of endotoxin to produce severe intravascular coagulation. The second dose (provocative dose) initiates the same release of platelet thromboplastin as did the first dose, but with the reticuloendothelial system blockaded, this thromboplastin is not cleared; most goes on to form thrombin and initiate conversion of fibrinogen to fibrin. This fibrin cannot be cleared by the blockaded RES and most becomes lodged in capillaries, particularly capillaries of renal glomeruli. The fibrinolytic system may not be capable of overcoming large amounts of fibrin formed in a short period of time. The end result may be fatal renal cortical necrosis.

SEPTIC SHOCK

The release of cytokines by macrophages reacting with bacterial products produced during sepsis produces septic shock. The major bacterial factor is the lipopolysaccharide of the outer layer of gram-negative bacteria, which is released upon lysis of the organism, known as **endotoxin**. Other bacteria toxins, such as the peptidoglycan of gram-positive bacteria (**exotoxin**) may also cause shock. These toxins react with macrophages and activate release of cytokines, mainly tumor necrosis factor (TNF), IL-1, IL-6, and IFN-γ. The cytokines, in turn, act on secondary cellular sites and produce fever or hypothermia, increased heart rate (tachycardia), increased breathing rate (tachypnea), and loss of blood pressure (shock). Endotoxin shock is produced in experimental animals by injection of endotoxin from gram-negative organisms, such as *Escherichia coli,* and clinically in humans with infections with gram-negative organisms. Endotoxin shock is different from the Shwartzman reaction in that no preparative injection is necessary; shock can be induced in many species (the Shwartzman reaction occurs in only man and rabbit); shock occurs with equal intensity at any age (young rabbits are much more sensitive than old rabbits to the Shwartzman reaction); thrombi are not prominent in endotoxin shock, which features hemorrhage and necrosis; and cortisone enhances the Shwartzman reaction but does not affect endotoxin shock. Treatment of endotoxin shock using monoclonal antibodies to endotoxin has met with mixed results, and treatment with monoclonal antibodies to TNF is now being tested (see Chapter 26). The reaction of exotoxins (super-antigens) with T cells and macrophages to produce toxic shock syndrome is covered in Chapter 16.

THE SHWARTZMAN REACTION AND PREGNANCY

A single injection of endotoxin in pregnant rabbits produces a generalized Shwartzman reaction. Bilateral renal cortical necrosis has been reported in septicemia following induced abortion in humans. Bilateral renal cortical necrosis in this circumstance represents a human equivalent of the generalized Shwartzman reaction due to endotoxemia during pregnancy. Pregnancy serves as the preparative step, because fibrinolytic activity and reticuloendothelial clearance are decreased during pregnancy. The occurrence of gram-negative septicemia during delivery or abortion serves as the provocative step, leading to hypotension and intravascular clotting. In addition, intravascular dissemination of amniotic fluid during delivery may activate fibrin formation. This may be followed by thrombocytopenia and hemorrhage or a typical generalized Shwartzman reaction with bilateral renal cortical necrosis. Fibrin deposition occurs within glomerular capillary loops within 48 hours of provocation. Hemorrhagic necrosis of the adrenals and/or renal cortical necrosis may occur 60 hours to 40 days later. However, most episodes of pregnancy-associated Shwartzman reaction do not progress to fatal renal cortical necrosis.

Amyloidosis

Amyloidosis refers to a heterogeneous group of diseases in which there is an extracellular tissue deposit of a hyaline microscopically amorphous material with a filamentous ultrastructure which gives green birefringence under polarized light after Congo-red staining. This property was first associated with staining of linear polysaccharides (ie, starch), and the name amyloid (starchlike) was applied by Rudolph

Virchow in 1851. Amyloid deposits are actually made up of protein, not cellulose as originally proposed. The proteinaceous deposits are very difficult to solubilize; thus, chemical analysis has been difficult. Tissue deposits build up because the reticuloendothelial and macrophage systems, as well as other cells, are unable to effect removal of the poorly degradable materials. In some cases, amyloid deposition is caused by the overproduction of precursor molecules of plasma proteins, which are incompletely catabolized and accumulate. In other cases, an altered form of a protein is produced that is more difficult to "turn over" than the normal protein. The major protein constituents of amyloid have three common features: (1) There is a serum precursor, (2) the protein has a high degree of antiparallel beta-sheet conformation, and (3) there is a distinctive ultrastructural appearance. The growing mass of amyloid fibrils associates with plasma and extracellular matrix proteins and proteoglycans to form amyloid deposits, which infiltrate the extracellular species of organs, destroying normal tissue architecture and function. The amyloidoses are complex diseases caused by pathologic conformational changes and polymerization, in which normally soluble precursors and converted into insoluble fibrils.

CLASSIFI-CATION

Amyloid deposition may affect different organs and give rise to many pathologic conditions (Table 10–1). The deposits may be generalized

TABLE 10–1. CLASSIFICATION OF SYSTEMIC AND LOCAL AMYLOIDOSIS

Type	Protein
Systemic Nonhereditary	
Primary and myeloma-associated	Immunoglobulin light-chain dimers
Secondary	HDL-SAA
Hemodialysis	β_2-Microglobulin
Systemic Hereditary	
*Familial Mediterranean fever	HDL-SAA
Familial amyloid polyneuropathy	Prealbumin variants
Systemic senile amyloidosis	Prealbumin varient–ILE 122
Local Cerebral	
Hereditary cerebral hemorrhage with amyloidosis	
Icelandic type	Cystatin C
Dutch Type	β-protein
Alzheimer disease and Down syndrome	β-protein
Transmissible spongioform encephalopathies	Protease-resistant protein
Local Endocrine	
Medullary carcinoma of the thyroid	Procalcitonin
Pancreatic	Calcitonin gene-related peptide

*Also found in nonhereditary form. (Modified from Castano EM, Frangione B: Biology of disease: Human amyloidosis, Alzheimer's disease, and related disorders. *Lab Invest* 58:122–132, 1988.)

or localized. Generalized nonhereditary amyloidosis is caused by the deposition of precursors of serum proteins and is associated with over-production. Generalized hereditary amyloidoses result from the production of a variant of prealbumin. Neuron-related proteins are found in localized cerebral amyloidoses and hormone-related proteins in endocrine amyloidosis. Disease is caused when deposits interfere with the normal function of an organ. In systemic amyloidosis, deposits in the liver, heart, or kidney may lead to failure of these organs. In cerebral amyloidosis, such as Alzheimer's disease, deposits in neurons lead to dementia. In others, such as hereditary cerebral hemorrhage with amyloidosis, deposits in cerebral vessels may cause recurrent cerebral hemorrhages. What chemical analysis has been possible has provided considerable insight into the pathogenesis of the different types of amyloidosis.

AMYLOIDO-GENIC PROTEINS

Systemic Amyloidosis

The four forms of amyloidogenic proteins found in systemic amyloidosis have been classified as AL, AA, AF, and AH. AL deposits are immunoglobulin light chains; AA deposits, protein AA; AF deposits, primarily prealbumin variants (F, familial); and AH, β_2-microglobulin (H, hemodialysis).

AL: Immunoglobulin Light Chains. Deposits of dimers of immunoglobulin light chains are found in primary amyloidosis and amyloid associated with multiple myeloma (a tumor of plasma cells that may make large amounts of immunoglobulin molecules). The dimers may consist of two variable halves of the light chain, a variable half and a complete light chain, or two complete light chains. Mixing V_Ls of some myeloma light chains (Bence Jones proteins) in vitro results in the formation of beta-pleated sheet structures characteristic of amyloid. Such structures are difficult to catabolize and may have an affinity to deposit in certain tissues, producing amyloidosis.

AA: Protein AA. Protein AA is related to the acute phase serum protein SAA. AA protein production by hepatocytes is stimulated by IL-1. Protein AA in tissue deposits of amyloid has a molecular weight of 8,500; that of SAA is 14,000. A proteolytic enzyme in macrophages clips off thirty to forty amino acid residues from the carboxyl end of SAA to produce protein AA. Protein AA then deposits in tissue, forming filamentous, poorly degradable amyloid. This form of amyloidosis is most likely caused by the increased production of SAA secondary to chronic inflammatory conditions such as rheumatoid arthritis, tuberculosis, bronchiectasis, leprosy, etc., or malignancies such as Hodgkin's lymphoma or renal cell carcinoma.

AH: β_2-Microglobulin. β_2-microglobulin is an 11.8-kDa part of the class I histocompatibility complex. High serum levels of β_2-microglobulin are found in renal failure and are not removed from the circulation by conventional dialysis membranes. Up to 70% of patients on chronic renal dialysis may develop deposits of amyloid in bone and synovium composed of intact normal β_2-microglobulin.

AF: Prealbumin Variants. Genetically determined amino acid substitutions in prealbumin are found in the group of familial amyloid polyneuropathies (FAP) and in systemic senile amyloidosis. FAP is recognized in different nationality groups. In Jews, there is substitution of methionine for valine at position 39 and isoleucine for phenylalanine at position 33. In patients of Swiss–German origin, there is substitution of serine for isoleucine at position 84. In Portuguese, Japanese, and Swedish families, there is methionine for valine at position 30. In systemic senile amyloidosis, there is isoleucine at position 122. It is possible that these genetic variants of prealbumin may aggregate abnormally in tissue or be resistant to proteolytic cleavage, leading to deposition in vessel walls and peripheral nerves, areas where normal mechanisms of tissue turnover may be limited.

Protein P. Protein P is a minor component ($< 10\%$) of most amyloid deposits and is related to the acute phase protein, C-reactive protein (see Chapter 8). Protein P is made up of a double pentamer composed of the MW-23,000 molecular subunits. C-reactive protein is a single pentamer. Protein P forms from aggregation of two C-reactive protein pentamers and can be seen by electron microscope as an 80-A doughnutlike structure. Protein P binds to many different ligands, including amyloid fibrils, fibronectin, and C_4-binding protein. This binding may be the reason protein P is found in amyloid deposits.

Heparan Sulfate Proteoglycan (HSPG). HSPG is a component of basement membrane that was first shown to be associated with protein AA deposition, but now has been found in four other forms of amyloid deposits: Alzheimer's disease; prion amyloids, such as Creutzfeld–Jakob disease; amyloid in type II diabetes; and in familial amyloidotic polyneuropathy. It is not clear if this is related to a disturbance in the synthesis of basement membrane, a passive absorption of HSPG by amyloid deposits, or a response provoked by amyloid deposition. HSPG, unlike other components of amyloid, is not found in the serum and does not appear to have a serum precursor.

Localized
Amyloidosis

Cystatin C. Cystatin C is a 12-kDa basic protein that is an inhibitor of cysteine proteases and is related to kininogens. The variant, which is found in amyloid fibrils in the walls of small arteries and arterioles in the cerebral cortex and leptomeninges, starts at position 11 of the normal protein and has glutamine instead of leucine at position 68. It has been identified in amyloid deposits in an autosomal dominant form of cerebral amyloidosis in Iceland.

β-Protein. β-Protein (beta amyloid protein [AB]) is a 4-kDa protein fragment of forty-two amino acids with a highly hydrophobic tail of fourteen residues found in the senile plaques of Alzheimer's disease and Down syndrome patients and in the vessel walls of patients with Dutch-type hereditary cerebral hemorrhage with amyloidosis. Amyloid β-protein deposition thus identifies a group of diseases with varied sites of deposition from primarily neuronal (dementia) to primarily vascular (cerebral hemorrhage). Deposits of β-protein undergo fibrillogenesis resulting in highly stable 5- to 10-nm filaments characteristic of amyloid. The precursor of β-protein is a fifty-six amino acid polypeptide that spans the cell membrane of many cell types (amyloid precursor protein [APP]). It has a large extramembranous portion and a small cytoplasmic domain. The forty-two amino acids of the β-protein include twenty-eight extracellular amino acids and the first eleven to fourteen amino acids of the hydrophobic transmembrane domain. The complete fifty-six amino acid precursor of β-protein may be a growth factor, but the abbreviated forty-two amino acid form is inactive, suggesting that the forty-two amino acid fragment may function to block the activity of the fifty-six amino acid molecule.

Protease-Resistant Protein (PrP). PrP is a poorly defined protein of MW 27- to 30-kDa found in amyloid deposits in the human transmissible spongioform encephalopathies (Creutzfeld–Jakob disease, Gerstmann–Strassler syndrome, and kuru), as well as in the sheep disease, scrapie. It has been suggested that this protein is a component of an infectious agent (prion) although it is expressed in both normal and infected brains.

PATHOGENESIS

The complete understanding of the pathogenesis of systemic amyloidosis remains elusive. Some common factors leading to the various forms of systemic amyloidosis include:

1. A circulating soluble precursor that includes an amyloidogenic primary structure; a proteolytic fragment that forms a beta-pleated sheet secondary structure and assembles into a fibrillary structure in tissue that is resistant to removal. In some cases, there are increased amounts of an amyloidogenic material (b_2-microglobulin) or aggregation of a precursor (protein P).

2. Increased serum levels of the precursor due to increased synthesis or decreased clearance or both.

3. Abnormal processing of the protein, such as prealbumin variants or immunoglobulin light chains, or incomplete degradation, such as for formation of protein AA from SAA.

The stimulus for the overproduction or abnormal production of some amyloid precursors may be the stimulation of liver and other tissues by cytokines (IL-1, IL-6) from macrophages. There appears to be a diversity of etiologic factors, leading to amyloid deposition. Deposition may result from a complication of inflammatory disease or malignancy, genetic defects, chromosomal abnormalities, or environmental factors. At this time, there is effective treatment for only one form of amyloidosis—the autosomal recessive disease, familial Mediterranean fever. Long-term treatment with colchicine can prevent the deposition of protein AA that otherwise causes early death due to renal failure.

Alzheimer's Disease

Alzheimer's disease is a progressive senile dementia of immense clinical importance. The pathologic hallmark of the lesions of Alzheimer's disease is the deposition of amyloid fibrils in senile plaques and in blood vessels in specific regions of the cerebral cortex. The plaques contain a mixture of proteins, but the most obvious feature is that the core of AD plaques contains insoluble β-protein. The Alzheimer's disease (AD) beta amyloid or A4 protein is derived from β-protein precursor (see above).

The gene for β-protein precursor is on chromosome 21, the same chromosome that is trisomic in Down syndrome, in which there is premature development of the neurologic lesions of Alzheimer's disease. Down syndrome patients with trisomy 21 are believed to produce larger amounts of β-protein because of gene dosage, as the gene for the protein precursor is located in or near 21q21. Point mutations in the β-protein precursor gene have been detected in two Swedish families with early onset AD and in a different location in a patient with hereditary cerebral hemorrhage of the Dutch type of amyloidosis. In the latter form of amyloidosis, deposition of β-protein is seen primarily in the walls of cerebral blood vessels, whereas in AD it is more prominent in neural plaques. The mutation in the Dutch disease occurs within the β-protein itself, whereas the mutation in the families with early onset AD is in the precursor molecule, two amino acid residues from the end of the β-protein. However, in the nonhereditary forms of Alzheimer's disease, there is no evidence that the β-protein gene is abnormal.

AD may be due to a genetically controlled increase in the amount of β-protein precursor that accumulates with aging because of an insidiously failing catabolic system or to aberrant function or metabolism of the β-protein precursor, most likely secondary to abnormalities in enzymes that process the precursor protein for secretion. Thus, research is now directed to the transcriptional, translational, and posttranslational events that might account for the progressive deposition of β-amyloid protein in AD. As a result of this, evidence has been obtained that accumulation of the β-protein may be derived from the precursor protein following uptake by the neuronal lysosomes. Lysosomes in neurons are small, intracellular vesicles where protein degradation normally occurs. In vitro, neurons release β-protein by cleavage of the extramembranous portion of the larger precursor molecule. The β-protein is then taken back into the cell by endocytosis, where it is normally degraded. However, if there is increased production, such as in the Swedish families, or an inability to break down the β-protein, either due to an abnormal β-protein or to defects in catabolism, gradual accumulation of the protein with aging and intracellular accumulation may occur, eventually leading to loss of the neuron. On the other hand, there is the opinion that β-amyloid is not the cause of the disease but the result of another mechanism of neuronal degeneration.

Summary

In this chapter, diseases caused by decreased clearance of poorly catabolizable proteins from the blood and tissues are presented. These are due to a failure of the cleansing system of the body—the reticuloendothelial system—to phagocytize and digest products of coagulation, inflammation, or metabolism. Failure to clear the bloodstream of products of coagulation leads to a condition known as disseminated intravascular coagulation (Shwartzman reaction), which can lead to multiple infarcts. Failure to clear tissues of proteins results in accumulation in tissue or cells known as amyloid. These accumulations can lead to organ failure. A particular form of amyloid deposition in the brain is the pathognomonic lesion of Alzheimer's disease.

Bibliography

RETICULO-ENDOTHELIAL SYSTEM

Heller JH, Gordon AS: The reticuloendothelial system. *Ann NY Acad Sci* 88, 1960.
Hershko A: Ubiquitin-mediated protein degradation. *J Biol Chem* 263:15237, 1988.
Stiffel C, Mouton D, Biozzi G: Kinetics of the phagocytic function of reticuloendothelial macrophages in vivo. In *Mononuclear Phagocytes*. Van Furth R (ed.). Oxford, Blackwell, 1970, 335.
Stuart AE: *The Reticuloendothelial System.* Edinburgh, Livingston, 1970.
Weigle WO, Dixon FJ: The elimination of heterologous serum proteins and associated antibody response in guinea pigs and rats. *J Immunol* 79:24, 1957.

SHWARTZMAN REACTION

Apitz KA: Study of the generalized Shwartzman phenomena. *J Immunol* 29:255, 1935.
Colman R, Robboy SJ, Minna JD: Disseminated intravascular coagulation: A reappraisal. *Annu Rev Med* 30:359, 1979.
Hjort PF, Rapaport SI: The Shwartzman reaction: Pathologic mechanisms and clinical manifestations. *Annu Rev Med* 16:135, 1965.

Mori W: The Shwartzman reaction: A review including clinical manifestations and proposal for a universal or single-organ third type. *Histopathology* 5:113, 1981.

Muller-Berghaus G: Pathophysiology of generalized intravascular coagulation. *Serum Thromb Hemostasis* 3:209, 1977.

Shwartzman G: *Phenomena of Local Tissue Reactivity.* New York, Hoeber, 1937.

SEPTIC SHOCK

Billiau A, Vandekercknove F: Cytokines and their interactions with other inflammatory mediators in the pathogenesis of sepsis and septic shock. *Eur J Clin Invest* 21:559, 1991.

Cerami A: Inflammatory cytokines. *Clin Immunol Immunopathol* 62:83, 1992.

Darville T, Giroir B, Jacobs R: The systemic inflammatory response syndrome (SIRS): immunology and potential immunotherapy. *Infection* 21:279–290 1993.

Johnson HM, Russell JK, Pontzer CH: Staphylococcal entertoxin superantigens. *Proc Soc Exp Biol Med* 198:765, 1991.

Wenzel RP: Anti-endotoxin monoclonal antibodies—a second look. *N Engl J Med* 326:1151, 1992.

AMYLOIDOSIS

Cohen AS, Connors LH: The pathogenesis and biochemistry of amyloidosis. *J Pathol* 151:1, 1987.

Glenner GG: Amyloid deposits and amyloidosis: The β-fibrilloses. *N Engl J Med* 302:1283,1333, 1980.

Glenner GG, Ein D, Eanes ED, et al.: Creation of "amyloid" fibrils from Bence Jones proteins in vitro. *Science* 174:712, 1971.

Husby G, Sletten K: Chemical and clinical classification of amyloidosis 1985. *Scand J Immunol* 23:253–265, 1986.

Kyle RA, Certz, MA: Systemic amyloidosis. *CRC Clin Rev Oncol Hematol* 10:49, 1990.

Myatt EA, Westholm FA, Weiss D, et al: Pathogenic potential of monoclonal immunoglobulin light chains: relationship of in vitro aggregation to in vivo organ deposition. *Proc Natl Acad Sci, USA* 91:3034–3038, 1994.

Puchtler H, Sweat F: A review of early concepts of amyloid in context with contemporary chemical literature from 1839 to 1859. *J Histochem Cytochem* 14:123, 1965.

Sipe JD: Amyloidosis. *Annu Rev Biochem* 61:947, 1992.

ALZHEIMER'S DISEASE

Cai X-D, Golde TE, Younkin SG: Release of excess amyloid β-protein from a mutant amyloid β-protein precursor. *Science* 259:514, 1993.

Castano EM, Frangione B: Biology of disease: Human amyloidosis, Alzheimer's disease, and related disorders. *Lab Invest* 58:122–132, 1988.

Goate A, Chartire-Harlin M-C, Mullan M, et al.: Segregation of a missense mutation in the amyloid precursor protein gene with familial Alzheimer's disease. *Nature* 349:704, 1991.

Haass C, Selkoe DJ: Cellular processing of β-amyloid precursor protein and the genesis of amyloid β-peptide. *Cell* 75:1039-1042, 1993.

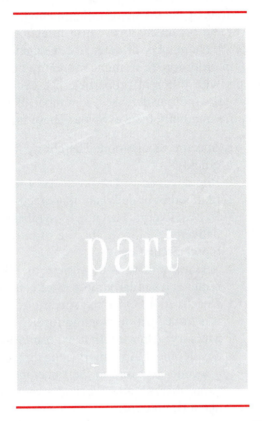

part

II

Immunopathology

Immune Effector Mechanisms

The manifestations of immunity in a living animal are expressed as variations of the theme of inflammation. The seemingly endless variety of the organisms that cause infectious diseases requires that we have a large number of defensive mechanisms to combat them.

In order for the immune system to be effective against infectious agents with different properties, life cycles, routes of infection, and ways to avoid our defenses, a number of important characteristics of specific immunity have evolved. These include:

1. Specific recognition: The ability to recognize foreign invaders quickly.
2. Rapid response: The products of the specific immune response (antibodies or cells) are manufactured within a very short time.
3. Fast delivery: The newly synthesized immune products are delivered rapidly to the site of infection by lymphatics and the blood circulation.
4. Versatility: The wide variety of potentially infectious agents requires a similar variety of effector mechanisms.
5. Deactivation: Once the specific response is no longer needed, it is turned off, preventing further tissue destruction.
6. Memory: After the first exposure, immunization results in the development of memory cells that can respond more rapidly to a second exposure to the same antigen. Immune memory prevents disease after second exposure to the same infectious agent (immunity).

Immuno-pathology

The specificity of antibody and specifically sensitized T-effector lymphocytes provides a means of directing the defensive force of inflammation directly to infecting foreign organisms. The immune response in this way provides immune effector mechanisms augmented by accessory inflammatory processes that protect us against specific infections. Antibody is generally operative against bacteria or bacterial products, whereas cellular reactivity is primarily against viral and mycotic organisms. However, we increasingly recognize instances in which the immune reaction of the host produces tissue damage (disease). The disease state produced by the destructive effect of immune reactions is termed **allergy** or **hypersensitivity**. Immunopathology is the study of tissue alterations produced by various types of hypersensitivity or allergic reactions, the subject of Part II of this book.

The terms "immunity" and "allergy" should be reserved for effects mediated through immune mechanisms. In a strict sense, some instances of altered reactivity as a result of a previous exposure are not reactions of allergy or immunity. These phenomena include the Shwartzman reaction (alteration in the state of blood coagulation), adaptive enzyme synthesis (substrate selection of enzyme production), anaphylactoid reactions (pseudoallergic reactions resulting from liberation of pharmacologically active agents that may also be liberated by allergic reactions), reactions to drugs caused by nonallergic physiologic hyperreactivity (idiosyncrasy), and other types of environmental adaptations (heat, cold, altitude, emotion) produced by nonimmune physiologic or psychologic mechanisms. In the next section, immune effector mechanism in causing tissue damage and disease will be presented. This will be followed by six additional chapters on immune disorders.

Classification

In the systemic study of disease, pathogenic changes are classified according to their anatomic location. In the study of diseases due to immune mechanisms, however, more than one organ system may be involved with the same process. Because the alterations in different organ systems caused by the same process have pathologic similarities, the lesions caused by immunopathologic reactions are best classified by the particular type of immunopathologic effector mechanism involved.

Until the 1960s, immune reactions were not classified according to mechanism but were presented as a bewildering list of peculiar lesions or diseases. The first working classification of four major immune mechanisms was introduced by Gell and Coombs in their classic textbook in 1963 as Type I–Type IV immune mechanisms (Table II–1). The classification of immune effector mechanisms used in this text includes seven general categories: **Inactivation** or **activation, cytotoxic, Arthus (immune complex), anaphylactic, cell-mediated cytoxicity, delayed hypersensitivity,** and **granulomatous.** These effector mechanisms are activated by the reaction of antibody or sensitized cells with antigens in vivo (Figure II–1).

TABLE II–1. CLASSIFICATION OF IMMUNE MECHANISMS

Gell and Coombs (1963)	Present
—	Inactivation or Activation
Type II	Cytotoxic or Cytolytic
Type III	Immune Complex (Arthus)
Type I	Atopic or anaphylactic
—	T-cell cytotoxic
Type IV	Delayed Hypersensitivity
—	Granulomatous Reactions

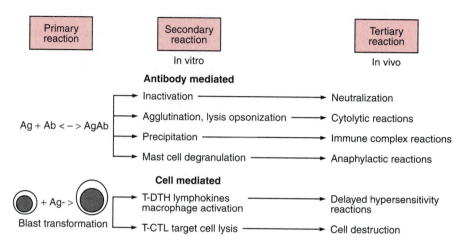

Figure II–1. Stages of Immune Reactions. Primary reactions refer to binding of antigen to antibodies or cells; secondary reactions refer to various phenomena which can be measured in vitro; tertiary effects are seen when immune effector mechanisms are activated in vivo.

ANTIBODY-MEDIATED MECHANISMS

The first four types of immunopathologic mechanisms are mediated by immunoglobulin antibodies. These reactions may be transferred by injection of antiserum from an immune animal into a nonimmune animal. The characteristics of the reactions are determined not only by the properties of the immunoglobulin molecules involved but also depend upon the nature and tissue location of the antigen and upon the accessory inflammatory systems that are called into play. Antibodies are able to inactivate biologically active molecules like toxins or hormones (**neutralization**), cause destruction of cells like red blood cells or bacteria (**cytotoxicity**), induce acute inflammatory reactions (**immune complex reactions**), and open up blood vessels to produce edema (**anaphylactic reactions**).

CELL-MEDIATED MECHANISMS

Cell-mediated reactions are not dependent upon antibody, but upon reaction of antigen with specifically sensitized cells (T_{CTL} or T_{DTH} lymphocytes). T_{CTL} recognize antigen in association with class I MHC markers and are usually CD8+. T_{DTH} cells recognize antigen in association with class II MHC markers and are usually CD4+. T_{CTL} are effective against viral-infected epithelial or solid tissue cells and kill target cells by direct transfer of cytotoxic factors or cell membrane alterations of the target cell. Activation of T_{DTH} cells leads to production and release of soluble factors (IFN-γ, IL-2, and other lymphokines) whose function is to attract and activate macrophages. The major mechanism of tissue damage is the phagocytosis and destruction of cells by macrophages. This mechanism is effective against intracellular parasites like leprosy bacilli, tubercle bacilli, and viruses that infect and multiply within macrophages. The products of the activated T_{DTH} cells "arm" the macrophages through the production of lysosomal enzymes so that they are able to kill and digest the intracellular parasites.

If macrophages are unable to eliminate the organisms completely or are unable to digest the material they phagocytose, masses of macrophages collect in the tissues and lead to space-occupying lesions (granulomas) that eventually interfere with normal tissue function. Granulomatous reactions are not separately classified in some systems but produce tissue lesions that are characteristic and clearly different from delayed hypersensitivity reactions or T_{CTL} destruction of target organs. Granulomatous reactions may be initiated by either antibody (immune complex) or cellular reactions with antigen and may also occur to nonimmunogenic material deposited in the body (ie, talc granulomas, urate crystals).

The "Double-edged Sword" of Immune Defense Mechanisms

Immune mechanisms reflect a "double-edged sword," cutting down our enemies with one edge and causing disease with the other edge. Some examples of protective and destructive effects of immune effector mechanisms are listed in Table II–2.

Much of what we recognize as immunopathology may result from artificial stresses put on a system that normally would not occur. The use of abnormally high doses of exogenous agents used in therapy and the delivery of these agents by unnatural routes (such as intravenously)

TABLE II–2. THE "DOUBLE-EDGED SWORD" OF IMMUNE REACTIONS

Immune Effector Mechanism	Protective Function "Immunity"	Destructive Reaction "Allergy"
Neutralization	Diphtheria, tetanus, cholera, endotoxin neutralization, blockade of virus receptors	Insulin resistance, pernicious anemia, myasthenia gravis, hyperthyroidism
Cytotoxic	Bacteriolysis, opsonization	Hemolysis, leukopenia, thrombocytopenia
Immune complex	Acute inflammation, polymorphonuclear leukocyte activation	Vasculitis, glomerulonephritis, serum sickness, rheumatoid diseases
Anaphylactic	Focal inflammation, increased vascular permeability, expulsion of intestinal parasites	Asthma, urticaria, anaphylactic shock, hay fever
Cell mediated cytoxicity	Destruction of virus infected cells, cancer cells	Contact dermatitis, auto-allergies, viral exanthems
Delayed hypersensitivity	Destruction of infected macrophages, tuberculosis, syphilis, leprosy	Auto-allergies, post-vaccinial encephalomyelitis, multiple sclerosis
Granulomatous*	Leprosy, tuberculosis, helminths, fungi, isolation of organisms in granulomas	Beryllosis, sarcoidosis tuberculosis, filariasis, schistosomiasis

*Granulomatous reactions, as other inflammatory lesions, may result from nonimmune stimuli, as well as from an immune reaction inactivated by antibody or by sensitized cells.

Modified from Sell S. Introduction to symposium on immunopathology: "Immune Mechanisms in Disease." Human Pathol 9:24–24, 1978.

may produce deleterious reactions such as anaphylaxis, serum sickness, transfusion reactions, and drug reactions. Tissue graft rejection is a protective response elicited by iatrogenic (physician-initiated) exposure to foreign tissue. However, there are many naturally occurring immune diseases, including autoimmune hemolytic anemia, erythroblastosis fetalis, hay fever, anaphylactic shock, polyarteritis nodosa, connective tissue diseases, poison ivy, etc. In many of these diseases, infectious agents are not the primary pathogenic event; although in some it is postulated that infections may initiate an "autoimmune" process that causes the disease. It may thus be said that the immune process is being used for the wrong purpose. Yet the very same processes that are responsible for the pathogenesis of these diseases are also essential for protective responses that are required for life.

Induction of Different Immunopathologic Mechanisms

Our understanding of how different types of immune responses are induced remains unclear. The immunoglobulin class of antibody and type of T cell (T_{CTL} or T_{DTH}) that is produced after immunogen recognition depends upon the type of immunogen processing and the nature of the helper T cell involved. A very brief working summary of this process is presented in Figure II–2. According to the classic model of antigen presentation for antibody responses, antigen is processed by follicular dendritic cells or B-cells that present the antigen to T-helper cells which produce interleukins/lymphokines that activate antigen reactive B-cells to proliferate and synthesize antibody. The current paradigm holds that different types of immune responses may be explained on the bases of two different T-helper cells. T-helper-2 (Th2) cells secrete lymphokines that drive B-cells to IgE and IgA antibody productions; T-helper-1 (Th1) cells secrete lymphokines that drive B-cells to produce IgG antibody. Thus, as originally presented, this model is useful for separating IgE and IgA from IgG immunoglobulin classes. The model has also been extended to separate antibody responses from delayed hypersensitivity responses (T_{DTH}). However, Th1 cells are implicated in induction of delayed-hypersensitivity as well as IgG antibody. If induction of both IgG antibodies and T_{DTH} employ Th1 cells, then another level of immune induction must be required to separate these responses. Separation of antibody from DTH most likely results from different antigen processing. Antibody responses occur in follicular zones of lymphoid organs after processing of antigen by dendritic cells or B-cells around which follicles form; DTH responses occur in the diffuse cortex of T-cell zones after processing of antigens by interdigitating dendritic (reticulum) cells. Cytotoxic T cells are produced after activation of CD8+ T-helper cells following antigen processing by any nucleated MHC class I positive cell. It is necessary to note that the above model is hypothetical and subject to change.

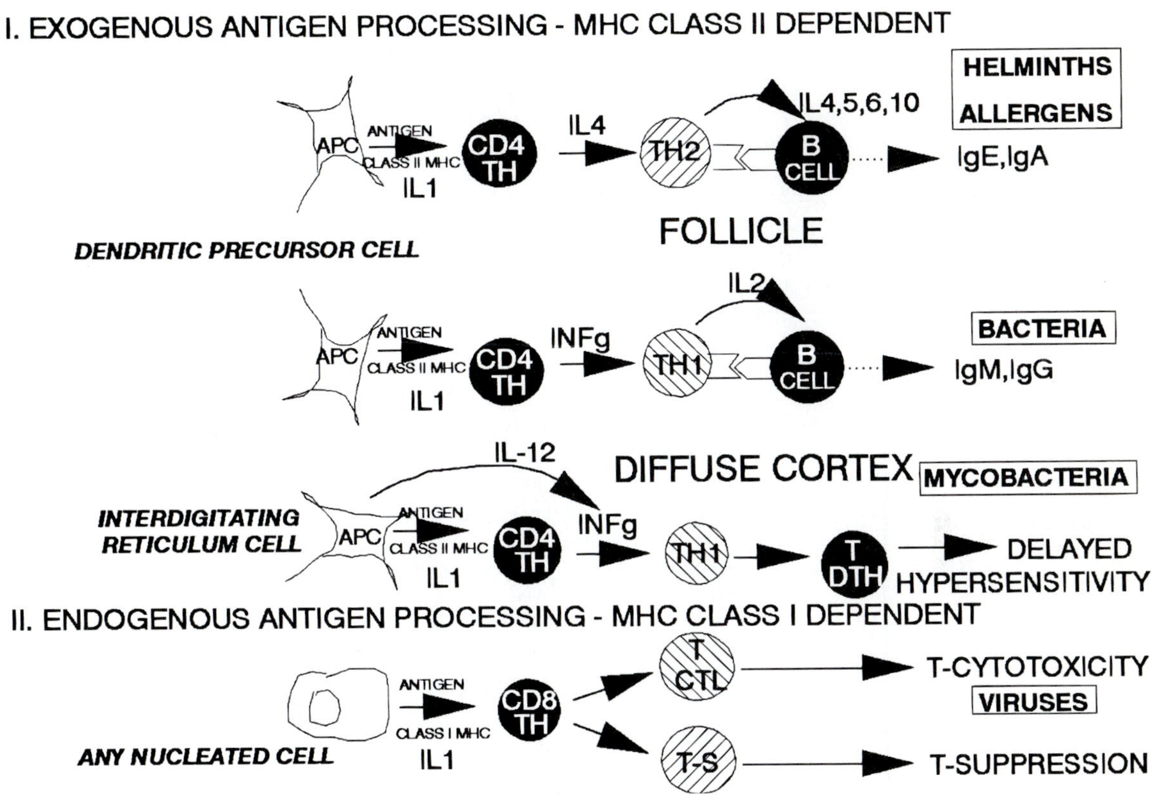

I. EXOGENOUS ANTIGEN PROCESSING - MHC CLASS II DEPENDENT

HELMINTHS
ALLERGENS

DENDRITIC PRECURSOR CELL

FOLLICLE

BACTERIA

INTERDIGITATING RETICULUM CELL

DIFFUSE CORTEX **MYCOBACTERIA**

DELAYED HYPERSENSITIVITY

II. ENDOGENOUS ANTIGEN PROCESSING - MHC CLASS I DEPENDENT

ANY NUCLEATED CELL

T-CYTOTOXICITY
VIRUSES

T-SUPPRESSION

Figure II–2. Exogenous Antigen Processing—MHC Class II Dependent. A simplified diagram depicting the presumptive role of antigen processing and T-helper cell subsets in different types of immune responses. IgE, IgA, and some IgG subclasses of antibodies result from antigen processing by Class II MHC+ dendritic cells that are located in follicles, presentation of antigen to CD4+ T-helper cells, activation of Th2 cells and differentiation of B-cells to produce IgE and IgA. IgE production is favored by IL-4 and IL-13; whereas IL-5 and TGF-β selects for IgA switching. IgG antibodies are produced by B-cells if this process involves the Th1 subset of helper cells instead of Th2. DTH also results from activation of Th1 cells, but DTH may result from antigen processing by interdigitating dendritic cells in the T-cell zones of lymph nodes. Cytotoxic CD8+ T-cells are produced following antigen processing by Class I MHC+ cells to CD+ helper cells. DTH cells are CD4+; CTL cells are CD8+.

Classification by Origin of Response and Source of Antigen

A second method of classification is based on identifying the source of the antigen and the origin of the immune response in relation to the affected individual.

This approach helps to understand the origins (etiology) of a given disease but does not address the immune mechanism (pathogenesis). In the system to be followed in Part II of this book, immune dis-

Classification of Allergic Diseases According to Source of Antigen and Origin of Response

---

I. Endogenous immune response to endogenous antigens
   A. Circulating antibody
      1. Autoimmune hematologic diseases
      2. Antibodies to tissue antigens in human diseases
   B. Cellular (delayed) sensitivity
      1. Experimental autoimmune diseases
      2. Human autoimmune diseases

II. Endogenous immune response to exogenous antigens
   A. Circulating antibody
      1. Anaphylactic-type reactions
      2. Atopic reactions
      3. Arthus reactions
   B. Cellular (delayed) sensitivity
      1. Tuberculin reaction
   C. Granulomatous hypersensitivity
      1. Berylliosis

III. Exogenous immune response to endogenous antigens
   A. Transfer of maternal antibody to fetus
      1. Erythroblastosis fetalis
      2. Neonatal leukopenia; thrombocytopenia
      3. Neonatal myasthenia gravis
   B. Experimental transfer of antibodies
      1. Masugi nephritis
   C. Experimental transfer of cells
      1. Graft versus host reaction

IV. Exogenous immune response to exogenous antigens
   A. Experimental transfer of antibody and antigens
      1. Passive anaphylaxis (Prausnitz–Kustner reaction)
      2. Passive Arthus reaction
   B. Experimental transfer of cells and antigens
      1. Tuberculin reaction
      2. Contact dermatitis

V. Endogenous immune response to complex antigens (hapten–protein)
   A. Circulating antibody
      1. Drug-induced blood dyscrasias
      2. Drug-induced lupus erythematosus
   B. Cellular sensitivity
      1. Contact dermatitis

Modified from lecture notes of Frank J. Dixon, M.D.

eases will be presented according to the predominant immune effector mechanism. Although this approach emphasizes the pathologic effect of the different mechanisms, the immune response cannot be simply compartmentalized in this manner. For most diseases, more than one immune mechanism is activated, perhaps at different times, and components of one mechanism may overlap with parts of another mechanism. This aspect of immunology will be discussed in more detail after presentation of each mechanism separately.

Bibliography

Austen KF, Cohn Z: Contribution of serum and cellular factors in host defense reactions. *N Engl J Med* 268:933, 1963.

Braude AI: Infection and immunity. In *Clinical Physiology.* Giallium A (ed.). New York, McGraw-Hill, 1957, 773.

Criep LH: *Clinical Immunology and Allergy.* New York, Grune and Stratton, 1962.

Gell PGH, Coombs RRA: *Clinical Aspects of Immunology,* 1st ed. Oxford, Blackwell, 1963.

Hirsch JG: Host resistance to infectious disease: A centennial. *Adv Host Defense Mech* 1:1, 1982.

Mosmann TR, Coffman RL. Heterogeneity of cytokine secretion patterns and functions of helper T cells. *Adv Immunol* 46:111, 1989.

Peltz G: A role for CD4+ T-cell subsets producing a selective pattern of lymphokines in the pathogenesis of human chronic inflammatory and allergic diseases. *Immunol Rev* 123:23, 1991.

Raffel S: *Immunity, Hypersensitivity, and Serology.* New York, Appleton–Century Crofts, 1953.

Roitt, IM: *Essential Immunology,* 1st ed. Oxford, Blackwell, 1971.

Romagnani S: Human TH1 and TH2 subsets: "Eppur si muove!" *Eur Cytokine Netw* 517–121, 1994.

Turk JL, Oort J: Germinal center activity in relation to delayed hypersensitivity. In *Germinal centers in Immune Responses.* Cottier J, Odortchenko N, Schindler R, Congden CC, (eds.). New York, Springer, 1967.

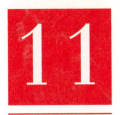

Inactivation/Activation of Biologically Active Molecules

Antibody to a hormone, hormone receptor, blood clotting factor, growth factor or enzyme, or drug may inactivate, activate, protect, or have no effect on the biologic function of these molecules. The nature of the disease caused by activation or inactivation depends upon the biologic function of the biologically active molecule or cell involved.

Antibodies to biologically active molecules are produced under two circumstances:

1. Breaking of tolerance with autoantibody production.
2. Immune response to a therapeutically administered hormone (insulin), enzyme, blood clotting factor, or drug that is recognized as a foreign antigen.

Antibody may neutralize or inactivate biologically active molecules by four major mechanisms (Fig. 11–1):

1. By direct reaction with the biologically active molecule, resulting in structural alteration of the molecule so that it is no longer active.
2. By causing increased catabolism of the antibody–antigen complex, effectively lowering the concentration of the biologically active molecules.
3. By reaction of antibody to cell surface receptors, causing blocking (steric hindrance), modulation (endocytosis), or destruction of the receptor, so that the cell is no longer able to respond to activating stimuli.
4. By attracting inflammatory cells that destroy the surface receptors (antibody-dependent cell-mediated cytotoxicity [ADCC]).

Mechanisms of Antibody-mediated Inactivation/Activation

INACTIVATION

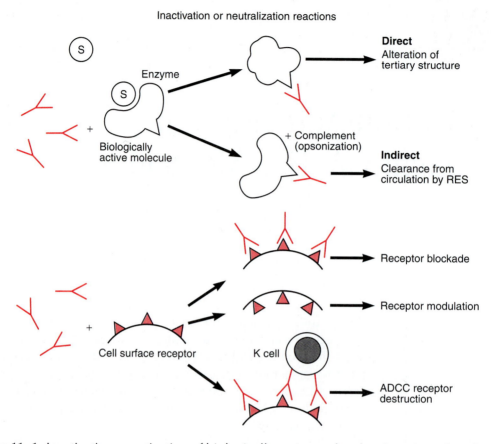

Figure 11–1. Inactivation or activation of biologically active molecules. Reaction of antibody with enzyme or other biologically active molecule may result in loss of biologic function due to steric hindrance of binding of the activating ligand with its receptor. However, the antigenic sites (epitopes) of an enzyme are usually located on a different part of the molecule than the substrate binding site. Inactivation may occur by alteration of the tertiary structure of the enzyme following reaction with antibody. This reaction affects the structure of the substrate binding site indirectly or inactivates the enzyme molecule. In vivo, either increased or decreased catabolism of an enzyme–antibody complex may occur. The biologic effect of neutralization depends upon the molecule neutralized. Antibodies to cell surface receptors may block or stimulate the receptor, or cause receptor modulation by endocytosis or destruction of the cell by antibody-dependent cell mediated cytotoxicity (ADCC).

The loss of receptor function and destruction of target cells in some tissues such as insulinitis, thyroiditis, atrophic gastritis, and myasthenia gravis are often associated with a lymphocytic infiltrate. This may be due to T-cell-mediated immunity (see Chapters 15 and 16), or autoantireceptors may direct ADCC.

Direct Inactivation

Antibodies may block the active site of a biologically active molecule or alter the conformation of the molecule so that it is no longer active. Biologically active molecules generally have one site that is necessary for biologic activity; localized in a small area of the whole molecule. An antibody reacting with or near this active site may block the reaction of the enzyme with its substrate. However, most antibodies that inactivate enzymes react with an epitope (antigenic site) quite distant from the biologically active site. Inactivation occurs by alteration of the tertiary structure of the molecule because of its reaction with antibody. Not all such reactions result in loss of substrate binding or inactivation. In fact, classic precipitin reactions with enzymes may occur with no apparent loss of activity in the precipitated enzyme, and antibodies may convert an inactive form of an enzyme to an active form (see below).

Not only is the site of antibody reaction important in neutralization of a biologically active molecule, but the effect of the antibody also depends upon other characteristics of the antibody–antigen reaction, such as the ratio of antibody to antigen, the strength of antibody–antigen binding, and the biologic properties of the antibody (eg, complement fixation, catalytic activity). Inactivation may be induced by the antibodies formed in one individual, whereas the antibodies formed in another individual may react with the same enzyme but not inactivate it.

Indirect Inactivation

In vivo, antigen–antibody complexes formed in antibody excess or at equivalence are rapidly cleared by the reticuloendothelial system due to formation of aggregated Fc regions of IgG or fixation of complement (macrophages have receptors for aggregated Fc or C_3b). However, not all antigen–antibody complexes are rapidly removed; some soluble complexes in antigen excess may continue to circulate. In some situations, binding of antibody to a hormone may actually produce a longer half-life, because bound molecules may be degraded more slowly than unbound molecules. This may lead to increased serum concentrations for the material involved but, paradoxically, a loss of biological function. On the other hand, such complexes may protect a hormone from catabolism, with later release of the active molecule (see below). The presence of such complexes may also lead to inflammatory lesions from the deposition of antibody–antigen complexes in vessels or renal glomeruli (see Immune Complex Reactions, Chapter 13).

Receptor Modulation

Antibodies may block or induce changes in cell surface receptors. The ability of cells to respond to activating stimuli may be lost because of reaction of antibody with the receptor. Antibodies to cell surface receptors may occupy the receptor (steric hindrance) or may induce endocytosis, stripping, or structural alteration of the receptor (receptor loss).

Antibody-dependent Cell-mediated Cytotoxicity (ADCC)	Antibodies reacting with cell surface receptors may induce the infiltration of inflammatory cells that secondarily destroy the receptors (ADCC). This is due to a reaction of K cells through Fc region receptors for antibodies bound to target cells. When IgG antibodies react with a target cell, the aggregated antibodies form altered Fc regions that bind to inflammatory cells.
ACTIVATION	Reaction of antibodies to a hormone, drug, or cell surface receptor may also **activate** or enhance the biologic function of the molecule. Through the use of monoclonal antibodies that recognize distinct epitopes on hormones, it has become clear that, on the one hand, an antibody to one site may inhibit activity, whereas antibody to another site may enhance activity, depending on the effect on the hormone itself or upon the effect on the binding of the hormone to its receptors.
Conformational Stabilization	Antibodies may act with a hormone directly but away from the active binding site and stabilize the active configuration of the molecule. The enzyme β-galactosidase exists in inactive and active conformers. Some antibodies to this enzyme are able to convert the inactive conformer to the active configuration. Presumably, reaction of the antibody with the inactive form of the enzyme results in an alteration of tertiary structure so that the active site becomes available.
Increased Binding Affinity	Antibodies, through cross-linking the molecule, may increase the affinity of binding and the activity of a hormone. The activity of epidermal growth factor (EGF) on the growth of fibroblasts in vitro may be increased with Fab_2 (bivalent), but not Fab (univalent) antibody, fragments to EGF. This is believed to be caused by conversion of low- to high-affinity binding between EGF and its receptor.
Receptor Selection	Antibodies may be able to redirect hormone binding from one receptor to another. A hormone may have more than one type of receptors on a cell or bind to receptors in different ways. Antibodies to one epitope on the hormone may block the ability of the hormone to react with one receptor and increase the binding to another receptor. Human growth hormone (hGH) has at least four distinct epitopes defined by monoclonal antibodies. A given antibody may enhance binding to one site,

while inhibiting binding to another site; in this way it blocks one activity while increasing another activity or redirecting the binding to a different tissue. One monoclonal antibody to growth hormone blocks activity in vitro by inhibiting binding to the target cells, yet enhances activity when injected into experimental animals.

Buffering

Antibodies may "protect" a hormone from degradation in vivo and prolong its activity by allowing "slow release" of the bound hormone. Most hormones are degraded rapidly by enzymes. Some antibodies are able to prevent the degradation of the hormone and prolong the survival of the hormone. So-called "superactive" forms of insulin appear to be protected by binding to serum albumin, and this "carrier" function may also be provided by antibody. Anecdotal cases of human diabetes that show a marked decreased requirement for insulin, as well as other patients who demonstrate enhanced effects of prolactin and thyroid-stimulating hormone, may be explained by this mechanism.

Receptor Activation

Antibodies may directly bind to the receptor for a hormone and activate the cells (eg, antithyroid receptor), because the antibody binding site mimics the structure of the activating ligand for the receptor (see below).

Examples of Antibody-mediated Inactivation/Activation

Some specific antibodies to biologically active molecules are listed in Table 11–1.

HORMONES

Insulin/Diabetes Mellitus

Diabetes mellitus is a general term for a heterogeneous group of diseases that have as a common denominator abnormalities in carbohydrate metabolism (Table 11–2), associated with a deficiency in the production or utilization of insulin. Insulin is an endocrine hormone produced by beta cells in the islets of Langerhans in the pancreas. Insulin specifically reacts with many other cells of the body through cell surface receptors and acts to stimulate transport and utilization of glucose for conversion to energy or for storage as glycogen in the liver or glycosides in fat cells. Diabetes results from impaired production or decreased utilization of insulin with resultant increase in blood glucose and related abnormalities of metabolism. Decreased insulin utilization occurs from impaired insulin secretion, loss of receptors or receptor

TABLE 11–1. DISEASES OF IMMUNE INACTIVATION/ACTIVATION

Disease	Antigen
Diabetes mellitus	Insulin
	Insulin receptor
	Islet cell cytoplasm (glutamic acid decarboxylase)
	Islet cell surface
Thyroid disease	
Hyperthyroidism	TSH receptor
Hypothyroidism	Triiodothyronine
Pernicious anemia	
Atrophic gastritis	Parietal cells
Megaloblastic anemia	Intrinsic factor
Infertility (induced)	Chorionic gonadotropin
	Estrogen, progesterone
Aplastic anemia	Erythropoietin
Chronic asthma	β-Adrenergic receptor
Myasthenia gravis	Acetylcholine receptor
Polyendocrinopathy	Multiple (adrenal, thyroid, parathyroid, gonads, pancreas, melanocytes)
Hemophilia, other blood diseases	Blood clotting factors (multiple)

response, or presence of blocking antibodies to insulin or to the insulin receptor (Fig. 11–2). About 20% of patients have "insulin-dependent" or type I diabetes (ie, the insulin receptors or responsive cells are normal, but insulin availability is low); the remaining 80% have "insulin-independent" or type II diabetes (insulin availability is normal, but the number of receptors is low).

TABLE 11–2. IMMUNOLOGIC FACTORS IN DIABETES MELLITUS

Type	Etiologic Factor
IMMUNE	
Type Ia juvenile onset	T cell- or ADCC-mediated destruction of beta cells; early, but not late, anti-islet cell antibody; HLA-DR3, -DR4 associated
Type Ib juvenile onset	T cell- or ADCC-mediated destruction of beta cells; both early and late islet cell antibody, associated with endocrinopathies
Insulin resistant	Anti-insulin antibodies in response to injection therapy
Insulin receptor (type II)	Autoimmune insulin receptor antibodies
NONIMMUNE	
Type II maturity onset	May develop insulin resistance
Secondary	Pancreatic disease (type III), hormonal (corticosteroid excess, etc.), drug-induced

Diabetes, from the Greek *dia* (through) and *bainein* (to go): To go through; a siphon.

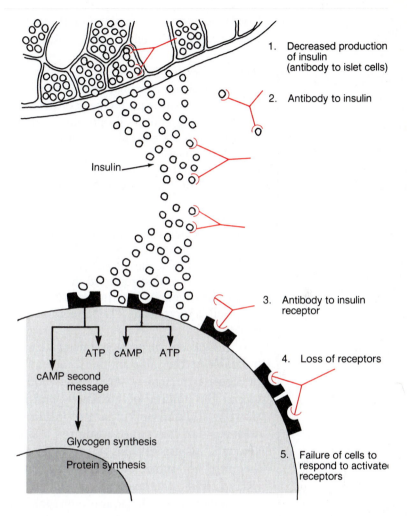

Insulin →

1. Decreased production of insulin (antibody to islet cells)

2. Antibody to insulin

3. Antibody to insulin receptor

4. Loss of receptors

5. Failure of cells to respond to activated receptors

ATP   cAMP   ATP

cAMP second message

Glycogen synthesis

Protein synthesis

Figure 11–2. Level of abnormality in diabetes. Antibody to insulin may block insulin action, and antibodies to receptors may block or modulate receptors. However, antibody to receptors is not the only way that loss of receptors may occur. Inflammation of islet cells is associated with autoantibody to islet cells and precedes juvenile-onset insulin-dependent diabetes. The islet cell destruction is caused by immune attack by T cells.

Both types of diabetes may have immunological origins. At least four different antibodies are associated with diabetes mellitus: to insulin, to islet cell cytoplasm (glutamic acid decarboxylase), to islet cell surface antigen, and to insulin receptors. In type I diabetes, there is a loss of beta cells in the pancreas as a result of immune attack early in life or there may be neutralizing antibodies to insulin. In type II diabetes, there may be loss of receptors secondary to antibody to receptors. However, most patients with type II diabetes have neither anti-insulin nor anti-receptor antibodies.

Antibodies to Insulin. Antibodies to insulin are often found in patients who are administered exogenous insulin, but most, but not all, such patients show no increase or decrease in insulin requirements. In 1938, Banting and his group observed an antibody-like neutralizer of insulin in a schizophrenic patient who had been receiving insulin shock treatment. Insulin resistance due to antibodies to foreign insulin sometimes occurred in diabetic patients receiving exogenous (eg, bovine or ovine) insulin for therapy. As antibodies develop, increasing doses of insulin may be required. In many cases, resistance to exogenous insulin derived from one species (ox) does not hold for insulin derived from another species (pig). Production of human insulin by gene-cloning techniques provides a less immunogenic molecule, but does not completely eliminate the possibility of antibody formation. Anti-insulin antibodies were first reported in 1970 in some patients who had never received exogenous insulin and who did not have islet destruction, but islet cell hyperplasia. This condition is termed "spontaneous hypo-glycemia."

Not all anti-insulins are neutralizing and not all insulins are neutralizable by the same antibody, indicating that even though the insulin molecule is relatively small, it has both overlapping and distinct epitopes. The binding of insulin by anti-insulin in vivo usually causes slowing of the disappearance of insulin from the bloodstream, that is, a longer half-life. Since insulin is a small antigen available in large amounts, insulin–anti-insulin complexes may not be cross-linked and therefore not subject to clearance by the reticuloendothelial system (RES). RES clearance is mediated by Fc or C_3b receptors on macrophages, which require aggregates of IgG or complement fixation. Such complexes may not be formed with antibodies to insulin unless the epitopes involved permit cross-linking. Insulin bound to antibody is catabolized at the rate of the antibody (IgG) and not at the rate of insulin. Therefore, instead of reducing the half-life of insulin, antibody to insulin actually prolongs the half-life, because the bound insulin is protected from degradation by insulinase in the liver. Although the antibody-bound insulin is prevented from exerting its biologic activity, release of the bound insulin from the antibody may allow it to be utilized. This phenomenon may result in a decrease in the amount of insulin required for therapy because of so-called "superactive" forms of bound insulin. Since antibodies to insulin may either decrease or enhance insulin activity, a close correlation between antibody titers and insulin requirement is usually not seen. Acute skin reactions and systemic anaphylactic shock may also occur if insulin is injected into a sensitive individual (see below). In addition, immune complexes of various antibody–antigen proportions may be formed. These may deposit in vessel walls or in renal glomeruli and induce immune complex reactions (see Chapter 13). The insulin–anti-insulin reaction has been adapted to provide a highly sensitive immunoassay for insulin.

Antibodies to Islet Cells. Autoantibodies to islet cell cytoplasm (beta cells) and/or islet cell surface antigens are associated with insulin-dependent (type I) juvenile onset diabetes mellitus, but the appearance of antibody in the serum *follows* the destruction of the beta cells in the islets (insulinitis). Antibodies to cow's milk albumin cross react with beta-cell surface proteins and are frequently found in patients with type I diabetes. Eighty percent of patients with recent onset autoimmune destruction of beta cells have antibodies to the cytoplasmic enzyme glutamic acid decarboxylase. In addition, antibodies to insulin receptors, insulin, proinsulin, glucagon, and several other peptide hormones may be found in patients with type I diabetes. The incidence of serum antibody drops markedly after onset of the disease so that after one year only about 20% of patients have detectable antibody.

The initial destruction of beta cells appears to be mediated by T-cell attack, not by antibody-directed mechanisms. In experimental animals, neonatal thymectomy can prevent diabetes in susceptible strains of mice, and the disease may be transferred with lymphocytes from animals with active disease. In humans, acute onset juvenile diabetes begins with lymphocyte infiltration of islets (lymphocytic insulinitis), and the actual immune-mediated destruction of the beta cells is caused by cell-mediated immunity. It is not clear which T-cell subpopulation is responsible; both CD4+ and CD8+ cells may be found in lesions. The pathogenic significance of antibodies to islet cell surface antigens is not known. Presumably, they could play an important role in the destruction of islets by an ADCC mechanism.

Recently, treatment with immunosuppressive drugs (ie, cyclosporine, azathioprine), antiinflammatory agents (corticosteroids, indomethacin) and monoclonal antibodies to T cells (CD3) has been shown to be effective in experimental models, and preliminary trials indicate that **immunomodulation** therapy of juvenile diabetes may be of value in preventing or limiting early destruction of the beta cells. For instance, in one study, the onset of juvenile diabetes was delayed in about one-third of patients by cyclosporine treatment if given within six weeks of onset. Juvenile diabetes shows a high relationship to certain histocompatibility types. It has been suggested that juvenile onset diabetes is a genetically controlled autoimmune reaction, perhaps triggered by a viral infection.

Thyroid Hormone/
Hypothyroidism

Most any of the common non-neoplastic diseases of the thyroid are immune in origin: Hypothyroidism, hyperthyroidism, and thyroiditis. A number of autoantibodies to thyroid antigens are found in normal individuals (particularly with aging) as well as associated with thyroid diseases (Table 11–3). Some of these have biologic effects and some do not. Antibodies to thyroid hormone or thyroid-stimulating hormone (TSH) may be responsible for hypothyroidism, whereas antibodies to the thyroid receptor for thyroid-stimulating hormone (TSH) may produce hyperthyroidism (Graves' disease). There is an associated swelling and inflammation of the orbit of the eye (Graves' ophthalmopathy). An amino acid sequence similarity between thyroglobulin and acetylcholinesterase opens the possibility that antithyroglobulin may react with epitopes common to thyroglobulin and the orbit of the eye (see below).

Antibody-dependent or cell-mediated immunity to thyroid antigens causes inflammation of the thyroid (thyroiditis) and may lead to destruction of the thyroid gland (see Chapter 21). Autoimmune thyroiditis may be induced in animals by immunization with thyroid hormone. The major feature of this disease is infiltration of the thyroid gland with mononuclear cells. The disease is believed to be mediated by specific T_{CTL}- or T_{DTH}-mediated inflammation, but could be caused by ADCC. In humans with chronic lymphocytic thyroiditis, autoantibodies to thyroid hormones may be found and may be responsible for hypothyroidism by binding thyroxine or triiodothyronine. Hyperthyroidism caused by antibodies to TSH receptors (Graves' disease) will be discussed below under Receptors.

Human Chorionic Gonadotropin (hCG), Estrogen, Progesterone/ Infertility

Antibodies to the hormones required to maintain pregnancy may prevent normal pregnancy. Antibodies to hCG have been reported in patients after hCG treatment of women with hypopituitarism, as well as in apparently normal individuals. These antibodies may explain the

TABLE 11–3. AUTOANTIBODIES TO THYROID ANTIGENS

Antigen	Effect of Antibody
Thyroxine and triiodothyronine	Blocks thyroid hormone action—hypothyroidism
TSH (Thyroid-stimulating hormone)	Blocks effect of TSH—hypothyroidism
TSH receptor	Stimulates receptor—hyperthyroidism (LATS) Inhibits TSH binding—hypothyroidism or both
Not defined (TSH-related)	Stimulates growth of thyroid cells
Cell surface antigen	Cytotoxic with lymphocytes (ADCC); associated with thyroiditis
Microsomal antigen	Cytotoxic with lymphocytes—thyroiditis
Thyroglobulin	Not clear; associated with thyroiditis; cross-reacts with acetylcholinesterase ? causing Graves' ophthalmopathy
Colloid antigen	Not known; associated with thyroiditis

TSH, thyroid-stimulating hormone; LATS, long-acting thyroid stimulator; ADCC, antibody-dependent cell-mediated cytotoxicity.

poor results of hCG therapy in some infertile women. In Rhesus monkeys active immunization with hCG or passive transfer of antibodies to hCG can effectively reduce the number of conceptions or cause early abortions. Anti-hCG apparently blocks the luteotropic support of the corpus luteum and may affect the development of the placenta or fetus as well. Trials of hCG immunization for selected populations in which more effective birth control is considered essential have been successful, and trials using different "vaccines" incorporating the β chain of hCG, which does not share epitopes with other hormones, are now underway.

Progesterone is the major hormone required for the establishment and maintenance of pregnancy. Antibodies to progesterone are of interest as a means of interruption of pregnancy. Passive transfer of monoclonal antibodies to progesterone shortly after conception blocks pregnancy in experimental animals. Women treated with oral contraceptive pills containing estrogenlike compounds may develop circulating antibody to ethylestradiol, which may be detected either as free antibody or in the form of circulating immune complexes. These women have a higher incidence of thrombosis than women who do not develop antibodies. Antibodies to zona pellucida antigens can be seen in both fertile and infertile women; it is not known if there are different epitopes that could explain the apparent lack of correlation.

Erythropoietin/
Anemia

Erythropoietin, produced by the kidney, stimulates the production of erythrocytes in the bone marrow. Erythropoietic inhibitors have been identified in the plasma of patients with refractory anemia, and it is possible that these patients may have an antibody that inhibits the action of erythropoietin.

RECEPTORS

Insulin Receptors

Antibodies to insulin receptors from different individuals recognize different antigenic determinants; some are associated with symptoms, and some are not. Autoantibodies to cell surface receptors for insulin may be found in patients with extreme insulin resistance. Most of these patients are female and also have a pigmented skin condition known as acanthosis nigricans. These antibodies inhibit the binding of insulin to cell surface receptors, thus interfering with the biological function of insulin. Anti-receptor antibodies are also found in patients treated with exogenous insulin, presumably because of formation of anti-idiotypes (anti-anti-insulin) that mimic part of the insulin ligand. Antibodies to insulin receptors may increase basal glucose oxidation of reactive cells in vitro, thus producing insulinlike effects. Receptor cross-linking appears to be required for antibody-included insulin receptor activation, as Fab univalent fragments will not activate. Presumably, insulin activation of the receptor is different from antibody-mediated activation, since insulin is univalent and cannot cross-link receptors. However, insulin reaction with receptors does cause aggregation of receptors presumably by perturbation of cytoskeletal elements.

Thyroid-stimulating (TSH) Hormone Receptors/Hyperthyroidism

Autoantibodies to TSH receptors that cause hyperthyroidism are termed long-acting thyroid stimulator (LATS). LATS has been shown to be an immunoglobulin antibody that can, on the one hand, inhibit the binding of TSH to human thyroid cell membranes, and, on the other hand, stimulate thyroid cyclic AMP and thyroid hormone release. Animals that are immunized with thyroid hormone not only produce blocking antibodies but also may produce a thyroid-stimulating globulin. Thus, either hyperthyroidism (Graves' disease) and hypothyroidism may result from an autoimmune response. The end result depends upon the degree of tissue damage and the type and amount of autoantibody produced. A distinct population of antithyroid autoantibodies is able to stimulate cyclic adenosine monophosphate (cAMP) and promote growth of thyroid cells in vitro. This antibody is also associated with enlargement of the thyroid in Graves' disease and not with other thyroid diseases. Thus, some anti-TSH receptors stimulate both production of thyroid hormone and growth of thyroid cells, whereas others stimulate only hormone production. Monoclonal antibody studies indicate that these epitopes are part of the ganglioside component of the receptor rather than the glycoprotein complement. There is a high association of hyperthyroidism with HLA-DR3 (about 60%) and those patients who are HLA-DR3-positive almost never go into remission whereas non-HLA-DR3 patients with Graves' disease frequently have remission.

Massive swelling of the extraocular muscles (Graves' ophthalmopathy) is frequently associated with hyperthyroidism. This reaction may progress rapidly and produce blindness. The cause of exophthalmos (bulging eyes) is not known. It has been hypothesized that there is cross-reactivity between the cell membrane of the eye muscles and some epitopes of the TSH receptor. Immune complexes may be present on extraocular muscle membranes. These could produce cell damage and lymphocytic infiltration, perhaps by ADCC. The chronic accumulation of glycosaminoglycans in the connective tissue that is characteristic of Graves' ophthalmopathy may be caused by chronic stimulation of fibroblasts by cytokines produced by lymphocytes. Treatment with immunosuppressive drugs (cyclosporine and low-dose prednisone) may control the inflammation of Graves' ophthalmopathy, or resistant cases may be treated with orbital irradiation and steroids.

Acetylcholine
Receptors/
Myasthenia
Gravis (MG)

MG is characterized by muscle weakness and easy fatigability; weakness is most prominent in the muscles of the face and throat. The disorder is the result of a functional abnormality in which the conduction of nerve impulses from the motor nerve to the muscle fiber is impaired (Fig. 11–3). Patients afflicted with this disease tire very easily; usually, they awaken with close to normal muscular function, but this deteriorates during the day. The clinical course is punctuated with remissions and exacerbations; total incapacitation and death from respiratory failure may occur.

Myasthenia gravis represents more than a single disease syndrome. A partial listing of some of the recognized syndromes is given in Table 11–4. Classical MG is associated with autoantibodies to the acetylcholine receptor; some variant syndromes have defects in neuromuscular transmission at other levels. The AChR is a neurotransmitter composed of a complex transmembrane protein formed by five polypeptide chains arranged as subunits consisting of two α and one each β, γ, and δ chains. An epitope located between amino acids 125 and 148 of the α chain contains a site that binds to ACh, and antibodies to this epitope are highly associated with experimental models of myasthenia. However, many human anti-AChRs bind to other epitopes and do not block binding of ACh to AChR. Impairment of neuromuscular transmission by these antibodies to AChR is accomplished by modulation of the AChR (internalization and degradation), often associated with lymphocytic infiltration. This modulation may be blocked by Fab fragments, indicating that cross-linking is required for AChR modulation or that aggregated Fcs are required for ADCC.

In autoimmune myasthenia gravis, the decrease in neuromuscular transmission in MG is associated with decreased AChR in the postsynaptic muscle membrane. Purified radiolabeled bungarotoxin binds to acetylcholine receptor (AChR). The amount of bungarotoxin binding

TABLE 11–4. SOME MYASTHENIA SYNDROMES

Type	Characteristics	Pathogenesis
Neonatal	Transient	Placental transfer of maternal anti-AChR
Adult I	Females under 40	Auto-anti-AChR (HLA-B8, DR3-associated)
Adult II	Males over 40	Auto-anti-AChR (HLA-A2-associated)
Ocular	Eyes only	Multiple
Congenital	Permanent	Multiple
Drug-induced	Transient, drug-induced (penicillamine)	Anti-AChR (HLA-DRI-associated)
Eaton–Lambert	Adults, cancer related	Autoantibody to presynaptic membrane
Engel's Disease	Mild, nonprogressive	Impaired acetylcholine packaging in neural end plate

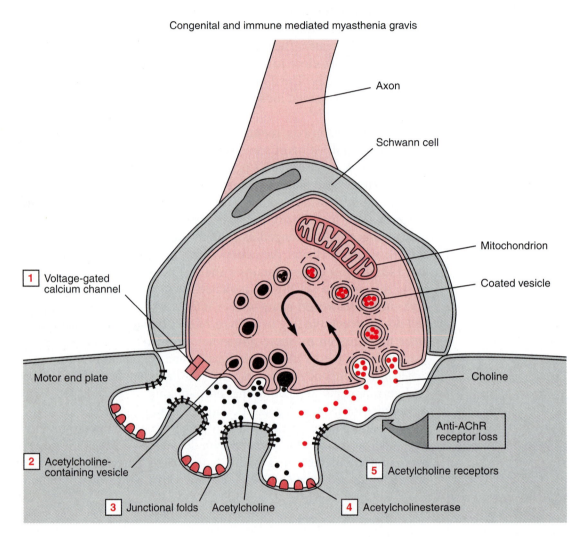

Figure 11–3. Neuromuscular transmission is mediated by acetylcholine (ACh) released from vesicles in the neuronal axon that bind to acetylcholine receptors (AChR) in the motor end plate. Acetylcholine is broken into choline and acetate by acetylcholinesterase, which inactivates ACh. Free choline reenters the neuron by endocytosis. ACh is produced in the vesicle from acetate and choline by choline acetyltransferase. ACh is released from vesicles that fuse with the cell membrane of the motor end plate. Congenital decrease in neuromuscular transmission may be impaired by (1) defects in voltage-gated calcium channels, (2) defects in ACh-containing vesicles, (3) defects in junctional folds, (4) decrease in ACh receptors, and (5) acetylcholinesterase levels in the synaptic cleft. Immune-mediated myasthenia gravis is caused by action of antibodies to AChR to block or cause loss of receptors.

sites is markedly decreased in muscle from MG patients, indicating a loss of AChR. The development of an experimental model of MG has provided a way to work out the autoimmune pathogenesis of MG. A syndrome with features almost identical to human MG has been produced by immunizing experimental animals with AChR from the electric eel (Fig. 11–4). AChR-immunized animals develop precipitating antibody to AChR, antibody to syngeneic muscle, and a flaccid paral-

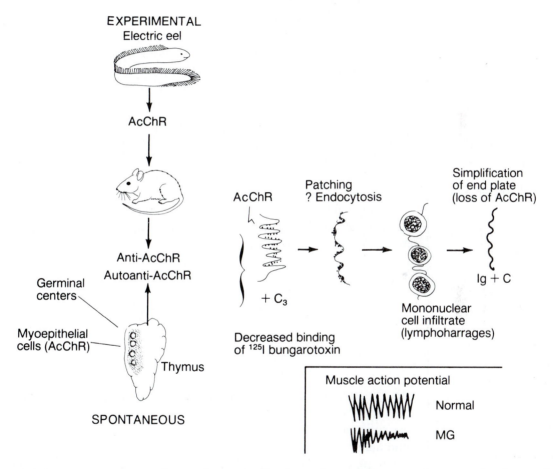

Figure 11–4. Comparison of experimental allergic and naturally occurring myasthenia gravis. Antibody to acetylcholine receptors (AChRs) may be induced in experimental animals by immunization with AChR from the electric eel or autologous AChR. Autoantibodies to AChR occur spontaneously in humans with myasthenia gravis. Both experimental animals and affected humans demonstrate progressive muscle weakness, a decrease in AChR, immunoglobulin, and complement deposition, and a mononuclear infiltrate at the neuromuscular junction. On restimulation, the muscle action potential reveals a rapid decline. The thymus of affected humans may contain germinal centers not normally found in the thymus. Since the thymus contains myoepithelial cells with AChR, it is possible that autoantibody production of AChR occurs in the thymus.

ysis that can be reversed by neostigmine, an agent that can also temporarily reverse the muscular weakness of patients with MG. Experimental allergic MG has also been produced by immunization with syngeneic muscle AChR in complete Freund's adjuvant.

Antibody to AChR could alter neuromuscular transmission in at least three ways. It may block or inhibit AChR activity, cause modulation of AChR from muscle membranes, or fix complement and cause destruction of the postsynaptic membranes either directly or by ADCC. A simple blocking or inhibition effect seems unlikely for the human disease, because most human anti-AChRs do not affect binding of bungarotoxin by AChR and do not alter the end-plate potential of neuromuscular junctions in vitro. As mentioned above, some epitopes of the major immunogenic region of the α chain of AChR are not involved in binding ACh. A decrease in AChR activities by modulation or immune destruction appears at this time to be more likely. The addition of immunoglobulin from myasthenic patients to mouse neuromuscular junctions leads to an accelerated degradation of the AChR receptors. Passive transfer of antibody to animals produces an acute MG syndrome associated with lymphocytic invasion of the motor end plate, suggesting ADCC.

Anti-idiotypic MG

Anti-idiotypic antibodies have been shown to be able to cause experimental myasthenia gravis. Anti-idiotypic antibodies to the AChR agonist trans-3,3'-bis[α-(trimethylammonia) methyl] azo benzene bromide (Bis Q) are able to cause MG:

Bis Q, a potent AChR agonist that binds to AChR, was conjugated to bovine serum albumin and antibodies to Bis Q induced in rabbits. The paratope of anti-Bis Q mimics the binding characteristic of AChR. Immunization of rabbits with anti-Bis Q resulted in anti-anti-Bis Q, which blocked binding of ACh to AChR and reproduced experimental MG (Fig. 11–5).

Antibodies to AChR have been demonstrated in over 90% of MG patients. Newborn infants of mothers with MG may be born with a temporary muscular weakness because of placental transfer of antibody from mother to fetus. Patients with other autoimmune diseases, such as systemic lupus erythematosus, Graves' disease, and thymoma, may also have antibody to AChR, and some of these patients develop clinical myasthenia gravis, suggesting that they had a latent or sub-

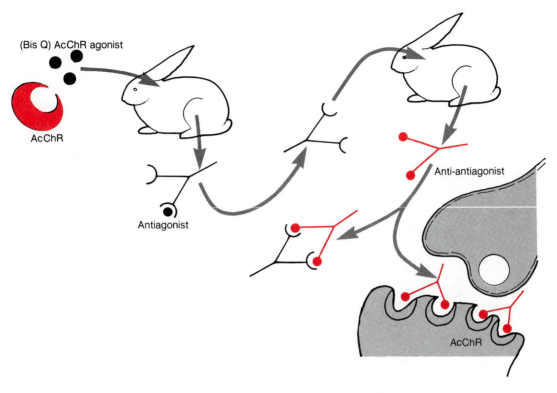

Figure 11–5. Production of myasthenia gravis by anti-idiotypic antibodies to anti-agonist antibody.

clinical form of MG. Therefore, most of the evidence supports the concept that human MG and experimental allergic MG are very similar and that the major pathogenesis of the disease is an antibody-mediated modulation of AChR.

In addition to anti-AChR, many myasthenics have a variety of other immune abnormalities. The serum of most myasthenics contains an antibody that binds to muscle fibers and epithelial reticular cells of the thymus. The level of this antibody does not always correlate to the severity of the disease. These muscle-binding antibodies could be a secondary effect of the disease or only an associated finding. Myasthenia is often associated with a peculiar thymic hyperplasia in which germinal centers are formed in the medulla of the thymus or with tumors of the thymus; thymectomy may lead to clinical improvement in these patients but may accelerate the disease in others. Treatment of severely myasthenic patients by plasmapheresis (to remove anti-AChR) and immunosuppressive drugs (to suppress anti-AChR production) have produced improved muscle reactivity in some patients. This improvement is associated with a fall in anti-AChR titers in serum. Recent trials with cyclosporine indicate a more prolonged beneficial effect than other immunosuppressive drugs.

The primary pathogenic role of antibodies to AChR does not explain all myasthenia syndromes (see Table 11–4). Rare congenital disorders of neuromuscular transmission have now been recognized that mimic autoimmune MG. Five levels of defects in neuromuscular transmission are recognized:

1. Decreased function of the voltage-gated calcium channel required to initiate vesicle release Lambert–Eaton Syndrome.
2. Impaired acetylcholine packaging caused by a reduction of vesicles in the neural end plate (Engel's disease).
3. Acetylcholinesterase deficiency.
4. Congenital paucity of synaptic clefts.
5. Defects of acetylcholine receptor function.

Extensive clinical and laboratory work-up is required to differentiate these syndromes from the autoimmune types. This is important since therapy appropriate for immune myasthenia may be harmful to patients with congenital myasthenia.

Antibodies to a neuromuscular junction antigen may also be pathogenic for amyotrophic lateral sclerosis. This disease causes severe debilitating neuromuscular disease with progressive compromise of arms, legs, speech, swallowing, and breathing. In an animal model of experimental autoimmune motor neuron disease there is loss of motor neurons, the disease may be transferred with serum, and Ig can be demonstrated within and on the cell membranes of lower motor neurons.

The Lambert–Eaton myasthenic syndrome occurs as a **paraneoplastic syndrome** in patients with small cell carcinoma of the lung and other cancers. Electrophysiologic findings indicate that the disorder is due to reduced ACh release from the motor nerve. IgG from patients with this syndrome can passively transfer the conduction disorder to experimental animals. Autoantibodies are directed to the presynaptic membrane and deplete the presynaptic membrane of active zones.

The stiff man syndrome is a rare disease characterized by fluctuating and progressive muscle rigidity and spasms associated with autoantibodies to gamma-amino-butyric acid (GABA) found on cells in the gray matter of the brain. It is hypothesized that these autoantibodies may cause the disorder by impairing the function of GABA-ergic neurons.

β-adrenergic Receptor/Asthma, Cardiomyopathy

The β-adrenergic catecholamine hormone receptor–adenylate cyclase complex functions to regulate the level of cAMP in essentially all cells, but in particular those involved in anaphylactic reactions, ie, mast cells and smooth muscle end organs (see Chapter 14). The "beta-blockade" theory of asthma proposes that chronic asthma is related to a decrease in β-adrenergic sensitivity in bronchial smooth muscle, mucous glands, mucosal blood vessels, and mast cells. Autoantibodies to β_2 (lung) adrenergic receptors have been found in some patients with hay fever and/or asthma. Receptor blockade by β-receptor antibodies raises the level of excitability of the end organ cells, setting the stage for chronic asthma.

In addition, autoantibodies to β-adrenergic receptors have been found in patients with dilated cardiomyopathy. These antibodies are directed to a specific epitope located in the second extracellular loop of the β_1-adrenergic receptor. These antibodies decrease the number of binding sites for β-adrenergic agonists and selectively downregulate the number of active binding sites on the membranes of myocardial cells, which is a characteristic of failing ventricular myocardium.

Dopamine Receptors/ Schizophrenia, Parkinson's Disease

It has been hypothesized that schizophrenia might be caused, at least in part, by autoantibodies to dopamine receptors. Dopamine receptors (D_2) are elevated in the brains of schizophrenics. Antipsychotic drugs effective in the treatment of schizophrenia block dopamine receptors. Thus, schizophrenia may be caused by overactivity of dopaminergic pathways. Dopamine receptor-stimulating autoantibodies have been suggested as a possible cause for overactivity. Antiserum to brain tissue evokes epileptic activity when applied topically to the cerebral cortex of animals, but a convincing role for autoantibodies in schizophrenia has not yet been demonstrated.

Associated with the pandemic of influenza between 1919 and 1926 was a variety of Parkinsonism disorders known collectively as Von Economo's encephalitis. It has been postulated that certain strains of influenza virus may have had an affinity for dopamine receptors, resulting in selective destruction of extrapyramidal neurons. However, in early Parkinson's disease, the dopamine receptor density is increased and patients respond well to dopamine mimetic medications.

Polyendocrinopathy

The autoimmune polyendocrinopathies, which feature two or more endocrine insufficiencies, have been divided into two groups: Type I and type II. Type I (Blizzard's syndrome) is very rare and presents almost always in childhood as Addison's disease, mucocutaneous moniliasis, and hypoparathyroidism, as well as one or more other additional endocrine abnormalities, skin lesions, and chronic active hepatitis. Type II (Schmidt's and Carpenter's syndrome) is seen in adults and features thyroiditis, Addison's disease, and insulin-dependent diabetes, often associated with pernicious anemia. The association of these diseases with circulating autoantibodies has stimulated the hypothesis that there is a loss of immune tolerance to endocrine hormones or receptors, perhaps through a depression of controlling suppressor T cells, resulting in autoimmune reactions to more than one endocrine system.

Autoantibodies to adrenocortical cells, parathyroid cells, thyroid microsomes, pancreatic islet cells and gastric parietal cells are often found. Shared epitopes on different endocrine organs have been demonstrated using monoclonal antibodies. It is also possible that a viral infection might stimulate such a polyspecific autoimmune reaction.

OTHER BIOLOGICALLY ACTIVE MOLECULES

Intrinsic Factor/Pernicious Anemia

Pernicious anemia is a disease in which there is an abnormality in the absorption of vitamin B_{12}. B_{12} is required for the normal maturation of all bone marrow precursors, so that failure of B_{12} absorption leads to a deficit in production of mature erythrocytes and to anemia. Absorption of B_{12} requires the action of a substance known as intrinsic factor, which is secreted by the lining cells of the stomach (parietal cells). Pernicious anemia is associated with two distinct antibodies. One reacts specifically with the parietal cells of the gastric mucosa. The presence of this antibody is almost invariably associated with a reduction in acid secretion, atrophic gastritis, and lymphocytic infiltration. Cellular reactions (delayed hypersensitivity) or ADCC are most likely responsible for atrophic gastritis.

The second antibody is to intrinsic factor. This antibody was first observed because of an acquired resistance to intrinsic factor in patients being treated for pernicious anemia. Anti-intrinsic factor antibody can be demonstrated to inhibit the binding of vitamin B_{12} to intrinsic factor and is associated with abnormalities of vitamin B_{12} absorption. Two types of anti-intrinsic factor antibody have been observed: (1) Blocking antibody, which prevents subsequent formation of vitamin B_{12}–intrinsic factor complexes and is associated with the presence of megaloblastic cells; and (2) binding antibody, which can be shown to bind to intrinsic factor but does not prevent bound intrinsic factor from subsequent combination with vitamin B_{12}. Intrinsic factor-blocking antibody appears to play a significant role in the pathogenesis of pernicious anemia.

Blood Clotting Factors/ Hemophilia

The clotting system requires the interaction of up to thirty different factors. Antibodies that may inactivate these factors have been reported (see Chapter 8). Antibodies to antihemophilic globulin frequently appear in hemophiliacs genetically lacking this globulin and are treated with infusions containing antihemophilic globulin. The hemophiliac recognizes the antihemophilic globulin as foreign. Similarly, individuals who lack other clotting components may develop antibody to the missing component when transfused. For reasons that are poorly understood, individuals with diseases such as lupus erythematosus, Sjögren's syndrome, tuberculosis, or hyperglobulinemia may also produce antibodies to clotting factors that complicate an already confusing clinical picture. Circulating antibodies to clotting factors have also been found in association with penicillin allergy. Finally, some individuals apparently produce circulating anticoagulants not associated with any known disease. The exact mechanism of action of antibodies to clotting factors is poorly understood. The clinical effect depends upon the particular factor or factors affected. Paradoxically, some antibodies to phospholipids may promote coagulation, perhaps by activation of platelets. In severe cases, treatment with immunosuppressive drugs, such as prednisone or cyclophosphamide, may reduce inhibitors of blood clotting factors, but care must be exercised because of possible toxicity.

Drugs

Antibodies to drugs may produce a number of different diseases, such as hemolytic anemias (see Chapter 12) and immune complex disease (see Chapter 13). Antibodies to drugs may also be used to treat drug overdoses. For instance, digoxin-specific $F(ab')_2$ antibody fragments have been used to reduce digitoxin levels rapidly in cases of digitoxin poisoning. Antibody inhibition may also affect the action of other drugs, such as steroids, chloramphenicol, morphine, oxytocin, and vasopressin.

Other Antibodies

Autoantibodies to vasopressin in rabbits produce diabetes insipidus. Antibodies to gluten may react with gluten bound to epithelial cells and damage intestinal epithelium by an ADCC mechanism causing sprue or celiac disease. Passive antibodies to gastrin have been used to induce serum gastrin levels in patients with the Zollinger–Ellison syndrome (intractable peptic ulcers caused by high gastrin levels). Sheep immunized with inhibin, a nonsteroid hormone found in ovarian follicular fluid that inhibits follicle-stimulating hormone (FSH) have an increased ovulation rate. This has resulted in increased fecundity in sheep in Australia. Autoantibodies to parathyroid hormone receptors are found in patients with secondary hyperparathyroidism. These antibodies block binding of hormone to receptors.

Ligands, Receptors, and Idiotypes

Antibodies, hormone receptors and enzymes have structural and functional similarities. Each type of molecule is organized into functional domains consisting of a specific ligand binding domain and a transmission domain. Reaction of the binding domain with ligand results in alteration of the transmission domain and activation of an effector system. Antibodies, hormone receptors and enzymes are able to distinguish a series of ligands (antigens) with similar structures and bind the

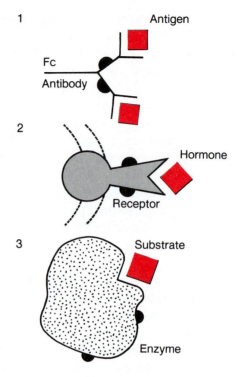

Figure 11–6. Similarities Between Antibodies, Hormone receptors, and Enzymes

   1. Recognition domain (paratope) that distinguishes fine structural differences.
   2. Functional domain (constant region).
   3. Recognition domains have similar binding properties for ligands and mechanisms of activation of cells through G proteins.

appropriate ligand with a high affinity (Fig. 11–6). Each have epitopes specific for the binding site, as well as epitopes on parts of the molecule away from the binding site.

Antibodies to receptors, enzymes, or other antibodies may react with ligand (antigen) binding-site epitopes or with nonbinding epitopes (Fig. 11–7). Antibodies that react directly with the binding site may mimic the structure of the natural ligand.

ANTI-IDIOTYPES AND LIGAND MIMICRY

The interrelationship of antibodies to ligands and receptors provides a network of related structures (Fig. 11–8). The paratope (antigen-binding site) of antibody to the ligand will mimic the receptor for the ligand. The anti-idiotype to the anti-ligand (anti-anti-ligand) will be a mirror-image of the receptor and mimic the ligand. Similarly, antibody to the receptor may mimic the ligand, and anti-idiotype to the anti-

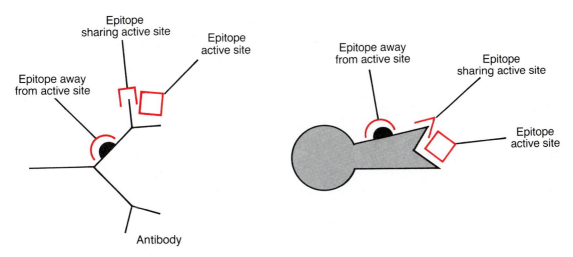

Figure 11–7. Antibodies to receptors may bind (1) the active site, (2) epitopes away from the active site, or (3) epitopes sharing part of the active site. Anti-idiotypes may react with (1) the active site of antibody, (2) epitopes away from the active site, or (3) epitopes sharing part of the active site.

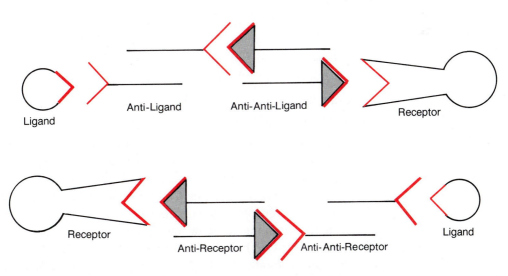

Figure 11–8. Relationship of ligand, anti-ligand, anti-idiotypes, receptor, anti-receptor, and anti-idiotypes. An immune response to a ligand may result in antibodies that mimic the receptor and anti-idiotypes that mimic the ligand; an immune response to the receptor may produce antibodies that mimic the ligand and anti-idiotypes that mimic the receptor.

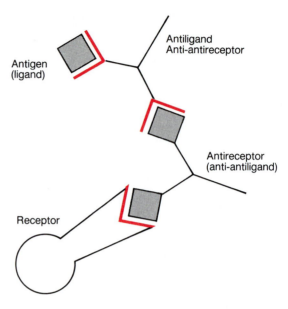

Figure 11–9. The ligand–antibody–receptor network. An immune response to a ligand may result in antibodies that mimic the receptor or the ligand (anti-anti-receptor). An immune response to a receptor may produce antibodies that mimic the ligand (anti-anti-ligand). Antibodies to the ligand may have paratopes that mimic the receptor. In this way, immune response to either ligand or receptor may produce inactivating or activating antibodies. Experimental animals immunized with insulin not only develop antibodies to insulin but also antibodies to the insulin receptor (anti-anti-insulin).

receptor (anti-anti-receptor) will mimic the receptor site for the ligand. In this way, a network of interactions may be completed (Fig. 11–9).

ANTI-IDIOTYPES AND DISEASE

Some examples of molecular mimicry between biologically active ligands and anti-idiotypic antibodies to anti-ligands are:

1. Anti-idiotypic antibodies against anti-insulin, containing the internal image of insulin, interact with the membrane-bound insulin receptor and mimic insulin action in vitro.
2. Anti-b-adrenergic ligand anti-idiotype antibodies bind to the β-adrenergic receptor and stimulate cyclase.
3. Rabbits immunized with rat–antihuman thyroid-stimulating hormone (TSH) antibodies produce anti-antibodies, which inhibit the binding of TSH to the TSH receptor (Fig. 11–10).
4. Antibodies to an agonist of the acetylcholine receptor mimic the binding characteristics of acetylcholine receptor, ie, the anti-agonist antibody binding site binds the same ligands as the receptor. An anti-idiotypic antibody to the anti-agonist causes myasthenia gravis (see above).

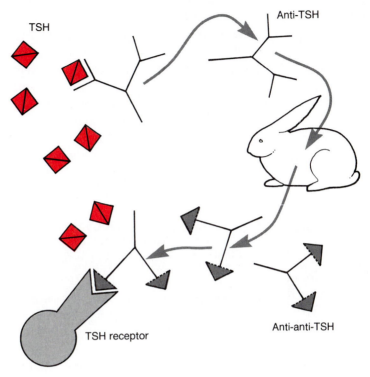

Figure 11–10. Production of TSH-blocking antibodies by immunization of rabbits with anti-TSH. Anti-idiotype to anti-TSH (anti-anti-TSH) reacts with TSH receptor and blocks TSH binding.

Neutralizing Antibodies— Cause and Effect

The presence of antibodies to a biologically active molecule in a patient with a given disease does not necessarily mean that the antibody actually causes the disease or is even responsible for any of the symptoms of the disease. Pierre Grabar has postulated that most autoantibodies are part of a physiological system of handling metabolic or catabolic products (transporters). Autoantibodies help in disposing of self materials, particularly if an unrelated event causes release of abnormally high amounts of tissue components. For example, massive tissue necrosis in an acute myocardial infarction results in release of intracellular antigens and triggers autoantibody formation. In this example, autoantibody formation occurs secondarily to cell necrosis and is not responsible for initiating this type of tissue damage. However, it has become increasingly apparent that the autoantibodies may produce disease as a primary mechanism or may cause resistance to therapy or other secondary effects. Autoimmune diseases caused by antibodies are covered in the individual chapters on immunopathogenic mechanisms and connective tissue diseases in Chapter 22.

Summary

Circulating antibodies to biologically active molecules may effectively inactivate or neutralize the activity of these molecules and thus produce deficiency diseases. On the other hand some autoantibodies may increase activity. Biologically active molecules that may be affected by antibodies include hormones, enzymes, growth factors, clotting factors, and cell surface receptors. Inactivation may occur by alteration of tertiary structure, blocking of active sites, or modulation of cell surface receptors. Autoantibodies to endocrine glands, hormones, or hormone receptors are the best understood examples of these activation or inactivation reactions.

Bibliography

**MECHANISMS
OF
INACTIVATION/
ACTIVATION**

Aston R, Cowden WB, Ada GL: Antibody-mediated enhancement of hormone activity. *Mole Immunol* 26:435, 1989.

Cinader B (ed.): *Antibodies to Biologically Active Molecules.* New York, Pergamon Press, 1967.

Rotman MB, Celada F: Antibody-mediated activation of a defective β-D-galactosidase extracted from an *Escherichia coli* mutant. *Proc Natl Acad Sci USA* 60:660, 1968.

Weigle WO: Fate and biological action of antigen–antibody complexes. *Adv Immunol* 1:283, 1961.

**DIABETES
MELLITUS**

Atkinson MA, Maclaren NK: Islet cell autoantibodies in insulin-dependent diabetes. *J Clin Investig* 92:1608–1616, 1993.

Banting FG, Franks WR, Gairns S: Anti-insulin activity of serum of insulin-treated patients. *Am J Psychiatry* 95:562, 1938.

Faustman D: Mechanisms of autoimmunity in type I diabetes. *J Clin Immunol* 13:1–7, 1993.

Karjalainen J, Martin JM, Knip M, et al.: A bovine albumin peptide as a possible trigger of insulin-dependent diabetes mellitus. *New Engl J Med* 327:302–307, 1992.

MacLaren N, Lafferty K: The 12th international immunology and diabetes workshop. *Diabetes* 42:1099–1104, 1993.

Rabinovich A: Immunoregulatory and cytokine imbalances in the pathogenesis of IDDM. *Diabetes* 43:613–621, 1994.

Vardi P, Brik R, Barzilai D: Insulin autoantibodies: Reflection of disturbed self-identification and their use in the prediction of type I diabetes. *Diabet/Metabol Rev* 7:209, 1991.

**THYROID
DISEASE**

Bahn RS, Heufelder AE: Role of connective tissue autoimmunity in Graves' ophthalmopathy. *Autoimmunity* 13:75–79, 1992.

Doniach D, Roitt IM: Autoimmunity in Hashimoto's disease and its implications. *J Clin Endocrin Metab* 77:1293, 1957.

Karlsson FA, Wibell L, Wide L: Hypothyroidism due to thyroid-hormone-binding antibodies. *N Engl J Med* 296:1146, 1977.

Ludgate M, Dong Q, Dreyfus PA, et al.: Definition, at the molecular level of a thyroglobulin-acetylcholinesterase shared epitope: Study of its pathophysiological significance in patients with Graves' ophthalmopathy. *Autoimmunity* 3:167, 1989.

McKenzie JM, Zakarija M: LATS in Graves' disease. *Recent Prog Horm Res* 33:29, 1977.

Mori T, Akamizu T, Kosugi S, et al.: Recent progress in TSH receptor studies with a new concept of autoimmune TSH receptor disease. *Endocrine J* 41:1–11, 1994.

Ochi Y, DeGroot LJ: Long-acting thyroid stimulator of Graves' disease. *N Engl J Med* 278:718, 1968.

hCG, ESTROGEN, PROGES-TERONE/ FERTILITY

Beaumont V, Lemort N, Beaumont JL: Oral contraception, circulating immune complexes, anti-ethirylestradial antibodies and theruliosis. *Am J Repro Immunol* 2:8, 1982.

Gupta SK, Singh V: Immunobiology of human chorionic gonadotropin. *Indian J Exp Biol* 26:243, 1988.

Musch K, Wolf AS, Lauritzen C: Antibodies to chorionic gonadotropin in humans. *Clin Chim Acta* 113:95, 1981.

Nasa HA, Chang CC, Tsong YY: Formulation of a potential antipregnancy vaccine based on the β-subunit of human chorionic gonadotropin. *J Rep Immunol* 7:151, 1985.

Wang MW, Whyte AK, Taussig MJ, et al.: Immunofluorescent localization, by use of anti-idiotypic antibody, of monoclonal antiprogesterone antibody in the mouse uterus before implantation. *J Reprod Fert* 86:211, 1989.

Wood DM, Liv C, Dunbar BS: Effect of alloimmunization and heteroimmunization with zona pellucida on fertility in rabbits. *Biol Reproduct* 25:439, 1981.

MYASTHENIA GRAVIS

Appel SH, Engelhardt JI, Garcia J, et al.: Immunoglobulins from animal models of motor neuron disease and from human amyotrophic lateral sclerosis patients passively transfer physiological abnormalities to the neuromuscular junction. *Proc Natl Acad Sci* 88:647, 1991.

Castleman B: Pathology of the thymus gland in myasthenia gravis. In *Thymectomy for Myasthenia Gravis*. Viets HR, Schwab RS (eds.). Springfield, IL, CC Thomas, 1960.

Dau P, Lindstrom JM, Cassel CK, et al.: Plasmapheresis and immunosuppressive drug therapy in myasthenia gravis. *N Engl J Med* 297:1134, 1977.

Engel AG: The investigation of congenital myasthenic syndromes. *Ann NY Acad Med* 681:425–434, 1993.

Fenichel GM: Clinical syndrome of myasthenia in infancy and childhood: A review. *Arch Neurol* 35:97, 1978.

Lennon VA, Lindstrom J, Seybold ME: Experimental autoimmune myasthenia: A model of myasthenia gravis in rats and guinea pigs. *J Exp Med* 141:1365, 1975.

Lopate G, Pestronk A: Autoimmune myasthenia gravis. *Hosp Pract* 28:55, 1993.

Smith RG, Appel SH: The Lambert–Eaton syndrome. *Hosp Pract* 27:57, 1992.

Solimena M, Folli F, Dennis-Domimi S, et al.: Autoantibodies to glutamic acid decarboxylase in a patient with stiff man syndrome, epilepsy, and type I diabetes mellitus. *N Engl J Med* 318:1012, 1988.

Sophianos D, Tzartos SJ: Fab fragments of monoclonal antibodies protect the human acetylcholine receptor against antigenic modulation caused by myasthenic sera. *J Autoimmunity* 2:777, 1989.

Strickroot FL, Schaeffer RL, Bergo HL: Myasthenia gravis occurring in an infant born of a myasthenic mother. *JAMA* 120:1207, 1942.

Valenzuela CF, Dowding AJ, Arias HR, et al.: Antibody-induced conformational changes in the torpedo nicotinic acetylcholine receptor: A fluorescent study. *Biochemistry* 33:6586–6594, 1994.

β-ADRENERGIC RECEPTORS

Courand PO, Lu BZ, Schmutz A, et al.: Immunologic studies of β-adrenergic receptors. *J Cell Biochem* 21:187, 1983.

Guillet JG, Chanet S, Hoeberke J, et al: Production and detection of monoclonal anti-idiotype antibodies directed against a monoclonal anti-β-adrenergic ligand antibody. *J Immunol Meth* 74:163, 1984.

Limas CJ, Goldenberg IF: Autoantibodies against cardiac β-adenoreceptors in human dilated cardiomyopathy. *Circ Res* 64:97, 1989.

Magnusson Y, Marullo S, Hoyer S, et al.: Mapping of a functional autoimmune epitope on the β_1-adrenergic receptor in patients with idiopathic dilated cardiomyopathy. *J Clin Invest* 86:1658, 1990.

Venter JG, Fraser CM, Harrison LC: Autoantibodies to β_2-adrenergic receptors: A possible cause of adrenergic hyporesponsiveness in allergic rhinitis asthma. *Science* 207:1361, 1980.

PERNICIOUS ANEMIA

Glass GBJ: Gastric intrinsic factor and its function in the metabolism of B_{12}. *Physiol Rev* 43:529, 1963.

Goldberg LS, Bluestone R, Steihm ER, et al.: Human autoimmunity, with pernicious anemia as a model. *Annu Intern Med* 81:372, 1974.

Irvine WJ: Immunologic aspects of pernicious anemia. *N Engl J Med* 273:432, 1965.

Jeffries GH, Sleisenger MH: Studies of parietal cell antibody in pernicious anemia. *J Clin Invest* 44:2021, 1965.

Kawashima K: Effects of gastric antibodies on gastric secretion. II. Effects of rabbit antibodies against rat gastric mucosa and gastric juice on gastric secretion in the rat. *Jpn J Pharmacol* 22:155–165, 1972.

Taylor KB, Roitt IM, Doniach D, et al.: Autoimmune phenomena in pernicious anemia: Gastric antibodies. *Br Med J* 2:1347, 1962.

ANTI-COAGULANTS

Hultin MB, Shapiro SS, Bowman HS, et al.: Immunosuppressive therapy of factor VIII inhibitors. *Blood* 48:94, 1976.

Margolius A, Jackson DP, Ratnoff OD: Circulating anticoagulants: A study of 40 cases and a review of the literature. *Medicine* 40:197, 1961.

Shapiro SS, Hultin M: Acquired inhibitors to the blood coagulation factors. *Semin Thromb Hemostasis* 1:336, 1975.

OTHER REFERENCES

Appel GB, Holub DA: The syndrome of multiple endocrine gland deficiencies. *Am J Med* 61:129, 1976.

Butler VP, Chen JP: Digitoxin specific autoantibodies. *Proc Nat Acad Sci* 57:71, 1967.

Gordon AS, Cooper GW, Zanjani ED: The kidney and erythropoiesis. *Semin Hematol* 4:337, 1967.

Jepson JH, Lowenstein L: Panhypoplasia of the bone marrow. I. Demonstration of a plasma factor with anti-erythropoietin-like activity. *Can Med Assoc J* 9:99, 1968.

Levitt MD, Cooperband SR: Hyperamylasemia from the binding of serum amylase by an 11S IgA globulin. *N Engl J Med* 278:474, 1968.

Seeman P: Dopamine receptors in human brain diseases. In *Dopamine Receptors*. Alan R. Liss, New York, 1987, 233.

Smolarz A, Roesch E, Lenz E, et al.: Digoxin-specific antibody (Fab) fragments in 34 cases of severe digitalis intoxication. *Clin Toxicol* 23:327, 1985.

Volpe R: The role of autoimmunity in hypoendocrine and hyperendocrine function. *Ann Intern Med* 87:86, 1977.

IDIOTYPES AND RECEPTORS

Courand PO, Strosberg AD: Anti-idiotypic antibodies against hormone and neurotransmitter receptors. *Biochem Soc Transact* 19:147, 1991.

Izadyar L, Friboulet A, Remy M, et al.: Monoclonal anti-idiotypic antibodies as functional internal images of enzyme active sites. Production of a catalytic antibody with a cholinesterase activity. *Proc Natl Acad Sci USA* 90:8876–8880, 1993.

Strosberg AD: Anti-idiotype and anti-hormone receptor antibodies. *Springer Semin Immunopath* 6:67, 1983.

Wasserman NH, Penn AS, Freimuth PI, et al.: Anti-idiotype route to antiacetylcholine receptor antibodies and experimental myasthenia gravis. *Proc Natl Acad Sci USA* 79:4810, 1982.

Yavin E, Yavin E, Schneider MD, et al.: Monoclonal antibodies to the thyrotropin receptor: Implications for receptor structure and the action of autoantibodies in Graves' disease. *Proc Natl Acad Sci* 78:3180, 1981.

CAUSE AND EFFECT

Grabar P: Hypothesis: Autoantibodies and immunological theories: An analytical review. *Clin Immunopath* 4:453, 1975.

12

Cytotoxic or Cytolytic Reactions

Cytotoxic or cytolytic reactions occur when antibody reacts with either an antigenic component of a cell membrane or an antigen that has become intimately associated with a cell. The reaction of antibody with the cell activates two complement-mediated pathways of cell death or lysis: (1) Activation of the complete cascade with insertion of membrane attack complexes and lysis of the target cell, or (2) aggregated immunoglobulin Fc regions and/or C3b receptor binding produces "immune adherence" of antibody-coated cells to phagocytic cells and phagocytosis (Fig. 12–1). An additional method of immunoglobulin binding is by passive adsorption to red cells of antibody–antigen complexes formed in the bloodstream with subsequent complement fixation and lysis. This mechanism has been identified with antibodies to drugs such an quinidine. Most destruction of affected blood cells occurs extravascularly by phagocytosis and destruction of antibody- or complement-coated cells in the spleen and liver, rather than by intravascular cell lysis. Blistering diseases of the skin are also mediated, in part, by cytolytic reactions.

Hemolytic Antibodies

Cytotoxic or cytolytic reactions are initiated by IgM or those IgG immunoglobulin subclasses that have the capacity to activate complement. Selected IgG subclasses bind complement better than others, eg, IgG_3, IgG_1. IgM is the most efficient complement-fixing antibody. One IgM antibody molecule reacting with a cell is sufficient to activate complement, whereas two IgG molecules in close apposition are required to produce an Fc region aggregate. Antibodies of the IgM class are approximately 600 times more efficient in fixing complement

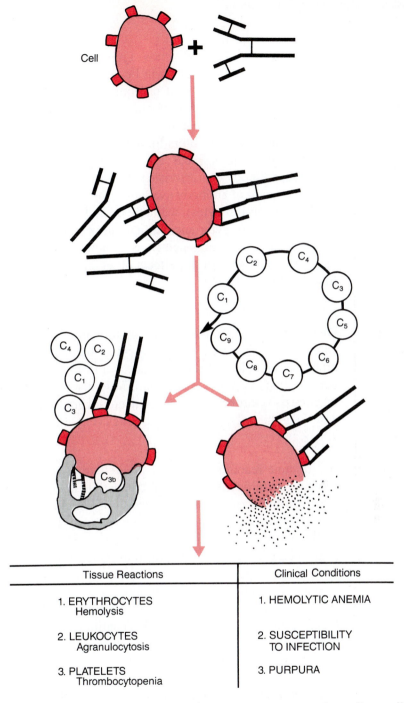

Tissue Reactions	Clinical Conditions
1. ERYTHROCYTES Hemolysis	1. HEMOLYTIC ANEMIA
2. LEUKOCYTES Agranulocytosis	2. SUSCEPTIBILITY TO INFECTION
3. PLATELETS Thrombocytopenia	3. PURPURA

Figure 12–1. Cytotoxic or cytolytic reactions. These reactions most often affect cellular elements in intimate contact with circulating plasma, such as erythrocytes, leukocytes, or platelets. Circulating humoral antibody reacts with antigens present on cell membranes. In vitro, through action of the complement system, the integrity of cell membrane is compromised and the cell lysed. The osmotic difference in intracellular and extracellular fluids causes release of intracellular fluids. In vivo, the cells coated with immunoglobulin antibody or complement are subject to phagocytosis and sequestration in the spleen and liver.

than antibodies of the IgG class. IgG-coated erythrocytes are cleared predominantly in the spleen via Fc and C_3b receptors, whereas IgM-coated cells are sequestered predominantly in the liver through C_3b receptors. Clearance of IgM-coated cells is entirely complement-dependent, whereas clearance of IgG-coated cells is not, since the clearing cells have receptors for aggregated Fcs.

The ultimate clinical effect depends upon the type of cell involved, antibody characteristics, the number of antigen sites per cell, and the amount of antibody available. The cells usually affected are red blood cells (erythrocytes), white blood cells, or platelets. The resulting diseases are hemolytic anemia, agranulocytosis, and thrombocytopenia; they are grouped together as immunohematologic diseases. An experimental model of the effects of an anti-red cell antibody is illustrated in Figure 12–2.

Immuno-hematologic Diseases

ERYTHROCYTES (ANEMIA)

Transfusion Reactions

Disease conditions arising from the immune destruction of red blood cells result from loss of erythrocyte function, from the damaging effects of the released cell contents, and from toxic effects due to antigen–antibody complexes formed. These disorders include transfusion reactions, erythroblastosis fetalis, acquired autoimmune hemolytic diseases, and hemolytic reactions to drugs (Fig. 12–3).

An immune reaction occurs when circulating antibody of host origin contacts erythrocytes from an incompatible donor. The red cells of an incompatible donor contain antigens not found on the recipient's cells (blood-group antigens). The donor antigen is exogenous and the immune response is endogenous. Blood group antigens are genetically controlled cell surface structures present on blood cells. An individual with blood type A has isoantibodies against type B erythrocytes. Isoantibodies are defined as antibodies to antigens within the same species. If this individual is transfused with type B blood, anti-B antibodies coat the B erythrocytes. This coating is also called sensitization. The sensitized cells may then be lysed by complement or destroyed in the spleen. Antibodies to blood group antigens are detected in vitro by their ability to agglutinate a selected panel of red cells expressing different blood group antigens.

Over fourteen human red blood cell antigen systems, which include over sixty different blood group factors, are known. (For more details on the carbohydrate structure of blood group antigens, see Chapter 30, Tumor Immunity p 901.) The ABO and Rh systems are the most important to identify for the routine transfusion service as these represent the majority of antibodies implicated in clinical transfusion reactions. The other antigens are less important clinically because of low antigenicity or low incompatibility frequency. Transfusion reac-

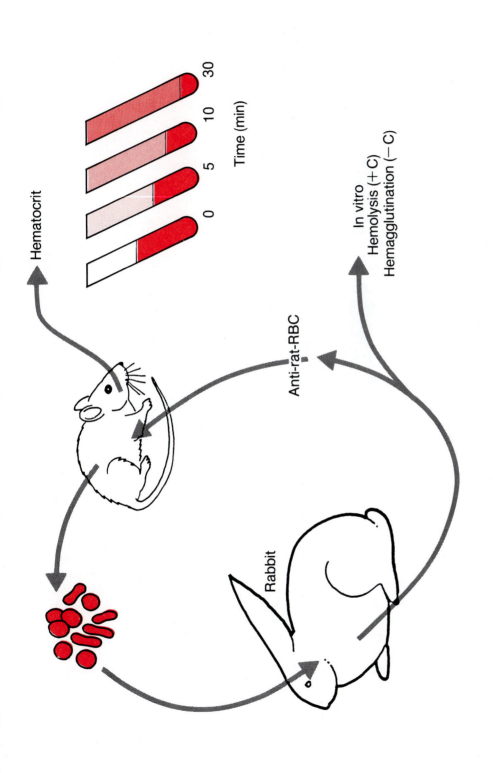

Figure 12–2. Experimental model of acute hemolytic reaction.

1. Rat RBC are injected into a rabbit to produce rabbit anti-rat RBC serum.
2. In vitro, this antiserum will lyse rat RBC in the presence of complement. If the antiserum is decomplemented, agglutination of the cells, but not lysis, occurs.

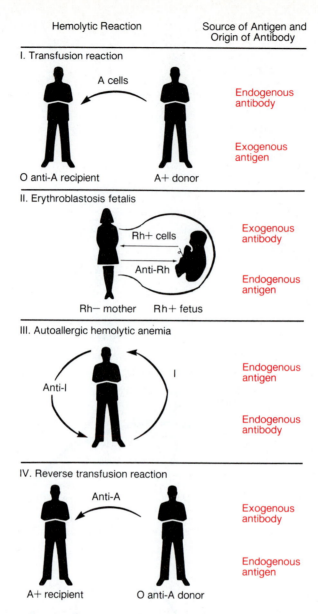

Hemolytic Reaction   Source of Antigen and Origin of Antibody

I. Transfusion reaction

A cells

O anti-A recipient   A+ donor

Endogenous antibody

Exogenous antigen

II. Erythroblastosis fetalis

Rh+ cells

Anti-Rh

Rh− mother   Rh+ fetus

Exogenous antibody

Endogenous antigen

III. Autoallergic hemolytic anemia

Anti-I   I

Endogenous antigen

Endogenous antibody

IV. Reverse transfusion reaction

Anti-A

A+ recipient   O anti-A donor

Exogenous antibody

Endogenous antigen

Figure 12–3. Hemolytic reactions. Shown are four types of hemolytic reactions caused by antibody-mediated complement activation in relationship to the origin of the antibody and the source of the antigen: I. *Transfusion reactions.* Erythrocytes from a donor (A+) that are antigenic for a recipient whose serum contains antibody to the donor's erythrocyte antigen (O anti-A) will be lysed upon transfusion, resulting in release of hemoglobin and a clinical syndrome known as a transfusion reaction. *Exogenous antigen–endogenous antibody.* II. *Erythroblastosis fetalis.* Rh+ erythrocytes cross the placenta and stimulate the production of antibody to Rh if the mother is not Rh+. These antibodies will cross back through the placenta to attack fetal erythrocytes. *Endogenous antigen–exogenous antibody.* III. *Autoimmune hemolytic anemia.* An individual becomes sensitized to the antigens of his own erythrocytes (autoantibody). *Endogenous antigen–endogenous antibody.* IV. *Reverse transfusion reaction.* Antibodies are transfused from a donor to a recipient whose red cells contain the antigen. This passively transferred antibody causes lysis of recipient red cells. *Endogenous antigen–exogenous antibody.*

tions are usually predictable from blood group typing, serum screening for antierythrocyte antibodies, or crossmatching. For blood typing, the red cells of an individual are tested in vitro for reaction with a panel of selected antisera that are known to react with given blood group antigens. For antibody screening, the serum of a potential recipient is tested in vitro with red cells from two to three donors who have been antigen typed and represent all of the common red cell antibodies among them. For crossmatching, the serum from a potential recipient is mixed with the cells of a potential donor. If agglutination occurs, the donor cells contain an antigen, the recipient has antibody to the antigen, and the donor cells cannot be used, even if there is no difference in ABO antigens or other detectable major blood groups. The potential for acute transfusion reactions due to the presence of preformed antibodies should be easily recognized and prevented by the appropriate cell typing, antibody screening, or crossmatch testing.

In some cases, delayed transfusion reactions may occur because of induction of an immune response in the recipient to transfused cells. The transfused donor cells may survive well initially, but after 3 to 14 days, hemolysis occurs because of the production of an antibody that was not detectable at the time of the initial crossmatch. This is most likely because of a secondary response in a patient previously primed but could also be because of a primary antibody response. The compatibility test relies on an agglutination end point and may, therefore, miss low concentrations of serum antibodies. Patients who receive multiple transfusions frequently develop antibodies to minor blood group antigens, and the incidence of hemolytic reactions in any given individual is related to the number of previous transfusions that have been given.

Erythroblastosis Fetalis

Erythroblastosis fetalis, or hemolytic disease of the newborn, is caused by maternal antibodies which cross the placenta and attack fetal erythrocytes. The Rh system of red cell antigens was first identified in 1939, and the first case of hemolytic disease of the newborn due to fetal–maternal Rh incompatibility was reported in 1941 by Philip Levine and his co-workers. The conditions for hemolytic disease exist when a pregnant woman lacks Rh antigens (Rh–) present in the fetus because of the contribution of paternal genes. An Rh– mother may become sensitized to Rh+ erythrocytes produced by the fetus. If the antibody formed by the mother crosses the placenta, it destroys the fetal erythrocytes (Fig. 12–4). Destruction of fetal erythrocytes occurs by the action of antibody and complement or by an antibody-dependent cell-mediated mechanism. Thus, red blood cells (RBCs) from infants with maternal anti-Rh may be coated with maternal antibody and killed by fetal lymphocytes or macrophages that react with the

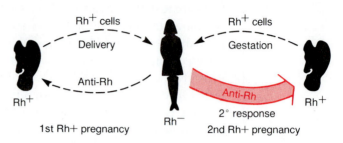

Figure 12–4. Erythroblastosis fetalis. Rh– mother carrying an Rh+ fetus. During first pregnancy, sensitization occurs. During subsequent pregnancy of a sensitized mother carrying an Rh+ fetus, anti-Rh antibodies may cross the placenta and react with fetal red cells. During the first pregnancy, small numbers of Rh+ fetal erythrocytes, usually insufficient for sensitization, cross the placenta. However, at delivery, a substantial number of Rh+ erythrocytes are released into maternal circulation. In a small percentage of Rh-incompatible pregnancies, this is sufficient to immunize the mother if the mother is not treated with passively administered anti-Rh antibody. During a second pregnancy, the small number of erythrocytes that reach the maternal circulation will induce a secondary antibody response in the mother to the Rh antigen. The maternal antibody is IgG and crosses the placenta to the fetus, where it acts on fetal erythrocytes, causing their destruction.

antibody on the RBC surface through Fc receptors (antibody-dependent cellular cytotoxicity [ADCC]).

Rh Antigens. The Rh antigenic system is a mosaic of genetically controlled specific antigenic determinants, which may serve as the targets for antibody from one individual to another, as in erythroblastosis fetalis or for antibody in the same individual toward his own red cells (autoimmune hemolytic anemia). In the case of erythroblastosis fetalis, in which antibodies produced by the mother act on fetal red cells, the antigen is endogenous (fetal antigen) and the immune response exogenous (maternal antibody) in respect to the affected individual, the fetus. Because of the proliferation of cells by the fetus in an attempt to make up for the destruction of fetal erythrocytes in the erythrocyte series, the spleen and liver continue to contain a large number of blood-forming precursor cells (extramedullary hematopoiesis), giving rise to the name erythroblastosis fetalis. Because of the marked destruction of red cells, high concentrations of one hemoglobin breakdown product—bilirubin—during the immediate neonatal period may lead to brain damage secondary to deposition of bilirubin in the brain (kernicterus).

Prevention of Rh Immunization. Hemolytic disease of the newborn is now a largely preventable disease. Prevention of immunization of Rh–

mothers carrying Rh+ fetuses is now commonly practiced by treating Rh− mothers, who have just delivered an Rh+ fetus, with passive antibody to Rh+ antigens. The observation that led to such a procedure was that protection against Rh immunization occurs if the fetus contains ABO blood group antigens not present in the mother (Fig. 12–5). Thus, if the blood of the fetus is A Rh+ or B Rh+ and the mother's blood is O Rh−, the mother develops anti-Rh antibodies less frequently than when the blood of the fetus is O Rh+ and the mother's is O Rh−, or when the blood of the fetus is A Rh+ and the mother's is A Rh−. The presence in the mother of antibodies to ABO group antigens on the fetal erythrocytes prevents immunization to the Rh antigens. In Rh incompatibility, fetal erythrocytes usually appear in the circulation of the mother in sufficient amounts to stimulate antibody production numbers at the time of delivery, and this is the time most Rh− mothers first become sensitized by Rh+ fetal cells. Because of the possibil-

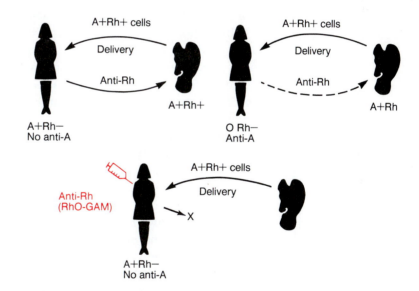

Figure 12–5. Prevention of Rh immunization by passive antibody. *Top*: Naturally occurring situation in which an ABO and Rh incompatibility are combined; sensitization of the mother to Rh+ antigens is significantly less than when there is an Rh incompatibility but no ABO incompatibility. The presence of antibody to fetal red cell A+ antigen in the non-A mother prevents sensitization to the Rh+ antigen, whereas the mother with no anti-A becomes sensitized to the Rh system. This observation was used as a rationale for passively transferring antibody to Rh to mothers who were Rh− and were carrying an Rh+ fetus. *Bottom*: Administration of anti-Rh at delivery significantly reduces the incidence of sensitization of the mother to the Rh system; erythroblastosis fetalis has thus become a preventable disease through the application of immunoprophylaxis.

ity that such sensitization could be prevented by passive transfer of anti-Rh antisera to Rh– mothers, trials were made on Rh– male volunteers. Passive transfer of anti-Rh serum along with Rh+ cells prevented immunization of these volunteers. Now adapted as a required procedure, the incidence of Rh immunization in subsequent pregnancies has been greatly reduced by the passive transfer of anti-Rh sera (or globulin) to an Rh– mother at the time of delivery of an Rh+ fetus. This prevention of an immune-mediated disease is considered by many to be one of the most important contributions of immunology to the prevention of human disease.

In addition, since sensitization may occur following spontaneous or therapeutic abortion of an Rh+ fetus in an Rh– mother, anti-Rh+ globulin should also be administered after abortion of an Rh+ fetus in an Rh– mother. Rare cases of sensitization may still occur, such as by the inadvertent transfusion of Rh+ blood to an Rh– woman and in a small number of instances when sensitization occurs during pregnancy prior to delivery. Antepartum administration of anti-Rh serum can even prevent those rare cases due to in utero sensitization of Rh– mothers by Rh+ babies prior to delivery. An interesting relationship is that of the Rh type of the grandmother on Rh sensitization. An increased incidence of sensitization is seen when the grandmother is Rh+, the mother Rh–, and the fetus Rh+ (about one in six mothers with this relationship will become sensitized). It appears that the Rh– mother may be primed or sensitized by Rh+ erythrocytes that crossed from the grandmother when the mother was a fetus, so that when she is exposed to Rh+ cells, there is a more rapid and intense response.

Treatment of Erythroblastosis Fetalis. In cases where Rh sensitization has occurred, the affected fetus may be treated by intrauterine transfusion of Rh– blood cells. Since the transfused blood does not have the Rh antigen, the erythrocytes will not be destroyed by maternal antibodies. However, this procedure has a high rate of complications and must be done only after amniocentesis, and analysis of amniotic fluid by optical density to determine the severity of the hemolytic process. Fluoroscopic and ultrasound examination of the fetal position are required in order to place the transfusion needle in the fetal abdomen. The transfused red cells eventually transverse the peritoneum and enter the fetal circulation. In less severe cases, the patient may be followed and transfusions delayed until after birth (exchange transfusion). Exchange transfusions are usually done to remove bilirubin and prevent kernicterus. If the fetal age is sufficient, labor is induced, when the risks of prematurity are less than the risk of intrauterine transfusion.

ABO Hemolytic Disease of Newborn. ABO hemolytic disease of the newborn is usually mild to minimal clinically, even if the mother's blood contains high titers of anti-A or anti-B antibodies and the fetus's blood is A, B, or AB. This may be because of three reasons: (1) Anti-A–anti-B antibodies are usually IgM and therefore do not cross the placenta; (2) ABO blood group antigens are widely distributed in the fetal tissues and the placenta, so that the effect upon fetal erythrocytes of any IgG anti-A or anti-B antibodies that may cross the placenta is diluted out because the antibodies react with many other tissue sites; and (3) ABO blood group carbohydrates are not fully expressed on fetal erythrocytes. In contrast, the Rh specificity is unique for erythrocytes, and the effect of anti-Rh antibodies that cross the placenta is concentrated on the fetal erythrocytes that have fully developed Rh antigens.

Acquired Autoimmune Hemolytic Disorders

Acquired autoimmune hemolytic disorders are caused by formation of antibodies to antigens present on the affected individual's own erythrocytes. Autoimmune hemolytic anemia (AIHA) may be differentiated from congenital metabolic hemolytic disorders by careful testing. The major difference between immune and congenital hemolytic diseases is that in the latter condition the erythrocytes are congenitally defective and do not survive normally in either the patient or a "normal" individual. In contrast, the erythrocytes are normal in patients with immune hemolytic disease and survive better in a "normal" recipient than in the patient. Therefore, congenital disease demonstrates an intracorpuscular defect; immune disease demonstrates an extra corpuscular defect. The extracorpuscular defect is an autoantibody. Intravenous infusions of immunoglobulin may produce rapid reversal of acute hemolytic episodes by blocking macrophage Fc receptors, and patients maintained on long term Ig treatment may be prevented from additional hemolytic attacks. There are two major forms of hemolytic disease caused by autoantibodies to red cells: Warm antibody-mediated and cold antibody-mediated, with rare patients having features of both. In a study of 1,834 patients with AIHA, 1,051 were idiopathic, and the rest associated with a variety of other diseases including cancer, infections, other autoimmune diseases, and other diseases.

Warm Antibody Disease. Warm antibody disease is almost always caused by IgG antibody that reacts with the patient's red cells. In two-thirds of the cases, the antibody reacts with Rh determinants. The antibody may appear without a known cause (idiopathic) but more frequently is associated with a collagen disease or with a lymphoproliferative disorder, eg, chronic lymphocytic leukemia. The patient's erythrocytes may be coated in vivo with IgG antibody, IgG and complement, or complement alone, when tested by the Coombs' technique (see below). The action of antibody and complement leads to destruction of the erythrocytes (hemolytic anemia), mostly after phagocytosis by reticuloendothelial cells, which have receptors which bind the Fc region of IgG and C_3b coating red blood cells. During active anemia, the spleen or liver sinusoids may be filled with red cells. Frank intravascular hemolysis by the complete complement sequence may also be observed. Treatment with corticosteroids may abort life-threatening acute hemolytic episodes. Steroids are believed to have at least three possible effects on autoimmune hemolytic anemia: (1) Decreased affinity of Fc receptor binding, (2) decreased phagocytic activity of the RES, and (3) decreased antibody production. Splenectomy is of some temporary value, but usually the anemia recurs even after the spleen is removed, indicating that the reticuloendothelial cells of other organs (eg, liver) can cause red cell destruction. The reason for the production of the autoantibody is not clear.

Cold Antibody Disease. Cold antibody disease is usually caused by antibodies of the IgM class that may react not only with red cells but also with other blood cells. Cold reactive antibodies may be found in patients with a viral infection or a lymphoproliferative disease. Cold antibody hemolytic disease occurs in two forms: Cold agglutinin disease and paroxysmal cold hemoglobinuria. In these disorders, the antierythrocytic antibody is not capable of binding to the red cell at 37°C but will do so at lower temperatures. When cells are coated by antibody in the cooler peripheral circulation and then warmed to core body temperature, complement components bind to the cell membrane and the cells are susceptible to lysis. At warm temperatures, the antibody comes off the cell so that complement may be detected on the affected cells in the absence of antibody. Hemolytic attacks occur on exposure to cold. The cold antibody binds to cells in the exposed areas of the body (skin). These cells are coated with complement and then destroyed on entering the bloodstream of warmer parts of the body.

Paroxysmal Cold Hemoglobinuria (PCH). PCH refers to the production of dark urine after exposure to the cold because of the presence of hemoglobin from lysed red cells. The antibody responsible was first recognized in 1904 and is referred to as Donath–Landsteiner (DL) antibody. Demonstration of the antibody requires two steps: First, the patient's serum is mixed with erythrocytes at 4°C; then, the mixture is warmed to 37°C, and lysis occurs upon warming. This type of antibody was classically found in patients with syphilis but may occur idiopathically or after a viral infection. The antibody is of the IgG class and the specificity is usually to blood group P.

Cold Agglutinin Disease. This disease is similar to PCH, but intense agglutination of red cells occurs in the cold, which is not the case with DL antibody. The antibody is a monoclonal or polyclonal IgM and is directed to the blood group I specificity. Mycoplasma infections have been associated with polyclonal anti-I formation, whereas monoclonal antibodies occur in lymphoproliferative diseases. Most patients with cold antibody hemolytic disease do well as long as they are kept warm and tolerate a chronic mild anemia with minimal disability. In fact, low titers of cold antibody are found in most normal adults and cause no apparent symptoms.

Hemolytic Reactions to Drugs

Hemolytic reactions to drugs may be activated by at least five mechanisms (Fig. 12–6).

1. **Hapten adherence**: Many drugs adhere to red cells and function as haptens. As such, the red cell–hapten complex induces an immune response, and cytotoxic reactions to the red cell or red cell–drug complex may occur. The exact mechanism of such a drug-induced hemolytic reaction depends upon the drug involved. *Penicillin* covalently binds to red cells, and the antibody formed reacts with the penicillin bound to the cell. Immunoglobulin can be demonstrated on the surface of affected cells by the direct Coombs' test. If the antibody is extracted from the red cell membrane, it will react only with cells preincubated with penicillin in an indirect Coombs' test.

2. **Immune-complex adsorption**: *Quinidine* administration can result in quinidine–antibody complexes that bind loosely to red cells. Antibody–quinidine complexes can dissociate from red cell surfaces and in complex form pass from one red cell to another. Destruction of red cells occurs as an "innocent bystander" reaction. Components of complement may be demonstrated on the affected cells in the absence of detectable antibody globulin.

3. **Auto-immunity**: *a-Methyl dopa* (aldomet) apparently induces alterations in lymphocytes so that the lymphocytes become "autoreactive". The antibody produced reacts with the patient's own red cells in the absence of bound drug. Normal erythrocytes are destroyed during a hemolytic drug reaction due to aldomet or quinidine, because the autoantibody of the antigen–antibody complex can bind to any red blood cell. In cases of hemolytic reactions to penicillin or quinidine, red cell

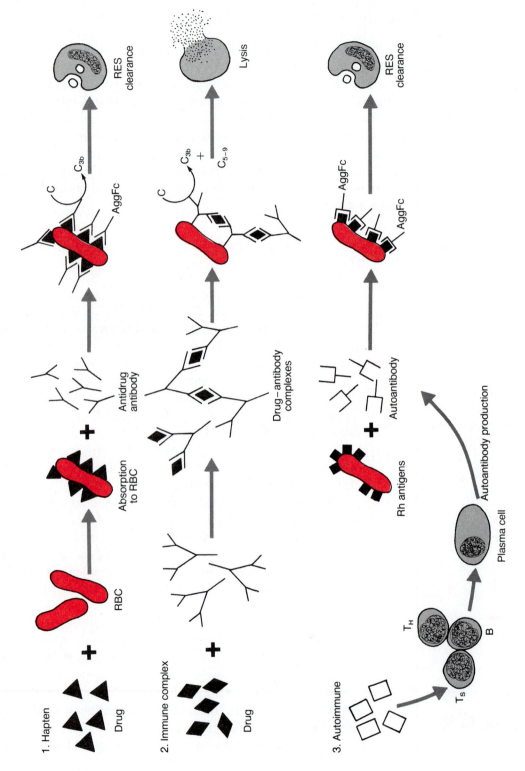

1. Hapten

Drug + RBC → Absorption to RBC + Antidrug antibody → AggFc — C → C₃ᵦ → RES clearance

2. Immune complex

Drug + → Drug–antibody complexes → AggFc — C → C₃ᵦ + C₅₋₉ → Lysis

3. Autoimmune

→ Tₛ / Tₕ / B → Plasma cell → Autoantibody production + Rh antigens + Autoantibody → AggFc / AggFc → RES clearance

340

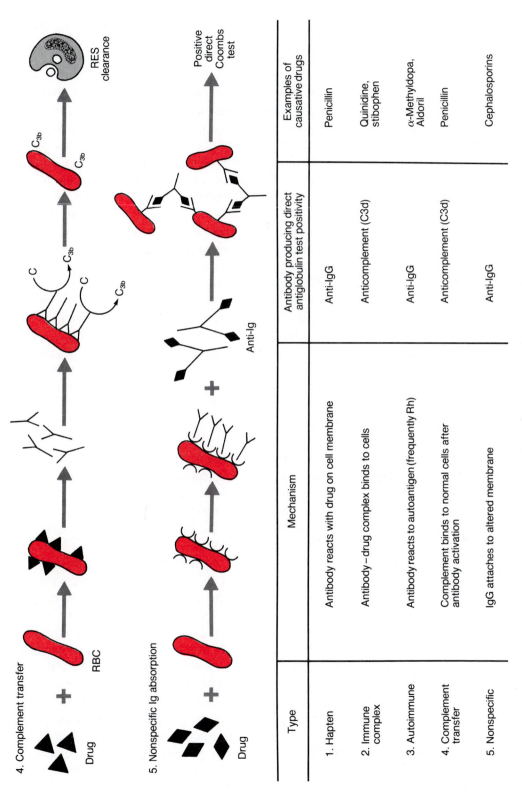

Type	Mechanism	Antibody producing direct antiglobulin test positivity	Examples of causative drugs
1. Hapten	Antibody reacts with drug on cell membrane	Anti-IgG	Penicillin
2. Immune complex	Antibody–drug complex binds to cells	Anticomplement (C3d)	Quinidine, stibophen
3. Autoimmune	Antibody reacts to autoantigen (frequently Rh)	Anti-IgG	α-Methyldopa, Aldoril
4. Complement transfer	Complement binds to normal cells after antibody activation	Anticomplement (C3d)	Penicillin
5. Nonspecific	IgG attaches to altered membrane	Anti-IgG	Cephalosporins

Figure 12–6. Mechanisms of drug-induced hemolytic drug reactions. (See text for details.)

destruction ceases soon after administration of the drug is stopped; a-methyl dopa hemolytic reactions may persist for as long as a year after the drug is stopped. In hemolytic reactions to quinidine and penicillin, the source of the antigen is exogenous (or a complex of exogenous hapten and host red cell), and the origin of the allergic response is endogenous. In hemolytic anemia due to a-methyl dopa, the antigen is endogenous and the origin of the allergic response is endogenous.

4. **Complement transfer**: During severe reactions, complement activated by reaction of antibodies to drugs on one cell may be passed into the fluid phase and bind to a second cell, leading to opsonization. Usually, activated complement components released into the fluid phase are rapidly inactivated in the blood. However, if large amounts of activated components are formed, transfer from one cell to another may occur.

5. **Nonspecific adsorption of proteins**: *Cephalosporins* alter the red cell membrane in a way that allows nonspecific protein absorption. Thus, patients on cephalosporins may have a positive Coombs' test without hemolytic anemia. In addition, patients on dialysis may have positive direct Coombs' tests because of antiformaldehyde antibodies. Formaldehyde is used to sterilize reusable dialysis equipment and is absorbed to the red cells during dialysis.

LEUKOCYTES (AGRANULO-CYTOSIS)

Antibody effects similar to those described above for erythrocytes may also occur with polymorphonuclear leukocytes resulting in loss of neutrophils (neutropenia or agranulocytosis). Most cases of agranulocytosis are secondary to a lack of proliferation of granulocytes in the bone marrow on a nonimmune basis, either congenital or drug-induced. Autoimmune neutropenia (AIN) accounts for about 10% of clinically recognized neutropenia. Two major forms of AIN are primary and secondary. Primary AIN is seen in children before three years of age. Secondary AIN occurs with the highest frequency between forty and sixty years of age, usually associated with autoimmune thrombocytopenia, connective tissue disease, or lymphoma. Antibodies to granulocytes in AIN are detected by immunofluorescence or agglutination. The bone marrow is normal or hypercellular, with a 50% reduction in mature neutrophils. The peripheral blood shows neutrophil counts around 250 cells/μL. Patients are affected by bacterial infections of the skin, upper respiratory tract, and middle ear. Treatment is usually symptomatic with antibiotics. Spontaneous remissions occur in most patients, and immune globulin or steroids may induce remission in prolonged cases. Hematopoietic growth factors are now being tested.

Neonatal
Leukopenia
(Alloimmune
Neonatal
Neutropenia
[ANN])

Low white cell counts in a neonate may be caused by destruction of fetal white blood cells coated by antibodies that cross the placenta from the mother after immunization of the mother to fetal leukocyte antigens. The neutrophil specific antigens are pleomorphic (at least eight have been identified) and may also be targets for autoimmune neutropenia of infancy and chronic idiopathic neutropenia in adults. Two antigens that have been identified as being associated with ANN: NA1 and NA2. They are located on the neutrophil Fc-γ receptor III (FcRIII). The mothers of such infants, otherwise normal, have granulocytes that lack FcRIII, and appear to identify FcRIII as a foreign molecule.

Drug-induced
Agranulocytosis

Destruction of a patient's own white blood cells may be caused by autoantibodies or by antibodies to certain drugs that adhere to white blood cells and function as haptens. Sulfapyridine and aminopyrine are two of the drugs that have been implicated.

The consequence of leukocyte destruction is a decreased ability to defend against infection. In some situations, drugs may have a direct nonimmune cytotoxic effect (idiosyncrasy), and some cases of agranulocytosis are caused by a congenital metabolic defect (see aplastic anemia, below). In nonimmune agranulocytosis, more than one line of leukocyte is usually involved; for instance, in some cases all leukocytes containing granules are destroyed or fail to develop. Antibodies to lymphocytes are found in a variety of human diseases, particularly in acquired immune deficiency syndrome (AIDS) (see Chapter 29), and may be associated with lymphocyte deficiencies.

PLATELETS

Immune reactions to platelets may cause destruction of platelets, with resulting purpura and other hemorrhagic manifestations. The word *purpura* (purple) describes hemorrhage into the skin and is easily recognized by the red or purple discoloration produced by the presence of extravasated red cells. The color is first red but becomes darker (purple) and fades to a brownish yellow as the red cells are destroyed or cleared from the site of hemorrhage by macrophages. Since platelets function to prevent such hemorrhages, a loss of platelets permits purpuric lesions to develop. An antiplatelet antibody can be demonstrated in about 60% of the affected individuals. Recent studies reveal that, in some diseases, antigen–antibody complexes cause thrombocytopenia. Currently, sensitive immunoassays are being developed that should increase the sensitivity of antiplatelet antibody tests. Thrombocytopenia may also occur congenitally or secondarily because of an increased splenic function (hypersplenism) or other nonimmune platelet consumptive disorders.

Posttransfusion Thrombocytopenic Purpura	Purpura after transfusion occurs as a result of the production of alloantibodies following transfusions of blood products containing allogeneic platelets. The cause of autologous platelet destruction is unclear. This reaction is very rare. It presents as an acute, severe thrombocytopenia occurring about one week after a transfusion. Antibodies to the platelet antigen PI^{A1} are invariably found; other platelet antibody specificities have rarely been implicated. Treatment consists of plasma exchange. This reaction is essentially seen only in women who have been pregnant, suggesting that sensitization may originally occur to platelet antigens from a fetus.
Neonatal Alloimmune Thrombocytopenia (NAIT)	NAIT occurs as a result of maternal IgG antibody to fetal platelet antigens contributed by the father, with thrombocytopenia occurring in the fetus when this antibody crosses the placenta. Most cases (50% to 90%) are due to antibodies to platelet antigen $P1^{A1}$, but at least 5 other platelet antigens have been implicated. The placentally transferred antibodies affect platelets in a way analogous to the effect of anti-Rh on red blood cells in hemolytic disease of the newborn. Although uncommon, bleeding may be severe with intracranial hemorrhage and permanent neurologic damage. Platelet transfusions may be very beneficial when the platelet count is very low, and at-risk pregnancies may be treated prophylactically by small weekly transfusions of antigen-negative platelets. NAIT can be distinguished from neonatal autoimmune thrombocytopenia by detection of normal levels of platelet-bound IgG on maternal platelets in NAIT.
Idiopathic Thrombocytopenic Purpura (ITP)	Acute ITP is more common in children than in adults. Most affected individuals have a history of infection (eg, rubella) occurring one to two weeks previously. The destruction of platelets may be due to antibodies to antigens of infectious agents adherent to platelets, to antibody–antigen complexes adsorbed to platelets (innocent bystander), or to antibodies to platelets altered by the infectious process. Platelets are destroyed rapidly when transfused into an affected individual. Chronic ITP is caused by the production of autoantibodies against altered or naturally occurring platelet antigens and is more common in adults. The chronic form is frequently associated with systemic lupus erythematosus or a lymphoproliferative disorder (leukemia, myeloma).
Quinidine (Sedormid) Purpura	Quinidine purpura is an example of a reaction to a drug acting as a hapten on the platelet surface.
	Treatment with Intravenous Immunoglobulin. In the early 1980s, it was discovered that intravenous immunoglobulin (IVIgG) was effective in treating immune thrombocytopenia. Although at least five dif-

ferent mechanisms have been suggested, the most important are non-specific blockade of the Fc receptor-mediated phagocytosis of platelets and suppression of inflammatory responses. Administration of IVIgG rapidly induces FcR blockade and a reduction in immunoglobulin production, perhaps by a feedback mechanism. The mechanism of the immunosuppression is not clear. Clinically, injection of 0.4 g/kg for 3 to 5 days is effective in reversing purpura associated with transfusion, alloimmune purpura, and ITP in pregnancy.

IMMUNE SUPPRESSION OF BLOOD CELL PRODUCTION

Aplastic anemia is a general term for failure of the bone marrow to produce blood cells. This condition is associated with virus infections, drugs, or pregnancy. The cause is not known but is believed to be due to "stem cell failure." Antibody to blood cell precursors may injure proliferating cells in the bone marrow, producing an aplastic anemia or agranulocytosis. Hematopoietic stem cells may have a variety of cell surface antigens, and cells in the erythrocyte, granulocyte, or lymphocyte line may carry differentiation antigens unique for the line. Thus, immune suppression may affect all cell lines or one cell line. Antibodies to stem cells have rarely been found spontaneously in man. Such antibodies to red or white cell precursors have been found associated with aplastic anemia, red cell aplasia, profound panleukopenia, and systemic lupus erythematosus. Thus, although rare, antibodies to blood cell precursors may produce a clinical picture similar to a metabolic defect in blood cell maturation (see also anti-erythropoietin, Chapter 11). However, the sera of most affected patients does not inhibit blood cell formation, but actually stimulates normal colony formation. It appears that aplastic anemia is a genetically determined "premalignant" abnormality of blood-forming cells. An immune reaction does occur to the abnormal cells but not to normal cells. If the immune reaction is strong, the abnormal cells are eliminated and acute severe aplasia results. If the immune response is weak, abnormal blood cell formation leads to a condition known as "myelodysplasia" with chronic pancytopenia. Immunosuppression does not cure the disease but leaves the patient with a fragile hematopoietic system that is prone to malignant transformation. On the other hand successful therapy with hematopoietic growth factors may be very beneficial in restoring blood cell formation (see Chapter 2).

Blistering Skin Diseases

Circulating antibodies that react with epidermal cell surface antigens result in complement activation and separation of the epidermal cells from each other or from their basement membrane, producing blisters (see Chapter 20). Three groups of cytotoxic skin diseases are recognized—pemphigus, pemphigoid, and herpes gestationis. Pemphigus is caused by antibodies that react with epithelial cell surface components that serve to hold the cells together (desmosomes) and produce intra-epithelial blistering lesions. Pemphigoid is caused by antibodies that react with the basement membrane of the skin, producing subepidermal blisters. The lesions may be accentuated by the inflammatory components of complement (C_3a and C_5a) which attract and activate polymorphonuclear cells (PMNs). The PMNs contribute to basement membrane destruction by release of lysosomal enzymes (see immune complex reactions, below). Herpes gestationis is a subepidermal blistering skin disease that usually starts during the second trimester of pregnancy and has a pathogenesis similar to pemphigoid. These lesions are presented in more detail in a separate chapter on immune skin diseases (see Chapter 20).

Other Cytotoxic Reactions

SPERM

Autologous or allogenic sperm is antigenic when injected into adults, and such immunization may decrease fertility in both females and males. Sperm antibodies are detected by binding assays and by their ability to agglutinate or immobilize sperm after inactivating complement in the serum by heating. The immobilizing sperm antigens are carbohydrates related to blood type -*i* or sialyl-*i,* having two or three repetitive Gal-Glu-NAc-structure substitutes, with sialic acid at a terminal Gal. Sperm antibodies may prevent fertilization by decreasing motility, by inhibiting migration through female genital secretions, or by blocking fusion of the gametes. Antibodies to sperm may occur in men who have had a vasectomy because of extravasation of immunogenic sperm, and these antibodies may affect fertility after reanastamosis of the spermatic cord (vasovasostomy), in spite of adequate postoperative sperm count. Antisperm antibodies are found more frequently in prostitutes than in normal age-matched control women. Women with sperm-immobilizing antibodies are frequently infertile and may require in vitro fertilization and embryo transfer to conceive. Intentional sperm immunization of women as a method for controlling pregnancy is possible but has not been considered practical because of possible deleterious effects of producing autoimmune reactions. Immunization of female animals with lactate dehydrogenase from testes produces highly specific antibodies and suppression of fertility.

AUTOIMMUNE DISEASES

Cytotoxic antibody may produce damage in allergic thyroiditis, allergic aspermatogenesis, and other autoimmune diseases, although it is generally believed that the primary mechanism of these diseases is cell-mediated immunity. Antibody-dependent cell-mediated reactions may also be involved (see Chapter 22, Autoimmune Diseases).

HOMOGRAFT REJECTION

In the 1950s, Chandler Stetson showed that specific antisera injected into a graft site may cause an acute "white" graft rejection. Although homograft rejection is usually mediated by sensitized cells (delayed sensitivity), antibody-mediated acute rejection is now recognized. Chronic graft rejection is caused by inflammation of the vessel lumen following activation of complement (see Chapter 13, Immune Complex Diseases).

FORSSMAN ANTIGEN

The Forssman antigen is a generic term for a family of carbohydrate antigens with overlapping specificities found in some plants (corn, spinach), some microorganisms (pneumococcus, *Shigella dysenteriae, Bacillus anthracis*), and some fish and animal tissues (carp, toad, chicken, horse, guinea pig, sheep, hamster, dog, cat, man). The injection of anti-Forssman serum into guinea pigs or chick embryos causes vascular damage and hemorrhage. The possibility of such a reaction occurring in humans is uncertain. For more information on the structure of Forssman antigen and its relationship to other carbohydrate antigens, see Chapter 30.

Detection of Circulating Cytotoxic Antibodies

PASSIVE TRANSFER (IN VIVO)

The effect of the antibody may be produced by passive transfer of serum-containing antibody into a normal recipient. If this antibody is associated with cellular injury, eg, platelet destruction in ITP, a specific cytopenia may develop.

COOMBS' TEST (IN VITRO)

Antibody to blood cells is detected in vitro by the ability of a serum to agglutinate or lyse the cells. In some cases, antibody does not result in agglutination unless a second antibody is added. Such nonagglutinating antibodies are termed "incomplete." Incomplete antibody in serum is detected by the indirect Coombs' test; incomplete antibody already on cells is detected by the direct Coombs' test. In the *direct* Coombs' test, target cells are already coated with incomplete antibody and/or complement. The addition of an antiserum containing antibodies directed against Ig or complement components then causes agglutination of the target cells. Thus, human Rh+ erythrocytes coated with incomplete anti-Rh antibody agglutinate when sheep antihuman immunoglobulin serum is added. For the *indirect* Coombs' test, serum containing incomplete antibody is added to uncoated target cells so that the antibody will bind to the test cells. The antibody-coated cells are then agglutinated by the addition of anti-immunoglobulin (second antibody). For detection of anti-Rh in serum, human Rh+ cells are added to human serum containing incomplete anti-Rh antibodies. These sensitized cells are agglutinated by sheep antihuman immunoglobulin serum (Fig. 12–7). In suspected Rh hemolytic disease of the newborn, both the direct and the indirect Coombs' tests must be done to rule out the presence of incomplete Rh antibodies. The direct test is usually positive for fetal erythrocytes coated with maternal anti-Rh, when free antibody is not present in the fetal serum. On the other hand,

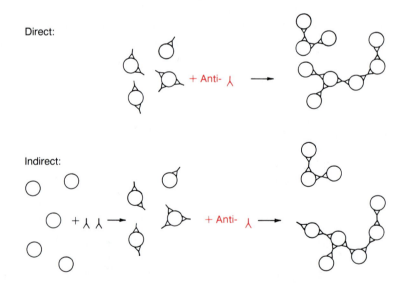

Figure 12–7. Coombs' antiglobulin tests. The Coombs' test for incomplete antibody to erythrocytes is carried out in two forms: Direct and indirect. Direct: Cells taken from the patient are coated with antibody in vivo and are agglutinated by the addition of anti-Ig, which reacts with the antibodies coating the cells. Indirect: The patient's serum contains free antibody that binds to but does not agglutinate erythrocytes added in vitro. Agglutination is accomplished by addition of a second antibody, which reacts with the first antibody (anti-Ig).

the mother's serum may contain anti-Rh antibody detectable by the indirect test; maternal serum added to fetal cells results in coating of the fetal Rh+ cells, which are then agglutinable by antibody to human IgG. The direct Coombs' test may also be used to reveal agglutination of a patient's own cells in acquired hemolytic anemia, thus demonstrating an incomplete autoantibody.

Summary

Cytotoxic or cytolytic reactions are caused by circulating antibody to cell surface structures with subsequent complement fixation. The cell surface antigens may be an integral part of the cell membrane or may be acquired by passive absorption. Reaction of antibody of the IgM or IgG class with the cell surface antigens results in activation of complement and destruction of the cell by complement-mediated lysis or by phagocytosis by macrophages with receptors for activated-complement components or aggregated immunoglobulin. Cells in contact with the circulating blood are most often the target cells; these include red blood cells, white blood cells, and platelets. The disease states are the result of a loss of the function of the affected cells. Examples of such diseases are hemolytic anemia, agranulocytosis, and thrombocytopenic purpura. In addition, epithelial cells of the skin may be targets of cytotoxic reactions leading to blistering skin diseases.

Bibliography

GENERAL

Atkinson JP, Frank MM: Studies of the in vivo effects of antibody: Interaction of IgM antibody and complement in the immune clearance and destruction of erythrocytes in man. *J Clin Invest* 54:339, 1974.

Boyle MDP, Borsos T: The terminal stages of immune hemolysis: A brief review. *Mole Immunol* 17:425, 1980.

Schreiber AD, Frank MM: Role of antibody and complement in the immune clearance and destruction of erythrocytes. II. Molecular nature of IgG and IgM complement-fixing sites and effects of their interaction with serum. *J Clin Invest* 51:583, 1972.

Wintrobe MM: *Clinical Hematology*, 7th ed. Philadelphia, Lea & Febiger, 1974.

TRANSFUSION REACTION

Race RR, Sanger R: *Blood Groups in Man*. Philadelphia, Davis, 1962.

Salmon C, Carton JP, Rouger P: *The Human Blood Groups*. New York, Masson, 1984.

Schmidt PJ: Transfusion Reaction: Status in 1982. *Clin Lab Med* 2:221, 1982.

Solanki D, McCurdy PR: Delayed hemolytic transfusion reactions: An often missed entity. *JAMA* 239:729, 1978.

Watkins WM: Genetics and biochemistry of some human blood groups. *Proc R Soc* (Lond) (Biol) 202:31, 1978.

ERYTHROBLASTOSIS FETALIS

Bowman JM: Fetomaternal ABO incompatibility and erythroblastosis fetalis. *Vox Sang* 50:104, 1986.

Clarke CA, Mollison PL: Deaths from Rh haemolytic disease of the fetus and new-born, 1877–1987. *J Roy Coll Phys Lond* 23:181, 1989.

Finn R, Clarke CA, Donohoe WTA, et al.: Experimental studies on the prevention of Rh haemolytic disease. *Brit J Med* 1:1486, 1961.

Gorman JG, Freda VJ, Pollack W: Prevention of Rhesus isoimmunization. *Clin Immunol Allergy* 4:473, 1984.

Hamilton EG: Intrauterine transfusion for Rh disease: A status report. *Hosp Pract* 13:113, 1978.

Levine P: Influence of ABO system in Rh hemolytic disease. *Hum Biol* 30:14, 1958.

Levine P: The discovery of Rh hemolytic disease. *Vox Sang* 47:187, 1984.

Levine P, Stetson R: An unusual case of intragroup agglutination. *JAMA* 113:126, 1939.

Szulman AE: The histologic distribution of the blood group substances in man as determined by immunofluorescence. III. The A, B, and H antigens in embryos and fetuses from 18 mm in length. *J Exp Med* 119:503, 1964.

Taylor JF: Sensitization of Rh-negative daughters by their Rh-positive mothers. *N Engl J Med* 276:547, 1967.

Voak D: The pathogenesis of ABO hemolytic disease of the newborn. *Vox Sang* 17:481, 1969.

AUTOIMMUNE HEMOLYTIC ANEMIA

Adams J, Moore VK, Issitt DD: Autoimmune hemolytic anemia caused by anti-D. *Transfusion* 13:214, 1973.

Cline MJ, Golde DW: Immune suppression of hematopoiesis. *Am J Med* 64:301, 1978.

Dacie JV, Wolledge SM: Autoimmune hemolytic anemia. *Prog Hematol* 6:1, 1969.

Donath J, Landsteiner K: Veber paroxysmale hamoglolunurie. *Much Med Wochenschr* 51:1590, 1904.

Frank M, Schreiber AD, Atkinson JP, et al.: Pathophysiology of immune hemolytic anemia. *Ann Int Med* 87:210, 1977.

Nissen C: Pathophysiology of aplastic anemia. *Acta Hematol* 86:57, 1991.

Petz LD, Garraty G: *Acquired Immune Hemolytic Anemias*. New York, Churchill–Livingston, 1980.

Sokol RJ, Booker DJ, Stamps R: The pathology of autoimmune haemolytic anaemia. *J Clin Pathol* 45:1047–1052, 1992.

Yomtovian R, Prince GM, Medof ME: The molecular basis for paroxysmal nocturnal hemoglobinuria. *Transfusion* 33:852–873, 1993.

DRUG-ASSOCIATED HEMOLYTIC REACTIONS

Ackroyd JF: Sedormid purpura, an immunologic study of a form of drug hypersensitivity. *Prog Allergy* 3:531, 1952.

Dausset J, Coutu L: Drug induced hemolysis. *Ann Rev Med* 18:55, 1967.

Dzik WH, Darling CA: Positive direct antiglobulin test result in dialysis patients resulting from antiformaldehyde antibodies. *Am J Clin Path* 92:214, 1989.

Kerr R-O, Cardamone J, Dalmasso AP, et al.: Two mechanisms of erythrocyte destruction in penicillin-induced hemolytic anemia. *N Engl J Med* 287:1322, 1972.

Lo Buglio AF, Jandl JH: The reaction of the alpha-methyldopa red cell antibody. *New Engl J Med* 276:658, 1967.

Molthan L, Reidenberg MM, Elchman MF: Positive direct Coombs' test due to cephalothin. *New Engl J Med* 277:123, 1967.

Petz LD, Fudenberg HH: Coombs-positive hemolytic anemia caused by penicillin administration. *New Engl J Med* 274:171, 1966.

Wolledge SM: Immune drug-induced hemolytic anemias. *Semin Hematol* 10:327, 1973.

**WBC
REACTIONS**

Bux J, Kissel K, Nowak K, et al.: Autoimmune neutropenia: Clinical and laboratory studies in 143 patients. *Ann Hematol* 61:249, 1991.

Dehoratius RJ: Lymphocytotoxic antibodies. *Clin Immunol* 4:151, 1980.

Madyastha PR, Glassman AB: Neutrophil antigens and antibodies in the diagnosis of immune neutropenias. *Ann Clin Lab Med Sci* 19:146, 1989.

Pisciotta AV: Immune and toxic mechanisms in drug induced agranulocytosis. *Semin Hematol* 10:279, 1973.

Shastri KA, Logue GL: Autoimmune neutropenia. *Blood* 81:1984–1995, 1993.

Stroncek DF, Sklubita KM, Plachta LB, et al.: Alloimmune neonatal neutropenia due to an antibody to the neutrophil Fc-γ receptor III with maternal deficiency of CD16 antigen. *Blood* 77:1572, 1991.

PLATELETS

Ackroyd JF: Sedormid purpura: An immunologic study of a form of drug hypersensitivity. *Prog Allergy* 3:531, 1952.

Aster RH: Posttransfusion purpura: Immunologic aspects and therapy. *N Engl J Med* 291:1163, 1974.

Baldini M: Idiopathic thrombocytopenic purpura. *N Engl J Med* 274:1245, 1302, 1360.

Cines DB, et al.: Immune thrombocytopenia purpura and pregnancy. *New Engl J Med* 306:826, 1982.

Fehr J, Hofmann V, Kappelar V: Transient reversal of thrombocytopenia in idiopathic thrombocytopenic purpura by high-dose intravenous gamma globulin. *New Engl J Med* 306:1254, 1982.

George JN, El-Harake MA, Raskob GE: Chronic idiopathic thrombocytopenia purpura. *N Eng J Med* 331:1207–1211, 1994.

Newland AC: The use and mechanisms of action of intravenous immunoglobulin: An update. *Brit J Haematol* 72:301, 1989.

Schiffer CA: Prevention of alloimmunization against platelets. *Blood* 77:1, 1991.

Skacel PO, Contreras M: Neonatal alloimmune thrombocytopenia. *Blood Rev* 3:174, 1989.

**OTHER
CYTOLYTIC
DISEASES**

Clines DB, Tomaski A, Tannenbaum S: Immune endothelial cell injury in heparin-associated thrombocytopenia. *N Engl J Med* 316:581, 1987.

Dondero F, Lenzi A, Lombardo F, et al.: Antisperm antibodies and assisted reproduction. In *Diagnosing Male Infertility*. Colpi GM, Pozza D, (eds.). Prog Reproduct Biol Med Basel, Karger 15:178, 1992.

Isojima S: Human sperm antigens corresponding to sperm-immobilizing antibodies in the sera of women with infertility of unknown cause: Personal review of our recent studies. *Human Repro* 4:605, 1989.

Li TX: Sperm immunology, infertility, and fertility control. *Obstet Gynecol* 44:607, 1974.

Naz RN, Menge AC: Antisperm antibodies: Origin, regulation, and sperm reactivity in human infertility. *Fertility and Sterility* 61:1001–1013, 1994.

Samuel T, Rose NR: The lessons of vasectomy: A review. *J Clin Lab Immunol* 3:77, 1980.

Stetson CA: The role of humoral antibody in the homograft rejection. *Adv Immunol* 3:97, 1963.

Taichman NS, Tsai C-C: Heterophile antibodies and tissue injury. II. Ultrastructure of dermal vascular lesions produced by Forssman antiserum in guinea pigs. *Int Arch Allergy* 42:78, 1972.

Waksman BH: Cell lysis and related phenomena in hypersensitivity reactions, including immunohematologic diseases. *Prog Allergy* 5:340, 1958.

COOMBS' TEST

Bohnen RF, et al.: The direct Coombs' test: Its clinical significance. Study in a large university hospital. *Ann Int Med* 68:19, 1968.

Coombs RRA, Mourant AE, Race RR: A new test for the detection of weak and "incomplete" Rh agglutinins. *Br J Exp Pathol* 26:255, 1945.

Coombs RRA, Roberts F: Antiglobulin reaction. *Br Med Bull* 15:113, 1959.

Gilliand BC, Leedy JP, Vaughn JH: The detection of cell-bound antibody on complement-coated human red cells. *J Clin Invest* 49:898, 1970.

13

Immune Complex Reactions

Immune complex reactions are caused by immunoglobulin antibody reacting directly with tissue antigens (usually basement membrane antigens), or by antibody reacting with soluble antigen in the blood to form soluble antigen–antibody complexes that deposit in tissues. Although these initiating events are different, the subsequent inflammatory reaction, mainly mediated by complement, is essentially the same (Fig. 13–1). IgG antibody reacting with tissue antigens accumulates to form aggregates in tissues. Soluble complexes, formed in the circulation by a single IgG molecule reacting with a soluble antigen, or antigens shed from cell membranes, form aggregates of IgG when two or more complexes from the blood deposit closely in tissue. These aggregated antigen–antibody complexes fix complement with activation of the anaphylactic and chemotactic activities of C_4a, C_3a, and C_5a. This results in the accumulation of neutrophilic polymorphonuclear leukocytes, which release lysosomal enzymes and reactive oxygen metabolites that cause destruction of the elastic lamina of arteries (serum sickness), basement membrane of the kidney glomerulus (glomerulonephritis), walls of small vessels (Arthus reaction), articular cartilage of joints (rheumatoid arthritis), or basement membrane of skin (pemphigoid).

The alternate pathway for complement activation, entered by activation of C_3 (the C_3 shunt; see Complement, Chapter 8) is active in the pathogenesis of some types of lesions that are similar to immune-complex-mediated lesions. Activation of either the classical or alternate pathway results in formation of C_3a and C_5a, production of complement chemotactic factors (mostly C_5a), accumulation of polymorphonuclear cells, and destruction of tissue. Complement mediators

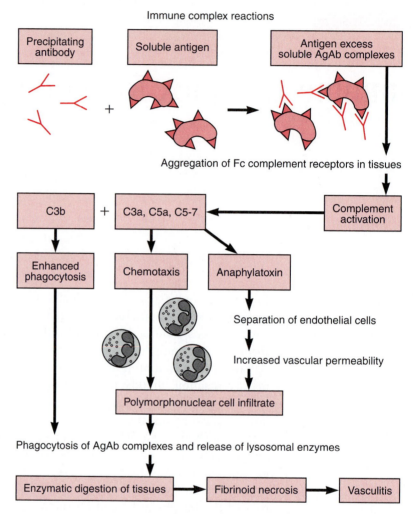

Figure 13–1. Immune complex reactions. Antibody (usually IgG) reacts with soluble antigens to produce soluble circulating immune complexes or with basement membranes (such as renal glomerular basement membrane). Antibody–antigen complexes causes activation of complement with formation of inflammatory (phlogistic) complement fragments. Fragments C_3a, C_4a, and C_5a (anaphylatoxin) cause constriction of vascular endothelium (increased vascular permeability). C_5a is also chemotactic for polymorphonuclear leukocytes, and C_3b enhances phagocytosis. Released lysosomal polymorphonuclear enzymes digest tissues, producing "fibrinoid" necrosis. Fibrinoid means "fibrinlike" and refers to the histologic appearance of the acellular amorphous areas produced by "digestion" of tissue by lysosomal enzymes that resemble the appearance of fibrin in clotted blood.

such as anaphylatoxin (C_4a, C_3a, and C_5a) may induce endothelial cell contraction and open cell junctions so that soluble complexes can deposit in basement membranes or inflammatory cells can enter into tissue spaces.

Arthus Reaction

The Arthus reaction is a dermal inflammatory response caused by the reaction of precipitating antibody with antigen placed in the skin (Fig. 13–2). It is named for Marcel Arthus, who first described it in 1903.

The reaction is characterized grossly by edema, erythema, and hemorrhage, all of which develop over a few hours, reaching a maximum in 2 to 5 hours or even later if the reaction is severe (Fig. 13–3).

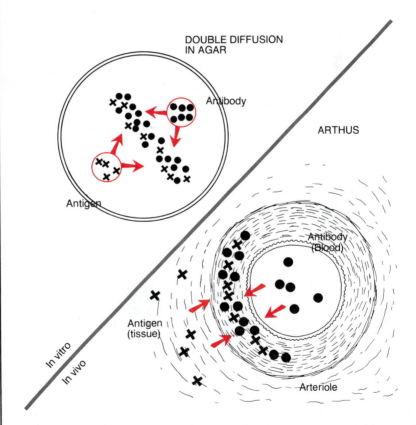

Figure 13–2. Comparison of double diffusion in agar precipitin reaction and Arthus reaction. When antibody and antigen are allowed to diffuse toward each other in agar, a precipitin band forms when the antigen and antibody concentration in the agar are in equivalence. Similarly, if antigen is injected into the skin it will diffuse toward the vessels. The major precipitin reaction occurs in the walls of small vessels, usually arterioles, where antibody in the circulation diffuses out to meet antigen diffusing in from the tissue.

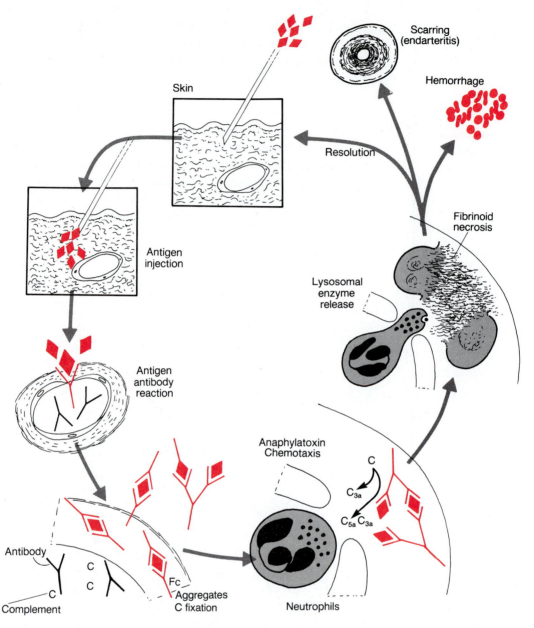

Figure 13–3. Steps in Arthus Reaction: (1) Injection of antigen into the dermis. (2) Diffusion of antigen in tissue to vessels. (3) Reaction of antigen with circulating antibody in wall of small arterioles. (4) Formation of antibody–antigen complexes, aggregation of Fc of antibody and activation of complement. (5) Contraction and separation of endothelial cells by C_3a, C_5a (anaphylatoxin), and attraction of neutrophils by C_5a and C_5a des-arg chemotactic factors. (6) Activation of neutrophils in vessel wall with release of lysosomal enzymes. (7) Digestion of vascular wall producing fibrinoid necrosis. (8) Resolution or scarring, depending on severity of reaction.

Histologically, vascular fibrinoid necrosis of the vessel wall and emigration of neutrophils and eosinophils are seen. If the reaction is severe, there is thrombosis with resulting ischemic necrosis and hemorrhage. This lesion is caused by the reaction of antigen with antibody forming microprecipitates in vessel walls or in adjacent tissue spaces and local activation of complement. Polymorphonuclear neutrophils (PMNs) infiltrate and attempt to phagocytose the complement-coated complexes. The PMNs discharge their lysosomal contents, and the oxygen radicals and lysosomal enzymes released produce damage to vascular walls and surrounding tissue. Clumping of cells and activation of the clotting system may result in occlusion of small vessels and ischemic necrosis.

Serum Sickness

Untoward systemic effects of the administration of serum from another species were noted by von Bering in 1891, when hyperimmune horse serum was introduced for the treatment of children with diphtheria. The syndrome of serum sickness was first described in detail by von Pirquet and Schick in 1905. It consisted of fever, arthritis, glomerulonephritis, and vasculitis appearing 10 days to 2 weeks following passive immunization with horse serum (ie, horse antitetanus toxin). The disease is the result of the production by the treated individual of circulating precipitating antibody to the injected horse serum (Fig. 13–4).

The lesions of serum sickness directly correlate with the presence of soluble immune complexes. In experimental models, the lesions of serum sickness appear at the time of immune elimination or when soluble complexes in antigen excess are present in the serum (Fig. 13–5). During a continuous infusion of a large amount of a soluble antigen, such as bovine serum albumin (BSA), into rabbits, there are three types of immune responses: (1) The production of no antibody to BSA (high dose tolerance) or the production of antibody in such small amounts that insufficient immune complexes are formed to produce serum sickness; (2) the production of large amounts of antibody, which form complexes with antigen in antibody excess that are cleared by the reticuloendothelial system and do not induce lesions; or (3) the production of a moderate amount of antibody, with formation of soluble antigen–antibody complexes in **antigen excess** that deposit in tissue and induce typical lesions of serum sickness. Antibody–antigen complexes formed in vitro and injected into animals may also produce lesions, but only if the complexes are formed in antigen excess. Immune complexes in antibody excess or equivalence are cleared by the reticuloendothelial system (RES) due to the presence of aggregated Fcs or C_3b. The phagocytic cells of the RES have receptors for aggregated Fcs and C_3b. However, soluble complexes in antigen excess (toxic complexes)

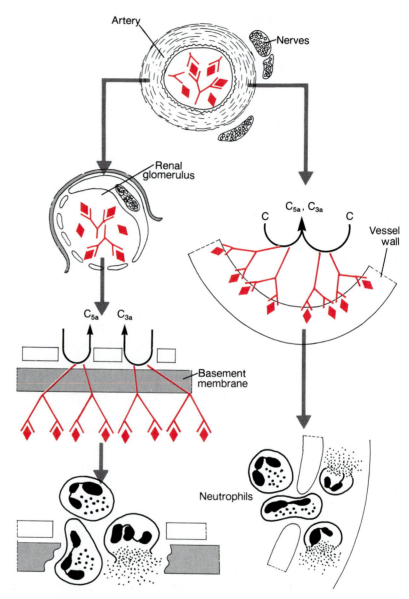

Figure 13–4. Steps in serum sickness: (1) Formation of soluble anti-body–antigen complexes in circulation. Such complexes do not fix complement because Fcs are not aggregated. (2) Soluble complexes pass through open endothelial spaces in glomeruli and deposit on epithelial side of basement membrane or deposit in walls of small arteries. Accumulation of complexes results in formation of aggregates of Ig, activating complement. (3) Neutrophils are attracted, pass into basement membrane or vessel wall, and release lysosomal enzymes causing destruction of basement membranes.

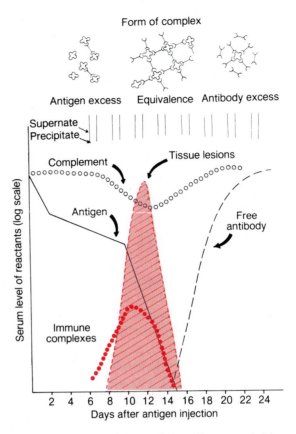

Figure 13–5. Comparison of antigen elimination, precipitin reaction, and serum complement levels during experimental serum sickness. Immune elimination of antigen follows production of antibody that binds to antigen in the circulation. When antibody first appears, there is an excess of antigen so that soluble immune complexes in antigen excess are formed. These complexes lodge in arteries, and in particular, in glomeruli where aggregates of immunoglobulin fix complement. This results in lesions of serum sickness and a fall in serum complement. As more antibody is produced, complexes in equivalence and then antibody excess are found. Since these complexes contain aggregated Fc regions of Ig, they will be cleared from the circulation by the reticuloendothelial system because of receptors on macrophages for aggregated Fc and C_3b.

are not cleared efficiently by the RES and deposit in vessels and glomeruli, where accumulation of complexes results in aggregation of Fcs and complement activation.

Horse serum contains at least thirty different, separate antigens, so that complexes of one or more of these antigens may be present in the circulation even though excess antibody or other free antigens may be present at the same time. In addition, different proportions of antibodies with different electrostatic charges may be formed. Some individuals may also produce reaginic (IgE) antibodies or a state of delayed hypersensitivity to some of the antigens in horse serum. The presence of different forms of immune complexes, as well as activation of different immune mechanisms can result in a very complicated clinical picture. In a recent study of thirty-five patients treated with antithymocyte globulin for bone marrow failure, over 80% developed fever, malaise, cutaneous eruptions, arthralgias, gastrointestinal complaints, headache, blurring of vision, arthritis and lymphadenopathy beginning one week after initiation of therapy and lasting for about 10 days after termination of therapy.

Immune Complexes in Infectious Diseases

Transient serum sickness-like episodes are frequently associated with infections. In many instances, antibody–antigen complexes may be demonstrated and the antigen may be identified as a component of the infectious agent. Immune complexes have been documented in glomerular or vascular deposits in animals infected with lymphocytic choriomeningitis virus, *Schistosoma mansoni*, leprosy bacilli, *Treponema pallidum*, and a number of other agents. In humans, vasculitis, glomerulonephritis, arthritis, and skin lesions may be associated with deposition of hepatitis antigen (HBsAg)–antibody complexes in patients with hepatitis B infection. Immune complexes may have a role in the inflammatory pulmonary lesions and serum sickness-like symptoms seen in cystic fibrosis patients with *Pseudomonas aeruginosa* lung infection. Chronic infectious endocarditis, during which there is continued release of organisms into the blood, features positive serum tests for immune complexes as well as a number of immune-complex-associated lesions, such as vasculitis, arthritis, and glomerulonephritis. In lepromatous leprosy, antibody production to leprosy antigens is associated with circulating immune complexes, rheumatoid factor auto-antimmunoglobulin and vasculitis (erythema nodosum leprosum), as well as renal disease. During chemotherapy, large amounts of leprosy antigens are released locally in the skin, and in the presence of antibodies to these antigens, a marked local acute necrotic neutrophil inflammation in the skin is often seen (type II leprosy reaction). Circulating immune complexes may also be found in high frequency in patients with recurrent infections in the absence of serum sickness-like lesions. The presence of immune complexes in the circulation does not necessarily correlate with lesions. The form of the complexes, the class of the antibody, and the properties of the antigen are each important factors, as well as the ability of the RES to remove immune complexes. Continued formation of immune complexes in equivalence or antibody excess may lead to RES blockade.

Glomerulo-nephritis

ACUTE GLOMERULO-NEPHRITIS

Inflammation of the glomeruli of the kidney is known as glomerulonephritis. The kidney is the organ most frequently affected by immune complex deposits. Lesions are caused either by deposition of antibody–antigen complexes formed elsewhere and deposited in the glomeruli, such as is seen in serum sickness, by shedding of antibody–antigen complexes from endothelial cells into the basement membrane, or by direct reaction of antibody with glomerular basement membrane or other antigens. To appreciate the nature of antibody-mediated glomerulonephritis, an understanding of the normal structure of the glomerulus and the form of deposition of antibody or immune complexes is necessary (Fig. 13–6). The nephron is the unit of the kidney that filters metabolites and electrolytes from the blood and produces urine. It is made up of glomerulus and tubule. An ultrafiltrate of the blood is produced in the glomerulus. The tubule collects this filtrate and resorbs electrolytes as urine passes into the collecting system. The glomerulus is made up of four principal cell types, each of which has a specific function: Endothelial cells, which line the glomerular capillary network; mesangial cells, which form a stalk that supports the basement membrane of the capillaries; and two types of epithelial cells—visceral and parietal. The mesangium is made up of cells of the reticuloendothelial system and is capable of phagocytosis of immune complexes. The visceral epithelial cells cover the external surface of the capillary basement membrane and, along with the parietal epithelial cells, which cover the inside of the capsule of the glomerulus, line the space in which the glomerular filtrate is collected. The critical feature of the glomerulus is that the capillary basement membrane is not completely covered by endothelial cells. This permits antibody-to-basement membrane or immune complexes to filter into the basement membrane. Complement activation (anaphylatoxin) or mast cell mediators may produce further separation by causing contraction of endothelial cells. In addition, the membrane attack complex (MAC) of complement may deposit in the basement membrane. If the MAC deposits are not lytically active, they are associated with a protein called clusterin. The exact pathologic role of MACs and clusterin in the glomerular basement membrane is not known, although it appears the lytically active MACS could contribute to glomerular damage and the MAC–clusterin deposits to membrane thickening.

Mechanisms

The lesions of immune complex glomerulonephritis are produced by alteration of the basement membrane by three mechanisms: (1) directly by the deposition of complexes, antibody, or complement, which cause changes in the electrostatic properties of the basement membrane and consequent leakage of serum proteins; (2) indirectly by complement-

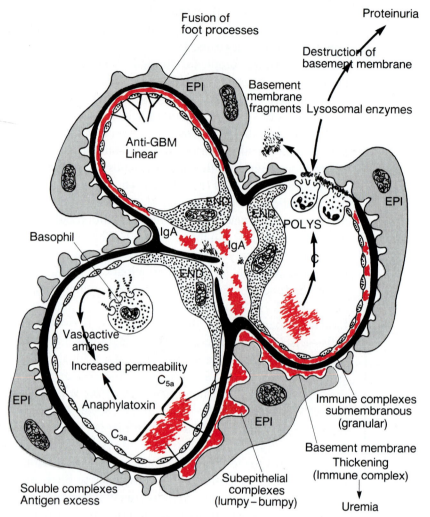

Figure 13–6. Pathogenesis of glomerulonephritis. Depicted is part of a glomerulus. The mesangial cells are located in the center and support the endothelial cells (ENDO), which line the inside of the basement membrane. There are gaps in the cytoplasm of the endothelial cells, which expose the basement membrane to blood components. The upper left part of the figure illustrates deposition of antiglomerular basement membrane antibody as a linear deposit of immunoglobulin on the endothelial side of the basement membrane. The upper right depicts deposition of soluble immune complexes on exposed basement membrane after contraction of endothelial cells by vasoactive amines or activation of anaphylatoxin. The lower left segment illustrates that the complexes may deposit as large clumps, distorting the foot processes of the endothelial cells. Dissolution of the basement membrane by release of lysosomal enzymes from polymorphonuclear leukocytes activated by complement or alterations in the electrostatic properties of the basement membrane by anti-GBM or immune complex deposition leads to leakage of proteins into the urine (proteinuria) (*upper right*). If more extensive destruction of the basement membranes occurs, cellular elements of the blood, as well as basement membrane fragments, may be detected in the urine. Prolonged accumulation of immune reactants leads to thickening of the basement membrane and fusion of the foot processes of epithelial cells. Clinically, this is expressed as a loss of the filtering capacity of the kidney and retention of toxic metabolites (uremia).

mediated attraction of polymorphonuclear leukocytes, which in turn release enzymes that digest the basement membrane; the lesions may resolve or progress into a chronic stage of inflammation with infiltration by mononuclear cells; and (3) long-term deposition of complexes may cause thickening of the basement membrane and fusion of the foot processes of the epithelial cells, leading to a loss of the filtering ability of the glomerulus. Dissolution of the basement membrane is associated with leakage of blood components into the urine (proteinuria, hematuria, nephrotic syndrome), whereas thickening of the basement membrane causes a loss in filtration capacity and uremia (uremic syndrome).

Role of Electrostatic Charge

The charge of the immune complex in the glomerular basement membrane in glomerulonephritis determines to a large extent the nature and location of the lesions. The basement membrane contains a large amount of sialic acid and is strongly negatively charged (anionic). The anionic membrane can be neutralized by deposits of cationic molecules. Neutralization of the charge of the basement membrane causes increased permeability to smaller serum proteins, such as serum albumin, which are also strongly anionic and usually repelled from the basement membrane. This increased permeability leads to proteinuria, which may occur without neutrophil-mediated basement membrane damage.

In experimental immune complex glomerulonephritis models, cationic antigens, in the form of soluble antigen or soluble immune complexes, tend to localize within or pass through the basement membrane, whereas complexes of anionic antigens deposit on the endothelial side (Fig. 13–7). In these models, the antibodies produced are heterogeneous in respect to charge; soluble immune complexes that deposit in the glomerular basement membrane are those that are formed from the most cationic population of antibodies. Thus, of the range of antibodies with different charges, a small proportion of cationic antibodies in immune complexes may be sufficient to mediate glomerular deposition. The charge of the complex is most important for the initial binding of complexes. After the initial binding, the complexes condense to form large deposits, and forces other than charge retain the complexes in the membrane.

Size and Solubility of Immune Complexes

In addition to charge, the size and solubility of immune complexes determines the type of glomerulonephritis (Table 13–1). There are two major types of complex deposition related to glomerular injury: Class I (transmembranous or diffuse) and class II (subendothelial–mesangial). Because of size, solubility, and charge, class I complexes pass

TABLE 13–1. CLASSIFICATION OF IMMUNE COMPLEX DISEASE

Location of Immune Complex Deposits	Proposed Nomenclature

I. Beneath epithelium
  A. At epithelial slits
  B. In subepithelial space
II. Subendothelial–mesangial
  A. In subendothelial space
  B. At lamina densa
  C. In mesangium/loop
	I. Class I deposit disease
	  A. Transmembranous glomerulonephritis
	  B. Transmembranous glomerulopathy
	II. Class II deposit disease
	  A. Endomembranous glomerulonephritis
	  B. Laminal glomerulonephritis
	  C. Mesangiopathic glomerulonephritis

into or through the basement membrane and deposit within the membrane or on the epithelial side of the membrane; class II complexes deposit on the endothelial side of the basement membrane or are phagocytosed by the mesangial system. Class I complexes are small, soluble antigen-excess complexes that usually deposit in small amounts over a long period of time, producing granular deposits of immunoglobulins or complement distributed diffusely along the basement membrane or at the epithelial slit membranes. In addition to deposition of complexes from the circulation, granular immune complex deposits are also formed when antibodies react with the surface antigens of the cells of the glomerular capillaries. The complexes containing plasma membrane antigens are shed between the endothelial cells and the glomerular basement membrane, where they form local granular deposits. Class II complexes are larger, less soluble complexes that accumulate in the subendothelial space or within the mesangium.

CHRONIC GLOMERULO-NEPHRITIS

Chronic glomerulonephritis (uremic syndrome) may be produced experimentally by repeated injections of small amounts of antigen into an appropriately immunized animal or by repeated injections of soluble complexes. The prolonged deposition of class I complexes leads to variable amounts of polymorphonuclear leukocyte infiltration and endothelial proliferation, but the most prominent result is progression

Figure 13–7. Effect of charge on immune complex localization in glomeruli. Cationic immune complexes (positively charged) preferentially localize in the glomerular basement membrane which is anionic (negatively charged) (A). Subepithelial localization may be explained by higher density of anions on the epithelial side of the basement membrane. Cationic free antigen may deposit in the basement membrane (B), and subsequent reaction with antibody leads to formation of immune complexes. Anionic complexes tend to be taken up by the mesangial cells (C) and are less pathogenic but may localize on the endothelial side of the basement membrane (D).

A. Soluble complexes—cationic antigen (subepithelial)

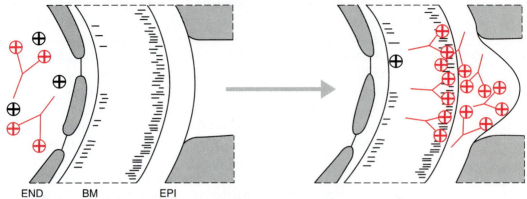

END   BM   EPI

B. Soluble cationic antigen (subepithelial & intramembranous)

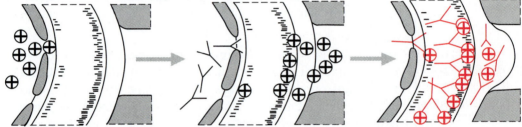

C. Anionic antigens or complexes (subendothelial)

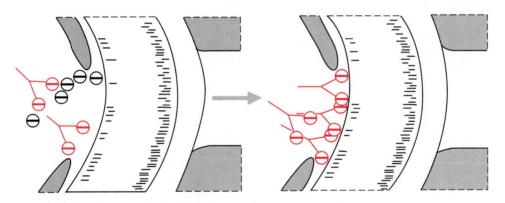

D. Soluble anionic antigen (mesangial)

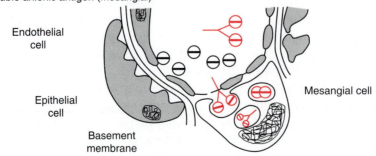

Endothelial
cell

Mesangial cell

Epithelial
cell

Basement
membrane

to marked thickening of the basement membrane and eventual scarring and destruction of the glomerulus. Cellular inflammation involving activation of lymphocytes, recruitment of macrophages, release of cytokines (TGF-B), and proliferation of endothelial cells leads to destruction of the glomerulus. This mechanism is responsible for the chronic membranoproliferative glomerulonephritis associated with various human diseases, such as lupus erythematosus (DNA–anti-DNA), diabetes mellitus (insulin–anti-insulin), and thyroiditis (Thyroglobulin–antithyroglobulin). In addition, the deposition of toxic complexes of antibody and viral antigens is responsible for some cases of human glomerulonephritis. Deposits of the tumor antigen, carcinoembryonic antigen (CEA), and antibody to CEA have been identified as being responsible for renal damage in some patients with colonic carcinoma. Rare instances of glomerulonephritis from the deposition of IgE antibody–antigen complexes may occur in atopic individuals.

ANTI-GLOMERULAR BASEMENT NEPHRITIS

Human and experimental animal glomerulonephritis may also be initiated by antibodies to glomerular basement membrane (anti-GBM) or to antigens on epithelial cells. The experimental model is known as experimental autoimmune glomerulonephritis (EAG); the human diseases caused by anti-GBM are poststreptococcal glomerulonephritis, Goodpasture's syndrome, and anti-GBM nephritis associated with vasculitis.

Experimental Autoimmune Glomerulonephritis

Experimental glomerulonephritis caused by autoantibodies to glomerular basement membrane (anti-GBM) may be induced by immunization of animals with glomerular basement membrane extracts in complete Freund's adjuvant. Anti-GBM first contacts and binds to antigens on the capillary side of the basement membrane and may be observed by immunofluorescence as a continuous thin layer along the membrane. Early in the course of anti-GBM disease, the antibodies deposit in a linear pattern, but with time reformation of the antibody–antigen complexes by rearrangement and condensation results in the formation of dense deposits. The reaction of antibody with the basement membrane results in the binding of complement, polymorphonuclear leukocyte infiltration, and basement membrane destruction. A transient form of the experimental disease may be passively transferred with serum from an affected animal on injection into a normal animal, but the antiserum donor must be nephrectomized several days prior to transfer. Nephrectomy is necessary to allow the accumulation of the antibody, because the nephritogenic antibody is absorbed in vivo by the glomerular tissue of the serum donor. Anti-GBM is responsible for Goodpasture's syndrome and may be pathogenic in poststreptococcal glomerulonephritis in humans (see below).

Nephrotoxic
Serum (Masugi)
Nephritis

Experimental glomerulonephritis may also be produced in animals by the passive transfer of xenogeneic antisera to glomeruli. For example, the passive transfer of rabbit anti-rat glomerulus serum to rats causes nephrotoxic serum nephritis. The nephritis consists of a biphasic response: (1) An acute transient proteinuria is observed as a result of the formation of complexes of rabbit antibodies and antigens present in rat glomerulus; and (2) after 10 days to 2 weeks, a potentially fatal chronic proliferative glomerulonephritis may develop. This second lesion is caused by the production of host (rat) antibodies to donor (rabbit) immunoglobulin. These rat antibodies react with the rabbit antiglomerular antibodies localized on the rat glomeruli, causing the second-phase lesions. The second-phase lesions feature production of tumor necrosis factor and other cytokines from macrophages in involved glomeruli.

Poststreptococcal
Glomerulo-
nephritis

The occurrence of acute glomerulonephritis in humans is associated with exposure to some strains of group A β-hemolytic streptococci. Such streptococcal strains have been termed nephritogenic. The acute infection usually presents as a sore throat and fever. There is a characteristic latent period following the onset of infection, during which no significant renal symptoms are observed. Acute post streptococcal glomerulonephritis is characterized by the onset of proteinuria and hematuria, which correspond in time with the appearance of host antibodies to streptococcal antigens. Immunofluorescence examination of affected kidneys reveals typical immune complex glomerulonephritis (described above); complement, immunoglobulins, and streptococcal antigens are found in glomeruli.

Several theories have been put forward to explain the pathogenic mechanisms for poststreptococcal glomerulonephritis:

1. Some staphylococcal products are toxic to glomeruli.
2. Antibodies to glomerular basement membranes include a GBM-deposited streptococcal antigen, a cross-reacting GBM antigen, or an altered GBM antigen.
3. Immune complexes of streptococcal antigens or autoantigens formed in the blood are deposited.

There is increasing evidence that poststreptococcal glomerulonephritis is caused by a cationic protein designated **nephritic strain-associated protein (NSAP)**, which is a plasminogen activator. The interaction between NSAP and plasminogen splits the C_3 molecule activating the alternate complement pathway, initiating inflammation in the glomerulus. Further progression of the disease might be a consequence of the deposit of antibody to the highly immunogenic NSAP trapped in the basement membrane or to basement membrane components.

Antibodies to all the major basement membrane macromolecules are present in sera from patients with poststreptococcal glomerulonephritis.

Goodpasture's Syndrome

The combination of pulmonary hemorrhage and glomerulonephritis is known as Goodpasture's syndrome. In severe cases, there is extensive intraalveolar hemorrhage and marked proliferative glomerulonephritis. Immunoglobulin and complement may be identified in the basement membrane of pulmonary alveoli and renal glomeruli. Antibody eluted from the kidneys of such patients binds to lung tissue, and antibody eluted from lung tissue binds to kidney. The shared antigen is the α3

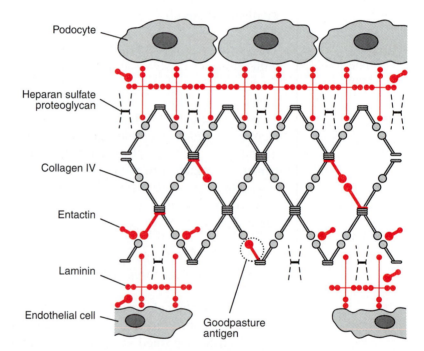

Figure 13–8. Schematic localization of Goodpasture antigen α3 chain of type IV collagen in glomerular basement membrane. The endothelial and epithelial surface of the glomerular basement membrane is lined with laminin; the membrane itself is composed of a scaffold of two subtypes of type IV collagen molecules (building blocks). Subtype A (classical) contains α1 and α2 chains; subtype B contains the α3 chain (Goodpasture antigen). The endothelial surface has a net negative charge; it repels negatively charged antibodies, but cationic antibodies pass into the membrane to react with Goodpasture antigen. Serum of patients with poststreptococcal glomerulonephritis may bind with any of the major components of the basement membrane. (Modified from Hudson et al.: Molecular architecture and function of basement membrane antigen. *Lab Invest* 61:256, 1989.)

chain of type IV collagen in the basement membrane, shared by lung and kidney (Fig. 13–8).

Anti-GBM Nephritis Associated with Vasculitis

Rare cases of rapidly progressive glomerulonephritis with evidence of systemic disease (including myalgia, arthritis, skin rash, and vasculitis) are seen in patient's with antiglomerular basement membrane antibodies and antibody to myeloperoxidase (antineutrophil cytoplasmic antibody [MPO-ANCA]). Pulmonary hemorrhage is seen in about half of these patients. The role of the ANCA in this disease is not clear, but patients with ANCA tend to have a better prognosis than those with rapidly progressive anti-GBM glomerulonephritis with only anti-GBM.

OTHER GLOMERULOP-ATHIES

Hypocomplementemic Glomerulonephritis

A chronic form of glomerulonephritis without evidence of Ig in the glomerulus but associated with low levels of serum complement has been termed **hypocomplementemic glomerulonephritis**. The etiologic mechanism has not been clearly established. Nonimmune activation of complement via the alternate pathway may lead to deposition of complement in renal glomeruli and produce glomerulonephritis. There may be a so-called C_3 nephritic factor, which acts like an antibody to altered C_3, resulting in chronic deposition of C_3 in the glomerulus and lowered serum levels of C_3. It is also possible that immune complexes may initiate the deposition of complement but be undetectable when the complement components are still active. C_3 receptors may be present on glomerular endothelial cells and serve to activate C_3 under some circumstances. In any case, glomerulonephritis associated with deposits of complement components without detectable immunoglobulin and lowering of the serum complement is known as hypocomplementemic glomerulonephritis.

IgA Nephritis

A usually, but not always, mild proliferative form of glomerulonephritis is associated with mesangial deposition of IgA, but more severe outcomes have now been recognized. IgA does not activate the classical complement pathway, and it stimulates macrophage phagocytosis rather than neutrophil activation. In contrast to IgG complex-related tissue damage, which is primarily mediated by neutrophils, IgA injury is predominantly mediated by macrophages. In addition, IgA antibody–antigen complexes are more negatively charged than IgG complexes and, after formation in the circulation, are cleared by the glomerular mesangial cells. The disease is usually a mild acute glomerulonephritis, with only a small proportion of patients progressing to renal failure. No specific antigens have yet been identified and no epidemiologic clues support an infectious agent. Mesangial IgA deposits have been found in patients with Henoch–Schönlein purpura, systemic lupus erythematosus, dermatitis herpetiformis, and viral hepatitis. The etiologic implications of such associations are not clear, although the presence of shared antigens between mesangium and cutaneous capillaries might account for the IgA deposits seen in Henoch–Schönlein purpura.

Henoch–Schönlein Nephritis

Henoch–Schönlein purpura is a unique form of immune-complex-mediated systemic vasculitis that involves the skin (purpura), kidneys (hematuria), and gastrointestinal tract (abdominal pain), and usually occurs in children below age 15. Clinically, urticarial and hemorrhagic lesions are the most prominent features and tend to occur around joints. Variations in the clinical syndrome include abdominal involvement with edema and hemorrhage into the gastrointestinal tract (Henoch's syndrome); joint involvement with effusion, swelling of the soft tissues, redness, and pain (Schönlein's syndrome); or renal lesions of focal proliferative glomerulonephritis. Granular deposits of IgA and C_3 are found in the walls of small vessels in intestine and skin, and in the glomerular mesangium. Polyanionic (negatively charged) immune complexes tend to localize in the mesangium, whereas polycationic (positively charged) complexes lodge in the basement membrane. It is possible that an abnormal mucosal immune response to negatively charged antigens may result in IgA complexes that preferentially lodge in the mesangium. Complement is then activated via the alternate pathway, leading to glomerular damage. This disease is self-limiting and does not lead to chronic renal disease.

TUBULAR DISEASE

Heymann Nephritis

Experimental immunization of rats with renal cortex extract may result in production of autoantibodies to the brush border of the proximal renal tubular cells, immune complex deposition on the epithelial side of the basement membrane, and vacuolization of the proximal tubular cells. The tubular cell damage may be caused by a cytotoxic effect of the antibody. The role of this mechanism in human disease is not clear at this time.

Experimental Allergic Interstitial Nephritis

Immune injury to renal tubules may be induced by immunization of experimental animals with whole kidney or an antigen from the basement membrane of the renal tubule. The lesion begins as a polymorphonuclear infiltrate but progresses to a chronic mononuclear infiltrate with atrophy and degeneration of the tubules. Linear deposits of IgG may be detected along the basement membrane of the proximal tubules. Immune-mediated interstitial nephritis may occur in association with collagen diseases or renal graft rejection in humans.

CLINICAL–IMMUNO-PATHOLOGIC CORRELATIONS IN GLOMERULO-NEPHRITIS

Glomerulonephritis may be caused by deposition of immune complexes formed elsewhere, by reaction of antibody directly with glomerular basement membrane antigens, or by the activation of complement by the alternate pathway. Each of these mechanisms may produce an identical clinical picture or pathologic lesion (Fig. 13–9). Clinically, glomerulonephritis is a syndrome with markedly variable expression; but the disease is classified clinically into acute, subacute, and chronic. The acute disease may include proteinuria, gross hematuria, oliguria or anuria, edema, azotemia, and rapid death because of renal failure. However, recovery from the acute disease occurs in over 99 percent of the cases. Adults may develop a more persistent subacute or chronic progression to renal failure. Pathologically, a variety of lesions may be seen in the glomeruli. During the acute stage, the lesions may be minimal (proteinuria associated with fusion of epithelial foot plates), necrotic (death of glomerular cells), infiltrative or exudative (glomeruli full of polymorphonuclear leukocytes), or hemorrhagic (red blood cells in glomeruli). Subacute glomerulonephritis is associated with proliferative (increased number of mononuclear cells or glomerular epithelial cells) or embolic (fibrin thrombi in glomerular capillaries) lesions. Chronic glomerulonephritis features membranous (thickening of glomerular basement membrane) or sclerotic (scarring of glomeruli) changes. Intermediate stages of the disease usually demonstrate an overlap of lesions.

Any of these lesions may be produced by one of the three basic immunopathologic mechanisms. The type of lesion depends upon the degree of injury produced in a given period of time, not upon the immunopathologic mechanism. Thus, the deposit of large amounts of immune complexes or of antibodies to the basement membrane in a short period of time will lead to infiltration of the glomerulus with a large number of polymorphonuclear leukocytes and extensive dissolution of the basement membrane. The dissolution permits proteins of large molecular weight to pass through the basement membrane. If larger segments of the basement membrane are destroyed, larger blood components such as erythrocytes will pass through the basement membrane, producing hematuria. The loss of protein leads to hypoproteinemia, decreased intravascular osmotic pressure, edema, and heart failure—the clinical picture of acute glomerulonephritis. The deposit of small amounts of immune complexes over long periods of time may produce some disruption of the basement membrane and leakage of serum proteins but mainly causes a build-up on or in the basement membrane, leading to thickening of the basement membrane and a

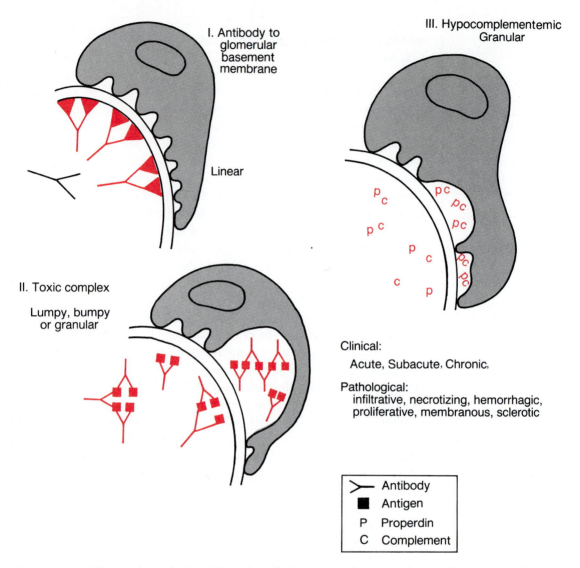

I. Antibody to glomerular basement membrane

Linear

II. Toxic complex

Lumpy, bumpy
or granular

III. Hypocomplementemic
Granular

Clinical:

Acute, Subacute, Chronic.

Pathological:
infiltrative, necrotizing, hemorrhagic,
proliferative, membranous, sclerotic

>—	Antibody
■	Antigen
P	Properdin
C	Complement

Figure 13–9. Glomerulonephritis: Clinical–pathologic correlations. The mechanisms of glomeru-lonephritis illustrated may produce a varied clinical and pathologic picture. **I.** Antiglomerular basement membrane antibody reacts with antigens on the lumenal side of the glomerular basement membrane and produces a linear deposition when examined by immunofluorescence. **II.** Soluble immune complexes formed elsewhere pass through the glomerular basement membrane and lodge on the epithelial side, producing lumpy–bumpy deposits or lodge within or on the endothelial side of the basement membrane as granular deposits. Granular deposit disease may also be produced from endothelial cell surface antigen–antibody complexes shed into the basement membrane. **III.** Complement in the absence of immunoglobulin may be detected as a granular deposit. Hypocomplementemic glomerulonephritis may be caused by a preceding immunoglobulin deposit or by the action of properdin, both of which may activate complement. No single mechanism produces a particular type of clinical picture or pathologic lesion, although hypocomplementemic glomerulonephritis is usually of the chronic variety. A capillary lumen, basement membrane endothelial cell foot plates, and an epithelial cell are illustrated. (Modified from illustration of C. Wilson, Scripps Clinic and Research Foundation, La Jolla, California.)

gradual loss of the filtering capacity of the glomeruli (membranous glomerulonephritis). This results in retention of nitrogen and waste products (azotemia) and gradual renal failure. It is not usually possible for the pathologist to be able to identify the immunopathologic mechanism responsible for a given case of glomerulonephritis by defining the histopathologic lesion. Identification of the mechanism requires immunofluorescent studies, serologic work-up, electron microscopy, and careful clinical documentation of the course of the disease.

HUMAN GLOMERULAR DISEASES

Human glomerulonephritis is classified by a combination of pathologic findings, clinical features, and course. A currently used classification is given in Table 13–2.

Vasculitis

Inflammation of vessels is a primary feature of many immune-complex-mediated diseases that are covered in different chapters in this book. The endothelial "Teflon-like" lining of the blood vessels usually repels white blood cells. This protective barrier becomes less effective when vasculitis develops, allowing the deposition of immune complexes on vascular endothelial surfaces, where they aggregate to fix complement, which, in turn, attracts and activates granulocytes. In 1990, the Diagnostic and Therapeutic Criteria Committee of the American College of Rheumatology published a classification of seven major vasculitic diseases (Table 13–3). In addition, vasculitis is associated with a large number of independent conditions, including infectious diseases; connective tissue disease malignancies; inflammatory diseases, such as Crohn's disease and cirrhosis; and as complications of atherosclerosis. There are definite associations between the size of the vessel and the underlying disease or syndrome. Each of these vascular lesions has a component of neutrophil infiltrate as well as lesions associated with other immune mechanisms. Often, the lesions are biopsied at a stage of development when the neutrophils have partially disintegrated. This is referred to as "leukoclastic vasculitis." Antineutrophil antibodies may form to proteases (C-ANCA, cytoplasmic immunofluorescence) or to myeloperoxidase (P-ANCA, perinuclear immunofluorescence) released from neutrophils and are used to help make the diagnosis of vasculitides, such as polyarteritis nodosa, Churg–Strauss syndrome, systemic vasculitis, Wegener's granulomatosis, and idiopathic concentric glomerulonephritis.

Major vascular diseases, such as polyarteritis nodosa and Wegener's granulomatosis, will be presented in more detail in other chapters. The presence of vasculitis in the early stages of the collagen vascular disease implies an important role for immune complexes in the pathogenesis of these diseases. Immune-complex-mediated vasculitis is often manifested in the skin. Because immune lesions in the

TABLE 13–2. SOME FORMS OF GLOMERULONEPHRITIS OF HUMANS

Type	Mechanism	Pathologic Findings
Post-infectious glomerulonephritis (human counterpart of acute serum sickness)	Immune complex	LM: Diffuse cellular proliferation, neutrophils EM: Subepithelial deposits ("humps")
Membranous nephropathy (human counterpart of chronic serum sickness)	Immune complex	LM: Diffuse basement membrane thickening EM: Subepithelial deposits, several, small
Minimal change disease	Immunological (exact mechanism unknown)	LM: Normal glomeruli EM: Effacement of epithelial cell foot processes
IgA nephropathy (Berger's disease)	Immune complex (IgA)	LM: Increase in mesangial matrix and cells EM: Electron-dense deposits in the mesangium
Goodpasture's disease	Antibasement membrane (kidney, lung)	LM: Crescentic glomerulonephritis EM: No evidence of deposits
Membranoproliferative GN (type I)	Immune complex	LM: Mesangial proliferation, basement membrane alteration EM: Split basement membranes, subendothelial deposits
Dense deposit disease (membranoproliferative GN, type II)	Alternate pathway of complement	LM: Mesangial proliferation, basement membrane alteration EM: Very dense material of unknown nature deposited in basement membranes

Abbreviations: LM, light microscopy; EM, electron microscopy; GN, glomerulonephritis. Note: These are basic characteristic features; variations occur in pathological and clinical findings.

Nephrotic syndrome: Proteinuria >3.5 g/24 h.

Nephritis: hematuria, red cell casts, hypertension.

skin may be used to compare different immunopathologic mechanisms, skin diseases due to immune complexes will be presented in a separate chapter (Chapter 20). Some rare vascular diseases with peculiar features will now be presented.

BEHÇET'S SYNDROME

Behçet's syndrome, rediscovered in 1937 by Hulusu Behçet, a Turkish dermatologist, was first described by Hippocrates. The disease consists of a clinical triad, which includes oral and genital aphthous ulcerations, vascular skin lesions, arthritis, and inflammation of the eye, for which an exact pathogenesis has not been determined. It is believed to be an immune complex disease. About half of the patients with this disease have a correlation with their disease activity and the level of circulating immune complexes. There is an increased incidence in individuals with HLA-B51. Positive delayed hypersensitivity skin reactions to streptococcal antigens and exacerbations of the disease in 15 of 85 cases given a

Immunofluorescence	Clinical Features	Prognosis
Coarse granular or lumpy–bumpy pattern in basement membranes (IgG, C3)	Acute nephritis	Good
Fine granular along basement membranes (IgG, C3)	Nephrotic syndrome	Slowly progressive (renal failure)
Negative or nonspecific	Nephrotic syndrome	Good
Positive in the mesangium (IgA, IgG, C3)	Hematuria Proteinuria	Usually good
Linear positivity along basement membranes (IgG, C3)	Acute renal failure, hemoptysis (lung hemorrhage)	Rapidly progressive (renal failure)
Granular irregular pattern in basement membranes (IgG, C3)	Variable (nephrotic syndrome, nephritis)	Progressive (renal failure)
Focal C3 (IgG and early-acting complement components absent)	Variable (nephrotic syndrome, nephritis hypocomplementemia)	Progressive (renal failure)

skin test has suggested that an immune reactivity to streptococcal antigens is responsible. About 25% of the patients develop arterial and venous large vessel disease, including arterial aneurysms and venous thrombosis.

KAWASAKI SYNDROME

Kawasaki syndrome (mucocutaneous lymph node syndrome) is similar to rheumatic fever (see Chapter 22) involving the heart (vasculitis and pancarditis) but with frequent involvement of the coronary arteries, leading to thrombosis, infarction, aneurysms, and scarring. The acute disease features fever, conjunctivitis, erythematous skin rash, mucous membrane ulcerations, edema, and lymphadenopathy.

HYPOCOMPLE-MENTEMIC VASCULITIC URTICARIAL SYNDROME

This syndrome includes urticaria, leukoclastic vasculitis, arthritis, and neurologic abnormalities. Laboratory findings are a low C_1q, C_4, C_2, and C_3, with normal C_1r and C_1s, C_{5-9}, and properdin. A 7S protein which precipitates C_1q is found (C_1q activating factor) and is believed to be responsible for complement activation.

TABLE 13–3. PATHOLOGIC OVERLAP IN SELECTED VASCULITIS SYNDROMES

	Polyarteritis Nodosa	Churg–Strauss Syndrome	Wegener's Granulomatosis
Vessels involved	Medium and small muscular arteries; sometimes arterioles	Small arteries and veins often arterioles and venules	Usually small arteries and veins; sometimes larger vessels
Sites involved	Visceral, cutaneous; infrequently cerebral and lung vessels	Upper and lower respiratory tract; viscera, heart, and skin	Upper and lower respiratory tract; often kidney; infrequently skin, heart, viscera, and skin
Type of vasculitis	Necrotizing, with mixed cells and few eosinophils; rarely granulomatous	Necrotizing or granulomatous, with mixed cells prominent eosinophils	Necrotizing or granulomatous, with mixed cells and occasional eosinophils
Special features	Focal segmental involvement; coexisting acute and healed lesions or normal and affected vessels; microaneurysms	Extravascular necrotizing granulomas with prominent eosinophils; may manifest as "limited form"	Geographic pattern of tissue necrosis and antineutrophil cytoplasmic antibodies; may manifest as "limited form"
Other comments	Vascular lesion in infants is indistinguishable from fatal Kawasaki disease	Most patients have asthma or history of allergy	Occurs in all ages, with a slight male preponderance; associated with HLA-DR2; may respond to antimicrobials

From LeRoy, EC: The Systemic Vasculitides. *Hospital Practice* 27:55, 1992.

GIANT CELL ARTERITIS

Giant cell arteritis features a granulomatous reaction (see Chapter 17) in and around the internal elastic lamina of the temporal artery. It is suspected that either there is an alteration in the elastic lamina leading to an immune response (perhaps due to solar radiation) or a congenital (perhaps HLA-D4-linked) disposition to development of an autoimmune response to elastin.

POSTCARDIAC BYPASS SYNDROME

Patients who have been on cardiac bypass develop fever, leukocytosis, and edema believed to be secondary to nonimmune-specific activation of C_3 to C_3a.

Hypersensitivity Vasculitis	Henoch–Schönlein Purpura	Giant Cell (Temporal) Arteritis	Takayasu's Arteritis
Arterioles and venules; often small arteries and veins	Arterioles and venules; often small arteries and veins	Vessels of all sizes	Elastic arteries and selected muscular arteries
Predominantly skin; less commonly viscera, heart, and synovium	Predominantly skin, gastrointestinal, kidney, and synovium	Predominantly temporal arteries; less often, any other vessels	Aorta, arch vessels, other major branches (coronary, renal, visceral), and pulmonary arteries
Leukocytoclastic or lymphocytic, with variable number of eosinophils; occasionally granulomatous	Leukocytoclastic, mixed cell or lymphocytic, with variable number of eosinophils	Granulomatous, with variable number of giant cells, sometimes only lymphoplasmacytic	Granulomatous, few giant cells in active phase and sclerosing fibrosis in chronic stage, with scanty infiltrate
May be associated with myocarditis interstitial nephritis, or hepatitis	IgA immune deposits	Affected extracranial large vessels Indistinguishable from Takayasu's arteritis; may form aneurysm or cause dissection	Aneurysmal in 20% may be segmental and cause rupture or dissection
Patients may have occult malignancy or history of drug or chemical allergy, vaccination	Predominantly children and young adults	Virtually all patients are over age 50; may be asymptomatic	Most common in women of childbearing age; more prevalent in Asia; important cause of renovascular hypertension in adolescents

ALEUTIAN MINK DISEASE

Aleutian mink disease is caused by the immune response to a persistent virus infection and offers an animal model for the relationship of the humoral immune response to the development of lesions found during a viral infection. The disease is characterized by a proliferation of lymphoid tissues, hypergammaglobulinemia, glomerulonephritis, hepatitis, and arteritis. There is an overproduction of IgG antibody and the formation of immune complexes because the humoral immune response is unable to control viral reproduction. This results in hyperplasia of IgG-forming cells, formation of antibody–virus complexes, and immune complex lesions of vasculitis and glomerulonephritis. The intracellular virus infection could possibly be controlled by the cellular reactivity of delayed hypersensitivity. However, for as yet undefined reasons, the affected mink produce a nonprotective, lesion-producing IgG antibody response. Thus, Aleutian mink disease is a prime example of the destructive effects of an immune response when the response is inappropriate (eg, humoral rather than cellular) (see also Leprosy, Chapter 17, and Chronic Mucocutaneous Candidiasis, Chapter 27). If the mink manifested a cellular rather than a humoral immune response to the virus, the disease in this form would not occur.

Other Immune Complex Diseases

In addition to the renal glomerulus, other organs of the body also contain capillary basement membrane exposed to circulating blood: The lung (see Goodpasture's Syndrome above), synovial capillaries, the choroid plexus of the brain, and the uveal tract of the eye. These organs are susceptible to antibasement membrane antibody attack and deposition of immune complexes.

CELLULAR INTERSTITIAL PNEUMONIA (CIP)

Immune complex deposition and subsequent inflammation may also cause interstitial inflammation in the lung. These lesions have been identified morphologically as an infiltration of the lung with different cellular elements. CIP is often found associated with various collagen diseases. Immunoglobulin and complement have been identified in the lungs of patients with active interstitial disease in a manner similar to an experimental systemic immune-complex-induced pneumonitis in rabbits. In addition, circulating immune complexes have been found in the serum of patients with interstitial pneumonias. A chronic form of interstitial pneumonia (diffuse fibrosis) is not associated with circulating immune complexes. This may be a later stage of CIP when complexes are no longer present or there may be a different pathogenesis. Patients with active stages of the disease (when immune complexes are present) are responsive to steroid therapy. The spectrum of interstitial pneumonias resembles the stages of glomerulonephritis described above. It is also possible that immune complex formation is secondary to, and not the cause of, cellular interstitial inflammation.

ARTHRITIS

Subsynovial capillaries are also a site for immune complex deposition. Transient arthritis is seen in many infectious diseases and is also often associated with collagen diseases. A classic example is the arthritis seen during acute attacks of rheumatic fever. It is likely that such transient arthritis episodes are due to immune-complex-initiated inflammation.

CHOROID PLEXUS DEPOSITION

The choroid plexus is a frequent site of immune complex deposition in experimental animals injected with immune complexes and with infections associated with circulating immune complexes. In humans, depositions of immune complexes in the choroid plexus are found in some diseases, such as systemic lupus erythematosus (SLE). In the choroid plexus, the endothelial cells are fenestrated so that, in contrast to other parts of the cerebral vasculature, there is not a tight blood–brain barrier. Immune complexes pass through the endothelial cells to lie between the endothelial and epithelial cells. The epithelial cells overlying the basement membrane are tightly joined and prevent increased filtration after complex deposition, such as is seen in renal glomeruli. The role of these immune complexes in producing neurologic symptoms of SLE remains undefined.

UVEITIS

Some forms of uveitis may be caused by deposition of immune complexes in the ocular basement membrane. In rabbits, circulating immune complexes may deposit in ocular tissue and be responsible for inflammation of the uveal tract (iris, ciliary body, and choroid). In humans, uveitis is associated with circulating immune complexes, and immune complexes have been detected in the aqueous humor of the anterior chamber of the eye. Thus, the uveal tract may also be a preferential site for immune complex deposition and subsequent inflammation. Other forms of uveitis may be caused by cellular autoimmunity to uveal antigens (see Chapter 21).

Evaluation of Circulating Immune Complexes (CIC)

There are a number of laboratory assays for immune complexes (Table 13–4). Since these assays depend upon different properties of immune complexes, different tests may give different results. It is recommended that at least three tests be used: C_1q binding, the Raji test, and monoclonal 19S rheumatoid factor with high reactivity to IgG in complex form. The interpretation of positive tests for circulating immune complexes is complicated. Many asymptomatic individuals have detectable CIC with no symptoms or lesions. However, in symptomatic individuals, the level of immune complexes often correlates with the severity of disease.

Summary

Immune complex reactions are caused by immunoglobulin antibody reacting with tissue antigens, by formation of antibody–antigen complexes that deposit in vessel walls or basement membrane of capillaries, or by antibodies that react with basement membrane antigens. Tissue destruction is mediated by lysosomal enzymes released from polymorphonuclear leukocytes attracted and activated by complement components (C_3a, C_5a). Acute lesions consist of tissue digestion by enzymes, whereas chronic lesions may be caused by deposition of large amounts of immune complexes or scarring. Typical diseases caused by this mechanism include serum sickness, glomerulonephritis, vasculitis, collagen diseases (see Chapter 22), and many types of skin eruptions (see Chapter 20). The antigens involved may be host tissue antigens (autoimmune reaction) or foreign (bacterial, viral) antigens.

TABLE 13–4. SOME TECHNIQUES FOR DETECTING IMMUNE COMPLEXES

Antigen specific:

    Isolation of complex (ie, anti-Ig precipitation) followed by specific identification of antigen.

Antigen nonspecific:

    Physical techniques

        Ultracentrifugation

        Sucrose gradient centrifugation

        Gel filtration

        Ultrafiltration

        Electrophoresis

        Polyethyleneglycol precipitation

    Biologic techniques

        Complement reactivity (C1q binding, PPT)

        C3 precipitation

        Antiglobulin (anti-IgG)

        Rheumatoid factors with specificity for IgG in complexes

    Cellular

        Platelet aggregation

        Release of enzymes from mast cells

        Rosette inhibition

        Raji cell (Fc receptor)

    Other

        Binding to staph A protein

Modified from Theofilopoulos, AN: *Evaluation and Significance of Circulating Immune Complexes in Progress in Clinical Immunology*, vol. 4. Schwartz, RS, ed. Grune & Stratton, 1980, 63.

Bibliography

IMMUNE COMPLEX INJURY

Cochrane CG: Immunologic tissue injury mediated by neutrophilic leukocytes. *Adv Immunol* 9:97, 1968.

Cochrane CG, Koffler D: Immune complex disease in experimental animals and in man. *Adv Immunol* 16:185, 1973.

Dixon FJ: The role of antigen–antibody complexes in disease. *Harvey Lect* 58:21, 1962.

Gotze O, Muller-Eberhard HJ: The C_3 activator system: An alternate pathway of complement activation. *J Exp Med* 134:905, 1971.

Hoiby N, Doring G, Schiotz PO: The role of immune complexes in the pathogenesis of bacterial infections. *Ann Rev Microbiol* 40:29, 1986.

Movat HZ: Pathways to allergic inflammation: The sequelae of antibody–antigen complex formation. *Fed Proc* 35:2435, 1976.

Oldham KT, Guice KS, Ward PA, et al.: The role of oxygen radicals in immune complex injury. *Free Radical Biol Med* 4:387, 1988.

Weigle WO: Fate and biological action of antigen–antibody complexes. *Adv Immunol* 1:283, 1961.

ARTHUS REACTION

Arthus M: Injections répétées de serum de cheval chez le lapin. *C R Soc Biol* (Paris) 55:817, 1903.

Cochrane CG: Mediators of the Arthus and related reactions. *Prog Allergy* 11:1, 1967.

Cochrane CG, Weigle WO, Dixon FJ: Factors responsible for decline of inflammation in Arthus hypersensitivity vasculitis. *Proc Soc Exp Biol* 101:695, 1959.

Crawford JP, Movat H, Ranadive NS, et al. Pathways to inflammation induced by immune complexes: Development of the Arthus reaction. *Fed Proc* 41:2583, 1982.

Gell PGH, Hinde IT: Observations on the histology of the Arthus reaction and its relation to other known types of skin hypersensitivity. *Int Arch Allerg* 5:23, 1954.

Humphrey JH: The mechanism of Arthus reactions. II. The role of polymorphonuclear leukocytes and platelets in reverse passive reactions in the guinea pig. *Brit J Exp Path* 36:283, 1955.

Opie EL: Pathogenesis of the specific inflammatory reaction of immunized animals (Arthus reaction). *J Immunol* 9:259, 1924.

Opie EL: The fate of antigen (protein) in an animal immunized against it. *J Exp Med* 39:659, 1924.

Rich AR, Follis RH: Studies on the site of sensitivity in the Arthus phenomenon. *Bull J Hopkins Hosp* 66:106, 1940.

SERUM SICKNESS

Bielory L, Gascon P, Lawley TJ, et al.: Human serum sickness: A prospective analysis of 35 patients treated with equine anti-thymocyte globulin for bone marrow failure. *Medicine* 67:40, 1988.

Dixon FJ, Vasquez JJ, Weigle WO, et al.: Pathogenesis of serum sickness. *Arch Pathol* 65:18, 1958.

Germuth FG: A comparative histologic and immunologic study on rabbits of induced hypersensitivity of serum sickness type. *J Exp Med* 97:257, 1953.

Kniker WT, Cochrane CG: Pathogenic factors in vascular lesions of experimental serum sickness. *J Exp Med* 122:83, 1965.

von Pirquet CF, Schick B: *Serum Sickness, 1905*. Schick B (trans.). Baltimore, Williams & Wilkins, 1951.

GLOMERULO-NEPHRITIS

Adler S, Baker P, Pritzl P, et al.: Effects of alterations in glomerular charge on deposition of cationic and anionic antibodies to fixed glomerular antigens in the rat. *J Lab Clin Med* 106:1, 1985.

Andres G, Brentjens JR, Caldwell PRB, et al.: Biology of disease: Formation of immune deposits and disease. *Lab Invest* 55:510–520, 1986.

Atkins RC, Holdsworth SR, Hancock WW, et al.: Cellular immune mechanisms in glomerulonephritis: The role of mononuclear leukocytes. *Springer Semin Immunopath* 5:269, 1985.

Batsford S, Oite T, Takamiya H, et al.: Anionic binding sites in the glomerular basement membrane: Possible role in the pathogenesis of immune complex glomerulonephritis. *Renal Physiol* 3:336, 1980.

Bresnahan BA, Wu S, Fenoy FJ, et al.: Mesangial cell immune injury: Hemodynamic role of leukocyte- and platelet-derived eicosanoids. *J Clin Invest* 90:2304–2312, 1992.

Burkholder PM: *Atlas of Human Glomerular Pathology*. Hagerstown, Harper & Row, 1974.

Costanza ME, Pinn V, Schwartz RS, et al.: Carcinoembryonic antigen–antibody complexes in a patient with colonic carcinoma and nephrotic syndrome. *N Engl J Med* 289:520, 1973.

Feintzeig ID, Dittmer JE, Cybulsky AV, et al.: Antibody, antigen, and glomerular capillary wall charge interactions: Influence of antigen location on in situ immune complex formation. *Kidney Int* 29:649, 1986.

Fouser LS, Michael AF: Antigens of the human glomerular basement membrane. *Springer Semin Immunopath* 9:317, 1987.

Gauthier VJ, Mannik M: A small proportion of cationic antibodies in immune complexes is sufficient to mediate their deposition in glomeruli. *J Immunol* 145:3348, 1990.

Gauthier VJ, Striker GE, Mannik M: Glomerular localization of preformed immune complexes prepared with anionic antibodies or with cationic antigens. *Lab Invest* 50:636, 1984.

Klassen J, Andres GA, Brennan JC, et al.: An immunologic renal tubular lesion in man. *Clin Immunol Immunopathol* 1:69, 1972.

Knisser MR, Jenis EH, Lowenthal DT, et al.: Pathogenesis of renal disease associated with viral hepatitis. *Arch Pathol Lab Med* 97:193, 1974.

Lampert PH, Dixon FJ: Pathogenesis of the glomerulonephritis of NZB/W mice. *J Exp Med* 127:507, 1968.

Lerner RW, Dixon FJ: Transfer of ovine experimental allergic glomerulonephritis (EAG) with serum. *J Exp Med* 124:431, 1966.

Nishikawa K, Guo Y-J, Miyasaka M, et al.: Antibodies to intercellular adhesion molecule-1/lymphocyte function-associated antigen-1 prevent crescent formation in rat autoimmune glomerulonephritis. *J Exp Med* 177:667–677, 1993.

Tipping PG, Leong TW, Holdsworth SR: Tumor necrosis factor production by glomerular macrophages in antiglomerular basement membrane glomerulonephritis in rabbits. *Lab Invest* 65:272, 1991.

Westberg NG, Naff GB, Boyer JT, et al.: Glomerular deposition of properdin in acute and chronic glomerulonephritis with hypocomplementemia. *J Clin Invest* 50:642, 1971.

POSTSTREPTO-COCCAL GLOMERULO-NEPHRITIS

Holm SE: The pathogenesis of acute poststreptococcal glomerulonephritis in new lights. APIMS 96:189, 1988.

Kefalides NA, Pegg MT, Ohno N, et al.: Antibodies to basement membrane collagen and to laminin are present in sera from patients with poststreptococcal glomerulonephritis. *J Exp Med* 163:588, 1986.

Zabriskie JB: The role of streptococci in human glomerulonephritis. *J Exp Med* 134:180, 1971.

IGA NEPHRITIS

D'Amico G: Idiopathic IgA mesangial nephropathy. *Nephron* 41:1, 1985.

Lowance DC, Mullins JD, McPhaul JS Jr: IgA-associated glomerulonephritis. *Int Rev Exp Pathol* 17:144–172, 1977.

Rifai A, Imai H, Oka D: IgA immune complexes and disease: An experimental perspective. *Pathol Immunopath Res* 5:278, 1986.

Stevenson JA, Leona LA, Cohen AH, et al.: Henoch–Schönlein purpura. *Arch Path Lab Med* 106:192, 1982.

Warren JS, Kunkel SL, Johnsom KJ, et al.: In vitro activation of rat neutrophils and alveolar macrophages with IgA and IgG immune complexes: Implications for immune-complex-induced lung injury. *Am J Pathol* 129:578, 1987.

GOOD-PASTURE'S DISEASE

Benoit FL, Rulon DB, Theil GB, et al.: Goodpasture's syndrome: A clinicopathologic entity. *Am J Med* 37:424, 1964.

Bruijn JA, Hoedemaeker PJ, Fleuren GJ: Pathogenesis of anti-basement membrane glomerulonephritis and immune complex glomerulonephritis: Dichotomy dissolved. *Lab Investig* 61:480, 1989.

DeGowin RL, Oda Y, Evans RH: Nephritis and lung hemorrhage: Goodpasture's syndrome. *Arch Intern Med* 111:62, 1963.

Hudson BG, Wieslander J, Wisdom BJ, et al.: Goodpasture's syndrome: Molecular architecture and function of basement membrane antigen. *Lab Invest* 61:256, 1989.

VASCULITIS

Arbesfeld SJ, Kurban AK: Behçet's disease. *J Am Acad Dermatol* 19:767, 1988.

Behçet H: Uber rez'diverende Aphtose durch ein Virus verursachte Geschwure am Mund, am Auge und an den Genitalein. *Dermatologische Wochenschrift* 105:1152, 1937.

Churg A, Churg J (eds.): *Systemic Vasculitides*. New York, Igaku–Shoin, 1991.

Goeken JA: Antineutrophil cytoplasmic antibody: A useful serologic marker for vasculitis. *J Clin Immunol* 11:161, 1991.

Gilliand BC: Vasculitis. *Immunol Allergy Clin N Am* 13:335–357, 1993.

Ferraro G, Meroni PL, Tincani A, et al.: Antiendothelial cell antibodies in patients with Wegener's granulomatosis and micropolyarteritis. *Clin Exp Immunol* 79:47, 1990.

Henson JB, Gorham JR: Animal model of human disease: Aleutian disease of mink. *Am J Pathol* 71:345, 1973.

Hunder CG, Lie JT, Goronzy JJ, et al.: Pathogenesis of giant cell arteritis. *Arth Rheum* 36:757–761, 1993.

International Study Group for Behçet's Disease: Criteria for diagnosis of Behçet's disease. *Lancet* 335:1078, 1990.

Koc Y, Gullu I, Akpek G, et al.: Vascular involvement in Behçet's disease. *J Rheumatol* 19:402, 1992.

LeRoy EC (ed.): *Systemic Vasculitis: The Biologic Basis*. New York, Marcel Dekker, 1992.

Lie JT: Illustrated histopathologic classification criteria for selected vasculitis syndromes. *Arth Rheum* 33:1074, 1990.

Michel BA: Classification of vasculitis. *Curr Opin Rheumatol* 4:3, 1992.

Mizushima Y: Recent research into Behçet's disease in Japan. *Int J Tiss Reac* 10:59, 1988.

Mizushima Y, et al.: Skin hypersensitivity to streptococcal antigens and the induction of systemic symptoms by the antigens in Behçet's disease: A multicenter study. *J Rheumatol* 16:506, 1989.

Penny R: Vasculitis: An approach for physicians. *Aust NZ J Med* 11:302, 1981.

Porter DD, Larsen AE, Porter HG: The pathogenesis of Aleutian disease of mink. I. Viral replication and the host antigen. *J Exp Med* 130:575, 1969.

OTHER IMMUNE COMPLEX DISEASE

Brentjens JR, O'Connel DW, Pawlowski IB, et al.: Experimental immune complex disease of the lung: The pathogenesis of a laboratory model resembling certain interstitial lung diseases. *J Exp Med* 140:105, 1974.

Buchmeier MJ, Oldstone MBA: Virus-induced immune complex disease: Identification of specific viral antigens and antibodies deposited in complexes during chronic lymphocytic choriomeningitis virus infection. *J Immunol* 120:1297, 1978.

Dreisin RB, Schwartz MI, Theofilopoulis AN, et al.: Circulating immune complexes in the idiopathic interstitial pneumonias. *N Engl J Med* 298:353, 1978.

Grey HM, Kohler PF: Cryoimmunoglobulins. *Semin Hematol* 10:87, 1973.

Lampert PW, Garrett R, Lampert A: Ferritin immune complex deposits in the choroid plexus. *Acta Neuropathol* (Berlin) 38:83, 1977.

Lampert PW, Garret RS, Oldstone MBA: Immune complex deposits in the choroid plexus. In *Birth Defects*, Original Article Series, vol. XIV, 1978, 237.

Liebow AA: Definition and classification of interstitial pneumonias in human pathology. *Hum Pathol* 8:1, 1975.

Maumenee AE, Silverstein AM (eds.): *Immunopathology of Uveitis*. Baltimore, Williams & Wilkins, 1964.

Rotter JI, Henner DC: Are these immunologic forms of duodenal ulcer? *J Clin Lab Immunol* 7:1, 1982.

**IMMUNE
COMPLEX
EVALUATION**

Delire M, Masson PL: The detection of circulating immune complexes in children with recurrent infections and their treatment with human immunoglobulins. *Clin Exp Immunol* 29:385, 1977.

Dernouchamps JP, Vaermau JP, Michaels J, et al.: Immune complexes in the aqueous humor and serum. *Am J Ophthalmol* 84:24, 1977.

Ploth DW, Fitz A, Schnetzler D, et al.: Thyroglobulin–antithyroglobulin immune complex glomerulonephritis complicating radioiodine therapy. *Clin Immunol Immunopathol* 9:327, 1978.

Ritzmann SE, Daniels JC: Immune complexes: Characteristics, clinical correlations, and interpretive approaches in the clinical laboratory. *Clin Chem* 28:1259, 1982.

Theofilopoulos AN: Evaluation and clinical significance of circulating immune complexes. *Prog Clin Immunol* 4:63, 1980.

Theofilopoulos AN, Dixon FJ: Immune complexes in human disease. *Am J Pathol* 100:531, 1980.

14

Atopic or Anaphylactic Reactions (Allergy)

The term **anaphylaxis** was coined by Portier and Richet in 1902 to indicate adverse reactions in dogs to a toxin derived from the sea anemone. They expected that repeated injections of the toxin would lead to a neutralization of the toxic effect by antibody, but instead found lethal responses to doses of the toxin that were previously innocuous. Although the word anaphylaxis literally means "without protection," the term as used by Portier and Richet implied a reaction that is the opposite of prophylaxis, a destructive rather than a protective reaction, as a result of previous exposure to an agent. Coca applied the term **atopy** in the 1920s for a variety of reactions in humans, at the time not yet described in other species. The origin of this term is from the Greek word *atopia*, meaning strangeness. These reactions are now included in the term "allergy." The word **allergy** was introduced by Von Pirquet in 1906 to designate "altered reactivity" as a result of previous exposure. The term allergy is now mostly used for atopic or anaphylactic reactions but is also used as a general term for reactions of discomfort of unknown origin. Although the association of seasonal allergic rhinitis (*catarrhous aestivus*) with grass pollen in England, and in the United States (*autumnal catarrh*) with ragweed, was reported in 1872, the name now applied to this group of diseases was not forthcoming until much later.

The effects produced by atopic or anaphylactic reactions are the result of a two-phase system initiated by mediators that are released by the reaction of antigen with effector cells passively sensitized by IgE antibody (Fig. 14–1). Antigens that elicit these responses are also called **allergens**. The **mast cell** (tissue) or **basophil** (peripheral blood) is the major effector cell for acute reactions, whereas T cells

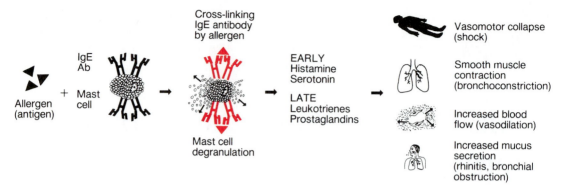

Figure 14–1. Atopic or anaphylactic reactions. Reaction of antigen (allergen) with reaginic antibody (IgE) fixed to effector (mast) cells causes release of pharmacologically active agents stored in cytoplasmic granules (degranulation of mast cells). These released mediators, primarily histamine and serotonin, cause contraction of endothelial cells and bronchial smooth cells and produce edema and bronchoconstriction. Cell-membrane-associated arachidonic acids also released from mast cells are converted to other inflammatory mediators—leukotrienes and prostaglandins—which are responsible for later stages of the reactions. The acute effects are termed anaphylactic, the more chronic effects, atopic.

TABLE 14–1. ALLERGIC SYMPTOMS: FIVE ORGAN SYSTEMS

Histamine Receptor	Reactive Tissue	Constriction	Dilation	Symptom
H_2	Vascular		X	Shock
H_1	Pulmonary	X		Asthma
	Gastrointestinal	X		Vomiting and diarrhea
	Genitourinary	X		Involuntary urination
	Endothelium	X		Edema

and eosinophils play important roles in persistent asthma (see Chapter 8).

Following reaction with allergens, mast cells release a number of biologically active substances, including histamine, heparin, and serotonin (early phase reaction), as well as arachidonic acid, which is converted by other cells into prostaglandins and leukotrienes responsible for the later phase inflammation reactions. The acute phase is characterized by immediate smooth muscle constriction or dilation. On the one hand, the smooth muscle of arterioles is stimulated to dilate by reaction of histamine with H_2 receptors (blocked by cimetidine), causing increased blood flow (erythema). On the other hand, the smooth muscle of pulmonary bronchi, gastrointestinal tract (asthma), and the genitourinary system (cramps and diarrhea), as well as endothelial cells (edema), are stimulated to contract by action of histamine on H_1 receptors (blocked by antihistamines) (Table 14–1). The effects of these agents include contraction of smooth muscle; increased vascular permeability; early increase in vascular resistance, followed by collapse (shock); and increased gastric, nasal, and lacrimal secretion. The type of lesion observed depends upon the dose of antigen, the route of contact with antigen, the frequency of contact with antigen, the tendency for a given organ system to react (shock organ), and the degree of sensitivity of the involved individual. This final factor may be genetically controlled or may be altered by environmental conditions (temperature), unrelated inflammation (presence of a viral upper respiratory infection), or the emotional state of the individual. Some of the reactions seen clinically are urticaria (wheal and flare, hives), hay fever, asthma, eczema, angioedema, and anaphylaxis.

The inflammatory properties of prostaglandins and leukotrienes are discussed in detail in Chapter 8. These mediators cause infiltration of polymorphonuclear leukocytes and other hallmarks of acute inflammation. Prostaglandin E (PGE) is a potent dilator of bronchial smooth muscle, whereas prostaglandin F (PGF) is a potent constrictor. Leukotriene-E4 (slow-reacting substance of anaphylaxis) causes later vasoreactions, whereas leukotriene-B_4 is chemotactic for acute inflammatory cells. The late phase occurs 6 to 12 hours after antigen exposure and is characterized by a more prolonged reaction involving infiltration by neutrophilic, eosinophilic, and basophilic polymorphonuclear cells, as well as lymphocytes and macrophages. This late phase causes an indurated, erythematous, painful reaction in the skin or, in the lung, a more prolonged deterioration in airflow as compared to the rapidly appearing wheal and flare skin reaction or asthma characterized by rapidly reversible bronchoconstriction in the immediate or early phase. A better understanding of the production, release, and effects of these mediators may lead to improved therapeutic approaches.

Acute reactions (wheal and flare, systemic shock) are generally referred to as anaphylactic; chronic recurring reactions (hay fever) are referred to as atopic. However, this distinction is not always made, and there is considerable overlap in the use of the terms atopy and anaphylactic. An atopic individual is one who is prone to develop this type of allergic reaction.

Chronic reactions, such as hay fever and persistent asthma, are accompanied by a lowering of the threshold to atopic stimuli. This hyperreactivity is associated with chronic tissue infiltration with mast cell, macrophages, T cells, B cells, and eosinophils. The increased numbers of inflammatory cells, as well as smooth muscle hyperplasia, set up conditions whereby lower levels of stimulation may trigger fits of sneezing or asthmatic attacks. One school of thought implies that Th_2 cell stimulation of eosinophil differentiation by IL-3, IL-5, and GM-CSF leads to production and release of leukotrienes (LTC_4/LTD_4)

and platelet-activating factors that contribute to the chronic inflammation in atopic conditions. However, the relative importance of this mechanism to those of the other possible mechanisms remains to be clarified. The role of non-IgE-mediated reactions in asthma will be presented in more detail below.

Allergens

ALLERGIC SENSITIZATION

The antigens that induce and elicit allergic reactions—allergens—have no unique features to distinguish them as a subset of antigenic molecules. Induction of IgE antibody appears to be favored by such things as route, dose, or presence of a modifying agent. Thus, inhalation or ingestion of an antigen predisposes to IgE formation as does low dose, or the use of adjuvants, such as alumina gel or *Bordetella pertussis*. The injected allergenic components of bee venom or mosquito bites also reach the immune system in very small doses, as do ingested allergenic compounds in foods. Inhaled allergens include pollen, fungi, dander, and dust, which are usually inhaled at very low doses. Larger pollen particulate allergens (20μm diameter) tend to deposit in the upper airway and produce allergic rhinitis (hay fever), whereas smaller particles are inhaled into the bronchi, where they may cause asthma.

Induction of IgE antibodies depends on the maturation of IgE-producing B cells after exposure to antigen. In the human, allergic sensitization to allergens, such as ragweed antigen, is associated with genetic factors (human lymphocyte antigen [HLA]). Immunologic factors which appear to determine if IgG or IgE B cells will be formed during induction of antibody formation are the relative balance of interleukins. This lymphokine balance is, in turn, related to the activation of different T-helper (Th) cell populations. There are two subpopulations of T_H cells: Th1 and Th2. Th1 cells secrete IL-2, IFN-γ, and lymphotoxin, but not IL-4; Th2 cells secrete IL-4, IL-5, IL-6, IL-13, but not IFN-γ. Th1 cell products drive B cells toward IgG production; Th2 cell products drive B cells to IgE and IgA production. IL-4 and IL-13 favor IgE production, IL-5 drives IgA production; IGF-β produced by CD8+ cells favors IgA production and inhibits IgE. Thus, activation of Th2 cells in preference to Th1 cells results in secretion of IgE rather than IgG antibodies. It is likely that IgE antibody production is determined by genetically controlled factors as well as dose, route, frequency of exposure, and presence of infections that act to direct antigen presentation to Th2 cells. The possibility of preventing allergies by inhibiting the synthesis of Th_2 type interleukins is now under active investigation.

CHEMISTRY OF ALLERGENS

Analysis of the pollen allergens in ragweed, as an example of a pollen allergen, indicates up to six different allergenic polypeptides with molecular weights from 5,000 to 38,000 (Table 14–2). There is little or no cross-reactivity among the pollens of different plants, but there may be extensive cross-reactivity within related species, such as with allergies to grass. Sequential (primary sequence) determinants appear to be relatively unimportant for most allergens. Conformational structures are recognized by IgE antibody so that denaturation of allergens results in loss of antibody binding. Cooking may greatly alter the allergenic potential of dietary allergens. Anaphylactic reactions to drugs are increasingly common and will be discussed below. **Allergoids** are allergens that have been chemically modified so that the allergenic reactivity has been greatly reduced, but the capacity to induce IgG antibody has been retained. Such modification has been attempted by formaldehyde, glutaraldehyde, and polyethylene glycol treatment. Allergoids have been shown to induce IgG antibodies in rodents, with little IgE antibody formation, but clinical trials in humans have not been successful.

NATURAL DISTRIBUTION OF ALLERGENS

Atopic reactions may occur to very unusual antigens. Systemic anaphylactic reactions have been unleashed by ingestion of beans, rice, shrimp, fish, milk, cereal mixes, potatoes, Brazil nuts, and tangerines. Men have complained about being allergic to their wives, but usually they are reacting to some component of makeup, hair spray, or other cosmetic agent. Rarely, women have developed systemic anaphylactic symptoms shortly after intercourse and appropriate tests demonstrate anaphylactic sensitivity to seminal fluid. Several such cases have been reported in which the allergy is an IgE-mediated reaction to a seminal plasma protein. About 10% of individuals who work with laboratory animals develop anaphylactic reactions to the dander or urinary and serum proteins from these animals that is severe enough to prevent them from further work with the animals. The incidence of such sensi-

TABLE 14–2. SOME PROPERTIES OF HIGHLY PURIFIED SHORT RAGWEED (*AMBROSIA ARTEMISIFOLIA*) ANTIGENS

Systematic Name	Original	Relative MW (MR)	No. Amino Acids	% Allergen in Dry Pollen
Amb aI	AgE	37,800	337	0.48
Amb aII	AgK	38,200	331	0.12
Amb aIII	Ra31	12,300	101	0.08
Amb aIV	RaIV(BPA-R)	22,800	189	0.1
Amb aV	RaV	4,990	45	0.3
Amb a VI	Ra6	11,500	108	0.12

tivity increases with the amount of contact with the animals. During the days of the cavalry, many officers and troops had to be discharged or moved to different tasks because of an allergic reaction to horse dander. As many as 20% of the cavaliers were involved. Documentation of allergic reactions of horses to humans has not been found. Laundry detergents containing allergenic enzymes derived from *Bacillus subtilis* caused severe symptoms to laundry detergent involving occasional unsuspecting users. With the widespread use of gloves for protection of health workers against AIDS, an increasing incidence of allergic reactions to latex has been seen.

Reaginic Antibody

IgE contributes less than 0.001% of the total circulating immunoglobulins, but has a major biologic effect as reaginic antibody. Reaginic antibody has a special ability to bind to skin or other tissues. The term **atopic reagin** was adopted to refer to the particular tissue-fixing antibody found in the serum of patients with hay fever and asthma. The original use of the word reagin was to designate the reacting serum component responsible for the Wassermann reaction. The Wassermann reagin is a peculiar serum reactant found in individuals infected with syphilis. The Wassermann reagin is demonstrable by its ability to combine with an antigen extracted from ungulate heart muscle (cardiolipin) and has no relation to anaphylactic or atopic reactions. It has been reported that atopic reaginic antibody may be found in all the major immunoglobulin groups (IgA, IgG, IgM). However, in essentially all cases, reagin is found only in IgE. It may be assumed that atopic or anaphylactic reactions in humans are due to IgE antibody.

IgE ANTIBODY

IgE antibody is termed "skin fixing" because it binds to mast cells in skin and sensitizes these cells to react to allergen. IgE anaphylactic antibodies have structures on the Fc piece of the molecule that fit receptors of the mast cell. There are two Fcε receptors—FcεRI and FCεRII. FcεRI is the highest-affinity Fc receptor known, is found only on mast cells and basophils, and is responsible for transmission of the mast cell degranulation signal upon reaction of Fc-bound IgE antibody with allergen. FcεRI is a tetramer and a member of the immunoglobulin supergene family. FcεRII is a low affinity receptor also found on macrophages, lymphocytes, eosinophils, and platelets. It is not well defined chemically and is believed to be involved in control of IgE synthesis and in ADCC-mediated parasite killing. The average number of FcεRIs on a mast cell is estimated to be 10,000 to 40,000. The number of FcεRI cell-bound IgE antibody molecules determines the sensitivity of mast cells to an allergen. However, the amount of mediators released from a given cell depends on enzyme systems that regulate the biochemical mechanisms of mediator release. Antigen cross-linking two adjacent IgE molecules on the cell surface initiates events leading to mediator release (see Fig. 8–5). Mediator release may also be initiated by cross-linking IgE on the cell surface by antibodies to IgE.

PASSIVE ANAPHYLAXIS

The reaginic activity of an immunoglobulin is determined by its ability to fix to skin of the same species. If serum from a sensitive individual is passively transferred to the skin of a normal recipient, the classic wheal-and-flare reaction can be elicited at this site upon application of the antigen (Prausnitz–Kustner test). In 1921, Carl Prausnitz (The Herr Professor) and Heinz Kustner (a medical student) reported the passive transfer of anaphylactic reactions both systemically and cutaneously by injection of serum from a patient sensitive to fish into a normal individual (Mr. Kustner). Because the antibody fixes to the skin, the transfer site may be tested up to 45 days later and still elicit a positive reaction. In contrast, with local passive transfer of nonreaginic IgG antibody (passive Arthus reaction), the skin site must be tested within a few hours in order to obtain a positive reaction before the non-skin-fixing IgG antibody diffuses away (Table 14–3).

The passive transfer of atopic or anaphylactic reactions may be accomplished by a variety of methods, all of which depend upon the ability of reagins or IgE antibodies to fix to tissue mast cells. Most of these methods are now used only in experimental animals.

1. For the local passive cutaneous anaphylaxis transfer (Prausnitz–Kustner) test, antibody-containing serum is injected into the skin and after an appropriate period of time (usually several days) the same skin site is challenged with antigen.
2. For systemic passive cutaneous anaphylaxis, either the antibody is injected intravenously and the antigen intradermally or the antibody is injected intradermally and the antigen intravenously.
3. Transfer of a systemic reaction (passive systemic anaphylaxis)

TABLE 14–3. PASSIVE TRANSFER OF ANTIBODY-MEDIATED SKIN REACTIONS

	Passive Cutaneous Anaphylaxis (Prausnitz-Kustner)	Passive Cutaneous Arthus
Days after Ab transfer	Up to 90	1–2
Time after Ag challenge	15 min	5–6 hrs
Reaction	Wheal and flare	Induration and erythema
Histology	Edema and congestion Spongiosis*	Vasculitis

*Spongiosis: Intercellular epidermal edema.

is best elicited by injection of the antibody intravenously, followed by injection of the antigen intravenously 24 hours later.

4. Reverse passive cutaneous anaphylaxis may be elicited if the antigen fixes to skin; in this instance the antibody does not require tissue-fixing capacities. For reverse reactions, the antigen is injected into the skin, and after a suitable period, the antibody is injected intravenously or at the same site. Reverse tests are useful for determining the skin-fixing properties of the immunoglobulins of one species for the skin of another species.

In most species studied, the antibody that fixes to the skin of the same species (eg, human reagin fixing to human skin) belongs to a special class of immunoglobulin with properties similar to human IgE. If a given antibody in a species fixes to the skin of individuals of the same species, it is termed **homocytophilic**. In some instances, the immunoglobulins that fit tissue receptors of another species belong to a class other than IgE. For instance, human IgG antibodies may fix to guinea pig skin, but IgA, IgM, or IgE does not fix to guinea pig skin. Immunoglobulins that fix to the skin of a species different from their source are termed **heterocytophilic**.

IgE (reaginic) antibody has other properties different from usual antibody—it does not fix complement in the usual manner and its skin-fixing capacity is heat-labile (56°C for 30 minutes). IgE antibody can precipitate with antigen if sufficient amounts of antibody can be obtained. However, the amount of IgE antibody present in the serum of a sensitive individual is usually too small to be detected by precipitation but can be detected by more sensitive techniques involving the anaphylactic response.

CLINICAL ANTIBODY TESTS (IN VIVO)

Because of the unusual properties noted above, there is no simple test for reagin. The most commonly used clinical test is the skin test. Suspected allergens are injected into the skin of an individual to test for cutaneous anaphylaxis. In this way, allergenic antigens may be identified. Skin testing must be done under careful supervision because systemic anaphylactic shock may be induced. Although the incidence of severe reaction is very low (approximately 1 fatality per 2 million doses per year in the United States), antianaphylactic drugs (eg, epinephrine) must be kept on hand for rapid use, if necessary. The local transfer of skin-fixing antibody may be used to demonstrate reaginic activity in serum (passive) cutaneous anaphylaxis. This is the basis of the Prausnitz–Kustner test. This test is no longer used because of the possibility of transmitting hepatitis or HIV infection.

Another in vivo test that is extremely sensitive is bronchoprovocation. Inhalation of small amounts of the allergen will elicit acute bronchospasm (asthma). This test is only done in well-controlled settings because of the obvious danger of inducing fatal anaphylaxis.

LABORATORY TESTS (IN VITRO)

In vitro laboratory tests for specific reaginic antibody include the Schultz–Dale test, histamine release by mast cells (degranulation), and the radioallergosorbent test (RAST). The radioimmunoabsorbent test (RIST) is used to measure total serum IgE.

Schultz–Dale Test

This test utilizes organs containing smooth muscle (guinea pig intestine or rat uterus) in an organ bath. When the organ is taken from a sensitized animal or incubated with serum from a sensitized individual, contraction will occur when the specific antigen is added. The extent of this contraction may be measured with a kymograph. Contraction may also be induced by the addition of mediators (histamine, leukotrienes).

Histamine Release

Histamine release from mast cells in vitro may be induced by contact of sensitized mast cells with antigen. The amount of histamine release may be determined spectrophotometrically or by morphologic observation of mast cell degranulation. Nonsensitized mast cells may be passively sensitized by incubation with reagin-containing serum. The passive leukocyte-sensitizing (PLS) activity of a given serum is determined by incubating a reaginic serum with blood leukocytes from nonallergic donors for about 2 hours. The cells are then washed and treated with antigen for 1 hour. The amount of histamine present in the supernate is then determined photometrically. The extent of histamine release is used as an index of the serum reagin content. The PLS activity of ragweed-sensitive individuals is highest in the early fall (during the pollen season) and lowest in summer just prior to the pollen season.

Radioallergosorbent Test (RAST)

This test depends upon the binding of IgE antibody to specific antigen and the subsequent binding of radiolabeled anti-IgE to the IgE antibody–antigen complex. Fluorescent and enzyme-labeled antibodies are also being used. The suspected antigen is first covalently bound to insoluble particles, or in the case of more commonly used clinical tests, to paper discs. The insoluble antigen is then added to samples of serum. Those sera containing antibodies to the antigen will have antibody immunoglobulin that binds to the insoluble antigen. Antibody of classes other than IgE may also bind so that excess insoluble antigen is used. Antigen fixed to paper or particles are incubated with test sera, washed and reacted with a labeled antibody to IgE. The labeled anti-IgE will bind to the IgE antibody, which is bound to the insoluble antigen. By determining the amount of labeled anti-IgE bound, an estimation of the IgE antibody to the specific antigen may be made. At present, the indiscriminate use of these tests to diagnose allergy has resulted in many false-positive results that do not correlate with in vivo testing. Reliable allergists conduct careful history taking and skin testing before attempting immunotherapy.

Radioimmuno-
absorbent Test
(RIST)

For total IgE, the radioimmunoabsorbent test (RIST) is most commonly used. Sera is added to anti-IgE-coated beads so that the IgE is bound to the beads. After washing, labeled anti-IgE is added. The amount of labeled anti-IgE bound is directly proportional to the amount of IgE in the unknown serum sample.

MEDIATOR RELEASE FROM MAST CELLS

Two types of mechanisms may operate for release of mediators from mast cells or basophils: Nonlytic, in which mast cell lysosomal membranes fuse with each other and with the cell surface membrane, resulting in release of lysosomal contents (degranulation); and lytic, in which antibody–antigen complexes on the surface of mast cells bind complement components and lyse the mast cell. Nonlytic release is the usual mechanism active in anaphylactic reactions involving reaginic antibody. The mast cell is not destroyed and granules reform. Lytic release provides a mechanism whereby cytolytic allergic reactions mediated by IgG or IgM may produce anaphylactic symptoms. The mechanism by which reaction of antigen with reaginic antibody on mast cells or basophils causes the release of mediators is described in Chapter 8 (see Fig. 8–5).

Genetics

One of the most fascinating questions about atopic diseases is why some individuals make an IgE response to the same antigen to which other individuals make an IgG response or no response. Whereas some of the differences may be explained by dose, route, and number of exposures, there has long been evidence that heredity plays a major role. In 1872, Wyman reported that allergies were higher in family members than in nonallergic families but that the expression of the allergy could differ (ie, asthma, allergic rhinitis, etc.). It was concluded later that children inherit an "allergic predisposition" about equally from both parents and that the prevalence of an allergic family history is about three times greater in allergic patients than in patients with a history of a nonallergic family.

Exposure is also critical. If a genetically allergic predisposed individual is not exposed to a given allergen, or a cross-reacting allergen, then the allergy will never become manifested. For instance, in primitive villages of Papua, New Guinea, a marked increase in mite allergy (asthma) correlated with the introduction of blankets that became infested with mites. Prior to this, mite allergy was not seen in this population.

The genetic regulation of atopic responses includes specific immune response control and overall IgE synthesis regulation. It is well known that control of specific immune responses is HLA-linked, and it has been reported that individuals of HLA type DW2 tend to form IgE antibodies to ragweed pollen extract. However, a clear relationship between the propensity to form allergic responses and HLA phenotype has not been convincingly demonstrated. The compounding variable of genetic control of mast cell numbers, mast cell distribution in tissues, and mediator release illustrate the multifactorial nature of the genetics of allergic reactions.

Similarly, overall IgE levels appear to be genetically controlled, but this control is not linked to HLA. The serum IgE concentrations of pairs of monozygotic twins are significantly more similar to each other than are the levels of otherwise comparable pairs of dizygotic twins. In addition, the concept of genetic control of basal IgE levels in man is supported by statistical analysis of serum IgE levels in normal adults. It is possible, although not yet established, that genetic control of the immune responses by immune response genes may extend to the IgE immunoglobulin class; certain individuals inherit genes that select an IgE antibody response to a given antigen rather than a response with another immunoglobulin class. Elevated serum IgE levels during the first year of life frequently occur in infants who develop atopic disease later, suggesting the early expression of a genetically controlled propensity of atopic individuals to produce IgE immunoglobulin.

Atopic Allergy

Atopic allergy is a term applied to a group of chronic human allergies to natural antigens, including asthma, hay fever, allergic rhinitis, urticaria (hives), eczema, serous otitis media, conjunctivitis, and food allergy. The mechanisms are essentially the same as those involved in systemic and cutaneous anaphylaxis. Anaphylaxis is included by many under the general term of "atopy."

CLINICAL FEATURES

The clinical features of atopic allergy are itching and whealing, sneezing, and respiratory embarrassment. The pathologic features include edema, smooth muscle contraction, and leukopenia. The pharmacologic characteristics are repeated episodes of histamine release and partial protection by antihistamines, as well as involvement of leukotrienes and prostaglandins. The type of reaction seen clinically depends upon four factors, described below:

Route of Access of Antigen

If contact occurs via the skin, hives (wheal and flare) predominate; if contact is via respiratory mucous membranes, asthma and rhinitis occur; if contact occurs via the eyes, conjunctivitis will predominate, or if through the ears, serous otitis media; if contact occurs via the gastrointestinal tract, food allergy, with cramps, nausea, vomiting, and diarrhea results.

Dose of Antigen

The rarity of death from most atopic allergies, in contrast to anaphylaxis, is most likely because of the dose and route of access of the antigen. In systemic anaphylaxis, inadvertent large doses of antigen are usually given intravenously; in atopic allergy, the doses are low, and contact is across mucous membranes. Such a conclusion is justified by the observation that anaphylactically sensitized guinea pigs exposed to small amounts of antigen by inhalation develop typical asthmatic symptoms. However, in highly sensitive individuals, minute doses of allergen may elicit fatal reactions, and in sensitized individuals injected with relatively large doses of allergen in the form of drugs, severe—sometimes fatal—anaphylactic reactions are likely.

"The Shock Organ"

Individual differences in reactivity depend upon individual idiosyncrasy, pharmacologic abnormality of the target tissue (increased numbers of mast cells or increased H receptors on target organs), or increased susceptibility of a given organ because of nonspecific irritation or inflammation. Many affected individuals commonly have an atopic reaction involving one organ system (asthma) without involvement of other organs.

Anaphylaxis

Anaphylaxis is edema and congestion that may occur locally (cutaneous anaphylaxis) or a systemic shock reaction (systemic anaphylactic shock).

CUTANEOUS ANAPHYLAXIS

Cutaneous anaphylaxis (urticaria, wheal and flare, hives) is elicited in a sensitive individual by skin test (scratch or intradermal injection of antigen). Grossly visible manifestations are: a pale, soft, raised wheal; pseudopods; and a spreading flare, reaching a maximum in 15 to 20 minutes and fading in a few hours. Itching is prominent early, there is edema, with essentially no cellular infiltration until 12 to 18 hours later. The mechanism is the same as in systemic anaphylaxis, but the reaction is localized because of antibody fixation in the skin and release of histamine or histaminelike substances into the skin, with local changes in vascular permeability. Cutaneous anaphylaxis should be differentiated from the Arthus reaction in terms of both time of appearance and morphology of the reaction (see Table 14–3).

SYSTEMIC ANAPHYLAXIS

Systemic anaphylaxis, or anaphylactic shock, is a generalized reaction elicited in a sensitized animal by the intravenous injection of antigen or in a human by natural exposure or iatrogenic injection of an allergen. It was discovered in 1902 following the injection of an extract of sea anemone into a dog. The injection was tolerated the first time but caused sudden death when injected into the same dog several weeks later. The use of horse serum as diphtheria antitoxin produced anaphylactic shock in humans, and resulted in a renewed interest in anaphylaxis. This interest has been renewed again by the number of such reactions to antilymphocyte globulin used to suppress transplantation rejection, to penicillin, and to other drugs, including chymopapain, used to digest the nucleus pulposus of herniated intervertebral disks. In highly sensitive individuals, a severe systemic reaction to small doses of the allergen placed on the skin (scratch or patch test) may occur. For this reason, the clinical allergist must be prepared to administer epinephrine (β-adrenergic stimulation) to any patient during skin testing. This counteracts the systemic effects of the anaphylactic reaction. The nature of the systemic reaction is species-dependent. In all species, bronchial and gastrointestinal smooth muscle contraction is prominent, as well as are increased permeability of small vessels, leukopenia, fall in temperature, hypotension, slowing of the heart rate, and decreased serum complement levels. However, different species have somewhat different fatal systemic anaphylactic reactions.

Guinea pig: Death occurs in 2 to 5 minutes, with prostration, convulsions, respiratory embarrassment, involuntary urination, defecation, itching, sneezing, and coughing. At autopsy, the lungs are inflated because of bronchiolar constriction with air trapping.

Rabbit: Death occurs in minutes; the course is similar in other respects to that in the guinea pig, except for the absence of respiratory difficulty. Autopsy shows right-heart failure attributed to obstruction of the pulmonary circulation.

Dog: Death occurs after 1 to 2 hours. There is a profound prostration with vomiting and bloody diarrhea, as well as liver engorgement from hepatic vein obstruction.

Rat: Death occurs in 30 minutes to 5 hours. There is congestion of the small intestine, and midzonal and periportal necrosis of the liver.

Man: Man exhibits a combination of the above reactions; death is not common but may occur upon exposure to high levels of the allergen. For instance, the description of systemic anaphylaxis by Prausnitz and Kustner after skin injection of fish muscle extract into a patient with fish allergy in 1921 is as follows:

"After half an hour: itching of the scalp, neck, lower abdomen, dry sensation in the throat; soon afterwards swelling and congestion of the conjunctivae, severe congestion and secretion of the respiratory mucous membranes, intense fits of sneezing, irritating cough, hoarseness merging into aphonia, and marked inspiratory dyspnoea. The skin of the entire body, especially the face, becomes highly hyperemic, and all over the skin of the body there appear numerous very itching wheals, 1 to 2 cm large, which show a marked tendency to confluence. Increased perspiration has not been noted. After about 2 hours heavy salivation starts and is followed by vomiting, after which the symptoms very gradually fade away. Temperature, cardiac and renal function have always been normal. After 10 or 12 hours all the symptoms have disappeared; only a feeling of debility persists for a day or so. After each attack there is a period of oliguria and constipation; this may be due to dehydration and vomiting."

Circulatory shock with dizziness and faintness may be the only manifestation, but collapse, unconsciousness, and death can occur within 16 to 120 minutes. There is obstruction and edema of the upper respiratory tract, laryngeal edema, and increased eosinophils in the sinusoids of the spleen and liver. Acute systemic anaphylaxis in man is often iatrogenic, ie, produced by injection of drugs (penicillin) or biologics (gamma globulin), but can occur naturally following insect (bee, wasp) stings.

Asthma

The word **asthma** is from the Greek *asthma*, meaning panting, a general term for difficulty in breathing. The problem was believed by Galen to be caused by secretions dripping from the brain into the lung: "Phlegm doth fall upon the lung." This, as well as other errors of Galen's concepts, were not disproved until the 17th century. Clinically, asthma must be differentiated from chronic bronchitis and emphysema. Asthma presents clinically as reversible acute respiratory distress from airway obstruction, presumably caused by constriction of the smooth muscles of the small bronchi and mucous secretion. Osler described presentation "with a distressing sense of want of breath and a feeling of great oppression of the chest. Soon the respiratory efforts become violent, and all of the accessory muscles are brought into play. In a few minutes the patient is in a paroxysm of the most intense dyspnea." After a gradual decline, the incidence of mortality due to asthma has been increasing since the mid-1980s. The reason for this increase is not clear. Some factors considered are air pollution or indoor living related to urban environment, overuse of β_2-agonists (see below), and changed therapy.

PREDISPOSING FACTORS

A number of factors predispose to development of allergic asthma, the most important being repeated exposure to the allergen. Other correlations with an allergic proclivity are listed in Table 14–4. There are at least two forms of asthma: One clearly mediated by the anaphylactic mechanism and one that is not mediated by known immune reactions. The immune-mediated (allergic) form is caused by the activation of effector cells (mast cells) sensitized by IgE antibody. Allergic asthma is termed extrinsic because of the clear identification of an exogenous eliciting antigen in most cases. The mechanism of activation of the nonallergic form of asthma is not well understood but is probably due to an imbalance of the physiologic control of smooth muscle tone (see Fig. 14-3 below). Immune mechanisms are not believed to be involved,

TABLE 14–4. FACTORS BELIEVED TO PREDISPOSE TO DEVELOPMENT OF ALLERGIC DISEASE

1. Heredity—positive family history (HLA-DW$_2$)
2. Prenatal effects (high cord blood IgE levels, prenatal exposure to allergens)
3. High postnatal IgE serum level
4. Birth during pollen season
5. Birth in urban environment
6. Stressful perinatal period
7. Early exposure to eggs, wheat, and bovine products (cows milk versus breast feeding)
8. Low serum IgA levels at three months of age
9. Low levels of T lymphocytes at three months of age
10. Early surgery or hospitalization
11. Exposure to animals, molds, tobacco smoke, and pollen
12. Frequent infections

Items 4, 5, 6, and 10 are questionable!

Modified from Johnston DE: Some aspects of the natural history of asthma. *Ann Allergy* 49:257, 1982.

and a specific eliciting antigen cannot be identified. Drugs that block β-adrenergic effects used for treatment of angina pectoris, cardiac arrhythmias, hypertension, glaucoma, migraine headache, and other diseases are contraindicated in patients with bronchial asthma.

Intrinsic asthma is manifested as chronic recurrent asthma attacks without a clearly identifiable exposure to an antigen. This may be because the antigen is just not detectable or because there is no antigen (nonimmune asthma). One possible explanation is that intrinsic asthma is caused by sensitivity to a chronic infecting organism, but proof of this hypothesis is lacking. Extrinsic allergic asthma is usually seasonal, although it is year-round in parts of the world where pollen allergens are present for most of the year (eg, Bermuda grass pollen in Southern California), or if nonpollen allergens such as animal dander are responsible. Occasional outbreaks of asthma may be associated with the sudden release of an allergen. Since 1981, twenty-six outbreaks of asthma have occurred in Barcelona, Spain, affecting 687 persons. The outbreaks have been traced to inhalation of soybean dust released during the unloading of soybeans at the city harbor. In contrast, intrinsic asthma occurs throughout the year without seasonal exception. A condition of intrinsic asthma may evolve from a background of seasonal asthma or from a nonatopic background of chronic bronchitis. In addition, a wide variety of agents has been identified as causing work-related asthma in selected populations (Table 14–5). For example, isocyanates, such as toluene diisocyanate used as an industrial solvent, may be the principal cause of occupational asthma in the Western world. IgE antibody has been detected in some affected workers. An increasing problem for medical workers is allergic reactions to latex

TABLE 14–5. AGENTS CAUSING ASTHMA IN SELECTED OCCUPATIONS

Occupation or Occupational Field	Agent
Laboratory animal workers, veterinarians	Dander, urine proteins
Food processing	Shellfish, egg proteins, pancreatic enzymes, papain, amylase
Dairy farmers	Storage mites
Poultry farmers	Poultry mites, droppings, feathers
Granary workers	Storage mites, aspergillus, indoor ragweed, grass pollen
Research workers	Locusts
Fish-food manufacturing	Midges
Detergent manufacturing	*Bacillus subtilis* enzymes
Silk workers	Silkworm moths and larvae
Plant Proteins	
Bakers	Flour amylase
Food processing	Coffee bean dust, meat tenderizer (papain), tea
Farmers	Soy bean dust
Shipping workers	Grain dust (molds, insects, grain)
Laxative manufacturing	Ispaghula, psyllium
Sawmill workers, carpenters	Wood dust (western red cedar, oak, mahogany, zebrawood, redwood, Lebanon cedar, African maple, eastern white cedar)
Electric soldering	Colophony (pine resin)
Cotton textile workers	Cotton dust
Nurses	Psyllium, latex
Inorganic Chemicals	
Refinery workers	Platinum salts, vanadium
Plating	Nickel salts
Diamond polishing	Cobalt salts
Manufacturing	Aluminum fluoride
Beauty shop workers	Persulfate
Welding	Stainless steel fumes, chromium salts
Organic Chemicals	
Manufacturing	Antibiotics, piperazine, methyldopa, salbutamol, cimetidine
Hospital workers	Disinfectants (sulfathiazole, chloramine, formaldehyde, glutaraldehyde)
Anesthesiology	Enflurane
Poultry workers	Aprolium
Fur dyeing	Paraphenylene diamine
Rubber processing	Formaldehyde, ethylene diamine, phthalic anhydride
Plastics industry	Toluene diisocyanate, hexamethyl diisocyanate, dephenylmethyl isocyanate, phthalic anhydride, triethylene tetramines, trimellitic anhydride, hexamethyl tetramine
Automobile painting	Dimethyl ethanolamine diisocyanate
Foundry workers	Reaction product of furan binder

From International Consensus Report on Diagnosis and Treatment of Asthma. NHLBI, US Dept. of Health and Human Services Pub. No. 92-3091, 1992.

resulting from increased use of latex gloves for protection against HIV transmission.

NONIMMUNE ASTHMA

Constriction of bronchial smooth muscle may be triggered by a variety of nonimmune mechanisms, including chemical irritation, change in temperature, physical activity, and emotional stress, as well as by a variety of respiratory infections. In cases of nonimmune asthma, no exogenous eliciting antigen can be identified, and no IgE antibodies may be demonstrated. One form is caused by exposure to aspirin and other nonsteroidal antiinflammatory agents through blocking of the cyclooxygenase pathway for metabolism of arachidonic acid and increased production of leukotrienes, which cause chronic airway inflammation and bronchial constriction. As stated above, it is believed that chronic inflammation with infiltration of the bronchial mucosa with inflammatory cells and hyperplasia of bronchial smooth muscle leads to a lowering of the threshold for a bronchospastic response to a variety of stimuli.

PATHOLOGIC CHANGES

A number of pathologic changes have been found in the lungs of patients with either type of asthma. In the acute attack, which may be fatal because of acute asphyxiation, there is marked constriction of the bronchi and occlusion of the bronchi with a particularly thick mucous secretion (mucous plugs). In chronic asthma, the pulmonary changes are:

1. Marked thickening of the basement membrane of the bronchial mucosa.
2. Hypertrophy of the bronchial smooth muscle.
3. Hypertrophy of the bronchial mucous glands.
4. Eosinophils, chronic inflammatory cells in the bronchial wall, with a substantial increase over normal in the number of mast cells.
5. The presence of mucous in the bronchi containing large numbers of eosinophilic leukocytes.

In addition, T cells are prominent in the lung of chronic asthmatics. The thickened basement membrane may contain deposits of IgG or IgM, but IgE has not been detected often. Eosinophil degranulation may contribute to epithelial desquamation. Other stigmata of chronic inflammation and airway obstruction not specific for asthma, including focal fibrosis and scarring, emphysema, and atelectasis, may be found in the periphery of the lung. Since repeated asthma attacks are also associated with increased susceptibility to pulmonary infections, some of the pathologic changes may be because of repeated bronchopneumonia. Mild asthmatics have histologic changes similar to those with severe asthma but to a lesser degree. It is now possible to follow patients with mild asthma using endobronchial biopsies and monitoring the degree of inflammation. If inflammation persists, treatment with antiinflammatory drugs may be warranted even though there are no immediate symptoms.

THERAPY

The increasing incidence of asthma has stimulated the formation of an international asthma management committee, which has recommended a six-part program treatment:

1. Educate patient to develop a partnership in asthma management.
2. Assess and monitor asthma severity with objective measures of lung function.
3. Avoid or control asthma triggers.
4. Establish medication plans for chronic management.
5. Establish plans for managing exacerbations.
6. Provide regular follow-up care.

This therapy program emphasizes three critical aspects of asthma: (1) Determining the extent of the disease and the motivation of the patient to control the manifestations; (2) to attempt to limit predisposing inflammation; and (3) to identify the specific allergen.

Specific therapy for asthma depends on whether or not a specific eliciting antigen can be identified. If it can, the best treatment is avoidance of the antigen. Immunotherapy by injection of the antigen in a manner that will change the reactivity of the patient may also be successful. Drugs that produce bronchodilation or that alter the state of activation of effector mast cells may be effective in both extrinsic and intrinsic allergy, and prompt administration by aerosol or injection may be required to prevent death in an acute attack. Inhibition of production of leukotrienes by 5-lipoxygenase inhibitors, such as A64077, may decrease airway hyperresponsiveness that predisposes to asthma attacks. Psychotherapy may be effective in some cases because the extent of a given attack may be increased by anxiety; the frequency of asthma is higher for individuals in emotional distress. Breathing exercises may reduce symptoms, especially in growing children. Intermittent short-term steroid therapy (up to 7 days) will produce dramatic relief of severe asthmatic symptoms (see below). On the other hand, long-term steroid administration may lead to secondary adrenal insufficiency, which at times of stress may be fatal in patients with otherwise severe but controlled asthma. In addition, all antiasthmatic medications have the potential to produce life-threatening reactions. For instance, aerosol bronchodilators (primarily β_2-adrenergic agonists) and theophylline together may produce significant cardiovascular effects. A more comprehensive discussion of the prevention and treatment of allergic reactions is presented below.

The following is recommended by the International Consensus Report on Asthma Treatment (NIH Pub. No. 92-3091, 1992):

1. Mild asthma: Inhalant β_2-agonist as needed; oral cromolyn.
2. Moderate asthma: Add antiinflammatory agents (Nedocromil); inhalant low-dose steroid as required; theophylline, if needed.
3. Severe asthma: High-dose steroids.

ALLERGIC ASPERGILLOSIS

An acute form of infective asthma may occur in persons with *Aspergillus* infection. *Aspergillus* is a mold, which may cause a pulmonary infection. A small number of individuals with pulmonary aspergillosis develop allergy to the infecting agent; this causes obstruction of the involved bronchi with mucous plugs (bronchopulmonary impaction). This disease is presented in more detail in Chapter 25.

Atopic Reactions

HAY FEVER (SEASONAL ALLERGIC RHINITIS)

Seasonal upper respiratory reactions to pollen are commonly referred to as hay fever. Perennial allergic rhinitis is caused by animal danders, house dust, house dust mites, and molds that cause a reaction in the nasal passages and eyes of affected individuals. In temperate climates, seasonal allergic rhinitis is caused by nonflowering, wind-pollinated plants. Larger pollen particles (>10 μm) are efficiently filtered out by the nasal mucosa and cause rhinitis, whereas smaller particles (< 1 to 2 μm) pass into the tracheobronchial tree and cause asthma. Hay fever symptoms include sneezing, nasal congestion, watery discharge from the eye, conjunctival itching, and cough with mild bronchoconstriction. Similar symptoms may be exhibited with **vasomotor rhinitis**, caused by parasympathetic hyperactivity, a foreign body, and infection—in particular, the common cold. The diagnosis is usually made by history of nasal itching, sneezing, nasal discharge, and difficulty breathing, particularly during the pollen season. A calendar of some common airborne allergens is shown in Table 14–6.

Examination of the allergic rhinitis patient may reveal a transverse wrinkle across the middle of the nose caused by the **allergic salute**. The allergic salute is delivered by placing the palm of the hand against the tip of the nose and pushing up. This is done to relieve the obstruction to the nasal air passages caused by allergic rhinitis. Pathologic changes are not extensive. Usually, there is edema of the submucosal tissue with an infiltration of eosinophils that is reversible. The degree of reaction and severity of symptoms are directly related to the amount of exposure to the allergen responsible. The lesion is caused by release of mediators from mast cells in the nasal mucosa,

TABLE 14–6. CALENDAR OF SOME COMMON AIRBORNE ALLERGENS IN A TEMPERATE CLIMATE.

Allergen	February	March	April	May	June	July	August	September
Alder, hazel	----------	----------						
Oak, ash, poplar		----------	----------					
Plane, birch			----------	----------				
Mixed grasses				----------	----------	----------		
Nettle					----------		----------	----------
Plantain, mugwort						----------	----------	
Cladosporium					----------	----------	----------	----------
Alternaria						----------	----------	----------
Ragweed							----------	----------

The timing of allergen exposure will vary with climate.

Modified from Howarth PH: Allergic rhinitis: A rational choice of treatment. *Respir Med* 83:179, 1989.

histamine, serotonin, eosinophil, and neutrophil chemotactic factors and mast cell proteases, as well as newly formed membrane-derived lipid mediators, such as prostaglandin-D_2 and other arachidonic acid metabolites (Table 14–7). These mediators produce vasodilation, mucosal edema, mucous secretion, stimulation of itch receptors, and reduction in the threshold for sneezing. The most effective approach to prevent allergic rhinitis is avoidance of the allergen, if possible. Repeated episodes of rhinitis leads to increased numbers of mast cells in the nasal mucosa and establishment of a state of nasal hyperresponsiveness to provoking stimuli. Treatment consists of antihistamines, H_1 receptor blockers (eg, Astemizole), adrenergic drugs which produce vasoconstriction (xylometazoline or oxymetazoline), disodium cromoglycate (reduces mast cell mediator release), and topical glucocorticoids administered by aerosol (beclomethasone, flunisolide, etc.). Steroids may take several days or a week to produce effects, but are usually more effective than disodium cromoglycate or antihistamines. Specific immunotherapy (see below) may be effective if the allergen has been identified and is available but is usually reserved for those patients whose symptoms are poorly controlled by optimal medical management. Psychological factors may determine the degree of discomfort considerably. Hay fever may progress to asthma but usually the severity of symptoms gradually diminishes with aging.

NASAL POLYPS

Nasal polyps are tumorlike masses that form in the nasal air passages, causing chronic airway obstruction and rendering nasal breathing very difficult or impossible. These masses can be removed surgically but usually recur promptly. The relationship between nasal polyps and allergic rhinitis is uncertain; they are frequently found in patients with perennial rhinitis. There is some evidence that chronic rhinitis and

TABLE 14–7. MEDIATORS AND SYMPTOMS OF ALLERGIC RHINITIS

Symptom	Pathology	Proposed Mediators
Pruritus	Sensory nerve stimulation	Histamine (H_1) prostaglandins
Obstruction	Mucosal edema due to vascular permeability and vasodilation	Histamine (H_1) kinins, LTC_4, LTD_4, LTE_4, TNF-α, neuropeptides (calcitonin gene-related peptide; substance P)
Sneezing	Sensory nerve stimulation	Histamine (H_1) LTC_4, LTD_4, LTE_4
Rhinorrhea	Mucous secretion	Histamine (muscarinic reflex), LTC_4, LTD_4, LTE_4, substance P, vasoactive intestinal polypeptide
Hyperreactivity and prolonged congestion	Late-phase reaction	Cytokines (IL-1, IL-5, IL-6, IL-8, and TNF-α), eicosanoids

Modified from White MV, Kaliner MA: Mediators of allergic rhinitis. *J Allerg Clin Immunol* 90:699–704, 1992.

sinusitis, as well as polyps, may be caused by bacterial allergy. Nasal polyps characteristically show marked edema, swelling of hydrophilic ground substance, and scattered eosinophilic infiltration. Eosinophilic polymorphonuclear leukocytes are associated with severe persistent allergic rhinitis, and it has been suggested that persistent contact with small amounts of antigen leads to the characteristic picture. The prolonged nature of the swelling may be explained by continued production of hydrophilic ground substance by tissue fibroblasts.

FOOD ALLERGY

Ingestion of allergens may lead to remarkable gastrointestinal (GI) reactions known collectively as food allergy. The relationship of the GI reaction to atopic sensitivity is not clear. Many individuals with positive skin reactions to an allergen react to ingestion of the allergen, whereas individuals with repeated episodes of vomiting or diarrhea that occur on eating a given food may not produce a skin reaction to the food. Food allergens are most likely to be those that survive the process of digestion (Table 14–8), or to drugs added to foods as preservatives. Allergy to cow's milk is the most frequently suspected GI reaction to food in infants. Milk contains over sixteen proteins that might be allergenic, and skin reactions to a number of these proteins occur in some sensitive children. It is thought that intact milk proteins are more likely to pass through the child's intestine than the adult's. In addition, unsuspected bovine food additives, such as penicillin, may be present in milk and elicit allergic reactions. Food allergy may lead to hypoproteinemia from the loss of protein in the GI tract and persistent diarrhea. Other manifestations of food allergy are extensive skin eruptions (urticaria or eczema) or systemic shock. Avoidance of the allergen is the primary therapy, and artificial diets are sometimes required to prevent food allergy reactions. Individuals with known severe food allergy

TABLE 14–8. SOME PURIFIED WATER-SOLUBLE FOOD ANTIGENS

Allergen	Source	MW	Composition	Characteristics
Antigen M	Codfish	12,328	113 amino acids to one glucose	A parvalbulin, chelates calcium acid and protease resistant
Antigen II	Shrimp	38,000	96% protein	Heat stable
Peanut I	Peanut		91% protein	acid and protease resistant
Trypsin inhibitor	Soybean	20,500	Polypeptide	acid and protease resistant

Modified from Metcalfe DD, Sampter M, Condemi JJ: Reactions to foods. In *Immunological Diseases*. Sampter M, et al. (eds.). Boston: Little, Brown, 1988, 1165.

should carry epinephrine and be instructed on how to use it if an anaphylactic attack is imminent. It has been recognized for many years that breast feeding results in a dramatic reduction in the incidence of food allergy in children, particularly allergic eczema.

INSECT ALLERGY

Atopic or anaphylactic reactions to insects may be divided into three types: Inhalant or contact reactions to insect body parts or products (mites) skin reactions (wheal and flare) to biting insects, and systemic shock reactions to stinging insects. Asthmatic or hay fever-like reactions may occur following airborne exposure of a sensitive individual to large numbers of insects or their body parts. This happens outdoors to insects that periodically appear in large numbers, such as locusts or grasshoppers, and indoors, more chronically, to beetles, flies, and spiders. IgE antibody in individuals with insect allergy reacts most frequently with gastrointestinal epithelium.

Bites

Biting insects may produce delayed hypersensitivity or acute wheal-and-flare skin reactions. A delayed reaction to insect bite may convert to an anaphylactic one with aging of the individual. The common reaction to a mosquito or flea bite is a localized cutaneous anaphylactic reaction. Although allergy may play a role, it is thought that local release of histamine triggered by the bite is the cause of such reactions. Delayed hypersensitivity reactions to mosquito bites may also occur. Serious effects of a reaction to biting insects may occur in parts of the world where large numbers of mosquitoes appear in waves; multiple mosquito bites to a sensitive individual may produce systemic effects.

Stings

Fatalities occur more frequently from stinging insects, such as bees and wasps. More people die each year as a result of being stung by an insect than from being bitten by a snake—about forty documented deaths in the United States per year. Deaths from stinging insects are caused by systemic anaphylaxis and usually occur within 1 hour of being stung. Therefore, immediate therapy is required. This may be provided by injection of epinephrine (see below). Immunotherapy may prevent subsequent severe reactions. People who raise bees may permit a bee to sting them and limit the amount of venom injected; by increasing the amount on subsequent stings, the degree of reaction to a larger dose becomes less. The amount of protein material injected in a sting is actually very small; about 50 μg for a honeybee and 2 to 20 μg for a wasp.

The venom of honeybees and wasps contains a number of biologically active agents, such as histamine, serotonin, and other biologic amines that directly produce vascular reactions, as well as phospholipase, hyaluronidase, and acid phosphatase. The peptides include melittin, which has a unique amipathic structure that incorporates into biomembranes; apamin, which blocks Ca^{++} dependent ion channels; and mast cell degranulating peptide, which causes release of histamine. The main ingredient of fire ant venom is phospholipase. The venom itself produces a marked acute and delayed inflammatory reaction that may be magnified by an allergic reaction to the venom. Most of the insect venom allergens are proteins of 20 to 50 kD and cross-react with similar proteins of other species (Table 14–9). It is possible that some susceptible people are sensitized to cross-reacting antigens and then react to minute doses of these antigens in insect venom.

Protective Role of Anaphylactic Reactions to Insects

It is not clear what survival advantage these acute allergic reactions to insect bites and stings provide. It has been postulated that the reaction induces immediate avoidance behavior and may limit the exposure of a bitten individual to a dose of a toxic venom that could be even more damaging. On the other hand, a systemic anaphylactic reaction to an insect sting may be interpreted as an immune mechanism that should be protective but is instead deleterious and potentially fatal.

TABLE 14–9. SOME ARTHROPOD ALLERGENS AND COMMON PROTEINS OF KNOWN SEQUENCE SIMILARITY OR ANTIGEN CROSS-REACTIVITY

Venom Allergens	Other Proteins
Honeybee phospholipase A_2	Bovine, porcine, and human pancreatic phospholipase A_2
Honeybee venom melittin	Calmodulin-binding protein, phospholipase A_2 stimulating protein
Hornet venom antigen 5	Tobacco and tomato leaf pathogenesis related protein
Major mite antigen	Human cathepsin B and other cysteine proteases
Midge antigen	Human hemoglobin alpha chain

Modified from King TP: Insect venom allergens. *Monogr Allergy* 28:84, 1990.

ATOPIC ECZEMA-ATOPIC DERMATITIS

In 1892, Brocq and Besnier described a familial, pruritic skin disease beginning in infancy and often occurring in association with hay fever and asthma. The term **atopic dermatitis** was coined by Wise and Sulzberger in 1933. Eczema refers to the weeping phase of early lesions; dermatitis refers to the more chronic dry, hyperkeratotic lesions. Atopic dermatitis is a chronic skin eruption of varied etiology that usually occurs in young individuals who develop atopic reactions (asthma or hay fever) at a later age. In children, the typical lesions are located in the antecubital and popliteal areas, with variable involvement of the neck, wrist, and ankles. The pathologic changes in the skin are consistent with those of a severe contact dermatitis (see Chapter 15). Erythema, papules, and vesicles are accompanied by intense pruritus. There is perivascular accumulation of mononuclear cells, followed by infiltration into the epidermis with epidermal spongiosis. As the affected child becomes older, thickening of the skin of the affected areas occurs (lichenification). Atopic dermatitis features thickened patches with frequent, acute itching episodes. Identification of an antigen that elicits the eczema is very difficult, but in some cases there is evidence that the antigens are those that also elicit other allergic reactions (pollen, house dust, animal dander). Atopic eczema is morphologically more like a reaction of cellular or delayed hypersensitivity but is discussed here because of its association with atopic conditions.

The pathogenic mechanism of atopic dermatitis remains unclear. Patients with atopic dermatitis will produce wheal-and-flare reactions when challenged with allergen, and this reactivity is IgE-mediated. On the other hand, cutaneous antigen exposure does not elicit the skin lesion characteristic of atopic dermatitis. Atopic dermatitis patients frequently have increased delayed hypersensitivity skin reactivity and decreased in vitro blast transformation responses to various test antigens; thus, it has been suggested that atopic dermatitis is caused by increased anaphylactic activity due to a lack of T-suppressor cells. The role of certain food allergies in accentuation of severe eczema has been found in double-blind food challenges.

An allergic etiology of all eczema must be questioned because typical eczema may occur in children with severe combined immune deficiency. Therefore, although proven eczema of atopic allergic origin exists, eczemalike (eczematoid) skin lesions may be produced in other ways. An abnormality in the activation, production, or inactivation of arachidonic acid metabolites has been considered as possibilities.

ASPIRIN INTOLERANCE

Aspirin, one of the world's most widely used drugs, was once generally thought to be almost completely devoid of undesirable effects when used within a therapeutic dose range. However, it is now known to be responsible for a variety of atopic and anaphylactic reactions, including asthma, rhinitis, nasal polyps, and even anaphylactic shock.

Aspirin intolerance may develop in children or appear in adults with no previous history of atopy. In adults, the symptoms of aspirin intolerance appear suddenly with a watery rhinorrhea, followed by development of nasal polyps, chronic asthma, and in some cases even shock reactions to ingestion of aspirin. The chronic asthma related to aspirin intolerance responds well to drug therapy, but, of course, avoidance of aspirin is the obvious treatment. This is easier said than done, because aspirin is included in many drug mixtures where it is unsuspected, and other cross-reacting haptens may elicit reactions in aspirin-sensitive individuals. Yellow food color number 5 contains such a related hapten. Desensitization to aspirin intolerance can be obtained by giving small doses of aspirin until symptoms disappear and then increasing dosage. This happens in all aspirin-sensitive individuals but is reversible and must be maintained by daily aspirin treatment.

Aspirin and widely different nonsteroidal antiinflammatory drugs (NSAIDs) act through a common pharmacologic mechanism, ie, inhibition of cyclooxygenase. The dose of drug required to elicit sensitivity is directly related to its ability to cause this inhibition. The present hypotheses regarding the mechanism of aspirin sensitivity are based on this action. One idea is that these drugs produce a relative deficiency in cyclooxygenase products, so that PGE_2 (bronchodilator) is produced relatively less than $PGF_{2\alpha}$ (bronchoconstrictor). Although such an imbalance in effect has not been demonstrated with aspirin treatment, this idea is supported by the recent observation that inhibition of thromboxane synthase, which does not decrease PGE_2 synthesis, does not induce asthma in aspirin-sensitive individuals. Another idea is that inhibition of the cyclooxygenase pathway diverts arachidonic acid metabolism to the 5-lipoxygenase pathway and production of bronchoconstrictive leukotrienes. This mechanism does not explain why aspirin sensitivity is limited to a subpopulation of asthmatic patients. Although an accepted mechanism has not yet been found, it appears likely that some individuals have an increased sensitivity to inhibition of cyclooxygenase, perhaps because of inflammation of the bronchi such as caused by a virus infection, that predisposes them to aspirin sensitivity. Further understanding of the interaction of cyclooxygenase inhibition and inflammatory cells, such as platelets, mast cells, and eosinophils may provide a better explanation of the mechanism of aspirin intolerance than is now available. See Chapter 19 for further discussion of aspirin intolerance.

Urticaria and Angioedema

Urticaria is a condition of red or pale, itchy, edematous swellings of the skin (hives), usually short-lived; **angioedema** is a more extensive swelling of the subcutaneous tissues and mucous membranes. Urticaria and angioedema may coexist and are believed to have similar mechanisms. The types of urticaria and angioedema may be arbitrarily classified as physical (see Anaphylactoid Reactions, below), immunological, hereditary, or idiopathic. Urticaria (hives) is usually due to release of mediators from mast cells as a result of allergen reacting with IgE-bound antibody, by bites of insects, by physical trauma (dermatographia), by exercise, heat, cold, sunlight, etc. Angioedema is a diffuse pale swelling of the skin or mucous membrane that may be associated with other forms of allergic reactions. Some of the more common physically induced urticarial and angioedema reactions are listed in Table 14–10. In some cases, these are caused by physical stimulation, inducing antigens that react with IgE; in others, there is increased numbers or sensitivity of mast cells or increased parasympathetic stimulation; in others, the etiology is not immunological or is unknown.

ANAPHYLAC-TOID REACTIONS

Any event causing histamine release may cause atopic symptoms that may be confused with a true allergic reaction. Anaphylactoid shock is produced in normal (nonimmune) animals by injection of a variety of agents capable of releasing histamine or activating arachidonic acid metabolism without the mediation of an antigen–antibody reaction.

TABLE 14–10. MAJOR URTICARIAL AND ANGIOEDEMATOUS REACTIONS INDUCED BY PHYSICAL STIMULI

Physical Agent	Immunological Findings	Pathophysiology
Cold		
Idiopathic	IgE-dependent passive transfer, ? Cold-induced skin antigen	Histamine, PDG_2, edema, urticaria
	IgG, IgM, auto-anti-IgE	
Cryoprotein	Cold-dependent autoantibodies	Anaphylatoxin, vasculitis, edema
Others	None consistent	Histamine, edema
Exercise		
Urticaria	Increased acetylcholine receptors (cholinergic)	Parasympathetic activation of cholinergic nerves, histamine, etc.
Anaphylaxis	? Food allergy	Increased lung mast cells, histamine
Heat	? Heat-induced autoantigen	Histamine, urticaria
Pressure		
Dermatographia	50% IgE-dependent	Histamine, increased mast cells
Delayed	None	Histamine, ? kinins, vasculitis
Solar	IgE transferrable non-IgE, complement activation	? Sun activated antigen, histamine, porphyrin photosensitization

The resulting clinical, physiologic, and pathologic picture is virtually indistinguishable from true anaphylaxis but is not produced by immune reaction. Physical agents (heat, cold), trauma (dermatographia), emotional disturbances, or exercise may evoke pharmacologic mechanisms that mimic allergic reactions. However, there is increasingly convincing evidence that most of these reactions are IgE-mediated. Dermatographia literally means "writing on the skin." Stroking the skin results in whealing at the contact points of the stroke. Pressure urticaria is closely related. Swelling may occur at the wrists or ankles if tight clothing is worn, or over the buttocks if the individual sits for long periods of time. Dermatographia and pressure urticaria may be caused by the release of anaphylactic mediators from mast cells by a degree of physical trauma that does not induce a reaction in normal individuals. In at least 50% of cases, passive-transfer studies have demonstrated an IgE-dependent mechanism. However, such a reaction may confuse the results of skin testing because a wheal may result from insertion of a needle alone. In some patients, a reaction to a physical agent may actually have an immune basis. A physical agent may cause release or production of altered tissue antigens to which a patient is sensitive. The reaction of idiopathic cold urticaria may be transferred with IgE from many patients, and it is possible that this reaction is caused by reaction of an IgE autoantibody to a cold-dependent skin antigen. Reactions to light (photoallergy) may be caused by agents activated by sunlight that are applied to the skin to form haptens. Such reactions are usually contact dermatitis reactions (see Chapter 15). Cholinergic urticaria is believed to be produced by an abnormal response to acetylcholine released from efferent nerves after emotional stress, physical activity, or trauma. Cholinesterase levels of the skin may be reduced in cholinergic urticaria, leading to prolonged survival of acetylcholine that may act to release histamine from tissue mast cells.

The clinical findings in an atopic reaction are often confused by associated nonimmune factors. Thus, asthma is frequently complicated by infection or bronchiectasis that may overshadow the allergic condition. The severity and duration of asthmatic attacks may be greatly influenced by psychologic conditions, and typical attacks may occur because of emotional stress with no known contact with an allergen. These anaphylactoid reactions may be mediated by nonimmunologic mediator release, an imbalance of the sympathetic nervous system or hyperreactivity of end organ smooth muscles.

HEREDITARY ANGIOEDEMA

Hereditary angioedema is a specific form of edema, first reported in 1882, that involves a defect in the ability to inactivate the first component of complement. Massive swellings may involve the eyelids, lips, tongue, and areas of the trunk. Involvement of the gastrointestinal tract may produce symptoms of acute abdominal distress, but the symptoms almost always disappear in a few days without surgical intervention. The most significant life-threatening complication is severe pharyngeal involvement, which may lead to asphyxia. The pathologic alteration is firm, nonpitting edema of the dermis and subcutaneous tissue, which can be differentiated from a wheal-and-flare reaction by the absence of erythema. In addition, antihistamines have no effect upon hereditary angioedema, and the lesions cause a burning or stinging sensation rather than itching.

Angioedema is inherited as an autosomal-dominant trait. Biochemically, there is a deficiency of C_1-esterase inhibitor (C_1-INH) or it is present in an inactive form. C_1-esterase is the active form of the first component of complement. If normal serum is incubated at 37°C, there is a gradual "spontaneous" loss of complement activity. In patients with angioedema, this spontaneous decrease may not occur due to a lack of C_1-INH. During attacks, the C_4 and C_2 levels in the serum are decreased, indicating that activation of the complement system is important in this phenomenon. The injection of C_1-esterase into the skin of normal individuals produces a wheal-and-flare reaction, but the injection of C_1-esterase into the skin of patients with angioedema produces a firm, nonpitting induration with no flare (localized angioedema). Production of the lesions of angioedema must involve factors other than lack of C_1-esterase inhibitor. C_1-INH is a γ-$_2$ neuroaminoglycoprotein that is a serine esterase inhibitor. It is not only effective on activated C_1 but also plasmin, activated Hageman factor (XIIa), and kallikrein. Thus, interactions of different inflammatory systems due to C_1-INH deficiency may be responsible for the clinical picture observed.

It has been claimed that attacks of hereditary angioedema may be terminated by the injection of fresh frozen plasma from normal individuals, presumably because of the presence of C_1-esterase inhibitors in such preparations. However, this observation has not been generally reproducible. Episodes of local angioedema may follow surgical procedures, such as dental extractions. It thus becomes important to prevent such attacks. Short-term administration of tranexamic acid does prevent these attacks. It is believed that tranexamic acid may inhibit plasmin-dependent conversion of the product of C_1, C_4, and C_2 interaction to a pathologically active peptide. Androgenic steroids raise the serum level of C_1-esterase inhibitor and is used extensively in postpubertal pediatric patients with angioedema. This reversal of C_1-esterase serum deficiency by drug therapy suggests a regulatory gene defect.

Immunotherapeutic Modification of Atopic Allergy: Hyposensitization, Desensitization, Tolerance, and Supression

Atopic or anaphylactic conditions may be treated by injection of small amounts of the offending allergen and increasing the amount of antigen over a protracted period of time. "Desensitization" therapy for hay fever was introduced in England in 1911 by L. Noon. He was following the lead of Pasteur, who had success in "vaccination" against infectious disease. Many farmers in England at that time developed severe reactions to hay during the harvest season and were unable to continue farming. Noon prepared aqueous extracts of hay, "immunized" the affected farmers, and obtained significant beneficial effects. The major factors contributing to successful immunotherapy are the proper antigen and adequate doses of the antigen. Immunotherapy for ragweed, for example, is successful largely because there is a known available major antigen (antigen E), an immune response to the antigen can be measured, and the skin tests are reproducible. In the case of asthma, these criteria are difficult to meet, and the efficacy of immunotherapy for asthma is questionable. During the application of inoculation therapy in office practice, frequently not enough of the allergen is given to be effective, but the placebo effect (estimated to be up to 30%) deludes the physician and patient that the low doses of allergen are effective. Controlled clinical trials demonstrate up to 70% effective use with high-dose immunotherapy for required allergy, but only 10% to 20% with low doses (the placebo effect). Effective immunotherapy has been accomplished using various preparations of plant antigens, insect venoms, cat dander and, more recently, fire ant toxin, but the proper antigens for immunotherapy of insect or animal dander reactions remain controversial. Purified allergen preparations must be used; "whole body" insect extracts are not effective.

The mechanism of the beneficial effect of immunotherapy of allergies is not always clear. Possible mechanisms include hyposensitization (blocking), desensitization, tolerance, and suppression (Fig. 14–2).

HYPO-SENSITIZATION

The production of blocking antibody is referred to as hyposensitization. Hyposensitization is a form of immune deviation. Immune deviation is the selective induction of one type of immune response instead of another by controlling the immunizing event. Hypothetically delivery of a potential allergen by a route other than inhalation, at doses higher than received by natural exposure or in a form other than small particles (eg, pollen) may favor a Th1 type helper response over a Th2 type response. In particular, decreasing the production of IL-4 and IL-13 by Th2 cells should block B-cell differentiation to IgE secreting cells. The question is how to accomplish this. It has been suggested that feeding areoantigens to infants of allergy prone families be tried to attempt to reduce the incidence of allergies later in life, but this

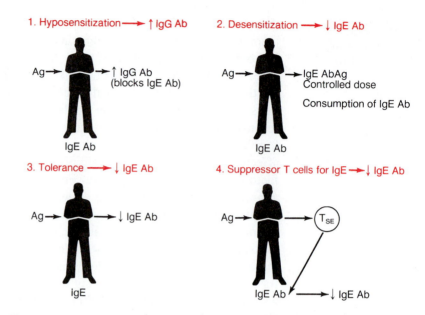

Figure 14–2. Immunotherapy of atopic allergies. Immunotherapy of atopic reactions by injection of the specific allergen is known to be effective, particularly for alleviation of the symptoms of hay fever. The mechanism of reduction of allergic symptoms is unclear. At least four possibilities are: (1) Hyposensitization, production of IgG blocking antibody; (2) desensitization, consumption of IgE antibody by repeated small doses of allergen; (3) tolerance, a loss or significant decrease in IgE antibody production to the allergen; and (4) production of suppressor T cells specific for IgE B cells. Another possible mechanism not yet identified as occurring due to specific immunotherapy is the production of nonspecific IgE that might block the effector cell receptors for IgE allergen-specific antibody.

approach remains highly theoretical. The observation that a mutant IL-4 protein inhibits IgE production in vitro and has led to the suggestion that mutant IL-4 or IL-12 proteins might be active in vivo.

In any case by careful immunization with the offending allergen it is often possible to induce the formation of nonreaginic, precipitating IgG antibody. Factors selecting against IgE production include high doses (1 mg versus 1 ng) of allergen; use of particulate antigens, such as alum precipitates; conjugation of antigens with polyethylene glycol; intramuscular or intraperitoneal injection of antigens, rather than aerosol exposure via mucous membranes; and the use of large carrier antigens, such as bacterial or parasitic extracts. Since the precipitation IgG antibody reacts with the same antigen as the reaginic antibody, the precipitating antibody will compete with the reaginic antibody in the reaction with antigen and help prevent atopic symptoms. The formation of precipitating antigen–antibody complexes may also produce tissue changes, but many more molecules of precipitating antibody reacting with antibody are needed to produce a reaction of clinical significance than molecules of reaginic antibody. Such blocking antibody may be demonstrated in vitro by its ability to inhibit the release of anaphylactic mediators from sensitized mast cells upon exposure to antigen and passive transfer of IgG antibody under controlled conditions reduces anaphylactic responses to be venom. However, in some individuals who have had a beneficial response to injection therapy, no blocking antibody is demonstrable. Another possibility is that IgA antibodies in nasal or bronchial secretions may block IgE-mediated reaction, but the small changes in mucosal IgA levels measured do not account for the marked beneficial effect seen. Thus, the decrease in sensitization of many individuals must be due to some other mechanism.

DESENSITIZATION

Desensitization may be produced by providing enough antigen in small doses to combine with the IgE antibody so that IgE antibody is not available for reactive tissue mast cells. Upon subsequent exposure to allergen, mediator release does not occur. Desensitization may occur with injection therapy for hay fever. Frequently, a series of injections of allergen bind the available antibody as it is produced without producing significant symptoms. With cessation of injections, continued IgE antibody production is able to overcome the antigen and become available for tissue sensitization.

TOLERANCE

Tolerance may be defined as the specific deletion of responding T or B cells for a given antigen. Specific deletion of responding cells has been difficult to demonstrate. However, it is possible that specific immunotherapy might produce a temporary loss of responsiveness by specific deletion. More recent experimental studies suggest that such lack of responsiveness is due to the action of T-suppressor cells.

SUPPRESSION

Suppressor T cells specific for IgE production have been found by several investigators using mouse model systems. Passive injection of IgE perinatally leads to long-term inhibition of IgE synthesis in mice. At first thought to be due to suppressor T cells for IgE but this effect has been shown to be caused by production of autoantibodies to IgE. IgE-suppressor T cells appear to control the degree of responsiveness of high and low IgE responder strains of mice, thus providing an explanation for the observation of the role of heredity in determining the class of immunoglobulin response to a given antigen. It is not clear whether the same phenomenon is being studied in these experimental systems, because some investigators find that the T-suppressor cells for IgE are antigen-specific, whereas others do not. T cells of humans have type 1 and type 2 histamine receptors. T cells bearing histamine type 2 receptors are activated by reaction with histamine to express suppressor function. This subclass of T cells appears to be lower than normal in allergic individuals, and allergic individuals are less able to generate histamine-induced suppressor activity. The role of this activity in controlling allergy is not known.

INCREASED SERUM IgE

The presence of high concentrations of an IgE that does not bind a particular antigen (nonantibody IgE) could saturate mast cell binding sites and prevent the functional sensitization of mast cells by IgE with specific antibody activity. This would be an IgE "blocking" effect, that is, nonantibody IgE blocking IgE antibody. Support for this concept comes from the observations that experimental animals with helminth infections who have high IgE serum concentrations have a decreased incidence of "allergic" reactions. On the other hand, in endemic areas of intestinal helminthiasis in Venezuela, there is a decreased incidence of allergies in rural populations as compared to urban populations, even though both have elevated IgE serum concentrations as compared to other populations. A final possibility that must be considered is a decrease in the threshold for activation of mast cells or decreased numbers of mast cells in effector organs, such as the bronchial and nasal submucosa, but the evidence for such changes is not consistent. **Hyperimmunoglobulin-IgE** is a clinical syndrome consisting of an immune deficiency manifested as dermatitis, very high serum levels of IgE, and recurrent staphylococcal infections of the skin and lung, associated with a defect in neutrophil chemotaxis. The role of the IgE in this syndrome is not clear, but it is possible that IgE or IgE–immune complexes may affect neutrophil function adversely.

Pharmacologic Control of Atopic Reactions

The severity of reaction by an anaphylactically sensitized individual upon exposure to the specific allergen depends not only upon the amount of allergen and reaginic antibody, but also upon the reactivity of mast cells, the excitability of the end organ (smooth muscle), and the effect of the autonomic nervous system (Fig. 14–3). Imbalance of these homeostatic control mechanisms explains how exposure to nonimmunologic stimuli, such as heat, cold, physical exercise, or light, may, in some individuals, serve to excite physiologic reactions that mimic allergic reactions (anaphylactoid reactions).

In fact, over 80% of asthma in adults is caused not by extrinsic antigen exposure but by physiologic imbalance of the responsive smooth muscle end organs. The concept of cyclic nucleotides as "second messengers" in controlling cellular responses has led to a theoretic appreciation of the mechanisms controlling anaphylactic reactions (β-adrenergic blockage theory of asthma). The role of physiologic control

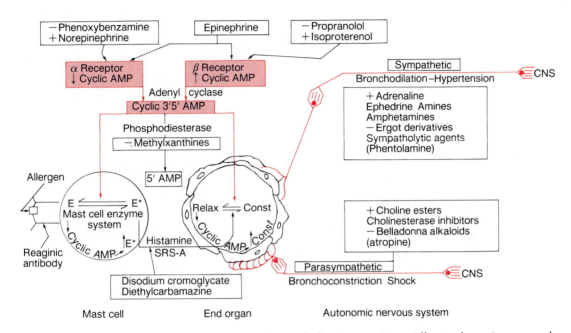

Figure 14–3. Pharmacologic control of atopic–anaphylactic reactions. Effects of atopic or anaphylactic reactions are mediated by biologically active mediators released by mast cells that affect end organ smooth muscle. The amount of mediators released and reactivity of end organ to mediators are controlled by cellular messenger systems. Mast cell sensitivity depends on the amount of reaginic antibody sensitizing the cell and on relative intracellular levels of AMP and cGMP. Cyclic AMP and cyclic GMP levels are controlled by adrenergic receptors. Simulation of α-receptors causes decrease of AMP, increase of cGMP, and increased reactivity; stimulation of β-receptors activates adenyl cyclase and produces increased AMP, decreased cGMP, and decreased reactivity. A similar mechanism is operative for end organ smooth muscle. Degree of mast cell and end organ excitability may be modified by pharmacologic agents that operate through adrenergic or autonomic systems. Cyclic AMP is broken down to 5'-AMP by phosphodiesterase, so that inhibition of phosphodiesterase activity by methyxanthines increases AMP and decreases sensitivity of mast cells and end organs. Epinephrine stimulates both α- and β-receptors but generally has pronounced ability to reverse acute allergic reactions at the usual therapeutic dose. Disodium cromoglycate and diethylcarbamazine inhibit histamine release from mast cells. Excitation of end organs is controlled by a balance of the autonomic nervous system. Parasympathetic effects are similar to anaphylactic effects (bronchial constriction, endothelial contraction, increased peristalsis, dilatation of bladder sphincter, etc.), whereas sympathetic effects are the opposite. Certain situations may result in temporary imbalance of these systems and increase severity of reaction, as in patients with chronic asthma.

in the severity of reaction to exposure to allergens was brought to the attention of allergists in the 1980s.

MAST CELLS

Control or sensitivity of mast cells to allergen (the amount of mediators released by sensitized mast cells following contact with allergen) is accomplished by balanced adrenergic receptors (α- and β-receptors) that control the cellular level of enzyme systems, such as methyltransferase phosphorylating enzymes and phospholipases, the activation of which leads to mediator release. Contact of the sensitized mast cell with antigen causes activation of the enzyme system and release of mediators (see Fig. 8–3). The amount of enzymes available is determined by the cellular level of cyclic AMP, which in turn is controlled by the stimulation of the α- and β-receptors. Stimulation of β-receptors activates adenyl cyclase, causes an increase in cAMP, and decreased reactivity, whereas activation of the α-receptors results in decreased cAMP and increases reactivity. Cyclic AMP is normally broken down to 5′-AMP by phosphodiesterase, so that inhibition of phosphodiesterase leads to increased cAMP and decreased reactivity. The extent of reaction of mast cells to antigen may be controlled by stimulating or blocking the controlling receptors. Norepinephrine stimulates α-receptors, which results in a decrease in cellular cAMP (increased enzymes and increased sensitivity to allergen), whereas isoproterenol stimulates β-receptors (decreased sensitivity to allergen). Phenoxybenzamine blocks both α- and β-receptors but has a more profound effect on β-receptors; selective stimulation may be achieved by the use of epinephrine combined with one of the blocking drugs. Methylxanthenes (theophylline) inhibit phosphodiesterase and thus prevent cAMP breakdown (decreased sensitivity to antigen). Two drugs block the release of mediators after contact of sensitized mast cell with allergen. The way that these drugs, diethylcarbamazine and disodium chromoglycate, inhibit histamine release is not known. Specific desensitization of sensitized cells occurs as patients treated with sodium cromolyn and challenged with antigen remain refractory to subsequent challenge with the same antigen, but not a different antigen, when retested after 5 hours.

END ORGAN SENSITIVITY

The unleashing of severe atopic reactions is not only controlled at the mast cell level but also depends upon the balance between homeostatic α- and β-end organ (smooth muscle) adrenergic receptors. The cAMP levels of the end organ cells may be controlled in a similar manner as described above for mast cells. Thus, stimulation of α-receptors leads to a decrease in cAMP and increased anaphylactic effects; stimulation of β-receptors leads to increased cAMP and decreased end organ effects. The β-adrenergic theory states that atopic individuals do not have the normal adrenergic end organ homeostatic mechanism. Activation of α-receptors in normal nonatopic individuals does not produce significant anaphylactic symptoms because such activation is counterbalanced by activation of the β-adrenergic system. Thus, in the terms of this theory, bronchial asthma is not primarily an immunologic disease but is due to an abnormality in the β-adrenergic end organ system. The marked beneficial effect of epinephrine upon anaphylactic symptoms is because of its apparent stimulation of end organ β-receptors and not because of its effect on mast cells.

THE AUTONOMIC NERVOUS SYSTEM

The excitability of the end organ smooth muscle (bronchial muscles, arterioles, gastrointestinal muscles) is also controlled by the autonomic nervous system and is maintained by a balance of sympathetic (adrenergic) and parasympathetic (cholinergic) effects. In general, parasympathetic effects are similar to anaphylactic effects (bronchial constriction, increased gastrointestinal peristalsis, dilatation of bladder sphincter, dilatation of arteries, pupil constriction), whereas sympathetic effects are the opposite (bronchial and pupil dilatation, arterial and sphincter constriction). In a normal individual, the effects of the two components of the autonomic system are usually in balance, with a tendency to sympathetic dominance. It is known that certain situations may result in a temporary imbalance of these systems. Thus, stimulation of the parasympathetic system by injection of Mecholyl or acetylcholine in a normal individual results in a temporary drop in blood pressure. Immediately after this effect, the individual may be hyperresponsive to sympathetic stimulation—so-called sympathetic tuning. A permanent imbalance may be produced in experimental animals by producing lesions in the pituitary. Ablation of areas of the anterior pituitary that reduces parasympathetic discharge protects against the lethal effects of anaphylaxis. Anaphylactically sensitized individuals may have a permanent imbalance of autonomic control that predisposes them to increased reactivity to mediator release. The shock organ effect (ie, selective reactivity of certain organs) may be explained by a local imbalance of autonomic effects. Anaphylactoid reactions may be overreactions of this balancing system induced by physiologic change. Because the autonomic nervous system is indirectly connected through neuronal synapses to higher areas of the brain, it is possible for emotional conditioning to effect the autonomic balance. Thus, emotional states may lead to parasympathetic tuning with resultant atopic or anaphylactic symptoms (cholinergic urticaria).

An imbalance of any or all of three levels—mast cells, end organ, or autonomic nervous system—may explain the increased sensitivity of atopic individuals to anaphylactic mediators. Atopic individuals injected with small doses of histamine have a much greater reaction than nonatopic individuals. It has been shown that the lymphocytes of atopic individuals have a decreased ability to respond to certain stimuli by increased AMP levels. Thus, atopic individuals may be unable to balance the effects of α stimulation or allergen contact.

AUTO-ANTIBODIES TO β-ADRENERGIC RECEPTORS

Some individuals with high risk for development of asthma have autoantibodies for β_2-adrenergic receptors. Since such antibodies might block β_2-adrenergic receptors, it is possible that this blockage could increase mast cell sensitivity to IgE-mediated degranulation (β_2-adrenergic receptor stimulation decreases mast cell sensitivity). Auto-anti-β_2-adrenergic receptors might also affect end organ responsiveness. At the time of this writing, only clinical correlations have been made, ie, such antibodies are found in 10% of severe asthmatics but not in sera of nonasthmatic individuals. Questions regarding the role that these antibodies play in the pathogenesis of asthma, how they arise (for instance, whether they are stimulated by therapy with synthetic β-adrenergic ligand), and whether or not they have any prognostic value, remain to be answered (see also Chapter 11).

Treatment of Atopic Allergy

Therapeutic procedures to prevent or decrease atopic reactions may be applied at the various levels of reaction: Contact with antigen, IgE receptor, sensitivity of the mast cell to stimulation, degranulation of mast cell, mast cell mediator activity, sensitivity of end organ cell, autonomic nervous system balance, and emotional state of the reactive individual (Fig. 14–4).

Drugs that counteract the effects of mast cell mediators upon target cells or decrease the release of mediators from mast cells are under active-development clinical investigation by pharmaceutical companies (Table 14–11). There is every reason to believe that new pharmacologic approaches will be able to decrease or inhibit allergic reactions with few or no side effects.

Protective Role of IgE

The protective role of atopic or anaphylactic reactions has been the subject of considerable speculation. The most popular hypothesis is that anaphylactic reactions serve to open small blood vessels via endothelial cell contraction and thus permit the exudation of other immunoglobulin classes of antibodies or inflammatory cells into the tissue containing the offending antigen, the "gate-keeper effect." Experimental support for this concept has been obtained. In immunized animals containing IgG anti-diphtheria toxin antibodies, the simultaneous injection of ragweed antigen and diphtheria toxin into the skin results in an increase in toxin neutralization if the skin site is prepared by previous sensitization with reaginic antibody for the ragweed antigen. It is concluded that the increased toxin-neutralizing capacity of the local skin sites in passively immunized animals is due to increased transudation of serum IgG antibody into the skin test sites.

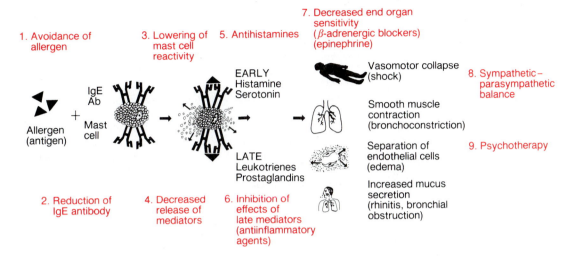

Figure 14–4. Levels of Possible Therapeutic or Preventive Intervention in Allergy.

(1) Avoidance of contact with the allergen is the most effective means of preventing atopic allergic reactions, thus removing antigen activation of IgE receptors. Avoidance is not always feasible, and other methods must be used.

(2) The availability of the IgE antibody may be reduced by hyposensitization, desensitization, tolerance or immune deviation (Th1 > Th2) as the result of injection therapy (see text).

(3) The sensitivity of the mast cell upon reaction of IgE receptors with allergen may be controlled by the amount of cyclic AMP available. This level may be affected by drugs as indicated in Figure 14–3. If mast cell cyclic AMP can be increased by the methods indicated above, the extent of mast cell mediator release upon reaction of sensitized cells with allergen may be decreased and atopic symptoms controlled.

(4) Two drugs—diethylcarbamazine and disodium chromoglycate—significantly decrease the release of mediators from mast cells upon contact with allergen.

(5) The effect of mast cell mediators may be partially controlled by drugs that interfere with histamine activity (antihistamines). The fact that antihistamines are only partially effective in decreasing atopic symptoms indicates that other mediators play an important role.

(6) The rapidly increasing understanding of the role of arachidonic acid metabolites in allergic reactions could well lead to more effective therapy. In particular, nonsteroidal antiinflammatory agents or agents that could control the balance of effects of PGE (bronchodilation) and PGF (bronchoconstriction) could have great potential beneficial effects. Steroids are used only as a last resort.

(7) The sensitivity of the end organ (smooth muscle) to atopic mediators also depends upon β-adrenergic control of cellular cAMP levels. If end organ cAMP can be increased, then atopic symptoms should be decreased.

(8) Sympathetic stimulation or parasympathetic blockade may also have a significant beneficial effect upon atopic reactions through the effect of the autonomic nervous system upon end organ excitability (see Fig. 14–3).

(9) It is well known that severity of atopic reactions (particularly asthma) depends upon the emotional state of the individual. Anxious or insecure patients have more severe symptoms than more secure or stable patients. Thus, the emotional state of the reactive individual should be evaluated and treated with psychotherapy, if necessary.

TABLE 14–11. PHARMACOLOGIC AGENTS USED IN TREATMENT OF MAST CELL-MEDIATED ALLERGIC REACTIONS

Class	Example	Mechanisms of Action	Result
Antihistamines	Diphenhydramine (H$_1$) Cimetidine (H$_2$)	Block action of histamine on H$_1$ or H$_2$ receptors in surrounding tissue	Block mediator effects on target organs
Beta-adrenergic drugs	Isoproterenol	Increase cAMP through activation of adenylate cyclase	Decrease mediator release; counteract mediator effects on target organs
Corticosteroids	Prednisone	Inhibit phospholipases, increase β-receptor number	Inhibit mediator synthesis, mediator secretion, chemotaxis, and cell adherence
Methylxanthines	Theophylline	Increase cAMP by inhibition of phosphodiesterase	Decrease mediator release; counteract mediator effects on target organs
Nonsteroidal antiinflammatory agents	Aspirin Indomethacin	Inhibit cyclooxygenase pathway	Inhibit prostaglandin production
Cromolyn-like drugs	Sodium cromolyn Doxantrazole	Inhibit phosphodiesterase; decrease Ca^{++} flux across mast cell membrane	Inhibit mediator release

Anaphylactic reactions also serve to protect the individual against intestinal parasites. Parasitic worm infestations are frequently associated with IgE antibody response. It has been postulated that gastrointestinal anaphylactic reactions may help expel intestinal parasites by acute severe diarrhea. Mechanisms of expulsion of intestinal parasites include: *Primary expulsion* of the first infection, which is associated with marked acute inflammation; and *rapid expulsion*, which is associated with increased intestinal motility, marked mucous secretion, hyperplasia of goblet cells, eosinophilic infiltrate, and mast cell hyperplasia. The histopathologic features of asthma and the rapid expulsion reaction share many similarities. It is also possible that the sneezing associated with acute asthma dislodges potential infectious agents from the lungs. Eosinophils may play a direct role in destruction of intestinal parasites through an ADCC mechanism. The major basic protein of eosinophils is not only cytotoxic for parasites but also can activate mast cell degranulation.

Finally, acute anaphylactic reactions may force the sensitized individual to avoid further exposure to the offending allergen. By avoiding exposure to the antigens, more prolonged extensive immune-mediated damage may be prevented. Avoidance may prevent formation of immune complex disease or delayed hypersensitivity to the same antigen, since anaphylactic reactions may be elicited by extremely small doses of an antigen.

Summary

Anaphylactic (acute) or atopic (chronic) reactions are caused by activation of mast cells via reaction of reaginic antibody fixed to the mast cell surface. Reaginic antibody belongs to a unique class of immunoglobulin, IgE, which has the capacity to bind to receptors on mast cells ("fix"). Mast cells are stimulated by reaction with allergen to release pharmacological agents stored in cytoplasmic granules (degranulation), such as histamine and serotonin, which produce acute reactions. In addition, arachidonic acid from membrane phospholipids is converted to leukotrienes and prostaglandins, which produce or cause later inflammatory lesions. These released mediators act on smooth muscle cells and endothelial cells, causing constriction. This, in turn, produces clinical symptoms because of bronchoconstriction (asthma), loss of intravascular fluid (edema, cutaneous anaphylaxis, shock), or chronic accumulation of mucous (hay fever, nasal polyps). The degree of reactivity of the system is controlled by a balance between adrenergic and cholinergic receptors, and the extent of these reactions may be controlled by drugs that affect this physiologic balance. Many allergic symptoms are believed to be the result of an imbalance of this controlling system rather than because of exposure to allergen. The extent of production of reaginic (IgE) antibody may be influenced by specific immunization (immunotherapy). The mechanism of action of immunotherapy remains poorly defined. Experimental models indicate that γ, δ T-suppressor cells specific for IgE production or selective activation of Th1 cells rather than Th2 cells may be active.

Anaphylactic reactions may serve a protective role in providing rapid egress of other antibodies or cells into sites of antigen deposition by inducing endothelial cell separation. However, allergic reactions cause problems for a large number of people and constitute the basis for the practice of a major clinical specialty—the allergist.

Bibliography

INTRODUCTION

Blackley CH: Experiments and researches on the causes and nature of catarrhous aestivus. London, Balliere, 1873.

Coca AF, Grove EF: Studies on hypersensitiveness. XIII. A study of the atopic reagins. *J Immunol* 10:445, 1925.

Corrigan CJ, Kay AB: T cells and eosinophils in the pathogenesis of asthma. *Immunol Today* 13:501, 1992.

DeJarnatt AC, Grant JA: Basic mechanisms of anaphylaxis and anaphylactoid reactions. *Immunol Allergy Clin N Am* 12:501, 1992.

Friedman MM, Kaliner MA: Human mast cells and asthma. *Am Rev Respir Dis* 135:1157, 1987.

Herxheimer H: The late bronchial reaction in induced asthma. *Int Arch Allergy Appl Immunol* 7:219, 1952.

Ishizaka T, Ishizaka K. Johansson SGO, Bennich H: Histamine release from human leukocytes by anti-E antibodies. *J Immunol* 102:884, 1969.

Lemanske RF, Kaliner M: Late-phase IgE-mediated reactions. *J Clin Immunol* 8:1, 1988.

Wyman M: Autumnal catarrh: Hay fever. Cambridge, MA, Hurd & Houghton, 1872.

ALLERGENS

Baldo BA (ed.): Molecular approaches to the study of allergens. Monograph. *Allergy*, vol. 28. Basel, Karger, 1988.

IVIS/WHO Allergen Nomenclature Subcommittee: Allergen nomenclature. Bull WHO 72:797–806, 1994.

Marsh DG, Goodfriend L, King TP, Lowenstein H, Platts-Mills TAE: Allergen nomenclature. *Clin Allergy* 18:201, 1988.

REAGINIC ANTIBODY

Bazaral M, Orgel HA, Hamburger RN: The influence of serum IgE levels of selected recipients, including patients with allergy, helminthiasis, and tuberculosis, on the apparent P–K titer of a reaginic serum. *Clin Exp Immunol* 4:117, 1973.

Ishizaka K, Ishizaka T, Hornbrook MH: Physicochemical properties of human reaginic antibody. IV. Presence of a unique immunoglobulin as a carrier of reaginic activity. *J Immunol* 97:75, 1966.

Keegan AD, Conrad DH: The receptor for the Fc region of IgE. *Springer Semin Immunopath* 12:303, 1990.

Metzger H: The receptor with high affinity for IgE. *Immunol Rev* 125:37, 1992.

Moller G (ed.): Immunoglobulin E. *Immunol Rev* 41:1, 1978.

Ownby DR: Allergy testing: In vivo versus in vitro. *Pediatr Clin N Am* 35:995, 1988.

Perelmutter L: IgG_4: Non-IgE-mediated atopic disease. *Am Allergy* 52:64, 1984.

Plaut, M: Antigen-specific lymphokine secretory patterns in atopic disease. *J Immunol* 144:4497, 1990.

Prausnitz C, Kustner H: Studies on sensitivity. *Zentralbl Bakteriol* (orig.) 86:160, 1921. English translation in Gell PGH, Coombs RRA: *Clinical Aspects of Immunology*. Philadelphia, Davis, 1963, 808.

Reid MJ, Lockey RF, Turkeltaub PC, Platts-Mills, TAE: Survey of fatalities from skin testing and immunotherapy 1985–1989. *J Allergy Clin Immunol* 92:6–15, 1993.

Ricci M, Rossi O: Dysregulation of IgE responses and airway allergic inflammation in atopic individuals. *Clin Exp Allergy* 20:601, 1990.

Sutton BJ, Gould HJ: The human IgE network. *Nature* 366:421–428, 1993.

GENETICS

Bazaral M, Orgel HA, Hamburger RN: Genetics of IgE and allergy: Serum IgE levels in twins. *J Allergy Clin Immunol* 52:211–244, 1974.

Cooke RA, VanderVeer A: Human sensitization. *J Immunol* 1:201, 1916.

Dowse GK, Turner KJ, Stewart GA, et al.: The association between *Dermatophagoides* mites and the increasing prevalence of asthma in village communities within the Papua, New Guinea highlands. *J Allergy Clin Immunol* 75:75, 1985.

Levine BB: Genetic control of reagin production in mice and man: Role of Ir genes in ragweed hayfever. In *Monographs in Allergy*, vol. 4. Goodfriend L, Sehon AH, Orange RP (eds.). Basel, Karger, 1969.

Orgel HA, Hamburger RN: Development of IgE and allergy in infancy. *J Allergy Clin Immunol* 56:296, 1975.

ATOPIC ALLERGY

Botham PA, Davies GE, Teasdale EL: Allergy to laboratory animals: A prospective study of its incidence and of the influence of atopy on its development. *Brit J Indust Med* 44:627, 1987.

Bubak ME, Reed CE, Yunginger JW, et al.: Allergic reactions to latex among health-care workers. *Mayo Clin Proc* 67:1075, 1992.

Ellis EF: Immunologic basis of atopic disease. *Adv Pediatr* 16:65, 1969.

Hunskaar S, Fosse RT: Allergy to laboratory mice and rats: A review of the patho-physiology, epidemiology, and clinical aspects. *Lab Animal Sci* 24:358–374, 1990.

Juliusson S, Pipkorn U, Karlsson G, et al.: Mast cells and eosinophils in the allergic mucosal response to allergen challenges: Changes in distribution and signs of activation in relation to symptoms. *J Allergy Clin Immunol* 80:898–909, 1992.

Levy DA, Charpin D, Pecquet D, et al.: Allergy to latex. *Allergy* 47:579–587, 1992.

Slavin RG, Lewis CR: Sensitivity to enzyme activities in laundry detergent workers. *J Allergy Clin Immunol* 48:262, 1971.

ANAPHYLAXIS

Austen KF, Humphrey JH: In vitro studies of the mechanism of anaphylaxis. *Adv Immunol* 3:1, 1963.

Bochner BS, Lichtenstein LM: Current Concept—anaphylaxis. *N Engl J Med* 324:1785, 1991.

Burks AV, Sampson HA, Buckley RH: Anaphylactic reactions after gamma globulin administration in patients with hypogammaglobulinemia: Detection of IgE antibodies to IgA. *N Engl J Med* 314:560, 1986.

Halpern BN, Ky T, Robert B: Clinical and immunological study of an exceptional case of reaginic type sensitization to human seminal fluid. *Immunology* 12:247, 1967.

James LP, Austen KF: Fetal systemic anaphylaxis in man. *N Engl J Med* 270:597, 1964.

Lamson RW: Fatal anaphylaxis and sudden death associated with the injection of foreign substances. *JAMA* 82:1091, 1924.

Parker CW: Allergic drug responses: Mechanisms and unsolved problems. *CRC Crit Rev Toxicol* 1:261, 1972.

Portier RH, Richet C: De l'action anaphylactique de certains venims. *C R Soc Biol* 54:170, 1902.

Quinke H: On acute localized edema of the skin. *Monatshefte Prakt Dermatol* 1:129, 1882.

Reunala T, Koskimies AI, Bjorksten F, et al.: Immunoglobulin E-mediated severe allergy to human seminal plasma. *Fertil Steril* 28:832, 1977.

Snell D: How it feels to die. *Life Magazine*, May 26, 1961.

Wall RT, Frank M, Hahn M: A review of 25 patients with hereditary angioedema requiring surgery. *Anesthesiology* 71:309, 1989.

Wicher K. Reisman RE, Arbesman CE: Allergic reaction to penicillin present in milk. *JAMA* 208:143, 1969.

ASTHMA

Aalbers R, Smith M, Timens W: Immunohistology in bronchial asthma. *Resp Med 87* (suppl. B):13–21, 1993.

Aas K: Heterogenity of bronchial asthma: Subpopulation or different stages of the disease. *Allergy* 36:3, 1981.

Anto JM, Sunyer J, Rodriguiz-Roisin R, et al.: Community outbreaks of asthma associated with inhalation of soybean dust. *N Engl J Med* 320:1097, 1989.

Beasley R, Burgess C, Crane J, et al.: Pathology of asthma and its clinical implications. *J Allergy Clin Immunol* 92:148–154, 1993.

Bienenstock J: Summing up: Present concepts and future ideas on immunoregulation of asthma. *Eur Respir J* 4:(suppl. 13)156S, 1991.

Buist AS: Asthma mortality: What have we learned? *J Allergy Clin Immunol* 84:275, 1989.

Chapman KR, Verbeek PR, Whie JG, et al.: Effect of a short course of prednisone in the prevention of early relapse after the emergency room treatment of acute asthma. *N Engl J Med* 324:788, 1991.

Frigas E, Gleich GJ: The eosinophil and the pathology of asthma. *J Allergy Clin Immunol* 77:527, 1986.

Hinson RFW, Moon AJ, Plummer NS: Bronchopulmonary aspergillosis. *Thorax* 7:317, 1952.

Karol MH, Jin R: Mechanisms of immunotoxicity to isocyanates. *Chem Res Toxicol* 4:402, 1991.

Lichtenstein LM, Austen KF: Asthma: Physiology, Immunopharmacology, and Treatment. New York, Academic Press, 1977.

Osler W: *The Principles and Practice of Medicine*. New York, Appleton & Low, 1892, 499.

Sheffer AL (chair): International consensus report on diagnosis and management of asthma. Bethesda, MD, US Dept. of Health and Human Services, Pub. No. 92-3091, 1992.

Stechschulte DJ: Leukotrienes in asthma and allergic rhinitis. *N Engl J Med* 323:1769, 1990.

Wardlaw AJ: *Asthma*. Bios Sci Publishers, Oxford, 1993.

Wilson SR, Scamagas P, German DF, et al.: A controlled trial of two forms of self-management education for adults with asthma. *Am J Med* 94:564–576, 1993.

HAY FEVER/ NASAL POLYPS

Howarth PH: Allergic rhinitis: A rational choice of treatment. *Respir Med* 83:179, 1989.

Mygind N, Nacierio RM: Allergic and nonallergic rhinitis: Clinical aspects. Orlando, FL, Saunders, 1993.

Raphael GD, Baraniuk JN, Kaliner MA: How and why the nose runs. *J Allergy Clin Immunol* 87:457, 1991.

Simmons FER: Allergic rhinitis: Recent advances. *Pediatr Clin N Am* 35:1053, 1988.

Winkerwerder WL, Gay LN: Perennial allergic rhinitis: An analysis of 198 cases. *Bull Johns Hopkins Hosp* 2:90, 1937.

FOOD ALLERGY

Aas K: The biochemistry of food allergens: What is essential for future research? In *Food Allergy*. Schmidt E (ed.). Nestlé Nutrition Workshop Series, vol 17. Vevry/Raven Press, New York, 1988, 1.

Frier S, Kletter B: Clinical and immunological aspects of milk protein intolerance. *Aust Paediatr J* 8:140, 1972.

Goldman AS, Sellars WA, Halpern SR, et al.: Milk allergy. II. Skin testing of allergic and normal children with purified milk proteins. *Pediatrics* 32:572, 1963.

Golert TM, Patterson R, Pruzansky JJ: Systemic allergic reactions to ingested antigens. *J Allergy* 44:96, 1969.

Hamburger RN: General strategies for prevention of atopic disease: A review of the current state of knowledge. In *Nutrition and Immunology*. Chandra RK (ed.). Newfoundland, St. John's, 1992, 335.

Hannuksela M. Haahtela T: Hypersensitivity reactions to food additives. *Allergy* 42:561, 1987.

Michaelsson G, Juhlin L: Urticaria induced by preservatives and dye additives in food and drugs. *Brit J Dermatol* 88:525, 1973.

Rowe AH, Rowe A Jr: *Food Allergy*. Springfield, IL, CC Thomas, 1972.

Savilahti E: Cow's milk allergy. *Allergy* 36:73, 1981.

Waldmann TA, Wochner RD, Laster L, et al.: Allergic gastroenteropathy: A cause of excessive gastrointestinal protein loss. *N Engl J Med* 276:761, 1967.

INSECT ALLERGY

Barr SE: Allergy to hymenoptera stings: Review of the world literature, 1953–1970. *Ann Allergy* 29:49, 1971.

Feinberg AR, Feinberg SM, Benaim-Pinto C: Asthma and rhinitis from insect allergies. *J Allergy* 27:437, 1956.

Feingold BF, Benjamini E, Michaeli D: The allergic response to insect bites. *Annu Rev Entomol* 13:137, 1968.

Frazier CA: *Insect Allergy*. St. Louis, Green, 1969.

Frazier CA: Biting insect survey: A statistical report. *Ann Allergy* 32:200, 1974.

Haberman E: Bee and wasp venoms. *Science* 177:314, 1972.

Killby VA, Silverman PH: Hypersensitive reactions in man to specific mosquito bites. *Am J Trop Med Hyg* 16:374, 1967.

King TP: Insect venom allergy. *Monogr Allergy* 28:84, 1990.

Perlman F: Stinging insect allergy: A historical sketch and confused state. *Ann Allergy* 39:285, 1977.

Reisman RE: Insect sting anaphylaxis. *Immunol Allergy Clin N Am* 12:535, 1992.

Shulman S: Insect allergy: Biochemical and immunochemical analyses of the allergens. *Prog Allergy* 12:246, 1968.

Zwick H, Popp W, Sertl K, et al.: Allergic structures in cockroach hypersensitivity. *J Allergy Clin Immunol* 87:626, 1991.

ATOPIC DERMATITIS

Blaylock WK: Atopic dermatitis: Diagnosis and pathology. *J Allergy Clin Immunol* 57:62, 1976.

Braathen LR: Atopic dermatitis. *Acta Dermato-Venereol*. Supplementum 1445, 1989.

Brocq L, Jacquet L: Notes pour servir à l'histoire des neurodermites: Du lichen circumscriptus des anciens auteurs, au lichen simplex chronique du M. le Dr. E. Vidal. *Ann Dermatol Syphilgr* 2:97, 1891.

Hanifin JM: Atopic dermatitis. *J Allergy Clin Immunol* 73:211, 1984.

Kay JW: Atopic dermatitis: An immunologic disease complex and its therapy. *Ann Allergy* 38:345, 1977.

McGready SJ, Buckley RH: Depression of cell-indicated immunity in atopic eczema. *J Allergy Clin Immunol* 56:393, 1975.

Rajka G: Atopic dermatitis. London, WB Saunders, 1975.

Wise F, Sulzberger MB: In *Year Book of Dermatology and Syphilogy*. Chicago, Year Book Medical, 1933, 59.

ASPIRIN INTOLERANCE

Abrishami MA, Thomas J: Aspirin intolerance: A review. *Ann Allergy* 39:28, 1977.

Falliers CJ: Aspirin and subtypes of asthma: Risk-factor analysis. *J Allergy Clin Immunol* 52:141, 1973.

Farr RS: Presidential message. *J Allergy* 45:321, 1970.

Fein BT: Aspirin shock associated with asthma and nasal polyps. *Ann Allergy* 29:589, 1971.

Sampter M, Beers RF Jr: Intolerance to aspirin. *Ann Intern Med* 68:975, 1968.

Szezklik A, Nizankowska E, Splawinski J, et al.: Effects of inhibition of thromboxane-A_2 synthesis in aspirin-induced asthma. *J Allergy Clin Immunol* 80:839, 1987.

Vanselow NA, Smith JR: Bronchial asthma induced by indomethacin. *Ann Intern Med* 66:568, 1967.

URTICARIA AND ANGIOEDEMA

Cohen G, Peterson A: Treatment of hereditary angioedema with frozen plasma. *Ann Allergy* 30:690, 1972.

Donaldson VH, Ratnoff OD, DaSilva WD, et al.: Permeability-increasing activity in hereditary angioneurotic edema plasma. *J Clin Invest* 48:642, 1969.

Ebken RK, Bauschard FA, Levin MI: Dermatographism: Its definition, demonstration, and prevalence. *J Allergy* 41:338, 1968.

Epstein JH: Photoallergy: A review: *Arch Dermatol* 106:741, 1972.

Grolnick M: An investigative and clinical evaluation of dermatographism. *Ann Allergy* 28:395, 1970.

Kaplan AP: Urticaria and angioedema. In *Inflammation: Basic Principles and Clinical Conditions*. Gallin JL, Goldstein IM, Snyderman R (eds.). New York, Raven Press, 1988, 667.

Leenutaphong V, Holze E, Plewig G: Pathogenesis and classification of solar urticaria: A new concept. *J Am Acad Dermatol* 21:237, 1989.

Sheffer AL, Austen KF, Gigli I: Urticaria and angioedema. *Postgrad Med* 54:81, 1973.

Wanderer AA, Maselli R, Ellis DF, et al.: Immunologic characterization of serum factors responsible for cold urticaria. *J Allergy Clin Immunol* 48:13, 1971.

IMMUNO-THERAPY

de Vries JE: Novel fundamental approaches to intervening in IgE-mediated allergic diseases. *J Invest Dermatol* 102: 141–144, 1994.

Haba S, Nisonoff A: Role of antibody and T cells in the long-term inhibition of IgE synthesis. *Proc Natl Acad Sci USA* 91:604–608, 1994.

Holt PG: Immunoprophylaxis of atrophy: Light at the end of tunnel? *Immunol Today* 15:484–489, 1994.

Ishizaka K: Cellular events in the IgE antibody response. *Adv Immunol* 23:1, 1976.

Ishizaka K: Regulation of IgE synthesis. *Ann Rev Immunol* 2:159, 1984.

Lee WY, Sehon AH: Suppression of reaginic antibodies with modified allergens. II. Abrogation of reaginic antibodies with allergens conjugated to polyethylene glycol. *Int Arch Allergy* 56:193, 1978.

Lightenstein LM, Levy DA: Is "desensitization" for ragweed hay fever immunologically specific. *Int Arch Allerg* 42:615, 1972.

Malling H-J, Weeke B: Position paper: Immunotherapy. *Eur J Allergy Clin Immunol* 14(suppl):8–35, 1993.

McMenamin C, Oliver J, Girn B, et al.: Regulation of T-cell sensitization at epithelial surfaces in the respiratory tract: Suppression of IgE responses to inhaled antigens by CD3+ TcR α^-/β^- lymphocytes (putative γ/δ T cells). *Immunol* 74:234, 1991.

Mosbech H, Weeke B: Does immunotherapy have a role in the treatment of asthma? *Clin Allergy* 16:10, 1986.

Noon L: Prophylactic inoculation against hay fever. *Lancet* I:1572, 1911.

Norman PS: Immunotherapy. *Prog Allergy* 32:318, 1982.

Ohman JL: Allergen immunotherapy in asthma: Evidence for efficacy. *J Allergy Clin Immunol* 84:132, 1989.

Reilly DT, Taylor MA, McSharry C, et al.: Is homoeopathy a placebo response? Controlled trial of homoeopathic potency, with pollen in hayfever as a model. *Lancet* II:881, 1986.

Stewart GE, Lockey RF: Systemic reactions from allergen immunotherapy. *J Allergy Clin Immunol* 90:567, 1992.

PHARMA-COLOGY OF ATOPIC REACTIONS

Beer DJ, Osband ME, McCaffery RP, et al.: Abnormal histamine-induced suppressor cell function in atopic subjects. *N Engl J Med* 306:454, 1982.

Church MK, Lowman MA, Pees PH, et al.: Mast cells, neuropeptides, and inflammation. *Agents Action* 27:8, 1989.

Fraser CM, Venter JC: Autoantibodies to β-adrenergic receptors and asthma. *J Allergy Clin Immunol* 74:227, 1984.

Gellhorn E: *Autonomic Imbalance and the Hypothalamus.* Minneapolis, University of Minnesota Press, 1957.

Goodfriend L, Sehon AH, Orange RP (eds.): *Mechanisms in Allergy: Reagin-mediated Hypersensitivity.* New York, Marcel Dekker, 1973.

Morley J (ed.): *Beta-adrenergic Receptors in Asthma.* Academic Press, New York, 1984.

Orange RP, Austen KF: Chemical mediators of immediate hypersensitivity. *Hosp Pract* 6:79, 1971.

Parker CW: Autoantibodies and β-adrenergic receptors. *N Engl J Med* 305:1212, 1981.

Robin GA, Butcher RW, Sutherland EW: *Cyclic AMP.* New York, Academic Press, 1971.

Sibley DR, Lefkowitz RJ: Molecular mechanisms of receptor desensitization using the β-adrenergic receptor-coupled adenylate cyclase system as a model. *Nature* 317:124, 1985.

Sutherland EW, Robinson GA, Butcher CW: Cyclic AMP. *Circulation* 37:279, 1968.

Szentivanyi A: The β-adrenergic theory of the atopic abnormality in bronchial asthma. *J Allergy* 42:203, 1968.

Wallukat G, Wollenberger A: Autoantibodies to β_2-adrenergic receptors with anti-adrenergic activity from patients with allergic asthma. *J Allergy Clin Immunol* 88:581, 1991.

Wasserman SI, Center DM: The relevance of neutrophil chemotactic factors to allergic disease. *J Allergy Clin Immunol* 64:231, 1979.

Willis T: *Pharmaceutic Rationales on the Operations of Mechanics in Humane Bodies.* London, Dring, 1984, 78–85.

TREATMENT OF ATOPIC ALLERGY

Berglund E, Svedmyr N: Asthma: Evaluation of drug therapy. *Scand J Resp Dis* 1011(suppl.):1, 1978.

Buckle DR, Smith H (eds.): Development of anti-asthma drugs. London, Butterworths, 1984.

Church MK, Warner JO: Sodium cromoglycate and related drugs. *Clin Allergy* 15:311, 1985.

Dahl R, Haahtela T: Prophylactic pharmacologic treatment of asthma. *Allergy* 47:588–593, 1992.

Kay AB, Austen KF, Lightenstein LM (eds.): *Asthma: Physiology, Immunopharmacology, and Treatment.* New York, Academic Press, 1984.

Orr TSC, Pollard MC, Gwilliam J, et al.: Mode of action of disodium cromoglycate: Studies on immediate-type hypersensitivity reactions using "double sensitization" with two antigenically distinct rat reagins. *Clin Exp Immunol* 7:745, 1970.

Platts-Mills TAE, Chapman MD: Dust mites: Immunology, allergic disease, and environmental control. *J Allergy Clin Immunol* 80:755, 1987.

PROTECTIVE ROLE OF ATOPIC REACTIONS

Moqbel R, Pritchard DI: Parasites and allergy: Evidence for a "cause-and-effect" relationship. *Clin Exp Allergy* 20:611, 1990.

Rothwell TLW: Immune expulsion of parasitic nematodes from the alimentary tract. *Int J Parasitol* 19:139, 1989.

Stebbings JH Jr: Immediate hypersensitivity: A defense against arthropods. *Perspect Biol Med* 17:233, 1974.

Soulsby EJL: The mechanism of immunity to gastrointestinal nematodes. In *Biology of Parasites.* New York, Academic Press, 1966.

Steinberg P, Ishizaka K, Norman PS: Possible role of IgE-mediated reactions in immunity. *J Allergy Clin Immunol* 54:359, 1974.

15

T Cell-Mediated Cytotoxicity

T$_{CTL}$, T$_{DTH}$, and
NK Cells

The term **cell-mediated immunity** was first used to refer to the effects of specifically sensitized lymphocytes after reaction with antigen or target cells in vitro. Cell-mediated immunity has been extended to two types of T cell-mediated effects in vivo: T-cell killing by cytotoxic T lymphocytes (T$_{CTL}$) and T cell-mediated delayed-type hypersensitivity (T$_{DTH}$) cells. T$_{CTL}$ lyse or "kill" target cells expressing specific antigens in vitro; T$_{DTH}$ cells release "lymphokines" with biologic activity after reaction with specific antigens in vitro. T-cell killing is initiated by a CD8+ subpopulation of specifically sensitized T$_{CTL}$, which react with cell surface antigens associated with class I major histocompatibility complex (MHC) markers and destroy the target cells. Delayed hypersensitivity is a local inflammatory reaction caused by the release of lymphokines from CD4+ T$_{DTH}$ cells that are induced through antigen processing in the context of class II MHC markers. The reason for the genetic restriction of recognition by T cells is not clear. However, functionally, T$_{CTL}$ may be induced by antigen processing in any nucleated cell (endogenous processing), whereas T$_{DTH}$ induction requires exogenous processing by class II MHC positive antigen presenting cells (macrophages/B-cells). MHC restriction is mediated by the receptors of T cells, which contain recognition sites for antigens only when seen in association with MHC molecules. Delayed hypersensitivity reactions are presented in the next chapter.

Upon reaction with antigens in association with class I MHC on tissue cells, T$_{CTL}$ are activated to kill the target cell. Professional CD8+ T$_{CTL}$s kill target cells through two distinct, but not mutually exclusive mechanisms, 1) granule exocytosis (perforin and granzymes) and by the Fas cell death system (Figure 15–1). **Granule exocytosis**: T$_{CTL}$s

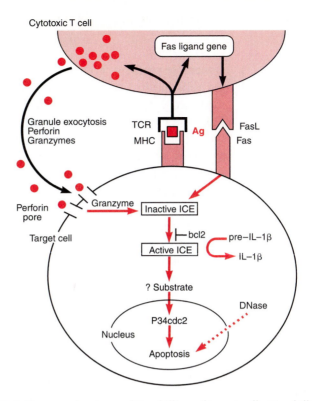

Figure 15–1. Two mechanisms of T_{CTL} killing of target cells. T_{CTL} killing is mediated through endogenous proteases in the target cell, such as interleukin 1β converting enzyme (ICE). Upon binding of the T_{CTL} receptor to antigen on class I MHC of the target cells T_{CTLS} activate the two killing systems: Fas ligand and granular (perforin and granzymes). Fas ligand on the T_{CTL} binds to and activates Fas (the death gene) on the target cell. Perforin reacts with the target cell membrane to produce "holes" in the membrane that permit granzymes to enter the cell. Upon entering the cytoplasm, granzymeB acts on a polyADPribose substrate, proYAMA to produce active YAMA. Active YAMA acts on an as yet know substrate to activate apoptotic mechanisms. Inactive intracellular ICE (interleukin 1β converting enzyme is converted to active ICE through the action of Fas in as yet unknown ways. The activation of ICE by Fas, is inhibited by the product of the bcl-2 gene. Conversion of pro-IL-1β to IL-1β by active ICE and the release of IL-1β signals adjacent cells of the impending death of the target cell. Activated ICE or YAMA appear to act on an as yet unidentified substrate essential for survival of the cell. This results in activation of p34[cdc2] kinase, entry of DNase into the nucleus, nuclear collapse and eventual cell death (apoptosis). There are many steps in this process that remain unclear. (Modified from Smyth MJ, Trapani JA: Granzymes: exogenous proteinases that induce target cell apoptosis. *Immunol Today* 16:202–206, 1995.)

contain multicomponent cytoplasmic granules containing cytolytic molecules such as perforin, proteoglycans and serine proteases (granzymes) which, in the presence of calcium, mediate lysis of target cells. These enzymes are also active in NK cell mediated killing and the mechanisms of cell lysis by T_{CTL} and NK cells appears to be very similar. However, some cytotoxic T_{CTL} cell line hybridomas lacking detectable perforin, granzymes and lytic granules are able to lyse target cells in vitro, suggesting still an additional mechanism(s) of T_{DTL}-mediated cytotoxicity. One additional mechanism is the Fas system.

Fas: The Fas gene codes for a cell surface receptor in the tumor necrosis factor receptor family that, when reacted with the Fas ligand (FasL), activates a "ready to go" cell death system. Activation of T-cytotoxic cells through the T-cell receptor leads to activation of the Fas ligand gene and expression of FasL on the surface of the T cell. Both CD8+ and CD4+(Th1) cells may express the FasL, but CD4+ cells do not express the granule system. Many cells including liver, heart, keratinocytes, express Fas, so that recognition of endogenous antigens through the TCR and class I MHC and activation of the FasL gene will activate the Fas death gene system. At the time of writing, the mechanism of Fas mediated death was not known.

The effectiveness of T_{CTL} killing is related to the expression of cell adhesion molecules, such as H-CAM (CD44) and α4β1-integrin (VLA-4), which determine the ability of the T_{CTL} to bind to target cells. The subset of δ CD4-8- T cells, which make up 1–2% of circulating T cells, may serve as an "early warning" rapid response T_{CTL} system, that acts to hold infections in check during the first few days after exposure. These cells are constitutively activated and can kill target cells *in vitro* without being activated by IL-2.

NK cells may also take part in what may be considered a mirror image of T_{CTL}-mediated cytolytic mechanisms. T_{CTL} cells recognize foreign peptides complexed to class I MHC and are activated to kill the cell; NK cells recognize class I MHC molecules complexed with self-protective peptides and do not kill the cells. Class I MHC expression by tissue cells protects against NK lysis by binding protective peptides, such as heat shock protein, elongation factor 2, histone H_3, and ribosomal proteins, which occupy a pocket in the MHC groove. Cells with abnormal MHC class I expression or insufficient protective peptide binding, such as tumor cells or cells infected with virus, are subject to lysis by NK cells. The conserved protective peptides appear to be similar to peptides encoded by infectious agents (eg, viruses), but the peptides produced by infectious agents have critical amino acid substitutions that do not confer protection. Upon infection, peptides from the infectious agent compete with self peptides for presentation by MHC molecules. Complexes of these peptides with MHC prevents self recognition by the NK receptor, rendering an infected cell susceptible to NK lysis. Although there is considerable interest in the adaptation of NK cells for tumor immunotherapy (see Chapter 30), it is not clear what role NK cells play during naturally occurring immune responses in vivo.

It was not until the mid-1960s that most immunologists began to consider cell-mediated immunity as an important immune mechanism.

Before that, essentially all that was known was the peculiar delayed hypersensitivity skin reaction that was elicited in certain infectious diseases, particularly tuberculosis, to extracts of organisms. It is now known that T-cell killing and/or delayed hypersensitivity are the major defense mechanisms against many infectious diseases, as well as the effector mechanisms in homograft rejections and many autoimmune diseases. CMI differs from the immune reactions mentioned previously in this text in that no humoral antibody is involved and reactivity cannot be transferred by serum, but only by cells; the time course of the development of the lesion is much prolonged; and the gross and microscopic appearance are different. Cell-mediated reactions feature infiltrations of tissues by mononuclear cells (lymphocytes and macrophages). The importance of cell-mediated immunity in infectious diseases has been brought to the forefront by the variety and number of opportunistic infections with viruses, protozoa, fungi, and mycobacteria in AIDS patients who have defective CD4+ T cell-mediated immunity (see Chapter 29).

T-Cytotoxic Reactions

The first appreciation of T-cytotoxic activity came from the recognition that T_{CTL} cells could "kill" specific target cells in vitro. The interaction of sensitized lymphocytes and target cells may be studied morphologically by observing the effect of sensitized lymphocytes on target cells growing in monolayers. Plaques or holes occur in the monolayer when sensitized lymphocytes are added. Sensitized lymphocytes surround the target cells and eventually cause their detachment from the monolayer. Figure 15–2 depicts the destruction of monolayer target cells. As long as the target cells remain attached to the monolayer, they appear to be viable; however, upon separation from the monolayer, the target cell undergoes morphologic alterations indicative of cell death. These alterations include vacuolization and disintegration of the cytoplasm and condensation of nucleus and cytoplasm. Although close contact between the sensitized lymphocytes and target cells occurs, the exact mechanism of target cell death remains unclear (see Fig. 15–1).

An identical type of interaction between lymphocytes and target cells may occur in vivo in tissue reactions mediated by lymphocytes. Figure 15–3 shows the pathologic changes occurring during the cell-mediated rejection of a renal allograft or development of experimental allergic thyroiditis. As in the target cell monolayer system, lymphocytes pass across the basement membrane of the renal tubule or the thyroid follicle. The T_{CTL} pass between the renal tubule cells or the thyroid follicular cells, causing them to separate from each other and from the basement membrane, eventually destroying the renal tubule or thyroid follicle cells. The basement membrane appears intact during the

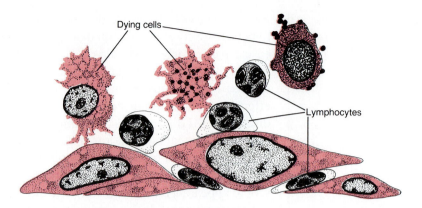

Figure 15–2. Reaction of sensitized lymphocytes with target cells in vitro. T lymphocytes from a sensitized donor infiltrate and surround monolayer target cells, seemingly without effect on viability or morphologic appearance of target cells. As a result of this infiltration, monolayer cells become separated from each other and from culture surface. Monolayer cells that retain contact with monolayer remain viable, but when separated from other monolayer cells, morphologic changes consistent with cell death occur. These alterations do not occur in tissue culture cells that become separated from the monolayer in the presence of normal lymphocytes. Fluids and washings taken from monolayers treated with sensitized lymphocytes cannot be used to initiate new cultures, whereas fluids or washings of cultures treated with normal lymphocytes can. DC, dead or dying cells separated from monolayers; L, lymphocytes; MTC, monolayer target cells. (Modified from Biberfield P, Holm G, Perlmann P: *Exp Cell Res* 52:672, 1968. Copyright Academic Press.)

development of the lesion. Infiltration of mononuclear cells, with separation, isolation, and destruction of target cells, is seen in contact dermatitis and viral exanthems, as well as in many autoimmune diseases and during tissue graft rejections.

CONTACT DERMATITIS

Contact allergy (contact eczema, dermatitis venenata) is exemplified by the common allergic reaction to poison ivy. It also occurs as an allergic response to a wide variety of simple chemicals in such things as ointments, clothing, cosmetics, dyes, rubber products, antiseptics, and adhesive tape, as well as metals such as nickel in sewing thimbles. The antigens are usually highly reactive chemical compounds capable of combining with proteins; they are also lipid-soluble and can penetrate the epidermis. The antigen often is an incomplete antigen (hapten) that combines with some constituent of the epidermis to form a complete antigen. Sensitization occurs by exposure of the skin once or repeatedly to sufficiently high concentrations of antigen to induce an

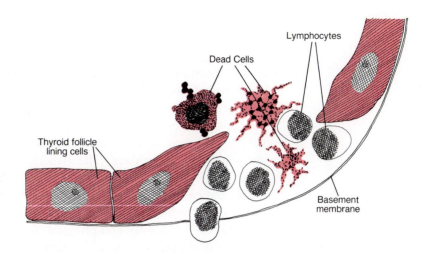

Figure 15–3. Reaction of sensitized lymphocytes with target cells in vivo (morphologic changes in experimental renal graft rejection or allergic thyroiditis). Changes similar to those observed in reactions of sensitized lymphocytes with tissue culture monolayers occur during renal homograft rejection or with thyroid follicle-lining cells in allergic thyroiditis. Mononuclear cells appear first in perivenular areas and then invade the stroma of the organ. Invasion of tubules or follicles follows. Lymphocytes appear to pass through basement membrane, separating renal tubule or thyroid follicle-lining cells from basement membrane and from other follicular cells. Death of lining cells occurs when these cells are isolated from basement membrane and from other tubule or follicular cells. DC, dead or dying cells; L, lymphocytes; TFC, thyroid follicle-lining cells. (Modified from Flax MH: *Lab Invest* 12:199, 1963. Copyright 1963, International Academy of Pathology.)

immune response. Langerhans' cells within the epidermis (see Chapter 3) are believed to play an important role in antigen processing and delivery of the antigen to the draining lymph node where sensitization takes place. In addition, epidermal keratinocytes express class I MHC antigens and may be able to present antigen directly to class I MHC-restricted T_{CTL} precursors.

Every person is susceptible if exposed to the antigen in sufficient amounts. For instance, poison ivy is not found in Great Britain. When native British are first exposed to poison ivy, they do not show the typical contact allergic reaction because they have not been sensitized. However, after a sensitizing exposure, poison ivy will elicit contact dermatitis.

A greater amount of antigen is needed for sensitization than for elicitation of skin reaction in an already sensitive individual. When United States soldiers moved into Japan after World War II, the military medical dispensaries noticed the widespread occurrence of a skin rash with the appearance of contact dermatitis. It was the distribution of the rash that was most unusual: It occurred on the elbows and buttocks. After diligent sleuthing, it was discovered that the bars and toilet seats of certain Japanese public establishments were coated with a lacquer made from the sap of a tree that contained small amounts of a substance closely related to the poison ivy antigen. The amounts of this related antigen were not great enough to sensitize the native Japanese, but were sufficient to elicit the characteristic dermatitis in the previously sensitized Americans. The American soldiers were sensitive because of previous exposure to poison ivy. Also related are the oleoresins of the cashew nut shell, the rind of the mango, the ginkgo tree fruit pulp, and Indian marking nut resin. All of these plants belong to the *Avacardiaceae* family and produce oleoresins called urushiol that cross-react in skin tests of sensitive patients.

The characteristic skin reaction is elicited in sensitized individuals by exposing the skin to the antigen (natural exposure, patch tests). The reaction is a sharply delineated, superficial skin inflammation, beginning as early as 24 hours after exposure and reaching a maximum at 48 to 96 hours (Fig. 15–4). It is characterized by redness, induration, and vesiculation. The reactions may take longer to reach a maximum than the tuberculin skin test (see below), because of the longer time required for the antigen to penetrate the epidermis, and persist for longer times, because of the time required to remove the antigen from the epidermis. Histologically, the dermis shows perivenous accumulation of lymphocytes and monocytes and some edema. The epidermis is invaded by these cells and shows intraepidermal edema (spongiosis), which progresses to vesiculation and death of epidermal cells. A histopathologically similar reaction may be observed in irritant contact dermatitis, in which there is chemical injury of epidermal cells not caused by an immune mechanism. In lesions, there is upregulation of the cell adhesion molecule ICAM-1 on keratinocytes that are associated with LFA-1 positive lymphocytes. Thus, these cell adhesion molecules may play an important role in the T_{CTL}–keratinocyte interaction.

It was once assumed that the lesion was the result of sensitization of the epidermal cells themselves. However, no reaction occurs when the local vascular supply is interrupted, and careful histologic study shows that infiltration of the epidermis with lymphocytes precedes the epidermal cell damage. Since antibody is not involved, it is clear that hematogenous cells are the carriers of sensitivity, and epidermal death is comparable to the destruction of parenchyma (ie, the cells bearing the antigen) in homograft rejection and cell-mediated autoimmune lesions. Sensitivity can be passively transferred with lymphocytes but not with antiserum. In addition, contact reactivity is suppressed by depleting the circulating lymphocytes in experimental animals by radiation or by specific antiserum to lymphocytes.

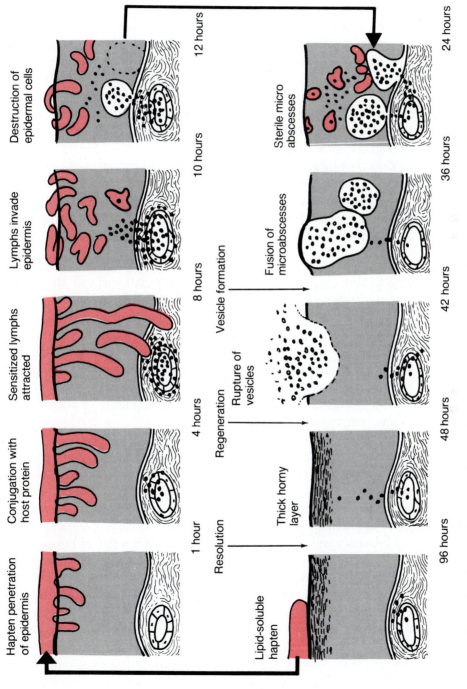

Figure 15–4. Evolution of contact dermatitis reaction. A contact-sensitizing hapten such as dinitrophenol or poison ivy oleoresin needs to be in either a lipid-solvent or lipid-soluble form in order to penetrate the epidermis. In so doing, the contact-sensitizing hapten joins to host proteins to become a complete antigen. In a sensitive individual, penetration of the epidermis brings the antigen into contact with specifically sensitized T_{CTL} cells that react with the antigen and initiate a cell-mediated reaction that destroys the epithelial cells.

The characteristics of the eliciting antigen determine the nature of the reaction. In poison ivy reactions, for example, because the lipid-soluble antigen is mainly present in the epidermis, it takes about two days for the reacting mononuclear cells (mainly lymphocytes but also macrophages) to invade from the dermis and react with the antigen. As a result of this invasion and reaction, epidermal cells are destroyed, and small foci (sterile microabcesses) are formed, eventually leading to vesicle formation that can be seen on the skin as small, fluid-filled blebs. Since all of the hapten may not be degraded in the vesicles, rupture of the vesicles by scratching may spread the antigen to uninvolved areas of the skin and provoke new reactions. Proliferation of the basal epidermal cells results in eventual sloughing of the affected epidermal cells. This process may take up to a week to ten days, depending on the amount of antigen present and the degree of sensitization of the individual. Poison ivy or poison oak oleoresin may remain stable in the dry state for long periods of time so that indirect exposure may occur from touching clothes, tools, or animals that are contaminated with dried plant resins.

TISSUE GRAFT REJECTION

Classic tissue graft rejection is usually caused by cell-mediated immunity to alloantigens, but antibody to donor antigens can also initiate complement-mediated injury. Both direct killing of target cells by CD8+ class I MHC-restricted T_{CTL} and release of lymphokines from CD4+ class II MHC-restricted T_{DTH} cells that attract and activate macrophages are involved in immune destruction of a tissue graft. In addition, humoral antibody can activate complement-mediated inflammation and destruction of a graft. Antibody-mediated graft rejection usually becomes important when cellular immunity is controlled by immunosuppressive therapy.

The immunopathologic events in tissue graft rejection are presented in more detail in Chapter 26. In the absence of immunosuppressive therapy, rejection of tissue grafts is associated with mononuclear cell infiltrate. For skin, kidney, and liver grafts, for example, the major target antigens are on differentiated epithelial cells—the squamous epithelium of the skin, the tubule-lining cells of the kidney, and the bile duct cells of the liver. Early histologic signs of rejection feature the infiltration of lymphocytes across the basement membrane into and between the epithelial cells with killing of individual keratinocytes, tubule cells, or bile duct cells. The major cellular infiltrate in the epithelial cells is made up of CD8+ cells; CD4+ cells are seen in the interstitial connective tissues. Cell-mediated rejection of the kidney, for example, is characterized by the infiltration of lymphocytes into the renal tubules (tubulitis). Interstitial infiltrates of mononuclear cells are not specific for graft rejection. Thus, the major mechanism of rejection of solid organs in untreated recipients is due to the cytotoxicity of T_{CTL} cells for epithelial cells.

Humoral antibody may contribute to rejection of a tissue allograft. Perhaps the first evidence that circulating antibody did play a role in graft rejection was provided by Chandler Stetson, who demonstrated an acute necrotic rejection of skin allograft when specific antiserum to the graft was injected directly into the site of the skin graft. The failure of any circulation to be established resulted in complete ischemic necrosis (*white graft rejection*). The interplay of antibody-mediated and cellular reactions in graft rejection is illustrated by the stages of rejection observed in human renal allografts (see Chapter 23).

VIRAL EXANTHEMS

Cell-mediated reactions to viral infections illustrate the "double-edged sword" of protective and destructive effects of immunity. Cell-mediated immunity (CMI) to viral antigens may be either protective by limiting viral infections or destructive by destroying functioning host cells that are expressing viral antigens. On the one hand, CMI is responsible for destruction of virus-infected cells and recovery from infections, such as measles, herpes simplex, and smallpox. On the other hand, CMI to viral antigens on vital host cells may lead to loss of tissue function, or viral infections may lead to reaction of CMI to self tissue antigens (autoimmunity).

An exanthem is a disease or fever associated with eruptive skin lesions. In 1907, von Pirquet observed that the local lesion following smallpox vaccination (vaccinia) consisted of a two-stage reaction. Early (first 8 days), there is a papular vesicular lesion because of the growth of the inoculated virus; later (8 to 14 days), an indurated erythematous reaction (take) follows. The take reaction corresponds to the development of CMI and is interpreted as evidence that protective immunity has been established. Similar lesions appear at the same time on different parts of the body, even though the different areas are inoculated with the virus at different times. Animal experiments have shown that protection against the virus is associated with T_{CTL} cells, and that the infective virus disappears from the local lesion when systemic CMI is maximal. The same concept was considered valid by von Pirquet for other viral exanthems (measles, varicella) in which multiple, disseminated lesions occur as a result of T_{CTL} reaction to viruses located at the sites of lesions. Some of the lesions of the viral exanthems may be modified by humoral antibody reacting with viral antigens to produce an Arthus-like reaction in the skin or T_{DTH} reaction producing delayed hypersensitivity reactions; however, T_{CTL}-mediated killing of virus infected cells is the major mechanism. Lesions are caused by destruction of infected epithelial cells.

SMALLPOX

Immunity to the smallpox virus is induced by stimulation of T_{CTL} cells. Vaccination against smallpox is accomplished by inoculation into the skin of a related virus (vaccinia) that usually produces only a local

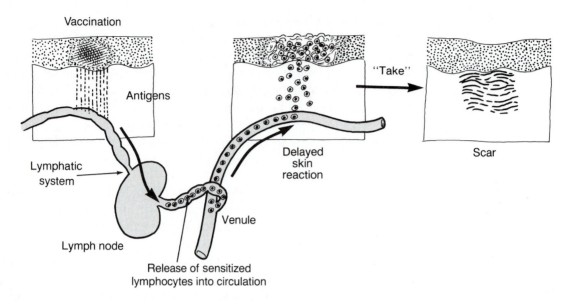

Figure 15–5. Vaccination against smallpox. Introduction of vaccinia virus into the skin results in proliferation of organisms in epithelial cells, followed by development of cytotoxic T cells and destruction of infected cells. Viral antigens are carried by lymphatics to draining lymph nodes where primary T-cell response results in production of sensitized cells. The sensitized cells return to attack virus-infected epithelial cells producing a take, ie, a necrotic delayed skin reaction. The take reaction indicates establishment of protective immunity to reinfection.

lesion. The local lesion, called a take, is produced by T-cytotoxic to vaccinia antigens, that are shared with the virulent smallpox virus. The "take" reaction consists of a focal necrotic reaction produced by infiltrating cytotoxic lymphocytes killing virus-infected epithelial cells (Fig. 15–5). Smallpox vaccination is presented in more detail in Chapter 26 (Vaccination).

AUTOIMMUNE DISEASE: THYROIDITIS

Thyroiditis is one of the most extensively studied experimental autoimmune diseases and is mainly mediated by T_{CTL} cells. It occurs 6 to 14 days following immunization of an experimental animal with thyroid extract or thyroglobulin in complete Freund's adjuvant. Evolution of the disease is presented in Figure 15–6. The lesion begins as a perivenous infiltration of lymphocytes, and destruction of the thyroid follicular epithelium is accomplished by the invasion of specifically sensitized cells similar to the lesion of contact dermatitis. Thus, the major effector mechanism for the disease appears to be T_{CTL}-mediated cytotoxicity. CD4+ cells are more active in passive transfer of the experimental disease, but CD8+ cells are found *in situ* in the lesions and are able to kill follicular cells in vitro. In active lesions, secretion of IFN-γ induces expression of ICAM-1 and class II MHC and

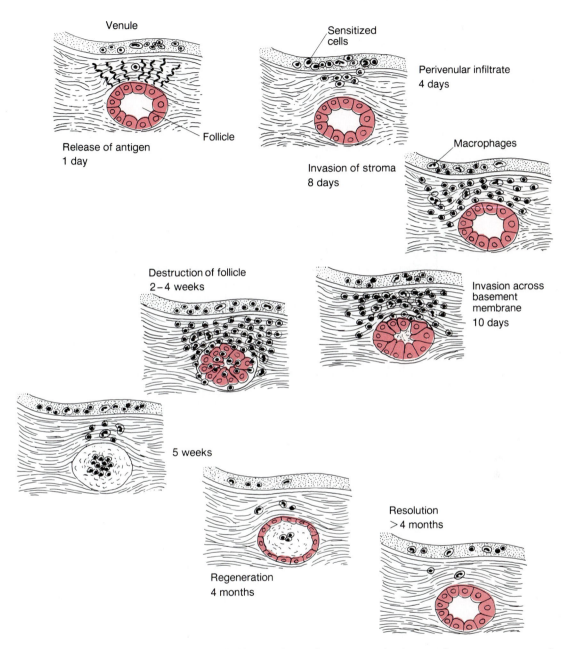

Figure 15–6. Evolution of experimental allergic thyroiditis (EAT). The lesions begin as perivascular infiltrates that extend through the interfollicular stroma to invade the follicular lining cells. Destruction of the lining cells occurs wherever mononuclear cells invade. Prior to destruction, the lining cells may enlarge and become more densely stained in histologic sections (Hurthle or Askanazy cells). After the follicular lining cells are destroyed, the follicles may be filled with mononuclear cells (Askanazy body). In EAT, the lesions always resolve, presumably because of regeneration of the follicular lining cells similar to that of epithelial cells after contact dermatitis.

ICAM-1 on thyroid cells. This may contribute to binding of T_{CTL} cells between ICAM-1 and $\alpha_1\beta_2$-integrin (LFA-1), and maintenance of the inflammatory response to autoantigens on thyroid cells by T_{DTH}. Of interest is the finding that about 20% of cancer patients treated with IL-2 or INF-α develop hypothyroid symptoms and evidence of autoimmune thyroiditis.

The experimental disease almost always resolves, although some instances of chronic lesions have been reported. The severity and course of the disease are not related to antibody titer, but do correlate with delayed hypersensitivity skin tests. In humans, **Hashimoto's thyroiditis**, a disease of unknown etiology, is characterized by intense lymphocytic infiltration and formation of lymphocytic follicles with prominent germinal centers. There are certain histologic similarities between Hashimoto's disease and experimental allergic thyroiditis, and there is a high incidence of antibodies in thyroglobulin and other thyroid antigens in patients with this disease.

The role of antithyroid antibodies in the pathogenesis of allergic thyroiditis remains unclear. Experimental thyroiditis may be transferred with both cells and antiserum in rabbits. Antibody may play a role in initiation of lesions by increasing the permeability of venules to lymphocytes, permitting the passage of sensitized cells, which make contact with the target cells. As covered in Chapter 11, antithyroid hormone antibodies may contribute to hypothyroidism, and antithyroid hormone receptor antibodies may cause hyperthyroidism (Graves' disease). Electron-dense deposits have been found in the follicular basement membrane of thyroids from patients with Hashimoto's disease that are similar to the deposits of immune complexes found in toxic complex glomerulonephritis. There is some evidence that circulating antibody may actually suppress the development of experimental allergic thyroiditis. In addition, circulating thyroglobulin–antithyroglobulin-soluble immune complexes may deposit out in the kidney and cause toxic complex glomerulonephritis. Also, antibody could direct an ADCC effect on follicular cells. "Natural" antibodies to thyroglobulin, found in the sera of normal individuals, react to a different region of the thyroglobulin molecule (region V) than do antibodies found in individuals with thyroid disorders (region II).

Summary

Cell-mediated immune reactions are initiated by reaction of specifically sensitized lymphocytes with antigen in tissues. Two major T-lymphocyte populations are involved: T_{CTL} killing of antigen-bearing target cells and T_{DTH} (delayed hypersensitivity). T_{DTH} cells release lymphocytic mediators when activated by antigen that produce tissue inflammation mainly by attracting and activating macrophages. Examples of T_{CTL}-mediated reactions presented in this chapter include contact dermatitis, viral exanthems (smallpox), tissue graft rejections and autoimmune diseases, such as thyroiditis. T-cytotoxic reactions are active in a number of other diseases, including skin lesions (see Chapter 20), autoimmune diseases (see Chapter 21), transplantation rejection (see Chapter 23), and infectious diseases (see Chapter 25), as well as playing a major role in tumor immunity (see Chapter 30).

Bibliography

T_{CTL}

Berke G, Rosen D: Mechanism of lymphocyte-mediated cytolysis: Functional cytolytic T cells lacking perforin and granzymes. *Immunology* 78:105–112, 1993.

Biberfield P, Holm G, Perlmann P: Morphologic observations on lymphocyte peripolesis and cytotoxic action in vitro. *Exp Cell Res* 52:672, 1968.

Flax MH: Experimental allergic thyroiditis in the guinea pig. II. Morphologic studies on the development of the disease. *Lab Invest* 12:199, 1971.

Liu C-C, Walsh CM, Young JD: Perforin: Structure and function. *Immunol Today* 16:194–201, 1995.

Lowrey DM, Hameed A, Lichenfeld MG, et al.: Isolation and characterization of cytotoxic granules from human lymphokine (IL-2)-activated killer cells. *Cancer Res* 48:4681, 1988.

Nomoto K, Yoshikai Y: Heat-shock protein and immunopathology: Regulatory role of heat-shock protein-specific T cells. *Springer Semin Immunopath* 13:63, 1991.

Rodiriques M, Nussenzweig RS, Romero P, et al.: The in vivo cytotoxic activity of CD8+ T-cell clones correlates with their levels of expression of adhesion molecules. *J Exp Med* 175:895, 1992.

Rosenau W, Moon HD: Lysis of homologous cells by sensitized lymphocytes in tissue culture. *J Natl Cancer Inst* 27:471, 1961.

Smyth MJ, Trapani JA: Granzymes: Exogenous proteases that induce target cell apoptosis. *Immunol Today* 16:202–206, 1995.

Versteeg R: NK cells and T cells: Mirror images? *Immunol Today* 13:244, 1992.

CONTACT DERMATITIS

Auerbuck R, Baer H: Comparison of potency of poison ivy extracts with synthetic pentadecylcatechols in sensitive humans. *J Allergy* 35:3, 1964.

Epstein E, Clairborne ER: Racial and environmental factors in susceptibility to Rhus. *Excerpta Med* 12:357, 1958.

Fisher AA: Allergic contact reactions in health personnel. *J Allergy Clin Immunol* 90:729–738, 1992.

Flax MH, Caulfield JB: Cellular and vascular components of allergic contact dermatitis. *Am J Path* 43:1031, 1963.

Foussereau J, Benezra C, Maibach HH: Occupational contact dermatitis: Clinical and chemical aspects. Philadelphia, WB Saunders, 1982.

Kalish RS, Johnson KL: Enrichment and function of urushiol (poison ivy)-specific T lymphocytes in lesions of allergic contact dermatitis to urushiol. *J Immunol* 145:3706, 1990.

Kalish RS, Wood JA, La Porte A: Processing of URUSHIOL (poison ivy) hapten by both endogenous and exogenous pathways for presentation to T cells in vitro. *J Clin Invest* 93:2039–2047, 1994.

Kligman AM: Poison ivy (Rhus) dermatitis: Experiment study. *Arch Dermatol* 77:149, 1958.

Kripke ML, Munn CG, Jeevan A, et al.: Evidence that cutaneous antigen-presenting cells migrate to regional lymph nodes during contact sensitization. *J Immunol* 145:2833, 1990.

Londei M, Lanb JR, Bottazzo GF, et al.: Epithelial cells expressing MHC class II determinants can present antigen to cloned T cells. *Nature* 312:639, 1984.

Spain WC, Newell JM, Meeker MG: The percentage of persons susceptible to poison ivy and poison oak. *J Allergy* 5:365, 1967.

Willis CM, Stephens CJM, Wilkinson JD: Selective expression of immune-mediated surface antigens by keratinocytes in irritant contact dermatitis. *J Invest Dermatol* 96:505, 1991.

Willis CM, Young E, Brandon DR, et al.: Immunopathologic and ultrastructural findings in human allergic and irritant contact dermatitis. *Brit J Dermatol* 115:305, 1986.

SMALLPOX

Behbehani AM: The smallpox story: Life and death of an old disease. *Microbiol Rev* 47:455, 1983.

Jenner E: An inquiry into the causes and effects of the variolae vaccine. London, Low, 1798.

Plotkin SA, Plotkin SL: Vaccination: One hundred years later. In *World's Debt to Pasteur*. New York, Liss, 1985, 83.

Ricketts TF, Byles JB: *The Diagnosis of Smallpox*, vol. 1. London, Cassell, 1908.

THYROIDITIS

Askanasy M: Pathologische-anatomische Beitrage zur Kenntnies des Morbus basedouri, insbesondere uber die dabie auftretende Muskelerkrankung. *Dtsch Arch Klin Med* 61:118–186, 1898.

Atkins MB, Mier JW, Parkinson DR, et al.: Hypothyroidism after treatment with interleukin-2 and lymphokine-activated killer cells. *N Engl J Med* 318:1557, 1988.

Bouanani M, Piechaczyk M, Pau B, et al.: Significance of the recognition of certain antigenic regions on the human thyroglobulin molecule by natural antoantibodies from healthy subjects. *J Immunol* 143:1129, 1989.

Flax MH: Experimental allergic thyroiditis in the guinea pig. II. Morphologic studies on the development of the disease. *Lab Invest* 12:119, 1963.

Hall R: Immunological aspects of thyroid function. *N Engl J Med* 266:1204, 1962.

Hamilton F, Black M, Farquharson MA, et al.: Spatial correlation between thyroid epithelial cells expressing class II MHC molecules and interferon-gamma–containing lymphocytes in human thyroid autoimmune disease. *Clin Exp Immunol* 83:64, 1991.

Hashimoto H: Zurkenntuissder lymphomatosen veranderung der schilddruse (Struma lymphomatosa). *Arch Klin Chir* 97:219, 1912.

Kalderon AE, Bogaars HA, Diamond I: Ultrastructional alterations of follicular basement membrane in Hashimoto's thyroiditis. *Am J Med* 55:485, 1973.

Roitt IM, Doniach D, Campbell PN, et al.: Autoantibodies in Hashimoto's disease (lymphodenoid goitre). *Lancet* 2:820, 1956.

Rose NR, Witebsky E: Studies on organ specificity. V. Changes in the thyroid glands of rabbits following active immunization with rabbit thyroid extracts. *J Immunol* 76:417, 1956.

Weigle WO: The induction of autoimmunity in rabbits following injection of heterologous or altered homologous thyroglobulin. *J Exp Med* 121:289, 1965.

Witebsky E, Rose NR, Terplan K, et al.: Chronic thyroiditis and autoimmunization. *JAMA* 64:1439, 1957.

16

Delayed Hypersensitivity

Delayed hypersensitivity reactions are variations on a theme of chronic inflammation (see Chapter 9). Specifically sensitized CD4+ Th1 (T_{DTH}) cells are attracted to gradients of antigen released from tissues and interact with activated endothelial cells through reaction of lymphocyte receptors L-selectin (Lam-1), $\alpha_4\beta_1$-integrin (VLA-4), $\alpha_L\beta_2$-integrin (LFA-1), and H-CAM (CD44), with E-selectin, VCAM-1, ICAM-1, and carbohydrates on endothelial cells (see Figure 9–6). Upon reaction with soluble antigens in tissues, sensitized T_{DTH} cells release lymphokines, such as tumor necrosis factor (TNF), interleukin-2 (IL-2), interferon-gamma (INF-γ), and other inflammatory initiating factors, which attract and activate macrophages (Fig. 16–1). In turn, activated macrophages produce TNF-α, IL-1, IL-6, and PGE_2 which contribute to the late phase of the DTH reaction, as well as phagocytose and digest cells and tissue debris. This reaction is particularly effective against intracellular parasites that can replicate within macrophages, such as mycobacteria. The products of activated T_{DTH} cells enable infected macrophages to destroy the organisms they harbor. Of particular importance is the ability of activated T_{DTH} cells to produce IFN-γ. Mice with inactive IFN-γ genes are particularly susceptible to parasites, such as *Mycobacterium bovis* and *Listeria monocytogenes*, which infect macrophages. T_{DTH}-activated macrophages are also effective against extracellular infections, such as fungi and syphilis. Both reactions may result in extensive tissue destruction.

Delayed hypersensitivity is an in vivo reaction, which cannot be duplicated in vitro. The delayed hypersensitivity reaction in tissue begins with a perivascular accumulation of lymphocytes and monocytes at the site where antigen is located. Evidence obtained using labeled, specif-

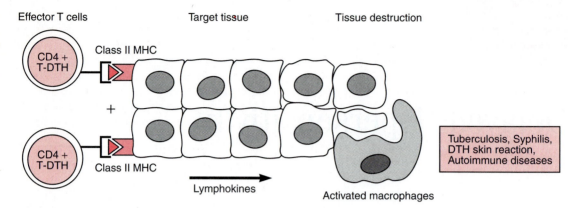

Figure 16–1. Delayed hypersensitivity reaction. Specifically sensitized T_{DTH} cells are activated by reaction with antigen to release interleukins (TNF, IL-2, INF-γ), which attract and activate macrophages. Activated macrophages produce TNF-α, IL-1, IL-6, and PGE_2 which contribute to the late phase of the DTH reaction, as well as phagocytose and digest cells and tissue debris. The activation of the macrophages is effective in clearing macrophages of intracellular infections, such as tuberculosis, leprosy, and leishmaniasis, as well as viral infections.

ically sensitized cells transferred to normal donors indicates that only a few of the infiltrating cells are specifically sensitized. The reaction of these few sensitized cells with the antigen in the tissue causes large numbers of unlabeled cells to infiltrate the area, with subsequent tissue destruction. The inflammatory response is induced and maintained by mediators derived from T_{DTH} lymphocytes (lymphokines). The role of lymphokines in inflammation is covered in Chapter 9. Destruction of infecting organisms or tissue is caused by macrophages. Specifically sensitized T_{DTH} cells are also activated to proliferate upon contact with antigen (blast transformation), resulting in an increased number of specifically sensitized cells, and mitogenic factors stimulate proliferation of nonsensitized cells.

The term "delayed" is applied because of the time course of the inflammatory skin reaction that follows intradermal injection of antigen into an individual who has been sensitized. The reaction takes several days to peak, in contrast to cutaneous anaphylactic reactions, which reach their peak in a few minutes, and the Arthus reaction, which occurs in hours. The term "tuberculin-type hypersensitivity" is used because for many years the study of this type of immune response was essentially the study of the delayed hypersensitivity immune response to tuberculin (proteins extracted from cultures of *Mycobacterium tuberculosis* and infection with tubercle bacilli.

T_{DTH} ACTIVATION AND SUPERANTIGENS

A group of toxins produced by various strains of *Staphylococcus aureus* and related toxins (Table 16–1) caused food poisoning, and one of the toxins is responsible for tampon-related toxic shock. These tox-

TABLE 16–1. DISEASES CAUSED BY SUPERANTIGENS

Superantigen/Toxin	Source	Disease
Staphylococcal enterotoxins	*S. aureus*	Food poisoning, shock
Toxic Shock Syndrome Toxin (TSST)	*S. aureus*	Toxic shock syndrome
Exfoliating toxins A and B	*S. aureus*	Scalded skin syndrome
Pyrogenic exotoxins A, B, and C	*S. pyogenes*	Rheumatic fever, scarlet fever
Mycoplasma arthritides supernatant	*M. arthritides*	Arthritis, shock

Modified from Marrack P, Kappler J: The staphylococcal enterotoxins and their relatives. *Science* 248:705, 1990.

ins are also called **superantigens** because they directly activate class MHC II-restricted T_{DTH} cells. These molecules are not processed to smaller peptides but bind to class II MHC molecules as whole molecules. The toxins/superantigens are intermediately sized proteins that bind to the Vβ region of the T-cell receptor in association with the class II DR protein, outside the peptide binding cleft (Fig. 16–2) and directly activate T cells. The most likely pathogenesis of symptoms is that the toxins produce massive T-cell stimulation and consequent release of T

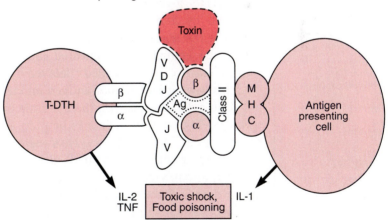

Figure 16–2. Hypothetical reaction of staphylococcal enterotoxin with class II MHC T-cell receptor. The toxins react with the class II MHC β chain, away from the antigen-binding grove and the Vβ chain of the T-cell receptor, acting as a clamp, to bring into close apposition the surfaces of the T-cell receptor and the MHC that would contact each other during T-cell recognition of antigen through conventional binding in the antigen grove of the MHC. J, D, V, chains of the cell receptor; α and β, chains of the MHC; Ag, antigen-binding grove of class II MHC; SA, superantigen.

cell-derived lymphokines such as IL-2 and TNF. Large amounts of these lymphokines released in the body cause the food poisoning/toxic shock reaction. It is also possible that toxins could stimulate macrophages through class II MHC binding, but experimental studies in mice that lack T cells but have normal macrophage activity indicate that activation of macrophages is not sufficient to produce disease. However, studies on human cells in vitro show not only that both monocytes and T cells are required, but also that the monocytes and T cells must be in contact with each other. Interleukin-1 (produced by macrophages) is elevated after toxin stimulation of human cells, but may not be sufficient to produce shock by itself.

DELAYED HYPERSENSITIVITY SKIN REACTION

The classic example of a delayed hypersensitivity skin test is the delayed-type tuberculin skin reaction (see Fig. 16–2). It is elicited in sensitive individuals by intradermal injection of tuberculoprotein antigens (PPD, OT). A delayed skin reaction to tubercle bacilli was noted in 1890 by Koch who injected live tubercle bacilli into guinea pigs previously infected with tuberculosis. Redness and swelling were noted 24 hours after injection. The lesion progressed to local tissue necrosis. This reaction was not observed in previously uninfected animals but could be demonstrated in infected animals using killed bacilli or extracts of the bacilli. The extract originally used was called old tuberculin (OT), a crude extract of cultures of tubercle bacilli. This was replaced by a more purified protein derivative (PPD) of cultures. Because the reaction occurred in hypersensitive animals, not in nonsensitized animals, and appeared much later after testing than the Arthus reaction, it was called "delayed hypersensitivity."

Following injection of antigen into the skin of an individual sensitive in a delayed manner, there is little or no reaction until after 4 to 6 hours. The grossly visible induration and swelling usually reach a maximum at 24 to 48 hours. Histologically, there is accumulation of mononuclear cells around small veins. Later, mononuclear cells may be seen throughout the area of the reaction with extensive infiltration in the dermis. Polymorphonuclear cells constitute fewer than one-third of the cells at any time, and usually few are present at 24 hours or later unless the reaction is severe enough to cause necrosis. There may also be infiltration and degranulation of basophils, perhaps contributing to the increased vascular permeability and edema observed. The CD4 and CD8 subsets of T cells in the perivascular areas are in the same ratio as in the peripheral blood, but the cells in the diffuse infiltrate in the dermis are predominantly CD4 T cells. The perivascular infiltrate may include nonspecifically attracted cells, whereas the diffuse infiltrate includes more specifically sensitized T_{DTH} cells.

The role of lymphocyte mediators in delayed hypersensitivity reactions may be delineated as follows: Upon contact with antigen, lymphocytes release migratory-inhibitory, skin-reactive, macrophage-specific chemotactic, and macrophage-activation factors, each of which serve to attract and hold macrophages in the reaction site. The number of specifically sensitized cells may be increased by lymphocyte-stimulating factors, which induces proliferation of lymphocytes. Cytotoxic factors may cause death of tissue cells in the reactive area; proliferative-inhibitory factor may inhibit nonlymphoid cell growth; and lymphocyte permeability factor may increase the magnitude of the inflammatory reaction by causing more cells to accumulate. (For a more detailed discussion of cytokines in inflammation, see Chapter 9).

The evolution of the delayed skin reaction is presented in Figure 16–3. This description incorporates the function of the lymphocyte mediators and macrophages. A simplified concept is that the lymphocyte initiates the reaction and the macrophage cleans it up.

CUTANEOUS BASOPHIL HYPERSENSITIVITY (CBH)

The term **cutaneous basophil hypersensitivity (CBH)** is used to denote a group of lymphocyte-mediated basophilic reactions that differ histologically from classic delayed-type reactions. Basophils may be found in a variety of cell-mediated reactions, including skin graft rejection, tumor rejection, reactions to viral infections, and contact allergy. CBH reactions require specifically sensitized lymphocytes. In contact dermatitis, infiltration of lymphocytes precedes basophils by at least 12 hours, probably releasing a lymphokine responsible for attracting basophils. The function of the basophilic infiltrate is not known but might serve as a phagocytic cell that supplements the macrophage.

The term Jones–Mote reaction originally referred to the reappearance of a delayed type of sensitivity to serum proteins after the development and regression of an Arthus reaction, noted in humans by Jones and Mote in 1934. This term was extended to cover the transient form of delayed skin reaction to protein antigens occurring prior to antibody production in experimental animals, a finding also previously observed in humans. With a better appreciation of the basophilic nature of these reactions, the term cutaneous basophil hypersensitivity has been applied. As an immunologic reaction, the significance of CBH-type reactions remains unclear. Since the presence of basophils in varying numbers has been described in human tuberculin as well as in Jones–Mote reactions, it may be that basophils are not really a distinguishing feature but are a variable constituent of delayed hypersensitivity reactions. Some experimental evidence suggests that tissue mast cells must be present in the dermis in order for antigens to elicit a DTH reaction. The mast cells may function to permit vasodilation and

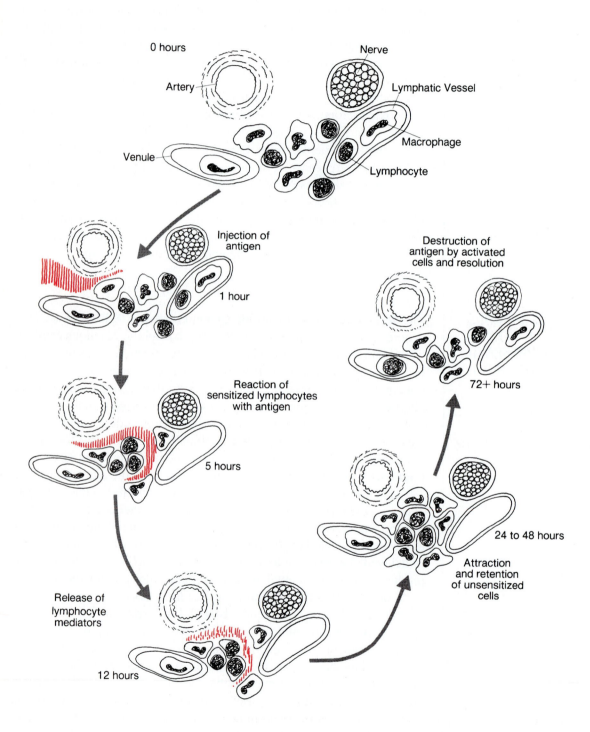

increased vascular permeability. However, typical DTH cutaneous reactions have been elicited in strains of mice lacking tissue mast cells.

TRANSFER FACTOR

In the 1950s, Lawrence reported that DTH reactions could be transferred from one individual to another with lysates from a population of highly sensitized lymphocytes, termed **transfer factor**. Previous passive transfer studies had required viable cells. Transfer factor is dialyzable, has a molecular weight of 10,000, is antigen specific, but is not genetically restricted. Transfer factor containing dialysates have been used to restore cell-mediated immunity in patients with a deficiency in CMI and to help control infections in patients with chronic mucocutaneous candidiasis. The chemical nature of transfer factor has not been adequately determined, and results of efficacy in different studies has led to considerable skepticism regarding the biological validity of transfer factor-mediated activity.

Delayed Hypersensitivity and Infection

For many years, the study of immunity was directed to the role of humoral antibody-mediated effects. During the 1960s, the importance of cell-mediated immunity in defense against viral, fungal, protozoal, and parasitic diseases became increasingly recognized. The opportunistic infections seen in the acquired immunodeficiency syndrome (AIDS) have driven home the significance of cellular immunity, especially DTH. The major immune deficit in AIDS is a lack of function of CD4+ T cells. Humoral antibody can prevent infections from first exposures, but once a virus infection has occurred, it will be combated by CMI. The effects of cell-mediated immunity in the pathogenesis of syphilis and viral infections (encephalomyelitis) will now be covered as an example of the "double-edged sword" of immunity. The role of T_{DTH} is also critical for the pathogenesis of tuberculosis. This will be covered in Chapter 17 (Granulomatous Reactions). See Chapter 25 for other examples of CMI in infectious immunity.

Figure 16–3. Evolution of the delayed skin reaction. In normal skin, lymphocytes pass from venules through the dermis to lymphatics, which return these cells to the circulation. Production of delayed skin reaction involves recognition of antigen by sensitized lymphocytes (T cells), immobilization of lymphocytes at the site, production and release of lymphocyte mediators, and accumulation of macrophages with eventual destruction of antigen and resolution of the reaction. This results in an accumulation of cells seen at 24 to 48 hours after antigen injection. Macrophages degrade the antigen. When the antigen is destroyed, the reactive cells are either destroyed or returned via the lymphatics to the bloodstream or draining lymph nodes. In this way, specifically sensitized lymphocytes may be distributed throughout the lymphoid system following local stimulation with antigen.

SYPHILIS

The tissue-clearing mechanism resulting in the healing of primary (chancre) and secondary syphilis lesions is T_{DTH}-mediated delayed hypersensitivity. The host–parasite relationship in syphilis has been the subject of study for 500 years, since syphilis was introduced into Europe by sailors returning with Columbus. By 1498, syphilis was ravaging Europe, killing up to 30% of infected individuals in the acute (primary) stage. The association of syphilis with sexual activity became readily apparent and is believed by some to have been the major factor in the change of sexual mores that occurred in the 16th and 17th centuries, giving rise to Puritanism. The social effects of syphilis in the 15th century resembles the effect of AIDS in the 20th century.

Natural History

The natural history of syphilis has changed, presumably as the less resistant population was killed off. Today we recognize primary, secondary, latent, and tertiary disease, each of which is determined largely by the immune response of the host. The evolution of the primary lesion, the chancre, the first clinical manifestation of primary syphilis, follows closely the pattern of a delayed hypersensitivity reaction in the skin. It lasts from one to five weeks, is initiated by sensitized T cells reacting with antigen, and is resolved by phagocytosis and digestion of organisms by macrophages (Fig. 16–4). Protection against reinfection may be partially mediated by antibody neutralization of organisms, but macrophages activated by a delayed hypersensitivity reaction appears to be the most effective way of killing the organism. Immunity to infection (chancre immunity) is established only by active infection for at least three months. The relative contribution of different immune mechanisms to "chancre immunity" is not clear at this time.

The skin and mucous membrane lesions of secondary syphilis, which appear 2 weeks to 6 months after primary infection also appear to be a delayed hypersensitivity reaction at sites of dissemination and replication of *Treponema pallidum*. The cellular reaction is similar to that of primary lesions, although plasma cells are more prominent. Although vasculitis has been described in secondary lesions, it is an exception to the rule. Thus, there is little evidence for immune complex-mediated vasculitis in syphilitic lesions. The lesions heal spontaneously, and the patient enters a period of latency.

In latent syphilis, there is no clinical evidence of infection. However, some *T. pallidum* survive the immune attack of the host and remain viable. There does not appear to be any abnormality of the immune system; indeed, persons with latent syphilis are resistant to reinfection; that is, they are immune, yet are infected (concomitant immunity).

The destructive lesions characteristic of tertiary syphilis are gran-

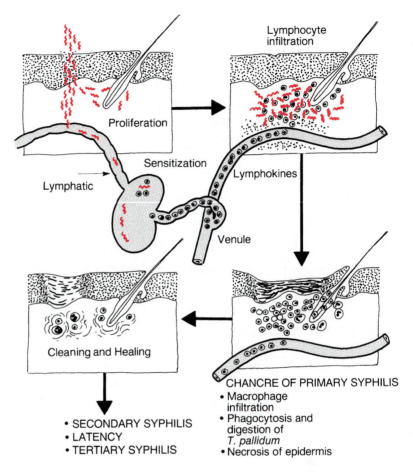

Figure 16–4. Progression of the primary chancre of syphilis. Infection with *Treponema pallidum* occurs by inoculation through abraded skin. Following inoculation, there is systemic dissemination of the organisms, as well as local proliferation at the site of infection. Hyperplasia of draining lymph nodes (lymphadenopathy) signifies an active immune response. Both sensitized cells and humoral antibody are produced. The primary lesion, which is a firm, elevated skin lesion with central necrosis, is a manifestation of a delayed hypersensitivity reaction. T cells infiltrate first, followed by macrophages, which phagocytose and destroy the infecting organisms. Viable organisms remain in "protective niches" in the body, giving rise to secondary, latent, and tertiary disease.

ulomatous reactions (gummas), which occur in areas where spirochetes apparently persist during latency (eg, brain, skin, bone, or viscera). As no differences in immune potential distinguish patients who develop tertiary disease from those who do not, it is not known why some patients move from latency to tertiary disease. Development of tertiary lesions could result either from an increased state of hypersensitivity causing more intense inflammation or from a decreased state of reactivity permitting organisms to proliferate and initiate a destructive reaction.

At present, no vaccine for syphilis is available. The major problem is that over 100 antigens have been identified in *T. pallidum*, but those that might be effective in induction of protective immunity have not been identified.

T_{DTH}-Mediated Autoimmune Disease

A number of autoimmune diseases are the result of delayed hypersensitivity. Because of the large number of these, they will be presented separately in Chapter 21. However, experimental allergic encephalomyelitis, the prototype autoimmune disease mediated by delayed hypersensitivity, is included here.

ENCEPHA-LOMYELITIS

Experimental allergic encephalomyelitis (EAE) is produced by the injection of central nervous system tissue incorporated into complete Freund's adjuvant, an immunization procedure that produces a high level of DTH. In rats, hind leg paralysis occurs after two to three weeks and is associated with a disseminated focal perivascular accumulation of inflammatory cells involving small veins or venules. The inflammatory cells, which accumulate within the vessel wall and in the perivascular space, are usually mononuclear, but polymorphonuclear leukocytes may be prominent in very acute reactions. Demyelination occurs in intimate association with the focal vasculitis and most likely is a result of the action of macrophages activated by specifically sensitized T_{DTH} cells; immune complex activation of polymorphonuclear neutrophils may be responsible for acute lesions. The antigen, encephalitogenic protein, has been studied extensively and the amino acid sequence determined. The major encephalitogenic determinant is a nonapeptide with the amino acid sequence Phe-Ser-Trp-Ala-Glu-Gly-Gln-Lys, the important amino acids being Trp and Gln. The astrocytes in the central nervous system (CNS) and Schwann cells in peripheral nerves are able to present antigen to T cells. Study of T-cell clones that are active in passive transfer of EAE indicate that the T-cell receptors employed for EAE are highly restricted, using only two Vα, one Jα, two Vβ, and two Jβ gene segments, and a highly conserved third hypervariable region, Vβ gene segment. Reactivity of the encephalogenic peptide with reactive T-cell clones can be blocked by anti-Vβ8 monoclonal antibody, suggesting that such an antibody may be used to treat demyelinating lesions. In the experimental model, immunization with the putative myelin basic protein peptide-binding region of the T-cell receptor produces cytotoxic T cells that react with the TCR of the encephalogenic T cell and prevent reaction of the encephalitogenic T cell with the myelin basic protein in vivo, blocking development of EAE.

Although the reaction of specifically sensitized cells with myelin antigen and subsequent attraction of macrophages is believed to be the major pathologic event (T cells are required to transfer the disease, and monoclonal antibodies to activated T cells block development of the disease in experimental animals), humoral antibody may also play an important effector role. The venules of the brain do not permit lymphocytes to pass through, as they do in other organs (blood–brain barrier). Humoral antibody may react with myelin antigens released from the brain normally or as the result of a viral infection. The antibody–antigen reaction may activate anaphylactic or complement mediators, causing contraction and separation of endothelial cells, thus permitting extravasation of lymphocytes into brain tissue (Fig. 16–5). In addition, demyelination may occur secondary to upregulation of expression of class I MHC antigens on oligodendrocytes without involvement of antibody or T cells. Transgenic mice expressing increased class I MHC antigens on oligodendrocytes have extensive demyelination in the brain and spinal cord without T-cell infiltrate.

The prominent tissue lesion is perivascular infiltration of the white matter of the brain and spinal cord with lymphocytes. Antigen-reactive T_{DTH} cells may first recognize myelin antigens on vascular cells at the blood–brain interface and release cytokines that activate the CNS endothelium to express cell adhesion and chemoattractant molecules. However, activated T cells appear to be able to cross the blood–brain barrier, whereas cells not in the activated phase do not. the phenotype of the cells in experimental lesions are mainly αβ-TCR+,CD4+ T cells. T-cell infiltration is followed by migration of macrophages into tissue containing myelinated nerve fibers and stripping of myelinated fibers by macrophages, culminating in phagocytosis and digestion of the myelin. Toxic products of activated T_{DTH} cells appear to have a role, as treatment of recipient mice with antibodies to lymphotoxin (IFN-β) and TNF-α prevents cell-mediated passive transfer of the disease.

The human disease takes three forms: Acute hemorrhagic encephalomyelitis, acute disseminated encephalomyelitis, and multiple sclerosis.

Acute
Hemorrhagic
Encephalomyelitis

This is a rare disease that shows necrosis and fibrin deposits within the walls of venules, hemorrhages through the venule walls with intense polymorphonuclear infiltration, and demyelination in areas of the infil-

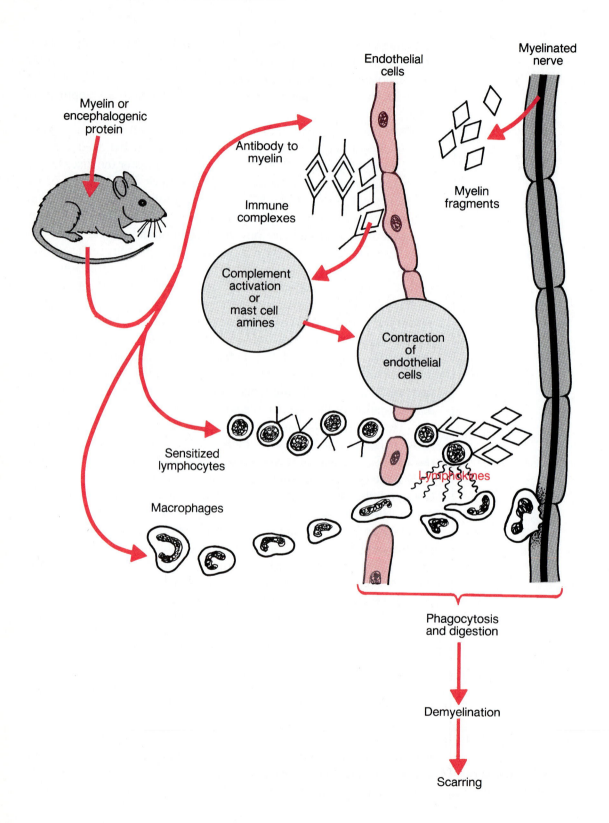

tration. This disease is similar to the acute forms of experimental allergic encephalomyelitis.

Acute
Disseminated
Encephalomyelitis

This has two variants. The form that was associated with rabies vaccination occurred 4 to 15 days following injection of killed rabies virus and was histologically identical to experimental allergic encephalomyelitis. The lesion was caused by an allergic reaction to the brain tissue used to culture the virus from which the vaccine is prepared. This type of vaccine has been replaced by one prepared from human tissue, and no proven case of postrabies inoculation encephalomyelitis has been reported since introduction of the new vaccine. The second type of acute disseminated encephalomyelitis occurs after smallpox vaccination or infection with rubella, varicella, or variola (see above). The clinical course of some cases suggest that acute hemorrhagic encephalomyelitis may progress to acute disseminated encephalomyelitis and then to multiple sclerosis.

Multiple Sclerosis
(MS)

This may be considered the end stage or chronic form of the encephalitides. There is a pathogenic similarity between MS and chronic EAE. However, animals who survive the acute stages of the experimental disease do not go on to develop the chronic scarring lesions typical of MS. Recently, it has been reported that mice with severe combined immunodeficiency disorder receiving mononuclear cells from the cerebral spinal fluid of MS patients developed demyelinated lesions. In addition, there is upregulation of vascular adhesion molecules for lymphocytes (ICAM-1 and H-CAM) on postcapillary venules in periplaque white matter. It is possible that the chronic lesions of MS are caused by stimulation of glial cell or fibroblast proliferation, following abnormal production or response to growth factors. (A "glial cell-stimulating factor" produced by lymphocytes has been de-

Figure 16–5. Pathogenic events in experimental allergic encephalomyelitis. Immunization of experimental animals with myelin or encephalogenic protein results in production of humoral antibody and specifically sensitized cells, which together lead to demyelination by macrophages. Antibody reacting with myelin released into circulation through endothelial venules in white matter (ie, myelinated area of brain and spinal cord) activates either anaphylatoxin (complement) or mast cell (IgE) degranulation. Contraction of endothelial cells opens up gaps in small venule walls. Sensitized small T_{DTH} lymphocytes move into white matter, react with myelin antigen, and release lymphocyte mediators. Macrophages, attracted and activated by these mediators, phagocytose and digest antibody-coated myelin or myelin affected by reaction with sensitized lymphocytes. If zones of demyelination are large, fibrosis will occur, and permanent loss of function will result.

scribed.) The lesions are multiple, sharply defined gray plaques that measure up to several centimeters in diameter and are composed of microglial cells, lymphocytes, and plasma cells, usually located around small veins. At later stages, scarring may obscure the small veins, and plaques may be found with no vascular component. One of the diagnostic features of MS is the presence of oligoclonal immunoglobulins in the cerebrospinal fluid. However, EAE may be consistently transferred with cells, but not with antiserum. Viral infections may produce an immunizing event leading to cellular sensitivity to myelin antigens.

Therapy is directed to limiting the progression of the disease. Treatment with corticosteroids and other antiinflammatory agents has not proved effective. Clinical trials are now underway using two drugs, interferon-β (IFN-β) and copolymer I (a synthetic polypeptide resembling myelin basic protein). Interferon may reduce the relapse rate, but the results are not yet conclusive. In animal experiments, synthetic peptides reduced the lesions of EAE. Although early results suggested that copolymer I treatment significantly reduced progression, similar effects were seen with placebo treatment. It is possible that in MS patients a positive attitude may be as effective as these specific treatments.

Experimental allergic neuritis is induced by the injection of peripheral nervous tissue in complete Freund's adjuvant. The lesions are limited to the peripheral nervous tissue; none are found in the central nervous system. The experimental disease is similar to a demyelinating syndrome that follows infection with certain microorganisms— the **Guillain–Barré syndrome**. It is postulated that there is immunological cross-reactivity between neural and viral antigens, resulting in breaking of tolerance to self neural antigens following a viral infection. The Guillain–Barré syndrome is an acute or subacute monophasic progressive ascending muscle weakness, usually self-limiting and reversible, but sometimes culminating in quadriplegia. Myelin destruction is confined to loci of nerve roots that are infiltrated by mononuclear inflammatory cells (demyelinating inflammatory polyradiculoneuropathy). Over 75% of affected patients have a well-documented antecedent infection, usually viral, but also mycoplasma, salmonella, or other bacterial infection. The Guillain–Barré syndrome also occurs after smallpox or rabies vaccination. A role for autoantibody in the pathogenesis is suggested by clinical improvement noted following plasmapheresis of treatment with antiidiotypic antibodies to presumptive antiperipheral nerve antigens.

An **experimental allergic sympathetic neuritis** may be induced by immunization with antigens obtained from sympathetic ganglia. The inflammatory lesions are limited to the sympathetic nervous system.

T_{CTL} and T_{DTH}— Tuberculosis

Because granulomas are a major feature of tuberculosis, the role of the immune response in the pathogenesis and protection to tuberculosis will be covered in Chapter 17. However, since T-cell-mediated immunity is paramount in tuberculosis, it is mentioned briefly here. Although the reaction to tuberculosis has been considered to be a classic example of a delayed hypersensitivity reaction, whereby T_{DTH} cells react with tubercular antigens and release lymphokines (IFN-γ, IL-2, etc.), which activate macrophages to kill tubercle bacilli that have been ingested by macrophages, there is new evidence that T_{CTL}-mediated cytotoxicity may be also called into play. T-cytotoxic cells may lyse incompetent macrophages that contain bacilli that they are unable to digest. The microorganisms are thus released into a toxic extracellular environment and made available for phagocytosis by fully competent macrophages. In this way, intracellular organisms that may persist in a protected niche are booted out and destroyed. Failure of this mechanism to operate may result in long-standing "latent" infections that may become reactivated by changing immune status with age or immunosuppressive therapy.

Summary

Delayed-type hypersensitivity (DTH) reactions are unleashed when antigens react with CD4+ T_{DTH}-sensitized cells. The tissue lesions are caused by macrophages that are attracted and activated through the release of lymphokines such as IFN-γ and IL-2. Activated macrophages phagocytose and destroy foreign organisms in protective responses but may also destroy host tissue cells in immunopathologic reactions. DTH reactions discussed as examples of this reactivity are delayed-type skin test (tuberculin) reactions, immune response to syphilis infection, and autoimmune encephalomyelitis. Both T_{CTL} and T_{DTH} activity are called into play in the intracellular infections with tuberculosis. Many other DTH-mediated protective and destructive effects are presented in other chapters.

Bibliography

Ameisen J-C, Meade R, Askenase PW: A new interpretation of the involvement of serotonin in delayed-type hypersensitivity: Serotonin-2 receptor antagonists inhibit contact sensitivity by an effect on T cells. *J Immunol* 142:3137, 1989.

Askenase PW, Van Loveren H: Delayed-type hypersensitivity: Activation of mast cells by antigen specific T-cell factors initiates the cascade of cellular interactions. *Immunol Today* 4:259, 1983.

Cohen S: Symposium on cell-mediated immunity in human disease. *Hum Pathol* 17:111–178, 1986.

Dalton DK, Pitts-Meek S, Keshav S, et al.: Multiple defects of immune cell function in mice with disrupted INF-γ genes. *Science* 259:1739–1742, 1993.

Dvorak HF, Galli SJ, Dvorak A: Cellular and vascular manifestations of cell-mediated immunity. *Hum Pathol* 17:112, 1986.

Dvorak HF, Mihm M Jr, Dvorak A, et al.: Morphology of delayed-type hypersensitivity reaction in man. I. Quantitative description of the inflammatory response. *Lab Invest* 31:111, 1974.

Ferreri NR, Millet I, Paliwal V, et al.: Induction of macrophage TNF-α, IL-1, IL-6, and PGE$_2$ production by DTH-initiating factors. *Cell Immunol* 137:389, 1991.

Galli SJ, Dvorak A: What do mast cells have to do with delayed hypersensitivity? *Lab Invest* 50:365, 1984.

Gell PGH, Benacerraf B: Delayed hypersensitivity to simple protein antigens. *Adv Immunol* 1:319, 1961.

Huang S, Hendriks W, Althage A, et al.: Immune response in mice that lack the IFN-γ receptor. *Science* 259:1742–1745.

Kelley VE, Naor D, Tarcic N, et al.: Anti-IL-2 receptor antibody suppresses delayed-type hypersensitivity to foreign and syngeneic antigens. *J Immunol* 137:2122, 1986.

Lawrence HS: The delayed type of allergic inflammatory response. *Am J Med* 20:428, 1956.

MacPhee MJ, Gordon J, Christou NV: Cells recovered from human DTH reactions: Phenotypic and functional analysis. *Cell Immunol* 151:80–96, 1993.

Peltz G: A role for CD4+ T-cell subsets producing a selective pattern of lymphokines in the pathogenesis of human chronic inflammatory and allergic diseases. *Immunol Rev* 123:23, 1991.

Raffel J, Newel JM: The "delayed hypersensitivity" induced by antigen–antibody complexes. *J Exp Med* 108:823, 1958.

Sell S, Weigle WO: The relationship between delayed hypersensitivity and circulating antibody induced by protein antigens in guinea pigs. *J Immunol* 83:257, 1959.

Simon FA, Rackeman FF: The development of hypersensitiveness in man. I. Following intradermal injection of the antigen. *J Allergy* 5:439, 1934.

Turk JL: *Delayed Hypersensitivity*. New York, Wiley, 1967.

Uhr JW: Delayed hypersensitivity. *Physiol Rev* 46:359, 1966.

Waksman BH: A comparative histopathological study of delayed hypersensitivity reactions. In *Cellular Aspects of Immunity*. Wolstenholme GEW, Connor CE (eds.). Boston, Little, Brown, 1960.

Waksman BH: Delayed hypersensitivity: A growing class of immunological phenomena. *J Allergy* 31:468, 1960.

SUPERANTIGENS

Cantor H, Crump AL, Raman VK, et al.: Immunoregulatory effects of superantigens: Interactions of staphylococcal enterotoxins with host MHC and non-MHC products. *Immunol Rev* 131:27–42, 1993.

Goodglick L, Braun J: Revenge of the microbes: Superantigens of the T- and B-cell lineage. *Am J Pathol* 144:623–636, 1994.

Herman A, Kappler JW, Marrack P, et al.: Superantigens: Mechanism of T-cell stimulation and role in immune responses. *Annu Rev Immunol* 9:745, 1991.

Janeway CA: Self superantigens. *Cell* 63:659, 1990.

Marrack P, Kappler J: The staphylococcal enterotoxins and their relatives. *Science* 248:705, 1990.

See RH, Kum WWS, Chang AH, et al.: Induction of TNF and IL-1 by purified staphylococcal toxic shock syndrome toxin-1 requires the presence of both monocytes and T lymphocytes. *Infect Immun* 60:2612, 1992.

TUBERCULIN TEST

Huebner RE, Schein MF, Bass JB: The tuberculin skin test. *Clin Infect Dis* 17:968–975, 1993.

Katz J, Kunofsky S, Krasnitz A: Variation in sensitivity to tuberculin. *Am Rev Resp Dis* 106:202, 1972.

Koch R: Weitere mittheilungen uberein Helmittel gegen Tuberculose. *Dtsch Med Wochenschr* 16:1029, 1890.

Youmans GP: Relation between delayed hypersensitivity and immunity in tuberculosis. *Am Rev Resp Dis* 111:109, 1975.

Zinsser H, Mueller JH: On the nature of bacterial allergies. *J Exp Med* 41:159, 1925.

CUTANEOUS BASOPHIL HYPERSENSITIVITY

Askanase PW, Atwood JE: Basophils in tuberculin and Jones–Mote delayed reactions of humans. *J Clin Invest* 58:1145, 1976.

Dvorak HF, Mihm MC Jr: Basophilic leukocytes in allergic contact dermatitis. *J Exp Med* 135:235, 1972.

Jones TD, Mote JR: The phases of foreign sensitization in human beings. *N Engl J Med* 210:120, 1934.

Mote JR, Jones TD: The development of foreign protein sensitization in human beings. *J Immunol* 30:149, 1936.

Richerson HB, Dvorak HF, Leskowitz S: Cutaneous basophil hypersensitivity: A new interpretation of the Jones–Mote reaction. *J Immunol* 103:1431, 1969.

TRANSFER FACTOR

Kirkpatrick CH: Transfer factor. *J Allerg Clin Immunol* 81:803, 1988.

Lawrence HS: The transfer in humans of delayed skin sensitivity to streptococcal M protein and to tuberculin with disrupted leucocytes. *J Clin Invest* 34:104, 1955.

SYPHILIS

Chesney AM: Immunity in syphilis. *Medicine* 5:463, 1926.

Dennie CC: *A History of Syphilis*. Springfield IL, CC Thomas, 1962.

Sell S, Norris SJ: The biology, pathology, and immunology of Syphilis. *Int Rev Exp Path* 24:203–276, 1983.

Turner TB, Hollander DH: *Biology of the Treponematoses*. Geneva, World Health Organization, 1957.

EXPERIMENTAL ALLERGIC ENCEPHALOMYELITIS, MULTIPLE SCLEROSIS, AND NEURITIS

Allen I, Brankin B: Pathogenesis of multiple sclerosis: The immune diathesis and the role of viruses. *J Neuropath Exp Neurol* 52:95–105, 1993.

Cross AH, Canella B, Brosnan CF, et al.: Hypothesis: Antigen-specific T cells prime central nervous system endothelium for recruitment of nonspecific inflammatory cells to effect autoimmune demyelination. *J Neuroimmunol* 33:237, 1991.

Deber CM, Reynolds SJ: Central nervous system myelin: Structure, function, and pathology. *Clin Biochem* 24:113, 1991.

Hickey WF: Migration of hematogenous cells through the blood–brain barrier and the initiation of CNS inflammation. *Brain Pathol* 1:97, 1991.

Hintzen RQ, Polman CH, Lucas CJ, et al.: Multiple sclerosis: Immunologic findings and possible implications for therapy. *J Neuroimmunol* 39:1, 1992.

Julien J, Ferrer X: Multiple sclerosis: An overview. *Biomed Pharmacother* 43:335, 1989.

Lampert PW: Mechanism of demyelination in experimental allergic neuritis: Electron microscopic studies. *Lab Invest* 20:127, 1969.

Lundkvist I, Van Doorn PA, Vermeulen M, et al.: Regulation of autoantibodies in inflammatory demyelinating polyneuropathy: Spontaneous and therapeutic. *Immunol Rev* 110:105, 1989.

Martin R, McFarland HF, McFarlin DE: Immunological aspects of demyelinating diseases. *Annu Rev Immunol* 10:153, 1992.

Paterson PY, Day ED: Current perspectives of neuroimmunologic disease: Multiple sclerosis and experimental allergic encephalomyelitis. *Clin Immunol Rev* 1:81, 1981.

Ropper AH: The Guillain–Barré syndrome. *N Engl J Med* 326:1130, 1992.

Ruddle NH, Bergman CM, McGrath KM, et al.: An antibody to lymphotoxin and tumor necrosis factor prevents transfer of experimental allergic encephalomyelitis. *J Exp Med* 172:1193, 1990.

Rudnick RA, Goodkin DE (eds.): Treatment of multiple sclerosis: Trial design, results, and future perspectives. New York, Springer-Verlag, 1992.

Saeki Y, Mima T, Sakoda S, et al.: Transfer of multiple sclerosis into severe combined immunodeficiency mice by mononuclear cells from cerebrospinal fluid of the patients. *Proc Natl Acad Sci USA* 89:6157, 1992.

Sobel RA, Kuchroo VK: The immunopathology of acute experimental allergic encephalomyelitis induced with myelin proteolipid protein: T-cell receptors in inflammatory lesions. *J Immunol* 149:1444, 1992.

Steiner I, Abramsky O: Immunology of Guillain–Barré syndrome. *Springer Semin Immunopathol* 8:165, 1985.

Urban JL, Kumar V, Knon DH, et al.: Restricted use of T-cell receptor V genes in murine autoimmune encephalomyelitis raises possibilities for antibody therapy. *Cell* 54:577, 1988.

Waksman BH: Experimental allergic encephalomyelitis and the "autoallergic" diseases. *Int Arch Allergy Appl Immunol* 14(suppl):1–87, 1959.

Yoshioka T, Feigenbaum L, Jay G: Transgenic mouse model for central nervous system demyelination. *Molec Cell Biology* 11:5479, 1991.

17

Granulomatous Reactions

The Nature of Granulomas

Granulomas are space-occupying chronic-inflammatory lesions. Granulomas (Fig. 17–1) are identified by of focal collections of reticuloendothelial cells in tissue, including macrophages, histiocytes, epithelioid cells, and giant cells, as well as lymphocytes and plasma cells surrounded by varying amounts of fibrous tissue. The characteristic epithelioid cell is derived from a macrophage and has a prominent eosinophilic amorphous cytoplasm and a large, oval, pale-staining nucleus with a sharp, thin nuclear membrane and large nuclei. These cells are called epithelioid because of their resemblance to epithelial cells. Granulomas progress from highly cellular reactions which are eventually replaced by fibrous scars (Fig. 17–2). Although it is not always possible using morphological criteria alone, these reactions should be differentiated from nonspecific chronic inflammatory reactions in which lymphocytes, plasma cells, and eosinophils accumulate.

Granulomatous reactions are cellular responses to irritating, persistent, and poorly soluble substances. These reactions are characteristically initiated by sensitized lymphocytes reacting with antigen but may also occur to poorly catabolizable antigen–antibody complexes that persist locally. However, not all granulomas have the origin in an immune response. Common granulomatous reaction are those surrounding insoluble suture material or around urate deposits in gouty lesions. Similar lesions may be induced by other foreign bodies. Antibody–antigen complexes may provide a stimulus for granuloma formation inflammation if the complex is insoluble and relatively indigestible. Antigen complexed to insoluble particles, such as latex beads, will produce granulomas when injected into immunized animals.

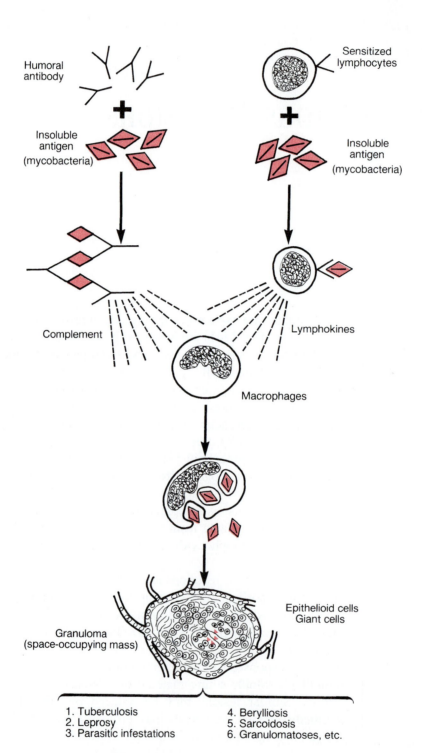

Figure 17–1. Granulomatous hypersensitivity reactions. Granulomatous reactions may be identified morphologically by appearance of reticuloendothelial cells, including histiocytes, epithelioid cells, giant cells, and lymphocytes arranged in a characteristic round or oval laminated structure called a granuloma. Hypersensitivity granulomas form as a variation of delayed hypersensitivity or antibody reactions. Sensitized lymphocytes react with antigens, releasing lymphokines which attract and activate macrophages. The activated macrophages are unable to "clear" the poorly degradable antigens, accumulate in the tissues, form epithelioid and giant cells, and organize into granulomas. Granulomas may also form in response to poorly degradable antibody–antigen complexes in tissue.

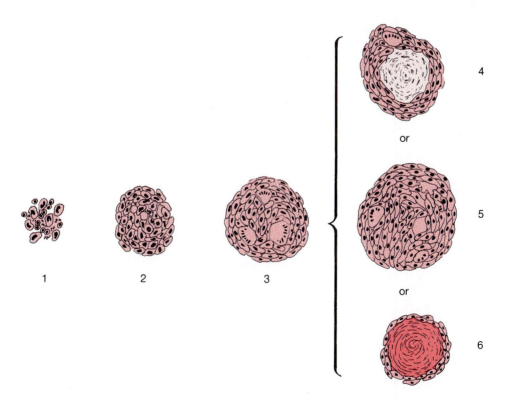

Figure 17–2. Progression of granulomas. (1) Granulomas begin as small collections of lymphocytes and macrophages which form around poorly degradable antigens, (2) macrophages change to epithelioid cells and become organized into a cluster of cells, and (3) further progression results in ball-like clusters of cells and fusion of macrophages into giant cells. Further progression may include: (4) Development of necrosis in the center as characteristic of chronic tuberculosis, (5) continued enlargement and replacement of normal tissue (progressive disease), or (6) fibrosis with scar formation, characteristic of "healed" sarcoidosis.

The origin of the most characteristic cell of granulomatous hypersensitivity reaction—the epithelioid cell—is from a phagocyte that has ingested foreign material but cannot digest and/or exocytose the material. Multinuclear giant cells form from fusion of macrophages or epithelioid cells. Granulomatous hypersensitivity reactions may evolve in weeks or even months due to the persistent nature of the stimulus. Several T-cell factors have been identified that modulate granuloma formation: (1) Interleukin-4 (IL-4) causes aggregation and fusion of macrophages, (2) interferon-γ (IFN-γ) causes inhibition of macrophage migration and fusion of monocytes, and (3) a suppressor factor has been reported to inhibit granuloma formation in experimental models. In addition, macrophage derived factors, including interleukin-1 (IL-1), stimulate fibrosis and scarring in granulomas.

Combinations of immune-mediated lesions in some granulomatous diseases indicates the involvement of different mechanisms in the production of the lesions (eg, toxic complex, anaphylactic, and granulomatous). Many diseases demonstrate both granulomatous reactions and vasculitis, varying from essentially pure granulomatous lesions to pure vasculitis (Fig. 17–3). "Allergic granulomatosis," or Churg–Strauss syndrome, includes necrotizing vasculitis, extravascular gran-

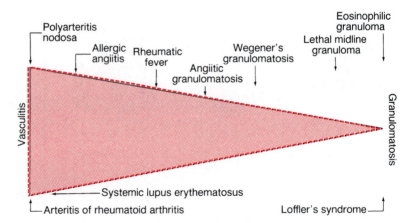

Figure 17–3. Spectrum of association of granulomatous reactions and vasculitis. The lesions of Loeffler's syndrome and eosinophilic granuloma are essentially granulomas; those of the vasculitis found with polyarteritis nodosa and collagen diseases are almost pure arteritis. On the other hand, a number of diseases such as some connective tissue diseases (see Chapter 22) and Wegener's granulomatosis, demonstrate a mixture of granulomatous reactions and vasculitis. In these lesions, which are difficult to classify, it is possible that the granulomatous reactions are secondary to tissue damage initiated by another mechanism.

ulomas, and tissue infiltration with eosinophils, which occur in a setting of bronchial asthma.

Granulomatous Diseases

Granulomatous hypersensitivity diseases include infectious diseases, such as tuberculosis, leprosy, and parasitic infestations; responses to known antigens, such as zirconium granuloma, berylliosis, and extrinsic alveolitis; and other diseases of unknown etiology in which epithelioid granulomas are the primary lesion. Epithelioid granulomas occur in other diseases, such as tertiary syphilis, fungus infections, and some foreign body reactions (eg, around urate deposits in gout or silica deposits in ruptured silicone gel implants). Granulomas are also a prominent feature of early asbestosis and silicosis.

Infectious Diseases

TUBERCULOSIS

Tuberculosis, "the white plague," has had a long and devastating relationship with mankind. The disease affected ancient humans. Lesions of tuberculosis have been found in Egyptian mummies, and the disease was described clinically in pre-Christian times. Until the discovery of antituberculosis drugs in the 1950s, tuberculosis was a major public health problem. In the early 1800s, mortality may have been as high as 1 in 100 adults per year in large American and European cities. The storyline in many novels revolved around the tragic end of the hero or heroine with fatal tuberculosis. The infectious nature of tuberculosis was discovered in 1882 by Robert Koch, who cultured the organism and satisfied his famous set of postulates (Table 17–1) to prove that the isolated organism caused the clinical manifestations of tuberculosis. The organism, now known as *Mycobacterium tuberculosis*, was first called Koch's bacillus. Eight years later, Koch announced that he had discovered a cure for tuberculosis. Koch claimed that injection of "tuberculin" could rapidly reverse advanced symptoms of tuberculosis. Within a few months, his spectacular claims were debunked and his reputation seriously damaged. Fortunately, we remember Koch's solid contributions and not his premature claims. Even though there was a gradual decline in the disease related to improved living standards,

TABLE 17–1. KOCH'S POSTULATES: A STATEMENT OF THE EXPERIMENTAL EVIDENCE REQUIRED TO ESTABLISH THE ETIOLOGIC RELATIONSHIPS OF A GIVEN MICROORGANISM TO A GIVEN DISEASE

1. The microorganism must be observed in every case of the disease.
2. It must be isolated and grown in pure culture.
3. The pure culture must, when inoculated into a susceptible animal, reproduce the disease.
4. The microorganism must be observed in, and recovered from, the experimentally diseased animal.

pasteurization of milk, vaccination of children with bacillus Calmette–Guérin (BCG), improved diagnostic and public health procedures, and isolation of infected individuals in sanatoria, most large cities in the first half of the 20th century still had entire hospitals dedicated to tuberculosis patients.

The dramatic effect of the antituberculosis drugs isoniazid in the early 1950s and rifampicin in the 1960s led to optimism that tuberculosis would finally be brought under control. However, in order to check the growth of the bacillus in infected individuals it was necessary to continue treatment for at least nine months. The biggest problem in attempts to eradicate tuberculosis was the tendency for patients to discontinue treatment when they began to feel better, allowing drug-resistant strains to develop. In the early 1990s, the incidence of tuberculosis has increased dramatically. Although at first primarily a disease of the elderly, the alcoholic, the drug user, the acquired immunodeficiency syndrome (AIDS) patient, and immigrants from third world countries, at the time of this writing, the disease is spreading gradually throughout the American population. The drugs once believed to be the means to eradicate tuberculosis are now relatively ineffective because of the emergence of drug-resistant strains. Patients who have been previously treated and then relapse are particularly likely to be harboring drug-resistant organisms.

Tuberculosis is the classic example of mixed protective and pathogenic effects of immune and nonimmune inflammatory reactions to a single agent. Primary infection begins by inhalation of a droplet containing a viable bacillus and implantation in the lung, usually in a lower lobe. This leads to a local infection (primary focus) of acute inflammation and to spread by drainage to the hilar lymph nodes and eventually to the blood (bacteremia). For pulmonary tuberculosis, four stages of infection may be identified at the cellular level. In stage 1, the bacillus is ingested by alveolar macrophages. The bacillus is usually destroyed by the macrophage; if not, it grows in the macrophage and eventually destroys it. At this stage $T_{\gamma\delta}$ cells may act on infected macrophages to kill them. It is estimated that only 3% to 5% of humans who contact the bacillus will progress to later stages of infection.

In stage 2, the bacilli grow logarithmically within immature macrophages that arrive from the blood stream. **Miliary tuberculosis** results from acute or reinfection blood-borne dissemination resulting in multiple small granulomas in many organs. However, these granulomas are poorly formed, being mostly made up of macrophages with few lymphocytes and epithelioid cells, and may contain large numbers of viable organisms. In miliary tuberculosis, cell-mediated immunity (CMI) to tuberculin antigens is often lacking, and the immune response is unable to check the spread of the infection with an often fatal outcome. CMI recovers in patients with miliary tuberculosis who are successfully treated with antibiotics.

In stage 3, the number of bacilli becomes stationary as their growth is inhibited by the immune response (bacteriostasis). In this stage, newly arriving immature macrophages may continue to support growth of the bacilli, whereas activated macrophages inhibit multiplication and destroy the organisms. Arrestment at this stage depends on the type of macrophage that predominates. If the infection is checked, the primary infection site and the hilar lesions heal by granuloma formation leading to formation of a **Ghon complex**. The Ghon complex consists of a healed granuloma or scar on the pleural surface of the middle lobes of the lung and granulomas in the draining hilar lymph nodes. The Ghon complex suggests that the patient resisted a previous tuberculosis infection by a granulomatous reaction.

In stage 4, bacilli multiply extracellularly in the center of granulomas protected from the host's immune defenses. The center of tubercular granulomas frequently becomes necrotic, resulting in a gross appearance similar to cheese. This is referred to as **caseous necrosis**, which may also occur in other granulomatous diseases but is most often seen in tuberculosis. Viable organisms may multiply to enormous numbers within the "protected niche" provided by the liquified center of a caseous granuloma. Rupture of the infected granuloma allows these viable organisms to enter the bronchial tree. The course of the infection then depends on whether or not the quantity of bacilli exceeds the capacity of the host's immune system to limit reinfection. Alterations in the host's immune response with aging or malnutrition may cause breakdown of the granuloma and allow auto-reinfection with persisting viable organisms (**reactivation tuberculosis**). This also provides a source for spreading the infection to others, as large numbers of viable tubercle bacilli may be released through coughing and provide an aerosol of potentially infective organisms for others.

Infection with tubercle bacilli may result in different types of immune responses, including nonspecific $T_{\gamma\delta}$ cytotoxic cells active during the first few days after infection, circulating antibody, T_{CTL} cells directed against infected monocytes, T_{DTH}-mediated classic delayed hypersensitivity, increased macrophage activity (immune phagocytosis), and granulomatous inflammation. Cell-mediated immunity is accepted by most as the main line of specific defense. There is little evidence that immunoglobulin antibody plays an important role. In the majority of cases, CMI to *M. tuberculosis* can be demonstrated by positive DTH skin tests to tuberculoproteins within 2 to 4 weeks after infection.

Both T_{CTL} and T_{DTH} are believed to play important roles in immunity to tuberculosis (Fig. 17–4). Infection is initiated by uptake of bacilli into macrophages. Key to the progression of the infection is the ability of the bacilli to replicate within the macrophages. In over 90% of infected individuals, bacilli are unable to replicate in infected macrophages. This effect may be due to rapid reaction of $T_{\gamma\delta}$ cells with infected macrophages. If infection persists, specific cell-mediated immunity is induced with production of specifically sensitized T_{DTH} and T_{CTL} cells. Specific T_{DTH} cells react with mycobacterial antigens and release mediators, such as IL-2, TNF, and INF-γ, which activate macrophages to digest the intracellular bacilli. T_{CTL} cells react with infected macrophages and lyse them. The released bacilli may then either be phagocytosed and destroyed by activated macrophages or reinfect immature macrophages. Four possible outcomes are cure with no residual lesions, cure with residual lesions (Ghon complex), arrest with healed granulomas, or progression with active granulomas.

Many believe the answer to how to control tuberculosis lies in finding ways to improve the effectiveness of the immune defenses to

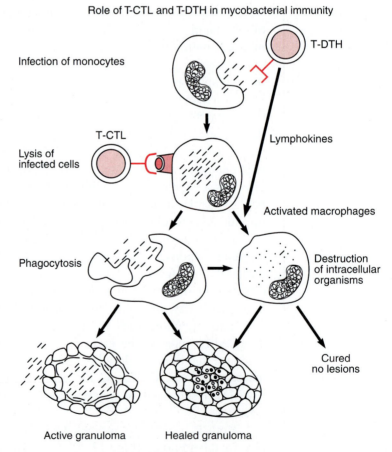

Figure 17–4. Postulated role of cell-mediated immunity to tuberculosis.

the infection. Individuals with depressed cell-mediated immunity are particularly susceptible. Previously, tuberculosis was noted in high incidence in the elderly and patients on immunosuppressive therapy; now AIDS patients are highly susceptible to progressive tuberculosis. New approaches to both therapy and prevention are urgently needed. One approach is to apply advances in molecular biology and tissue culture to identify and clone the genes responsible for the production of the protective epitopes of *Mycobacterium tuberculosis* and to introduce these into specifically designed vectors to produce vaccines that might provide protective immunity. Regardless of the availability of new medical approaches, reinstitution of stringent isolation procedures, careful supervision of antibiotic treatment, and public health-directed education may be the most effective measures.

LEPROSY

Leprosy is another mycobacterial infection clearly known since biblical times. The clinical features of leprosy depend on the immune reaction of the infected individual; a form of **immune deviation**, in which some individuals express predominantly cell-mediated immunity and others express predominantly humoral immunity. The immune characteristics of different clinical classifications of leprosy are presented in Table 17–2.

At one pole of the leprosy spectrum, patients have little more manifestation of the disease than one or more well-defined erythematous or hypopigmented anesthetic plaques or macules on the skin. This is the high-resistance or **tuberculoid** form. Histologic examination reveals sarcoidlike dermal granulomatous lesions with prominent Langhans' giant cells, epithelioid cells, and many lymphocytes. Few, if any, *Mycobacterium leprae* organisms can be found in the tissues. Because of a tendency to involve peripheral nerves with loss of sensory function, this is also known as the anesthetic form. The neural fibrosis appears to be related to production of fibroblastic stimulatory factors by activated macrophages. Affected individuals may develop secondary traumatic injury due to loss of pain sensation. There is hyperplasia of the paracortical areas of the lymph nodes, a prominent delayed skin reaction to injection of lepromin, and little or no humoral antibody to mycobacterial antigens.

At the other pole of the clinical spectrum is **lepromatous leprosy**. This form is the low-resistance type. It is known as the **nodular** form because of a prominence of skin and lymph node involvement and gross nodule formation. There is massive infiltration of tissues with large macrophages filled with numerous mycobacteria. There is extensive skin involvement that can produce marked disfigurement (leonine faces). The cellular infiltrate in the dermis is separated from the basal layer of the skin by a band of foamy macrophages (Virchow cells)

TABLE 17–2. IMMUNOLOGIC CHARACTERISTICS OF LEPROSY

Characteristics	Form of Leprosy		
	Tuberculoid	Borderline	Lepromatous
M. leprae in tissues	– or ±	+ or + +	+ + + +
Granuloma formation	+ + + +	+ + +	–
Lymphocytic infiltration	+ + +	–	–
Lymph node morphology:			
Paracortical lymphocytes	+ + + +	+ +	–
Paracortical histiocytes	–	+ +	+ + + +
Germinal center formation	+	+ +	+ + + +
Plasma cells	±	+	+ + +
Lepromin test	+ + +	–	–
Delayed hypersensitivity, per cent reactivity to:			
Dinitrochlorobenzene	90	75	50
Hemocyanin	100	100	100
Antimycobacterial antibodies (% patients with precipitins in serum)	11–28	82	95
Autoantibodies in serum (%)	3–11		30–50
Immune complex disease (erythema nodosum leprosum)	–	±	+ + +

Key: – to ++++ indicates extent of the observation noted.

Modified from Turk JL, Bryceson ADM: Immunological phenomena in leprosy and related disease. *Adv Immunol* 13:209, 1971.

filled with acid-fast organisms (Grenz zone). The lymph nodes of lepromatous patients have hyperplastic germinal centers, yet the cell-mediated immune defense against these organisms is diminished. The paracortical areas have a paucity of lymphocytes and are often filled with large macrophages containing organisms. There are few, if any, lymphocytes in the tissue lesions, the lepromin skin test is negative, and antibodies to mycobacterial antigens are common (see Table 17–2). In addition, patients with lepromatous leprosy develop a number of autoantibodies, most likely because of polyclonal B-cell responses in this form of the disease. Antibodies to cross reacting antigens between human skin and *M. leprae* have been identified and may play a role in this chronic destruction of the skin seen in this disease. In addition, the production of antinuclear factor and rheumatoid factor (anti-Ig) may cause rheumatic manifestations.

The spectrum of leprosy includes many patients who have characteristics that are essentially mixtures of the tuberculoid and lepromatous forms. Between the two polar forms of the disease are intermediate forms, progressing from the paucibacillary (tuberculoid) form to the multibacillary (lepromatous) form: TT—full tuberculoid →

BT—borderline tuberculoid → BB—borderline → BL—borderline lepromatous → LL—full lepromatous. The manifestations of *M. leprae* infection are therefore quite variable and range from severe tissue destruction to only local depigmented areas of the skin. This latter form is frequently found in the natives of Baja California. Europeans tend to be resistant; South Americans develop little immune response but frequently manifest only depigmented skin, while South East Asians are prone to develop progressive lepromatous leprosy.

The protective function of granulomatous reactivity is exemplified by the spectrum of reactions to *M. leprae* in leprosy. Resistance is associated with granuloma formation and a high degree of delayed hypersensitivity, whereas low resistance is associated with lack of granuloma development and prominence of antibody formation. The position that a given patient occupies on the clinical spectrum frequently changes. A shift from a lepromatous form to a tuberculoid form is associated with a definite clinical improvement.

When the bacterial load diminishes, tissues that contain residual organisms undergo hypersensitivity reactions. There is swelling and erythema of skin lesions associated with fever. The skin lesions show infiltration with lymphocytes. The foamy macrophages lose their content of organisms and become more epithelioid. Although patients with polar tuberculoid or polar lepromatous leprosy usually remain in their part of spectrum, frequent shifts in the borderline groups occur. Effective chemotherapy frequently precipitates a reversal reaction. Chemotherapy of leprosy with 4:4-diaminodiphenylsulphone may produce a reduction in the antigenic load and permit poorly reactive patients to express a granulomatous reaction.

In order to produce an effective granulomatous reaction, both macrophages and T cells are required. Cytologic analysis indicates segregation of T_{DTH} cells within the aggregate of macrophages and T_{CTL} cells in the mantle of tuberculoid granulomas, whereas T_{DTH} and T_{CTL} cells are admixed among the undifferentiated macrophages of lepromatous lesions. The formation of a tuberculoid granuloma appears to require activated T_{DTH} cells, which produce soluble factors that activate macrophages to kill the intracellular organisms and stimulate giant cell formation. Granulomas from tuberculoid leprosy contain large numbers of cells containing IL-1β, TNF-α, and TNF-γ. Without this lymphokine-mediated activation of macrophage killing, the infected macrophages serve as the permissive cell for proliferation of the organisms. In lepromatous leprosy, T_{CTL} may not be able to act against *M. leprae*, which are protected by their intracellular location, and the few T_{DTH} cells present are unable to produce sufficient interleukins to activate the infected macrophages to kill the bacilli they harbor.

The development of a granuloma is mediated through the action of T_H (helper) and T_S (suppressor) cells on T_{DTH} activity. T cells from patients with lepromatous leprosy fail to respond to *M. leprae* antigens in vitro and not only fail to produce IL-2, but also do not express IL-2 receptors. There is compelling evidence, both in experimental and human leprosy, that there is activation of a T-cell suppressor mechanism to explain the immune deviation responsible for the lack of cell-mediated immunity in lepromatous leprosy. In lepromatous lesions, the CD4/CD8 ratios are markedly reduced when compared to lesions of tuberculoid leprosy. Addition of blood lymphocytes from patients with lepromatous leprosy to cultures of lymphocytes from patients with tuberculoid leprosy greatly reduces the mitogen response to *M. leprae* antigens. Secretion of a "suppressor factor" that inhibits development of granulomas has been reported. In borderline lepromatous leprosy, removal of CD8+ cells can partially restore the mitogen response; however, in polar lepromatous leprosy, the lymphocytes fail to respond even when CD+ (suppressor) cells are removed. Thus, suppressor T cells cannot account for the entire lack of CMI in lepromatous leprosy; a deletion of leprosy-specific CD4+ T_{DTH} cells also occurs.

The macrophages of lepromatous leprosy patients have a decreased capacity for destroying various target cells, as well as other microorganisms (decreased cell-mediated immunity), and decreased IL-1 production. Treatment of mice with agents that increase the phagocytic and metabolic activity (digestive capacity) of macrophages will prevent the development of experimental infection. Leprosy infection is always limited in normal mice but assumes a more virulent course in thymectomized or antilymphocyte serum-treated mice who have depressed cell-mediated immunity. Patients with lepromatous leprosy have a decreased capacity to respond to a variety of cell-mediated reactions, including mitogen activation of lymphocytes, sensitization to contact-sensitivity agents, and decreased production of lymphokines.

The **lepromin test** is a skin reaction to extracts of *M. leprae*. It consists of a two-stage reaction. The first is a typical delayed hypersensitivity reaction that occurs 24 to 48 hours after injection of the antigen (the Fernandez reaction); the second (Mitsuda reaction) appears between 2 and 4 weeks after testing and is an indurated skin nodule caused by the formation of a granuloma. This reaction is over 4 mm in diameter and usually ulcerates. The 24- to 48-hour Fernandez reaction is positive in a large number of persons who have no history of ever contacting leprosy. This is probably because of exposure to cross-reacting antigens of other bacteria. Therefore, the lepromin reaction cannot be used to indicate active or acute infection with *M. leprae*. The clinical importance of the lepromin test in determining the reactivity of infected patients is as a prognostic test. A positive Mitsuda granulomatous reaction is associated with high resistance to the infection and good prognosis, but is difficult to evaluate.

Better laboratory tests are being developed to aid in the diagnosis of leprosy. Attempts to use so called *M. leprae*-soluble antigens (MLSAs) as skin test antigens have had limited success, as about 50% of cases of tuberculoid leprosy are negative using these antigens. Serologic tests include a fluorescence (FLA-ABS), enzyme-linked immunosorbent assay (ELISA), and ELISA inhibition test. The ELISA-based tests measure antibody to a *M. leprae*-specific terminal disaccharide (PGL_1) or to specific epitopes on different protein antigens. These are consistently positive in lepromatous leprosy (multibacillary form) but negative in tuberculoid leprosy (paucibacillary form).

Erythema nodosum leprosum is an immune complex-mediated vascular skin reaction (Arthus reaction) found in patients with lepromatous leprosy and antibody to mycobacterial antigens. Crops of red nodules appear in the skin and last for 24 to 48 hours. These may be associated with systemic manifestations, such as arthritis, inflammation of the eye or testes, pain along nerves, fever, and proteinuria. The lesions in the skin show a fibrinoid vasculitis with polymorphonuclear infiltrate. The frequent occurrence of these reactions during chemotherapy suggests that they are related to the release of mycobacterial antigens and deposition of immune complexes in affected tissues. Similar lesions may also be seen in patients with progressive tuberculosis (erythema nodosum tuberculosum). One final feature of lepromatous leprosy worthy of mention is the high incidence of autoantibodies. These include antinuclear factor, rheumatoid factor, antithyroglobulin antibodies, and false-positive serologic tests for syphilis. Most of these autoantibodies do not appear to produce lesions or symptoms in affected patients. The high incidence of autoantibodies in leprosy may be because of an adjuvant effect of the organisms, continued tissue destruction-releasing potential autoantigens, or altered activity of suppressor cells.

PARASITIC INFECTIONS

The role of granulomatous reactions in the protective and immunopathologic processes of infectious diseases is presented in Chapter 25. Granulomatous reactions occur in response to many parasitic infections, particularly those from certain helminths. Schistosomiasis and filariasis will be mentioned briefly here. In infestations with *Schistosoma mansoni*, the eggs are released into the portal bloodstream and lodge in the portal veins of the liver. Here the eggs evoke a severe granulomatous inflammatory reaction that may gradually increase and lead to extensive fibrosis of the portal areas (pipestem fibrosis). If the liver involvement is severe, collateral circulation around the portal system develops as the portal radicals in the liver become obstructed. The eggs may then pass from the portal system through collateral channels to the pulmonary arteries, resulting in multiple small granulomatous lesions resembling miliary tuberculosis (pseudotubercles). The eggs of other schistosomes (*S. hematobium* and *S. japonicum*) are deposited in large numbers in the subepithelial connective tissue of the urinary bladder. A severe granulomatous reaction may occur, resulting in obstruction of urinary flow. The extent of granulomatous inflammation may actually decrease in chronic infection, at least in experimental animals. This amelioration of the disease state is termed modulation, and may occur because of an active suppressor mechanism mediated by both cellular and humoral systems.

The adult worms of *Wuchereria bancrofti* (filaria) reside in the larger lymphatic channels, particularly those of the extremities. In some persons, the presence of these worms evokes an extensive granulomatous inflammatory reaction that causes obstruction to lymphatic flow. This obstruction may lead to massive swelling (lymphedema) of the involved area (elephantiasis). Only a small number of individuals with filaria infestation develop this complication, and it is believed that those persons who do not develop clinical manifestations do not have granulomatous sensitivity to the organism. Therefore, although the granulomatous reaction leads to death and isolation of the offending agent, it is definitely deleterious to the host.

Granulomatous Response to Known Antigens

ZIRCONIUM GRANULOMAS

Some six months following the marketing of stick deodorants containing zirconium salts, individuals were observed with axillary granulomas. The injection of zirconium into the skin of such patients resulted in the delayed appearance of a typical epithelioid granuloma. Further studies have clearly implicated zirconium as the causative agent. Some type of hypersensitivity was suspected because only relatively few individuals who used such deodorants actually developed lesions. Lesions no longer occurred when the use of zirconium was discontinued.

BERYLLIOSIS

Two forms of lung disease are associated with inhalation of beryllium: An acute chemical inflammation, caused by heavy exposure; and a chronic progressive pulmonary disease, following low exposure, featuring multiple small noncaseating granulomas, first reported in 1946. The conclusion that a type of hypersensitivity is involved in the latter is based on the observations that only a small number of the exposed individuals actually develop the disease and that there may be a delay of months or years from the time of exposure to the development of berylliosis. Beryllium was once used for the manufacture of fluorescent light bulbs, and many exposed individuals remained symptomless. Beryllium is no longer used for this purpose, and the disease has been greatly reduced. Berylliosis has been reported more recently following low exposure in precious-metal refining. Beryllium is still used in the aircraft industry. Cases have been reported following exposure to levels previously believed to be safe. The chronicity of the disease may also be due to the fact that beryllium tends to remain in the tissue indefinitely. It has been reported that patients with berylliosis give positive patch test reactions with the antigen, but the validity of this observation has been questioned. Further studies have shown that beryllium is an active inducer of contact (delayed-type) sensitivity. A more relevant test is the production of granulomas upon intradermal application of beryllium in patients with berylliosis. Application of beryllium in a patch test most likely does not stimulate a granulomatous reaction, which requires deposition of the eliciting antigen in tissues. The lymphocytes of patients with berylliosis will transform in vitro upon exposure to beryllium sulfate, further suggesting that cellular sensitization to beryllium occurs. Zirconium, as well as beryllium, may bind serum proteins and function as a hapten in the production of contact sensitivity. However, the relation of this mechanism to the development of granulomas remains obscure. Berylliosis may be considered an example of hypersensitivity pneumonitis.

HYPERSENSITIVITY PNEUMONITIS (EXTRINSIC ALLERGIC ALVEOLITIS)

Allergic reactions to organic dusts, bacteria, or mold products in the lung are believed to be causative in a certain type of interstitial pneumonitis, termed by Pepys **extrinsic allergic alveolitis** (Table 17–3). Frequently, the diagnosis is made after acute respiratory distress develops 4 to 12 hours after exposure to an eliciting "antigen." With repeated exposure, progressive pulmonary fibrosis (farmer's lung) occurs with the main tissue lesion being granulomatous; however, the frequent coexistence of other types of reactions, such as anaphylactic, toxic complex, or delayed may produce a complex clinical and pathologic picture in a given patient. The pathologic reaction is mixed, but inflammation of the alveolar walls is the primary feature, usually consisting of epithelioid cell granulomas. Plasma and lymphoid cell infiltration (high ratio of CD8+/CD4+ T cells) may also be prominent, and granulomas are not always present. In fact, a variety of lymphoid cell infiltrates and inflammatory reactions may be found in the lung, suggesting that a mixture of different types of immune or allergic reactions may be manifested at any given time. In many cases, precipitating antibodies may be demonstrated to test antigens. However, vasculitis is not a prominent feature, although there are notable exceptions. Patients

TABLE 17–3. SOURCE AND TYPE OF ANTIGEN-PRODUCING EXTRINSIC ALLERGIC ALVEOLITIS

Disease	Source of Antigen	Antigen Against Which Precipitating Antibody Is Present
Farmer's lung	Moldy hay	*Micropolyspora faeni, Thermoactinomyces vulgaris*
Bagassosis	Moldy bagasse*	*T. vulgaris*
Mushroom-worker's lung	Mushroom compost	*M. faeni, T. vulgaris*
Fog-fever in cattle	Moldy hay	*M. faeni*
Suberosis	Moldy oak bark, cork dust	Moldy cork dust
New Guinea lung	Moldy thatch dust	Thatch
Maple-bark pneumonitis	Moldy maple-bark	Cryptostroma (Coniosporium)
Malt-worker's lung	Moldy barley, malt dust	*Aspergillus clavatus Aspergillus fumigatus*
Bird-fancier's lung	Pigeon/budgerigar/parrot/ hen droppings	Serum protein, droppings
Pituitary snuff-taker's lung	Heterologous pituitary powder	Serum protein, pituitary antigens
Wheat-weevil disease	Infested wheat flour	*Sitophilus granarius*
Sequoiosis	Moldy sawdust	*Graphium Aureobasidium pullulans* (pullularia)
Mollusk shell pneumonitis	Mollusk shell dust	Pearl oyster shells
Cheese-washer's lung	Moldy cheese	Penicillin spp.

*Residue of sugar cane after extraction of syrup.

Modified from Pepys J: Hypersensitivity diseases of the lungs due to fungi and organic dusts. *Monogr Allergy*, vol. 4, Basel/New York, Kar-ger, 1969.

with these chronic pulmonary diseases often have acute attacks of asthma on exposure to the antigen; these may be caused by the existence of anaphylactic antibodies. Experimental hypersensitivity pneumonitis models in animals also support a combined role of immune complexes and CMI in the pathogenesis of this disease.

Diseases of Unknown Etiology

SARCOIDOSIS

Boeck's sarcoidosis is a systemic, noncaseating, granulomatous process of unknown etiology, prominently involving the lymph nodes, lungs, eyes, and skin, with lesions that may be indistinguishable from those of tuberculosis, fungus infections, or other granulomatous hypersensitivity reactions. The term "sarcoid" was coined by Caesar Boeck in 1899 for the skin lesions; later, systemic involvement was recognized by Schaumann in 1917. The clinical presentation of sarcoidosis may masquerade as acute rheumatoid arthritis, tuberculosis, erythema nodosum, or Crohn's disease, but usually appears as pulmonary masses and bilateral hilar adenopathy on a chest x-ray of a young adult black male with dyspnea. More recently, there appears to be an increase in older women. Berylliosis and sarcoidosis may be almost identical in their clinical presentation. About 80% of patients with sarcoidosis will resolve spontaneously; 20% will progress without treatment and 5% will die from complications of the disease. Rarely, sarcoidosis will present in an explosive picture by the appearance of erythema nodosum, polyarthritis, iritis, and fever (Lofgren's syndrome), but the onset is usually insidious, with lesions often being found in asymptomatic individuals. Progressive loss of pulmonary function is the major cause of disability and death; sudden death from sarcoid lesions in the conducting system of the heart is a rare, but recognized, possibility. Corticosteroids are the drugs of choice, but should not be used unless disease progression is noted. The serum levels of angiotensin-converting enzymes are elevated in patients with sarcoidosis and may be used to monitor disease activity. Sarcoidosis is noted for its geographic prevalence in the southeastern United States and its relative rarity in the western United States. The highest incidence is in Sweden, where 64 persons per 100,000 have radiologic evidence of the disease. In the 1960s, this geographic distribution was used to argue effectively that sarcoidosis was caused by an "allergy" to pine pollen, which contains acid-fast waxy material similar to *Mycobacterium tuberculosis*. However, a number of studies showed that a variety of infectious agents and fatty acids could produce granulomas in experimental animals identical to those of sarcoidosis. The nonspecificity of granuloma production led to dismissal of the pine pollen hypothesis.

A cutaneous granulomatous reaction may be elicited 3 to 4 weeks after the subcutaneous injection of crude extracts of spleen or lymph nodes from patients with sarcoidosis. This test was first reported in 1935 by Williams and Nickerson but has become known as the Kveim–Sitzbach reaction. The specificity of this reaction and its use as a diagnostic test is controversial. The diagnostic accuracy of the Kveim test depends on the preparation of "antigen" used; new extracts must be tested on known positive and negative controls before being used to test patients suspected of having sarcoidosis.

An infectious agent is suspected, but as yet no specific agent has been identified. The characteristic noncaseating granuloma is not pathognomonic; identical histopathologic lesions may be seen with mycobacterial and fungal infections, brucellosis, mineral dust exposure, hypersensitivity pneumonitis, and Wegener's granulomatosis. The granuloma has a central zone with tightly packed cells, including epithelioid cells, macrophages, and giant cells, surrounded by a peripheral zone with more loosely arranged mononuclear cells. The giant cells may contain concentrically laminated basophilic structures (Schaumann bodies), and smaller spindle-shaped inclusions with radiating spines (asteroid bodies) may be found at the outer edge of the central zone of the granuloma. The granuloma ultimately resolves, leaving no morphologic lesion, or undergoes fibrosis and contraction. The lesions are believed to be caused by T-cell activation leading to accumulation, fusion, and epithelioid changes in macrophages, but the "antigen" responsible for the T-cell activation has not been identified. Patients with sarcoidosis generally exhibit a depression of delayed-type hypersensitivity and increased levels of circulating antibody. The relationship of these findings to the disease process remains unclear but suggests an imbalance in the immune system, with a relatively incompetent T-cell system. This could be because of a redistribution of T cells in the inflammatory process or to an inherent loss of T-cell activity (see Chapter 27). The reason for the polyclonal activation of B cells is not known but may be secondary to production of interleukins by activation of T-helper cells during granuloma formation or to a form of immune deviation. Helper T cells (CD4+) predominate early in the disease, but suppressor T cells (CD8+) predominate during regression of the granulomas. Recently $T_{\gamma\delta}$ cells have been reported to be elevated in the blood and lung of patients with sarcoidosis. Could it be that hyperactivity of this nonspecific "early warning system" is part of the pathogenesis of sarcoidosis?

WEGENER'S GRANULO-MATOSIS

Wegener's granulomatosis is a triad of granulomatous arteritis, glomerulonephritis, and sinusitis. The presentation of the disease is variable, and glomerulonephritis may or may not be present. The granulomas may be disseminated but are usually prominent in the lungs, nasal and oral cavities, and spleen. The granulomatous lesions are destructive and contain fibroblastic proliferation, necrosis, and prominent Langhans' giant cells. This disease may be related to polyarteritis nodosa, and some authors have called it polyarteritis of the lungs or a type of hypersensitivity angiitis. However, the lesions of Wegener's granulomatosis are distinctive enough to warrant a separate diagnosis. An unusual finding is granulomatous glomerulonephritis, believed to be caused by a reaction to fibrin mixed with immune complexes in gaps in Bowman's capsule, leading to destruction of Bowman's capsule and a surrounding granulomatous inflammation. The natural history of the disease is invariable rapid progression with destruction of the upper respiratory system. Treatment with low dose cyclophosphamide combined with alternate-day corticosteroids has led to a high rate of temporary remissions, but relentless progression occurs in some patients. In some cases, exacerbation of the disease is closely associated with infections, and treatment of the infection with antibiotics may be associated with remission of the granulomatous lesions. The relation of Wegener's granulomatosis to other necrotizing granulomatous processes, such as midline lethal granuloma of the face, is not clear. No infectious agent has been consistently isolated from patients with any of these diseases.

Antibodies to neutrophils, antineutrophil cytoplasmic antibodies (ANCA), have been found in patients with Wegener's granulomatosis. Two types of antineutrophil antibodies are recognized—cytoplasmic ANCA (cANCA) and perinuclear ANCA (pANCA). cANCA reacts with proteinase-3 and gives a diffuse staining of the cytoplasm of neutrophils; pANCA reacts with myeloperoxidase and gives perinuclear pattern. cANCA has a sensitivity of 78% to 96% for Wegener's but is not diagnostic, as positive cANCA is also found in other related diseases, such as polyarteritis nodosa, rapidly progressive glomerulonephritis, and Churg–Strauss syndrome. Rising cANCA titers are highly suggestive of relapse. pANCA is found in patients with disease limited to the kidneys, especially idiopathic concentric glomerulonephritis, whereas cANCA predominates in patients with respiratory disease. Although a pathogenic role for ANCA is not established, it is possible that infections (such as pneumonitis) cause degranulation of neutrophils and release of lysosomal enzymes that elicit an autoimmune response. Excessive stimulation of neutrophils by ANCA and the proteolytic effects of released lysosomal enzymes may then cause endothelial damage and tissue necrosis.

GRANULO-MATOUS HEPATITIS

Circumscribed granulomas consisting of epithelioid cells surrounded by plasma cells and lymphocytes may be seen in the liver and are associated with a variety of diseases, including sarcoidosis, histoplasmosis, tuberculosis, cirrhosis, lymphomas, Wegener's granulomatosis, immune deficiency diseases, and malignant tumors. However, in a substantial number of patients, no specific disease association occurs (**idiopathic granulomatous hepatitis**). It is likely that the reaction represents an allergic reaction to a drug or response to an unidentified infectious agent.

REGIONAL ENTERITIS

Regional enteritis is a peculiar chronic inflammatory lesion of unknown etiology related to ulcerative colitis (see Inflammatory Bowel Disease, Chapter 21). The primary feature is thickening and scarring of the intestinal wall that may occur at any level of the gastrointestinal tract but usually involves the terminal ileum. Histologically, the inflammatory changes vary from those consistent with a delayed hypersensitivity reaction (dense infiltration of mononuclear lymphoid follicles often containing germinal centers) to those of granulomatous hypersensitivity (typical epithelioid granulomas with prominent giant cells, essentially identical to the pulmonary lesions of sarcoidosis). The lesions appear to begin as accumulations of lymphocytes and plasma cells around intestinal crypts. Later, macrophages are seen associated with destruction of the crypt (**crypt abscess**), followed by formation of epithelial cells and then granulomas (Fig. 17–5). The T-cell ratios in

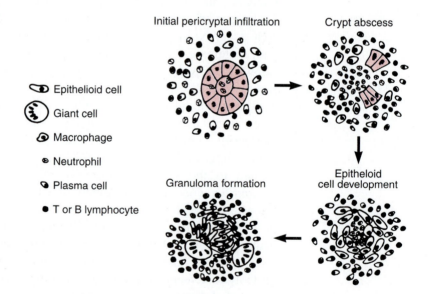

Figure 17–5. Sequence of tissue changes in evolution of granulomas in regional enteritis. Lesions begin with pericryptal mononuclear cell infiltration. This is followed by destruction of the epithelial cells (crypt abscess). Macrophage reaction converts the lesion to a granuloma. (Modified from Schmitz-Moorman P, Becker H: Histologic studies on the formal pathogenesis of the epithelial cell granuloma in Crohn's disease. In *Recent Advances in Crohn's Disease*, Pera AS, et al. (eds.). The Hague, Martinus Nijhoff, 1981, 76.)

mature lesions are 2:1 CD4+/CD8+, about the same as in control tissues. The mononuclear inflammation of regional enteritis may be the result of the development of delayed hypersensitivity to soluble antigens in the diet, and the granulomatous inflammation may be due to the development of granulomatous hypersensitivity to insoluble antigens in the diet, but no causative antigen has yet been identified.

SILICONE GRANULOMAS

Considerable controversy has arisen over the effect of rupture of silicone gel breast implants and development of local and systemic lesions. There is no clear documentation that the incidence of systemic lesions is increased in women who have received breast implants as compared to age-matched controls. Although granulomatous reactions may occur around ruptured implants, most ruptured implants remain silent and are discovered at mammography or at surgery for implant exchange. Physical findings consistent with implant rupture include nodules, decreased breast size, asymmetry, tenderness and compressibility. Migration of silica out of a ruptured implant may result in local granulomas and infrequently in systemic granulomatous lesions, but the frequency of these complications is unknown.

Immune Deficiency Diseases

GRANULO-MATOUS DISEASE OF CHILDREN

Granulomatous disease of children consists of chronic pulmonary disease, recurrent suppurative lymphadenitis, and chronic dermatitis with scattered granulomas in many organs. This disease is due to a defect in nicotinamide-adenine dinucleotide phosphate (NADPH) that prevents the phagocytic cell from producing free radicals necessary to kill bacteria following phagocytosis (see Chapter 27, Immune Deficiency Diseases). This results in formation of nonallergic granulomas which consist of collections of large macrophages in affected tissues.

Protective Functions of Granulomatous Reactions

The formation of a granuloma is a way that the body deals with substances that it finds difficult to eliminate by the usual process of phagocytosis and digestion by macrophages. The fixed macrophages within tissues and the monocytes that infiltrate sites of inflammation are primarily scavenger cells that are able to break down most infectious agents, as well as foreign bodies and residua of inflammation, by an array of toxic effector molecules and hydrolytic enzymes (see Chapter 9). It is ironic that a number of infectious agents, including protozoa, bacteria, fungi, mycobacteria, and viruses, actually preferentially infect and replicate within these same cells. Complex signals generated through the products of activated T cells, as well as other cytokines, induce a state of activation in the infected cell that kills the intracellular parasites. In addition, T_{CTL} cells that react with antigens of the infecting organisms expressed on macrophages may attack and kill infected cells, with subsequent destruction of the extracellular organisms by phagocytosis and digestion by other-activated macrophages. The major killing mechanism of activated macrophages may be through generation of nitrogen oxides derived from L-arginine.

Granulomas form because of the sometimes massive load of organisms or poorly digestible breakdown products of the organisms. When the system is functioning, activation of macrophages by cytokines prevents proliferation of the infecting organisms, and the infection may be cleared early on with little residual evidence in the tissues that infection ever occurred. Positive DTH skin tests provide evidence of previous infection in some individuals with no evidence of disease. However, if the infecting organisms are allowed to multiply, the macrophage system may be faced with an incredible clean-up job, and continued survival and multiplication of some organisms may continue even when there is massive destruction of most of the infecting agents. This results in a sometimes lifelong, life and death struggle between the host and the infection. Prolonged chemotherapy may hold replication of the organisms in check and allow the immune response to get the upper hand. However, if therapy is stopped too soon or the immune system is weakened by age, immunosuppressive drugs, or other infections, recurrence of active infection is the expected course.

Summary

Granulomatous reactions are characterized by the accumulation of oval collections of modified mononuclear cells in tissue. The typical tissue lesion contains large mononuclear cells that look like epithelial cells (epithelioid cells), multinucleated giant cells, lymphocytes, and plasma cells. Granulomatous reactions may be a variant of delayed hypersensitivity reactions to insoluble antigens, but also frequently occur in association with vasculitis or in response to nonantigenic foreign bodies. It is likely that poorly degradable antigens or insoluble antibody–antigen complexes produce granulomas, whereas soluble complexes cause vasculitis or glomerulonephritis. The mechanism of granulomatous reactivity is not clear but the inability of macrophages to digest antigens is believed to be a major pathogenic feature. Granulomatous tissue reactions serve to isolate infectious agents, such as tubercle bacilli, leprosy bacilli, or parasites. Deleterious effects of these reactions occur because of the displacement of normal tissue by granulomas and healing by fibrosis, leading to a loss of normal function.

Bibliography

GENERAL

Adams DO: The granulomatous inflammatory response. *Am J Pathol* 84:164–192, 1976.

Bently AG, Phillips SM, Kaner RJ, et al.: In vitro delayed hypersensitivity granuloma formation: Development of an antigen-coated bead model. *J Immunol* 134:4163, 1985.

Boros DL: *Basic and Clinical Aspects of Granulomatous Disease.* New York, Elsevier/North Holland, 1981.

Chambers TJ, Spector WG: Inflammatory giant cells. *Immunobiol* 161:283, 1982.

Epstein WL: Granulomatous hypersensitivity. *Prog Allergy* 11:36, 1967.

Langhans T: Veber Riesenzellen mit mandestandigen kernen in Tuberkeln und die fibrose form des tuverkels. *Virchams Arch Pathol Anat Physiol Kim Med* 42:382, 1868.

McInnes A, Rennick DM: Interleukin-4 induces cultured monocytes/macrophages to form giant multinuclear cells. *J Exp Med* 167:598, 1988.

Muller J: Ueber den feineren bau formen der krankhaften geschwulste. Berlin, 1838.

Perrin PJ, Phillips SM: The molecular basis of granuloma formation in schistosomiasis. I. A T cell-derived suppressor effector factor. *J Immunol* 141:1714, 1988.

Spector WG, Heesom N: The production of granulomata by antigen–antibody complexes. *J Pathol* 98:31, 1969.

Sutton JS, Weiss L: Transformation of monocytes in tissue culture into macrophages, epitheloid cells, and multinucleate giant cells. *J Cell Biol* 28:303, 1966.

Turk JL: The role of delayed hypersensitivity in granuloma formation. *Res Monogr Immunol* 1:275, 1980.

TUBERCULOSIS

Burke DS: Of postulates and peccadilloes: Robert Koch and vaccine (tuberculin) therapy for tuberculosis. *Vaccine* 11:795–804, 1993.

Collins FM: Antituberculous immunity: New solution to an old problem. *Rev Infect Dis* 13:940, 1991.

Dannenberg AM: Delayed-type hypersensitivity and cell-mediated immunity in the pathogenesis of tuberculosis. *Immunol Today* 12:228, 1991.

Donerty PC: The function of $T_{\gamma\delta}$ cells. *Brit J Haematol* 81:321, 1992.

Freerksen E, Rosenfeld M: *Leprosy–Tuberculosis Eradication: Principles, Practical Implementation.* Amsterdam, Excerpta Medica, 1980.

Glassroth JG, Robins AG, Snider DE: Tuberculosis in the 1980s. *N Engl J Med* 302:1441, 1980.

Hsu KHK: Thirty years after isoniazid: Its impact on tuberculosis in children and adolescents. *JAMA* 251:1283, 1984.

Kaufmann SHE: Immunity against intracellular bacteria: Biologic effector functions and antigen specificity of T lymphocytes. *Curr Top Microbiol Immunol* 138:141, 1988.

Kumararatne DS, Pithie A, Drysdale P, et al.: Specific lysis of mycobacterial antigen-bearing macrophages by class II MHC-restricted polyclonal T-cell lines in healthy donors or patients with tuberculosis. *Clin Exp Immunol* 80:314, 1990.

Orme IM, Miller ES, Roberts AD, et al.: T lymphocytes mediating protection and cellular cytolysis during the course of *Mycobacterium tuberculosis* infection. *J Immunol* 148:189, 1992.

Rich AR: *The Pathogenesis of Tuberculosis.* Springfield, IL, CC Thomas, 1951.

Weissler JC: Tuberculosis—immunopathogenesis and therapy. *Am J Med Sci* 305:52–65, 1993.

LEPROSY

Alpert DA, Weissman MH, Kaplan R: The rheumatic manifestations of leprosy (Hansen disease). *Medicine* 59:442, 1980.

Arnoldi J, Gerdes J, Flad HD: Immunohistologic assessment of cytokine production of infiltrating cells in various forms of leprosy. *Am J Pathol* 137:749, 1990.

Band H: Interleukin-1: A possible mediator of neural fibrosis in leprosy. *Med Hypothesis* 20:143, 1986.

Britton WJ: Leprosy 1962–1992: Immunology of Leprosy. *Trans Royal Soc Trop Med Hyg* 87:508–514, 1993.

Fine PEM: Immunological tools in leprosy control. *Int J Leprosy* 57:671, 1989.

Garcia-de la Torre I: Autoimmune phenomena in leprosy, particularly antinuclear antibodies and rheumatoid factor. *J Rheumatol* 20:900–903, 1993.

Kaplan G, et al.: An analysis of in vitro T-cell responsiveness in lepromatous leprosy. *J Exp Med* 162:917, 1985.

Naafs B, Kolk AHJ, Roel AM, et al.: Anti-*Mycobacterium leprae* monoclonal antibodies cross-react with human skin: An alternative explanation for the immune responses in leprosy. *J Invest Dermatol* 94:685, 1990.

Sieling PA, Abrams JS, Yamamura M, et al.: Immunosuppressive roles for IL-10 and IL-4 in human infection: In vitro modulation of T cell responses in leprosy. *J Immunol* 150:5501–5511, 1993.

Skinsnes OK: Immunopathology of leprosy: The century in review—pathology, pathogenesis, and the development of classification. *Int J Leprosy* 41:329, 1973.

Turk JL, Bryceson ADM: Immunologic phenomena in leprosy and related disease. *Adv Immunol* 13:209, 1971.

OTHER GRANULO-MATOUS INFECTIONS

Baker RD (ed.): The pathologic anatomy of mycoses: Human infection with fungi, actinomycetes, and algae. New York, Springer–Verlag, 1971.

Binford CH: Histoplasmosis: Tissue reactions and morphologic variations of the fungus. *Am J Clin Pathol* 25:25, 1955.

Marcial-Rojas RA (ed.): Pathology of protozal and helminthic diseases. Baltimore, Williams & Wilkins, 1971.

Vanek J, Schwartz J: The gamet of histoplasmosis. *Am J Med* 50:89, 1971.

Warren KS: Modulation of immunopathology and disease in schistosomiasis. *Am J Trop Med Hyg* 26:113, 1977.

BERYLLIUM DISEASE

Barna BP et al.: Immunologic studies of experimental beryllium lung disease in the guinea pig. *Clin Immunol Immunopathol* 20:402, 1981.

Cullen MR, Kominsky JR, Rossman MD, et al.: Chronic beryllium disease in a precious-metal refinery: Clinical, epidemiologic, and immunologic evidence for continuing risk from exposure to low-level beryllium fume. *Am Rev Resp Dis* 135:201, 1987.

Deodhar SD, Barna B, Van Ordstrand HS: A study of the immunologic aspects of chronic berylliosis. *Chest* 63:309, 1973.

Denardi JN, Van Ordstrand HS, Curtis GH, et al.: Berylliosis. *Arch Industr Hyg* 8:1, 1953.

Hardy HL, Tabershaw IR: Delayed chemical pneumonitis occurring in workers exposed to beryllium compounds. *J Ind Hyg Toxicol* 28:2693, 1946.

Kanared DJ, Wainer RA, Chamberlin RI, et al.: Respiratory illness in a population exposure to beryllium. *Am Rev Resp Dis* 108:1295, 1973.

Kreiss K, Miller F, Newman LS, et al.: Chronic beryllium disease—from the workplace to cellular immunology, molecular biology, and back. *Clin Immunol Immunopathol* 71:123–129, 1994.

Tepper LB, Hardy HL, Chamberlin RI: *Toxicity of Beryllium Compounds*. Amsterdam, Elsevier, 1961.

HYPERSENSI-TIVITY PNEUMONITIS

Larson G: Hypersensitivity lung disease. *Annu Rev Immunol* 3:59, 1985.

McCombs RP: Diseases due to immunologic reactions in the lungs. *N Engl J Med* 286:1186–1245, 1972.

Nicholson DP: Bagasse worker's lung. *Annu Rev Resp Dis* 97:546, 1968.

Orriols R, Manresa J-M, Aliaga J-L, et al.: Mollusk shell hypersensitivity pneumonitis. *Ann Int Med* 113:80, 1990.

Pepys J: Hypersensitivity diseases of the lungs due to fungi and organic dusts. In *Monographs in Allergy*, vol. 4, Kallos P, Hasek M, Interbitzen TM, Miescher P, Waksman BH (eds.). Basel, Karger, 1969.

Richardson HB: Immune complexes in the lung: A skeptical review. *Surv Synth Path* 3:281, 1984.

Solley GO, Hyatt RE: Hypersensitivity pneumonitis induced by penicillin species. *J Allergy Clin Immunol* 65:65, 1980.

ALLERGIC GRANULO-MATOSIS

Alarcon-Segovia D, Brown AL: Classification and etiologic aspects of necrotizing angiitis: An analytic approach to a confused subject with a critical review of the evidence for hypersensitivity in polyarteritis nodosa. *Mayo Clin Proc* 39:205, 1964.

Bhathena DB, Migdal SD, Julian BA, et al.: Morphologic and immunohistochemical observations in granulomatous glomerulonephritis. *Am J Pathol* 126:581, 1987.

Chumbley LC, Harrison EC Jr, Deremee RA: Allergic granulomatosis and angiitis (Churg–Strauss syndrome): Report and analysis of 30 cases. *Mayo Clin Proc* 52:477, 1977.

Churg J, Strauss L: Allergic granulomatosis, allergic angiitis, and polyarteritis nodosa. *Am J Pathol* 27:277–301, 1951.

Churg J: Allergic granulomatosis and granulomatous vascular syndromes. *Ann Allergy* 21:619, 1963.

Fahey JL, Leonard E, Churg J: Wegener's granulomatosis. *Am J Med* 17:168, 1954.

Gross WL, Schmit WH, Csernok E: ANCA and associated diseases: Immunologic and pathogenetic aspects. *Clin Exp Immunol* 91:1–12, 1993.

Hagen EC, Ballieux BEPB, Daha MR, et al.: Fundamental and clinical aspects of anti-neutrophil cytoplasmic antibodies (ANCA). *Autoimmunity* 11:199, 1992.

Hoffman GS, Kerr GS, Leavitt RS, et al.: Wegener granulomatosis: An analysis of 158 patients. *Ann Int Med* 116:488–498, 1992.

Leavitt R, Fauci A, Bloch D, et al.: The American College of Rheumatology 1990 criteria for the classification of Wegener's granulomatosis. *Arthritis Rheum* 33:1101, 1990.

Liebow AA: The J. Burns Amberson Lecture: Pulmonary angiitis and granulomatosis. *Am Rev Resp Dis* 1081:1, 1973.

Oreo GA: Wegener's granulomatosis. *Arch Dermatol* 81:169, 1960.

SARCOID

Balbi B, Moller DR, Kirby, Holroyd K, Crystal RG: Increased numbers of T lymphocytes with $T_{\gamma\delta}$ antigen receptors in a subgroup of individuals with pulmonary sarcoidosis. *J Clin Invest* 85:1353, 1990.

Boeck C: Multiple benign sarkoid of the skin. *J Cutan Genit Urin Dis* 17:543, 1899.

Cummings MM: An evaluation of the possible relationship of pine pollen to sarcoidosis (a critical summary). In *Proceedings of the Third International Conference on Sarcoidosis*. Lafres S, (ed.). *Acta Med Scand* 425(Suppl):48, 1964.

Israel HL, Goldstein RA: Relation of Kveim antigen reaction to lymphodenopathy. Study of sarcoidosis and other diseases. *N Engl J Med* 284:345, 1971.

Iwai K, Tachibana T, Takemura T, et al.: Pathologic studies on sarcoidosis autopsy. I. Epidemiologic features of 320 cases in Japan. *Acta Pathol Jap* 43:372–376, 1993.

James DG, Williams WJ: Sarcoidosis and other granulomatous disorders. Philadelphia, WB Saunders, 1985.

Kveim A: En ny og spesifik Kulan-reackjon ved Boeck's sarcoid. *Nord Med* 9:169, 1941.

Schaumann J: Studies of lupus pernio and its relationship to sarcoidosis and tuberculosis. *Ann Dermatol Venereol* 6:356, 1917.

Siltzbach LE: The international Kveim test study, 1960–1966. In *Proceedings of the Fourth International Conference on Sarcoidosis*. Turial T, Chabot J (eds.). Paris, Masson and Cie, 1967, 201–213.

Williams RH, Nickerson DA: Skin reactions in sarcoid. *Proc Soc Exp Biol Med* 33:403, 1935.

REGIONAL ILEITIS

Crohn BB, Ginzburg L, Oppenheimer GD: Regional ileitis: A pathologic and clinical entity. *JAMA* 99:1323, 1932.

Janowitz HD, Sachar DB: New observations in Crohn's disease. *Ann Rev Med* 27:269, 1976.

Sartor RB, et al.: Granulomatous entercolitis induced in rats by purified cell wall extracts. *Gastroenterol* 89:587, 1985.

SILICONE

Williams CW: Silicone gel granulomas following compressive mammography. *Aesthetic Plast Surg* 15:49–51, 1991.

GRANULO-MATOUS DISEASE OF CHILDREN

Berendes H, Bridges RA, Good RA: A fetal granulomatosis of childhood: The clinical study of a new syndrome. *Mini Med* 40:309, 1957.

Gallin JI, et al.: Recent advances in chronic granulomatous disease. *Ann Int Med* 99:657, 1983.

Johnston RB, Baehner RL: Chronic granulomatous disease: Correlation between pathogenesis and clinical findings. *Pediatrics* 48:730, 1971.

Landing BH, Shirkey HS: A syndrome of recurrent infection and infiltration of viscera by pigmented lipid histiocytes. *Pediatrics* 20:431, 1957.

18

Interplay of Inflammatory and Immunopathologic Mechanisms

In any inflammatory reaction, both immune and "nonimmune" mechanisms may be activated. In the preceding chapters, the distinguishing characteristics of each individual immune-mediated pathogenic mechanisms has been emphasized. However, in many immune disease processes, more than one immune mechanism may be playing a part sequentially, at the same time, or both. In addition, nonimmune systems may contribute to either increase or decrease the effect of immune-specific mechanisms. The clinical manifestations and pathologic lesions associated with a given immune-mediated disease are not only determined by more than one mechanism, but different mechanisms share common components of the inflammatory process, such as cytokine release or upregulation of adhesion molecules.

Nonimmune Inflammation

Inflammation may be activated by nonimmune factors such as tissue necrosis (infarct), release of bacterial products, or trauma. Such stimuli may activate complement, kinin, coagulation, or mast cell inflammatory mediators, as well as cell cause upregulation of vascular adhesion molecules, leukocyte selectins and integrins, and/or cytokines that are also activated by immune effector mechanisms (see Chapters 8 and 9). The tissue manifestations may include acute or chronic inflammatory changes that in some cases are indistinguishable from the lesions caused by immune mechanisms. Chronic nonimmune inflammation in the skin may be manifested by a perivascular mononuclear infiltrate that looks like a delayed hypersensitivity reaction; "nonimmune" granulomatous reactions to foreign bodies may be very similar, if not identical, to granulomatous "hypersensitivity" reactions activated by immune mechanisms.

Immune Inflammation

Histologic similarities between lesions of immune- and nonimmune-mediated inflammation are not surprising, since the same basic inflammatory mechanisms are utilized, and immunization often results in production of different classes of antibody, as well as cellular immunity to the same antigens. CD4+ T-helper cells not only produce factors that help B cells make antibody but also are precursors for T_{DTH} cells. In addition, different immune mechanisms share some of the same inflammatory mediators, or one immune mechanism may activate another through cross-stimulation of the effectors. In serum sickness, over fifty serum protein antigens are potentially available to react with different antibodies or T cells. Anaphylactic and cell-mediated lesions, as well as immune complex lesions, often coexist in the acute phase of serum sickness.

The reaction of an antibody with an antigen in vivo may result in activation of more than one immune mechanism. For example, immune complex-like inflammatory reactions may activate or be activated by each of the other immune mechanisms (Fig. 18–1). Antibody reacting with a biologically active antigen may not only cause neutralization but also lead to the formation of soluble immune complexes and immune complex lesions. In fact, neutralization reactions may be considered as a specialized form of immune complex reaction wherein the biologic activity of the antigen adds an additional dimension to the effects of an antibody–antigen reaction. Binding of antibody–antigen complexes to red cells may result in their destruction by activation of complement (the innocent bystander reaction), and soluble complexes released by lysed cells may contribute to an immune complex effect. The activation of complement or release of enzymes from polymorphonuclear neutrophils as a result of an immune complex reaction may cause mast cell lysis and activation of anaphylactic mechanisms. The reaction of immune complexes with platelets may induce serotonin release, which causes increased vascular permeability and upregulation of cell adhesion molecules, and polymorphonuclear infiltrate, with subsequent tissue damage, followed by lymphocytic and macrophage invasion and further inflammation or healing.

Anaphylactic mediators released from mast cells may cause separation of endothelial cells, exposing the basement membrane and thus forming foci where immune complexes can lodge and initiate basement membrane damage by an Arthus mechanism or allow sensitized cells, T_{CTL} or T_{DTH} cells, to pass through the vessels into tissue spaces. Both immunoglobulin antibody and sensitized cells may play a role in the lesions seen in autoimmune diseases such as thyroiditis, encepha-

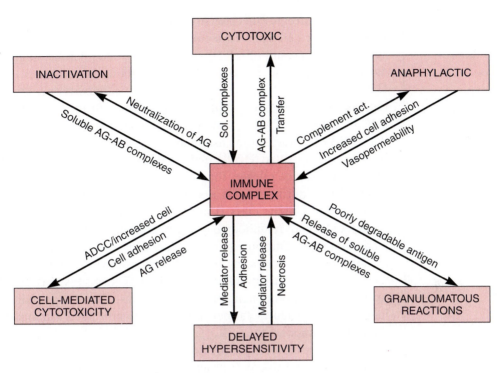

Figure 18–1. Possible interactions of immune complex and other immunopathologic mechanisms. See text for description.

lomyelitis, or orchitis. Upregulation of adhesion molecules on endothelial cells in the brain as a result of formation of myelin–antimyelin complexes leads to lymphocyte margination and emigration of mononuclear cells into the brain.

The role of immune complex reactivity, cell-mediated immunity, macrophage activation, and chronic proliferative response in the pathogenesis of a progressive lesion is illustrated by rheumatoid arthritis (see Chapter 22). Chronic immune complex-mediated injury leads to mononuclear cell proliferation and activation of pannus formation by macrophage products. Immune complex vasculitis may lead to upregulation of cell adhesion molecules and lymphocyte infiltration characteristic of cell-mediated reactions. Tissue damage or cell destruction caused by T-cell cytotoxicity or DTH may activate cytokines that attract and activate polymorphonuclear cells. The formation of poorly degradable antibody–antigen complexes may initiate granuloma formation, whereas tissue antibody or breakdown products produced by granulomatous reactions may lead to toxic complex glomerulonephritis. Granulomatous lesions frequently occur in association with immune complex vasculitis and/or anaphylactic type reactions.

Other allergic mechanisms may also interact. Complement-induced mast cell lysis (cytotoxic reaction) may cause anaphylactic symptoms as a result of release of mediators, and pharmacologic mediators and vascular reactions may contribute to cytotoxic effects. Cytotoxic antibody may contribute to cell-mediated tissue destruction (eg, aspermatogenesis); antibody-dependent cell-mediated cytotoxic cells or cytotoxic factors released by activated lymphocytes may produce lysis of cells. Chronic asthmatic lesions are characterized by infiltration with activated T cells that lower the threshold for reactivity by increased cytokine release. Interleukin-1 (IL-1) released from activated macrophages during a DTH reaction upgrades expression of adhesion molecules and MHC class II antigens on endothelial cells, leading to granulocyte and lymphocyte margination, respectively. Lymphocyte mediators may contribute to the evolution of a granulomatous reaction by attracting and activating macrophages; release of lymphocyte-stimulating factors from granulomatous inflammatory sites may contribute to the cellular component of such reactions. Finally, granulomatous lung diseases (such as farmer's lung) frequently have asthmatic (anaphylactic) components.

Granulomatous inflammation may increase the number of mast cells present, and tissue destruction by anaphylactic mechanisms may contribute to granuloma formation. Mixtures of vasculitis, glomerulonephritis, cellular lesions, and granulomas, such as seen in Wegener's granulomatosis and some infectious diseases, are among the most complex diseases to analyze from the immunopathologic standpoint.

Interaction of Immune and Nonimmune Inflammation

Other systems, such as the blood clotting and the kinin systems, may be activated during the evolution of an inflammatory reaction that also involves allergic reactions. For example, the role that Hageman factor (factor XII of the blood sequence) plays in involvement of other systems is illustrated in Chapter 8. Conversion of plasminogen to plasmin produces activation of complement that may induce lytic or inflammatory reactions. Kinins increase vascular permeability and may expose basement membranes for toxic complex deposition. Reaction of α_2-macroglobulin with prekallikrein forms a temperature-sensitive complex that produces increased capillary permeability and chronic inflammation in the skin. Complement may be activated by nonimmunologic mechanisms (see Alternate Pathway of Complement, Chapter 8).

Interaction of these "nonimmune" inflammatory mechanisms with allergic (immune) mechanisms may make it very difficult to evaluate the role of different immune mechanisms responsible for an inflammatory processes taking place in a given patient. However, it is critical for diagnosis and therapeutic decisions to identify the type of inflammatory or immunopathologic reactions responsible for disease in a given patient. In most cases, nonimmune inflammatory reactions or the clotting system are activated secondary to tissue damage caused by immunopathologic mechanisms, and successful treatment may be directed to both the primary immunopathologic and the secondary inflammatory process.

Bibliography

Cochrane CG: Immunologic tissue injury mediated by neutrophilic leukocytes. *Adv Immunol* 9:97, 1968.

Johnston MG, Hay JB, Movat HZ: The role of prostaglandins in inflammation. *Curr Top Pathol* 68:259, 1979.

Kimball ES: *Cytokines and Inflammation*. Boca Raton, FL, CRC Press, 1991.

Lampert PW: Mechanism of demyelination in experimental allergic neuritis: Electron microscopic studies. *Lab Invest* 20:127, 1969.

Lasser EC, Lyon SG, Negrete S: Alpha$_2$-macroglobulin–kallikrein complex: A temperature-sensitive mediator in contact system-induced inflammation with a potential role in late and delayed hypersensitivity responses. *Int Arch Allergy Appl Immunol* 96:134, 1991.

Marx JL: The leukotrienes in allergy and inflammation. *Science* 215:1380, 1982.

Movat HZ: The kinin system and its relation to other systems. *Curr Top Pathol* 68:111, 1979.

Owen CH, Bowie EJW: *The Intravascular Coagulation–Fibrinolysis Syndromes in Obstetrics and Gynecology*. Kalamazoo, MI, Upjohn, 1976.

Ratnoff O: The interrelationship of clotting factors and immunologic mechanism. In *Immunology*, Good RA, Fisher DW (eds.). Stanford, CT, Sinaver, 1971, 135.

Ryan GB, Majno G: Acute inflammation: A review. *Am J Pathol* 86:247, 1977.

Scibner DJ, Fahrney D: Neutrophil receptors of IgG and complement: Their roles in the attachment and ingestion phases of phagocytosis. *J Immunol* 116:892, 1976.

Stossel TP: Phagocytosis. *N Engl J Med* 290:761, 774, 833, 1974.

Waksman BH: The distribution of experimental autoallergic lesions: Its relation to the distribution of small veins. *Am J Pathol* 37:673, 1960.

Wilkinson PC, Lackie JM: The adhesion, migration, and chemotaxis of leukocytes in inflammation. *Curr Top Pathol* 68:47, 1979.

19

Drug Allergy

The untoward or undesirable effects of a drug may be from over-dosage, intolerance, idiosyncrasy, side effect, secondary effect, or from an allergic reaction to the drug (Table 19–1). In general, drug-induced toxicities may be classified into those that are intrinsic (ie, due to the chemical properties of the drug) or extrinsic (due to a peculiar reaction of the treated individual). Extrinsic toxicities are caused by idiosyncrasies or by allergic reactions. Drug allergies may be classified, on the basis of the immune mechanism involved, as neutralization or inactivation, cytotoxic, atopic or anaphylactic, immune complex (Arthus), T-cytotoxic, delayed hypersensitivity, or granulomatous reactions. In some instances, it is very difficult to differentiate drug allergy from idiosyncrasy. For instance, phenacetin may induce hemolytic anemia in patients with glucose-6-dehydrogenase deficiency, which closely resembles allergic hemolytic anemia but is not due to antibody. Unless tests for antibody, such as the Coombs' test, are positive, it may be impossible to prove an immune pathogenesis. Even if antibody is present, it does not necessarily prove that the patient's symptoms are due to an antibody to the drug.

Allergic reactions to drugs, therefore, include one or more of the immune mechanisms listed in Table 19–2. A given patient may express drug resistance due to neutralization or clearance of antigen–antibody complexes. The capacity of antibodies to drugs to neutralize the thera-peutic effect of the drug has not received much attention yet may be responsible for treatment failure. Clearly, antibodies may cause resis-tance to antibiotics, insulin, blood clotting factor replacement, or other replacement therapy. In some instances antibody neutralization of a drug may be used to treat an overdose. The passive transfer of Fab_2

494

TABLE 19–1. CLASSIFICATION OF DRUG REACTIONS

Type	Definition
Overdose	Normal reaction to too much of the drug
Intolerance	Increased sensitivity to normal doses of the drug
Idiosyncrasy	Qualitatively abnormal pharmacologic response, not a result of the normal pharmacologic effect
Side effect	Normal, but not desired effect of a drug
Secondary effect	Normal, undesired effect of a drug as a result of producing the desired effect
Allergic reaction	Reaction mediated by immune response to the drug

antibody is effective in treatment of arrhythmias secondary to digitalis toxicity. Autoantibodies have been shown to inhibit a variety of other effector molecules, including steroid hormones, catecholamines, histamine, serotonin, morphine, oxytocin, and vasopressin. Hemolytic reactions to drugs are presented in more detail in Chapter 12.

Historically, the first conception of an allergic reaction to a "drug" was the recognition of serum sickness following administration of horse antidiphtheria toxin serum to humans with diphtheria. Serum sickness-like symptoms include fever, joint pains, urticaria, and proteinuria (immune complex nephritis). The most striking allergic drug reaction is anaphylactic shock, which occurs within a few seconds or minutes after exposure; less severe anaphylactic symptoms include urticaria and wheezing. Later urticarial reactions may be seen 2 to 48 hours after exposure.

TABLE 19–2. ALLERGIC REACTIONS TO DRUGS

Mechanism	Examples	
Neutralization	Resistance to therapy	Insulin, blood clotting factors, cancer chemotherapeutic agents, penicillin
Cytolytic	Hemolysis, thrombocytopenia, agranulocytosis, purpura	Penicillin, quinidine, α-methyl-dopa, quinine
Immune complex	Exanthematous skin rashes, serum sickness, vasculitis, lupus syndrome, nephritis	Penicillin, serum, insulin, hydralazine, isoniazid, sulfa drugs, vaccines
Anaphylactic	Shock, urticaria, asthma, angioedema	Penicillin, antibiotics, cancer chemotherapeutic agents, vaccines
T-cytotoxic	Contact dermatitis	Penicillin, antibiotics, metals
Delayed hypersensitivity	Toxic epidermal necrosis, cytokine release syndrome	Penicillin, antibiotics, etc., monoclonal antibodies
Granulomatous	Granulomatous vasculitis, hepatitis	Penicillin, etc.

The most common allergic drug reactions are manifested in the skin: Exanthematic, erythematous, and maculopapular rashes; urticaria; angioedema; serpiginous lesions; contact dermatitis; erythema multiforme; erythema nodosum; purpura; eczema; and fixed eruptions. Fixed eruptions appear in the same area of the skin each time the responsible drug is administered and may be macular, eczematous, or bullous. The mechanism involved in fixed eruptions may be delayed hypersensitivity—immune complex or anaphylactic—but, for as yet unknown reasons, the reaction occurs in the same place. Renal reactions associated with drug reactions include interstitial nephritis, tubular necrosis, membranous nephritis polyarteritis and acute glomerulonephritis. Any allergic mechanism, including systemic delayed hypersensitivity and granulomatous reactions, may be found as a reaction to penicillin. Other drug allergies are described in Chapters 11 through 17 in relationship to the immunopathologic mechanisms activated.

Sensitization to Drugs

Since drug allergies are manifestations of immunologic responses, these reactions have the character of the immune mechanism(s) activated (Table 19–3). Although a clinical reaction is not usually seen after the first exposure; often, sensitization may occur because of exposure in food or another environmental source not realized by the patient. In addition, if drug therapy is continued over several weeks, or as in the case of serum sickness, if the drug persists in the body for several weeks, sensitization to the drug may occur during the period of first exposure. Re-exposure results in a much more rapid and intense reaction and requires much less of the drug. Administration of the drug at low doses, under carefully controlled conditions in an attempt to induce the suspected reaction, is the most clinically reliable test for an allergic reaction. The most common reactions are to antibiotics, such as semisynthetic penicillins, sulfa drugs, and erythromycins (Table 19–4). Other common agents are corticotropin and incompatible blood transfusions. The incidence of an allergic reaction to a drug in a patient without a previous history is less than 3% for drugs even with the highest rates.

TABLE 19–3. CHARACTERISTICS OF ALLERGIC DRUG REACTIONS

1. No response to first exposure; can be re-elicited once individual is sensitized.
2. Reaction elicited at doses far below therapeutic dose.
3. Manifestations reflect allergic mechanism and not pharmacologic action of drug.
4. Only a small number of treated individuals develop allergic response.
5. Specific antibodies or lymphocytes reactive with drug demonstrable.

The mechanism of drug sensitization to large polypeptides is similar to that of other complete antigens (immunogens). However, most drugs are molecules of less than seven amino acids, have molecular weights of less than 1 kD, and are not complete antigens. For the development of drug allergy, some mechanism of covalent binding of the drug to an immunogenic carrier must occur. Such reactions are readily accomplished in vitro in the laboratory, but how this occurs in vivo is not clear. It is possible that some drugs may be metabolized in vivo to active intermediates that combine with host proteins, but this has not yet been clearly established as being chemically important. The best example of sensitization to drugs is penicillin.

Penicillin Allergy

Antibiotics are the drugs that most frequently cause allergic reactions (Table 19–4). Allergy to penicillin will be presented to exemplify antibiotic hypersensitivity. Penicillin is probably the most thoroughly studied drug responsible for producing allergic reactions, not only because it is so widely used, but also because it produces a relatively high rate of sensitization. The reported frequency of anaphylactic reactions to penicillin is from 1 to 10/100,000 injections. Recent increases in the number of cases of gestational syphilis have stimulated interest in penicillin allergy, since penicillin is the only treatment for syphilis that reaches the fetus. The penicillin molecule contains a number of structures that can combine with amino, hydroxy, mercapto, disulfide, or histidine groups on macromolecules due to generation of a number of metabolites (Fig. 19–1). Most studies indicate that sensitization is due to the presence of preformed polymers, high-molecular-weight aggregates, or impurities present in the manufactured penicillin preparations. In addition, presensitization to penicillin may occur from contamination of penicillin in food, particularly milk or milk products from cattle fed with grain containing penicillin. Penicillin is also present in a number of vaccines and could be responsible for sensitization via this vector.

Experimental studies have shown that a high epitope density (over thirty determinants per carrier molecule) is needed to induce an IgE antibody response to substituted serum albumin in rabbits, and similar densities are needed to induce delayed hypersensitivity to haptens on autologous carriers in guinea pigs. Thus, it is unlikely that such immunogenic molecules could be manufactured from small drug haptens and that sensitization to drugs occurs in vivo in this manner. In fact, tolerance to free haptens may be more easily induced than an immune reaction. Penicillin itself may be immunogenic in animals when administered in adjuvants such as complete Freund's adjuvant or together with *Bordetella pertussis*. Complete immunogens are pro-

TABLE 19–4. ALLERGIC AND TOXIC REACTIONS TO SOME COMMONLY USED ANTIBIOTICS

Drugs	Disease	Contraindications	Untoward and Allergic Reactions
AMEBICIDES			
Chloroquine	Malaria, amebiasis	Psoriasis, pregnancy, G6PD deficiency	Shock, pleomorphic skin reactions, nausea, vomiting (hemolytic anemia)
ANTIBACTERIALS			
Nitrofurantoin	Urinary tract infections, enterococci, *S. aureus, E. coli*	Impaired renal function, pregnancy	Anaphylaxis, fever, pulmonary edema, exfoliative dermatitis, multiple skin reactions, asthma, hepatitis, anemia, etc.
Penicillin	Many bacterial infections	Hypersensitivity	Multiple skin rashes, serum sickness, anaphylaxis, hemolytic anemia, leukopenia, neuropathy, etc.
Trimethoprim–sulfamethoxazole	Broad spectrum	Hypersensitivity, pregnancy	Skin eruptions, serum sickness, anaphylaxis, arthralgia, myocarditis anemia, thrombocytopenia, hepatitis diarrhea, polyneuritis, Stevens–Johnson, etc.
Tetracycline	Gram negatives, *Rickettsia,* mycoplasma, enterococci, etc.	Hypersensitivity, pregnancy, infants	Nausea, vomiting, renal toxicity, enterocolitis, skin eruptions, anaphylaxis, angioedema, pericarditis, SLE, serum sickness, hemolytic anemia, thrombocytopenia, neutropenia, eosinophilia, etc.
Cephalosporin	Broad spectrum, streptococci, *S. aureus, H. influenzae,* etc.	Hypersensitivity, impaired renal function	Pseudomembranous colitis, urticaria, skin rashes, eosinophilia
Gentamicin, kanamycin (aminoglycoside)	Broad spectrum	Hypersensitivity	Nephrotoxicity, neurotoxicity, various skin rashes, lethargy, anaphylaxis, fever, nausea, vomiting, anemia, alopecia, agranulocytosis
Chloramphenicol	Broad spectrum, used only when others are ineffective	Hypersensitivity, pregnancy, lactation	Bone marrow depression, nausea, vomiting, neurotoxicity, anaphylaxis, vasculitis, skin rashes
Erythromycin	Broad spectrum	Hypersensitivity	Nausea, vomiting, mild skin eruptions, anaphylaxis
Vancomycin	Gram-positive bacteria	Hypersensitivity	Nausea, fever, macular rashes, anaphylaxis, neutropenia, myalgia

ANTIFUNGALS			
Griseofulvin	*Microsporum, Epidermophyton, Trichophyton*	Liver disease, porphyria, hypersensitivity	Multiple skin rashes, urticaria, nausea, granulocytopenia, glomerulonephritis
Myastatin	*Candida*	Hypersensitivity	Relatively nontoxic; diarrhea, vomiting at high doses
MYCOBACTERIALS			
Isoniazid	Tuberculosis	Hypersensitivity	Hepatitis, peripheral neuropathy, neurotoxicity, nausea, vomiting, agranulocytosis, skin eruptions, vasculitis, SLE, rheumatoid arthritis
Rifampicin	Tuberculosis, *Neisseria*	Hypersensitivity, pregnancy	Various skin rashes, hepatitis, hemolytic anemia, thrombocytopenia, renal failure, nausea, vomiting
Streptomycin	Tuberculosis, various bacteria	Hypersensitivity, pregnancy	Vertigo, nausea, vomiting, fever, various skin rashes, hemolytic anemia, anaphylaxis, thrombocytopenia, agranulocytosis
Dapsone	Leprosy	Anemia, G6PD deficiency, hypersensitivity	Multiple cutaneous reactions, hemolytic anemia, neuropathy, nausea, vomiting, vertigo, SLE, glomerulonephritis
ANTIVIRAL			
Adenine arabinoside	Herpes simplex, herpes zoster	Hypersensitivity	Nausea, vomiting, anorexia, encephalopathy, mild skin rashes
Acyclovir	Herpes	Hypersensitivity	None (ointment), inflammation of injection site (IM)
HELMINTHS			
Piperazine	*Ascaris*, pinworm	Impaired liver or renal function, hypersensitivity	Neurotoxicity, nausea, vomiting, fever, skin rashes, arthralgia
Thiabendazole	*Strongyloides, Ascaris*	Hepatic or renal dysfunction, hypersensitivity	Neurotoxicity, nausea, vomiting, leukopenia, various skin rashes, Stevens—Johnson, mild abdominal discomfort, nausea, rare skin rash
Praziquantel	Schistosomiasis	Hypersensitivity, eye lesions	Mild malaise, rare urticaria

G6PD, glucose-6-phosphate dehydrogenase; SLE, systematic lupus erythematosus.

Data extracted from *Physician's Desk Reference*, Oradell, NJ, Medical Economics Company, 1985.

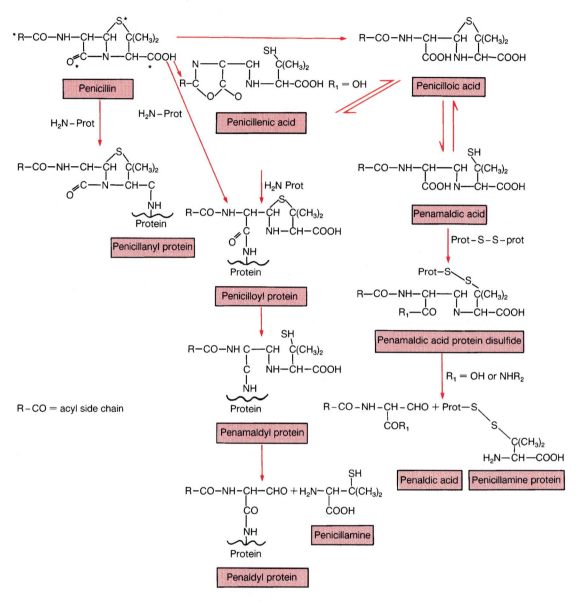

Figure 19–1. Reactive sites of the penicillin molecule and penicillin-derived antigens. Asterisks indicate the reactive sites of the parent penicillin compound. Major metabolic derivatives include penicilloyl (formed by reaction of the α-lactam carbonyl). Homopolymers may be formed by reaction of penicilloyl with aminopenicillin; aminopenicillins contain an amino group that can react with the β-lactam carbonyl of penicilloyl. The penamidyl and penadyl determinants are formed from penicilloyl and may bind to proteins but are of limited importance clinically. S-penamaldate conjugates are formed from penicilloic and penillaic acids, which are included in minor determinants in penicillin preparations. The use of ester prodrugs of penicillin allows the formation of penicilloyl derivatives. The penicilloyl determinant is considered to make the major contribution to penicillin allergy. Once sensitization has occurred to one haptenic form, cross-reactivity allows elicitation of an allergic reaction with other penicillin derivatives.

duced by conjugation of penicillin with host proteins as a result of an adjuvant induced granuloma or by penicilloylation of adjuvant components. However, high-molecular-weight contaminants or homopolymers are much more immunogenic than purified penicillin under any circumstances and are more likely to provide the immunogenic stimulus.

The route of application of penicillin is also important as a factor in sensitization. Intravascular and intramuscular exposure produces a low incidence of sensitization. However, topical application, particularly over an inflamed area, or nasal inhalation, is associated with a much higher incidence of sensitization. This may be due to an adjuvant effect of the inflammation or to formation of immunogenic conjugates by bacterial metabolism of penicillin or to action of inflammatory mediators.

The allergic manifestations of penicillin include each of the immunopathologic mechanisms. Neutralization is not usually recognized, as it is not usually discriminated from simple treatment failure, and granulomatous reactions are rare but can occur. The incidence of other reactions to penicillin are given in Table 19–5. Pseudoallergic reactions due to release of bacterial toxins as the result of lysis of bacteria after penicillin treatment or secondary to inflammatory mediators may be responsible for a large number of penicillin reactions. The Jarisch–Herxheimer phenomenon, in which fever, chills, skin rash, edema, lymphadenopathy, and headache appear during the treatment of syphilis, is most likely due to the release of microbial "toxins" or antigens and will subside as penicillin treatment is continued. This is not caused by an allergic reaction to penicillin but is due to the effects of release of microbial substances secondary to penicillin therapy.

One of the most striking reactions to penicillin is toxic epidermal necrosis (see Chapter 20). This reaction is characterized by erythema and detachment of skin resembling extensive scalding. It is an acute, life-threatening reaction. There is separation of the epidermis at the basal layer in the detached areas and necrosis and dyskeratosis of cells in the erythematous areas. Such patients demonstrate a positive delayed

TABLE 19–5. FREQUENCY OF ALLERGIC REACTIONS TO PENICILLIN

Mechanism	Percent of Penicillin Allergies
Hemolytic (lysis)	0.5
Immune complex (fever, vasculitis)	20
Anaphylactic (shock, urticaria)	10
Cellular (dermatitis, toxic epidermal necrosis)	0.5
Skin eruptions (exanthems, erythema multiforme, purpura)	69

skin test or lymphocyte transformation to penicillin or to other drugs (phenobarbital, phenylbutazone) associated with this lesion. This is believed to represent an intense delayed reaction to the responsible drug.

Cases of suspected penicillin sensitivity are best tested by skin testing. However, many patients that give a positive skin test to penicilloyl-lysine, the most frequently used test antigen, do not manifest a systemic reaction when injected under controlled conditions with large (over 1,600,000 units) doses of penicillin. In addition, a negative skin test does not always rule out a positive systemic reaction to a larger dose. Even when symptoms consistent with an allergic reaction are obvious, it may be difficult to identify by antibody or skin testing the presence of immune reactivity. Therefore, the results of skin testing must be interpreted with caution relative to an individual patient. If the test to penicilloyl-lysine is negative, reactions to other minor antigenic determinants must be tested using benzylpenicillin. In skin test reactive patients, approximately 70% will demonstrate a wheal and flare reaction, 20% an Arthus reaction, and 10% a delayed reaction. If antibiotic treatment is required, another drug should be given in order to avoid a possibly serious allergic response to penicillin. Third-generation cephalosporins appear to have only a slight risk of reactions in penicillin-allergic individuals, in contrast to earlier cephalosporins. However, in some instances, the nature of an infectious disease is such that no drug, other than penicillin, will be effective, yet the patient that requires treatment is allergic to penicillin.

If penicillin is considered essential, desensitization may be attempted. This is done by injecting small doses of penicillin (10 units) subcutaneously and gradually increasing the dose at twenty-minute intervals over a six-hour period to 400,000 units intramuscularly. Such patients usually tolerate this procedure, but care must be taken to treat anaphylactic shock. After desensitization, penicillin therapy may be continued for at least six weeks. The mechanism for desensitization is not clear. Desensitized patients become skin test negative but demonstrate no change in IgE or IgG antibodies to penicillin.

Allergic Reactions to Cancer Chemotherapeutic Agents

Although clearly less frequent than allergic reactions to antimicrobial agents, the increased use of chemicals to treat cancer has led to an increased recognition of reactions to the drugs used. The reactions to some of the more frequently used chemotherapeutic drugs are given in Table 19–6. In most instances, allergic reactions to most of these drugs are infrequent or very rare. The polypeptide L-asparaginase is the drug most likely to produce an allergic reaction, with a 1% mortality rate due to anaphylactic shock. A history of previous use, intravenous administration, and use without other drugs (prednisone, 6-mercapto-

TABLE 19–6. ALLERGIC REACTIONS TO CANCER CHEMOTHERAPEUTIC AGENTS

Drug	Type of Reaction	Risk
L-asparaginase	Anaphylactic, neutralization, immune complex, hemolytic (very rare)	Appreciable
Cisplatin	Anaphylactic, nonspecific release of vasoactive agents, hemolytic	Appreciable
Melphalan	Anaphylactic	Appreciable (IV), infrequent (oral)
Methotrexate	Anaphylactic, immune complex	Infrequent
Bleomycin	Pyrogen release from neutrophils	Infrequent
Cyclophosphamide	Anaphylactic	Infrequent
Cytosine arabinoside	Anaphylactic, immune complex	Very rare
Chlorambucil	Anaphylactic	Very rare
Hydroxyurea	Pyrogen release	Very rare
5-Fluorouracil	Anaphylactic	Very rare
Mitomycin	Anaphylactic	Very rare

Modified from Weiss RB: Hypersensitivity reactions to cancer chemotherapy. In *Toxicity of Chemotherapy*. Perry MC, Yarbro JW (eds.). New York, Grune & Stratton, 1984.

purine, and/or vincristine) are factors that increase the risk of allergic reactions to L-asparaginase. The presence of IgG antibodies to L-asparaginase reduces the effective level of the drug, protecting against an anaphylactic reaction but reducing its effectiveness through a neutralization reaction.

Some drugs produce anaphylactoid reactions due to effects on mast cells directly and not mediated through IgE antibody. Anaphylactic reactions due to IgE antibody, as well as anaphylactoid reactions due to direct release of vasoactive mediators from mast cells, have been found in 1% to 25% of cisplatin recipients, but no deaths from cisplatin allergy have been reported. Cisplatin may also be associated with neutralization and hemolytic reactions. Anthracyclin antibiotics (daunorubicin, doxorubicin, and aclarubicin) may produce severe anaphylactoid reactions on the first exposure, including shock or cardiac arrhythmias, due to direct action on mast cells.

Unsuspected Drug Reactions to Contaminants

Clinically, reactions often are not to a drug itself but to a contaminating substance in the drug preparation used. Certain vaccines produced in tissue culture may contain trace amounts of penicillin. Many other similar situations have been identified. For instance, in insulin allergy, the reaction may not be to insulin but to zinc in the insulin preparation.

Some patients develop reactions to insulin, manifested by delayed-type hypersensitivity (DTH) reactions at the injection site. Usually, these are self-limiting and resolve with continued insulin use. Cases of persistent reactions may be handled by changing to another insulin preparation. However, some patients have persistent reactions to different insulin preparations due not to insulin but to zinc present in different insulin preparations.

Autoimmune Reactions Induced By Drugs

A number of diseases caused by drugs are due to the induction of autoantibodies (Table 19–7). Prominent among the drugs responsible for autoimmunity are penicillin and gold salts. Syndromes resembling systemic lupus erythematosus (SLE) are induced by several drugs, including hydralazine, procainamide, isonicotinic acid, and penicillamine (see Chapter 22). The fully developed clinical picture includes arthritis resembling rheumatoid arthritis, fever, skin rashes, hepatomegaly, splenomegaly, and lymphadenopathy. The mechanism of drug-induced SLE is not clear. Antibodies to the drugs have not been shown to cause the syndrome. Antinuclear antibodies are found in many of these patients, suggesting that drug-induced alterations lead to sensitization to nuclear antigens. Since the syndrome goes away when the drug is withdrawn, it appears that drugs may alter nuclear components and that this process is irreversible.

TABLE 19–7. AUTOIMMUNE DISEASES INDUCED BY DRUGS

Inducing Drug	Disease
D-penicillamine, possibly gold salts	Myasthenia gravis
α-methyldopa, L-dopa, captopril, cefalexin, mefenamic acid, penicillins	Autoimmune hemolytic anemia
Aminopyrine, captopril, cefalexin, chloral hydrate, chlorpromazine, gold salts, mercurial diuretics, indomethacin, penicillins, sulfapyridine, thiouracils, tolazoline	Granulocytopenia
Gold salts, D-penicillamine	Immune-complex glomerulonephritis
D-penicillamine	Goodpasture's syndrome
D-penicillamine	Pemphigus
Gold salts, griseofulvin, hydralazine, phenytoin practolol, D-penicillamine, procainamide, thiouracil, others	Systemic lupus erythematosus
Halothane, tienilic acid	Chronic active hepatitis (virus)

Modified from Gleichmann E, Kimber I, Purchase IFH: Immunotoxicity: Suppressive and stimulatory effects of drugs and environmental chemicals on the immune system. *Arch Toxicol* 63:257, 1989.

TABLE 20–1. CYTOKINES PRODUCED BY HUMAN KERATINOCYTES IN VITRO

Interleukins	IL-1α, IL-Iβ, IL-6, IL-8
Colony-stimulating factors	IL-3, GM-CSF, G-CSF, M-CSF
Interferons	IFN-α, IFN-β
Tumor necrosis factor	TGF-α, F-β
Transforming growth factors	TGF-α, TGF-β
Growth factors	PDGF, FGF

Modified from Bos JD, Kapsenberg ML: The skin immune system: Progress in cutaneous biology. *Immunol Today* 14:75, 1993.

T cells in the skin express phenotypes of activated or memory-T cells, thus the skin contains T cells that appear to be highly trained and ready for action (frontline troops). The presence of E-selectin (ELAM-1) on the dermal endothelial cells may act as an adhesion molecule for skin homing of memory-T cells. In many infectious and immune diseases, one of the features is perivascular cuffing of inflammatory cells in the skin.

FUNCTIONS OF THE SIS

The effector function of the SIS is realized by a combination of signals from keratinocytes that prepare the dermal perivascular units for specific and nonspecific responses to injury. Langerhans' cells and dermal dendritic cells are well situated to contact and process antigens that enter through the skin. The perivascular unit provides chemoattractive and adhesion molecules that signal inflammatory cells to enter the skin. Dermal T cells are situated to provide a rapid response to recall antigens and initiate cell-mediated immunity. Dermal macrophages are activated to phagocytose and clear away products of inflammation, as well as provide proliferation signals to dermal fibroblasts and endothelial cells for repair. It is not surprising that the skin is the site of immune reactions representing all of the major immunopathologic mechanisms.

The skin is the largest organ of the body and the most common site for manifestations of immune reactions. Immune skin lesions may be classified by the different immunopathologic mechanisms, such as the cytotoxic destruction of epidermal cell contacts in pemphigus, immune complex-mediated vasculitis, the acute wheal and flare or hive reaction of cutaneous anaphylaxis, or delayed skin reactions and intraepithelial T_{CTL} effects of cell-mediated immunity. A listing of skin diseases is given in Table 20–2 and Figure 20–1.

Inactivation or Activation

There is no direct example of neutralization or inactivation as primarily responsible for a skin lesion. However, pretibial myxedema is a secondary manifestation of hyperthyroidism (Graves' disease) and

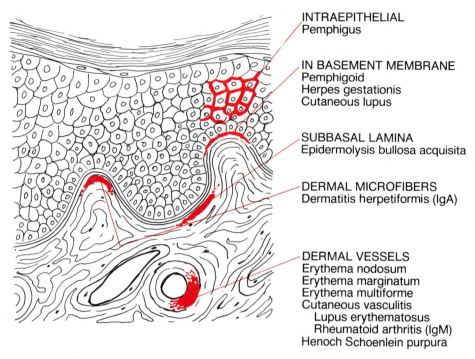

INTRAEPITHELIAL
Pemphigus

IN BASEMENT MEMBRANE
Pemphigoid
Herpes gestationis
Cutaneous lupus

SUBBASAL LAMINA
Epidermolysis bullosa acquisita

DERMAL MICROFIBERS
Dermatitis herpetiformis (IgA)

DERMAL VESSELS
Erythema nodosum
Erythema marginatum
Erythema multiforme
Cutaneous vasculitis
    Lupus erythematosus
    Rheumatoid arthritis (IgM)
Henoch Schoenlein purpura

Figure 20–1. Diagrammatic representation of lesion location and deposits of immunoglobulin, complement cell infiltrates in some skin diseases.

appears to be related to the level of long-acting thyroid stimulator (LATS), which is an autoantibody that stimulates thyroid hormone receptor. Pretibial myxedema is a nonpitting, brawny, plaquelike swelling of the pretibial area, ankles, or feet that has the appearance of orange skin and is seen in about 2% of patients with Graves' disease. The pathogenesis of pretibial myxedema is not known.

Cytotoxic or Cytolytic Reactions

Cytotoxic effects of antibodies to epithelial cell or basement membrane antigens produces separation and destruction of the cells. The basal layer of the epidermis, the basement membrane, and the subdermal connective tissue are connected by a complex of proteins (Fig. 20–2). Abnormalities or alterations of these connecting proteins produces spaces or bullae either in the epidermal layer or at the basement membrane. These diseases are caused by antibodies that react with the proteins that connect the basal cells to the basement membrane, maintain the integrity of the basement membrane or connect the basement membrane to the dermis, or by inherited deletions or abnormalities in these proteins (Table 20–3).

TABLE 20–2. IMMUNE MECHANISM IN SOME SKIN DISEASES

Disease	Lesion	Association	Immune Mechanism
Cytotoxic Lesions			
Pemphigus	Intraepithelial bullae	Autoallergic diseases	Autoantibody to epithelial cell surfaces
Pemphigoid	Subepidermal bullae	Neoplasm, autoallergy	Autoantibody to basement membrane
Dermatitis herpetiformis	Subepidermal bullae	Gluten enteropathy (sprue)	IgA and complement deposition in dermal microfibers and basement membrane (auto–antibody or immune complex)
Herpes gestationis	Subepidermal bullae	Pregnancy	Properdin, C3 and IgG in basement membrane (auto–antibody or immune complex)
Epidermolysis bullosa	Subepidermal bullae	Other autoimmune diseases	Autoantibody to basement membrane
Psoriasis	Corneum parakeratosis, acanthosis	Rheumatoid arthritis	Autoantibody to keratin
Cutaneous lupus	Basement membrane degeneration sub–cutaneous vasculitis	Systemic and discoid lupus	Autoantibody to BM or immune complex deposition
Vitiligo	Melanocytes, depigmentation	Autoallergic diseases	Antibody to melanocytes
Alopecia areata	Loss of hair	Endocrinopathy	Antibody to capillary of endothelium hair bulb
Vascular Lesions (immune complex)			
Erythema nodosum	Subcutaneous vasculitis	Infection, SLE	Immune complex
Erythema marginatum	Subcutaneous vasculitis	Rheumatic fever	Immune complex (π anaphylactic)
Erythema multiforme	Subcutaneous vasculitis	Drug reaction	Immune complex
Cutaneous vasculitis	Subcutaneous vasculitis	Infection	Immune complex
Anaphylactic Reactions			
Cutaneous anaphylaxis	Wheal-and-flare	Mosquito bite Allergic reaction	IgE-mediated mast cell Degranulation-histamine
Giant urticaria	Wheal	Allergy	IgE
Angioedema	Nonpitting edema	—	C1 inhibitor deficiency
Delayed Hypersensitivity Lesions			
Contact dermatitis	Vesiculation, induration, spongiosis	Poison ivy, poison oak	Delayed hypersensitivity
Viral exanthems	Vesiculation, induration, spongiosis	Measles, smallpox, etc.	Delayed hypersensitivity
Tuberculin test	Perivascular mononuclear cell infiltrate, induration	Tuberculosis	Delayed hypersensitivity
Syphilis (chancre)	Perivascular and diffuse mononuclear cell infiltrate	Syphilis	Delayed hypersensitivity
Granulomatous lesions			
Zirconium granulomas	Axillary granuloma	Stick deodorants	Granulomatous hypersensitivity
Tuberculoid leprosy	Cutaneous granulomas	Leprosy	Granulomatous hypersensitivity
Sarcoidosis	Granulomas	Sarcoid	Granulomatous hypersensitivity

Modified from Sell S: in Jordan, RE (ed.) Mechanisms of immune–mediated injury in the skin. *Immunologic Disease of the Skin.* Norwalk, Appleton & Lange, 1991, 87-100.

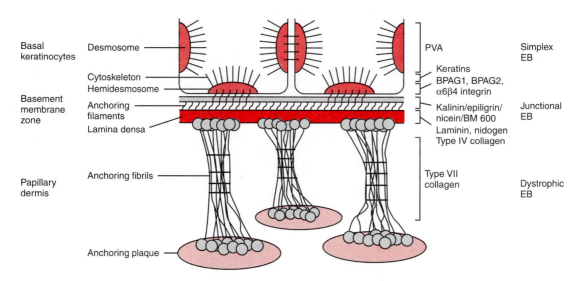

Figure 20–2. Schematic drawing of the connecting structures of the skin. Depicted are basal cells overlying the papillary dermis with the basement membrane separating them. Morphologic structures are shown on the left; the proteins making up these structures are shown on the right. Modified from Uitto J, Christiano AM: Molecular genetics of the cutaneous basement membrane zone: perspectives on epidermolysis bullosa and other blistering skin diseases. *J Clin Invest* 90:687-692, 1992.

TABLE 20–3. LEVEL OF LESIONS AND CONNECTING PROTEINS IN BLISTERING SKIN DISEASES

Disease	Tissue Level	Proteins
Antibody-mediated acquired diseases		
Pemphigus vulgaris	Intraepidermal, suprabasilar	Cadherin (PV antigen)
Pemphigus foliaceous	Intraepidermal, superficial	Desmoglein I (cadherin)
Bullous pemphigoid	Lamina lucida	BP Ag1 and/or BP Ag 2
Herpes gestationis	Lamina lucida	BP Ag 2
EB acquisita	Sub-lamina densa	Type VII collagen
Heritable diseases		
EB simplex	Basal keratinocytes	Keratins 5 and 14
EB junctional	Lamina lucida	Anchoring filament proteins
EB dystrophic	Sub-lamina densa	Type VII collagen
Epidermolytic hyperkeratosis	Intraepidermal, suprabasilar	Keratins 1 and 10

BP Ag1 is now designated type XVII collagen; BP Ag2 is a noncollagenous intracellular protein; also involved in attachment of basal cells to the basement membrane is epithelial cell specific integrin ($\alpha_6\beta_4$).

PEMPHIGUS AND PEMPHIGOID

Pemphigus and pemphigoid are skin lesions caused by denudation of the epidermis. In pemphigus, the epidermal cells separate above the basal layer, resulting in either formation of large fluid-filled spaces (pemphigus vulgaris) or stripping of the upper (horny and granular) layer of epidermis (pemphigus foliaceous). In pemphigoid, separation occurs between the basal layer of the epidermis and the dermis, leading to the formation of subepidermal bullae. Antibodies to cell surface or intraepithelial antigens, most likely to adhesion molecules in the stratified epithelium, are found in the sera of patients with pemphigus; in contrast, antibodies to the subepidermal basement membrane are found in patients with pemphigoid. Thus, pemphigus antibodies attack the epithelial cells in the stratified layers, leading to their separation from each other, cell death, and bullae formation, whereas pemphigoid antibodies attack the basement membrane, separating the epidermis from the dermis and producing subepidermal bullae. In bullous pemphigoid, there is also infiltration of neutrophils and eosinophils, indicating that complement-mediated inflammation is also involved in these lesions.

Evidence that antiepithelial autoantibodies cause the lesions includes the following facts: The patient's own immunoglobulin binds to his skin cells; both IgG and complement are demonstrable in the lesions, and the site of the lesion (either intraepithelial or subepithelial) is directly related to the site of Ig binding in pemphigus and pemphigoid. Although it has been suggested that antibodies in these lesions may activate epithelial proteases, most evidence indicates an antibody-mediated complement-dependent cytotoxicity mechanism. Lesions similar to those of the human may be induced by injection of pemphigus antibodies into monkey mucosa, and antiepidermal cell surface antibody from pemphigus patients detaches viable epidermal cells from tissue culture dishes. Several clinical courses are recognized, from rapidly fatal to relatively benign. Corticosteroid and immunosuppressive therapy have been highly efficacious in severe cases. Successful therapy not only reverses the skin lesions but also causes a reduction in the titer of autoantibodies. Pemphigoid lesions are frequently associated with other autoimmune diseases and antitissue antibodies.

DERMATITIS HERPETIFORMIS AND GLUTEN SENSITIVE ENTEROPATHY (SPRUE, CELIAC DISEASE)

Dermatit herpetiformis is a blistering skin lesion with papillary edema, microabscesses containing polymorphonuclear cells in dermal papillae, and subepidermal blisters. There may be intense burning and itching. Immunoglobulin A and complement are prominent in microfibers in the dermal papillae and some patients have a bandlike granular deposition of IgA and complement in the dermal papillae along the epidermal basement membrane. IgA activates complement by the alternate pathway, and C_3 is regularly found in areas of IgA deposition. Patients with celiac disease have a high incidence of IgA antibody to endomyosin. There are also IgA antibodies to gliadin and reticulin but at a lower incidence. Endomyosin is the intermyofibril substance of smooth muscle. Patients with dermatitis herpetiformis usually have sprue, a gluten-sensitive enteropathy (GSE) (ie, an inability to absorb nutrients from the gastrointestinal tract) and increased amounts of gastrointestinal IgA. Gluten is a gelatinous protein found in wheat and other grains. Elimination of gluten from the diet frequently results in reversal of the gastrointestinal lesions as well as the skin lesions. The IgA antibodies to gliadin and reticulin completely disappear on withdrawal of gluten from the diet, whereas antiendomyosin persists. These antibodies are all directed against the connective tissue of surface of smooth muscle cells. It is postulated that gluten protein activates production of IgA antibodies in the gut-associated lymphoid tissues (GALT). With villous atrophy of the gut because of GSE, more gluten is absorbed and more IgA antibodies are produced and released into the circulation. IgA antibodies may then circulate and deposit preferentially in the dermal microfibers in the skin because of its mucosal origin or genetically determined characteristics.

HERPES GESTATIONIS

Herpes gestationis is a rare, blistering skin disease associated with pregnancy and the postpartum period. The skin lesions are large subepidermal bullae. C_3 and properdin have been identified in the epidermal basement membrane, indicating that the alternate pathway of complement is activated. However, IgG may be identified by more sensitive techniques, and a more recent interpretation is that IgG antibody is involved but may not be identified by the usual immunofluorescent techniques. The antigen-binding specificity of the IgG deposited remains unknown.

EPIDER-MOLYSIS BULLOSA ACQUISITA

Epidermolysis bullosa acquisita is a rare skin disease characterized by blisters and extreme fragility of the skin due to subepidermal bullae similar in appearance to bullous pemphigoid. There are two major forms—hereditary and acquired. In the hereditary forms, separation may occur between the basal cells and the basement membrane (simplex form), within the basement membrane (junctional form), or below the basement membrane (dystrophic form). The hereditary forms of epidermolysis bullosa appear to be caused by genetic abnormalities in the proteins that join the basal keratinocytes to the basement membrane and the basement membrane to the dermis. For the acquired form, as in bullous pemphigoid, linear depositions of immunoglobulin and complement are seen along the dermal–epidermal junction. However, by immune-electron microscopy, these depositions are localized below the sub-basal lamina-anchoring fibril zone of the basement membrane, whereas in bullous pemphigoid, the deposits are localized within the lamina lucida. The autoantibody in this disease is directed to type VII procollagen (anchoring fibrils).

LUPUS ERYTHEMA-TOSUS

The skin lesions associated with lupus erythematosus (LE) are quite variable. The term "lupus" refers to the wolflike appearance of individuals with the full-blown facial rash. In chronic discoid lupus, there is extensive accumulation of keratin in hair follicles (keratotic plugging). The epidermis is atrophic and there is a patchy mononuclear cell infiltrate near the hair follicles. In systemic lupus erythematosus (SLE) the epidermis is atrophic, with dissolution of the basal layer (liquefaction degeneration). There is less inflammatory filtrate, usually limited to a perivascular cuffing, and less keratotic plugging than seen in discoid lupus. There may be small vacuoles within, above, and below the basement membrane, and marked thickening of the basement membrane occurs in chronic lesions. Immunoglobulin and complement are found in the walls of blood vessels and at the dermal–epidermal junction. The characteristic lesion is described as a band of immunoglobulin at the dermal–epidermal junction and may be seen prior to development of anti-nuclear antibodies. Granular depositions of immunoglobulin and/or complement may help predict those patients with glomerulonephritis, even in those patients where the skin is not involved clinically. It is likely that in lupus deposition of anti-nuclear antibody–antigen complexes occurs in epidermal basement membrane, as well as in renal glomerular basement membrane, but autoantibodies to basement membrane of the skin are also present.

VITILIGO

Vitiligo is seen as sharply delineated patches of depigmentation of the skin that occur in various sizes and shapes. Histologically, all that can be identified is an absence of melanin pigment, although melanocytes are present in normal numbers. The occurrence of vitiligo is associated with autoimmune diseases and a variety of autoantibodies. Autoantibodies to melanin are seen in some patients with vitiligo, and complement deposits have been found. Therefore, an autoimmune etiology of vitiligo is postulated. However, loss of melanocytes could be due to a metabolic defect in melanocytes, deficiency in an unidentified melanocyte growth factor, or lack of a melanocyte receptor.

ALOPECIA

Alopecia is a loss of hair in either circumscribed areas (alopecia areata) or in the entire body (alopecia totalis). There is a loosely arranged nonspecific inflammatory infiltrate around the lower third of the hair follicle. Later, the hair follicle becomes atrophic and the inflammatory infiltrate disappears. An association between alopecia and endocrine disease has been noted. An antibody that reacts with the capillary endothelium of the hair bulb has been reported to be eluted from lymphocytes in these patients, suggesting an antibody-dependent cell-mediated mechanism.

Immune Complex Reactions

Immune complex reactions are responsible for a variety of vascular reactions in the skin. Most lesions are secondary to deposition of immune complexes in dermal vessels.

ERYTHEMA NODOSUM

The lesions of erythema nodosum are painful red nodules that appear bilaterally on the shins. The lesions occur predominantly in women in the fall and winter months. Their appearance is usually associated with an infection, a reaction to a drug, or a granulomatous disease, such as sarcoidosis. In particular, erythema nodosum is associated with SLE and leprosy (erythema nodosum leprosum). The major pathologic finding is a subcutaneous vasculitis featuring a polymorphonuclear infiltrate of small veins or arterioles. It is generally believed that erythema nodosum is caused by an immune complex allergic reaction. The skin reactions usually fade and do not require treatment.

ERYTHEMA MARGINATUM

Erythema marginatum is an uncommon feature of rheumatic fever. Classic erythema marginatum is described as a bright pink, ringlike lesion that spreads irregularly through a pale skin. It is flat and is not pruritic or painful. The center fades as the peripheral pink edge spreads. The lesions change appearance quite rapidly (in hours or even minutes) and may fade and reappear within a few minutes. It is associated with cardiac involvement and may go on intermittently for months, even when all other signs of rheumatic fever are gone. The pathology is not well documented, although a nonspecific perivascular mononuclear infiltrate is sometimes seen. The lesions may be mediated by the vasomotor activity of anaphylatoxin, as well as by inflammatory cells. Erythema chronicum migrans, which resembles erythema marginatum, follows a tick bite introducing the *Borrelia* organism responsible for Lyme disease.

ERYTHEMA MULTIFORME

Erythema multiforme lesions may vary from a mild skin eruption consisting of erythematous or edematous flat plaques to widespread eruptions with bullous formation and extensive sloughing of the surface of the skin, involvement of the mucous membranes of internal organs, and rapid progression to death (Stevens–Johnson syndrome). The skin lesions consist of large circular macules or papules with a central blue depression and an elevated red periphery. The variety of types of lesions is reflected in the term erythema multiforme. Vesicles and bullae may occur and new crops of lesions may appear in the center fading plaques, resulting in a targetlike appearance. These eruptions usually resolve in a few weeks but a mortality rate of up to 20% occurs with the more severe form of the disease. Lesions begin in the dermal vessels with an extensive lymphocytic infiltrate; edema fluid accumulates, leading to formation of a cavity of fluid and inflammatory cells lying between the dermis and epidermis (subepidermal bullae). Necrosis of epidermal cells may occur in the absence of inflammatory cell infiltrate. The occurrence of the disease is associated with infections and the use of certain drugs. Evidence of an allergic reaction includes:

1. A latency period of 10 to 12 days between initial exposure to a drug and development of the disease.
2. The appearance of lesions in a few hours on second exposure to the drug.
3. Recurrence of the disease after subsequent exposure to the offending drug.
4. Changes in the small blood vessels consistent with the allergic vasculitis.
5. Positive skin tests with a suspected antigen that elicit the cutaneous lesion.

No circulating autoantibodies to epidermal or dermal antigens have been demonstrated, and Ig and complement are not present in the lesions. It is suspected that erythema multiforme is an immune complex reaction, but the mechanism of production of this disease is still unclear. Severe cases are benefitted by corticosteroid treatment.

CUTANEOUS VASCULITIS IN INFECTIOUS DISEASES

A variety of skin lesions may be associated with infections, such as viral hepatitis, infective endocarditis, infectious mononucleosis, and a number of bacterial infections, particularly streptococcal and pseudomonal. In some cases, immunoglobulin and complement have been identified in cutaneous vessels, and circulating immune complexes are present. Often, these patients have glomerular or pulmonary lesions as well.

Anaphylactic Reactions

Wheal and flare reactions and urticarial skin eruptions are common occurrences, not only on contact with allergens but also during the course of infectious diseases or drug treatment.

MASTOCYTOSIS

Mastocytosis is a mixed group of diseases in which there is a marked increase in the number of mast cells in tissues. Mastocytosis may occur as a localized lesion in the skin or as a systemic disease (Table 20–4). The initial report in 1889 of the typical lesions of mastocytosis

TABLE 20–4. CLASSIFICATION OF MASTOCYTOSIS

I. Indolent mastocytosis
   A. Skin only
      Urticaria pigmentosa
      Diffuse cutaneous mastocytosis
   B. Systemic
II. Mastocytosis associated with hematologic diseases
III. Mast cell leukemia
IV. Lymphadenopathic mastocytosis with eosinophilia

Modified from Metcalfe DD: Classification and diagnosis of mastocytosis. *J Invest Dermatol* 96:2S, 1991.

described the production of a wheal by stroking the skin over a localized skin lesion. Lesions may be solitary or disseminated, indolent or progressive, benign or malignant, depending on the location and progression of the disease, but all have tissue infiltration with mast cells as a result of disorders of mast cell and basophil proliferation. The preponderance of symptoms are due to the release of mast cell mediators and include flushing episodes, whealing, and anaphylaxis.

CUTANEOUS ANAPHYLAXIS

Cutaneous anaphylaxis (urticaria, wheal and flare, hives) is an IgE antibody–allergen activated mast cell-mediated skin reaction consisting of erythema; itching; a pale, soft, raised wheal; pseudopods; and a spreading flare, reaching a maximum in 15 to 20 minutes and fading in a few hours. The reaction is a vascular response to release of histamine or histamine-like substances into the skin with local changes in vascular permeability. A typical example of cutaneous anaphylaxis is a mosquito bite caused by histamine release from mast cells as a toxic reaction to mosquito saliva (see Chapter 14).

GIANT URTICARIA

Giant urticaria is manifested by the widespread development of firm, raised wheal-like lesions over large areas of the skin. They are superficial, erythematous, and intensely pruritic, with raised serpiginous edges and blanched centers. Individual lesions last about 48 hours, but new eruptions may appear for an indefinite period. Although allergic mechanisms may be operative, identification of an eliciting allergen is not possible in most instances, and nonimmunologic stimuli, such as heat, cold, or sunlight, frequently initiate urticarial lesions. However, in some instances, the lesions of cold urticaria can be transferred with serum factors—either IgM, suggesting the involvement of a cryoimmunoglobulin, or IgE, indicating that an IgE-mediated reaction can cause giant urticaria.

ANGIOEDEMA

Angioedema is a hereditary deficiency of C1-esterase inhibitor (C1-INH) that allows extensive edema and swelling upon activation of C1. The lesion may involve the eyelids, lips, tongue, and areas of the trunk. Involvement of the gastrointestinal tract may produce symptoms of acute abdominal distress, but the symptoms almost always disappear in a few days without surgical intervention. The most significant life-threatening complication is severe pharyngeal involvement, which may lead to asphyxia. The pathologic alteration is firm, nonpitting edema of the dermis and subcutaneous tissue, which can be differentiated from a wheal-and-flare reaction by the absence of erythema.

HYPOCOMPLE-MENTEMIC VASCULITIC URTICARIAL SYNDROME

A 7S protein that precipitates C1q (C1q-activating factor) is believed to activate complement and produce urticaria, leukoclastic vasculitis, arthritis, and neurologic abnormalities.

ATOPIC DERMATITIS (AD)

The diagnosis of AD is based on three findings: (1) A focal or generalized maculopapular pruritic skin rash on the flexural area of the extremities and the face and neck, (2) a chronic or chronic-relapsing course, and (3) a family history of asthma or eczema. Patients with AD have the following immune dysfunctions: Elevated serum IgE, positive wheal-and-flare skin tests to many antigens, reduced responsiveness to contact allergens, and lack of DTH reactivity to intradermally administered microbial antigens. The skin lesions are infiltrated by activated CD4+ Th_2 type IL-4–producing T cells, IgE-bearing dendritic reticular cells, and macrophages. One of the effects of IL-4 is to upregulate the $Fc\epsilon II$ receptor on mononuclear cells. Although the pathogenesis of these lesions remains unclear, it is thought that they may be caused by effector mononuclear cells bearing $FC\epsilon II$ receptors through IgE antibody binding and activation by antigens. A relative imbalance of Th_2 over Th_1 activity is believed to contribute.

Cell-Mediated Reactions

Skin reactions mediated by sensitized cells can be divided into those primarily due to T_{CTL} cells and those mediated by T_{DTH} cells. Contact dermatitis and viral exanthems will be presented as reactions mainly mediated by T_{CTL} cells, which cross into the epidermis and cause death of epithelial cells. The tuberculin skin test and the primary chancre are presented as examples of reactions initiated by T_{DTH} cells, which release lymphokines that attract and activate macrophages. Although these represent examples of the different effector arm of cell-mediated immunity, clearly both effector arms may be active in different degrees in other reactions.

T-CYTOTOXIC REACTIONS

Contact Dermatitis

Contact dermatitis, or contact allergy, is exemplified by the common allergic reaction to poison ivy. The characteristic skin reaction is elicited in sensitized individuals by exposing the skin to the oleoresins of poison ivy or poison oak. The reaction is a sharply delineated, superficial skin inflammation, beginning as early as 24 hours after exposure and reaching a maximum at 48 to 96 hours. It is characterized by redness, induration, and vesiculation, caused by the invasion of T_{CTL} cells into the epidermis, where they react with antigen on epidermal cells and kill them. In active lesions, keratinocytes have a marked increased expression of ICAM-1 associated with LFA-1–positive lymphocytes in the epidermis.

Viral Exanthems

The early (first 8 days) papular vesicular lesion of cutaneous viral infections (ie, measles) is most likely caused by the growth of the virus, and the later (8 to 14 days) inflammatory reaction (rash) is caused by T_{CTL} invasion and destruction of virus-infected epidermal cells. Similar lesions appear at the same time on different parts of the body, even though the different areas are inoculated with the virus at different times. See Chapter 15 for more details.

Delayed Hypersensitivity Reactions

TUBERCULIN TEST

The classic delayed-type tuberculin skin reaction is elicited in sensitive individuals by intradermal injection of tuberculoprotein antigens (PPD, OT). Redness and swelling occur 24 hours after injection. Because the reaction requires prior sensitization and occurs much later after testing than cutaneous anaphylaxis or the Arthus reaction, it is called a delayed hypersensitivity reaction. Specifically sensitized T_{DTH} cells react with the antigen in the tissue and release lymphokines that attract and activate macrophages, and the activated macrophages phagocytose and digest the antigen (see Chapter 16).

SYPHILIS

The chancre, the primary lesion of syphilis, is a delayed hypersensitivity reaction to organisms in the skin. It lasts from 1 to 5 weeks, is initiated by sensitized T_{DTH} cells reacting with antigen, and is resolved by phagocytosis and digestion of organisms by macrophages. Infection with *Treponema pallidum* occurs by inoculation through abraded skin.

The skin and mucous membrane lesions of secondary syphilis, which appear 2 weeks to 6 months after primary infection, appear to be mixed delayed hypersensitivity and antibody-mediated immune complex reactions at sites of dissemination and replication of *T. pallidum*. The cellular reaction is similar to that of primary lesions. Many systemic effects of secondary syphilis may be the result of immune complexes or cytokine release.

PSORIASIS

Psoriasis is a chronic, brownish, scaly, sharply demarcated skin lesion associated with arthritis. Psoriasis is characterized by an abnormality in keratinization, with elongation of dermal papillae, epidermal proliferation, parakeratosis (imperfect keratinization), and intraepithelial collections of polymorphonuclear leukocytes. The pathogenesis is believed to be caused by an exaggerated cytokine response to injury (Table 20–5). There is immunoglobulin deposition in the epidermal layer, which has a characteristic intracellular and diffuse staining pattern in the stratum corneum. A pathogenic role of stratum corneum antibody is implied but not established in psoriasis. Many normal individuals apparently have such autoantibodies, and the antibody may be able to gain access to the stratum corneum only because of an as yet undefined abnormality in psoriatic individuals. Multiple human lymphocyte antigens (HLAs), particularly HLA-CW6, have been associated with psoriasis.

TOXIC EPIDERMAL NECROLYSIS

Toxic epidermal necrolysis (TEN) is a drug-induced, acute, life-threatening reaction in which there is extensive shedding of the skin. In some cases, DTH skin reactions to the suspected drug have been found. CD8+ T cells have been reported to be the predominant cell type in the necrotic lesions; CD4+ cells are found in the underlying dermis. It is postulated that TEN is caused by T_{CTL} cell destruction to drug or metabolites of drugs localized in the skin. The lesions of TEN have many features in common with the skin lesions of graft-versus-host reaction.

TABLE 20–5. POSTULATED PATHOGENIC STEPS IN PSORIASIS

1. Inflammation stimulates release of IL-1, leukotriene, prostaglandin, histamine.
2. Dermal dendritic cells respond to these mediators by production of TNF-α.
3. TNF-α stimulates epidermal endothelial cells to express adhesion molecules (ICAM, VCAM and ELAM).
4. TNF-α stimulates keratinocytes to release IL-8.
5. IL-8 attracts T cells, which pass through activated endothelial cells.
6. T cells infiltrate the epidermis and release INF-γ.
7. INF-γ activates keratinocytes to release monocyte chemotactic and activating factors.
8. Activated monocytes accumulate and release more TNF-α.
9. TNF-α increases ICAM expression on keratinocytes, which allows T cells to bind and produce TGF-α.
10. TGF-α and IL-8 stimulate keratinocyte proliferation and angiogenesis typical of psoriasis.

Granulomatous Reactions

Granulomatous lesions in the skin result from the accumulation of macrophages and reactive fibrosis to poorly degradable phagocytosed debris. The reactions may be initiated by antibody to T cells reacting with antigen or to foreign bodies that are not immunogenic. The characteristic lesion is a space-occupying mass of epithelioid macrophages with varying amounts of lymphocytic infiltration and fibrosis.

GUMMA

The destructive lesions characteristic of tertiary syphilis are granulomatous reaction (gummas), which occur in areas where spirochetes apparently persist during latency (eg, brain, skin, bone, or viscera).

ZIRCONIUM GRANULOMAS

Stick deodorants containing zirconium salts may induce axillary granulomas in apparently sensitized individuals. Lesions no longer occurred when the use of zirconium was discontinued.

LEPROSY

The clinical features of leprosy were presented in detail in Chapter 17. At one pole of the leprosy spectrum, there are prominent granulomatous lesions with epithelioid cells and many lymphocytes, and few, if any, *Mycobacterium lepra* organisms in the tissues (tuberculoid leprosy). At the other pole of the clinical spectrum, there is massive infiltration of tissues with large, foamy macrophages filled with numerous mycobacteria with few lymphocytes and limited fibrosis (lepromatous leprosy).

SARCOIDOSIS

Boeck's sarcoidosis is a systemic granulomatous process prominently involving the lymph nodes, lungs, eyes, and skin, with lesions that may be indistinguishable from those of tuberculosis, fungus infections, or other granulomatous hypersensitivity reactions. A cutaneous granulomatous reaction may be elicited 3 to 4 weeks after the subcutaneous injection of crude extracts of sarcoid lymph nodes in patients with sarcoidosis (Kveim reaction). The specificity of this reaction and its use as a diagnostic test are questionable.

Disorders of Coagulation

A common manifestation of lesions of small vessels in the skin is purpura. Purpura refers to purple lesions caused by extravasation of blood. Purpura is caused by inflammatory lesions of blood vessels, such as "palpable purpura" found in association with immune complex vasculitis in the skin (see Chapter 13) or by thrombosis of dermal vessels. **Purpura fulminans** is a sudden onset of massive bleeding into the skin, followed by necrosis, and is often fatal. The bleeding is secondary to necrosis of endothelial cells. The lesion is initiated by the development of microvascular thrombosis, such as is associated with disseminated intravascular coagulation, particularly with endotoxin. Cytokines, such as IL-1 and TNF, are released by inflammatory cells exposed to endotoxin, and attraction of granulocytes followed by release of lysosomal enzymes further contributes to the necrotic reaction. This may be considered an extensive cutaneous Shwartzman reaction.

Summary

Immune-mediated cutaneous lesions are illustrative examples of diseases caused by different immunopathologic mechanisms. Cytotoxic reactions produce blistering diseases; immune complex reactions, vascular lesions; anaphylactic reactions, whealing lesions; cell-mediated reactions, chronic infiltrative diseases; and granulomatous reactions, destructive mass lesions of the skin. In addition, many other disease processes, such as disorders of coagulation, are manifested in the skin. Thus, the skin is a "window" through which immunopathologic processes may be viewed.

Bibliography

GENERAL

Jordon, RE: *Immunologic Diseases of the Skin.* Norwalk, CT, Appleton & Lange, 1991.
Stone J: *Dermatologic Immunology and Allergy.* St. Louis, CV Mosby, 1985.

SKIN IMMUNE SYSTEM (SIS)

Bergstresser PR: Immunology and skin disorders. *Drug Develop Res* 13:107, 1988.
Bos JD, Kapsenberg ML: The skin immune system: Progress in cutaneous biology. *Immunol Today* 14:74, 1993.
Cumberbatch M, Kimber I: Dermal TNF-α induces dendritic cell migration to draining lymph nodes, and possibly provides one stimulus for Langerhans' cell migration. *Immunol* 75:257, 1992.
Steinman RM: The dendritic cell system and its role in immunogenicity. *Annu Rev Immunol* 9:271, 1991.
Streilein JW: *Skin Immune System.* Boca Raton, FL, CRC Press, 1990.
Walsh LJ, Lavker RM, Murphy GF: Determinants of immune cell trafficking in the skin. *Lab Invest* 63:592, 1990.

NEUTRALI-ZATION

Hamberger J: The various presentations of thyroiditis: Diagnostic considerations. *Ann Int Med* 104:219, 1986.

CYTOTOXIC REACTIONS

Anhalt GJ, SooChan K, Stanley JR, et al.: Paraneoplastic pemphigus: An autoimmune mucocutaneous disease associated with neoplasia. *N Engl J Med* 323:1729, 1990.
Beutner EH, Jordon RE, Shorzelski TP: The immunopathology of pemphigus and bullous pemphigoid. *J Invest Dermatol* 51:63, 1968.
Bödvarsson S, Jónsdóttir I. Freysdóttir J, et al.: Dermatitis herpetiformis: An autoimmune disease due to cross-reaction between dietary glutenin and dermal elastin? *Scand J Immunol* 38:546–550, 1993.
Bor S, Feiwel M, Chanarin I: Vitiligo and its aetiological relationship to organ specific autoimmune disease. *Br J Dermatol* 81:83, 1969.
Chorezelski TP, Von Weiss JF, Lever WF: Clinical significance of autoantibodies in pemphigus. *Arch Dermatol* 93:570, 1966.
Clark WH, Reed RJ, Mihm MC: Lupus erythematosus: Histopathology of cutaneous lesions. *Hum Pathol* 4:157, 1975.

Cochran REI, Thompson J, MacSween RNM: An autoantibody profile in alopecia totalis and diffuse alopecia. *Br J Dermatol* 95:61, 1976.

Diaz LA, Calvauico NJ, Tomasi TB Jr, et al.: Bullous pemphigoid antigen: Isolation from normal human skin. *J Immunol* 118:455, 1977.

Farb RM, Dykes R, Lazarus GS: Anti-epidermal cell surface pemphigus antibody detaches viable epidermal cells from culture plates by activation of proteins. *Proc Natl Acad Sci USA* 75:459, 1978.

Flowers FP, Sherertz EF: Immunologic disorders of the skin and mucous membranes. *Med Clinics N Am* 69:657, 1985.

Hall RP: Dermatitis herpetiformis. *J Invest Dermatol* 99:873, 1992.

Hertz KC, Gazze LA, Kirkpatrick CH, et al.: Autoimmune vitiligo: Detection of antibodies to melanin-producing cells. *N Engl J Med* 297:634, 1977.

Holubar K, Konrad K, Stingl G: Detection by immunoelectron microscopy of immunoglobulin G deposits in skin of patients with herpes gestationis. *Br J Dermatol* 96:569, 1977.

Jordon RE, Heine KG, Tappeiner G, et al.: The immunopathology of herpes gestationis: Immunofluorescence studies and characterization of "HG factor". *J Clin Invest* 57:1426, 1976.

Karpati S, Amagai M, Prussick R, et al.: Pemphigus vulgaris antigen, a desmoglein type of cadherin, is localized within keratinocyte desmosomes. *J Cell Biol* 122:409–415, 1993.

Korman NJ, Eyre RW, Klaus-Kovtun V, et al.: Demonstration of an adhering-junction molecule (plakoglobulin) in the autoantigens of pemphigus foliaceus and pemphigus vulgaris. *N Engl J Med* 321:631, 1989.

Krogh HK, Tonder O: Immunoglobulins and antiimmunoglobulin factors in psoriatic lesions. *Clin Exp Immunol* 10:623, 1972.

Katz SI, Strober W: The pathogenesis of dermatitis herpetiformis. *J Invest Dermatol* 70:63, 1978.

Langhof HV, Feverstein M, Schabinski G: Antimelanin antibody in vitiligo. *Hautarzt* 5:209, 1965.

Lever WF: Pemphigus. *Medicine* 32:1, 1953.

Norris DA, Kissinger RM, Noughtom GM, et al.: Evidence for immunologic mechanisms in human vitiligo: Patients' sera induce damage to human melanocytes in vitro by complement-mediated damage and antibody-dependent cellular cytotoxicity. *J Invest Dermatol* 90:783, 1988.

Ortonne J-P, Bose SK: Vitiligo: Where do we stand? *Pigment Cell Res* 6:61–72, 1993.

Pedro SD, Dahl MV: Direct immunofluorescence of bullous systemic lupus erythematosus. *Arch Dermatol* 107:118, 1973.

Provost TT, Tomasi TB Jr: Evidence for the activation of complement via the alternate pathway in skin diseases. II. Dermatitis herpetiformis. *Clin Immunol Immunopathol* 3:178, 1974.

Schultz JR: Pemphigus acantholysis: A unique immunologic injury. *J Invest Derm* 74:359, 1980.

Stanley JR: Pemphigus and pemphigoid as paradigms of organ-specific, autoantibody-mediated diseases. *J Clin Invest* 83:1443, 1989.

Uitto J, Christiano AM: Molecular genetics of the cutaneous basement membrane zone: Perspectives on epidermyolysis bullosa and other blistering skin diseases. *J Clin Invest* 90:687, 1992.

Volta U, Molinare N, Fusconi M, et al.: IgA antiendomysial antibody test: A step forward in celiac disease screening. *Dig Dis Sciences* 36:752, 1991.

Woolfson H, Finn OA, Mackie RM, et al.: Serum antitumor antibodies and autoantibodies in vitiligo. *Br J Dermatol* 92:395, 1975.

Yaoita H, Briggaman RA, Lawley TJ, et al.: Epidermolysis bullosa acquisita: Ultrastructural and immunological studies. *J Invest Dermatol* 76:288, 1981.

IMMUNE COMPLEX REACTIONS

Bedi TR, Pinkus H: Histopathologic spectrum of erythema multiforme. *Br J Dermatol* 95:243, 1976.

Claxton RC: Review of 31 cases of Stevens–Johnson syndrome. *Med J Aust* 50:963, 1963.

Fletcher MWC, Harris RC: Erythema exudativum multiforme (Mebra)–bullous type. *J Pediatr* 27:465, 1945.

Hall RP: Dermatitis herpetiformis. *J Invest Dermatol* 99:873–881, 1992.

Shelley WB: Herpes simplex virus as a cause of erythema multiforme. *JAMA* 201:153, 1967.

Starr JC, Brasher CW: Erythema marginatum preceding hereditary angioedema. *J Allergy Clin Immunol* 53:352, 1974.

Tan EM, Kunkel HG: An immunofluorescent study of the skin lesions in systemic lupus erythematosus. *Arthr Rheum* 9:37, 1966.

Thomas BA: The so-called Stevens–Johnson Syndrome. *Br J Med* 1:1393, 1950.

Weiss TD, Tsai CG, Baldassare AR, et al.: Skin lesions in viral hepatitis: Histologic and immunofluorescent findings. *Am J Med* 64:269, 1978.

ANAPHYLACTIC REACTIONS

Frank MM, Gerland JA, Atkinson JP: Hereditary angioedema: The clinical syndrome and its management. *Ann Int Med* 84:580, 1976.

King TP: Insect venom allergens. In Molecular approaches to the study of allergens. *Monogr Allergy.* Baldo BA (ed.). 28:84–100, Basel, Karger, 1990.

Metcalf DD: Classification and diagnosis of mastocytosis: Current status. *J Invest Dermatol* 96:2S, 1991.

Sagher F, Even-Paz Z: Mastocytosis and the mast cell. Chicago, Year Book, 1967.

Sheffer AL, Austen KF, Gigli I: Urticaria and angioedema. *Postgrad Med* 54:81, 1973.

Zeiss CR, Burch FX, Marder RJ, et al.: A hypocomplementemic vasculitic urticarial syndrome. *Am J Med* 60:867, 1980.

Takigawa M, Skakmoto T, Nakayama F, et al.: The pathophysiology of atopic dermatitis. *Acta Derm Venereol* 176(suppl.):58–61, 1992.

CELL-MEDIATED REACTIONS

Arnason BG, Waksman BH: Tuberculin sensitivity: Immunologic considerations. *Adv Tuberc Res* 13:1, 1964.

Chase MC. Developments in delayed type hypersensitivity, 1950–1975. *J Invest Dermatol* 67:136, 1976.

Miyauchi H, Hosokawa H, Akaeda T, et al.: T-cell subsets in drug-induced toxic epidermal necrolysis: Possible pathogenic mechanism induced by CD8+ T cells. *Arch Dermatol* 127:851, 1991.

Murphy GF, Guillen FJ, Flynn TC: Cytotoxic T lymphocytes and phenotypically abnormal epithelial dendritic cells in fixed cutaneous eruptions. *Human Pathol* 16:1264, 1985.

Nicholoff B, Karabin G, Barker J, et al.: Cellular localization of IL-8 and its inducer, TNF-α in psoriasis. *Am J Pathol* 138:129, 1991.

Polak L: Immunological aspects of contact sensitivity. *Monogr Allergy* 15:1, 1979.

Saurat JH: Cutaneous manifestation of graft-versus-host disease. *Int J Dermatol* 20:249, 1981.

Sell S, Norris SJ: The biology, pathology and immunology of syphilis. *Int Rev Exp Pathol* 24:203, 1983.

Schlaak JF, Buslav M, Jochum W, et al.: T cells involved in Pemphigus vulgaris belong to the Th1 subset. *J Invest Dermatol* 102:145–149, 1994.

Sontheimer RD, Gilliam JN: Immunologically mediated epidermal cell injury. *Springer Semin Immunopathol* 4:1, 1981.

Turk JL: *Delayed Hypersensitivity*, 2nd ed. Amsterdam, Elsevier–North Holland, 1975.

Wong RL, Winslow CM, Cooper KD: The mechanisms of action of cyclosporin A in the treatment of psoriasis. *Immunol Today* 14:69, 1993.

Willis CM, Stephens CJM, Wilkinson JD: Selective expression of immune-associated surface antigens by keratinocytes in irritant contact dermatitis. *J Invest Dermatol* 96:505, 1991.

GRANULOMAS

Epstein WL: Granulomatous inflammation in the skin. In *Pathology of Granulomas.* Ioachim HL (ed.). New York, Raven, 1983, 21–59.

Shelley WB, Hyrley HJ: The allergic origin of zirconium deodorant granuloma. *Br J Dermatol* 70:75, 1958.

Travis WD, Balogh K, Abraham JD: Silicone granulomas. *Hum Pathol* 16:19, 1985.

Turk JL, Bryceson ADM: Immunological phenomena in leprosy and related diseases. *Adv Immunol* 13:209, 1971.

DISORDERS OF COAGULATION

Adcock DM, Brozna J, Marlar RA: Proposed classification and pathologic mechanisms of purpura fulminans and skin necrosis. *Semin Thromb Hemostasis* 16:333, 1990.

Henoch E: Ueber purpura fulminans. *Berl Klin Wochenschr* 24:8, 1887.

Spicer TE, Rau JM: Purpura fulminans. *Am J Med* 61:566, 1976.

21

Autoimmunity—Cell-mediated Autoimmune Diseases

Autoimmune diseases are caused by a damaging effect of an endogenous immune response to an endogenous antigen (self antigen). Normally, the immune system of our bodies is able to distinguish our own tissue antigens (self) from foreign tissue antigens (nonself) (Chapter 6). The essential mechanism of autoimmunity is the failure of the immune system to recognize its own tissues as self and to react to self as a foreign antigen. When the hypothetical results of an autoimmune attack to self were first considered by Paul Ehrlich at the turn of the century, he considered the outcome so disastrous that he introduced the term "horror autotoxicus" for such a possibility. Sir MacFarlane Burnett, in work for which he shared the Nobel Prize with Sir Peter Medawar in 1960, called the immune cells responsible for autoimmunity "forbidden clones." He postulated that these forbidden clones of reactive immune cells should normally be eliminated during development (neonatal tolerance). We now recognize that autoimmune responses are not unusual and in many individuals autoantibodies may be found without manifestations of an autoimmune disease. Some autoantibodies may be a normal part of the regulation of the immune system or take part in the turnover and catabolism of effete molecules. On the other hand, a large number of diseases caused by autoimmunity are now recognized. Myasthenia gravis, acquired hemolytic anemia, idiopathic thrombocytopenic purpura, experimental allergic glomerulonephritis, and lupus erythematosus are examples of autoimmune diseases caused by humoral autoantibodies. Juvenile diabetes mellitus and rheumatoid arthritis are diseases in which both humoral antibodies and cell-mediated immunity play a role. These diseases have been covered in earlier chapters or, in the case of rheumatoid arthritis and other rheumatologic diseases, will be covered in Chapter 22. Many other autoimmune diseases are the result of cell-mediated immunity, initiated by specifically reactive CD4+ T_{DTH} cells and/or CD8+ T_{CTL} cells. For instance, demyelinating diseases are caused by T_{DTH} activation of macrophages which phagocytose and destroy myelin (see Chapter 16); destruction of thyroid epithelial cells is due to invasion and interaction with T_{CTL} cells, which kill the thyroid follicle cells (see Chapter 15). In this chapter, the diseases caused by cell-mediated autoimmunity will be presented following a brief review of tolerance and autoimmunity.

Tolerance and Autoimmunity

Self tolerance is the specific lack of an immune response to self antigens that usually is established during embryonic development of the immune system. Autoimmunity results from a termination of natural tolerance to self. When there is a loss or a lack of tolerance to a self antigen, autoantibodies or cell mediated-immunity to self antigens results. We now know that during development of the immune system, immunologically competent cells to self antigens are produced, but these are eliminated or controlled by the mechanisms of tolerance. There are three major mechanisms for the induction of self tolerance: **Clonal deletion**, elimination of autoreactive cells; **clonal anergy**, nonresponsiveness of autoreactive cells; and **suppression**, functional inhibition of autoreactive cells. The first two mechanisms are caused by events related to antigen (tolerogen) recognition during development (**central tolerance**); other mechanisms, such as suppression, act after immune cells have achieved competence (**peripheral tolerance**). More is known about the induction of tolerance in T cells than in B cells. (See Chapter 6 for a more thorough discussion of thymic selection of the T-cell repertoire.)

T-CELL TOLERANCE AND AUTOIMMUNITY

Central Tolerance

The specificity of recognition of individual T cells is determined during their maturation in the thymus. Prothymocytes are produced in the bone marrow and do not express T-cell receptors (TCRs) until after they undergo maturational development in the thymus. The development of maturity in TCR+ thymocytes involves interactions with self major histocompatibility complex (MHC) molecules on thymic stromal cells (see Chapter 6). In the thymus immature thymocytes develop both CD4 and CD8 and are referred to as **double-positive thymocytes** (CD4+CD8+). Later, these give rise to **single-positive thymocytes** (either CD4+CD8− or CD4−CD8+), which leave the thymus and localize in thymus-dependent areas in the lymph nodes, spleen, and other lymphoid organs. When a cell that has matured in the thymus is able to function in the periphery, it is called a thymus-derived cell.

Peripheral Tolerance

Clonal anergy may be induced in peripheral lymphoid organs after development of T cells by a defect in T-cell signaling. Activation of T cells requires two signaling events, one through the antigen-specific receptor and one through the receptor for the costimulatory self MHC receptor. In the absence of the latter signal, the T cell not only does not make a complete response but enters a state of anergy in which it is incapable of being activated and does not produce interleukins or proliferate upon stimulation. If the T-cell antigen receptor of cells in a cloned T-cell line is occupied at the same time that interleukin-2 (IL-2) reacts with the IL-2 receptor, the cell is blocked from entering the cell cycle and becomes anergic.

Suppressor mechanisms could also cause peripheral unresponsiveness of T cells. Recently, it has been shown that CD8+ T_{CTL} may be induced that react specifically with peptides on the T-cell receptor. These "suppressor" or "regulatory" T cells may be able to control the production or reaction of CD4+ T_{DTH} with specific antigens. It has been suggested that immunization of animals with TCR containing the endogenous TCR peptide to induce specifically reactive regulatory T cells to the autoimmune effector T cells might be used to downregulate autoimmune reactions.

B-CELL TOLERANCE

The mechanisms of B-cell tolerance are understood less well than those of T-cell tolerance (see Chapter 4). Tolerance in B cells may reflect an absence of B-cell reactivity (deletion or anergy), failure of functional T-cell help, T cell-mediated suppression or control of specific antibody production by B cells. B-cell development and tolerance also takes place at the central or peripheral level. At the central level, a "preimmune" repertoire of B-cell clones is generated by variable diversity joining regions of immunoglobulin genes recombinations that occur in the developing bone marrow or liver B-cell populations. This gives rise to B-cell populations that produce low-affinity antibodies. At the peripheral level, contact of these preimmune B cells with specific antigen in the presence of helper T cells results in selective and reiterative clonal expansion of B cells that produce high affinity antibody through **somatic mutation**. Since most preimmune B-cell clones express "antibodies" with low affinity, it is unlikely that self-reactive B cells could be eliminated at this level unless the self-reactive antigens are present in very high levels. Clonal deletion may occur if preimmune low-affinity B cells encounter large amounts of antigen early in their development in the bone marrow or liver (high dose tolerance). Clonal anergy or functional inactivation may be induced in mature high-affinity peripheral B cells by contact with low amounts of antigen (low dose tolerance).

Functional lack of antibody production may occur to T-dependent antigens if there is a lack of T-cell help. It has been shown experimentally that T cells are more easily tolerized and remain tolerant for longer periods of time than B cells, so that the failure to produce a specific antibody response may not be due to inherent B-cell tolerance but to tolerance in T-helper cells. It is possible for T-helper cells reactive to an immunogenic epitope on an antigen molecule to deliver activation signals to B cells reactive to an epitope on the same molecule to which the T cell is tolerant. Finally, B cells may not respond because of T-suppressor activity or to idiotype network control. In any case, *self-reactive B cells appear to be a normal component of the immune system and can be stimulated by a number of ways to produce autoreactive antibodies*. It appears that most self antigens that are reactive to autoantibodies do not appear in the developing fetus until after the initial development of the immune system. The production of low levels of low affinity self-reactive antibodies may pose little risk for autoimmune disease. Low levels of self-reactive antitissue antibodies are present in most elderly individuals with no evidence of autoimmune disease. For example, low affinity anti-double–stranded DNA antibodies are not associated with lesions, whereas high-affinity anti-dsDNA is believed to be pathogenic for some forms of systemic lupus erythematosus (SLE). On the other hand, tolerance may be more easily induced in "high-affinity" B cells, perhaps through processing of antigen in the absence of helper T cells.

The CD5+ B Cell and Autoimmunity

The T cell-associated antigen CD5, found on all T cells, is expressed on activated B cells associated with autoantibody formation. CD5+ B cells are increased in patients with rheumatoid arthritis and SLE, as well as in autoimmune strains of mice and in normal mice following induction of autoantibodies. Increased numbers of CD5+ B cells are also found following bone marrow transplantation, and the cells making up chronic lymphocytic leukemia are surface Ig+ B cells expressing CD5. Once thought to be a separate subpopulation of B cells, there is now evidence that CD5 expression reflects activation of B cells in vivo, and that there is not a special subpopulation of B cells responsible for autoimmunity.

Breaking Tolerance and Induction of Autoimmunity

Experimental and clinical observations have led to identification of at least eight possible ways that natural unresponsiveness to self antigens may be abrogated, leading to autoimmunization. This is called **breaking tolerance**.

1. Altered self antigens. William Weigle has shown that in the normal adult animal, B cells may lose tolerance to self antigens while T cells are still tolerant, and that humoral autoimmune responses may be induced by bypassing specific T-helper cells. Altered self molecules may be recognized by T cells as foreign when complexed to foreign antigens. Drugs may act as haptens, binding to self molecules so that they are recognized by T cells. T cells reacting to the hapten/carrier are able to provide help to B cells, which recognize the self epitopes of the carrier component of the hapten–self protein molecule presented on the T cell. This mechanism is responsible for drug-induced autoimmune hemolytic anemias (see Chapter 12). Virus may also incorporate host proteins into their capsule (pseudotypes). Viral pseudotypes may serve as haptens in breaking tolerance to self antigens.

2. Polyclonal B-cell activation. Infections, adjuvants, and endotoxins (lipopolysaccharides) may cause release of interleukins that stimulate proliferation and differentiation of B cells, bypassing the need for specific T-cell help. This may nonspecifically activate production of autoantibodies by nontolerant B cells.

3. Release of sequestered antigens. Tissue damage from injury or infections may cause release of host molecules not usually presented to the immune system, or partial degradation of self molecules may expose epitopes not normally seen in the native molecule.

4. Loss of suppression. Suppressor or regulatory T cells may prevent T-cell help or suppress B-cell proliferation and differentiation. The severity of autoimmune disease in some experimental models may be greatly reduced by passive transfer of "suppressor" cells from syngeneic animals who have recovered from acute autoimmune diseases. Administration of anti-Ia, which induces suppression of delayed hypersensitivity reactions, can prevent induction of experimental autoimmune diseases by activation of suppressor cells. T-suppressor cells may prevent presentation of antigen, block the function of T-helper cells, inhibit proliferation of B cells, or block differentiation of B cells to plasma cells.

5. Molecular mimicry. Tolerance may be broken because of the sharing of epitopes between foreign immunogens and self molecules. Antigens of bacteria or viruses may have amino acid sequences or conformational structures that induce immune responses to self antigens. Digested peptide fragments of viral and other alien antigens are often homologous to host proteins after processing in antigen presenting cells. An example of molecular mimicry that will be presented in more detail in the next chapter is rheumatic fever (see Chapter 22). The causative agent, β-hemolytic streptococcus, shares several epitopes with human tissues, the most important being cardiac myosin.

Coxsackievirus and myosin also share a common epitope, as do hepatitis B virus and myelin basic protein.

6. Heat shock proteins. Heat shock proteins (hsp) are highly conserved peptides found on many different cells, both prokaryotic and eukaryotic. Heat shock proteins are major targets for cell-mediated immunity. $T_{\gamma\delta}$ cells preferentially react with hsp. In influenza virus infections, the $T_{\alpha\beta}$ cell that mediates the immune response to human influenza viruses induces high levels of hsp65 expression in activated macrophages, which in turn stimulates reactive $T_{\gamma\delta}$ cells. Cytokines from activated $T_{\gamma\delta}$ cells maintain macrophage activation and provides protection against secondary bacterial infections during the process of recovery from influenza. Although normally a protective mechanism, it has been postulated that reaction of $T_{\gamma\delta}$ cells with hsp from microorganisms and subsequent production and release of cytokines may be a critical step for development of rheumatoid arthritis and other cell-mediated autoimmune diseases.

7. Idiotypic network interactions. Autoantiidiotypic antibodies have been found in a number of experimental and human autoimmune diseases (see Chapter 11). Some antiidiotypes may also react with bacterial or viral antigens. The idiotope of an antiviral antibody may react with the cellular receptor for the virus. Patients with myasthenia gravis in remission may have an antiidiotypic antibody that reacts with anti-acetylcholine receptor antibody. Antiidiotypic antibodies have been found in patients with SLE, Sjögren's syndrome, rheumatoid arthritis, hyperthyroidism, multiple sclerosis, etc. Antiidiotypic antibodies may cause or ameliorate symptoms of autoimmune diseases (see Chapter 22 for autoantibodies in connective tissue diseases).

8. Control of somatic mutation. A defect in regulation of somatic mutation of B cells may lead to the production of high-affinity antibodies responsible for connective tissue diseases, such as SLE. High affinity anti-dsDNA is found in mice and humans with SLE, whereas low-affinity anti-dsDNA is found in many clinically normal individuals. This has raised the possibility that there may be some difference in the control of somatic mutation of B cells in SLE-susceptible individuals, resulting in the production of high-affinity antibodies.

Comparison of Experimental and Human Autoimmune Diseases

Autoimmune lesions are produced in experimental animals by immunizing an individual with constituents of its own tissues. Humoral antibody-induced disease is produced when the autoantibodies react with self antigens, neutralizing the function of the antigen (myasthenia gravis), causing lysis of cells (autoimmune hemolytic anemia), or producing immune complex mediated inflammation (see Lupus Erythematosus, Chapter 22). Cell-mediated autoimmune disease is caused by reaction of specifically self-reactive T_{CTL} or T_{DTH} cells with tissue antigen. When the hypersensitive state appears, inflammatory reactions occur where antigen is situated. Cell-mediated lesions have been produced by immunization with tissues, such as lens, uvea, central nervous system myelin, peripheral nervous system myelin, thyroid, adrenal, testes, and salivary gland. Antibody has been produced, but no lesions observed, with breast, pancreas, and other tissues. Cell-mediated lesions are irregularly distributed in regions of high antigen concentration (the white matter of the central nervous system in experimental allergic encephalomyelitis). Local inflammatory reactions occur around small veins and consist of lymphocytes, histiocytes, and other mononuclear cells. Necrosis, hemorrhage, and polymorphonuclear leukocyte infiltration occur only in very severe reactions and only in some species. Parenchymal destruction is coexistent with inflammation (ie, demyelination, destruction of uvea pigment). Byron Waksman has stressed that within the involved tissue, the lesion distribution is determined by blood–tissue barriers. There is a high correlation between the sites at which lesions appear and the passage of injection of large colloids, such as trypan blue, from the blood into the tissues. Thus, in the testes, the most severe (though, not the only) involvement is in the epididymis and the rete testes, both areas provided with numerous veins that permit passage of trypan blue.

Experimental cell-mediated autoimmune diseases are of great interest because they provide useful models for the human diseases of unknown etiology listed in Table 21–1. The human diseases in general are chronic relapsing processes, since the antigen is consistently present in the tissues and the hypersensitive state may persist or be boosted from time to time by further immunization. The acute monocyclic disease may result from allergic reactions to viruses or to combinations of bacterial products and tissues. The morphologic similarity of the acute infection-related human lesions to the experimental autoimmune lesions is evidence that the same hypersensitivity response is involved in the production of lesions in both instances, even though the antigens may be different.

Cell-mediated Autoimmune Diseases

ENCEPHALO-MYELITIS AND MULTIPLE SCLEROSIS

Experimental allergic encephalomyelitis (EAE) is manifested by demyelination as a result of the action of macrophages activated by specifically sensitized CD4+ T_{DTH} cells. Immunization with myelin basic protein (MBP) induces highly restricted T-cell receptor recognition of an immunodominant epitope on MBP. In animals that recover from EAE, specific regulatory T cells that recognize a single immunodominant TCR peptide can be identified. However, in progressive disease, additional epitopes and T-cell populations take part in the response. This is called **determinant spreading** and is believed to be an important factor in determining the course of the disease. The

TABLE 21–1. RELATION OF CELL-MEDIATED EXPERIMENTAL AUTOIMMUNE DISEASES TO HUMAN DISEASES

Experimental Disease	Tissue Involved	Histologically Similar Human Disease	
		Acute Monocyclic	Chronic Relapsing
Allergic encephalomyelitis	Myelin (CNS)	Postinfectious encephalomyelitis	Multiple sclerosis
Allergic neuritis	Myelin (PNS)	Guillain–Barré polyneuritis	
Phacoanaphylactic endophthalmitis	Lens		Phacoanaphylactic endophthalmitis
Allergic uveitis	Uvea	Postinfectious iridocyclitis	Sympathetic ophthalmia
Allergic orchitis	Germinal epithelium	Mumps orchitis	Nonendocrine chronic infertility
Allergic thyroiditis	Thyroglobulin	Mumps thyroiditis	Subacute and chronic thyroiditis
Allergic sialoadenitis	Glandular epithelium	Mumps parotitis	Sjögren's syndrome
Allergic adrenalitis	Cortical cells		Cytotoxic contraction of adrenal
Allergic gastritis	Gastric mucosa		Atrophic gastritis
Experimental allergic nephritis	Glomerular membrane	Acute glomerulonephritis	Chronic glomerulonephritis

CNS, central nervous system; PNS, peripheral nervous system.
Experimental Allergic Nephritis is caused by antibody to glomerular basement membrane.

Modified from Waksman BH: *Int Arch Allergy Appl Immunol* 14(suppl.), 1959.

prominent tissue lesion is perivascular infiltration of the white matter of the brain and spinal cord with lymphocytes. This is followed by migration of activated macrophages into tissue containing myelinated nerve fibers by lymphokines released from the T_{DTH} cells. The activated macrophages strip off, phagocytose, and digest myelin from the axons, resulting in loss of nerve function. Multiple sclerosis is considered to have a similar pathogenesis. See Chapter 16 for a detailed discussion of the role of DTH in these diseases. Destruction of neurons associated with an antibody to neuronal nuclei (anti-Hu) is a rare complication of neoplastic disease.

EYE

Anterior Chamber-associated Immune Deviation

The anterior chamber of the eye is a specialized zone in regard to determination of the type of immune response. Humoral antibody and T_{CTL} (cytotoxic) responses to intraocular antigens are active as defensive mechanisms against infectious agents, whereas T_{DTH} (delayed hypersensitivity) reactions cause immune damage to the eye. The immune integrity of the eye is maintained by the anterior chamber and is called anterior chamber-associated immune deviation. Delayed hypersensitivity reactions to foreign antigens in the eye, which enlist nonspecific host defense mechanisms of great intensity, destroy vision through "innocent bystander" disruption of the precise anatomic arrangements of the visual axis. The "overkill" of DTH may not result in permanent damage in other organs, but the eye is not able to resolve inflammatory reactions and restore vision because of destruction of the anatomic relationships. Intraocular immunization induces systemic stimulation of humoral antibody and T_{CTL} activity, but also appears to induce T-suppressor cells for T_{DTH}. This suppression of DTH upon intraocular immunization is extended systematically so that there is less effective defense against infections originating in the eye, such as herpes simplex, and to intraocular tumors, such as malignant melanomas. Antibody and T-cytotoxic activity appear to be adequate to maintain defense against most pathogens that enter the eye without compromising vision. However, this is a "dangerous compromise" as suppression of delayed hypersensitivity may be critical in allowing progression of some infections and cancers arising in the eye.

Phacoanaphylactic Endophthalmitis

The lens was probably the first tissue to which an autoimmune reaction was recognized in 1903. Experimental lesions have been produced by scratching the lens of rabbits previously sensitized to lens material. The cornea becomes vascularized and infiltrated with mononuclear cells. Because the lens is not vascularized, specifically sensitized cells cannot come into contact with the antigen (lens) unless there is some release of the antigen into the anterior chamber of the eye or other tissue spaces. This is why scratching the lens is necessary to induce the lesion. The disease is not related to circulating antibody, and no lesions are produced by washing the anterior chamber of the eye with large amounts of antibody. An infrequent complication of cataract extraction is an intraocular inflammatory (presumably autoimmune) reaction. In some cases, the inflammation may extend to involve the unoperated eye.

Uveitis

Uveitis is caused by autoreactivity of CD4+ T_{DTH} cells against uveal self antigens with destruction mediated by activated macrophages. Lesions similar to human disease can be produced in experimental animals by injection of uveal tissue in complete Freund's adjuvant (experimental allergic uveitis). Lesions are focal, involve mainly the uvea and retina, and include vasculitis, mononuclear cell infiltrate, and granuloma formation leading to retinal detachment. A human condition, known as **sympathetic ophthalmia**, is an inflammatory lesion of the uveal tract that appears 2 to 6 weeks after a perforating wound of the eye and affects both the injured and normal eye. Other forms of uveitis are associated with the collagen-vascular diseases. Pain, photophobia, and blurred vision result. The early lesions are focal inflammatory infiltrations of lymphocytes in the choroid, usually related to small veins. As early as 1910, it was proposed that this disease represented an allergic response to uveal antigens. If an individual loses sight in one eye because of injury, the eye is usually removed as soon as possible because the incidence of inflammation occurring in the remaining eye is directly related to the length of time the damaged eye is allowed to remain in situ. Two major autoantigens have been characterized, identified as retinal binding proteins: A 136,000 MW protein which has multiple pathogenic epitopes, including one that has been characterized to be an 8-amino-acids peptide (RTATAAEE) located at amino acid positions 521 to 540; and a 45-kDa protein with a 14-aa pathogenic peptide.

EAR

Autoimmune Inner Ear Disease

Experimental allergic labyrinthitis can be induced in guinea pigs by immunization with cochlear tissue in complete Freund's adjuvant. There are perivascular infiltration by round cells, edema, hemorrhage, spiral ganglion degeneration, and hearing loss. In humans, a chronically progressive bilateral sensorineural hearing loss that responds to immunosuppressive therapy is believed to be caused by an autoimmune reaction in the inner ear (McCabe's syndrome).

Cogan's Syndrome

Cogan's syndrome is a disease of young adults featuring acute interstitial keratitis (inflammation of the cornea) and disturbances of the ear (vastibuloauditory dysfunction) manifested by nausea, vomiting, ringing in the ear, and vertigo. This syndrome often occurs in association with collagen-vascular diseases. The onset of the syndrome has a clear association with a preceding upper respiratory infection. There is a prompt response to steroid therapy. The etiology of the lesions is not known, but it has been suggested that a local inflammatory reaction mediated by autoantibodies or antibodies to an infectious agent might be responsible.

ORCHITIS/ OOPHORITIS

Focal perivenous accumulations of lymphocytes and macrophages occur 8 to 14 days after sensitization of experimental animals with testes or spermatozoa in complete Freund's adjuvant. The inflammatory infiltrate is found primarily in the vascular areas of the testes (epididymis) and causes progressive damage of germinal cells, leading to aspermatogenesis. Complement-fixing, sperm-immobilizing, skin-sensitizing antibody may be demonstrated in the serum. The destruction of seminiferous tubules is associated with a mononuclear infiltrate, while spermatic ducts have a polymorphonuclear reaction with IgG and C_3 deposits present. Therefore, antibody and cell-mediated immunity are both active in this form of allergic aspermatogenesis. Experimental autoimmune orchitis has been transferred using CD4+ T cells. More recently, autoimmune orchitis has been induced in certain strains of mice by two or three subcutaneous injection of viable syngeneic testicular germ cells with use of any adjuvants or immunopotentiators. In this model, there is no epididymitis, despite a marked orchitis and hypospermatogenesis. The major inflammation is by CD4+ T cells, but there are also deposits of immunoglobulin on the basement membrane. Autoimmune oophoritis is a very rarely diagnosed condition in which there is intense T-lymphocytic infiltration around the developing ovarian follicles. Primordial follicles are spared, and the intensity of infiltration increases with follicular maturation.

Mumps orchitis is a human disease that occurs approximately 14 days after mumps parotitis. The histologic picture is very similar to that of the experimental disease. It has not been possible to demonstrate viruses in the testes of patients with mumps orchitis. Therefore, it appears likely that mumps orchitis may serve to release sequestered antigens or altered testicular proteins, leading to autoimmunization.

Thyroiditis

Autoimmune inflammation of the thyroid has been discussed in Chapter 15 as an example of T_{CTL}-mediated inflammation. Experimentally the disease is induced by immunization with thyroid antigens and features lymphocytic infiltration of the thyroid follicles. The "spontaneously" occurring human disease is known as Hashimoto's thyroiditis (see Chapter 15 for more details).

SIALOADENITIS (SJÖGREN'S SYNDROME) (SICCA COMPLEX)

Sialoadenitis is an inflammation of the salivary glands. Mononuclear inflammatory lesions have been reported in experimental animals following the injection of salivary gland tissue in complete Freund's adjuvant. However, the validity of these observations is questionable, and the autoimmune nature of such lesions is not well established. The human disorder, consisting of dryness of the eyes (keratoconjunctivitis sicca) and dryness of the mouth (xerostomia) may occur alone (primary Sjögren's syndrome) or be associated with connective tissue diseases (rheumatoid arthritis, systemic lupus erythematosus, or scleroderma) and is included in the list of collagen-vascular diseases. See Chapter 22 for more information.

ADRENALITIS AND MULTIPLE ENDOCRINE DEFICIENCY

Immunization of animals with adrenal tissue in complete Freund's adjuvant or lipopolysaccharide leads to mononuclear cell infiltration and necrosis of the adrenal cortex that can be transferred by spleen cells from immunized syngeneic animals. Most cases of adrenal insufficiency in man (Addison's disease) are secondary to endocrine, infectious, or neoplastic processes. However, a type of adrenal insufficiency, primary cytotoxic contraction, is of unknown origin and may be a correlate of experimental autoimmune adrenalitis. Complement-fixing antibody has been found in some patients with Addison's disease. Autoantibodies to endocrine glands are also associated with other endocrine gland deficiencies, including hypothyroidism, hypogonadism, and diabetes, as well as hypoadrenalism and lymphocytic hypophysitis. It is not clear in each case what role cell-mediated immunity and/or antibody inactivation has in these endocrine diseases. Sensitized autoimmune T cells may cause destruction of the glandular cells, and antibody may inactivate the hormonal product.

GASTRO-INTESTINAL TRACT— INFLAMMATORY BOWEL DISEASE (IBD)

Ulcerative Colitis and Crohn's Disease

Crohn's disease and ulcerative colitis are chronic destructive inflammatory diseases of unknown etiology involving the bowel—so-called inflammatory bowel disease (IBD). Ulcerative colitis primarily involves the colon; Crohn's disease may involve the colon, the small intestine, or both. The clinical characteristics of both are abdominal pain and diarrhea. In ulcerative colitis, there are superficial mucosal ulcers, vascular congestion, edema, hemorrhage, a mixed infiltration of polymorphonuclear leukocytes, activated T and B lymphocytes, plasma cells, and eosinophils. In Crohn's disease, the inflammatory infiltrate frequently contains granulomas and extends through all layers of the bowel wall rather than being confined to the mucosa and submucosa as in ulcerative colitis. The lesions of IBD have been described as similar to those of graft-versus-host lesions in the colon of experimental animals. Associated with IBD are hypergammaglobulinemia, a prevalence of atopic sensitivities, a prominent occurrence of other autoimmune diseases, antibodies to colonic tissue, and increased levels of some cytokines. However, the antibody is not cytotoxic in vitro, and "anticolon" antibodies are frequently found in individuals without IBD. In addition, the cytotoxic capacity of intestinal lymphocytes is less than that of peripheral blood lymphocytes, and there is no evidence that intestinal lymphocytes from IBD patients have increased killing for intestinal epithelial cells. Specific colon antigens to which an autoimmune response might be directed have not been identified, and etiologic agents for these diseases have not been convincingly demonstrated. Although there are higher rates for IBD in family members than in the general population, there is no clear correlation with human lymphocyte antigens (HLAs) except for the high association of HLA-B27 in patients with IBD and ankylosing spondylitis. It has been postulated that ulcerative colitis may be due to a failure to control normal cell turnover by withdrawal of kcl-2 or over expression of b53 leading to increased apoptosis of colonic epithelial cells. **Auer's colitis** is a hemorrhagic necrotic lesion of the colon, with a cellular infiltrate at the base of the crypts and perivascular polymorphonuclear leukocyte accumulation produced experimentally by the injection of antigen (egg albumin) into the colonic cavity of sensitized rabbits (Arthus reaction).

Autoimmune Gastritis

Autoimmune inflammation of the stomach is an infrequent lesion in humans, but when it occurs, it is often associated with other autoimmune diseases. This disease was first recognized by the identification of autoantibodies to intrinsic factor and gastric parietal cells in patients with pernicious anemia (see Chapter 12). There is a high association of gastritis with the parietal cell antibody. Autoimmune gastritis may be induced in experimental animals by immunization with crude gastric mucosal antigens. Gastric parietal cell and chief cell destruction is associated with marked mucosal lymphocytic infiltration, and cell transfer studies indicate that T cells are the primary mediators of the lesions. Infection with *Helicobacter pylori* is the major cause of chronic gastritis in humans, but this infection is not highly associated with autoimmune gastritis.

Intestinal Villous Atrophy

An extremely rare intractable diarrhea and membranous glomerulonephritis in children appears to be caused by an autoantibody to small intestinal mucosa and renal epithelial cells. There is a common 55-kDa antigen in small bowel and kidney with which the antibody reacts.

LIVER DISEASE (CHRONIC ACTIVE HEPATITIS)

Although direct evidence for the involvement of immune mechanisms in the initiation or progression of human liver diseases is controversial, considerable circumstantial evidence is available to implicate cell-mediated immunity in chronic active hepatitis, primary biliary cirrhosis, and some types of reactions to drugs causing jaundice and viral hepatitis (see above), as well as alcoholic liver disease. These presumptive findings include diffuse (polyclonal) hypergammaglobulinemias; tissue lesions containing lymphocytes and plasma cells consistent with a cell-mediated cytotoxic reaction; a depression of serum complement at some stages of the disease; a demonstration of immunoglobulin and complement in some early lesions; an association with other allergic diseases, such as lupus erythematosus, Sjögren's syndrome, and scleroderma (lupoid hepatitis); a beneficial response to drugs that cause depressed immune response; the presence of a variety of autoantibodies; and cloned CD4+ T-cell lines from patients with chronic active hepatitis that are activated by liver cell membranes antigens. Antibodies can be demonstrated by immunofluorescence to bind to the nuclei, ductular cells, and mitochondria of the liver and to smooth muscle cells. Of particular interest is the antimitochondrial antibody found in most patients with primary biliary cirrhosis. Despite its description almost 30 years ago, an etiologic or pathogenic role has not yet been demonstrated. More recently, antibodies to nuclear envelope proteins have been found in patients with autoimmune hepatitis (lamins A/B/C), hepatitis B with hepatitis C coinfection (lamin C only), or primary biliary cirrhosis (lamin B receptor or gp210). These antibodies give rimlike nuclear staining patterns by immunofluorescence. At this time, it is more likely that the autoantibodies found in patients with inflammatory liver disease are a result of the destruction and not a cause of the lesions.

Chronic active hepatitis may have at least four etiologies: Autoimmune, hepatitis virus-associated, cryptogenic, and drug-induced. A classic finding is the destruction of individual liver cells surrounded by mononuclear inflammatory cells ("piecemeal necrosis") at the edge of inflammation of portal areas. This lesion is most easily explained by the reaction of T_{CTL} cells with antigens on liver cells. An immune role for T_{CTL} cells in alcoholic cirrhosis has also been suggested. The lesions of congenital biliary cirrhosis, which occurs in very young infants, are similar to those seen in liver transplants that have been rejected. The primary lesion is a segmental and focal mononuclear inflammation of the bile ducts, with a predominance of CD8+ cytotoxic T cells. It has been suggested that congenital biliary cirrhosis may be caused by an "autoimmune" reaction to bile ducts or by a rejection of fetal bile ducts by maternally derived lymphocytes.

Halothane is an anesthetic agent that has some very desirable properties but produces liver disease similar to viral hepatitis. This reaction rarely, if ever, occurs upon the first exposure to halothane but is induced only on subsequent exposures, suggesting that a sensitization event occurs. The destructive lesions are associated with a mononuclear infiltrate similar to that seen in other delayed hypersensitivity reactions. It is possible that halothane acts like a hapten with affinity for a liver protein that leads to a contact dermatitis-like reaction in the liver.

Animal models for autoimmune liver disease (experimental allergic hepatitis) through the induction of liver injury by immunization with liver extract have not accurately reproduced the human disease, although mild inflammatory lesions may be observed in some immunized animals. In experimental autoimmune hepatitis in rats, induced by immunization with liver homogenates in complete Freund's adjuvant, there is a marked infiltration of the portal zone of the liver with CD8+ lymphocytes, and these cells are cytotoxic for liver cells in vitro.

HEART— IDIOPATHIC CARDIO- MYOPATHY

Autoimmune reaction to the heart is exemplified by antibody-mediated rheumatic heart disease (see Chapter 25) and the development of anti-heart antibodies associated with postinfarction syndrome, following cardiac surgery (postpericardiotomy syndrome), or with idiopathic cardiomyopathy. The presence of these heart-reactive antibodies reflects an ongoing chronic inflammatory response, and diffuse or perivascular mononuclear infiltrates may be seen in the heart muscle. Antibodies to heart muscle include sarcolemma/myolemma, and contractile elements and mitochondria. Autoreactive lymphocytes have been demonstrated in patients with cardiomyopathy and viral myocarditis. Antibodies to heart-specific epitopes of contractile proteins (myosin, actin, tropomyosin, and troponin), are particularly attractive candidates for functional myocardial disorders. In an experimental model of myocarditis induced by immunization with cardiac myosin, destruction of heart muscle is associated with infiltration of CD4+ T_{DTH} cells and macrophages, and production of IL-1 and tumor necrosis factor (TNF) promotes postinfectious autoimmune myocarditis after coxsackie infection of mice. However, a clear documentation of a significant pathogenic role for autoimmune mechanisms in human cardiomyopathies has not been achieved. Autoantibodies to cholesterol are present at varying levels in all normal human sera, and it has been proposed that these may actually inhibit development of atherosclerosis. Under normal circumstances, antibodies to lipids are harmless because the target lipid antigens are cryptic and not available for reaction with native molecules.

PERIODONTAL DISEASE

Periodontal disease is a chronic inflammatory and proliferative reaction of the gums surrounding the teeth that may be at least partially caused by delayed hypersensitivity reactions, ie, lymphokine-mediated inflammation and proliferation. The disease begins as a marginal inflammation of the tissue surrounding the teeth (gingivitis) with a predominant lymphocytic infiltrate. The supporting collagen fibers of the gingiva are destroyed and an extensive reactive proliferation of the epithelial cells occurs. Subepithelial inflammation may extend into the marrow of the bone of the jaw leading to bony resorption and eventual loss of teeth in the involved zones. The antigens responsible may be oral bacterial products, tissue breakdown products, or dietary material. Periodontal disease is a result of poor dental hygiene and the best preventive action is keeping the oral cavity clean. The lymphocytic infiltrate in periodontal disease may change from predominantly T cell to predominantly B cell as the form of the disease becomes more aggressive. The lesions of severe periodontal disease regress if the patient is treated with immunosuppressive therapy. This effect on periodontal disease has been noticed in patients with cancer or with a transplanted organ who have received immunosuppressive agents; gingival inflammation subsides while the patient is being treated.

ADJUVANT DISEASE

Following the injection of complete Freund's adjuvant alone into rats, lesions may be found in joint synovia, colon, and skin, which resemble human diseases of unknown but suspected immune origin. The joint lesions are similar to those of Reiter's syndrome and resemble, but are not identical to, those of rheumatoid arthritis. The lesion of rheumatoid arthritis is a villous or papillary thickening of synovial membrane and a vascular granulation tissue (pannus) that may erode the articular surface of the involved joint. The lesions of rheumatoid arthritis include both immune complex and cellular (delayed hypersensitivity) reaction components (see Chapter 22). In mouse models, epitopes on type II and type XI articular collagen have been shown to have arthritogenic capacity; immunization with type II collagen produces a set of pathogenic T cells that recognize a single 12-amino-acid epitope.

HEAT SHOCK PROTEINS AND AUTOIMMUNE DISEASE

Adjuvant Arthritis

One of the major antigens responsible for autoimmunity in adjuvant arthritis is heat shock protein 65 (hsp65), a member of the "chaperonin" family. Chaperonins are proteins that react with unfolded protein molecules in the body and by so doing prevent the hydrophobic regions from disrupting cell function. There is a strong epitope (aa 180-188) on mycobacterial heat shock protein, and T-cell clones that are stimulated by this epitope also react with cartilage proteoglycan. Preimmunization with the strong epitope peptide can actually suppress the later development of arthritis, indicating that this epitope may be both disease-inducing and disease-protective, depending on the type of T-cell response—T-effector or T-regulatory. There is no such cross-reactive epitope on human hsp65! The epitope on cartilage has not yet been characterized. Children with juvenile rheumatoid arthritis (RA) have T cells that recognize the cross-reactive epitope, but those of adult RA patients do not. Immunization of susceptible mice with hsp65 in Freund's incomplete adjuvant does not induce adjuvant arthritis, but this immunization can protect against the arthritis induced using complete Freund's adjuvant.

Insulin-dependent Diabetes Mellitus

T-cell reactivity to hsp65 has also been shown to be the mechanism of destruction of the beta cells of the pancreas in strains of mice with spontaneous insulin-dependent diabetes mellitus (IDDM). In addition, immunization of strains of mice that do not develop IDDM spontaneously with hsp65 in oil will induce the disease, and IDDM can be transferred using T-cell lines reactive to hsp65. The epitope is different from that found to be active in adjuvant arthritis. In the experimental IDDM model, it is possible to induce T-suppressor cells for expression of IDDM by immunization of young mice with irradiated inactivated anti-hsp65 T cells.

From the above observations, it is postulated that there are immunodominant epitopes on the hsp65 protein that cross-react with mycobacterial hsp65. Autoimmunity is induced directly to these epitopes by mycobacterial infections or autoimmunity is stimulated to noncross-reactive epitopes on host hsp65. In most individuals the autoimmunity is controlled by antiidiotype networks, but in others the normally benign process progresses to autoimmune disease.

Treatment of Autoimmune Diseases

In general, the treatment of cell-mediated autoimmune diseases has not been satisfactory. Drugs such as corticosteroids, alkylating agents (cyclophosphamide, etc.), and antimetabolites have had little effect. (See Chapter 28 for a systematic approach to immunosuppressive therapy.) Cyclosporine has had some beneficial effect in T cell-mediated diseases, such as psoriasis, uveitis, type 1 diabetes, and primary biliary cirrhosis, but has no clear effect on antibody-mediated diseases. FK506 has had a more pronounced effect on experimental T cell-mediated diseases, such as uveoretinitis, thyroiditis, type I diabetes, arthritis, etc., and clinical trials are now underway to determine effectiveness in human disease. Administration of cytokines that may modulate inflammation, such as TGF-β, and monoclonal antibodies to inflammatory cytokines, such as anti-TNF, have been partially successful in suppressing experimental autoimmune encephalomyelitis, but potential long-term complications must be addressed before these approaches could be tested in clinical trials.

Three recent experimental approaches are directed toward the T-cell receptor: Monoclonal antibodies to T-cell receptors, T-cell receptor vaccines, and blocking the costimulatory signal for T-cells. Antibodies to the T-cell receptor (Anti-TCR, anti-CD4, and anti-CD3) have shown some promise in experimental models and limited clinical trials, but positive effects are found in only about 25% of patients, and there are some serious side effects. In addition, it is difficult to control the dosage due to host immune response to the administered mouse monoclonal antibodies.

Vaccination using specific TCR peptides appears to be successful in inducing specific T-suppressor cells. In EAE, immunization with peptides derived from the TCR of encephalogenic T cells that react with myelin basic protein induces immune response to the TCR that modulate the activity of the effector T cells. Immunization against the TCR induces regulatory CD8+ T_S cells that react with the TCR on the autoreactive CD4+ encephalogenic T_{DTH} cells and suppresses their activity. Suppression in this model can be transferred using CD8+ cells that are cytotoxic for the CD4+ T_{DTH} encephalogenic cells.

Activation of T cells may be inhibited not only by blocking the reaction of antigen with TCR but also by blocking the costimulatory signal. Activation of antigen-reactive T cells requires two signals—one through the TCR binding to antigen on an antigen-presenting cell (APC), and the other a costimulatory signal, through binding of CD28 on the T cell to B7 on the APC. CTLA-4 is a T-cell surface antigen that also binds to B7 on the APC and has a higher affinity for binding to B7 than does CD28. Recently, this ligand has been linked to immunoglobulin to produce a new drug called CTLA4Ig, which binds to B7 on the APC but blocks binding of CD28, the T-cell receptor for B7. CTLA4Ig inhibits T-cell activation by blocking the costimulatory reaction of B7 with CD28. In experimental models of antibody production and xenogeneic pancreatic islet cell transplantation, CTLA4Ig has been shown to have powerful immunosuppressive effects.

Summary

Autoimmune diseases are caused by an immune reaction to an individual's own tissues. The primary cause is a loss of tolerance to one's own tissue antigens (see Chapter 6). Autoimmune lesions may be caused by each of the seven immune effector mechanisms or by mixtures of these mechanisms. Diseases caused by cell-mediated autoimmune responses are presented in this chapter. Those caused by antibody have been presented under each mechanism in earlier chapters or will be covered in the next chapter. Many autoimmune lesions involving solid tissue are mediated by cell-mediated immunity. These include postinfectious encephalomyelitis, multiple sclerosis, thyroiditis, and endocrinopathies, chronic active hepatitis, Sjögren's syndrome (salivary and lacrimal glands), chronic rheumatoid arthritis, and other diseases. These lesions are initiated by reaction of sensitized T cells (T_{CTL} or T_{DTH}) with antigen and often involve tissue destruction by immune-activated macrophages. Humoral immune reactions may play an important role in opening blood vessel barriers to allow sensitized T cells to enter tissues. The effect is destruction of solid organs related to infiltration with mononuclear cells, particularly around vessels (perivascular). Many of these diseases are self-limited. This may be because of eventual dampening of the autoimmune response by immune control mechanisms. Nonspecific immunosuppression has had little effect on the progression of these diseases. Recently developed experimental approaches directed to interfering with activation of T cells may hold promise for controlling cell-mediated autoimmune diseases.

Bibliography

TOLERANCE
AND
AUTOIMMUNITY

Blackman M, Kappler J, Marrack P: The role of the T-cell receptor in positive and negative selection of developing T cells. *Science* 248:1335, 1990.

Brostoff SW, Howell MD: T-cell receptors, immunoregulation, and autoimmunity. *Clin Immunol Immunopathol* 62:1–7, 1992.

Burnet FM: A reassessment of the forbidden clone hypothesis of autoimmune disease. *Aust J Exp Biol Med Sci* 50:1, 1972.

Coutinho A, Kazatchkine M (eds.): Autoimmunity: Physiology and disease. New York, Wiley–Liss, 1993, 474.

Diamond B, Katz JB, Paul E, et al.: The role of somatic mutation in the pathogenic anti-DNA response. *Annu Rev Immunol* 10:731, 1992.

Dighiero G, Lymberi P, Guilbert B, et al.: Natural autoantibodies constitute a substantial part of normal circulating immunoglobulins. *Ann NY Acad Sci* 475:135, 1986.

Doherty PC, Allan W, Eichelberger M, et al.: Heat-shock proteins and the Tγδ-cell response in virus infections: Implications for autoimmunity. *Springer Semin Immunopathol* 13:11, 1991.

Ehrlich P: On autoimmunity with special reference to cell life. *Proc Roy Sci Bio* (Lond) 66B:424, 1900.

Fowlkes BJ, Ramsdell F: T-cell tolerance. *Current Biol* 5:873–879, 1993.

Goodnow CC, Adelstein S, Basten A: The need for central and peripheral tolerance in the B-cell repertoire. *Science* 248:1373, 1990.

Kroemer G, Carlos Martinez A: Cytokines and autoimmune disease. *Clin Immunol Immunopathol* 61:275, 1991.

Kronenberg M: Self-tolerance and autoimmunity. *Cell* 65:537, 1991.

Kunkel HG, Tan EM: Autoantibodies and disease. *Adv Immunol* 4:231, 1964.

Nakamura MC, Nakamura RM: Contemporary concepts of autoimmunity and autoimmune diseases. *J Clin Lab Anal* 6:275, 1992.

Ohno S: Many peptide fragments of alien antigens are homologous with host proteins, thus canalizing T-cell responses. *Proc Natl Acad Sci USA* 88:3065, 1991.

Ramsdell F, Fowlkes BJ: Clonal deletion versus clonal anergy: The role of the thymus in inducing self-tolerance. *Science* 248:1342, 1990.

Rodey GE: Antiidiotypic antibodies and regulation of immune responses. *Transfusion* 32:361, 1992.

Rose NR, Mackey I: *The Autoimmune Diseases*. Orlando, FL, Academic Press, 1985.

Sakashi T, Eishi Y: Developmental expression of autoimmune target antigens during organogenesis. *Immunology* 74:524, 1991.

Schwartz RH: A cell culture model of T-lymphocyte clonal anergy. *Science* 248:1249, 1990.

Shirai T, Hirose S, Okada T, et al.: CD5+ cells in autoimmune disease and lymphoid malignancy. *Clin Immunol Immunopathol* 59:173, 1991.

Shoenfeld Y, Isenberg D: *The Mosiac of Autoimmunity*. New York, Elsevier, 1990.

Stollar BD: Autoantibodies and autoantigens: A conserved system that may shape a primary immunoglobulin gene pool. *Molec Immunol* 28:1399, 1991.

Waksman BH: Autoimmunization and the lesions of autoimmunity. *Medicine* 41:93, 1962.

Weigle WO: Recent observations and concepts in immunological unresponsiveness and autoimmunity. *Clin Exp Immunol* 9:437, 1971.

Weigle WO: Analysis of autoimmunity through experimental models of thyroiditis and allergic encephalomyelitis. *Adv Immunol* 30:159, 1980.

Werner-Favre C, Vischer TL, Wohlwend D, et al. Cell surface antigen CD5 is a marker for activated human B cells. *Eur J Immunol* 19:1209, 1989.

ENCELPHALO-MYELITIS

Kumar V, Sercarz EE: The involvement of T-cell receptor peptide-specific regulatory CD4+ T cells in recovery from antigen-induced autoimmune disease. *J Exp Med* 178:909–916, 1993.

Rosenblum MK: Paraneoplasia and autoimmunologic injury of the nervous system: The anti-HU syndrome. *Brain Pathol* 3:199–212, 1993.

EYE–EAR

Chan C-C, Caspi RR, Ni M, et al.: Pathology of experimental autoimmune uveoretinitis in mice. *J Autoimmunity* 3:247, 1990.

Cogan DC: Syndrome of nonsyphilitic interstitial keratitis and vestibuloauditory symptoms. *Arch Ophthalmol* 33:144, 1945.

Davis JL, Chan C-C, Nussemblatt RB: Immunology of intermediate uveitis. In *Intermediate Uveitis*. Boke WRF, Manthey KF, Nussenblatt RB (eds.). Basel, Karger, 1992, vol. 23, 71–85.

Donoso LA, Merryman CF, Sery T, et al.: Human interstitial retinoid-binding protein: A potent uveitopathogenic agent for the induction of experimental autoimmune uveitis. *J Immunol* 143:79, 1989.

Easom HA, Zimmerman LE: Sympathetic ophthalmia and bilateral phacoanaphylaxis: A clincopathologic correlation of the sympathogenic and sympathizing eyes. *Arch Ophthalmol* 72:9, 1964.

Faure JP: Autoimmunity and the retina. *Curr Top Eye Res* 2:215, 1980.

Harris JP: Experimental autoimmune sensorineural hearing loss. *Laryngoscopy* 97:63, 1987.

Haynes BF, Kaiser-Kupper MI, Mason P, Fauci AS. Cogan syndrome: Studies in thirteen patients, long-term follow up, and a review of the literature. *Medicine* 59:426, 1980.

McCabe BF: Autoimmune inner ear disease. In *Immunology of the Ear*. Bernstein J, Ogra P (eds.). New York, Raven Press, 1987, 427.

Melchers F: Immunity and autoimmunity—with special reference to inner ear diseases. *Adv Otorhinolaryngol* 46:17, 1991.

Merryman CF, Donoso LS, Zhang X, et al.: Characterization of a new, potent, immunopathogenic epitope in S-antigen that elicits T cells expressing $V\beta_8$ and $V\alpha_2$-like genes. *J Immunol* 146:75, 1991.

Meyers-Elliott RH: Autoimmunity and the retina: Experimental autoimmune uveitis. In *Developmental Immunology: Clinical Problems and Aging*. New York, Academic Press, 1982.

Silverstein AM, O'Conner GR (eds.): *Immunology and Immunopathology of the Eye*. New York, Masson, 1979.

Strelein JW: Immune regulation and the eye: A dangerous compromise. *Federation of American Societies for Experimental Biology J* 1:199, 1987.

Wakefield D, Schrieber L, Penny R: Immunological features in uveitis. *Med J Aust* 1:229, 1982.

ORCHITIS

Brown PC, Glynn LE: The early lesion of experimental allergic orchitis in guinea pigs: An immunological correlation. *J Pathol* 98:277–282, 1969.

Itoh M, Hiramine C, Tokunaga Y, et al.: A new murine model of autoimmune orchitis induced by immunization with viable syngeneic testicular germ cells alone. II. Immunohistochemical findings of fully developed inflammatory lesion. *Autoimmunity* 10:89, 1991.

Mahi-Brown CA, Tung KSK: Activation requirements of donor T cells and host T-cell recruitment in adoptive transfer of murine experimental autoimmune orchitis (EAO). *Cell Immunol* 124:368, 1989.

Somerville JE, Iftikhar M, O'Sullivan JF, et al.: Autoimmune oophoritis: An incidental finding. *Path Res Pract* 189:475–477, 1993.

Teuscher C: Experimental allergic orchitis in mice. II. Association of disease susceptibility with the locus-controlling *Bordetella pertussis*-induced sensitivity to histamine. *Immunogenetics* 22:417, 1985.

Tung KSK, Unanue ER, Dixon FJ: The immunopathology of experimental allergic orchitis. *Am J Pathol* 60:313, 1970.

Waksman BH: A histologic study of the autoallergic testis lesion in the guinea pig. *J Exp Med* 109:311, 1959.

SJÖGREN'S SYNDROME

Adamson TC: Immunologic analysis of lymphoid infiltrates in primary Sjögren's syndrome using monoclonal antibodies. *J Immunol* 130:203, 1983.

Anderson LG, Tarpley TM, Talal N, et al.: Cellular versus humoral autoimmune responses to salivary gland in Sjögren's syndrome. *Clin Exp Immunol* 13:335, 1973.

Boss JH, Sela J, Ulmansky M, et al.: Experimental immune sialoadenitis. *Isr J Med* 24:15, 1975.

Hadden WB: "Dry mouth", or suppression of the salivary buccal secretions. *Trans Clin Soc Hand* 21:176, 1888.

Manthorpe R, Frost-Larson K, Isager H, et al.: Sjögren's syndrome: A review with emphasis on immunologic features. *Allergy* 36:139, 1981.

Sjögren H: Zur Kenntnis der keratoconjunctivitis sicca (keratitis filiformus) bee hypofunction der tranendrusen. *Acta Ophthalmol* (KbH) 11:1, 1933.

ENDOCRI-NOPATHIES

Christy NP, Holub DA, Omasi T: Primary ovarian, thyroidal, and adrenocortical deficiencies simulating pituitary insufficiency, associated with diabetes mellitus. *J Clin Endocrinol* 22:155, 1962.

Edmonds M et al.: Autoimmune thyroiditis, adrenalitis and oophoritis. *Am J Med* 54:782, 1973.

Fuji Y, Kato N, Kito J, et al.: Experimental autoimmune adrenalitis: A murine model for Addison's disease. *Autoimmunity* 12:47, 1992.

Irvine WJ: Immunologic aspects of premature ovarian failure associated with idiopathic Addison's disease. *Lancet* 2:883, 1968.

Levine S, Wenk EJ: The production and passive transfer of allergic adrenalitis. *Am J Pathol* 52:41, 1968.

Muir A, Schatz DA, MacLaren NK: Autoimmune Addison's disease. *Springer Semin Immunopathol* 14:275–284, 1993.

Ozawa Y, Shishiba Y: Recovery from lymphocytic hypophysitis associated with painless thyroiditis: Clinical implications of circulating antipituitary antibodies. *Acta Endocrinol* 128:493–498, 1993.

Strickland RG: Pernicious anemia and polyendocrine deficiency. *Ann Int Med* 70:1001, 1969.

Toivanen P, Toivanen A: Does *Yersinia* induce autoimmunity? *Int Arch Allergy Immunol* 104:107–111, 1994.

Van de Casseye M, Gepts W: Primary (autoimmune?) parathyroiditis. *Virchows Arch Pathol Anat* 361:257, 1973.

Volpe R (ed.): *Autoimmune Diseases of the Endocrine System*. Boca Raton, FL, CRC Press, 1990.

Werdelin O, Witebsky E: Experimental allergic rat adrenalitis: A study on its elicitation and lymphokinetics. *Lab Invest* 23:136, 1970.

GASTROINTESTINAL DISEASE

Broberger O, Perlmann P: Autoantibodies in human ulcerative colitis. *J Exp Med* 110:657, 1959.

Brynskov J, Nielsen OH, Ahnfelt-Ronne I, et al.: Cytokines in inflammatory bowel disease. *Scand J Gastroenterol* 27:897, 1992.

Colletti RB, Guillot AP, Rosen S, et al.: Autoimmune enteropathy and nephropathy with circulating antiepithelial cell antibodies. *J Pediatr* 118:858, 1991.

Crohn BB, Ginzburg L, Openheimer GD: Regional ileitis: A pathologic and clinical entity. *JAMA* 99:1323, 1932.

Eigenbrodt ML, Eigenbrodt EH, Thiele DL: Histologic similarity of murine colonic graft-versus-host disease (GVHD) to human GVHD and inflammatory bowel disease. *Am J Pathol* 137:1065, 1990.

MacDermott RP, Stenson WF: Alterations of the immune system in ulcerative colitis and Crohn's disease. *Adv Immunol* 42:285, 1988.

Markesich DC, Sawai ET, Butel JS, et al.: Investigations on etiology of Crohn's disease: Humoral immune response to stress (heat shock) proteins. *Digest Dis Sci* 36:454, 1991.

Rabin BS, Rogers SJ: Cell-mediated immune model of inflammatory bowel disease in the rabbit. *Gastroenterol* 75:29, 1978.

Raedler A, Schreiber: Immunology of ulcerative colitis. *Hepatogastroenterol* 36:213, 1989.

Strickland RG: The Sydney system: Autoimmune gastritis. *J Gastroenterol Hepatol* 6:238, 1991.

LIVER DISEASE

Berg PA, Klein R: Mitochrondrial antibodies in primary biliary cirrhosis. *J Hepatol* 15:6, 1992.

Chedid A, Medenhall CL, Moritz TE, et al.: Cell-mediated hepatic injury in alcoholic liver disease. *Gastroenterol* 105:254–266, 1993.

Doniach D: Autoimmune aspects of liver disease. *Br Med Bull* 28:145, 1972.

Galbraith RM, Fudenberg HH: Autoimmunity in chronic active hepatitis and diabetes mellitus. *Clin Immunol Immunopath* 8:116, 1977.

Kohda H, Sekiya C, Kanal M, et al.: Flow cytometric and functional analysis of mononuclear cells infiltrating the liver in experimental autoimmune hepatitis. *Clin Exp Immunol* 82:473, 1990.

Krawitt EL, Wiesner RH (eds.): *Autoimmune Liver Disease*. New York, Raven Press, 1991.

Mackay IR, Popper H: Immunopathogenesis of chronic hepatitis: A review. *Aust NZ J Med* 1:79, 1973.

Paronetto F, Sagnelli E: Immunologic observation in chronic active hepatitis: A disease of different etiologies. *Pathobiol Ann* 10:157, 1980.

Popper H, Paronetto F: Problems in immunology of hepatic diseases. *Hepatogastroenterol* 31:1, 1984.

Subcommittee on the National Halothane Study: Summary of the National Halothane Study: Possible association between halothane anesthesia and postoperative hepatic necrosis. *JAMA* 197:775, 1966.

Uzunalimoglu B, Yardley JH, Boitnott JK: The liver in mild halothane hepatitis. Light and electron microscopic findings with special reference to the mononuclear cell infiltrate. *Am J Pathol* 61:457, 1970.

Walker JG, Doniach D, Roitt IM, et al.: Serologic tests in diagnosis of primary biliary cirrhosis. *Lancet* I:827, 1965.

Wen L, Peakman M, Lobo-Yeo A, et al.: T cell-directed hepatocyte damage in autoimmune chronic active hepatitis. *Lancet* 336:1527, 1990.

Worman HJ, Courvalin J-C: Autoantibodies against nuclear envelope proteins in liver disease. *Hepatology* 14:1269, 1991.

HEART DISEASE

Alving CR, Swartz GM: Antibodies to cholesterol, cholesterol conjugates, and liposomes: Implications for atherosclerosis and autoimmunity. *Crit Rev Immunol* 10:441, 1991.

Beisel KW: Immunogenic basis of myocarditis: Role of fibrillary antigens. *Springer Semin Immunopathol* 11:31, 1989.

Kodama M, Zhang S, Hanawa H, et al.: Immunohistochemical characterization of infiltrating mononuclear cells in the rat heart with experimental autoimmune giant cell myocarditis. *Clin Exp Immunol* 90:330, 1992.

Llane JR, Neumann DA, Lafond-Walker A, et al.: Role of IL-1 and tumor necrosis factor in coxsackievirus-induced autoimmune myocarditis. *J Immunol* 151:1682–1690, 1993.

Maisch B, Trostel-Soeder R, Stechemesser E, et al.: Diagnostic relevance of humoral and cell-mediated immune reactions in patients with acute viral myocarditis. *Clin Exp Immunopathol* 48:533, 1984.

PERIODONTAL DISEASE

Horton JE, Oppenheim JJ, Mergenhagen SE: A role for cell-mediated immunity in the pathogenesis of periodontal disease. *J Periodontol* 45:351, 1974.

Nisengard RJ: The role of immunology in periodontal disease. *J Periodontol* 48:505, 1977.

Seymour GJ, Cole KL, Powell RN: Analysis of lymphocyte populations extracted from chronically inflamed human periodontal tissue. I. Identification. *J Periodont Res* 20:47, 1985.

Tollefsen T, Saltvedt E, Koppang HS: The effect of immunosuppressive therapy on periodontal disease in man. *J Periodont Res* 13:240, 1978.

ADJUVANT DISEASE— ARTHRITIS

Cohen IR: Autoimmunity to chaperonins in the pathogenesis of arthritis and diabetes. *Annu Rev Immunol* 9:567, 1991.

Cremer MA, Terato K, Seyer JM, et al.: Immunity to type XI collagen in mice: Evidence that the $\alpha3(XI)$ chain of type XI collagen and the $\alpha1(II)$ chain of type II collagen share arthrotigenic determinants and induce arthritis in DBA/1 mice. *J Immunol* 146:4130, 1991.

Katz H, Piliero SJ: A study of adjuvant-induced polyarthritis in the rat with special reference to associated immunological phenomena. *Ann NY Acad Sci* 147:515, 1969.

Pearson CM: Development of arthritis, periarthritis, and periostitis in rats given adjuvant. *Proc Soc Exp Biol Med* 91:95, 1956.

Rosenthale ME, Capetola RJ: Adjuvant arthritis: Immunological and hyperalgesia features. *Fed Proc* 41:2577, 1982.

Stuart JM, Townes AS, Kang AH: Collagen autoimmune arthritis. *Immunol Rev* 2:199, 1984.

Waksman BH, Pearson CM, Sharp JT: Studies of arthritis and other lesions induced in rats by injection of mycobacterial adjuvant. II. Evidence that the disease itself is a disseminated immunological response to exogenous antigen. *J Immunol* 85:403, 1960.

TREATMENT

Bach J-F: *Monoclonal antibodies and peptide therapy in autoimmune diseases.* New York, Marcel Dekker, 1993.

Brostoff SW, Howell MD: T-cell receptors, immunoregulation and autoimmunity. *Clin Immunol Immunopathol* 62:1, 1992.

Bryskov J, Freund L, Norby-Rasmussen S, et al.: Final report on a placebo-controlled, double-blind, randomised, multicentre trial of cyclosporine treatment in active chronic Crohn's disease. *Scand J Gastroenterol* 26:689, 1991.

Lenschow DJ, Zeng Y, Thistlethwaite JR, et al.: Long-term survival of xenogeneic pancreatic islet grafts induced by CTLA4Ig. *Science* 257:789, 1992.

Linsley PS, Wallace PM, Johnson J, et al.: Immunosuppression in vivo by a soluble form of the CTLA-4 T-cell activation molecule. *Science* 257:792, 1992.

Racke MKS, Dhib-Jalbut S, Canella B, et al.: Prevention and treatment of chronic relapsing experimental allergic encephalomyelitis by $TGF_{\beta 1}$. *J Immunol* 146:3012, 1991.

Ruddle NC, Bergman M, McGrath KM, et al.: An antibody to lymphotoxin and tumor necrosis factor prevents transfer of experimental allergic encephalomyelitis. *J Exp Med* 172:1193, 1990.

Thompson AW, Starzl TE: FK506 and autoimmune disease: Perspective and prospects. *Autoimmunity* 12:303, 1992.

Zhang J, Raus J: T-cell vaccination in autoimmune diseases. *Human Immunol* 38:87–96, 1993.

22

Autoimmune Diseases II—Diffuse Connective Tissue (Collagen–vascular, Rheumatoid) Diseases

Connective Tissue Diseases

Connective tissue diseases are presented as a separate chapter because of their clinical importance and because they represent a major group of diseases caused by autoimmunity. The diffuse connective tissue diseases include rheumatoid arthritis, systemic lupus erythematosus (SLE), Sjögren's syndrome, polymyositis (dermatomyositis) and progressive systemic sclerosis (scleroderma). These diseases were previously termed collagen-vascular diseases or rheumatoid diseases. The term "collagen-vascular" was used because of lesions believed to be in the collagen of connective tissues and the association with vascular lesions. The term "rheumatoid" was used because of the use of the general term *rheumatism* used to cover a number of diseases now known to be different, particularly rheumatic fever and skeletal tuberculosis.

RHEUMATOID DISEASE

Rheumatoid diseases got their name because of the resemblance of these diseases to rheumatic fever. Rheumatic fever is an acute systemic disease also caused by immune complex mechanisms that includes inflammation of the heart (carditis), joints (polyarthritis) and skin (erythema marginatum); the development of subcutaneous nodules; and involuntary movements of muscles (chorea, St. Vitus' dance). These findings occur in a variety of combinations that together permit the diagnosis of rheumatic fever. Rheumatic fever occurs as a sequel to certain group A β-hemolytic streptococcal infections. The inflammatory lesions are caused by deposition of immune complexes, believed to be of host antibody–streptococcal origin, as well as by "autoantibodies" to host tissue antigens induced by cross-reacting epitopes between some streptococcal antigens and host tissue (molecular mimicry). Rheumatic fever is presented in more detail in Chapter 25. The term "rheumatologist" in reference to physicians who diagnose and treat patients with rheumatoid diseases was introduced by Comroe in Philadelphia in 1940.

COLLAGEN DISEASE

In 1942, Klemperer coined the term "collagen disease" for this group of diseases because they had in common a morphologically similar lesion in collagen—fibrinoid necrosis, an increase in ground substance with swollen, fragmented collagen fibers and necrosis, resulting in a structureless eosinophilic area resembling fibrin in appearance. The concept that one disease could affect the function of many organs was revolutionary at the time. The discovery of rheumatoid factor and the lupus erythematosus cell in 1948, as well as the application of cortisone for therapy in 1949, led to major advances in understanding the connective tissue diseases. We now think that many of the lesions of the connective tissue diseases are caused by immune complex-mediated mechanisms, but other mechanisms, particularly cell-mediated hypersensitivity, may also contribute, in particular for Sjögren's syndrome.

CONNECTIVE TISSUE DISEASE

Each of the connective tissue diseases has its own pattern of clinical features, time course, location of lesions, autoantibody reactivities, and immunopathologic mechanisms. Rheumatoid arthritis mainly affects joints; Sjögren's syndrome, the exocrine glands; polymyositis, the skeletal muscle; and scleroderma, the dermal and submucosal connective tissue. SLE has a multiplicity of autoantibodies and a wide spectrum of tissue involvement. As depicted in Figure 22–1, there is considerable overlap of pathologic features within the connective tissue disease group, and a given patient may have features of several of the connective diseases (overlap syndromes). Many individuals with a connective tissue disease have angiitis or glomerulonephritis, immunoglobulin abnormalities, and autoantibodies with varied specificities of reactivity, including falsely positive tests for syphilis. Some of the protean manifestations of syphilis, and other chronic infectious diseases, are not unlike many of the features of the connective tissue diseases and may be the result of autoimmune reactions caused by alteration of host tissue or allergic reactions to the infecting organisms located in host tissue. Similarly, the lesions seen in the connective tissue diseases may result from allergic reactions to as yet undetected infectious agents.

The variable clinical and pathologic features of the connective tissue diseases may be the result of the operation of different types of allergic reactions with different degrees of severity at different times, directed toward different antigenic specificities with different tissue locations. The interplay of these variables could produce varying clin-

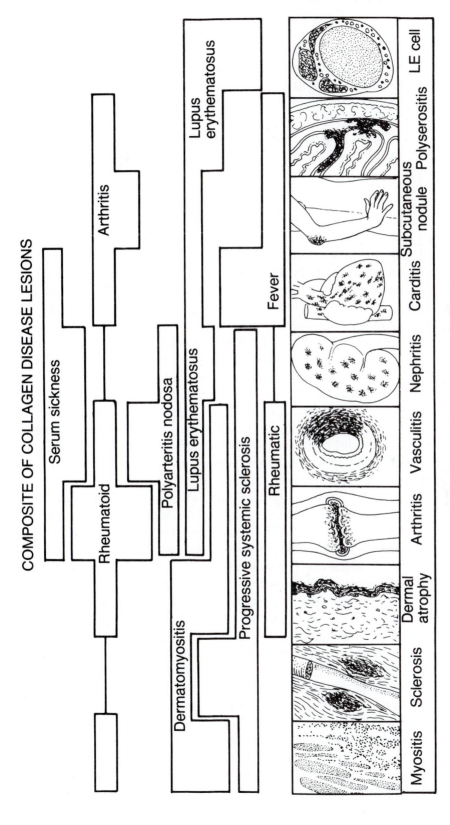

COMPOSITE OF COLLAGEN DISEASE LESIONS

Figure 22–1. Pathologic features of connective tissue diseases. The lesions associated with connective tissue diseases. The lesions associated with each disease is indicated by the thickness of the boxes (top). Serum sickness is included because its characteristic lesions (vasculitis, glomerulonephritis, myocarditis, and arthritis) are also found in the connective tissue diseases. This suggests a primary role for immune complex mechanisms in connective tissue disease.

553

ical pictures during the course of a disease in a given individual. For further information, the reader is referred to the "Primer on the Rheumatic Disease" published by the Arthritis Foundation, Atlanta, Georgia. The disease polyarteritis nodosa (PAN) will be presented first. Although PAN is not officially a connective tissue disease, it is included here to illustrate the features of a multiorgan disease caused by immune complex vasculitis.

Polyarteritis Nodosa (PAN)

DIAGNOSIS

PAN illustrates the multiorgan nature of a disease primarily affecting arteries. The clinically apparent lesions of PAN consist of multiple foci of localized infarcts affecting almost any organ or combination of organs in the body. Inflammation of small and medium-sized arteries results in thrombosis and obstruction of blood flow, leading to many areas of necrosis and scarring. There is characteristically necrosis of a portion of the arterial wall with sparing of the remaining wall. The necrotic segment may become distended due to intraarterial pressure, resulting in the formation of microaneurysms, giving rise to the term "nodosa," hence polyarteritis nodosa. Microaneurysms (pseudo-aneurysms) may be seen in the medium-sized arteries of the liver and kidney by angiography. Initially, symptoms may include malaise, fatigue, fever, myalgias, muscle weakness, and pain in different locations. Renal involvement with glomerulonephritis or vasculitis is common. Inflammation of the arteries of the heart or brain may cause myocardial or cerebral infarcts.

The arterial lesion is similar to that seen in serum sickness arteritis, and immunoglobulin may be identified in the areas of fibrinoid necrosis. The role of this immunoglobulin in the production of the lesion is unclear. The immunoglobulin may be antibody that is reacting with antigen that is part of the vessel wall; it may be part of an antigen–antibody complex formed in the circulation and deposited in the vessel wall, or the immunoglobulin may be nonspecifically absorbed to an arterial lesion evoked by an unrelated mechanism.

Complexes of viruses and immunoglobulin appear to be responsible for a considerable number of the cases of polyarteritis nodosa. There is a high association of polyarteritis nodosa with hepatitis B antigenemia, suggesting that polyarteritis occurring naturally may be due to an immune response to viral hepatitis infection with HBV antigen release. The association of polyarteritis with drug administration also suggests that some cases of polyarteritis may be caused by an immune response to drugs administered for therapy of other diseases. In addition, polyarteritis nodosa has been reported rarely in patients undergoing hyposensitization for allergic diseases (asthma), perhaps because of the production of complement fixing IgG antibody to the allergen.

Only about half of the cases of histologically proven polyarteritis nodosa survive over five years. Early and vigorous treatment with corticosteroids and cyclophosphamide may significantly improve the prognosis, but this has not been documented in a controlled study.

Rheumatoid Arthritis (RA)

Rheumatoid arthritis is a systemic syndrome in which chronic inflammation of the joints initiated by autoantibodies and maintained by cellular inflammatory mechanisms is the major feature. The autoantibodies are directed to self-immunoglobulin determinants (rheumatoid factor). The formation of immune complexes in the joint spaces leads to activation of complement and destructive inflammation (see below). The acute phase is followed by a DTH-type chronic inflammation. Chronic RA is believed to be driven by macrophages after initiation by T_{DTH} cells. T_{DTH} cells are present in large numbers in rheumatoid synovium, and cytotoxic T cells may contribute to chronic articular damage. However, the major cytokines found in the joint are macrophage-derived, such as IL-1, TNF-α, GM-CSF, and IL-6, whereas T_{DTH} cell factors (IL-2, INF-γ) are present in only very small amounts. Thus, the pathogenesis of RA involves a complex interplay of immune complex and DTH reactions.

DIAGNOSIS

The precise diagnosis of mild rheumatoid arthritis is difficult, as evidenced by the criteria established by a committee of the American Rheumatism Association (Table 22–1). The most common symptoms include a symmetric arthritis usually involving the small joints of the hands or feet and the knees. The arthritis is the result of an inflammatory synovitis that begins as a chronic inflammatory infiltration but usually proceeds to destructive inflammation and proliferation (pannus), eroding the articular surface. The synovia becomes hyperplastic and filled with lymphocytes and plasma cells, and prominent germinal center formation is seen as the disease progresses. Muscle wasting and the formation of subcutaneous nodules (see below) are found in about 20% of patients. Serositis, myocarditis, vasculitis, and peripheral neuropathy may also be found. Many attempts have been made to measure the progression of RA using mechanical and electrical instruments, laboratory tests, radiologic changes, and clinical measurements, such as discomfort and disability. It appears that the best predictor of the prognosis for RA is loss of function as determined clinically. In the classic case of seropositive nodular erosive disease, functional disability occurs early and continues to worsen, despite treatment, to severe functional loss within 10 years.

TABLE 22–1. THE 1987 REVISED CRITERIA FOR THE CLASSIFICATION OF RHEUMATOID ARTHRITIS (TRADITIONAL FORMAT)*

Criterion	Definition
1. Morning stiffness	Morning stiffness in and around the joints, lasting at least 1 hour before maximal improvement
2. Arthritis of 3 or more joint areas	At least 3 joint areas simultaneously have had soft tissue swelling or fluid (not bony overgrowth alone) observed by a physician. The 14 possible areas are right or left PIP, MCP, wrist, elbow, knee, ankle, and MTP joints
3. Arthritis of hand joints	At least 1 area swollen (as defined above) in a wrist, MCP, or PIP joint
4. Symmetric arthritis	Simultaneous involvement of the same joint areas (as defined in 2) on both sides of the body (bilateral involvement of PIPs, MCPs, or MTPs is acceptable without absolute symmetry)
5. Rheumatoid nodules	Subcutaneous nodules, over bony prominences, or extensor surfaces, or in juxtaarticular regions, observed by a physician
6. Serum rheumatoid factor	Demonstration of abnormal amounts of serum rheumatoid factor by any method for which the result has been positive in <5% of normal control subjects
7. Radiographic changes	Radiographic changes typical of rheumatoid arthritis on posteroanterior hand and wrist radiographs, which must include erosions or unequivocal bony decalcification localized in or most marked adjacent to the involved joints (osteoarthritis changes alone do not qualify)

*For classification purposes, a patient shall be said to have rheumatoid arthritis if he/she has satisfied at least 4 of these 7 criteria. Criteria 1 through 4 must have been present for at least 6 weeks. Patients with 2 clinical diagnoses are not excluded. Designation as classic, definite, or probable rheumatoid arthritis is *not* to be made.

From Arnett FC, Edworthy SM, Bloch DA, et al.: The American Rheumatism Association 1987 revised criteria for the classification of rheumatoid arthritis. *Arth Rheum* 31:315, 1988.

RHEUMATOID FACTOR

One of the diagnostic features of rheumatoid arthritis is rheumatoid factor (RF), a circulating autoantibody with reactivity to immunoglobulins. RF was discovered in 1940 by Waaler, who observed the agglutination of immunoglobulin-coated sheep red blood cells by factors in human sera. Historically, three general reactive specificities were recognized: (1) To xenogeneic immunoglobulins (rabbit, horse), (2) to allogeneic immunoglobulins (denatured human IgG), or (3) to autologous immunoglobulins (the patient's own IgG). Rheumatoid factor usually is an IgM (19S) antibody that reacts with one or more of the above antigens, although IgG rheumatoid factors are also found in some cases. The formation of RF is the result of an immune response by the host to one or more specific antigenic determinants present in his own immunoglobulins. RF is usually detected by agglutination of particles (erythrocytes, latex) coated with IgG; it also reacts with antigen–antibody complexes. RFs most often react with antigenic groupings of IgG that are buried in the native molecule and may be shared with Igs of other species. These antigenic specificities may be revealed by unfolding of the IgG molecule due to various denaturing processes or to the reaction of IgG antibody with antigen. RFs may also react with genetically controlled isoantigens (allotypes) located on immunoglobulins. The specificity of RFs produced by synovial tissue may be different from that reflected in the serum. The major antigenic determinant for synovial fluid RF appears to be in the CH3 domain of the IgG3 molecule. The significance of this is not clear.

Reaction of RF with IgG occurs in vivo and is believed to be the initiating factor for the early lesions associated with rheumatoid arthritis. Necrotizing arteritis is especially likely to evolve in patients with high titers of RF, presumably caused by deposition of immune complexes in vessels. In most cases, rheumatoid factor (anti-IgG) forms large complexes with IgG in vivo. These complexes are cleared from the circulation by the reticuloendothelial system with no further tissue damage. In rare cases, the rheumatoid factor–immunoglobulin complexes are soluble at body temperature but can be precipitated from the patient's serum by cooling (cryoglobulins). Patients with cryoglobulins are more apt to develop secondary vascular lesions than those without cryoglobulins. Some cryoimmunoglobulins are not immune complexes but abnormal Igs found in the sera of patients with connective tissue diseases and patients with lymphoproliferative disorders. These "monoclonal" cryoimmunoglobulins do not cause the significant vascular and glomerular lesions found with the immune complex (mixed) cryoimmunoglobulins.

Since RA occurs in the joint, it seems reasonable that the pathogenic important RF for arthritis is in the synovium and not in the serum. The titers of RF in serum do not correlate closely with the occurrence or severity of arthritis. Pertinent noncorrelative findings are that RF is found in some normal individuals, RA may occur in agammaglobulinemic individuals, and the infusion (transfer) of large amounts of RF to a normal individual causes no noticeable lesions. However, in several studies, RF in the sera predated the appearance of RA. In addition, the serum levels of RF do correlate well with the appearance of subcutaneous nodules, the presence of deforming arthritis, and the incidence of systemic disease.

PATHOGENESIS

The role of antibody and cellular immune mechanisms in RA is depicted in Figure 22–2. The acute inflammatory process is initiated by an immune complex reaction, but in progressive RA it resembles a chronic cell-mediated immune reaction. Although most of the serologic findings do not support an etiologic role for serum RF in the

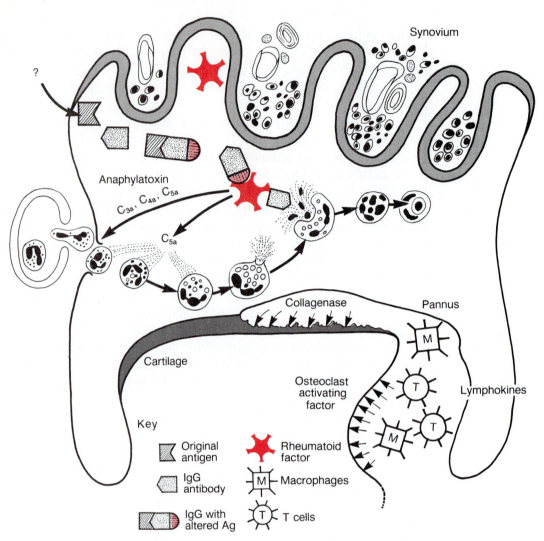

Figure 22–2. Current concepts of the pathogenesis of rheumatoid arthritis postulate that an as yet unidentified antigen (infectious agent, host autoantigen) present in the joint cavity stimulates the production of an antibody. Antigen–antibody complexes are formed that produce an alteration in the tertiary structure of the antibody revealing new or buried antigenic determinants. These determinants in turn stimulate the production of another antibody, rheumatoid factor, (IgM or IgG), which can react with IgG. Complexes form in the synovial fluid and activate complement components, which attract polymorphonuclear leukocytes. A proliferation of lymphocytes and plasma cells in the synovial lining tissue converts the synovium into a lymphoid organ, which produces rheumatoid factor that is released locally into the synovial fluid. T_{DTH} lymphocytes in the synovium are activated to produce lymphokines that attract and activate macrophages. Activated macrophages and lymphocytes secrete cytokines that upregulate expression of cell-adhesion molecules on endothelial cells and synovial fibroblasts. Macrophages also produce osteoclast-activating factor and other activation factors that lead to destruction of adjacent bone. Hyperplasia of granulation tissue and inflammatory cells occurs and extends as a mass (pannus) over the articular cartilage. The pannus produces collagenase and elastase that destroys the joint cartilage. This pannus may progress to form a scar in the joint that leads to immobilization.

pathogenesis of RA, observations on synovial fluid (the fluid of the articular cavity) indicate an immune complex RF autoimmune mechanism for the early inflammation of RA and cell-mediated immunity for the chronic disease. The formation of immune complexes of RF and altered host immunoglobulins in the joint initiates immune complex-mediated inflammation. The synovial fluid aspirated from patients with active RA contains immune complexes, and the polymorphonuclear leukocytes in such fluids may have complexes of RF and IgG in their cytoplasm (RA cells). There is also a selective lowering of complement components in the synovial fluid during active RA. The synthesis of complement components by synovial inflammatory tissue may also contribute to the severity of the early stage of arthritis. Eventually, the synovium is converted into a lymphoid organ containing germinal centers and T-cell domains mimicking the structure of a lymph node.

The chronic stage of RA is cell-mediated, with involvement of T cells, macrophages, endothelial cells, cytokines, and cell adhesion molecules as well as fibroblasts and osteoclasts. The phenotype of synovial T-cell infiltrates during active inflammation is predominantly CD3+ $T_{\gamma\delta}$ cells. The function and role in pathogenesis of this particular type of T cell has not been determined. The major immune mechanism is through macrophage activation. There is local production of IL-2, IL-6, granulocyte-monocyte colony-stimulating factor (GM-CSF), TNF-α, and TGF-β, presumably from activated T cells; IL-1, TNF-α, IL-6, IL-8, macrophage colony-stimulating factor (M-CSF), platelet-derived growth factor (PDGF), TGF-β, and osteoclast-activating factors from activated macrophages, as well as factors from fibroblasts and endothelial cells in the synovium, including arachidonic acid metabolites, vasoactive amines, platelet-activating factor, and endothelin-1. TGF-β is a strong chemoattractant for granulocytes and may be a major factor in recurrent acute inflammation in the joint. The production of IL-1 by activated macrophages during early synovial inflammation appears to induce development of postcapillary venules with high endothelium (HEV), not found in normal synovium. The HEVs and capillaries of the synovium contain increased ELAM-1 and VCAM-1, thus increased adhesiveness for inflammatory cells. IL-1, TNF-α, and INF-γ activate synovial fibroblasts and macrophages to express increased ICAM-1, which may promote lymphocyte adhesion through LFA-1 (see Chapter 9). T-lymphocytes may also bind to synovial lining cells through VLA-4 binding to VCAM-1 and VLA-5 (fibronectin). IL-1 also stimulates synovial cells to secrete collagenase, neutral proteases, plasminogen activator, and prostaglandin E2, as well as chrondrocytes to secrete collagenase, proteoglycase, and neutral proteases. IL-1 also directly activates osteoclasts to effect bone resorption. Endothelin-1 stimulates proliferation of fibroblasts and smooth muscle cells. Thus, the process of chronic inflammation is activated, leading to production and release of lymphokines and cytokines, upregulation of cellular adhesion molecules, activation of endothelial cells and macrophages, cartilage and bone destruction, and scarring, resulting in loss of function and deformation of the involved joints. Activation of synovial cells, chrondrocytes, and osteoclasts by IL-1 and TNF may be the major pathway for cartilage destruction and bone remodeling. Transgenic mice carrying and expressing the TNF gene develop an inflammatory arthritis similar to RA.

Rheumatoid nodules are granulomatous collections of mononuclear cells, primarily consisting of palisading macrophages surrounding a central area of fibrinoid necrosis. Rheumatoid nodules are prominent in the skin but may form in any tissue of the body. In the lung, rheumatoid nodules are worsened or exacerbated by tissue injury, such as produced by silica exposure in hard coal miners (Caplan's syndrome). Nodules are believed to form around inflamed blood vessels. The central necrotic areas contain fibrin, immunoglobulins, and complement. Thus, it is thought that nodules represent chronic destruction and scarring from a previous immune complex-mediated vasculitis.

ETIOLOGY

The relative roles of a transmissible agent and genetic factors in the etiology of RA is still open for speculation. Rheumatoid arthritis was first described by Landre-Beauvais 200 years ago. Studies of remains of American Indians for arthritic changes have led to the hypothesis that RA may have been a disease localized to certain areas of the New World, later spreading to the Old World (Europe) after exposure to New World inhabitants. A search for an infectious agent initiating RA has yielded a number of possibilities, but as yet there is no clear identification of an etiologic agent. Streptococci, diphtheroids, mycoplasma, and clostridia each have been proposed and later discarded because of lack of evidence. The presence of human T-lymphotropic virus-1 (HTLV-1)-related proteins in cells in rheumatoid synovium suggests a possible retroviral agent. There is stronger evidence that the Epstein–Barr (EB) virus may be associated with rheumatoid arthritis. EB virus is believed to be the causative agent for infectious mononucleosis and lymphoid tumors in humans (Burkitt's lymphoma) (see Chapter 24). The sera of patients with RA contain antibody activity to a nuclear antigen found in only B-cell lymphoid cell lines that have been transformed (immortalized) by EB virus. This antigen is not the same as the EB virus antigen found in Burkitt's lymphoma and has been termed rheumatoid arthritis-associated nuclear antigen (RANA). An EBV protein shares the same five amino acids as the HLA-Dw4, four of five of DR4 (Dw14) and DR1 molecules, which are implicated in genetic susceptibility to RA (see below), suggesting that molecular mimicry may be a mechanism. However, a direct etiologic relationship between EB virus infection and RA has not been demonstrated, but further studies on this possibility are underway. Any postulated infectious etiology must include a mechanism that leads to the stimulation of B cells to produce autoreactive RF.

CLINICAL COURSE

The clinical course of rheumatoid arthritis is quite variable; in some cases, there is rapid progression to severe disability, and in others, a prolonged progressive course, leading to moderate, little, or no joint deformity. Spontaneous remissions and exacerbations occur frequently and make evaluation of therapy difficult. RA may shorten life and can lead to total disability in about 10% of the cases. Inflammation of the heart, small or medium vessels, and lung (diffuse interstitial pulmonary fibrosis) is infrequent but may occur and is believed to be part of the rheumatoid process.

THERAPY

Therapy is directed toward controlling pain, reducing inflammation, and preventing severe deformities by active physical therapy or orthopedic surgery. The general approach is to move through stages of therapy. Salicylates and other nonsteroidal antiinflammatory agents are usually the first drugs used and may have a beneficial effect, but are not effective for many patients. The synovium of rheumatoid arthritics contains mast cells and macrophages. Mast cells release arachidonic acids, and macrophages process arachidonic acid to prostaglandins. Prostaglandins are present in high concentrations in rheumatoid synovium and are believed to contribute to the disease. Salicylates or other cyclooxygenase inhibitors may function to reduce prostaglandin synthesis in synovial tissues. Second-line drugs include gold, hydroxychloroquine, penicillamine, and sulfasalazine. These have become known as "remission-inducing" drugs, but this is almost certainly an overstatement. There is controversy regarding the beneficial effects of these drugs, and amelioration of symptoms may only last for a few months. When these drugs are no longer effective, immunosuppressive therapy, especially methotrexate, has been applied in severe cases. Corticosteroids may provide temporary relief of pain but do not effectively control the disease. It is becoming increasingly clear that this "pyramid therapy" is not working, and better effects may be obtained by using stronger drugs earlier in the disease. More recently, use of monoclonal antibodies directed to CD4+ T cells or to interruption of different factors believed to be important in the progression of the disease, such as IL-1, TNF-γ, CD5, IL-2R, and ICAM-1, have resulted in clinical improvement in about 25% of patients. Despite the various drugs and regimens used, therapy is still unsatisfactory. Surgical restoration is very effective in some cases, restoring much of the function of deformed hands. Physical therapy can help minimize pain and improve functional activity.

HLA ASSOCIATIONS

Genetic susceptibility was originally demonstrated by RA clusters in families, and there is a higher concordance of RA in monozygotic than in dizygotic twins. Genetic predisposition to RA is associated with HLA-DR4 in Caucasians and HLA-DR1 in other ethnic groups. HLA-DR4 subtypes Dw4, Dw14, and Dw15 predispose to RA, whereas Dw10 and Dw13 do not. These subtypes contain only a few amino acid differences in the third hypervariable region of the HLA-DR4 beta chain. HLA-DR1 shares the same third hypervariable region as the Dw14 subtype of DR4. The critical shared epitope of the RA subtypes appears to be on a combining site for the T-cell antigen receptor. Thus, these Class II MHC subtypes may present processed antigen, perhaps altered host Ig, to helper T cells in a manner that results in the abnormal autoimmune response inherent to the etiology of RA.

Spondylo–arthropathies and HLA-B27

The spondyloarthropathies include three joint diseases: Ankylosing spondylitis, Reiter's syndrome (RS), and psoriatic arthritis, similar to rheumatoid arthritis, in which the interarticulating joints of the spine are involved (sacrolitis or spondylitis). These are also called "seronegative arthritides" because there is a lack of rheumatoid factor or antinuclear antibodies. The occurrence of these diseases is clearly associated with HLA-B27 (Table 22–2). Ankylosing spondylitis is chronic inflammation, fibrosis, and ossification of the articulations of the spine that occurs in young adults. More than 90% of patients with ankylosing spondylitis are HLA-B27 positive. Reiter's syndrome, or reactive arthritis, is an acute peripheral arthritis, nongonococcal urethritis, and conjunctivitis that characteristically develops two to four weeks after an infection with *Shigella, Salmonella, Yersinia, Campylobacter,* or *Chlamydia* infection. Antigens from the triggering organisms can be demonstrated in synovial fluid leukocytes and macrophages, but viable microorganisms are not present. Chlamydia has emerged as the primary pathogen for Reiter's syndrome. Antibodies against the chlamydia 57 kDa heat shock protein have been found in the sera and spinal fluid of RS patients after chlamydial infection. The significance of this observation is not clear. Seventy-five percent of cases are HLA-B27. Patients with psoriasis and inflammatory bowel disease without joint disease generally do not show a higher frequency of HLA-B27 than the normal population, but approximately 50% of those with spondylitis associated with psoriasis or inflammatory bowel disease carry HLA-B27.

TABLE 22–2. SPONDYLOARTHROPATHIES ASSOCIATED WITH HLA-B27

Characteristic	Disorder				
	Ankylosing Spondylitis	Reactive Arthritis[a]	Juvenile Spondyloarthropathy	Psoriatic Arthropathy	Enteropathic Arthropathy
Sacroiliitis or spondylitis[b]	100%	<50%	<50%	20%	10%
Peripheral arthritis[c]	25%	90%	90%	95%	90%
Gastrointestinal inflammation	Common, usually asymptomatic	Common, often asymptomatic	Not known	Uncommon	All
Skin and nail involvement	Rare	Most	Uncommon	All	Uncommon
Genitourinary involvement (males only)	Uncommon	Most	Uncommon	Uncommon	Rare
Eye involvement[d]	25%	Common	Common	Occasional	Occasional
Cardiac involvement	<5%	5%-10%	Not known, probably rare	Rare	Rare
Usual age of onset (years)	18–40	18–45	7–18	20–50	15–50
Sex prevalence	Males 3:1	Males 3:1[e]	Males 10:1	Equal	Equal
Type of onset	Gradual	Acute	Variable	Variable	Gradual
Role of infectious agents	Unknown	Definite trigger	Unknown	Unknown	Unknown
Prevalence of HLA-B27[f]	>90%	60%-80%	80%	50%[g]	50%-75%[g]

[a]Includes Reiter's syndrome, classically defined as the triad of arthritis, conjunctivitis, and urethritis.

[b]Inflammation in the spine or sacroiliac joints.

[c]Inflammation in joints of the extremities.

[d]Predominantly conjunctivitis in reactive arthritis; iritis with the other disorders.

[e]Male to female ratio is 10:1 if venereally acquired; 1:1 if enteropathically acquired.

[f]Caucasians of northern European extraction only. General prevalence in this population is 6%-8%. Some variation seen in other populations, but the basic associations with HLA-B27 are seen worldwide.

[g]Frequency elevated only in those with spondylitis or sacroiliitis.

From Hammer RE, Maika SD, Richardson JA: Spontaneous inflammatory disease in transgenic rats expressing HLA-B27 and human B_2m: An animal model of HLA-B27 associated human disorders. *Cell* 53:1099, 1990.

Mechanisms to explain the association of spondylitis and HLA-B27 are not known at this time. Three hypothetical possibilities include: (1) Selective class I MHC antigen processing by HLA-B27 to CD8+ cytotoxic T cells, (2) the use of B27 as a receptor for arthritic factors released by arthritis-related organisms, and (3) molecular mimicry between bacterial antigens and host B27 residues. Six identical residues on B27 and *Klebsiella pneumoniae* have been identified. In support of these hypotheses is the finding that transgenic rats expressing HLA-B27 and human β2-microglobulin spontaneously develop inflammatory lesions similar to human spondyloarthropathies. Recently, six subtypes of HLA-B27 based on amino acid substitutions have been identified. One of these, B2703, is not associated with spondyloarthropathies, whereas the others are. This finding explains why the previous lack of correspondence between spondylo-arthropathies and B27 in Gambian blacks, who carry a relatively high (up to 3%) incidence of B2703. Peptides from gram-negative enteric microorganisms specifically bind to HLA-B27 and may provide an immune stimulation for a subset of T-cell receptors.

Systemic Lupus Erythematosus (SLE)

Systemic lupus erythematosus (SLE) is a multiorgan disease caused by autoantibodies produced to a wide variety of the patient's own nuclear, cytoplasmic, and cell membrane antigens. Most, but not all, of the lesions can be explained by the effects of formation of circulating immune complexes or autoantibody that deposit in different organs. This disease appears most frequently in women of childbearing age but can occur at any age.

DIAGNOSIS

The classical presentation of a young woman with a "butterfly rash" on the upper cheeks, history of recent sun sensitivity, pleuropericarditis, arthritis, fever, fatigue, seizures, and nephrotic syndrome, occurs in only a few patients. However, these findings illustrate the major features of the disease. The fatal form is a rapidly advancing systemic disease featuring high fever, skin rash, nephritis, polyarthritis, polyserositis (pleural, pericardial, and peritoneal effusions), and central nervous system symptoms. With more sensitive diagnostic techniques (mainly tests for antinuclear antibodies), milder forms of SLE have been recognized that may include only a remitting arthralgia, myalgia, and malaise. Degrees of severity between these extremes are common, and the clinical course is usually characterized by spontaneous remissions and exacerbations. The diagnosis and classification of SLE in a given patient are based on the results of a series of clinical findings and laboratory tests (Table 22–3).

PATHOGENESIS

Most of the lesions of SLE are related to autoantibodies, and the primary mechanism is immune complex-mediated inflammation. The heterogeneity of clinical, pathologic, and laboratory abnormalities suggests more than one simple pathogenesis, but the leading player is believed to be anti-double–stranded DNA. The major pathologic changes of SLE most frequently involve the skin and kidney, but systemic vasculitis may lead to symptoms relating to any organ of the body. The lesions reflect the progression of immune complex vasculi-

TABLE 22–3. THE 1982 REVISED CRITERIA FOR CLASSIFICATION OF SYSTEMIC LUPUS ERYTHEMATOSUS*

Criterion	Definition
1. Malar rash	Fixed erythema, flat or raised, over the malar eminences, tending to spare the nasolabial folds
2. Discoid rash	Erythematous raised patches with adherent keratotic scaling and follicular plugging; atrophic scarring may occur in older lesions
3. Photosensitivity	Skin rash as a result of unusual reaction to sunlight, by patient history or physician observation
4. Oral ulcers	Oral or nasopharyngeal ulceration, usually painless, observed by a physician
5. Arthritis	Nonerosive arthritis involving 2 or more peripheral joints, characterized by tenderness, swelling, or effusion
6. Serositis	a) Pleuritis—convincing history of pleuritic pain or rub heard by a physician or evidence of pleural effusion *OR* b) Pericarditis—documented by ECG or rub or evidence of pericardial effusion
7. Renal disorder	a) Persistent proteinuria greater than 0.5 grams per day or greater than 3+ if quantitation not performed *OR* b) Cellular casts—may be red cell, hemoglobin, granular, tubular, or mixed
8. Neurologic disorder	a) Seizures—in the absence of offending drugs or known metabolic derangements; e.g., uremia, ketoacidosis, or electrolyte imbalance *OR* b) Psychosis—in the absence of offending drugs or known metabolic derangements, e.g., uremia, ketoacidosis, or electrolyte imbalance
9. Hematologic disorder	a) Hemolytic anemia—with reticulocytosis *OR* b) Leukopenia—less than 4,000/mm^3 total on 2 or more occasions *OR* c) Lymphopenia—less than 1,500/mm^3 on 2 or more occasions *OR* d) Thrombocytopenia—less than 100,000/mm^3 in the absence of offending drugs
10. Immunologic disorder	a) Positive LE cell preparation *OR* b) Anti-DNA: antibody to native DNA in abnormal titer *OR* c) Anti-Sm: presence of antibody to Sm nuclear antigen *OR* d) False positive serologic test for syphilis known to be positive for at least 6 months and confirmed by *Treponema pallidum* immobilization or fluorescent treponemal antibody absorption test
11. Antinuclear antibody	An abnormal titer of antinuclear antibody by immunofluorescence or an equivalent assay at any point in time and in the absence of drugs known to be associated with "drug-induced lupus" syndrome

* The proposed classification is based on 11 criteria. For the purpose of identifying patients in clinical studies, a person shall be said to have systemic lupus erythematosus if any 4 or more of the 11 criteria are present, serially or simultaneously, during any interval of observation.

From Tan EM, et al.: The 1982 revised criteria for the classification of systemic lupus erythematosus. *Arth Rheum* 25:1271, 1982.

tis and may involve arterioles, venules, and sometimes larger arteries and veins. The early lesions are characterized by granulocyte infiltration, leukoclasia, and periarteriolar edema; later lesions are characterized by mononuclear cell infiltration and fibrinoid necrosis. The kidney lesions also reflect stages of immune complex disease and vary from mild to severe glomerular inflammation, which may progress to chronic glomerulonephritis. The most common lesions are proliferation and/or membranous glomerulonephritis. Chronic deposition of immune complexes may result in marked thickening of the basement membranes seen in histologic sections as so-called wire loops. Hyaline thrombosis and hematoxylin bodies (nuclear debris deposited in tissue—the tissue equivalent of the lupus erythematosus cell) are also classic findings. Glomerular crescent formation and sclerosis indicate poor prognosis. The pathogenesis of lupus nephritis is due to the deposition of immune complexes (see Glomerulonephritis, Chapter 13), but there may also be direct binding of anti-DNA antibodies to renal antigens.

In addition to the kidney, other major organs involved are the skin, spleen, heart, and brain. The characteristic skin lesions are patchy atrophy, hyperkeratosis, and lymphocytic infiltration of the epidermis and collagen degeneration of the dermis, both of which occur more frequently in areas of the skin exposed to sunlight, as well as leukoclastic vasculitis. The spleen may have a marked periarteriolar fibrosis described as "onion skin" to reflect the layering of fibrous tissue around the arterioles. Scattered focal thickening, necrosis, and fibrosis of medium-sized arterioles may be found in many different organs. Nonbacterial verrucous endocarditis (Libman–Sacks endocarditis) are ovoid sterile vegetations on the undersurface of the heart valves or chordae tendineae. These are composed of fibrin and fibrous tissue-containing platelets, lymphocytes, and plasma cells. The vegetations are usually 1 to 4 mm in diameter but can become quite large and serve as a source for emboli to the brain or even to the coronary arteries. Vasculitis in the brain may cause a variety of neurologic symptoms.

ANTINUCLEAR ANTIBODIES

A major diagnostic advance in SLE was first the recognition of the lupus erythematosus cell by Hargraves in 1948, and later the identification of specific antinuclear antibodies. The lupus erythematosus (LE) cell is a polymorphonuclear neutrophil that has phagocytized nuclear material. Its formation depends upon the presence of an antibody capable of reacting with nucleoprotein. When whole anticoagulated peripheral blood from a patient with SLE is incubated in vitro, this antibody reacts with the nuclei of lymphocytes. The swollen nuclear material is then phagocytized by polymorphonuclear neutrophils in the peripheral blood, and LE cells are formed (Figure 22–3).

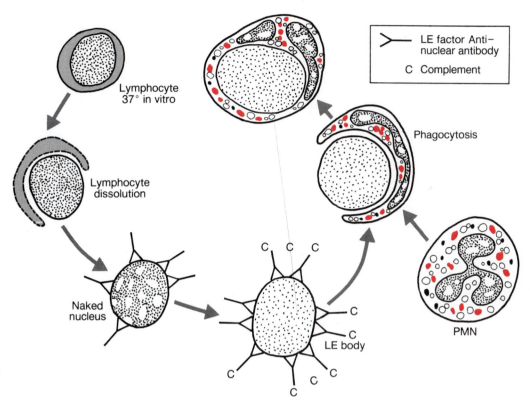

Figure 22–3. Formation of LE cell. LE cells are polymorphonuclear leukocytes that have phago-cytosed the nuclei of lymphocytes by coating the nuclei with antibody. This takes place at 37°C upon incubation of the whole blood of a patient with SLE who has antibody to nucleoprotein or other nuclear antigens. Lymphocytes break up, and lymphocyte nuclei become coated with anti-body (LE factor), swell, and are phagocytosed by polymorphonuclear leukocytes. LE cells may also be formed by phagocytosis of the nuclei of cells other than lymphocytes.

A variety of antinuclear antibodies have been identified in the sera of patients with SLE, and identification of these has replaced the LE cell test in the clinical laboratory. These include anti-DNA, antinu-cleoprotein, antinuclear membrane proteins, antihistones, antiacidic nuclear proteins, antinucleolar DNA, and antibodies to fibrous or par-ticulate nucleoprotein (Table 22–4). The immunofluorescent staining pattern observed when serum from a patient with SLE is allowed to bind to tissue nuclei provides some clues to diagnosis. The localization of the bound immunoglobulin is determined by addition of fluorescent-labeled antibody to immunoglobulin (indirect fluorescent antibody test). Four major patterns are seen: Nuclear rim (antimembrane pro-teins), speckled (antiacidic nuclear proteins), nucleolar (antinucleolar DNA), and homogeneous (not antigenically specific) (Table 22–5).

TABLE 22-4. SOME REACTIVITIES OF ANTINUCLEAR ANTIBODIES

Type of Antibody	Disease in Which Antibodies Seen	Characteristic of Antigenic Determinants	Nuclear Pattern Observed by Indirect Immunofluorescent Test
Antibody to DNA			
1. Reacts only with double-stranded DNA	Characteristic of SLE; correlates with nephritis	Double-strandedness of DNA essential	Rim and/or homogeneous
2. Reacts with both double- and single-stranded DNA	High levels in SLE; lower levels in other rheumatic diseases	Related to deoxyribose, purines, and pyrimidines, but not dependent on double helix	Same as No. 1
3. Reacts only with single-stranded DNA	Rheumatic, nonrheumatic diseases	Related to purines and pyrimidines, with ribose or deoxyribose equally reactive	Not detected on routine screen; special treatment necessary
Deoxynucleoprotein, soluble form	LE cell antibody in SLE, drug-induced LE	DNA—histone complex necessary: dissociated components are nonreactive	Rim and/or homogeneous
Histone	SLE, drug-induced SLE	Different classes of histones may have different determinants	Homogeneous and/or rim
Sm	Highly diagnostic of SLE	U1-RNP, U2, U4-6	Speckled
Nuclear RNP (Mo)	High levels in mixed connective tissue disease; lower levels in other rheumatic diseases	U1-RNP (RNA-splicing enzymes)	Speckled
Ribosomal P	Highly diagnostic of SLE; correlates with psychosis	Ribosome P protein	Cytoplasmic
Scl-70	Highly diagnostic of scleroderma	Extractable antigen, topoisomerase I	Speckled
Ku	20% of all connective tissue diseases	DNA binding protein	Speckled
SS-A (Ro)	High prevalence in Sjögren's syndrome sicca complex (40%); lower prevalence in other rheumatic diseases (SLE 25%)	Chemical nature unknown	Negative
SS-B (La) (Ha)	High prevalence in Sjögren's syndrome sicca complex (20%); lower prevalence in other rheumatic diseases (SLE 10%)	Extractable antigen, transcription termination factor for pol III	Speckled
PM-Scl	High prevalence in myositis and scleroderma overlaps	Chemical nature unknown	Nucleolar
RNA Polymerase I, II, III	Scleroderma	RNA Polymerase I, II, III	Nucleolar
U3-RNP (fibrillarin)	Scleroderma	Splicing enzymes	Nucleolar
Centromere	High prevalence in mild scleroderma (CREST syndrome)	Centromere antigens (CENP-B)	Discrete centromeric staining
Jo-1	Highly specific for polymyositis	Histidyl tRNA synthetase	Cytoplasmic or nuclear
Mi-2	Specific for dermatomyositis	Chemical nature unknown	Speckled

Abbreviations: ANA, antinuclear antibodies; DNA, deoxyribonucleic acid; RNA, ribonucleic acid; LE, lupus erythematosus; RNP, ribonuclear protein; RA, rheumatoid arthritis; Sm, Smith; Scl, scleroderma; SS, Sjögren's syndrome.

Table contributed by Frank Arnett, University of Texas Medical School, Houston.

TABLE 22–5. NUCLEAR STAINING PATTERNS OBSERVED IN PATIENTS WITH CONNECTIVE TISSUE DISEASES

Staining Pattern	Major Disease Association	Specificities of Antibody
Rim	SLE	Nuclear membrane protein
Speckled	SLE, scleroderma, other connective tissue diseases	Ribonucleoprotein
Nucleolar	Scleroderma, Sjögren's syndrome	U3-RNP, RNA polymerase I, Pm-Scl
Homogeneous	SLE, Sjögren's syndrome, rheumatoid arthritis	Nucleoprotein, unknown

The association of antibodies of different specificities with the connective tissue diseases is shown in Table 22–4.

Patients with SLE may have a number of serologic abnormalities in addition to antinuclear antibodies. These include antibodies to basement membranes of the skin, to red blood cells (positive Coombs' test), antibodies to phospholipids involved in blood clotting (lupus anticoagulant), antibodies to lymphocytes (usually to T-suppressor cells), falsely positive serologic reactions for syphilis, and antibodies to cytoplasmic antigenic components. These "autoantibodies" may be responsible for some SLE lesions and for associations of SLE with other connective tissue disease (Table 22–6).

Antiphospholipid antibodies (APAs) (the lupus anticoagulant, cardiolipin, VDRL for syphilis) are associated with vascular thrombosis in the brain and elsewhere and deposition of fibrin and platelet thrombi in the heart valves (Libman–Sacks endocarditis, see above). Although called lupus anticoagulant, APAs may be found in individuals without SLE and produce the primary APA syndrome, which is defined by the presence of antiphospholipid and any or all of the following clinical events: recurrent thrombosis, recurrent fetal losses, thrombocytopenia, and livedo reticularis. APAs were first identified by Wassermann in 1906, when serum from patients with syphilis was mixed with saline extracts of liver. The reactive antigen was later identified as cardiolipin. The antigens in cardiolipin are negatively charged phospholipids (phosphatidyl choline, phosphatidyl serine, sphingomyelin, etc.), resulting in identification of a family of antiphospholipid antibodies with different specificities. The common feature of these antibodies is their reactivity with cell membrane phospholipids on platelets and endothelial cells, activating vasospasm (livido reticularis) and coagulation (thrombosis).

Antibody to Ro (SSA) antigen may cause a transient annular erythematous skin rash or permanent heart block in neonates of mothers with antibody to Ro (SSA) antigen due to passive transfer of antibody from mother to fetus. This may occur when the mother is asympto-

TABLE 22–6. AUTOANTIBODIES IN SYSTEMIC LUPUS ERYTHEMATOSUS (SLE) AND OTHER CONNECTIVE TISSUE DISEASES

	SYSTEMIC LUPUS ERYTHEMATOSUS	
Organ Involvement	Associated Autoantibodies	Proposed Mechanisms
Glomerulonephritis	Anti-dsDNA Anti-Ro (SS-A) Other (?)	Immune complex
Cerebritis (psychosis), seizures, infarction	Antineuronal Antiribosomal P Antiphospholipid	Antibody-mediated Immune complex vasculitis Vascular thrombosis
Dermatitis	Anti-Ro (SS-A) Anti-DNA Others (?)	Immune complex Antibody dependent cytotoxicity (?)
Libman–Sacks endocarditis Heart block in neonates	Antiphospholipid Anti-Ro (SS-A)	Endocardial thrombosis Antibody-mediated
Red blood cell	Anti-RBC	Antibody-mediated
Lymphocyte	Antilymphocyte	Antibody-mediated
Platelet	Antiplatelet	Antibody-mediated
Arthritis, serositis	?DNA	Immune complex
	SJÖGREN'S SYNDROME	
Exocrine glands (eyes, nose, mouth, skin, GI lungs, GU)	Antisalivary gland Antisweat gland Other Auto-Abs	Infiltration by lymphocytes and plasma cells Antibody-mediated Cell-mediated
Extra-glandular (vasculitis)	Anti-Ro (SS-A) Anti-La (SS-B)	Immune complex
	POLYMYOSITIS (DERMATOMYOSITIS)	
Skeletal muscle	Anti-Jo1, Mi, Pm-Scl, RNP	Cell-mediated ADCC
	PROGRESSIVE SYSTEMIC SCLEROSIS (SCLERODERMA)	
Severe skin and visceral fibrosis	Anti-Scl-70	Immune attack of unknown kind on endothelium of arterioles and capillaries with proliferative endarteritis
Mild disease (CREST syndrome)	Anticentromere	

Modified from the lecture notes of Dr. Frank Arnett, University of Texas, Houston.

matic. Anti-Ro reactivity is also seen in "subacute cutaneous lupus erythematosus," a subgroup of SLE patients with prominent photoaggravated skin rash and musculoskeletal pains but who do not usually develop significant systemic disease.

Anti-Sm antibodies are highly specific for the diagnosis of SLE, but probably do not play a critical role in the pathogenesis. Anti-Sm antibodies include antibodies to U1 small nuclear RNP (U1 snRNP) and small cytoplasmic RNP (scRNP), as well as U2, U4 to U6 small nuclear RNP (snRNP), that are ribonuclear protein particles involved in splicing of precursor messenger RNA during posttranscriptional regulation of gene expression. These antibodies, as well as anti-La and Ro react with RNPs of infectious agents, such as human cytomegalovirus RNA. The reason that antibodies to these antigens, as well as to the nucleosome, are highly diagnostic of SLE is not known. The continuing subclassification of lupus patients according to the predominant autoantibodies promises to lead to more precise diagnosis and prognosis of the disease, as well as give clues to the pathogensis.

The membranous glomerulonephritis of SLE may contain deposits of immunoglobulin and DNA; both granular and linear deposits of Ig have been observed. Immunoglobulin and complement may also be detected in the vascular lesions of the spleen and other organs, and in the basement membrane of skin and along the dermal–epidermal junction of grossly normal-appearing skin (positive lupus band test). These latter antibodies are associated with liquefication necrosis of the basement membrane of the skin and subendothelial deposits in the basement membrane of renal glomeruli. In addition, antibodies to lymphocyte antigens that cross-react with neurons may be found in lupus erythematosus sera, and immune complexes are frequently found in the basement membrane of the choroid plexus (see above). The relationship of these to the central nervous system (CNS) symptoms associated with lupus erythematosus remains unclear.

ETIOLOGY

The etiology of naturally occurring SLE remains unsolved. Although it is clear that the major signs and symptoms are caused by autoantibodies, the reasons why these autoantibodies are produced is not so clear. There appear to be both genetic and environmental factors.

The genetic factors (Table 22–7) include the tendency to produce high antibody responses in general, as well as to produce antibodies to

TABLE 22–7. GENETIC FEATURES OF SYSTEMIC LUPUS ERYTHEMATOSUS

Features	Examples
1. Inheritance of autoimmune predisposition	Increased familial incidence of SLE (10% to 12%) Concordance in identical twins (70%) Family members develop other autoimmune diseases or produce autoantibodies
2. Androgens suppress expression, estrogens promote expression	Female:male ratio of 10:1
3. Multiple genes involved	Associated with complement deficiencies (C4, C2, C1r, C1s), MHC class II alleles, correlate with different autoantibodies
4. Independent predisposing factors	Inherited tendency to produce antibody

particular nuclear antigens, to have reduced clearance of immune complexes, or to have impaired DNA repair. Hormonal factors are implicated as androgens tend to protect against SLE. Bacterial or viral infections may stimulate the immune system to produce autoantibodies either nonspecifically through polyclonal B-cell activation or specifically to nuclear antigens through molecular mimicry. There may be an imbalance of humoral immunity similar to that described for New Zealand black (NZB) mice (see below). This leads to abnormal antibody formation to a variety of antigens, including host molecules. Multiple MHC and non-MHC genes appear to predispose to this imbalance. There is an increased incidence of HLA-DR2 and/or HLA-DR3, as well as inherited deficiencies of complement due to null alleles at complement C4 loci. The frequency of certain autoantibodies is related to HLA types (HLA-DQ1/DQ2 heterozygotes, anti-Ro (SSA), HLA-B8 and DR3, anti-La (SSB), HLA-DR4, and antinuclear RNP (Sm). There does not appear to be a linkage between SLE and polymorphisms at the heavy- and light-chain genes, as no differences in restriction endonuclease fragments in the germline immunoglobulin heavy-chain or kappa-chain variable regions have been detected between healthy individuals and lupus patients.

The role of environmental factors in SLE has attracted much attention, but there is no clear etiologic agent yet identified. Some drugs (see below) have been shown to cause symptoms similar to SLE. Many infectious agents have been accused, but none have been convicted. Analyses of the antibodies to dsDNA, believed to be key to the pathogenesis of SLE, indicate that they are not germline-encoded but antigen-driven, indicating that the autoantibody response in SLE is initiated by antigen exposure. Elevated levels of plasma nucleic acids are found in lupus patients, and these nucleic acids have a striking homology with the gag-pol overlap region of HIV-1, leading to the hypothesis that a retrovirus infection may lead to induction of autoantibodies to DNA. In support of this is the observation that the snRNPs which react with antibody in SLE sera have remarkable sequence homology with p30gag sequences of several oncoviruses. The most acceptable explanation at the present time is that an abnormal humoral antibody response to an infection leads to formation of antibodies that cross-react with a wide variety of human tissues in individuals who are genetically predisposed to produce autoantibodies.

DRUG-INDUCED LUPUS ERYTHEMA-TOSUS

In recent years, the features of SLE have appeared in patients receiving certain drugs. The important difference between drug-induced SLE and naturally occurring SLE is that the drug-induced symptoms usually disappear upon discontinuation of the drugs. Drugs that are associated with SLE include diphenylhydantoin, isoniazid, hydralazine, and procainamide, used for the treatment of epilepsy, tuberculosis, hypertension, and cardiac arrhythmias, respectively. Other drugs produce SLE-like syndromes less frequently. The mechanisms of induction of drug associated SLE-like syndromes are not yet fully understood. Patients with hydralazine-induced SLE may have antibodies to hydralazine as well as antibodies to native DNA. In contrast, procainamide induces antibodies to denatured DNA, presumably because of complexes of the drug and host DNA; antibodies to native DNA or to procainamide alone are not produced. Procainamide acts by stabilization of cell membranes. It may bind to erythrocyte surfaces, alter red cell membranes, and produce immunogenic membrane fragments that lead to autoantibody formation and a Coombs'-positive hemolytic anemia. Hydralazine and isoniazid may form reactive intermediate radicals that inactivate and alter DNA, producing immunogenic DNA fragments. The induction of autoantibodies or formation of drug–antibody toxic complexes results in drug-induced SLE-like syndromes; different drugs may act by different mechanisms.

TREATMENT

Treatment of SLE is generally designed to reduce both the inflammatory reaction of the disease and the amount of pathogenic antibodies. Treatment for mild or moderate manifestations of SLE include avoidance of the sun, rest, and aspirin or other nonsteroidal anti-inflammatory drugs (NSAIDs), as well as effective emotional support. Foods containing psoralens, such as celery, parsnips, figs, and parsley, as well as alfalfa sprouts, which contain L-canavanine, should be avoided. Two agents are used for life-threatening episodes: Corticosteroids and immunosuppressive drugs (azathioprine, cyclophosphamide), and in some cases, a combination of the two. The protocol used for steroid treatment calls for high initial doses (1 mg/kg/day) with tapering after 7 to 10 days when fulminant disease manifestations are controlled. Steroid therapy not only prolongs the lives of patients with severe SLE but also significantly changes the character of the syndrome. Prior to steroid therapy, patients frequently died of an acute crisis; now the disease is more protracted, and chronic renal or neurologic problems cause death. Lower doses of steroids and anti-inflammatory drugs may control symptoms in patients with less severe disease. Effective therapy reduces the acute symptoms (fever, joint pain, others) and reverses the immunologic abnormalities. The intensity of therapy depends upon the severity of the disease and the degree of response, which may vary considerably from patient to patient. Mild forms of the disease with skin lesions, but without major organ involvement, may be controlled by hydroxychloroquine (200 to

400 mg/day). Two important prognostic indicators are the severity of renal disease (a creatinine greater than 3.0 mg/dL) and the presence of antibodies to skin basement membrane (lupus band test). These are associated with a poor prognosis. Patients with acute disease that responds to steroids should have steroids withdrawn as soon as possible. The major deleterious effect of steroids is a decrease in immune defensive reactions, resulting in susceptibility to a variety of opportunistic infections (secondary immune deficiency). Although the present therapy considerably improves the prognosis and condition of patients with SLE, it is far from satisfactory. At least 90% of well-managed SLE patients have at least a ten-year survival, but over 50% of those with renal or neurologic involvement die within ten years of the onset of symptoms. Plasmapheresis does not improve the clinical outcome over standard therapy.

"LUPUS MICE"

New Zealand black (NZB) mice, F_1 hybrids of NZB mice, and some other inbred mouse strains spontaneously develop lesions similar to human SLE and serve as animal models of lupus erythematosus. The NZB inbred mouse strain was developed by Marianne Bielchowsky in New Zealand in the 1950s for cancer research. These mice were found to respond immunologically quite differently from other mouse strains. After immunization with a variety of exogenous antigens, NZB mice produce abnormally high humoral antibody responses but less intense, delayed (cellular) hypersensitivity than other mice. The "lupus" strains of mice spontaneously develop a number of immunopathologic abnormalities, including a Coombs'-positive hemolytic anemia, SLE and rheumatoid-like factors, hypergammaglobulinemia, circulating immune complexes, and glomerulonephritis. The thymi of NZB mice develop germinal centers with aging; germinal centers are not normally found in the thymus but sometimes occur in humans with myasthenia gravis. Other lupus mouse strains have atrophy of the thymic cortex. The development of these immunologic abnormalities occurs after about 4 to 6 months of age. Female mice develop more severe abnormalities than male mice, and at an earlier age.

The reason for development of "lupus" in these mice is not clearly understood but appears to depend on multiple factors, including genetically controlled tendencies to abnormally high antibody responses associated with virus infections. Multiple immune controlling factor abnormalities have been described, including polyclonal B-cell activation, decreased T-suppressor cell activity, increased T-helper cell activity, antilymphocyte antibodies, increased complement activation, and increased T-killer cell activity. A constellation of these incompletely understood factors appears to contribute to the lupus erythematosus disease syndrome in these mice.

Sjögren's Syndrome (Sicca Complex)

DESCRIPTION

Sjögren's syndrome is inflammation of the salivary glands (sialoadenitis) and lacrimal (tear) glands. This causes decreased secretions and symptoms of dry mouth and difficulty in swallowing (xerostomia) and sore eyes (keratoconjunctivitis sicca), resulting in the sensation of a sandy foreign body in the eye. The name Sjögren's syndrome pays homage to the description of nineteen women with keratoconjunctivitis sicca and xerostomia by Henrick Sjögren in 1933. Earlier descriptions of xerostomia were most likely recorded by Hadden in 1888 and keratoconjunctivitis sicca by Mikulicz in 1892. Clinically, there is swelling of the lacrimal and salivary glands. If the parotid gland alone is involved, the eponym Mikulicz's syndrome has been used. The inflammation is mononuclear with features consistent with cell-mediated immune destruction of glandular tissue. Lymphocytes and plasma cells infiltrate the salivary and lacrimal glands, and fibrosis, acinar atrophy, and proliferation of the myoepithelial cells of the ducts may lead to obstruction. In small lesions, B cells predominate, and germinal centers may be seen; in large lesions, T cells are found centrally and B cells peripherally. Similar findings may be observed in the mucosal glands of the pharynx and larynx, and the submucosal glands of the esophagus, trachea, and bronchi.

ASSOCIATIONS

Sjögren's syndrome (SS) may occur alone (primary SS) or be associated with connective tissue diseases, such as rheumatoid arthritis, systemic lupus erythematosus, or scleroderma (secondary SS). It is associated with HLA-B8 and HLA-DR3 MHC types. Precipitating and complement-fixing antibody to salivary gland tissue has been found associated with the disease, as have other serologic abnormalities, such as antinuclear antibodies (anti-Ro [SSA], 50%; Anti-La [SSB], 20%), rheumatoid factor, and antibodies to thyroglobulin. There is a close relationship between the presence of anti-Ro (SSA) antibody and the co-occurrence of Sjögren's syndrome and SLE. Patients with anti-Ro–positive SS for many years may suddenly develop SLE. On the other hand, SLE patients with anti-Ro tend to have prominent cutaneous SLE (psoriasiform cutaneous lupus) for many years and suddenly develop SS. The overlap disease tends to occur in older patients and in association with the HLA-DR3 MHC phenotype. The mechanism responsible for the clinical expression of disease in the anti-Ro(SSA) patients with SS/SLE is not known.

PATHOGENESIS

It is postulated that Sjögren's syndrome (SS) may be initiated by immune complexes in the salivary gland and the chronic disease maintained by cell-mediated immunity, similar to what occurs in the articular (joint) space in rheumatoid arthritis. The presence of antibodies to salivary ducts is associated with less cellular infiltrate in the salivary glands of patients with SS when these lesions are compared to those of patients who lack this antibody. Thus, antibody to salivary gland ducts may block cellular-mediated tissue destruction or could contribute to inflammation through an antibody-dependent cell-mediated (ADCC) mechanism. It is more likely, however, that a major component of SS or sialoadenitis in humans is caused by a toxic immune complex mechanism (vasculitis is increasingly recognized in lesions). The salivary gland normally serves as a site for production of secretory antibody responsible for local defense. In experimental autoimmune sialoadenitis, as well as in the human disease, there is substantial infiltration of the glandular tissue with plasma cells and local synthesis of large amounts of immunoglobulin with rheumatoid factor activity. Thus, the initial inflammation may be caused by immune complexes formed from antibody produced locally, and the chronic destructive inflammation maintained by cell-mediated immunity. Mononuclear inflammatory lesions have been reported in experimental animals following the injection of salivary gland tissue in complete Freund's adjuvant, but the relationship of this experimental disease to the human disease is not clear. The mononuclear infiltrate in SS may become so pronounced that the term **benign lymphoepithelial lesion** or **pseudolymphoma** has been applied. Extensive lymphoid infiltrates may also be seen in the lung, kidney, or skeletal muscle. Occasionally, these pseudolymphomas progress to frank B-cell lymphoma. The differential diagnoses of pseudolymphoma and malignant lymphoma may be very difficult, but pseudolymphomas are polyclonal and malignant lymphomas usually monoclonal.

TREATMENT

Sjögren's syndrome is usually a benign disease in which conservative treatment involving fluid replacement, such as eye drops and frequent ingestion of water, is effective. If pseudolymphoma lesions become large, immunosuppressive agents or corticosteroids may shrink them. The malignant lymphomas that develop require aggressive lymphoma therapy, depending on the location and extent of disease.

Inflammatory Myopathies (Dermatomyositis/ Polymyositis)

The inflammatory myopathies include three major disease groups: Polymyositis, dermatomyositis, and inclusion-body myositis (Table 22–8). The first case of classic dermatomyositis was reported by Wagner in 1886. The characteristic symptom of all three is muscle weakness of insidious onset. The major feature is diffuse muscle damage manifested by swelling, pain, and weakness associated with a perivascular and/or interstitial infiltrate of lymphocytes. Symptoms of this disease complex may also include an erythematous skin rash (in dermatomyositis), mild arthritis, and progressive muscular weakness, each of which may occur with a different degree of severity. The primary lesion is in muscle and consists of a degeneration of muscle fibers (myositis).

DIAGNOSIS

Four clinical or laboratory abnormalities are used to make the diagnosis and are found in most patients:

1. Progressive symmetrical muscle weakness.
2. Electromyography demonstration of short duration, small polyphasic potentials, fibrillation potentials, and bizarre, high-frequency, repetitive discharges.
3. Muscle biopsy showing muscle degeneration, mononuclear cell infiltration, and phagocytosis of muscle fibers.
4. Elevated muscle enzymes in the blood: The activity of the disease process may be followed by detection of enzymes (especially creatinine phosphokinase) released from affected muscle tissue. In addition, the characteristic dermatitis (erythematous, scaly rash on the face, neck, elbows, knees; a heliotrope periorbital discoloration; and Grotton's papules, scaly erythema-

TABLE 22–8. CHARACTERISTIC OF INFLAMMATORY MYOPATHIES

Characteristic	Dermatomyositis	Polymyositis	Inclusion-body Myositis
Age at onset	Children and adults	>18 years	>50 years
Skin rash	Yes	No	No
Pathogenic mechanism	Immune complex	T_{CTL}	T_{CTL}
Associated conditions			
Connective-tissue diseases	Scleroderma and mixed CTD	Yes	Yes, in 15% of cases
Systemic autoimmune diseases	Infrequently	Frequently	Infrequently
Malignant conditions	Sometimes	No	No
Viruses	Not clear	HIV, HTLV-I	Not clear
Parasites, bacteria	No	Yes (protozoa, nematodes, etc.)	No
Drugs	Yes (penicillamine, tryptophan)	Yes	Yes
Familial	No	No	Yes, in some cases

Modified from Dalakas MC: Polymyositis, dermatomyositis and inclusion-body myositis. N Engl J Med 325:1487, 1991.

tous flat plaques over the dorsum of the hands) are seen in dermatomyositis. In general, a poor prognosis is indicated by older age, an associated malignancy, and involvement of respiratory muscles.

PATHOGENESIS

The pathogenesis of dermatomyositis is due to activation of complement by the immune complex mechanisms, whereas that of polymyositis and inclusion-body myositis is destruction of muscle by cytotoxic T cells. In dermatomyositis, the inflammatory lesions are predominantly perivascular and are predominantly B cells and CD4+ T cells. Complement deposits in the capillaries is the earliest and most specific lesion and precedes mononuclear cell infiltration, and destruction of muscle occurs by microinfarction. In contrast, the cellular infiltrate of polymyositis and inclusion-body myositis are primarily in the connective tissue fascicles surrounding individual muscle fibers (not perivascular), and the predominant cell infiltrate is CD8+. Destruction of individual muscle fibers is by the action of T_{CTL} cells. There is increased expression of class I MHC, which is recognized by T_{CTL} cells, further supporting the pathogenic role of cytotoxic lymphocytes. Inclusion-body myositis also features granular inclusions containing whorls of membranes, which are dissolved by the usual process of paraffin embedding. An experimental disease—experimental allergic myositis with features similar to polymyositis—may be produced in animals by immunization with xenogeneic muscle tissue in complete Freund's adjuvant.

AUTO-ANTIBODIES

A number of antinuclear and anticytoplasmic autoantibodies have been found in myositis patients. However, there is no consistent pattern that permits them to be used for diagnosis, and their role in pathogenesis is doubtful. One antibody, JO-1, directed against histidyl-tRNA synthetase is found in 50% of patients with lung involvement (see Table 22–4).

THERAPY

The disease frequently has remissions and exacerbations, but the natural course is progressive. Corticosteroid therapy provides effective relief, and death from progressive muscular weakness producing respiratory failure occurs rarely. Nonsteroidal immunosuppressive drugs (cyclophosphamide, cyclosporine) have been reported to induce remissions in some steroid-resistant cases, but the response is generally disappointing.

SHULMAN'S SYNDROME

Shulman's syndrome (diffuse fascitis with eosinophilia) is a very rare disease consisting of diffuse fascitis of rapid onset, hypergammaglobulinemia, and eosinophilia associated with scleroderma-like lesions with firm, taut skin and flex in contractures. There is often a dramatic response to prednisone therapy. There is an absence of Raynaud's phenomena or visceral involvement but immune-mediated aplastic anemia and/or thrombocytopenia may occur. Immunoglobulin and C3 are localized in the affected fascia.

Mixed Connective Tissue Disease/ Overlap Syndromes

In 1972, G.C. Sharp described a syndrome characterized by features of different rheumatic diseases that has been designated mixed connective tissue disease, now also referred to as "overlap syndromes." These patients have a variety of the clinical features of connective tissue diseases, which overlap with systemic lupus erythematosus. Thus, patients with SLE may develop features of dermatomyositis, rheumatoid arthritis, and scleroderma, including arthritis and arthralgia, Raynaud's phenomena, myositis, serositis, splenomegaly, anemia, leukopenia, hyperglobulinemia, and glomerulonephritis. As mentioned above, a group of Sjögren's syndrome patients will develop SLE and a group of SLE patients will develop Sjögren's syndrome. In addition, patients with SLE may manifest multiple sclerosis, autoimmune thyroiditis, autoimmune hemolytic anemia, and diabetes mellitus. The mixed connective tissue disease group is defined by a very high speckled antinuclear antibody (ANA) titer and antibodies to ribonuclear protein (RNP). However, there are patients with similar symptoms who lack this finding. Another way of looking at these groups is that they appear to be part of the overall spectrum of SLE.

Thrombotic Micro- angiopathies

This group of syndromes, while not included in the connective tissue (CT) disease group, has vascular lesions that must be differentiated from CT lesions. The thrombotic microangiopathies include hemolytic-uremic syndrome (HUS), thrombocytopenic purpura (TTP), and peripartum HUS. The disorders are mainly secondary to thrombocytopenia (deceased number of blood platelets) and include hemolytic anemia, hemorrhagic skin lesions (purpura), and central nervous system signs and symptoms secondary to thrombosis. TTP usually occurs in adults and has a high mortality rate if not treated, whereas HUS occurs in young children and postpartum women, is usually self-limiting, and features renal failure, which is rare in TTP. Autopsy of TTP patients reveals widespread thrombotic occlusion of arterioles and capillaries by hyaline masses that are usually located beneath the endothelium. The central nervous system symptoms are presumably due to microvascular occlusions. The anemia is microangiopathic—secondary to mechanical destruction of erythrocytes by physical trauma of contact with the altered vascular walls. The etiology of the vascular lesions is unknown, but they may be caused by a form of toxic complex or autoantibody deposits leading to focal fibrinoid necroses and hyaline scarring or by activation of the clotting mechanism by toxic complexes.

Summary

Connective-tissue (collagen-vascular) diseases represent a number of diseases believed to be caused by autoantibodies and mediated primarily by immune complex mechanisms, but chronic progressive diseases are driven by cell-mediated immunity. These diseases are polyarteritis nodosa, rheumatoid arthritis, systemic lupus erythematosus, Sjögren's syndrome, dermatomyositis, and progressive systemic sclerosis (scleroderma). The shared lesions include fibrinoid necrosis, glomerulonephritis, and vasculitis. Other immune effector mechanisms (neutralization, cytotoxic and granulomatous reactions) play a pathogenic role in some lesions seen in these diseases, but most of the major acute manifestations are due to immune complex reactions and chronic stages caused by cell-mediated immunity. The etiology of these diseases is not known. Most hypotheses include the possibility of a genetically determined immune reaction to some infectious agent, but none has been clearly identified. There is clear evidence of inherited tendencies and HLA association in the case of rheumatoid arthritis and SLE. The symptoms may be quite variable with many very mild limited cases but, unfortunately, also many severe life-threatening ones. Fulminate manifestations may be controlled by antiinflammatory drugs or steroids, but chronic progression is usual in severe cases.

Bibliography

GENERAL

Benedek TG: A century of American rheumatology. *Ann Int Med* 106:304, 1987.
Bigazzi PR, Reichlin M: *Systemic Autoimmunity*. New York, Marcel Dekker, 1991.
Bland EF: Rheumatic fever: the way it was. *Circulation* 76:1190, 1987.
Farid NR: *The Immunogenetics of Autoimmune Diseases*. Boca Raton, FL, CRC Press, 1990.
Klemperer P: The concept of collagen diseases in medicine. *Am Rev Resp Dis* 83:331, 1961.
Klemperer P, Pollack AD, Baehr G: Diffuse collagen disease: Acute disseminated lupus erythematosus and diffuse scleroderma. *JAMA* 119:331, 1942.

POLYARTERITIS NODOSA

Alarcon-Segovia D, Brown AL: Classification and etiologic aspects of necrotizing antigitides: An analytical approach to a confused subject with a critical review of the evidence for hypersensitivity in polyarteritis nodosa. *Mayo Clin Proc* 39:205, 1964.

Gocke DJ, Hsu K, Morgan C, et al.: Association between polyarteritis and Australia antigen. *Lancet* 2:1149, 1970.

Kussmaul A, Maier R: Ueber eine bisher nicht beschriebene eigenthumliche Arterienerkrankung (periarteritis nodosa), die mit Morbus Brightii and rapid fortschreitender allgemeiner Muskellahmung einhergeht. *Dtsch Arch Klin Med* 1:484, 1866.

Mackel SE: Treatment of vasculitis. *Med Clin N Am* 66:941, 1982.

McCombs RP: Systemic "allergic" vasculitis: Clinical and pathological relationships. *JAMA* 194:1059, 1965.

Moskowitz RW, Baggenstoss AH, Slocumb CH: Histopathologic classification of periarteritis nodosa: A study of 56 cases confirmed of at autopsy. *Proc Mayo Clin* 38:345, 1963.

Phanuphak P, Kohler PF: Onset of polyarteritis nodosa during allergic hypersensitization treatment. *Am J Med* 68:479, 1980.

Rich AR, Gregory JE: The experimental demonstration that polyarteritis nodosa is a manifestation of hypersensitivity. *Johns Hopkins Med J* 72:63, 1943.

Rose GA, Spencer H: Polyarteritis nodosa. *Quart J Med* 26:43, 1957.

Trepo CG, Thivolet J, Prince AM: Australia antigen and polyarteritis nodosa. *Am J Dis Child* 123, 390, 1972.

RHEUMATOID ARTHRITIS

Arnett FC: Immunogenetics and arthritis. In *Arthritis and Allied Conditions*. McCarty DJ (ed.). Lea & Febiger, Philadelphia, 1986, 405.

Arnett FC, Edworthy SM, Bloch DA, et al.: The American Rheumatism Association: 1987 revised criteria for rheumatoid arthritis. *Arthritis Rheum* 31:315, 1988.

Bellamy N: Prognosis in rheumatoid arthritis. *J Rheumatol* 18:1277, 1991.

Brennan FM, Londei M, Jackson AM, et al.: T cells expressing γ/δ chain receptors in rheumatoid arthritis. *J Autoimmun* 1:319, 1988.

Chin JE, Winterrowd GE, Krzesicki RF, et al.: Role of cytokines in inflammatory synovitis: The coordinate regulation of intercellular adhesion molecule-1 and HLA class I and II antigens in rheumatoid synovial fibroblasts. *Arth Rheum* 33:1776, 1990.

Dayer JM, Graham R, Russel G, et al.: Collagenase production by rheumatoid synovial cells: Stimulation by a human lymphocyte factor. *Science* 195:181, 1977.

Dinther-Jannsen ACHM, Kraal G, Soesbergen RM, et al.: Immunohistological and functional analysis of adhesion molecule expression in the rheumatoid synovial lining layer. Implications for synovial lining cell destruction. *J Rheumatol* 21:1998–2004, 1994.

Felson DT, Anderson JJ, Boers M, et al.: The American College of Rheumatology preliminary core set of disease activity measures for rheumatoid arthritis clinical trials. *Arch Rheum* 36:729–740, 1993.

Furst DE, Weinblatt ME: *Immunomodulators in the Rheumatic Diseases*. New York, Marcel Dekker, 1990.

Gregerson PK, Silver J, Winchester RJ: The shared epitope hypothesis: An approach to understanding the molecular genetics of susceptibility to rheumatoid arthritis. *Arch Rheum* 30:1205, 1987.

Hammer RE, Maika SD, Richardson JA, et al.: Spontaneous inflammatory disease in transgenic rats expressing the HLA-B27 and human $\beta_2 m$: an animal model of HLA-B27-associated human disorders. *Cell* 53:1099, 1990.

Hay EM: Rieter's syndrome and reactive arthritis. *Brit J Rheumatol* 30:474, 1991.

Hill AV, Allsopp CE, Kwaitkowski D: HLA class typing by PCR: HLA-B27 and an African B27 subtype. *Lancet* 337:640-642, 1991.

Inman RD: Arthritis and enteritis: An interface of protean manifestations. *J Rheumatol* 14:406, 1987.

Jacobs MR, Haynes BF: Increase in $TCR_{\gamma\delta+}$ lymphocytes in synovia from rheumatoid arthritis patients with active synovitis. *J Clin Immunol* 12:130, 1992.

Jalkanen S, Steere AC, Fox RI, et al. A district endothelial cell recognition system that controls lymphocyte traffic into inflamed synovium. *Science* 233:556, 1986.

Keffer J, Probert L, Cazlaris H, et al.: Transgenic mice expressing human tumor necrosis factor: A predictive genetic model of arthritis. *EMBO J* 10:4025, 1991.

Kremer JM, Phelps CT: Long-term prospective study of the use of methotrexate in the treatment of rheumatoid arthritis. *Arth Rheum* 35:138, 1992.

Kurosaka M, Ziff M: Immunoelectron microscopic study of the distribution of T-cell subsets in rheumatoid synovium. *J Exp Med* 158:1191, 1983.

Lipsky PE, Davis LS, Cush JJ, et al.: The role of cytokines in the pathogenesis of rheumatoid arthritis. *Springer Semin Immunopathol* 11:123, 1989.

Mellbye OJ, Forre O, Mollnes TE, et al.: Immunopathology of subcutaneous rheumatoid nodules. *Ann Rheumat Dis* 50:909, 1991.

Mertens AV, de Clerck LS, Moens MM: Lymphocyte activation status, expression of adhesion molecules and adhesion to human endothelium in rheumatoid arthritis. *Res Immunol* 145:101–108, 1994.

Mizel S, Dayer JM, Krane SM, et al.: Stimulation of rheumatoid synovial cell collagenase and prostaglandin production by partially purified lymphocyte-activating factor (interleukin-1). *Proc Nat Acad Sci* 78:2474, 1981.

Moore TL, Dorner RW: Rheumatoid factors. *Clin Biochem* 26:75–84, 1993.

Mooreland LW, Heck LW, Sullivan W, et al.: New approaches to the therapy of autoimmune diseases: Rheumatoid arthritis as a paradigm. *Am J Med Sci* 395: 40–51, 1993.

Pincus T, Wolfe F: Treatment of rheumatoid arthritis: Challenges to traditional paradigms. *Ann Int Med* 115:825, 1991.

Rosenbaum JT: Acute anterior uveitis and spondyloarthropathies. *Rheumat Dis Clin N Am* 18:142, 1992.

Rothschild BM, Woods RJ: Symmetrical erosive disease in archaic Indians: The origin of rheumatoid arthritis in the new world. *Semin Arth Rheum* 19:278, 1990.

Scofield RH, Warren WL, Koelsch G, et al.: A hypothesis for the HLA-B27 immune dysregulation in spondyloarthropathy: Contributions from enteric organisms, B27 structure, peptides bound by B27, and convergent evolution. *Proc Natl Acad Sci USA* 90:9330–9334, 1993.

Short CL, Bauer W, Reynolds WE: *Rheumatoid Arthritis*. Cambridge, MA, Harvard University Press, 1957.

Starkebaum G: Review of rheumatoid arthritis: Recent developments. *Immunol Allergy Clin N Am* 13:273–289, 1993.

Vaughn JH: Pathogenic concepts and origins of rheumatoid factor in rheumatoid arthritis. *Arth Rheum* 36:1–6, 1993.

Wicks I, McColl G, Harrison L: New perspectives on rheumatoid arthritis. *Immunol Today* 15:533–556, 1994.

Williams RC: Rheumatoid factors: Historical perspective, origins, and possible role in disease. *J Rheumatology* 19(suppl. 32):42, 1992.

Wilske KR, Healy LA: Challenging the therapeutic pyramid: A new look at treatment strategies for rheumatoid arthritis. *J Rheumatol* 17(suppl. 25):4, 1990.

Yu DT, Choo SY, Schaack T: Molecular mimicry in HLA-B27-related arthritis. *Ann Int Med* 111:1182, 1989.

Ziff M: Emigration of lymphocytes in rheumatoid synovitis. *Adv Inflam Res* 12:1, 1987.

Zvaifler NJ: Immunoreactants in rheumatoid synovial fluid. *J Exp Med* 134:2765, 1971.

Zvailfer NJ: Rheumatoid synovitis. An extravascular immune complex disease. *Arth Rheum* 17:297, 1974.

SYSTEMIC LUPUS ERYTHEMATOSUS

Arnett FC: HLA and genetic predisposition to lupus erythematosus and other dermatologic dermatologic disorders. *J Am Acad Dermatol* 13:472, 1985.

Asherson RA, Hughes GRV: The expanding spectrum of Libman Sacks endocarditis: The role of antiphospholipid antibodies. *Clin Exp Rheumat* 7:225, 1989.

Baart de la Faille H: Lupus therapy. *Clin Investig* 72:749–753, 1994.

Bick RL: The antiphospholipid-thrombosis syndromes. *Am J Clin Pathol* 100: 477–480, 1993.

Blomgren SE: Drug-induced lupus erythematosus. *Semin Hematol* 10:345, 1973.

Bluestein HG, Zvaifler NJ: Brain-reactive lymphocytotoxic antibodies in the serum of patients with systemic lupus erythematosus. *J Clin Invest* 57:509, 1976.

Cheatum DE, Hurd ER, Strunk SW, et al.: Renal histology and clinical course of systemic lupus erythematosus: A prospective study. *Arth Rheumat* 16:670, 1973.

David-Bejar KM: Subacute cutaneous lupus erythematosus. *J Invest Dermatol* 100:2S–8S, 1993.

Deng J-S, Bair LW, Shen-Schwarz S, et al.: Localization of Ro (SS-A) antigen in the cardiac conduction system. *Arth Rheumat* 30:1232, 1987.

Foster MH, Cizman B, Madio MP: Nephritogenic autoantibodies in systemic lupus erythematosus: Immunochemical properties, mechanisms of immune deposition, and genetic origins. *Lab Investig* 69:494–507, 1993.

Freese E, Sklarow S, Freeze EB: DNA damage caused by antidepressive hydrazines and related drugs. *Mutat Res* 5:343, 1968.

Gilliam JN, Cheatum DE, Hurd ER, et al.: Immunoglobulin in clinically uninvolved skin in systemic lupus erythematosus: Association with renal disease. *J Clin Invest* 53:1434, 1974.

Gourley MF: Systemic lupus erythematosus: Disease management. *Springer Semin Immunopathol* 16:281–294, 1994.

Hahn BH, Sharp GC, Irwin WS, et al.: Immune responses to hydralazine and nuclear antigens in hydralazine-induced lupus erythematosus. *Ann Intern Med* 76:365, 1972.

Hargraves MM, Richmond H, Morton R: Presentation of two bone marrow elements: The "tart" cell and the "LE" cell. *Mayo Clin Proc* 23:25, 1948.

Harley JB, Scofield RH: Systemic lupus erythematosis: RNA-protein autoantigens, models of disease of disease heterogeneity, and theories of etiology. *J Clin Immunol* 11:297, 1991.

Harvey AM, Shulman LE, Tummey A, et al.: Systemic lupus erythematosus: Review of the literature and analysis of 138 cases. *Medicine* 33:291–437, 1954.

Hughes GRV, Asherson RS, Khamashta MA: Antiphospholipid syndrome: Linking many specialties. *Ann Rheum Dis* 48:355, 1989.

Kalden JR, Hermann M: Autoimmune diseases in humans, eg, autoimmune rheumatic diseases. *Intervirology* 35:176–185, 1993.

Kalden JR, Winkler TH, Herrman M, et al.: Pathogenesis of SLE: Immunopathology in man. *Rheumatol Int* 11:95, 1991.

Koffler D, Schur PH, Kunkel HG: Immunological studies concerning the nephritis of systemic lupus erythematosus. *J Exp Med* 126:607, 1967.

Lampert PW, Oldstone MBA: Host immunoglobulin G and complement deposits in the choroid plexis during spontaneous immune complex disease. *Science* 180:408, 1973.

Lord PCW, Rothschild CB, DeRose RT, et al.: Human cytomegalovirus RNAs immunoprecipitated by multiple systemic lupus erythematosus antisera. *J Gen Virol* 70:2383, 1989.

Luciano A, Rothfield NF: Patterns of nuclear fluorescence and DNA-binding activity. *Ann Rheum Dis* 32:337, 1973.

McCurdy DK, Bick M, Gatti RA, et al.: Autoantibodies in systemic lupus erythematosus. *Dis Markers* 10:37–49, 1992.

McNeil HP, Chesterman CD, Krilis SA: Immunology and clinical importance of antiphospholipid antibodies. *Adv Immunol* 46:193, 1991.

Ray E, Brezis M, Rosenmann E, Eliat D: Anti-DNA antibodies bind directly to renal antigens and induce kidney dysfunction in the isolated perfused rat kidney. *J Immunol* 142:3076, 1989.

Siegel M, Lee SL, Peress NS: The epidemiology of drug-induced systemic lupus erythematosus. *Arth Rheumat* 10:407, 1967.

Steinberg AD: Concepts of pathogenesis of systemic lupus erythematosus. *Clin Immunol Immunopathol* 63:19, 1992.

Tan EM, Chan EKL, Sullivan KF, et al.: Antinuclear antibodies (ANAs): Diagnostically specific immune markers and clues toward the understanding of systemic autoimmunity. *Clin Immunol Immunopathol* 47:121, 1988.

Tan EM, Cohen AS, Fries JF, et al.: 1982 revised critical for classification of systemic lupus erythematosus. *Arth Rheumat* 25:1271, 1982.

Triplett DA: Antiphospholipid antibodies: Proposed mechanisms of action. *Am J Repro Immunol* 28:211–215, 1992.

Winfield JB, Mimura T: Pathogenic significance of antilymphocyte autoantibodies in systemic lupus erythematosus. *Clin Immunol Immunopathol* 63:13, 1992.

SJÖGREN'S SYNDROME

Adamson TC: Immunologic analysis of lymphoid infiltrates in primary Sjögren's syndrome using monoclonal antibodies. *J Immunol* 130:203, 1983.

Anderson LG, Cummings NA, Asofsky R, et al.: Salivary gland immunoglobulin and rheumatoid factor synthesis in Sjögren's syndrome: Natural history and response to treatment. *Am J Med* 53:456, 1972.

Anderson LG, Talal N: The spectrum of benign to malignant lymphoproliferation in Sjögren's syndrome. *Clin Exp Immunol* 9:199, 1971.

Anderson LG, Tarpley TM, Talal N, et al.: Cellular-versus-humoral autoimmune responses to salivary gland in Sjögren's syndrome. *Clin Exp Immunol* 13:335, 1973.

Hadden WB: On "dry mouth," or suppression of the salivary buccal secretions. *Trans Clin Soc Hand* 21:176, 1888.

Mikulicz J: Concerning a peculiar symmetrical disease of the lacrimal and salivary glands (original published in 1892). In *Medical Classics*. Baltimore, Williams & Wilkins, 1937, vol. 2, 137–186.

Provost TT, Talal N, Harley JB, et al.: The relationship between anti-Ro (SS-A) antibody-positive Sjögren's syndrome and anti-Ro (SS-A) antibody-positive lupus erythematosus. *Arch Dermatol* 124:63, 1988.

Sjögren H: Zur Kenntnis der keratoconjunctivitis sicca (keratitis filiformus bee hypofunction der tranendrusen. *Acta Ophthalmol* 11:1, 1933.

DERMATO-MYOSITIS

Bohan A, Peter JB: Polymyositis and dermatomyositis. *N Engl J Med* 292:344, 403, 1975.

Dalakas MC: Polymyositis, dermatomyositis, and inclusion-body myositis. *N Engl J Med* 325:1487, 1991.

Dawkins RL: Experimental myositis associated with hypersensitivity to muscle. *J Pathol Bacteriol* 90:619, 1965.

Kissel JT, Mendell JR, Rammohan KW: Microvascular deposition of complement membrane attack complex in dermatomyositis. *New Engl J Med* 314:331, 1986.

Mastaglia FL, Ojeda VJ: Inflammatory myopathies. *Ann Neurol* 17:215, 317, 1985.

Salmeron G, Greenberg D, Lidsky MD: Polymyositis and diffuse interstitial lung disease: A review of the pulmonary histopathologic findings. *Arch Intern Med* 141:1005, 1981.

Wagner E: Ein Fall von acuter Polymyositis. *Dtsch Arch Klin Med* 11:241, 1886.

PROGRESSIVE SYSTEMIC SCLEROSIS (SCLERO-DERMA)

Brautbar N, Vojdani A, Campbell AW: Silicone implants and systemic immunological disease: Review of the literature and preliminary results. *Toxicol Indust Health* 8:231–237, 1992.

Cathcart MK, Krakauer RS: Immunologic enhancement of collagen accumulation in progressive systemic sclerosis. *Clin Immunol Immunopathol* 21:128, 1981.

Claman HN, Jafee BD, Huff JC, et al.: Chronic graft-versus-host disease as a model for scleroderma. *Cell Immunol* 94:73, 1985.

Feghali CA, Bost KL, Boulware DW, et al.: Mechanisms of pathogenesis in scleroderma. I. Overproduction of interleukin-6 by fibroblasts cultured from affected skin sites of patients with scleroderma. *J Rheumatol* 19:1207, 1992.

LeRoy EC, Black C, Fleischeajer R, et al.: Scleroderma (systemic sclerosis): Classification, subsets, and pathogenesis. *J Rheumatol* 15:202, 1988.

Meehan R, Spencer R: Systemic sclerosis. *Immunol Allergy Clin N Am* 13:313–334, 1993.

Sollberg S, Peltonen J, Uitto J, et al.: Elevated expression of β_1 and β_2 integrins, intercellular adhesion molecule-1, and endothelial leukocyte adhesion molecule-1 in the skin of patients with systemic sclerosis of recent onset. *Arth Rheum* 35:290, 1992.

Stastny P, Stembridge VA, Vischer T, et al.: Homologous disease in the adult rat, a model for autoimmune disease. I. General features and cutaneous lesions. *J Exp Med* 118:635, 1963.

Tuffanelli DL, Winkelman RK: Systemic scleroderma: A clinical study of 727 cases. *Arch Dermatol* 84:359, 1961.

MIXED CONNECTIVE TISSUE DISEASE

Alarcon-Segovia D: Mixed connective tissue disease: A decade of growing pains. *J Rheumatol* 8:535, 1981.

Sharp GC, Irvin WS, Tan EM, et al.: Mixed connective tissue disease: An apparently distinct rheumatic disease syndrome associated with a specific antibody to an extractable nuclear antigen. *Am J Med* 52:148, 1972.

Smolen JS, Chused TM, Leiserson WM, et al.: T cell subsets in systemic lupus erythematosus (SLE): Correlation with clinical features. *Am J Med* 289:139, 1985.

THROMBOTIC THROMBO-CYTOPENIA PURPURA

Antes EH: Thrombotic thrombocytopenic purpura: A review of the literature with a report of a case. *Ann Intern Med* 48:512, 1958.

Brain MC, Neame PB: Thrombotic thrombocytopenic purpura and the hemolytic-uremic syndrome. *Semin Thromb Hemost* 8:186, 1983.

Breckenridge RT, Moore RD, Ratnoff OD: A study of thrombocytopenia: New histologic critical for the differentiation of idiopathic thrombocytopenia and thrombocytopenia associated with disseminated lupus erythematosus. *Blood* 30:39, 1967.

23

Transplantation

Introduction

The replacement of the lost function of a diseased organ by transplantation of a healthy organ from one individual to another has been considered as a possibility for many years but in practice has become clinically useful only during the last 30 years (Table 23–1). Now transplantation can be used to supply a missing gene, as well as to replace a diseased organ. Transplantation of a number of solid organs, including kidney, liver, heart, and lung; sheets of skin; and cell suspensions, such as bone marrow, pancreatic islet cells, and fetal brain cells has met with different levels of clinical success. The practical obstacles to transplantation are the availability of donor organs and the cost. A national system of organ procurement has been established but still falls short of meeting the needs of identified recipients. The expense of organ transplantation adds greatly to the national health costs. In 1992, the costs of an individual organ transplant at a Houston hospital with a major transplant service were: $55,000 (kidney); $163,000 (heart), plus $30,000 for the first year follow-up; and $234,000 for liver (*The Houston Post*, December 30, 1992). The number of solid organ transplantations has increased 262% during the last ten years. This increase is driven both by the improved clinical success and by the willingness of third-party payers to reimburse hospitals and physicians for these services. As a result, more transplant centers are created and supply exceeds demand. The main biologic obstacle to successful transplantation is control of immune rejection of the transplanted organ or cells and prevention of infections. This requires extensive follow-up of transplant patients, involving hundreds of hours of professional care and hundreds of laboratory tests.

TABLE 23–1. A BRIEF HISTORY OF CLINICAL TRANSPLANTATION

1942	Skin grafts in war casualties
1954	First kidney transplant in identical twins
1962	First successful kidney transplant in unrelated individuals
1965–75	Discovery of HLA system and development of tissue typing
1975	25,000 kidney transplants worldwide
1978	Introduction of cyclosporine
1981	4,885 kidney, 62 heart, and 26 liver transplants
1987	8,967 kidney, 1,512 heart, and 1,182 liver transplants

Graft Rejection

Graft rejection is principally determined by differences in the histocompatibility antigens between the donor and the recipient, mainly antigens of the major histocompatibility complex. The genetics of the HLA system are covered in Chapter 5. Control of the rejection reaction is accomplished by matching donor and recipient, as well as by immunosuppressive treatment of the recipient. Immunosuppression is covered in Chapter 28. Complications of immunosuppression include drug toxicity, opportunistic infections, and increased rates of neoplasia, particularly lymphomas. Thus, clinical deterioration of a patient with a tissue graft may be due to rejection, infection, neoplasia, or failure of the transplanted tissue. In this chapter, the immune aspects of transplantation will be emphasized.

SENSITIZATION

The mechanism of delivery of immunogenic tissue antigens that sensitize recipients to graft antigens remains incompletely understood. Immunogens for skin, as well as other solid organ grafts, may be provided by delivery of antigen to draining lymph nodes, by migration of antigen-presenting macrophages (such as Langerhans' cells of the skin) or by "passenger lymphocytes." Passenger lymphocytes are lymphocytes in the grafted tissue that migrate to draining lymph nodes where they provide a strong immunogenic signal. On the other hand, class I MHC antigen-containing cells in solid organs, such as hepatocytes or activated epithelial cells, are also strongly immunogenic and are able to stimulate alloreactive T_{CTL} cells directly without exogenous antigen processing (endogenous antigen processing).

GRAFT ADAPTATION

Graft adaptation refers to the concept first reported by Woodruff that "transplants become less vulnerable to rejection as time goes on, and after a certain critical period, are capable of surviving in the face of a high degree of immunity in the recipient, which they would not have been able to withstand earlier in their life history." When treatment of immunosuppressed mice that have skin grafts surviving for up to 30 days is discontinued, the graft may still survive, whereas a second graft from the same donor will be rejected after 10 to 12 days. The mechanism of graft adaptation is not well understood. It may be that passenger lymphocytes responsible for rejection have been depleted in the prolonged graft or that vascularization of the graft with recipient endothelial cells provides a barrier to sensitized cells.

GRAFT FACILITATION

Graft facilitation is prolonged graft survival mediated by humoral antibody that blocks cell-mediated immunity (CMI). This paradoxical situation was first recognized in the 1930s, when it was noted that prior immunization to tumor tissue might increase the incidence and growth of tumors in allogeneic recipients that otherwise would regard the tumor as a foreign graft. This phenomenon was termed **tumor enhancement** (see Chapter 30). Later, it was noted that grafts of normal tissues would survive longer if the animal was preimmunized to produce circulating humoral antibody to allograft antigens rather than CMI, or if humoral antibody was passively transferred to the recipient. This effect was termed **graft facilitation**. The enhancement/facilitation effect may suppress other effects of CMI, such as graft-versus-host reactions, rejection of fetal tissues by the mother, and autoimmune diseases.

The enhancement/facilitation effect of antibody interferes with a potential rejection reaction mediated by sensitized cells. The process of graft rejection may be divided into three phases: Afferent, central, and efferent. Afferent refers to the delivery of antigen to the immune cells recognizing it; central refers to antigen processing and immunization, culminating in production of specifically sensitized cells; and efferent refers to the delivery of the sensitized cells to the target tissue, the reaction of those cells with target cell antigens, and destruction of the target cell by the sensitized killer cells. At present it is impossible to select one mechanism as the most important; it is likely that more than one mechanism is operative in a given situation. In particular, blocking antibodies may mask antigenic sites so that they are not available to recognition cells (afferent effect) or to effector cells (efferent effect). Interference with effector cells by masking of target cell antigens is supported by the finding that humoral antibody to a target cell may block immune attack by T_{CTL}s *in vitro*. In addition, blocking antibodies or complexes of blocking antibodies and antigen, may react directly with reacting or sensitized cells to block either the induction or expression of CMI.

The Major Histocompatibility Complex (MHC) and Tissue Transplantation

Historically, the major importance of identification of the products of the MHC involved their role in human tissue transplantation. Transplants between identical twins are not rejected, whereas rejection occurs where there are differences at the MHC. Tissue grafts from one genetically different individual to another (allografts) require suppression of the immune response if graft is to survive. Delineation of the role of MHC molecules in antigen processing has focused broader attention on the immune function of MHC molecules (see Chapter 5).

DONOR RECIPIENT MATCHING IN HUMAN TRANSPLAN-TATION

Graft survival in humans is related to the degree of histocompatibility differences between donor and recipient. Better tissue matching of recipient and donor combined with less vigorous immunosuppression is considered to be the best practical approach to prolong transplant survival. Extensive serologic testing is now done in attempts to match donor and recipient histocompatibility antigens. Specific molecular probes for DNA sequences of the MHC and development of technology for applying high-resolution genetic fingerprinting techniques to tissue typing give promise to improve donor–recipient matching in the future. Perhaps each individual will be typed at birth and this information used not only in transplant programs but also for legal identification. However, since it is now clear that the transplantation antigen recognized by T cells are not the MHC surface molecules themselves, but endogenous peptides located in the antigen-presenting groove of the MHC, a different tissue typing approach directed to identification of allotypes of these peptides, may provide more definitive tissue typing information.

Histo-compatibility Antigens

Histocompatibility antigens are those cellular determinants specific for each individual of a species that are responsible for immune rejection when attempts are made to transfer or transplant cellular material from one individual of the same species to another. Identical twins are the only known human individuals who share all histocompatibility antigens. The chances for an identical match in related individuals who are not identical twins is estimated to be 1 in 50,000. Perhaps the most familiar example of histocompatibility antigens is the ABO blood group system. The A and B antigens are found not only on erythrocytes but also on other tissue cells. Therefore, no attempt to transfer solid organs from one individual to another should be made across a known AB blood group difference. However, other histocompatibility antigens are obviously important, because matching of the ABO or other erythrocyte antigen systems between donor and recipient is not enough to provide a compatible relation.

During the 1960s, many attempts were made to develop tests for histocompatibility antigens and matching tests for potential donors and recipients. Tests that have been used to select organ donors include the mixed lymphocyte culture reaction (MLR) and the analysis and matching of histocompatibility antigens by serologic tests. The in vitro systems are not only useful for matching donors and recipients of grafts but provide a means of evaluating immunologic recognition and its significance.

Mixed Lymphocyte Reactions (MLRs). MLRs occur in cultures of mixtures of lymphocytes from two genetically different individuals. DNA synthesis and proliferation of the lymphocytes is stimulated by their interaction. The MLR is of historic interest. It is no longer used clinically for tissue matching but has contributed greatly to our understanding of the interactions of genetically different lymphocyte populations. The degree of stimulation in an MLR correlates to the degree of histocompatibility difference between the lymphocyte donors. This is a two-way test (a crossmatch test), because the lymphocytes of each donor interact with each other. The test can be made one-way by preventing the response of one set of lymphocytes of the organ donors by treatment with radiation or an antimetabolite, such as mitomycin C (one-way MLR). This gives an estimate of the rejection response of a potential recipient (living cells) against the cells of a potential organ donor (the treated cells). Stimulation is measured by an increase in DNA synthesis occurring 5 to 7 days after interaction in culture that is not seen when the cells of only one individual are cultured (control). The ability to store lymphocytes in vitro in liquid nitrogen freezers permits tissue typing even when a given donor is no longer living.

Although it was first suspected that MLR reactions depended upon the class I MHC antigens defined by humoral antibodies (see below), it is now known that extent of DNA synthesis in a mixed lymphocyte reaction is mostly dependent upon the class II gene products. The cell that responds in the MLR is a T_{DTH} cell that responds by proliferation and secretion of lymphokines. The stimulator cell containing the class II MHC antigens to which the responding T_{DTH} cell reacts is a macrophage or B cell. The class I specificities may stimulate mixed lymphocyte reactions weakly or increase the extent of class II-induced reactions, but for practical purposes, MLRs are caused by class II differences. A second aspect of the mixed lymphocyte reaction is the generation of T_{CTL} cells that react specifically with the class I region markers of the stimulator cells. These cells are generated from CD8+ precursor cells; the T_{DTH} cells that proliferate in the mixed lymphocyte reaction are CD4+. Thus, CD8+ T_{CTL} killing is directed to class I MHC markers; CD4+ T_{DTH} MLR proliferation response to class II MHC products. T_{CTL} cells appear later after initiation of MLR than does the proliferation of T_{DTH} cells as a result of the interaction of T_{CTL} precursors with class I MHC antigens and effects of lymphokines released from CD4+ T_{DTH} cells on CD8+T_{CTLs}.

Serologically Defined Histocompatibility Tests. The identification of histocompatibility antigens for tissue matching in the laboratory depends upon the serologic (antibody-mediated) recognition of MHC products on lymphocytes. Class I MHC are shared by lymphocytes and solid tissue; class II MHC are on macrophages, B cells, and some activated epithelial cells, but not on most epithelial cells. The identification of a given antigen on a lymphocyte can be determined by the ability of an antiserum to react with the antigen, activating complement and causing the death of the lymphocytes.

Alloantisera that reacted with lymphocytes were recognized as long as 60 years ago, but the significance of such antibodies in regard to histocompatibility was not readily apparent. Antibodies in human sera to human lymphocytes are found in patients with certain diseases, such as lupus erythematosus, in multiparous women and in patients receiving multiple blood transfusions. In retrospect, these latter situations were due to genetically controlled differences in MHC specificities among human individuals (allotypy). In the 1950s, the reaction patterns of such antisera with lymphocytes from a number of different individuals were first realized. For instance, some antisera reacted with lymphocytes from essentially the same donors in a panel (eg, twenty of fifty donors), whereas other antisera reacted with the lymphocytes of different donors. The reaction patterns observed were extremely complicated and, it seemed, unresolvable. However, in the early 1960s, Van Rood introduced computer analysis of the reaction patterns, a method that was soon adopted by others. This resulted in resolution of the reaction patterns of many different antisera. In the mid-1960s, a number of individuals who had been testing such antisera held a series of conferences at which many of the problems involving detection techniques and reaction patterns were compared, and the basis for human lymphocyte antigen (HLA) testing was established.

HLA Testing and Graft Survival

HLA antigens provide a means of identifying individuals who have similar or identical tissue antigens and who are less likely to reject tissue grafts. Using skin grafts, it was observed that grafts between identical twins would survive indefinitely; whereas grafts between unrelated HLA, nonidentical individuals would be rejected within about 10 days. Grafts between HLA-matched unrelated individuals lasted only slightly longer than those between HLA-nonidentical unrelated individuals, whereas grafts between HLA-identical siblings survived 20 to 40 days. Thus, although HLA matching was very important for graft survival, more than HLA antigen matching is required to select a histocompatible donor. At least two other factors must be considered—other HLA loci and minor histocompatibility loci (non-HLA antigens). Standard tissue typing can only take into account detectable specificities. Matches presently classified as identical indicate only identity at the known HLA loci; nonidentity at another locus might explain some of the lack of correlation of matching to graft survival.

Transplantation studies in mice have resulted in the concept of strong and weak histocompatibility antigens, and at least eleven histocompatibility systems have been identified in the mouse. The MHC system is termed the **strong histocompatibility system** because organ grafts between individual mice differing in antigenic specificities controlled by the MHC evoke strong rejection reactions. If organ donor and recipient are matched for the MHC but differ in one of the other systems, rejection is not as rapid or as severe. Therefore, these histocompatibility antigen systems are called weak. It is apparent that weak histocompatibility systems are also present in man but remain to be defined. Rejections due to difference in weak histocompatibility antigens can be more readily controlled by immunosuppressive therapy than can differences in strong histocompatibility antigens.

The clinical experience in regard to HLA matching for renal and other tissue graft survival has consistently improved graft survival. An example is the data compiled in 1983, presented in Figure 23–1. The survival of grafts reflects the histocompatibility differences (MHC and others) as well as other factors (complicating diseases, infection, etc.). The difference between survival of renal grafts between identical twins and between HLA-identical siblings probably reflects non-MHC complications and indicates that non-MHC differences contributed to 15% of transplant failures. The difference between HLA-identical siblings and HLA-nonidentical siblings at one year suggests that MHC differences also contributed 15% to transplant failure.

Additive effects of MHC plus non-MHC alloantigens probably account in large part for the higher failure rate in unmatched cadaver donors than in living related donors. There appears to be a good correlation between selective matching between class I MHC (HLA-A, -B, and -C) and class II (HLA-DR, -MT, and -DQ) matching and graft survival. Results reported by the London Transplant Group indicate that selective matching HLA-DR plus HLA-B, or HLA-MT (DRw52/53) plus HLA-B is not only practical but also provides long-term survival without cyclosporine treatment. Matching at HLA-DQ does not improve results. HLA typing has not had as great an influence on transplantation programs in the United States, as has controlled immunosuppression. In fact, the feeling among some transplant surgeons in the United States is that HLA matching may be unnecessary. However, after sharing of donor kidneys that were matched for six HLA antigens on a national basis beginning in 1989, it is estimated that there has been a 5% to 10% improvement in graft outcome. With better serologic and molecular testing, as well as HLA peptide and conformational epitope matching now underway, it is hoped that even better survival will be achieved. However, as mentioned above, further refinement of serologically defined MHC epitopes may not be rewarding. Since T cells recognize histocompatibility differences based on endogenous peptides presented on MHC molecules and not MHC molecules themselves, characterization of the allotypic differences in these molecules may be much more rewarding.

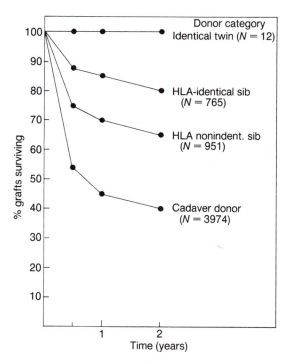

Figure 23–1. Survival times of kidney allografts among people of different genetic relationships ranging from identical twins to unrelated individuals (cadaver donors). From Hildemann WH: *Tissue Antigens* 22:1–6, 1983. Because of better matching and more controlled immunosuppressive regimens, the survival of renal grafts has improved since the time these data were available, but these earlier data show more clearly the effect of tissue matching. At the present time, the ten-year expected survival rates for kidneys from HLA-matched siblings, one haploype-matched related donors, and cadaver donors are 74%, 51%, and 40% respectively. The effects of matching have been largely superseded by controlled immunosuppression.

Xeno-transplantation

Transplantation of organs of other species to man would solve the current critical shortage of donor organs. However, xenografts are usually rejected within minutes or hours after transplantation. A 15 day old baby who received a baboon heart because hers had a lethal defect died after 35 days. In 1992 a 35 year old man lived for 2.5 months after a baboon heart transplant and then died not from tissue rejection, but from infection. In 1995 a committee of the Institute of Medicine was set up to examine again the possibility of transplantation of baboon or swine organs to humans, and by the time this book is published it is likely that clinical trials will have started. Because baboon organs will never be numerous enough to fill the need for organs scientists hope that eventually it will be possible to use genetically altered organs from swine. Pig organs come in all sizes; pigs can be raised in pathogen-free environments and pig heart, liver, and pancreas function similarly to man. The drawback is that swine organs are rejected within minutes when placed in a human (antibody and complement mediated hyperacute rejection). Research is directed to protect swing organs from the action of antibodies and complement by inserting protective genes for complement such as decay accelerating factor, membrane cofactor protein, and CD59.

Pathology of Graft Rejection

SKIN GRAFTS

The pathology of rejection reactions is perhaps best illustrated by the behavior of two skin grafts from the same donor to the same recipient, with the second graft placed about one month after the first graft (Fig. 23–2). *First-set rejection*: During the second or third day following the first grafting procedure (first-set rejection), revascularization begins and is complete by the sixth or seventh day. A similar response is observed for autografts, synografts, allografts, or xenografts, in that each type of graft becomes vascularized. However, at about one week, the first signs of rejection appear in the deep layers of the allograft or xenograft. A perivascular (perivenular) accumulation of mononuclear cells occurs similar to those seen in the early stages of a tuberculin skin reaction. The infiltration steadily intensifies, and edema is grossly visible. Migration of lymphocytes into the epithelial layer of the skin is associated with separation and death of epithelial cells. T_{CTL} cells are the major effector cells for epithelial cell destruction, whereas lymphokines released by T_{DTH} cells may contribute to the vascular inflammation and thrombosis. Monoclonal antibodies to lymphocyte function-associated antigen-1 (LFA-1) block interaction between T_{CTL} cells and target cells in vitro, and in vivo administration prolongs skin graft survival. At about 10 days, thrombosis of the involved vessels occurs, with necrosis and sloughing of the graft. This entire process usually requires 11 to 14 days and is called a first-set rejection. The synograft or autograft does not undergo this process but remains viable with little or no inflammatory reaction. *Second-set rejection*: When a second graft is transplanted from the same genetically unrelated donor who provided the rejected first graft, a more rapid and more vigorous rejection occurs (second-set rejection). For the first 3 days after transplant, the second-set graft looks essentially the same as the first graft. However, vascularization is abruptly halted at 4 to 5 days, with a sudden onset of ischemic necrosis. Because the graft never becomes vascularized and the blood supply is cut off by the second-set rejection, there is little chance for cellular infiltration to occur. The primary target for the second-set rejection appears to be the capillaries taking part

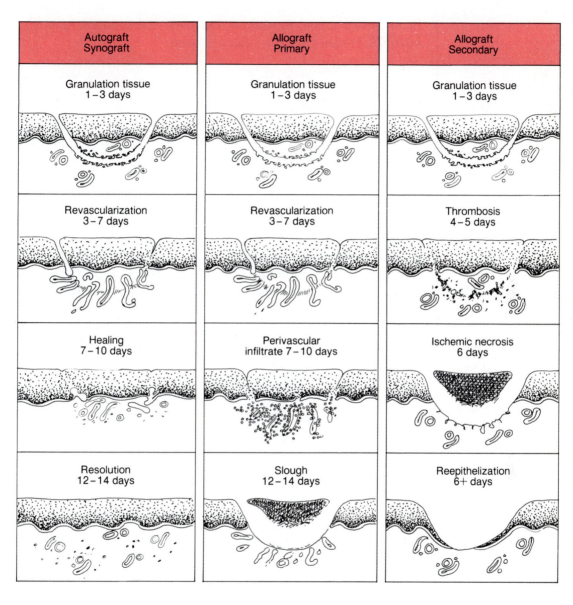

Autograft Synograft	Allograft Primary	Allograft Secondary
Granulation tissue 1 – 3 days	Granulation tissue 1 – 3 days	Granulation tissue 1 – 3 days
Revascularization 3 – 7 days	Revascularization 3 – 7 days	Thrombosis 4 – 5 days
Healing 7 – 10 days	Perivascular infiltrate 7 – 10 days	Ischemic necrosis 6 days
Resolution 12 – 14 days	Slough 12 – 14 days	Reepithelization 6+ days

Figure 23–2. Stages of skin graft rejection. The type of rejection of an allogeneic skin graft depends upon immune reactivity. An autograft or synograft will "take", that is, survive and heal into the grafted site. An allograft to an unsensitized individual will be rejected after a stage of vascularization by a mononuclear cell infiltrate. An allograft to a sensitized recipient will not become vascularized and will be rejected by ischemic necrosis within a few days after transplantation (See text for details.)

in revascularization. Essentially the same events follow grafting of other solid organs, such as kidney or heart.

RENAL GRAFTS

The effect of specific antibody and of sensitized cells in allograft rejection is illustrated by different stages of rejection of kidney grafts recognized in man. The possible fates of renal allografts are depicted in Figure 23–3 and Table 23–2.

First-Set Rejection (Acute Rejection)

The morphology of renal graft rejection across major histocompatibility barriers in untreated recipients is entirely consistent with classic cellular mechanisms. The main feature is the accumulation of a mononuclear cell infiltrate. Within a few hours, small lymphocytes collect around small venules; later, many more mononuclear cells appear in the stroma. After a few days, these mononuclear cells are much more varied in structure, with many small and large lymphocytes, immature blast cells, and more typical mature plasma cells. Both T_{CTL} and T_{DTH} cells are active, but many non-T cells are also present. Irreversible graft injury is associated with activation of infiltrating cells and secretion of IL-2. HLA class I reactive CD8+ T_{CTL} cells react

TABLE 23–2. STAGES OF RENAL ALLOGRAFT REJECTION

Type of Rejection	Principal Target	Primary	Secondary Mechanism
Hyperacute rejection	Vascular endothelium	Antibodies to alloantigens (especially HLA and ABO) from previous sensitization, ?Also T cell	Complement, neutrophils, and coagulation system, leading to acute vascular insufficiency
Acute rejection			
Cellular allograft rejection	Vascular endothelium Tubular epithelium Other cells	HLA class I reactive T8 cells HLA class II reactive T4 cells May act via lymphokines or direct cytotoxicity	Monocytes/macrophages, basophils, other granulocytes, clotting system (chiefly nonthrombotic); small vessel injury; ischemic and direct cytotoxic injury
Fibrinoid allograft arteritis	Arterial endothelium	Humoral antibody cytotoxic to cells in vessel wall	Complement, clotting system, neutrophils
Chronic rejection			
Chronic allograft arteritis	Arterial endothelium and media	Probably combination of T cell- and antibody-mediated injury damage	Scarring, organization of mural thrombi, intimal proliferation, superimposed hypertension
Chronic allograft interstitial nephritis	As for cellular allograft rejection	Repeated episodes of cellular allograft rejection or with a much slower pace	As for cellular allograft rejection plus ischemia from chronic allograft arteritis

From Russell PS: Transplantation of solid organs. In *Immunological Diseases*, 4th ed. Sampter M, et al., (eds.). Boston, Little, Brown, 1988.

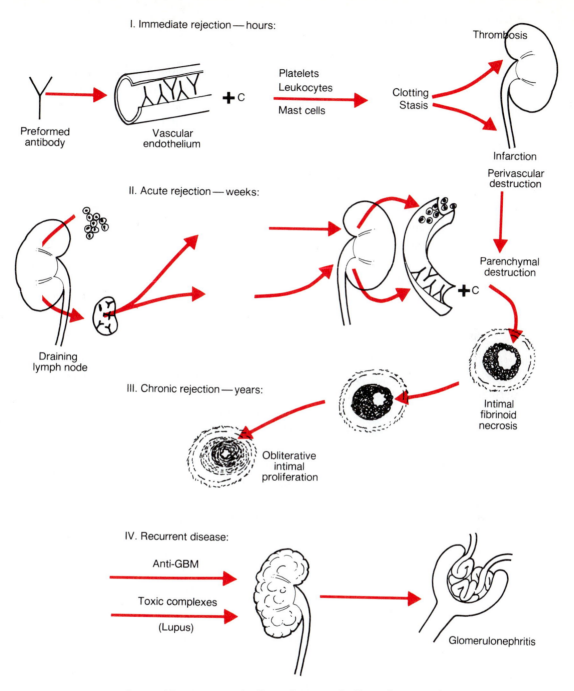

I. Immediate rejection — hours:

Preformed antibody

Vascular endothelium

+C

Platelets
Leukocytes
Mast cells

Clotting
Stasis

Thrombosis

Infarction

Perivascular destruction

II. Acute rejection — weeks:

Draining lymph node

+C

Parenchymal destruction

Intimal fibrinoid necrosis

III. Chronic rejection — years:

Obliterative intimal proliferation

IV. Recurrent disease:

Anti-GBM

Toxic complexes

(Lupus)

Glomerulonephritis

Figure 23–3. Some fates of human renal allografts. Renal allografts are subject to immune rejection as well as to recurrence of the original disease. Long term uncomplicated survival essentially only occurs with completely matched donor and recipient, such as with identical twins. Immune rejection may be caused by either antibody or cell-mediated reactions. Immediate rejection is caused by reaction of performed antibody with vascular endothelium and activation of the clotting system. Acute rejection is caused mainly by mononuclear cell infiltration ($T_{CTL \text{ mediated tubulitis}}$). Chronic rejection occurs as a result of continuing low-grade endarteritis because of long-term deposition of antibody or immune complexes. Recurrence of the original disease may occur if the predisposing cause is not controlled.

against vascular endothelium, as well as tubular epithelial class I MHC antigens. T_{CTLs} invade of the renal tubular cells, with isolation, separation, and death of these cells occurring in a way very similar, if not identical, to that described for the effects of T_{CTL} cells on tissue culture monolayers and thyroid follicular cells during thyroiditis. The interstitial tissue of the rejecting kidney accumulates large quantities of fluid (edema). Finally, the afferent arterioles and small arteries become swollen and occluded by fibrin and white cell thrombi. Occasionally, these vessels show fibrinoid necrosis and contain immunoglobulins and complement consistent with deposition of antibody–antigen complexes. Therefore, the first-set renal allograft rejection by an untreated recipient occurs primarily via cellular mechanisms, although there is evidence that humoral antibody may contribute. For practical purposes, infiltration of the renal tubules by lymphocytes (tubulitis) is the most important criterion used for diagnosis of acute rejection.

Second-set Renal Graft Rejection (Hyperacute Rejection)

A second renal allotransplant from the same donor who provided the first graft is rejected much more rapidly (within 1 to 3 days). There is little mononuclear cell infiltrate, presumably because adequate circulation necessary for the accumulation of blood mononuclear cells is never established. Morphologically, the main features are destruction of peritubular capillaries and fibrinoid necrosis of the walls of the small arteries and arterioles. The glomeruli may contain intercapillary deposition of fibrin clots similar to those observed in the systemic Shwartzman reaction. By 24 hours, there is widespread tubular necrosis, and the kidney never assumes functional activity. Perfusion of a renal homotransplant with plasma from an animal hyperimmunized against the donor of the kidney produces a similar reaction. Therefore, the hyperacute second-set rejection of renal allograft is mediated by preformed circulating antibodies. This type of rejection has been observed in humans when grafting was attempted across ABO blood group types. A renal allograft from a B or A to an O recipient may lead to complete failure of circulation in the graft. There is distention and thrombosis of afferent arterioles and glomerular capillaries with sludged red cells, presumably owing to the action of cytotoxic antiblood group antibodies upon blood group antigens located in the vasculature of the grafted kidney.

Late Rejection

Immunosuppressive therapy (see Chapter 28) is very effective in controlling allograft rejection, and the use of immunosuppressive agents has resulted in a prolonged survival of human renal allografts. At the time of this writing, nearly all clinical immunosuppressive regimens for renal grafting were cyclosporine based but use of FK5O6 is replacing cyclosporine (See Chapter 28). Antilymphocyte antibody induction therapy with delayed administration of cyclosporine is used to avoid cyclosporine toxicity to the kidney. Rejection crises are treated with high-dose glucocorticoids. Such therapy appears to be effective in suppressing the development of rapid rejection but does not eliminate later rejection. Some patients with renal allografts survive for many years before rejection results in loss of function of the transplant. Morphologically, the major finding in such late-rejected kidneys is a marked intimal proliferation and scarring of the walls of medium-sized arteries. The appearance is much like that of healed or late-stage polyarteritis nodosa. This late proliferative obliterative endarteritis is the result of a chronic antibody-mediated toxic complex reaction causing scarring of the intima of the arteries.

Recurrent Disease

An important factor in the survival of a renal transplant is the original disease that caused renal failure. The most frequent diseases for which renal transplantation is done include diabetic renal disease, pyelonephritis, and glomerulonephritis. Of these, patients with diabetes (usually males) generally have less success following transplantation than do patients without diabetes. Patients with pyelonephritis will have recurrence of pyelonephritis if the factors predisposing to pyelonephritis are still present. Those recipients whose renal failure resulted from glomerulonephritis may develop glomerulonephritis in the transplanted kidney, but in practice this rarely occurs, indicating that the original situation producing glomerulonephritis is no longer present. In diabetes and other diseases associated with chronic deposition of immune complexes, recurrent glomerulonephritis will occur if production of the complexes is not controlled. For instance, recurrence of immune complex nephritis is to be expected in patients with lupus nephritis if the immune complexes are still present.

Solid Organ Transplantation in Humans

KIDNEY

The success of renal grafts serves as the prototype for the clinical transplantation of solid organs. Over 95% of patients receiving renal grafts are alive after one year and 80% at five years. However, there are a number of reasons why renal transplantation is more successful than transplantation of other organs, such as the heart, liver, lung, and pancreas. Short-term preservation of the kidney up to 72 hours (by law 48 hours in the United States and 72 hours in Europe) can be accomplished by perfusion and cooling; preservation of the other organs is only possible for shorter periods of time. The operative procedure is not as difficult; the kidney does not have to be placed in the same anatomic position as the original kidney, and the connections of vessels and ureter are easier to do than the more complicated connections of the other organs. Hemodialysis provides a reliable long-term back-up to hold patients before transplant or to carry patients through episodes of failure. Donor organs are much more readily available; living donors can be used, in contrast to heart, lung, or most liver transplants. The use of sibling or parent donors is superior to the use of cadaver donors for graft survival. However, most kidneys come from cadaver donors. Although the survival rate for recipients of unrelated cadaver donors is not as good as that of related donors, cadaver donors are much easier to obtain. Transplantation can be done across MHC barriers and a functional kidney maintained for longer periods by immunosuppressive therapy. Immunosuppression with cyclosporine, antilymphocyte monoclonal antibody (to CD3) and other drugs has worked out better for kidney grafts than for other organs. Although cyclosporine itself has nephrotoxic side effects that may contribute to failure of graft function, this may be controlled by monitoring blood levels of cyclosporine, and there is no evidence of long-term deterioration of renal function due to cyclosporine nephrotoxicity.

Hemodialysis was introduced to control renal failure in the 1960s, but dialysis depended on the use of inlaying catheters to maintain circulation, required repeated visits to the dialysis center, and produced a number of uncomfortable effects, including weight gain, infections, and mood changes related to the time between dialysis. However, the availability of dialysis as a temporary means of support had much to do with the rapid development of allografting as the treatment of choice for some types of renal failure. It costs $36,000 for a year of hemodialysis, compared to $55,000 plus follow-up for a renal transplant patient.

Presensitization to HLA antigens will affect survival of renal and other transplants. Clearly, if a recipient has antibody to HLA antigens prior to transplantation, acute antibody-mediated rejection may occur. Recipients with antibody to donor antigens (presensitized) have lower (47%) graft survival rates than patients without antibody to donor antigens (57%). For this reason, blood transfusions to potential recipients have been generally avoided. However, more recent evidence indicates better graft survival in recipients who have had multiple exposures to donor HLA antigens (but are crossmatch negative). Thus, 44% one-year renal graft survival is found in patients who have received no blood transfusions, 58%, 60%, and 64%, respectively, in patients who have received 1 to 4, 5 to 9, and 10 or more units of blood before the transplantation procedures.

HEART

Heart transplantation has emerged during the last 15 years as an acceptable therapy for end-stage heart disease caused by cardiomyopathy, coronary artery disease, valvular lesions, and refractory dysthrythmias. Earlier poor survival rates limited cardiac transplantation to a few experimental centers. However, survival rates have increased significantly. The number of heart transplants is now approximately 2,500 per year with a 72% five-year actuarial survival rate. Improved survival is related to recipient selection, donor–recipient matching, and patient management, particularly more carefully controlled immunosuppressive posttransplant therapy reducing the death rate due to infection. Infectious complications accounted for over 50% of patient deaths during the early era of heart transplantation. Accelerated coronary atherosclerosis is the limiting factor for long-term survival of cardiac transplants. Immune-mediated inflammation of the coronaries may induce macrophage accumulation and smooth muscle migration through the internal elastic lamina. In addition, cytokines, such as IL-1 and TNF-β, can disrupt β-adrenergic signal transduction and agonist stimulation of contractility.

Acute cardiac rejection reactions may be diagnosed by endocardial biopsy, particularly of the right ventricle. Hyperacute rejection within hours of transplantation is rare and is characterized by interstitial hemorrhages and edema due to plugging of small vessels by platelet aggregates and erythrocytes, presumably due to reaction of preformed antibodies to vascular endothelium. Hyperacute rejection necessitates rapid retransplantation, if the patient is to survive. Cell-mediated rejection is graded by the degree of mononuclear infiltrate as mild, moderate, or severe, and as focal or diffuse. Grading of the rejection reaction may increase the chances of successfully treating patients by intensive immunosuppression before rejection is advanced. With cyclosporine treatment, 60% to 70% of patients will have complete resolution of a mild to moderate acute rejection by the second week. Experimental studies have shown that persistence of activated CD4+ cells (T_{DTH}) results in inflammatory endothelial proliferation that precedes infiltration of CD8+ T_{CTL} cells that mediate cytotoxic destruction of cardiac myocytes. Immunosuppressive treatment may prevent this development. The major impediment to clinical application of heart transplants is the availability of donor organs. Development of artificial hearts genetically engineered or animal organs that bypass this problem is actively being pursued. However, only short-term survival with artificial hearts has been obtained. Even short-term survival may increase the possibility of eventually finding a donor by prolonging the life of potential recipients.

LIVER

The effectiveness of liver transplantation has also increased substantially as a result of better patient selection, better controlled immunosuppression and better postoperative management procedures. The most important factor in the increased functional survival of orthotopic liver allografts is the use of cyclosporine of FK506 immunosuppression.

More than 18,000 liver transplants have been done in 160 centers worldwide. Since 1980, life expectancy for one year following liver transplantation has increased from 25% to 75%. Preliminary results indicate even better results using the new immunosuppressive drug FK506. Liver transplantation has become the preferred alternative to medical management of end-stage liver disease. Essentially any primary liver failure can be treated by transplantation. The major contraindications are complicating extrahepatic disease, active alcohol or drug use, HBsAg positivity, portal vein thrombosis or prior hepatobiliary surgery, and age greater than 60 years. Liver transplantation as a treatment for alcoholic liver disease is based on an estimate of the recipient for future abuse. After psychiatric evaluation, patients who are judged likely to abstain from alcohol and have favorable medical and surgical indicators may be considered reasonable candidates for liver transplantation. The most important factors now limiting liver transplantation are the cost and the availability of donor livers. As with other transplantation approaches, the number of well-trained liver transplant surgeons now exceeds the availability of donor organs. Extensive networks have been organized to identify potential donors, obtain donor organs, and deliver them to undersupplied transplant centers. However, it is doubtful that any public health service system can support liver transplantation on a large scale.

Acute rejection of the liver occurs in about 80% of cases at 5 to 15 days after transplantation. Laboratory assay of blood levels of liver enzymes does not accurately relate to the degree of liver rejection as determined by histologic analysis of biopsies. During the first 3 or 4 months after transplantation, the best means of identifying significant pathologic conditions in liver allografts is by biopsy. Rejection is recognized by mixed mononuclear inflammation primarily in the portal zone of the liver, cholestasis by bile staining in the central zone of the liver and the presence of bilirubin in dilated canaliculi, ischemia by confluent necrosis, hepatitis by parenchymal disorganization and focal necrosis of hepatocytes. The four major causes of early liver allograft losses in one study were:

Primary graft nonfunction	30%
Ischemic injury of graft	10%
Acute rejection	10%
Vascular complications	27%

Survival curves of liver graft patients are characterized by an early and steep decline with most deaths occurring during the first postoperative month. This is reflected in the loss of grafts due to nonfunction, ischemia, and vascular complications, with acute rejection causing only 10% of early graft loss. The bile ducts have been shown to express class I MHC antigens at a much higher level than parenchymal liver cells. Thus, acute rejection appears to be directed against the ductular cells by CD8+ T_{CTL} cells. However, during chronic liver rejection, there is increased expression of class I antigens on hepatocytes and a more diffuse mononuclear cell infiltrate, as well as endophlebitis of middle and large-sized hepatic arteries. Chronic rejection features progressive loss of bile ducts, the **vanishing bile duct syndrome**, manifested by increasing cholestasis. This is seen in about 25% of liver transplant patients and is unresponsive to immunosuppressive therapy.

PANCREAS

In general, major organ transplantation of kidney, heart, liver, or lung is only undertaken when the alternative is death. Pancreas transplantation is being increasingly used for treatment of complications of type 1 insulin-dependent diabetes (retinopathy, renal failure, neuropathy, and arterial disease) and has become routine for uremic diabetic patients. Diabetic renal failure is now treated by a combined pancreas/kidney transplant with associated immunosuppression. However, most experts believe that currently there is a very limited place for pancreas or islet transplantation. Systematic experimental studies of transplantation of pancreatic islets for treatment of experimental diabetics in animals has provided data that the approaches worked out could be successfully applied to man. The following factors are important:

1. Development of automated techniques for preparation of a suspension of isolated islet cells from pancreatic tissue.
2. Transplantation into an accessible site, such as a peritoneal envelope on the omentum or infusion into the portal vein.
3. Removal of "passenger lymphocytes" by cultivation in vitro or treatment of islet cell preparations with anti-class II MHC antibody. (Islet cells do not express class II antigens, whereas passenger lymphocytes do.) This procedure has not been found to be required for successful islet cell transplantation in humans.
4. Matching of donor and recipient for class II MHC antigens.

Prior to 1985, pancreatic islet transplantation in human clinical trials was found to be safe but unfortunately not successful. The major problem was obtaining sufficient numbers of isolated islet cells. Procedures have now been developed to obtain 100,000 to 500,000 human islet cells by automated collagenase digestion perfusion and gradient centrifugation. Transplantation is accomplished by injection into the portal vein, which usually results in survival of the islet cells in the recipient liver. In diabetic recipients of renal transplants, who are already receiving immunosuppression for the renal graft, a pancreas transplant may provide significant benefits in management of the diabetes and possible amelioration of secondary effects of diabetes. Application of pancreas transplants to the general diabetic population now depends on the development of a benign antirejection protocol since the complications of immunosuppression (cyclosporine, azathioprine, and prednisone) are greater than those of insulin replacement therapy. Islet cell transplantation may be the choice of therapy for individual diabetic patients who are labile or who have problems in management that exceed those of immunosuppression. As of 1993 over 6,000 pancreas transplants had been performed worldwide, and two-thirds of these were simultaneous kidney/pancreas transplants. Of the remaining one-third, half were pancreas transplants after a kidney grant, and half were pancreas transplants alone. Most pancreas transplants are from unrelated cadaver donors, but some have been from living related donors after hemipancreatectomy to obtain donor tissue. The effect of hemipancreatectomy on the donor does not appear to be significant, but the long-term effects of this procedure are not known. HLA matching has a marked effect on graft survival, with more than 90% one-year survival for grafts with 0-1 HLA-A, -B, or -D mismatch, but only 56% for those mismatched are 2-3 antigens. Changes in technique and management have improved one-year graft survival from 20% in the 1980s to over 90% at the time of this writing; for combined kidney/pancreas grafts, 80% had functioning kidney grafts and 70% were insulin independent.

Transplantation of the pancreas as a solid organ is now being attempted, but the results as of the time of this writing are not yet promising enough for general application. Transplantation of the vascularized pancreas for replacement of islet function carries the additional burden of cotransplantation of undesired acinar tissue. Approximately 800 vascularized pancreas transplants are done each year worldwide. The most widely used procedure includes anastomosis of the donor duodenum to the urinary bladder to provide drainage of the pancreatic duct. This results in recurrent cystitis and urethritis in approximately 50% of the recipients. However, satisfactory long-term results have been obtained and some centers recommend combined kidney-vascularized pancreas grafts for type I diabetics with end-stage renal disease.

LUNG

Until the last few years lung transplantation had limited success but now has become a realistic possibility for selected patients with end-stage lung disease. From 1963 to 1973, at least 36 lung transplants were done worldwide with only three patients surviving more than one month and none longer than 10 months. At one medical center, from 1988 to 1991, the actuarial survival of 69 lung transplant recipients for one year was 79%. Single lung transplants survive slightly better than double lung transplants. Currently, success has been achieved for patients with chronic obstructive pulmonary disease, emphysema, cystic fibrosis, and primary pulmonary hypertension. Infection and rejection are the major causes of transplant failure. Rejection correlates with the number of CD3+, CD8+, CD25+ cells in transbronchial biopsies. In addition, late-occurring obliterative bronchiolitis caused by CMI to donor bronchial epithelium, presumably by reaction of T_{CTL} cells with class I MHC on bronchial lining cells, has been reported in about one-third of patients who survive for more than 4 months.

Combined heart-lung transplantation (HLT) has been attempted over 500 times prior to 1989 and has leveled off at about 200 per year. The principal indications are pulmonary hypertension and congenital heart defects. However, isolated lung transplantation has become more in favor for pulmonary hypertension and other diseases for which heart/lung transplants were attempted. The major advantage of HLT is the ability to transplant organs to patients with combined cardiopulmonary disease. The survival rates for HLT has risen at one center to 78% at one year and 70% at two years, a significant improvement over previous rates. Infection is the leading cause of death, accounting for 48% of early postoperative failures and 74% of overall deaths. The overall survival is 55% at five years. This difficult approach remains experimental and is only carried out in a few transplant centers. Lung and heart/lung transplantation remain experimental procedures, with major problems of organ procurement, patient selection, and posttransplant maintenance.

PARATHYROID

Autotransplantation of parathyroid glands into the forearm musculature has been used following parathyroidectomy for parathyroid hyperplasia. This permits replacement of portions of the gland into easily accessible areas, where their function can be monitored and controlled.

NEURAL

The possibility of brain transplantation has titillated the imagination of science fiction writers for many years, and mammalian neural transplantation in experimental animals has recently been demonstrated to be feasible. The brain is an immunologically privileged site so that the usual graft rejection mechanisms may not be active in neural transplantation. In experimental models, it has been possible to transplant neuronal cells to reenervate damaged zones of the host brain. In these studies, small grafts of fetal brain cells can be placed in zones of damage induced in the brain. Small groups of only a few thousand cells are able to restore some neuroendocrine deficits, cognitive disorders, and motor dysfunctions in young adult rodents, and neuroendocrine cells can integrate into brains of aged rodents and improve behavioral performance.

Human applications of neural transplantation are directed toward correction of neurotransmitter defects in Parkinson's disease or

Alzheimer's disease. In Parkinson's disease, patients lose dopamine-producing cells in a part of the brain called the substantia nigra. Theoretically, these cells could be replaced using fetal brain cells, and preliminary results demonstrate some benefit in patients given fetal ventral mesencephalic implants. Although in one study only 5% to 10% of the cells injected into four patients with Parkinson's disease survived, three of the four patients had improved mobility. Although many questions remain unanswered, the results of three recent studies have resulted in cautious optimism that this approach will eventually work, and a large clinical trial is now underway. Other possible uses are to restore some function in patients with Alzheimer's disease and to replace defects in damaged spinal cord by transplantation of fetal spinal cord cells, which stimulate growth of host axons and reconstitution of synaptic complexes within the transplant. Lifting of the ban on the use of fetal tissue for research in the United States should result in an acceleration of the clinical development of these approaches. In animals, transplantation of the photoreceptor layer of the retina has been successful in restoring retinal degeneration.

DIAGNOSIS OF GRAFT REJECTION

One of the critical factors in long-term survival of a graft is the ability of the physician to predict when a rejection episode may occur. Increased immunosuppressive therapy can usually reduce the effects of such an episode, but the effectiveness of this therapy is directly related to how long the rejection reaction has been going on. It is important to be able to monitor transplant patients for possible rejection reactions. The most important methods for diagnosing transplant rejections are listed in Table 23–3.

The impact of clinical transplant programs on clinical pathology laboratories at transplant centers is extensive. Implementation of a transplant program at a midwestern center resulted in a 200% increase in procedure volume and an additional $9 million in charges for laboratory tests.

FACTORS AFFECTING GRAFT SURVIVAL

The survival rates for organ transplants have steadily increased over the last 15 to 20 years (Table 23–4). The survival of a functioning solid organ graft is dependent upon multiple factors, including the original disease and condition of the recipient, tissue matching, organ source, time between organ removal from the donor and placement in the recipient, effectiveness of organ preservation techniques, choice of immunosuppressive treatment, and surgical skill. However, from a pragmatic standpoint, the most important factors for successful grafting are careful pretransplant work-up and conditioning, and thorough and painstaking posttransplant follow-up of the patient by his physicians, including psychiatric counseling. Recently, local (regional) immunotherapy has been directed to eliminating infiltrating lympho-

TABLE 23–3. METHODS USED TO EVALUATE TRANSPLANT FUNCTION OR REJECTION

Transplant	Clinical Tests of Organ Function	Radiological Methods	Gross Physiological Assessment	Biopsy
Kidney	Creatinine, BUN, urine Na$^+$ conc. +++	Scan, ultrasound, angiogram ++	Urine output, blood pressure +++	+++
Heart	Enzyme determinations ± ±	±	Blood pressure, heart sounds ++	++++
Liver	Enzymes, bilirubin +++	Scans, cholangiogram ++	Bile production, jaundice ++	++
Heart-lung	Enzymes ++	Chest film +	As for heart transplant ++	++++
Pancreas	Glucose levels, levels in urine of C-peptide fragment of insulin ++	Scans +	±	±
Lung	±	++	++	±

Interpretation: Applicability and success of each approach ± to + + + +.

From Russell PS: Transplantation of solid organs. In *Immunological Diseases*, 4th ed. Sampter M, et al., (eds.) Boston, Little, Brown, 1988.

cytes that may mediate graft rejection by maintaining a high drug level within the grafted organ. Regional immunosuppression is accomplished by infusion of drugs, such as cyclosporine, into blood vessels that supply the organ (renal artery, portal vein) or as aerosols into the lung. Because of the nature of the data, the fact that transplantations are done at many different centers, and the presence of multiple uncontrolled variables, many of the results reported on human organ transplantation are difficult to evaluate. The increasing success of solid organ transplantation is a tribute to the immense research effort that

TABLE 23–4. SURVIVAL RATES FOR TRANSPLANTED SOLID ORGANS

Organ	Percent Survival at Month After Transplantation	
	1 Year	5 Years
Kidney (HLA-matched)	95	85
Kidney (HLA-mismatched)	80	75
Heart	80	72
Liver	75	39
Lung/Heart–lung	79	55
Pancreas	70	—

has gone into advancing transplant technology. For the major organs—kidney, liver, heart, and lung—the technical limitations of transplantation are well on the way to resolution. However, wider application of this technology is and will be limited by social and economic considerations, and above all by the availability of donor organs.

ORGAN PROCUREMENT

The National Organ Transplantation Act of 1984 established a federally funded network for organ procurement and transplantation, which functions as a nonprofit private organization called the United Network for Organ Sharing (UNOS). This organization keeps a record of all candidates for cadaveric organ transplants. At any given time, there is a list of over 25,000 potential recipients, which is matched by far fewer organ donors (5,000). The organ donation process consists of eight steps: Donor identification, referral, evaluation, consent, management, recovery of organs, allocation, and follow-up. An attempt is made to provide HLA-matched donor organs with the most desirable recipients. In addition, methods of preserving organ viability in vitro have allowed organs to be maintained ex-corpora for several days permitting transportation of the organ prior to transplantation. However, since the need for organs far exceeds the availability of donors, many patients may never be able to have the transplant they need.

Bone Marrow (Stem Cell) Transplantation

A growing number of hematologic diseases, including aplasias, leukemias, and lymphomas, are being successfully treated by bone marrow transplantation to replace the loss of hematopoietic cells. For leukemias and lymphomas, bone marrow is used to restore the loss of hematopoietic tissue following ablative irradiation. In some forms of previously fatal leukemias and aplasia, two-year disease-free survival exceeds 60%. Bone marrow transplantation by intravascular infusion is much simpler to carry out than transplantation of solid organs, and since donor cells may be obtained by bone marrow aspiration, it is usually easy to find a living related donor. However, the complications that result from graft-versus-host disease (GVHD) and its subsequent treatment represent a major problem. Since it is now possible to isolate stem cells from peripheral blood using stem cell markers, this source of Stem cells is replacing bone marrow in many situations.

GRAFT-VERSUS-HOST REACTIONS

Transfer of cell populations such as bone marrow, which contain immunocompetent lymphocytes, may lead to a reaction of the transferred cells to antigens of the recipient. This is called a graft-versus-host (GVH) reaction. GVH reactions occur when immunocompetent cells from an allogenic or xenogeneic donor are transferred to a recipient whose own immune responsiveness has been impaired by immunosuppression or neoplastic disease, or because of immature development. GVH reactions may occur rarely after blood transfusions, usually in children under 18 years of age, with evidence of immunosuppression. The transferred cells colonize in the recipient, recognize host tissue antigens as foreign, and react to them. The immunoreactive cells responsible for the GVH reaction are the mature T cells present in the bone marrow. Some components of GVH may include reaction of residual host cells to the grafted cells. When the lymphoid tissue of the recipient is not completely destroyed, regeneration of the host immune system in the presence of donor cells may result in a state of mutual tolerance of grafted and recipient cells. Individuals whose tissues contain cells of more than one genotype are called **chimeras**. A chimera is a fire-spouting monster of Greek mythology with a lion's head, goat's body, and serpent's tail. In lymphoid cell chimeras, the recipient maintains both its own and the donor lymphoid components—an interesting condition in which two separate immune and hematopoietic systems coexist and may react against each other.

Wasting Disease

The reaction of grafted immune cells to host antigens and vice versa produces a disease known as GVH disease, secondary disease, or wasting disease (Table 23–5). Acute GVHD usually occurs 20 to 100 days after transplantation and is fatal in 10% of the affected individuals. Acute GVHD consists of two pathologic processes: Infiltration of tissues, especially the skin, intestine, spleen, and liver, with proliferating lymphocytes, resulting in hepatosplenomegaly, diarrhea, and a scaly contact dermatitis-like skin lesion; and loss of immune reactivity with susceptibility to opportunistic infections. The major reaction appears to be by CD4+ T_{DTH} cells to class II MHC antigens on lymphoid cells, activated epithelial cells in the skin and intestine, and bile duct cells. Proliferating host cells may make a major contribution to the lymphoid hyperplasia, and it is the host's MHC class II+ lymphopoietic tissue that bears the brunt of the attack by the transferred cells. Hyperplasia of the spleen and other lymphoid organs is followed by atrophy, presumably because the grafted cells have attacked and destroyed the host's lymphoid tissue. A variety of causative factors may contribute to

TABLE 23–5. FINDINGS IN ACUTE AND CHRONIC GRAFT-VERSUS-HOST DISEASE

Organ	Acute	Chronic
Skin	Erythroderma, rash, desquamation, inflammation of hair follicles and basal cells	Sclerodermalike skin atrophy papulosquamous dermatitis, dyspigmentation, alopecia
Liver	Elevated bilirubin and liver enzymes, periportal inflammation	Cholestatic disease with biliary cirrhosis
GI tract	Diarrhea, ileus, inflammation at base of crypts	Destruction of mucosa with intestinal strictures
Lymphoid	Delayed immunologic recovery	T and B cell deficiencies, opportunistic infections

the severity of GVHD, including effects of antineoplastic drugs or total body irradiation (for treatment of leukemias or lymphomas), medications used for treatment of GVHD, and infectious complications and antimicrobial therapies. Veno-occlusive disease of the liver occurs in up to 20% of cases. Chronic GVHD may lead to sclerodermalike skin lesions and liver lesions resembling primary biliary cirrhosis. The success of bone marrow transplantation depends largely on controlling the extent of the GVH reaction and preventing opportunistic infections from loss of the recipient's immune system.

Hybrid Resistance

Hybrid resistance refers to the failure of inbred parental bone marrow cells to induce GVHD in lethally irradiated F_1-recipient mice. Since the F_1 hybrid immune system shares only one MHC haplotype with the homozygous parent, parental cells are able to recognize F_1 cells, but F_1 cells should not react against the parent homozygous cells. Thus, the parental cells should survive and produce GVHD. Parental bone marrow cells are rejected by a multistep process involving an antigen, termed Hh-1, linked to H-2D region that is only expressed in the homozygous condition. The hybrid resistance reaction involves two steps. First, a radioresistant CD4-CD8-CD5+ cell in the F_1 hybrid recognizes the Hh-1 antigen and stimulates macrophages to secret IFN-α/β. The IFN activates a natural killer cell that specifically kills parental cells bearing Hh-1 antigens using an antibody-dependent recognition mechanism. Expression of the Hh-1 antigen is associated with the homozygous haplotype; heterozygous mice do not express this Hh-1 antigen. Since the F_1 recipients are heterozygous and the parental mice are homozygous, the radioresistant F_1 T cells are able to initiate the hybrid resistance response.

CLINICAL BONE MARROW TRANSPLANTATION

The objective of bone marrow transplantation is to replace hematopoietic stem cells. Bone marrow grafts have been used to treat patients with aplastic anemia (failure of blood cell production), severe combined immune deficiencies (see Chapter 27), or patients with leukemia treated with irradiation or ablative chemotherapy (see Chapter 24). Although these diseases are the subjects of later chapters in this book, the principles of bone marrow transplantation will be covered here. With careful follow-up, excellent results are obtained in most of the cases of aplastic anemia or immune deficiency if an HLA identical sibling donor is used. Similarly, bone marrow failure following accidental irradiation can be treated with bone marrow transplantation. Irradiation leads to failure of blood cell production and reduction in immune function.

Leukemia

In leukemias, bone marrow transplantation is used to "rescue" patients following irradiation and/or chemotherapy. Irradiation or doses of chemicals sufficient to cause potentially curative reduction in leukemic cell mass frequently result in death by infection or bleeding secondary to loss of bone marrow function, ie, loss of production of white cells and platelets. This can be circumvented by transfer of bone marrow from a healthy donor. Unless an identical twin is available, some degree of GVH reactivity seems inevitable. If possible, autologous bone marrow obtained during remission may be stored, treated with monoclonal antibodies to try to remove any residual leukemia cells, and reinfused back into the patient after ablative treatment for recurrence.

Bone marrow transplantation (BMT) following radiation and chemotherapy treatment of leukemia has had increasing success (Table 23–6). For instance, approximately 25% of patients with acute nonlymphocytic leukemia will have long-term disease-free survival after intensive chemotherapy alone. Of the 75% who do not have long-term remission after chemotherapy, one-third will go into long-term remission after ablative therapy and bone marrow transplantation. Chemotherapy alone is ineffective against chronic myelogenous leukemia, but BMT after radiation leads to long-term remission in 25% to 65% of cases.

The therapeutic process starts with conditioning, the administration of high-dose chemotherapy or irradiation or both to eliminate the malignant cell population, as well as host cells that might react against the transplanted cells. This is followed by transplantation of bone marrow and supportive care of the patient against infection and bleeding. Support includes administration of antibiotics and transfusions of platelets and red blood cells, as well as transfusions of granulocytes in some cases.

Prevention of Graft-versus-host Reactions

Efforts in improving bone marrow transplantation have centered on ways to reduce the severity of the GVH reaction yet provide sufficient bone marrow stem cells to reconstitute the irradiated recipient. In

TABLE 23–6. PERCENTAGES OF LONG TERM DISEASE-FREE SURVIVAL OF LEUKEMIA PATIENTS TREATED WITH CHEMOTHERAPY ALONE, OR WITH BONE MARROW TRANSPLANTATION (BMT) AFTER FAILURE OF CHEMOTHERAPY

Type of Leukemia	Chemotherapy Alone	BMT after Failure
Acute nonlymphocytic	25%	25%
Acute lymphocytic	20%	30%
Chronic myelogenous	0[*]	20–65%[†]

[*] Approximately 10 complete remissions have been reported using interferon.
[†] 20% if treated during blast crisis; 65% if treated during chronic phase.

most remissions, a transient GVH reaction occurs and the treated individual demonstrates both host and donor cells after the reaction (chimerism). Thus, there is a delicate balance between removing the alloreactive cells and preserving the stem cells. In numerous clinical trials, a variety of methods have proved to be at least partially feasible in reducing the reactivity of the donor cells to the host. Since it is the mature T cells in the marrow that are responsible for the GVH reaction, the approach has been to remove these cells. For clinical application, fresh bone marrow preparations to be used for transplantation are purged of mature T cells with anti-CD6 monoclonal antibody and complement. This procedure significantly reduces the severity of GVHD.

Mild GVHD is expected and is not treated. Treatment of moderate to severe acute GVHD consists of antilymphocyte preparations, cyclosporine, high-dose steroids, and azathioprine in various combinations. Infection is the most common cause of death because immunosuppression is both a component of the disease and the effect of therapy. Abnormalities of T cells, B cells, macrophages, and neutrophils have been found, and responses to immunization with new antigens are severely impaired. The entire immune system is affected and the cellular interactions required for induction and expression of immunity are dysfunctional. As time passes, the balance and regulation of the immune system are restored. Antibiotics are used to cover infections but may also contribute to the manifestations of GVHD. Recovery is dependent upon stem cells in the donor bone marrow repopulating the hematopoietic and lymphopoietic systems with recapitulation of neonatal development of the immune system over a one- to two-year period. Early after bone marrow transfer, primitive functions, such as CD8+ T_{CTL}-mediated cytotoxicity and suppression, are predominant, and T_{DTH} and T-helper cell functions are inhibited. This stage may be necessary for the donor cells to become established.

Transplant
Leukemia

A particularly interesting and perplexing observation has been that in a few cases of leukemia treated by whole-body irradiation and bone marrow from an HLA-matched sibling of the opposite sex, the donor's blood cells became established but subsequently became leukemic. This could be because of excessive antigenic stimulation of donor cells in a foreign environment; an abnormal homeostatic mechanism in the recipient that also applies to donor cells; fusion of donor and recipient cells, resulting in transfer of donor chromosome markers to recipient leukemic cells; transmission of an agent (oncogenic virus) from host to donor cells; or the presence of an oncogenic virus in the donor cells that was not expressed in the donor. In some cases, Epstein–Barr virus has been demonstrated in the leukemic cells.

Self-recognition

An additional factor in determining the effectiveness of stem cell transfers is the necessity of self-recognition of T and B cells in order for cooperation to occur. Unless donor and recipient are adequately HLA-matched, it is possible that the T and B cells that develop from the engrafted donor stem cells may not be able to cooperate. At first glance, it would seem that after transfer, a given population of stem cells from both the developing T and B cells would be of donor origin. However, in experimental systems, the ability of T cells to recognize self depends not on the origin of the pre-T (stem) cell but on the thymic environment in which T-cell maturation takes place (adaptive differentiation). Thus, if type X stem cells, containing both T- and B-cell precursor potential, are engrafted into a type Y recipient, the type X pre-T cells will mature in the environment of the type Y thymus and acquire the capacity to recognize Y and not X as self. On the other hand, the type X pre-B cells will mature as type X cells. The person so reconstituted will have X-type T cells that recognize Y and cannot cooperate with X-type B cells.

Gene Transfer
Therapy

In the last few years, the availability of retroviral techniques for transferring specific genes with high efficiency into various cell types has permitted the development of methods for specific gene replacement. The cells of choice for gene transfer therapy are stem cells, such as the hematopoietic stem cell found in bone marrow or peripheral blood. DNA-mediated gene transfer using viruses, such as adenoviruses, SV40, adeno-associated viruses, or herpes simplex have not been shown to transduce or transfect hematopoietic cells effectively. Hepatocytes, endothelial cells, muscle cells, keratinocytes, and fibroblasts have all been suggested as potentially useful cells for gene transfer; however, hematopoietic Stem cells are considered best for such transfer as it contains self-renewing stem cells and because it is easy and relatively safe to obtain. Auto-logous hematopoietic stem cells may be isolated in a highly purified state from the peripheral blood by using monoclonal antibodies (to CD34) after mobilization of marrow stem cells by growth factor treatment. These stem cells may then be transfected with the appropriate gene, expanded in vitro, and reinjected into the donor to replace a missing gene. Such "gene transfer therapy" has been used to replace missing enzymes in severe combined immunodeficiency caused by adenosine deaminase deficiency, and is now being developed for many other genetic diseases. Table 23–7 lists some of the diseases that have been cured or in which symptoms have dramatically improved after bone stem cell transfer of transfected cells. Use of more primitive embryonic stem cells for gene transfer of other diseases, using modified genes to correct a specific gene defect, requires more efficient methods of gene targeting. The use of genetically engineered cells for tumor therapy is discussed in Chapter 30.

TABLE 23–7. DISEASES SUCCESSFULLY TREATED BY GENE TRANSFER USING HEMATOPOIETIC STEM CELLS

Disease	Gene Defect
Red Cells	
β-Thalassemia	β-Globin
Lymphocytes	
ADA deficiency	Adenosine deaminase
PNP deficiency	Purine nucleotide phosphorylase
Monocytes and neutrophils	
Chronic granulomatous disease	Cytochrome b, β chain
Leukocyte adhesion deficiency	CD18 β subunit
Lysosomal storage diseases (mostly macrophages)	
Gaucher's disease	Glucocerebrosidase
Mucopolysaccharidosis I	α-L-iduronidase
Niemann–Pick type B	Sphinogomyelinase
Metachromatic leukodystrophy	Arylsulfatase A

Modified from Karlsson S: Treatment of genetic defects in hematopoietic cell function by gene transfer. *Blood* 78:1481, 1991.

PREGNANCY: A TOLERATED GRAFT

THE FETUS AS A GRAFT

Since the fetus acquires half of its genetic endowment from the father, it is a **semiallogeneic** tissue graft from the immunologic view of the mother. The potential reaction of the maternal immune response in pregnancy to fetal antigens has been the subject of extensive investigation and speculation. Except for matings within inbred strains of animals, a fetus in utero is a graft of tissue containing transplantation antigens to which the mother can react. Paternal histocompatibility antigens are present on spermatozoa and are represented in fetal tissue. In spite of this potential for immune rejection as an allograft, the fetus is not usually affected. The fetus survives a longer time in the uterus than other foreign tissue grafts, and gestation is terminated by nonimmune events. In fact, there is statistical evidence from human studies that HLA differences between parents may increase fetal survival. In addition, histocompatible gestations have smaller birth weights and placental sizes than histoincompatible gestations. Thus, HLA differences may actually contribute to fetal survival; HLA sharing may adversely affect pregnancy outcome. Cytokines, such as IL-1, TNF-α, IFN-γ, and CSFs may actually aid blastocyst attachment and placentation. However, increased spontaneous abortion rates may be associated with specific MHC haplotypes or antigens. There is evidence for a spontaneous abortion susceptibility region (SAR) in, or linked to, the HLA region on chromosome 6. The relationship of this SAR to immune interactions between mother and fetus is not clear.

Whereas in general it has been impossible to induce a GVH reaction by immunization of the mother to fetal antigens, such runting can be observed under special circumstances. Female rats of one strain who rejected skin grafts from another produced runted (GVHD) offspring if mating to fathers of the other strain took place at the time of rejection of the graft. If rejection of the graft took place two weeks prior to mating, runting was not observed. Runting is believed to be due to the presence of large numbers of lymphoid cells sensitized to fetal antigens at a time when no humoral antibody is present and the fetus is particularly susceptible to a GVH reaction; rejection of a graft two weeks prior to mating does not interfere with pregnancy. Thus, fetal rejection may occur if the mother has large numbers of specifically reactive T cells to fetal antigens at critical times during gestation.

MECHANISMS OF TOLERANCE OF FETAL GRAFTS

The means by which the fetus avoids immune reaction is not fully understood. The following mechanisms have been proposed:

1. Paternal antigens are not present on embryonal or fetal tissue. This is certainly not true. Although histocompatibility antigens are present on postnatal cells in higher amounts than on fetal cells, tissue antigens have been demonstrated on embryonal and fetal cells at essentially all stages of development and are present in sufficient amounts to be killed by sensitized lymphocytes in vitro and in vivo.
2. The fetus is not rejected because half of its histocompatibility antigens are common with those of the mother. This is also not true because a mother will reject skin grafts of fetal skin and surrogate mothers will support ova from unrelated parents when transplanted in utero.
3. The mother does not become immunized to fetal tissues during pregnancy, ie, is tolerant. This is unlikely because mothers will develop antibodies to fetal antigens; one of the common sources of HLA typing sera is multiparous women. In addition, a significant hypertrophy of the draining lymph nodes occurs during pregnancy. Furthermore, protection is afforded to the fetus even if the mother is preimmunized to fetal tissues by injection of paternal antigens or rejection of paternal skin graft prior to pregnancy.
4. The uterus is an immunologically privileged site. Skin grafts from F_1 or paternal strains will be rejected if placed in the uterus of an histoincompatible female even if the recipient is hormonally prepared and the uterus has undergone a decidual reaction (ie, the uterus is hormonally prepared for acceptance of a fertilized ovum). In addition, delayed hypersensitivity reactions can be elicited in the uterus by injection of antigen into the uterus of a sensitized animal. However, pregnancy may alter the immune cell composition of the uterus. Decidua

618   IMMUNOLOGY/IMMUNOPATHOLOGY AND IMMUNITY

(uterine lining) from early pregnancy contain high numbers of Tγd+ cells which have selective downregulation of the TCR/CD3 complex and decreased alloreactivity to fetal tissues. It is postulated that these Tγd cells may act as specific suppressor cells for fetal graft rejection.

5. The production of blocking antibody prevents cellular reactivity to fetal antigens. It is well known that mothers will produce antibody to fetal antigens during pregnancy. The production of humoral antibody by the mother against paternal antigens on the fetus may enhance fetal viability (**pregnancy facilitation**). The placentas of F_1 mice are larger than those of inbred mice. Maternal preimmunization against paternal antigens enhances this effect. In humans, the incidence of spontaneous abortions is higher in couples who share MHC markers as compared to those who don't, and antibodies to paternal class II MHC are absent in the sera of spontaneous aborters. By these mechanisms, maternal immunostimulation may result in protection against T cell-mediated graft rejection of the fetus and actually stimulate growth of the fetus and placenta.

6. A factor (soluble serum protein) may be produced during pregnancy that interferes with immune effector mechanisms. Such proposed immunosuppressive factors include alpha-fetoprotein, pregnancy-associated proteins, alpha-regulatory globulin, etc. The support for immunosuppression is based on the effects of addition of these proteins to in vitro cultures. However, conflicting results have been obtained and a suppressive role in vivo has not been convincingly demonstrated. A suppressive effect on immune induction is not likely because pregnant animals are not immunosuppressed. In fact, in mice, pregnancy significantly increases the level of immunoglobulin-secreting cells in lymph nodes draining the uterus, and immune responses to injected antigens and mitogens are increased over normal. However, it is possible that a suppressive factor might function locally at the fetal–maternal interface to block effector mechanisms.

7. The early development of immune competence by the fetus in utero may provide a protective response for the immune elimination of the small number of maternal lymphocytes that get across the placenta. Fetal liver-derived lymphoid progenitors are largely Tγd cells that can rise to CD8+ T-cell lines, which are cytotoxic for maternal class I MHC antigens on T-cell lines. Under carefully defined conditions, the passive transfer of cells from unrelated strains of mice immunized against the parental strain will produce runting of the offspring while no GVH reaction occurs in the mother. It is suggested that the passively transferred cells crossed the placenta and produced a

GVH reaction in the fetuses that were not yet sufficiently immunologically competent to reject the specifically sensitized transferred cells; but the mother, who was immunologically mature, did reject the transferred cells. In humans, most instances of neonatal GVHD are associated with an immune deficiency of the fetus. There is speculation that the high incidence of lymphomas in children may be related to production of subclinical runt disease caused by maternal lymphocytes that infiltrated the fetus during pregnancy and were not eliminated by an immune response of the fetus. The high incidence of "autoimmune" reactions found in patients with lymphomas and leukemias suggests that the individual's lymphoid system may be responding to self antigens; perhaps this represents stimulation of maternally derived sequestered lymphocytes and is a GVH reaction.

8. The placenta serves as a barrier to immunization and to maternal immune cells. The fetus is contained in a fluid-filled cyst of fetal origin, the amniotic sac, which separates the mother from the fetus except at the point of attachment of the placenta. At this point, fetal tissue (the trophoblast) actually invades the endometrial wall of the uterus and comes into direct contact with the maternal circulation. Trophoblastic tissue is not rejected if transplanted into sites outside the uterus. In fact, the developing fetus may actually be maintained in the abdominal cavity outside of the uterus until nonimmune complications develop (ectopic pregnancy). Trophoblastic cells do not contain H, A, or B blood group antigens; the endothelium of the vessels of the placenta and umbilical cord have only the basic H structure. In contrast, the endothelial cells of the fetus have a high amount of these antigens. The lack of ABH antigens in the trophoblast prevents attack by maternal AB isoantibodies. The trophoblastic cells contain a large amount of glycocalyx, a cell coating of carbohydrate that masks transplantation antigens and repels lymphocytes. However, small numbers of maternal lymphocytes do cross the placenta, but evidently not in sufficient numbers to cause rejection of the fetus. That the placenta may contain lymphocytes that might attack the fetus is supported by the finding that placental size and lymphocyte content is increased in proportion to the degree of immunity of the mother to the fetus. It is possible that the placental tissue may contain histocompatibility antigens distributed in such a way that specifically sensitized lymphocytes react with placental tissue with minimal effect on placental function but are prevented from passing into the fetal circulation. There appear to be regulatory mechanisms that suppress the synthesis of both class I and class II MHC antigens in the placenta.

Maternal lymphocytes that do cross the placenta may not be reactive to fetal tissue antigens. Passively transferred antibody to fetal tissues is rapidly absorbed from the maternal circulation, most likely by the placenta. Thus, the placenta may act not only to provide a simple banner but also to remove and inactivate immune reactants.

Thus, although considerable controversy remains, the most likely explanation for the survival of the semiallogeneic fetal graft is the **placenta**. The placenta serves as a selective barrier between the mother and the fetus. Other mechanisms that have not been ruled out as playing a role, but are less likely, include immunologic immaturity of the conceptus; selective and local immunosuppression; some qualitative difference in the immune response of the mother during pregnancy, which promotes rather than hinders fetal survival; and reactivity of fetal immune cells to maternal cells that cross the placenta. There does not appear to be an immunologic explanation for the natural termination of pregnancy after nine months. This is most likely an endocrinologically determined event.

Summary

Transplantation of tissues from one genetically different individual to another (allograft) is subject to cell-mediated and antibody-directed graft rejection. The major mechanism is CMI against major histocompatibility antigens, and in some instances humoral antibody may actually protect a graft from cellular rejection (graft facilitation). Transplantation rejection can be controlled by chemical immunosuppression or by matching the major histocompatibility antigens of the donor tissue to those of the recipient. Suppression of CMI allows for long-term survival of solid tissue grafts, but chronic rejection may be caused by antibody-mediated scarring of blood vessels. In the last few years, the introduction of new immunosuppressive agents (ie, cyclosporine and PK506) has led to a much better prognosis for kidney, heart, liver, and other organ grafts. The major limitation to the clinical application of solid organ transplantation is the availability of donor organs.

Transplantation of bone marrow to replace diseased or lost stem cells may lead to an immune reaction of the graft against host tissues (graft-versus-host reaction). A number of techniques have been developed to control this reaction. Hematopoietic Stem cell transplantation has had increasing success in the treatment of immune deficiencies and leukemia treated with otherwise lethal radiation.

During pregnancy, immune rejection of the fetus is mainly prevented by the barrier of the placenta, but a number of other mechanisms may play a role.

Bibliography

GRAFT REJECTION/ GENERAL

Flye MW: *Principles of Organ Transplantation*. Philadelphia, WB Saunders, 1989.

Koene RAP: The role of adaptation in allograft acceptance. *Kidney Int* 35:1073, 1989.

Lafferty KJ, Prowse SJ, Simeonovic CJ, et al.: Immunology of tissue transplantation: Return to the passenger leukocyte concept. *Ann Rev Immunol* 1:143, 1983.

Manning DD, Reed ND, Shaffer CF: Maintenance of skin xenografts of widely divergent phyogenetic origin on congenitally athymic (nude) mice. *J Exp Med* 138:488, 1973.

Markin RS: The impact of transplantation on the clinical laboratory: Experience at the University of Nebraska with bone marrow and liver transplantation. *Arch Pathol Lab Med* 116:1004, 1992.

Pober JS, Collins T, Gimbrone MA, et al.: Inducible expression of class II major histocompatibility complex antigens and the immunogenicity of vascular endothelium. *Transplant* 41:141, 1986.

Salvatierra O, Perkins HA, Amend W, et al.: The influence of presensitization on graft survival rate. *Surgery* 81:146, 1977.

Sibley RK: Pathology and immunopathology of solid organ graft rejection. *Transplant Proc* 21:14, 1989.

Stetson CA: The role of humoral antibody in the homograft rejection. *Adv Immunol* 3:97, 1963.

Van Rood JJ, Claas FHJ: The influence of allogeneic cells on the human T and B cell repertoire. *Science* 248:1388, 1990.

MHC AND ORGAN TRANSPLAN- TATION

Amos DB, Kostyu DD: HLA-A central immunological agency of man. *Adv Human Genet* 10:137, 1980.

Bodmer JG, Marsh SCE, Albert ED, et al.: Nomenclature for factors of the HLA system, 1994. *Tiss Antigens* 44:1–18, 1994.

Cheigh JB, Chami J, Stenzl KH, et al.: Renal transplantation between HLA-identical siblings: Comparison with transplants from HLA-semi-identical donors. *N Engl J Med* 296:1030, 1977.

Colombani J: Changing the name of the major histocompatibility complex. *Res Immunol* 143:411, 1992.

Dausset J: The major histocompatibility complex in man. *Science* 213:1469, 1981.

Festenstein H, Doyle P, Holmes J: Long-term follow-up in London Transplant Group recipients of cadaver renal allografts: The influence of HLA matching on transplant outcome. *N Engl J Med* 314:7, 1986.

Leivestad T, Sodal G, Bratilie A, et al.: Role of HLA matching in cadaveric renal transplantation: Influence of improved serologic HLA-DR typing. *Transplant Proc* 25:220–221, 1993.

Lindahl KF: Minor histocompatibility antigens. *Trends Genet* 7:219, 1991.

Morris PJ: Histocompatibility antigens and transplantation over twenty years. *Immunol Lett* 21:25, 1989.

Smith SL: *Tissue and organ transplantation: Implications for Professional Practice*. St. Louis, Mosby-Year Book, 1990.

Terasaki PI: Histocompatibility testing in transplantation. *Arch Pathol Lab Med* 115:250, 1991.

Terasaki PI, Takemoto S, Park MS, et al.: HLA epitope matching. *Transfusion* 32:775–786, 1992.

Van Rood JJ, Eernisse JG: The detection of transplantation antigens in leukocytes. *Prog Surg* 7:217, 1967.

GRAFT FACILITATION

Casey AE: Experimental enhancement of malignancy in the Brown–Pearce rabbit tumor. *Proc Soc Exp Biol Med* 29:816, 1932.

Feldman JD: Immunological enhancement: A study of blocking antibodies. *Adv Immunol* 15:167, 1972.

Hellstrom KE, Hellstrom I: Immunological enhancement as studied by cell culture techniques. *Ann Rev Microbiol* 24:213, 1970.

Kaliss N: Immunological enhancement of tumor homografts in mice: A review. *Cancer Res* 18:992, 1958.

Voisin GA: Immunological facilitation: A broadening concept of the enhancement phenomenon. *Prog Allergy* 15:328, 1971.

XENOGRAFTS

Lu CY, Khair-El-Din TA, Dawidson IA, et al.: Xenotransplantation. *FASEB J* 8:1122–1130, 1994.

Nowak R: Xenotransplants set to resume. *Science* 266:1148–1151, 1994.

PATHOLOGY

Hammond EH (ed.): Solid organ transplantation. Orlando, WB Saunders, 1994.

SKIN GRAFTS

Balner H: Skin grafting in monkeys and apes. *Transplant* 8:206, 1969.

Berlin PJ, Bacher JD, Sharrow SO, et al.: Monoclonal antibodies against human T-cell adhesion molecules: Modulation of immune function in nonhuman primates. *Transplant* 53:840, 1992.

Mayer TG, Bhan AK, Winn HJ: Immunohistochemical analysis of skin graft rejection in mice: Kinetics of lymphocyte infiltration in grafts of limited immunogenetic disparity. *Transplant* 46:890, 1988.

Nakamura H, Grees RE: Graft rejection by cytotoxic T cells. *Transplant* 49:453, 1990.

RENAL GRAFTS

Almond PS, Gillinghan KJ, Sibley R, et al.: Renal transplant function after ten years of cyclosporine. *Transplant* 53:316, 1992.

Balch CM, Diethelm AG: The pathophysiology of renal allograft rejections: A collective overview. *J Surg Res* 12:350, 1972.

Barry JM: Immunosuppressive drugs in renal transplantation: A review of the regimens. *Drugs* 44:554, 1992.

Cameron JS: Glomerulonephritis in renal transplants. *Transplant* 34:237, 1982.

Chapman JR: Renal transplantation: An effective therapy in the 1990s. *Med J Aust* 157:315–317, 1992.

Flye MW: Renal transplantation. In *Principles of Organ Transplantation*. Flye W (ed.). Philadelphia, WB Saunders, 1989, 264–293.

Guttmann RD: Long-term problems of renal transplantation. *Transplant Proc* 24:1741–1743, 1992.

Kirk AD, Ibrahim MA, Bollinger RR, et al.: Renal allograft-infiltrating lymphocytes. *Transplant* 53:329, 1992.

Monaco AP: Clinical kidney transplantation in 1985. *Transplant* 17:5, 1985.

Porter KA, Dossitor JB, Marchioro WD, et al.: Human renal transplants. I. Glomerular changes. *Lab Invest* 16:153–181, 1967.

Papaport FT, Cortesni R: The past, present, and future of organ transplantation, with special reference to current needs in kidney procurement and donation. *Transp Prac* 17(suppl. 2):3, 1985.

Showstack J, Katz P, Amend W, et al.: The effect of cyclosporine on the use of hospital resources for kidney transplantation. *N Engl J Med* 321:1086, 1989.

Stratta RJ, Oh C-S, Sollinger HW, et al.: Kidney retransplantation in the cyclosporine era. *Transplant* 45:40, 1988.

Waltzer WC, et al.: Etiology and pathogenesis of hypertension following renal transplantation. *Nephron* 42:102, 1986.

HEART

Baldwin JC, Shumway NE: Cardiac transplantation. *J Cardiol* 74:39, 1985.

Billingham ME, Cary NRB, Hammond ME, et al.: A working formulation for the standardization of nomenclature in the diagnosis of heart and lung rejection: Heart rejection study group. *J Heart Transplant* 9:587, 1990.

Bishop DK, Shelby J, Eichwald EJ: Mobilization of T lymphocytes following cardiac transplantation. *Transplant* 53:849, 1992.

Carrel A, Guthrie C: The transplantation of veins and organs. *Amer Med* 10:1101, 1905.

Ettinger NA, Trulock EP: Pulmonary considerations of organ transplantation. III. *Am Rev Resp Dis* 144:433, 1991.

Haller JD, Cerruti MM: Heart transplantation in man: Compilation of cases. II. *Am J Cardiol* 24:554, 1969.

Kriett JM, Kaye MP: The registry of the International Society for Heart Transplantation: Seventh official report—1990. *J Heart Transplant* 9:323, 1990.

Lange LG, Schreiner GF: Immune cytokines and cardiac disease. *Med J Aust* 157:145–151, 1992.

O'Connell JB, Bourge RC, Costanzo-Nordin MR, et al.: Cardiac transplantation: Recipient selection, donor procurement, and medical follow-up. A statement for health professionals from the committee on cardiac transplantation of the Council on Clinical Cardiology, American Heart Association. *Circulation* 86:1061, 1992.

Shumway NE: Recent advances in cardiac transplantation. *Transp Prac* 75:1223, 1983.

Valantine HA: Long-term management and results in heart transplant recipients. *Cardiol Clin* 8:141, 1990.

PANCREAS

Allen RDM: Transplantation of the endocrine pancreas in 1992. *Med J Aust* 157:623, 1992.

Baker CF, Frangipane LG, Silvers WK: Islet transplantation in genetically determined diabetes. *Am Surg* 186:401, 1977.

Eckoff DE, Sollinger HW: Pancreatic and component transplantation for type I diabetes. *Clin Immunol Newslet* 12:129–133, 1992.

Hering BJ, Browatzki CC, Schultz A, et al.: Clinical islet transplantation: Registry report, accomplishments in past and future research needs. *Cell Transp* 2:269–282, 1993.

Lacy PE, Davie JM: Transplantation of pancreatic islets. *Ann Rev Immunol* 21:183, 1984.

Nakhleh RE, Sutherland DER: Pancreas rejection: significance of histopathologic findings with implications for classification of rejection. *Am J Surg Pathol* 16:1098, 1992.

Pyzdrowski KL, Kendall MK, Halter JB: Preserved insulin secretion and insulin independence in recipients of islet autografts. *N Engl J Med* 327:220, 1992.

Ricordi C: Pancreatic islet cell transplantation. CRC Press, Boca Raton, FL, 1992.

Ricordi C, Tzakis AG, Carroll PB, et al.: Human islet isolation and allotransplantation in 22 consecutive cases. *Transplant* 53:407, 1992.

Robertson RP: Pancreas transplantation in human with diabetes mellitus. *Diabetes* 40:1085, 1991.

Sutherland DER: Pancreas transplantation: Indication and outcomes. *Acta Diabetol* 28:185, 1992.

Sutherland D, Gruessner A, Moudry-Munns K: International pancreas transplant registry report. *Transplant Proc* 26:407–411, 1994.

LIVER

Bismuth H, Farges O, Samuel D, et al.: Past, present, and future in liver transplantation immunosuppression. *Transplant Proc* 24:85, 1992.

Doyle HR, Marino IR, Jabbour N, et al.: Early death or retransplantation in adults after orthotopic liver transplantation. *Transplant* 57:1028–1036, 1994.

Fennell RH, Shikes RH, Vierling JM: Relationship of pretransplant hepatobuliary disease to bile duct damage occurring in the liver allograft. *Hepatology* 3:84, 1984.

Henley KS, Lucey MR, Appelman HD, et al.: Biochemical and histopathologic correlation in liver transplant: The first 180 days. *Hepatology* 16:688, 1992.

Hockerstedt K: Liver transplantation: Present results and problems. *Ann Med* 24:365, 1993.

Kamada N: The immunology of experimental liver transplantation in the rat. *Immunology* 55:369, 1985.

Lucey MR, Beresford TP: Alcoholic liver disease: To transplant or not to transplant? *Alcohol & Alcoholism* 27:103, 1992.

Maddrey WC, Van Thiel DH: Liver transplantation: An overview. *Hepatology* 8:948, 1988.

Quiroga J, Colina I, Demetris AJ, et al.: Cause and timing of first allograft failure in orthotopic liver transplantation: A study of 177 consecutive patients. *Hepatology* 14:1054, 1991.

Vierling JM, Fennell RH: Histopathology of early and late human hepatic allograft rejection: Evidence of progressive destruction of interlobular bile ducts. *Hepatology* 5:1076, 1985.

Wood RP, Ozaki CF, Katz SM: Liver transplantation: The last 10 years. *Surg Clin N Amer* 74:1133–1153, 1994.

HEART–LUNG

De Blic J, Peuchmaur M, Carnot F: Rejection in lung transplantation: An immunohistochemical study of transbronchial biopsies. *Transplant* 54:639, 1992.

Griffith BP, Hardesty RL, Trento A, et al.: Heart–lung transplantation: Lessons learned and future hopes. *Ann Thorac Surg* 43:6, 1987.

Griffith BP, Paradis IL, Zeevi A, et al.: Immunologically mediated disease of the airways after pulmonary transplantation. *Ann Surg* 208:371, 1988.

McCarthy PM, Starnes VA, Theodore J, et al.: Improved survival after heart–lung transplantation. *J Thorac Cardiovasc Surg* 99:54, 1990.

Shennib H, Adoumie R, Noirclerc M: Current status of lung transplantation for cystic fibrosis. *Arch Int Med* 152:1585, 1992.

Tanoue LT: Lung transplantation. *Lung* 170:187, 1992.

Trulock EP, Cooper JD, Kaiser LR, et al.: The Washington University–Barnes Hospital experience with lung transplantation. *JAMA* 266:1943, 1991.

NEURAL

Dunnett SB: Neural transplants as a treatment for Alzheimer's disease? *Psychol Med* 21:825, 1991.

Freed WJ: Neural transplantation: A special issue. *Exp Neurol* 122:1–4, 1993.

Freed CR, Breeze RE, Rosenberg NL, et al.: Survival of implanted fetal dopamine cells and neurologic improvements 12 to 46 months after transplantation for Parkinson's disease. *N Engl J Med* 327:1549, 1992.

Gage EH, Fisher LJ: Intracerebral grafting: A toll for the neurobiologist. *Neuron* 6:1, 1991.

Lindvall O, Brundin P, Widner H, et al.: Grafts of fetal dopamine neurons survive and improve motor function in Parkinson's disease. *Science* 247:574, 1990.

Rosenfeld JV, Kilpatrick TJ, Barlett PF: Neural transplantation for Parkinson's disease: A critical appraisal. *Aust NZ J Med* 21:477, 1991.

Silverman MS, Hughes SE: Photoreceptor transplantation in inherited and environmentally induced retinal degeneration: Anatomy, immunohistochemistry, and function. In *Inherited and Environmentally Induced Retinal Degeneration.* New York, NY. Liss, 1989, 687.

Sladek JR, Gash DM: *Neural transplants.* New York, NY. Plenum, 1984.

Tessler A: Intraspinal transplants. *Ann Neurol* 29:115, 1991.

Spencer DD, Robbins RJ, Naftolin F, et al.: Unilateral transplantation of human fetal mesencephalic tissue into the caudate nucleus of patients with Parkinson's disease. *N Engl J Med* 327:1541, 1992.

Widner H, Tetrud J, Rehcrona S, et al.: Bilateral fetal mesencephalic grafting in two patients with parkinsonism induced by 1-methyl-4-phenyl-1,2,3,6-tetrahydrophridine (MPTP). *N Engl J Med* 327:1556, 1992.

CORNEA

Elliot JH: Immune factors in corneal graft rejection. *Invest Ophth* 10:216, 1971.

Khodadoust AA, Silverstein AM: The survival and rejection of epithelium in experimental corneal transplants. *Invest Ophth* 8:169, 1969.

Young E, Stark WJ, Predergast RA: Immunology of corneal allograft rejection: HLA-DR antigens on human corneal cells. *Invest Ophth* 26:571, 1985.

GRAFT SURVIVAL

Gruber SA: The case for local immunosuppression. *Transplant* 54:1, 1992.

Zenti M, Conforti A, Fabbi A, et al.: Regional immunosuppression for the prevention of solid organ allograft rejection: A better idea? *J Immunol Res* 3:139, 1991.

ORGAN PROCUREMENT

Cortesini R, Alfani D (eds.): World cooperation in transplantation: First society for organ sharing. *Transp Proc* 23:1–2707, 1991.

National Organ Transplantation Act, P.L. 98-507, sec. 273, 1984.

Phillips MG: *UNOS: Organ Procurement, Preservation and Distribution in Transplantation.* Richmond, VA, William Byrd, 1991.

Schaeffer MJ, Alexander CD: U.S. system for organ procurement and transplantation. *Am J Hosp Pharm* 49:1733, 1992.

GRAFT-VERSUS-HOST REACTIONS

Cabaniols J-P, Bolonakis-Tsilvakos I, Cibotti R, et al.: Mechanism of hybrid resistance: The role of a natural antibody in parental bone marrow cell rejection. *J Immunol* 146:860, 1991.

Cudkowicz G, Mennett M: Peculiar immunobiology of bone marrow allografts. II. Rejection of parental grafts by resistant F_1 hybrid mice. *J Exp Med* 134:1513, 1971.

Daley P, Wroblewski JM, Kaminsky SG, et al.: Genetic control of the target structure recognized in hybrid resistance. *Immunogenetics* 26:21, 1987.

Deeg HJ, Storb R: Graft-versus-host disease: Pathophysiologic and clinical aspects. *Ann Rev Med* 35:11, 1984.

Ferrara JLM, Deeg HJ: Graft-versus-host disease. *N Engl J Med* 324:667, 1991.

Kelemen E, Szebeni J, Petrányi GG: Graft-versus-host disease in bone marrow transplantation: Experimental, laboratory, and clinical contributions of the last few years. *Int Arch Allergy Immunol* 102:309–320, 1993.

Simonsen M: Graft-versus-host reactions: Their natural history and applicability as tools of research. *Prog Allergy* 6:349, 1962.

Snover DC: Acute and chronic graft-versus-host disease: Histopathologic evidence for two distinct pathogenic mechanisms. *Human Pathol* 15:202, 1984.

Wick MR, Moore SB, Gastineau, DA, Hoagland, HC: Immunologic, clinical, and pathologic aspects of human graft-versus-host disease. *Mayo Clin Proc* 58:603-612, 1983.

BONE MARROW TRANSPLAN-TATION

Blomquist MD, Boggards M, Guerra-Hanson IC, et al.: Monoclonal anti-T cell (T_{12}) antibody treatment of graft-versus-host disease in severe combined immunodeficiency: Targeting of antibody and activation of complement on CD8+ cytotoxic T-cell surfaces. *J Allergy Clin Immunol* 87:1029, 1991.

Bortin MM, Horowitz MM, Rowlings PA, et al.: 1993 progress report from the International Bone Marrow Transplant Registry. *Bone Marrow Transplant* 12:97–104, 1993.

Congdon CC: Radiation injury: Bone marrow transplantation. *Annu Rev Med* 13:203, 1962.

Deeg HJ, Storb R, Thomas ED: Bone marrow transplantation: A review of delayed complications. *Brit J Hematol* 57:185, 1984.

Ettinger NA, Trulock EP: Pulmonary considerations of organ transplantation. II. *Am Rev Respir Dis* 144:213, 1991.

Gale RP, Armitage JO, Butturini A: Is there a role for autotransplants in acute leukemia? *Bone Marrow Transplant* 4:217, 1989.

Genogzian M, Edwards CL, Vodopick HA, et al.: Bone marrow transplantation in a leukemic patient following immunosuppression with antithymocyte globulin and total body irradiation. *Transplantation* 15:446, 1972.

Greenbaum BH: Transfusion-associated graft-versus-host disease: Historical perspectives, incidence, and current use of irradiated blood products. *J Clin Oncol* 9:1889, 1991.

Klumpp TR: Immunohematologic complications of bone marrow transplantation. *Bone Marrow Transplant* 8:159, 1991.

Leibundgut K, Hirt A, Lüthy AR, et al.: Autotransplants with peripheral blood stem cells and clinical results obtained in children. *Eur J Pediat* 152:546–554, 1993.

Lenarsky C, Parkman R: Bone marrow transplantation for the treatment of immune deficiency states. *Bone Marrow Transplant* 6:361, 1990.

Lum LG, Ueda M: Immunodeficiency and the role of suppressor cells after human bone marrow transplantation. *Clin Immunol Immunopathol* 63:103, 1992.

Mathe G, Schwarzenberg L, Amiel JL, et al.: Immunogenetic and immunologic problems of allogeneic haematopoietic radio-chimeras in man. *Scand J Haematol* 4:193, 1967.

McGovern JJ Jr, Russell PS, Atkins L, et al.: Treatment of terminal leukemic relapse by total-body irradiation and intravenous infusion of stored autologous bone marrow obtained during remission. *N Engl J Med* 260:675, 1959.

Sakamoto H, Michaelson J, Jones WK, et al.: Lymphocytes with a CD4+CD8-CD3- phenotype are effectors of experimental cutaneous graft-versus-host disease. *Proc Natl Acad Sci USA* 88:10890, 1991.

Shearer WT, Ritz J, Finegold MJ, et al.: Epstein–Barr virus-associated B cell proliferations of diverse clonal origins after bone marrow transplantation in a 12-year-old patient with severe combined immune deficiency. *N Engl J Med* 312:1151–1159, 1985.

Slavin RE, Santos GW: The graft-versus-host reaction in man after bone marrow transplantation: Pathology, pathogenesis, clinical features, and implications. *Clin Immunol Immunopathol* 1:472, 1973.

Soiffer RJ, Dear K, Rabinowe SN, et al.: Hepatic dysfunction following T cell-depleted allogeneic bone marrow transplantation. *Transplant* 52:1014, 1991.

Taliaferro WH, Taliaferro LG, Jaroslow BN: *Radiation and Immune Mechanisms.* New York, Academic Press, 1964.

Thomas ED: Marrow transplantation for malignant diseases. *J Clin Oncol* 1:517, 1983.

Thomas ED, Bryant JI, Buckner CD, et al.: Leukemic transformation of engrafted bone marrow. *Transplant Proc* 4:567, 1972.

Thomas ED, Storb R, Clift RA, et al.: Bone marrow transplantation. *N Engl J Med* 292:832, 895, 1975.

Vallera DA, Blazar BR: T-cell depletion for graft-versus-host disease prophylaxis. *Transplantation* 47:751, 1989.

GENE TRANSFER

Apperley JF, Williams DA: Gene therapy. Current status and future directions. *Br J Haematol* 75:148, 1990.

Boggs SS: Targeted gene modification for gene therapy of stem cells. *Int J Cell Cloning* 8:80, 1990.

Karlsson S: Treatment of genetic defects in hematopoietic cell function by gene transfer. *Blood* 78:2481, 1991.

Krauss JC: Hematopoietic stem cell gene replacement therapy. *Biochem Biophys Acta* 1114:193–207, 1992.

Lehn PM: Gene therapy using bone marrow transplantation. *Bone Marrow Transplant* 1:243, 1987.

Miller AD: Progress toward human gene therapy. *Blood* 76:271, 1990.

Williams DA, Lemischka IR, Nathan DG, et al.: Introduction of new genetic material into pluripotent haematopoietic stem cells of the mouse. *Nature* 310:476, 1984.

FETOMATERNAL RELATIONSHIP

Billingham RE, Beer AE: Reproductive immunology: Past, present, and future perspects. *Biol Med* 27:259, 1984.

Chaouat G: *Immunology of Pregnancy*. Boca Raton, FL, CRC Press, 1992.

Clark DA: Controversies in reproductive immunology. *Crit Rev Immunol* 11:215, 1991.

Dresser DW: The potentiating effect of pregnancy on humoral immune responses of mice. *J Reprod Immunol* 20:253, 1991.

Gill TJ: Immunity and pregnancy. *CRC Crit Rev Immunol* 5:201, 1985.

Hill JA: Cytokines considered critical in pregnancy. *Am J Reprod Immunol* 28:123–126, 1992.

Hunziker RD, Wegmann TG: Placental immunoregulation. *CRC Crit Rev Immunol* 6:245, 1986.

Mincheva-Nilsson L, Hammarstrom S, Hammarstrom M-L: Human decidual leukocytes from early pregnancy contain high numbers of γδ+ cells and show selective downregulation of alloreactivity. *J Immunol* 149:2203, 1992.

Ober C: The maternal–fetal relationship in human pregnancy: An immunogenic perspective. *Exp Clin Immunogenet* 9:1, 1992.

Szulman AE: The A, B, and H blood group antigens in the human placenta. *N Engl J Med* 286:1028, 1972.

Wegmann TG, Carlson GA: Allogenic pregnancy as immunoabsorbent. *J Immunol* 119:1659, 1977.

24

Lymphoproliferative Diseases

Immunoproliferative (lymphoproliferative) diseases include both inflammatory (self-limited, reversible) and malignant (progressive) increases in numbers of cells belonging to lymphoid cell populations (lymphocytes and macrophages). The term **malignant lymphoma** was first proposed by Billroth in 1871, to differentiate malignant tumors from inflammatory reactions or benign hyperplasia. The suffix "-oma" means mass (or lump), thus lymphoma means an increase in mass of a lymphoid organ. According to the standard nomenclature for cancer, malignant tumors of lymphoid cells should be called "lymphosarcomas" to indicate their malignant nature, and benign lymphoid tumors should be called lymphomas. However, in practice, the term lymphoma is used for malignant tumors. Leukemia means "white blood." In patients with cancers of the circulating white blood cells, the large numbers of malignant leukemic white blood cells give the normally red blood a whitish color. Thus, lymphoma is used for malignant proliferation of white cells in lymphoid organs, and leukemia is used for malignant increases in white cells in the blood.

Lymphomas and leukemias are progressively growing tumors that mimic in appearance normal lymphoid cells. Until recently, classification and understanding of these diseases were based mainly on morphologic observations and clinical correlations. The identification of cell surface markers for different lymphocyte populations has led to a much better understanding of lymphocyte differentiation and to reclassification of immunoproliferative diseases on the basis of T cell, B cell, or macrophage (histocyte) lineage. This reclassification, in conjunction with investigations with animal models of lymphoproliferation, is being applied to give a better appreciation of these diseases in humans.

Older classifications are confusing because the terminology presumed a cell type of origin on the basis of morphology, which may not have been valid. For instance, the terms "reticulum cell sarcoma" and "histiocytic lymphoma," implying a macrophage origin, were used for tumors that are now known to express B-cell markers. These are now classified as poorly differentiated forms of diffuse B-cell lymphoma.

Lymphoid Tissue Structure and Lymphoproliferative Disease

MATURATION OF BLOOD-FORMING CELLS

To understand the morphology, growth patterns, manifestations, and tissue distribution of the human lymphoproliferative diseases, the localization of normal lymphoid cells in lymphoid organs and phenotypic markers reflecting differentiation of lymphocytes must be considered (see Chapters 2 and 3). A diagram of the normal maturation of blood cells, including lymphocytes and other blood cell lineages, and the putative site of the block in differentiation is illustrated in Figure 24–1. The precursors of lymphoid cells arise mainly in the bone marrow. Before maturation, these cells do not express T- or B-cell markers but differentiate into cells that migrate to other lymphoid organs. A block in the differentiation of malignant lymphocytes results in the accumulation of large numbers of relatively homogeneous, less mature cells. As a result of the differentiation block, cells in a given lineage that normally would differentiate into cells that would die to make way for newly formed cells (terminally differentiate), do not die and continue to accumulate in tissues. This results in the "forcing out" of normal cells leading to loss of function of blood cells and disease manifestations, such as anemia (loss of red blood cells), bleeding (loss of platelets), susceptibility to infection (loss of lymphocytes and granulocytes), and wasting.

TISSUE LOCALIZATION OF LYMPHOID CELLS

In this chapter the emphasis is on tumors of the lymphoid cells, ie, lymphocytes and monocytes (macrophages). Most human lymphocytic tumors (lymphomas) are of B-cell lineage; but tumors of T cells and macrophages also occur frequently. Tumors of lymphoid cells usually are first located in lymphoid organs in areas where cells of the same lineage are normally found (Fig. 24–2). T-cell precursors circulate to the thymus, develop into mature T cells, and then migrate from the thymus to localize in T-dependent zones (lymph node paracortex, spleen periarteriolar sheath, etc.) in peripheral organs. B cells arise in bone marrow

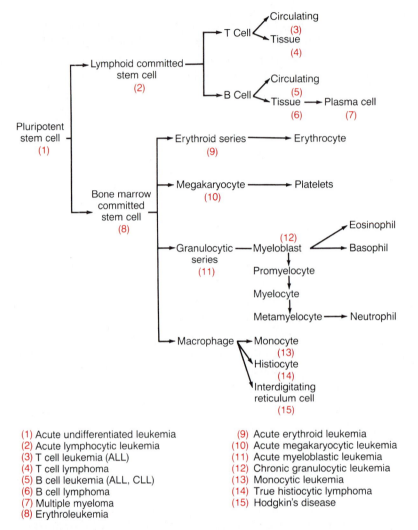

(1) Acute undifferentiated leukemia
(2) Acute lymphocytic leukemia
(3) T cell leukemia (ALL)
(4) T cell lymphoma
(5) B cell leukemia (ALL, CLL)
(6) B cell lymphoma
(7) Multiple myeloma
(8) Erythroleukemia

(9) Acute erythroid leukemia
(10) Acute megakaryocytic leukemia
(11) Acute myeloblastic leukemia
(12) Chronic granulocytic leukemia
(13) Monocytic leukemia
(14) True histiocytic lymphoma
(15) Hodgkin's disease

Figure 24–1. Maturation of blood-forming cells and postulated site of maturation arrest in lymphomas and leukemias. Pluripotent stem cells are present in the bone marrow and give rise to other cell types by differentiation to "end" cells. Mature cells in each series normally die at the same rate as new cell types in each series are produced, resulting in a relatively constant number of each cell type. In lymphomas and leukemias differentiation of a given cell lineage is arrested so that increasing numbers of a given cell type appear. This process is not normally reversible by physiological mechanisms, although it may be controlled by chemotherapy. ALL, acute lymphocytic leukemia; CLL, chronic lymphocytic leukemia. (See Chapter 4 for a detailed description of the development of the immune system.)

or fetal liver and localize in B-cell zones (lymph node follicles, spleen follicles), with mature immunoglobulin-producing plasma cells found in medullary zones (lymph node medulla or splenic red pulp cords). Macrophages are found in follicular zones and are also prominent in medullary zones. In addition to these, a substantial proportion of cells

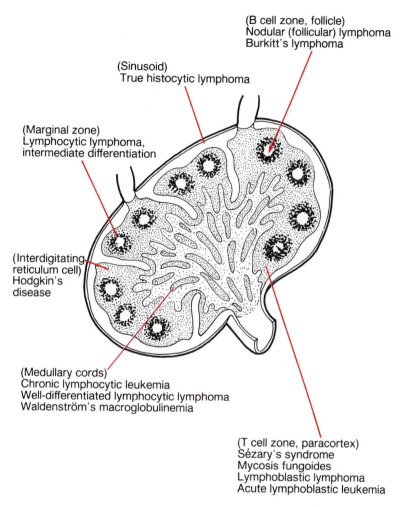

(B cell zone, follicle)
Nodular (follicular) lymphoma
Burkitt's lymphoma

(Sinusoid)
True histocytic lymphoma

(Marginal zone)
Lymphocytic lymphoma,
intermediate differentiation

(Interdigitating
reticulum cell)
Hodgkin's
disease

(Medullary cords)
Chronic lymphocytic leukemia
Well-differentiated lymphocytic lymphoma
Waldenström's macroglobulinemia

(T cell zone, paracortex)
Sézary's syndrome
Mycosis fungoides
Lymphoblastic lymphoma
Acute lymphoblastic leukemia

Figure 24–2. Structure of lymph node and origin of lymphomas. Drawing of lymph node illustrating anatomic localization of B cells (follicles), T cells (diffuse, paracortex, and deep cortex), and macrophages (medullary cords). B-cell tumors arise in the cortex and are often follicular in structure but sometimes diffuse. T-cell lymphomas arise in the paracortex and deep cortex and are always diffuse. Tumors of macrophages arise in the medulla and are diffuse. In general, the structure of the tumors reflects the normal morphology of the cell type from which it arises. (Modified from Mann RS, Jaffe ES, Berard CW: Malignant lymphomas: A conceptual understanding of morphologic diversity. *Am J Pathol* 94:105–192, 1979.)

without markers (null cells) are found at different tissue sites. Of particular importance is the fact that some lymphoid cells normally circulate and are found in peripheral blood. One of the major differences between lymphomas and leukemias is the lack of cell surface homing markers on leukemic cells that react with endothelial cells. Thus, these cells do not "home" to lymphoid organs as do cells of lymphomas.

Nonmalignant Lympho-proliferation

Physiologic stress may result in reversible increased production of a given cell type (hyperplasia). When production exceeds terminal differentiation, the number of cells will increase. At high altitudes the production of erythrocytes will increase, resulting in higher numbers of erythrocytes; during a chronic infection, production of granulocytes will increase. With removal of the stimulus for hyperplasia, production will return to normal and the number of cells dying will exceed production until previous cell numbers are reached.

Benign (nonmalignant) hyperplasia of lymphoid tissue usually occurs in response to inflammatory stimuli or infections. Both benign and malignant lymphoproliferative diseases may present with enlarged lymph nodes or spleen associated with fever, so that it is often not a simple matter to differentiate benign from malignant lymphadenopathy or splenomegaly (enlarged lymph nodes or spleen). If an obvious source of infection is present, such as inflamed tonsils associated with cervical lymphadenopathy, and if this responds to appropriate therapy by antibiotics, malignancy may be considered unlikely. However, if in doubt it is advisable to obtain a lymph node biopsy to rule out malignancy. If an invasive procedure is to be performed, every effort should be made to obtain a satisfactory diagnostic tissue specimen. It is important to obtain the largest nodes accessible to the surgeon, not just some nodal tissues, because frequently not all nodes in a group will be involved. Histologically, inflammatory hyperplasias are not monoclonal or limited to one cell type, as are most lymphomas. The cells involved will be a mixture of T, polyclonal B, and null, as well as polymorphonuclear cells and macrophages. Malignant tumors demonstrate a relative uniformity of cell type and replacement of normal structures, whereas hyperplasias contain a mixture of cell types and an exaggeration of normal structure.

SUPPURATIVE LYMPHADENITIS

Suppurative lymphadenitis is an inflammatory reaction in the lymph node draining a zone of acute infection. Usually, polymorphonuclear leukocytes are found early after onset; macrophages appear later. The basic structure of the lymph node is not altered. Tonsillitis is a form of suppurative lymphadenitis.

POSTVACCINIAL AND VIRAL LYMPHADENITIS

The lymph nodes draining the site of vaccination (tetanus, diphtheria, and others) or viral infection show a mixed cellular response, particularly an increased paracortical component with a large number of blast cells and, in some instances, even giant cells. In some cases, it may be very difficult to distinguish this response from malignant lymphomas by histologic examination. These responses are also seen in immunized animals and represent primarily a T-cell proliferative response of lymphoid tissue to antigenic stimulation or viral infection.

AIDS-RELATED LYMPH-ADENOPATHY

Generalized enlargement of lymph nodes has been noted to precede the appearance of opportunistic infections characteristic of the AIDS syndrome. (See Chapter 29 for a more detailed description of AIDS.) AIDS is caused by the human immunodeficiency virus (HIV). HIV infects helper T cells, as well as other cell types, particularly dendritic monocytes. Histologically, the nodes in pre-AIDS show polyclonal follicular (B-cell) and diffuse (T-cell) hyperplasia. As the disease progresses, there is a mixture of hyperplasia and hypoplasia in the same node. Finally, marked lymphocyte depletion is seen in lymph nodes in fatal AIDS and is believed to represent the end-stage lesion. The findings are qualitatively similar to those seen in other viral infections, such as infectious mononucleosis, but are often more extensive. A true lymphoma may be a late manifestation of HIV infection. These are usually undifferentiated or Burkitt's type B-cell lymphomas; T-cell lymphomas are not found in increased frequency in AIDS patients (see Chapter 29).

DRUG-INDUCED LYMPH-ADENOPATHY

Ingestion of anticonvulsant drugs (diphenylhydantoin, mephenytoin) may lead to a lymphoid cell reaction that mimics lymphoma, including skin rash, fever, and lymphadenopathy. There may be loss of normal architecture with a pleomorphic cell infiltrate, including blasts, eosinophils, neutrophils, and plasma cells. Without the clinical history of drug exposure, differentiation from lymphoma may be very difficult; the term pseudolymphomatous lymphadenitis has been used to emphasize the resemblance of these lesions to lymphoma.

SINUS HISTIOCYTOSIS WITH MASSIVE LYMPH-ADENOPATHY (ROSAI–DORFMAN DISEASE)

Massive cervical lymphadenopathy, fever, and leukocytosis may be associated with dilation of lymph node subcapsular and medullary sinusoids that become filled with proliferating histiocytes, which phagocytose normal lymphocytes. This may persist for some years but is entirely self-limited. The etiology is unknown, but most likely represents a response to a chronic inflammatory or antigenic stimulus.

LYMPHO-DERMATITIS (DERMATOPATHIC LYMPHADENITIS)

Lymphadenopathy may occur with a variety of infectious diseases, such as tuberculosis, sarcoidosis, cat scratch disease, various dermatologic conditions, and following injection of radiographic contrast media (lymphangiography). Usually, the enlarged lymph nodes show some form of inflammation, including granulomas, histiocytosis, follicular hyperplasia, and polymorphonuclear exudation.

GIANT LYMPH NODE HYPERPLASIA

Giant lymph node hyperplasia (Castleman's disease) is a benign, usually localized lesion of unknown etiology. There are two varieties: Hyaline vascular and plasma cell. The hyaline vascular type consists of small follicles containing hyalinized blood vessels in the center.

Between the follicles is a mixture of capillaries and lymphoid cells. The plasma cell variety has sheets of plasma cells in the interfollicular tissue. The lesions are usually mediastinal but may occur in other locations, such as mesentery or axillary. Most of the proliferating cells are polyclonal B cells. It is often difficult to distinguish the lesions of Castleman's disease from those secondary to inflammation. The plasma cell variety of Castleman's disease is found in patients with rheumatoid arthritis. In addition, some patients with typical features of Castleman's disease lesions develop systemic symptoms, and similar lesions are found associated with AIDS, Wiskott–Aldrich syndrome, and in nodes draining cancer sites.

INFECTIOUS MONO-NUCLEOSIS

Infectious mononucleosis (IM) is a benign lymphoproliferative disease related to the malignant B-cell tumor, Burkitt's lymphoma. It is common in young adults, sometimes reaching epidemic proportions when young adults from different backgrounds and for the most part, different sexes, are placed together, as in college (kissing disease). It is caused by infection with Epstein–Barr (EB) virus, the virus that is also found with Burkitt's lymphoma and nasopharyngeal carcinoma. These diseases may represent different racial or environmentally determined responses to the same infectious agent, but such a relationship has not been critically established. The symptoms of infectious mononucleosis follow an incubation period of about 20 to 30 days and consist of fatigue, general malaise, and loss of appetite. Occasionally, high fever, lymphadenopathy, pharyngitis, and hepatosplenomegaly are found, all of which usually last for a few weeks. There may be polyclonal B-cell proliferation. Antibodies to EB virus antigens appear in the serum of patients during the course of the disease.

Mononucleosis refers to the presence of an abnormally large number of immature mononuclear cells in the peripheral blood. These are large lymphocytes with enlarged nuclei and abundant cytoplasm (atypical lymphocytes). Sometimes autologous rosettes with the patient's red blood cells are formed. Some of the atypical cells have properties of T cells (they form rosettes with sheep RBC, react with anti-T-cell sera), whereas others have B- or null-cell markers. Atypical lymphocytes of infectious mononucleosis may be immunocompetent cells reacting immunologically to EB virus infection. These atypical lymphocytes have been shown to actively synthesize DNA, and it is postulated that they represent heterogeneous T and B blast cells responding to antigens; they are not infected proliferating cells. In contrast, the proliferating (EBV-infected) cells of Burkitt's lymphoma are usually, but not always, homogeneous (monoclonal) B-cell populations. Heterogeneous atypical lymphocytes are also found in the blood after organ transplantation or immunization, in patients with rheumatoid or autoimmune disease, in association with malignant tumors, during drug reactions, and in the presence of other bacterial or viral infections. Although it is tempting to speculate that infectious mononucleosis is a benign form and that Burkitt's lymphoma is a malignant form of EB virus infection, absolute proof of this relationship has not been obtained.

Permanent cell lines are relatively easy to obtain using the blood lymphocytes of patients with infectious mononucleosis. These cell lines are invariably infected with EB virus and often have chromosome $8 \rightarrow 14$ translocations. The cells are usually diploid and display monoclonal surface and cytoplasmic immunoglobulin (B cells). The cells that grow out are infected B cells and not the atypical lymphocytes seen in peripheral blood. The EB virus infects only B cells, apparently because a receptor for the virus is related to the C3 receptor found on B cells and not on T cells. T cells from patients with IM are often able to kill B-cell lines expressing EB viral antigens. Atypical T lymphocytes may actually be a cytotoxic reactive cell to infected B cells. Very rarely is infectious mononucleosis a fulminant fatal disease similar to acute lymphoblastic leukemia, and IM features a polyclonal instead of monoclonal increase in "transformed" B cells. It may be that in this acute form of the disease, multiple cells are undergoing transformation at about the same time, resulting in more than one type of B cell in the tumor. In the absence of the immune mechanisms of T-cell cytotoxicity, these cells might proliferate rapidly and produce an overwhelming diffuse lymphoproliferative disease. EBV-positive tumors have developed in some immunosuppressed patients who receive bone marrow transplants, presumably because of the unrestricted growth of the EBV-infected donor cells in the immunosuppressed recipient.

Human Lymphomas

Human lymphomas are cancer of lymphoid cells: T cells, B cells, macrophages, or null cells (cells without markers). The major clinical classification is divided into two types—non-Hodgkin's and Hodgkin's lymphoma—because the response to the therapy and clinical course of Hodgkin's diseases and other lymphomas is critically different. The cellular origin of Hodgkin's disease has been the subject of controversy, but recent evidence suggests that these tumors arise from a particular macrophage subpopulation, the interdigitating reticulum cells (see below), whereas non-Hodgkin's lymphomas are usually derived from lymphocytes. Also of critical importance is the characterization of the growth potential and clinical course as acute or chronic.

NON-HODGKIN'S LYMPHOMAS

Classification

Three major findings determine the ability to predict the growth behavior of a malignant lymphoma, non-Hodgkin's type: The pattern of tissue replacement, the morphology of the cells, and the extent of organ involvement. A general principle of neoplastic disease is that cancer tissue is a caricature of the normal tissue from which it arises. Lymphomas are tumors of lymphoid organs, and the morphologic structure reflects the lymphoid cell organ. The most useful working morphologic classification of non-Hodgkin's lymphomas reflect this relationship.

Nodular or Diffuse. The major morphologic differentiation of non-Hodgkin's lymphomas is nodular (follicular) or diffuse. Nodular lymphomas reflect the morphology of lymphoid follicles and are composed of B cells. Diffuse lymphomas reflect the structure of the diffuse cortex of lymph nodes and appear as sheets of cells without follicular structure and may be of B cell, T cell, null cell, or true histiocytic (macrophage) origin. Nodular tumors have a much better prognosis than diffuse tumors.

Cell Structure. The second major morphologic feature is the size of the cells that make up the tumor. The size of the cells within a tumor are a reflection of the number of cells in the growth cycle. Resting cells are usually small, whereas cells in the cell cycle enlarge as RNA and DNA are synthesized. Therefore, the size of the cells in a given lymphoma is an indication of the growth fraction, ie, the proportion of actively proliferating cells. Tumors made up of small cells have a better prognosis than tumors made up of large (undifferentiated) cells. Tumors made up of a mixture of large, intermediate, and small cells have an intermediate prognosis.

Organ Involvement. The third major prognostic factor is the extent of organ involvement by the tumor. This is known as clinical staging and will be described in more detail below. In general, the more organs that are involved with lymphoma cells when the diagnosis is made, the poorer the prognosis.

Rappaport System

The morphologic features are incorporated into the classic classification of non-Hodgkin's lymphomas proposed by Henry Rappaport in 1956 (Table 24–1). In this classification, histiocytic refers to a large lymphocytic type of tumor, now known usually to be composed of B cells and not histiocytes. Rappaport used the term "histiocytic lymphoma" because the large cells looked like tissue histiocytes. Over the

TABLE 24–1. MORPHOLOGIC CLASSIFICATION OF NON-HODGKIN'S LYMPHOMAS

Topography	Nodular or Diffuse
Cell type	Lymphocytic, well differentiated
	Lymphocytic, poorly differentiated
	Histiocytic* (reticulum cell sarcoma)
	Mixed histiocytic and lymphocytic
	Undifferentiated (blast)

* Histiocytic refers to large cells and does not necessarily imply macrophage origin.

Modified from Rappaport H, et al.: *Cancer* 9:792, 1956.

last thirty years, this classification has provided a valuable method of evaluating non-Hodgkin's lymphomas. Although there have been a number of attempts to "improve" on this classification, the general rule is that patients with tumors of small cells do better than patients with tumors of large cells, and patients with nodular tumors do better than those with diffuse tumors. In 1982, a reclassification called "The Working Formulation" was devised by an international group of authorities. Since then, a number of different classifications have been proposed, none of which has received universal acceptance. In this chapter, a simplified classification of B-cell, T-cell, and macrophage tumors will be used.

B-cell Tumors

These include 90% of chronic lymphocytic leukemia, several kinds of nodular or diffuse lymphoma, and tumors of plasma cells (eg, multiple myeloma). The cells of these tumors reflect their B-cell origin by expressing either cell surface immunoglobulin, cytoplasmic monoclonal immunoglobulin, rearranged Ig genes, or cell surface markers of B-cell lineage. These may all be considered to be tumors arising from cells at different stages of B-cell development and thus reflect the tissue distribution and surface characteristics of normal B cells at similar stages. The incidence of B-cell tumors is much higher in elderly individuals (50 to 70 years of age) than in people younger than 50 years of age. B-cell tumors may arise because of a lack of control by the appropriate suppressor cells. Thus, a loss of T-cell control of B-cell proliferation with aging may result in uncontrolled B-cell proliferation. Monoclonal immunoglobulins are sometimes found in other diseases, such as with nonlymphoid tumors, and in elderly persons. The significance of these elevations remains uncertain. The presence of a monoclonal immunoglobulin (gammopathy) in an otherwise normal person suggests that covert myeloma is present and will become manifest if the person lives long enough (see below).

B-cell
Lymphomas

Two major forms of B-cell lymphoma are recognized topographically—follicular and diffuse. Either follicular or diffuse B-cell lymphomas may contain small and large lymphocytes in different proportions and are usually found in lymph nodes, spleen, or gastrointestinal tract. The growth pattern of follicular lymphomas mimics the nodular arrangement of cells in lymphoid follicles—thus, the designation of follicular or nodular.

Follicular Center Cells. In 1971, Lukes and Collins attempted to refine the cellular classification of non-Hodgkin's lymphomas. They recognized that the cells of most non-Hodgkin's lymphomas resembled cells seen in germinal centers and postulated that these cells represented different stages of the cell cycle of B cells, whether the lymphoma was nodular or diffuse. This concept is presented in Figure 24–3. Most non-Hodgkin's lymphomas are of B-cell type, and the idea

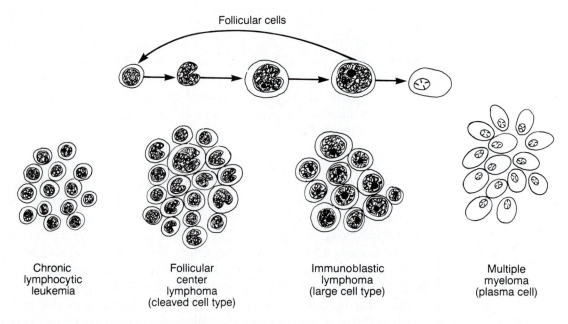

Figure 24–3. Histologic features of B-cell lymphomas as related to morphology of B cells. During the cell cycle, B cells change from small round cells to large "blast" cells and divide to form small cells. Differentiation results in production of plasma cells. The nucleus of the early activated B cell is cleaved, whereas those of the small resting cell and the cells in later stages of B cell differentiation are not cleaved. Chronic lymphocyte leukemia represents a maturation arrest at the small noncleaved stage, multiple myeloma at the plasma cell stage, follicular lymphomas at the activated B-cell stage (cleaved), and large cell lymphomas at the immunoblastic B-cell stage (large noncleaved cells). Modified from Lukes RJ, Collins RD: Lukes–Collins classification and its significance. (*Cancer Treatment Reports* 61:971–979, 1977; and Taylor CR: Classification of lymphoma. *Arch Pathol Lab Med* 102:549–554, 1978.)

that the morphology of these tumors reflects the cell cycle position of the majority of the cells in the tumor is probably correct. Lukes and Collins also postulated that the shape of the nuclei of the cells ("cleaved or not cleaved") of a lymphoma reflected the stage of maturation of the cells in the tumor, and that there is evolution of B-cell lymphomas from small cleaved → large cleaved → small noncleaved → large noncleaved, associated with progression to more malignant behavior. Unfortunately, the fine morphologic characteristics used in this classification are subject to subtle changes in tissue fixation and processing and are not easily defined, even by experienced pathologists. Thus, the reproducibility of this classification at different centers has not been uniform. In the 1970s, a number of classification systems of non-Hodgkin's lymphomas was proposed, generating considerable debate and confusion. These classifications, while still useful, have largely been superseded by the use of other cellular markers, but morphologic classification of small, large, intermediate, and mixed-cell type is still critical in determining the prognosis of lymphoma. Small-cell types progress very slowly. Large-cell types progress more rapidly but respond better than small cell-types to chemotherapy. Unfortunately, they frequently develop resistance to chemotherapy and are often fatal.

Tissue Pattern. In contrast to normal lymph follicles, which are found in the cortex of a lymph node, neoplastic follicles are found throughout the node with obliteration of the normal node architecture (Fig. 24–4).

Normal follicle   Follicular lymphoma

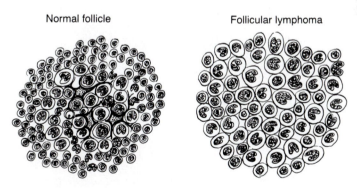

Figure 24–4. Patterns of normal polyclonal and neoplastic B-cell follicles. Normal secondary or germinal centers contain a mixture of different cell types, including not only polyclonal B cells but also macrophages and T cells, and are surrounded by a rim of polyclonal cells. On the other hand, malignant B-cell tumors may form follicles or replace the node structure diffusely with a homogeneous cell type. Malignant follicles are made up of cells of a single clonal line, do not contain T cells or macrophages, and are not surrounded by a rim of polyclonal cells. Malignant follicles efface the other components of the lymph node (paracortex, medulla) and extend diffusely into adjacent tissue with loss of the structure of capsule and subcapsular sinus, whereas these areas, although relatively less conspicuous, are preserved in nonmalignant hyperplasia.

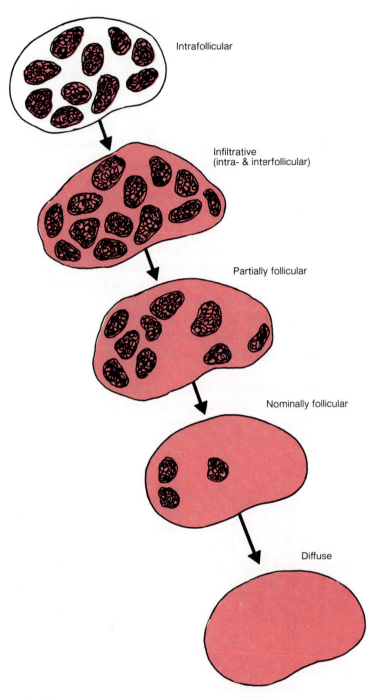

Figure 24–5. B-cell lymphoma exists in variations from follicular to diffuse patterns. Increased malignancy or the progression toward more aggressive tumor is associated with a change from more follicular to more diffuse, as well as with cell size and morphology. Small, cleaved, follicular tumors have the best prognosis. Large, noncleaved, diffuse tumors have the worst prognosis. Approximately 30% of patients followed carefully demonstrate progression from less to more malignant forms.

Diffuse B-cell lymphocytic lymphoma consists of small to medium-sized lymphocytes, which diffusely infiltrate and replace lymph node and spleen structures. The variations in follicular and diffuse patterns of B-cell lymphomas and the progression from follicular to diffuse are illustrated in Figure 24–5. Analysis of the immunoglobulin genes of diffuse and follicular areas in a given lymphoma indicate that diffuse B-cell tumors represent tumor progression by a single clone of malignant cells. Diffuse large-cell lymphomas are made up of large cells, sometimes resembling reticulum cells or macrophages, which replace lymphoid organs as sheets of malignant cells. This tumor has a much worse prognosis than the diffuse lymphocytic lymphoma, which consists of small cells. Fine tuning of the cellular morphology of diffuse B-cell tumors permits more accurate prognosis. For example, intermediate lymphocytic lymphoma (ILL) has cytologic features and a prognosis that lie between those of small lymphocytic lymphoma and diffuse, small, cleaved-cell lymphoma.

Phenotypic Markers. The stage of maturation arrest in the B-cell lineage may be deduced from the phenotypic expression of immunoglobulins produced by B-cell tumors and rearrangements of immunoglobulin genes or by expression of developmentally related cell surface markers (Fig. 24–6). The major distinguishing feature of B-cell tumors is monoclonality, ie, the presence or production of only one class of immunoglobulin and/or one light-chain type by all the cells of the tumor. In contrast, the B cells or plasma cells that make up normal or benign lymphoproliferation are mixtures of cells with different Ig

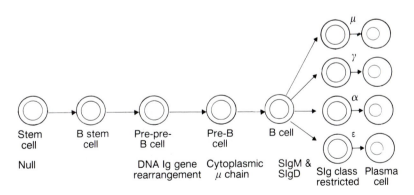

Figure 24–6. Stages of maturation arrest in B-cell lymphomas. The designation of B-cell lineage in leukemia or lymphoma may be deduced from the presence of rearranged IgG genes (pre-pre-B cell), the presence of cytoplasmic μ-chain in the absence of surface Ig (pre-B cell), the presence of surface immunoglobulin restricted to one class (monoclonal), or the presence of plasma cells restricted to one class and one light chain.

classes and light chains. A simple test for monoclonality is immune labeling of tissue for kappa and lambda light chains of immunoglobulin. If all of the cells contain one light-chain type, then the criterion for monoclonality is met. If some cells express kappa chain and others lambda chain (usually a 60:40 ratio), then polyclonality is established.

Ig Gene Rearrangements. Rearrangements of immunoglobulin genes may be used to differentiate B-cell tumors from non-neoplastic proliferation, T-cell tumors, or nonlymphoid tumors that resemble B-cell tumors morphologically. As described in Chapter 4, the first step in B-cell differentiation that can be detected is rearrangement of the immunoglobulin genes. First, genes encoding the heavy chain rearrange beginning with the diversity region (D), then the joining region (J) and the variable region (V). The DNA between these segments is deleted. The second event is rearrangement between the V and J region of the kappa light chain and then after both kappa genes are rearranged, the lambda light-chain genes rearrange. B-cell lymphoma rearrangements can be differentiated from normal polyclonal rearrangements by the presence of a single band on polyacrylamide gel fractionation of DNA digested with appropriate restriction enzymes. Selected enzymes cut the DNA at specific points in the sequence of bases. Polyclonal DNA contains multiple gene arrangements that produce a diffuse, nondistinct pattern when labeled with a specific cDNA probe for the Ig gene probe (Fig. 24–7). In contrast, the DNA from a

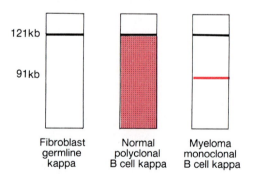

Figure 24–7. Autoradiography of polyacrylamide gel electrophoresis of BamHI restriction endonuclease fragments of DNA from fibroblasts (germline), normal B cells (polyclonal), and B-cell lymphoma tissue (monoclonal). The presence of kappa region sequences is detected using a radiolabeled cDNA for kappa light chain. Monoclonal rearranged kappa genes appear as a single tight band compared to the rearranged germline genes. BamHI will produce many different-sized fragments because of digestion occurring at different positions in the Ig gene polyclonal fragments, and these fragments yield a diffuse pattern.

clonal proliferation will be cleaved at the same site, giving rise to discrete bands. In this manner, clonal B cells that make up only 2% to 5% of a heterogeneous tissue sample may be detected, and diagnosis of lymphoma within a mixture of polyclonal cells can be made accurately. In addition, undifferentiated carcinomas or atypical hyperplasia of lymphocytes can be differentiated from B-cell lymphomas. An unexpected finding is that some B-cell leukemias have rearranged T-cell receptor genes. However, the nature of the T-cell receptor gene in B-cell tumors does not correlate with response to therapy.

B-cell Differentiation Markers. B-cell surface markers identified by monoclonal antibodies to lymphocyte differentiation markers may also be used to evaluate the stage of differentiation of B-cell lymphomas and leukemias (Fig. 24–8). By international agreement, the differentiation markers on lymphoid cells are termed "cluster designations" or "clusters of differentiation" (CD) (see Appendix B). A CD number refers to a group of epitopes identified by a set of monoclonal antibodies that is present on a subset of lymphocytes. These epitopes are markers of normal differentiation or activation states but also appear on leukemia and lymphoma cells.

So far, classification of B-cell lymphomas by phenotypic markers has not contributed greatly to determination of prognosis or choice of therapy. In general, expression of markers of mature B cells is associated with better prognosis and expression of markers of immature B cells with poor prognosis. For instance, expression of CD23, a marker of late B-cell differentiation, and the lack of early B-cell differentiation markers, such as CD38, indicate longer disease-free survival than vice versa. The expression of CD markers on B cells frequently disobeys the differentiation patterns. Thus, CD21 and CD23, markers of different stages of normal differentiation, are often found on the same tumor cells. Unfortunately, analysis of CD expression does not provide better prognostic information than conventional histology or clinical features. An exception to this is the proliferation antigen called Ki67. Monoclonal antibody to Ki67 reacts with a nuclear antigen expressed during the cell cycle but not on resting cells. In a recent comparison to histologic grading, the percentages of Ki67-positive cells correlated to grade as follows:

Grade	Ki67-positive	Examples
Low	14%	Small cell, follicular
Intermediate	43%	Mixed, follicular
High	58%	Large cell, diffuse

Multiple Myeloma. The final step in differentiation of B cells is the plasma cell that synthesizes and secretes immunoglobulin. Tumors of

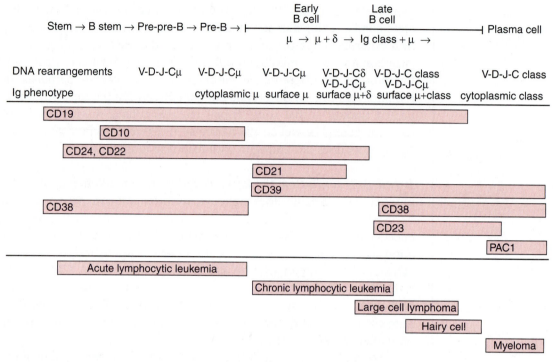

Figure 24–8. Expression of CDs during B-cell development and on B-cell tumors. The expression of CD markers during development is as follows:

1. Stem cell—CDs 19 and 38; sometimes CDs 22 and 24; no Ig gene rearrangements; no Ig expression.
2. Pre-pre-B cell—gain of CD 10; VDJCμ rearrangement; no Ig expression.
3. Pre-B cell—same CDs as above; VDJCμ rearrangement; cytoplasmic μ chain.
4. Early B cell—loss of CD 10 and 38, gain of CD 21 and 39; μ or μ and δ surface positive.
5. Late B cell—loss of CD 21, gain of CDs 23 and 38; VDJC class gene rearrangements, μ, γ, ε, or δ surface positive.
6. Plasma cell—loss of CDs 19, 22, 23, and 24; gain of PCA1 (Plasma Cell Antigen); cytoplasmic Ig of a single class.

In this figure, the expression of these markers on various B-cell tumors is indicated at the bottom of the figure.

plasma cells almost always arise in the bone marrow and are termed multiple myeloma because of many sites (multiple) of masses (-oma) of the tumor cells found in the bone marrow (myelo-). The cells of multiple myeloma are plasma cells that usually contain or secrete a single type of immunoglobulin molecule (monoclonal). These may belong to any of the major immunoglobulin classes and may, but usually do not, demonstrate antigen-binding capacity. A variant form of myeloma that produces IgM and that has slightly different morphologic and clinical features is termed Waldenstrom's macroglobulinemia.

Monoclonal immunoglobulin refers to a uniform, homogeneous, molecular species of immunoglobulin, in contrast to the heterogeneous array of immunoglobulins present in sera of normal persons. This homogeneous immunoglobulin is often referred to as myeloma paraprotein. Electrophoretic or immunoelectrophoretic analysis of sera from myeloma patients reveals a characteristic peak of protein in about 80% of cases (myeloma spike). The myeloma proteins are usually complete immunoglobulin molecules. In some cases, one part of the molecule (eg, light chain or heavy chain) may be produced in excess or may be the only myeloma paraprotein found. The light-chain paraprotein is usually rapidly cleared from the circulation by filtration through the kidney and appears in the urine as Bence Jones protein. Bence Jones protein (light chains) classically precipitates in acidified urine when heated to 50° to 60°C, and redissolves at 100°C (see also Chapter 30). Free excess heavy chains may also be the only secreted myeloma paraprotein identified in the serum of affected patients (H-chain disease). In about 1% of cases, no myeloma paraprotein can be detected, even though myeloma plasma cells are present in the bone marrow and contain monoclonal immunoglobulin. Kappa light chains are present in myeloma proteins at a slightly higher frequency than lambda type (55% vs. 45%), and patients with kappa-type myeloma proteins tend to have longer survival. The degree of elevation of a paraprotein in a given patient may be used to monitor therapeutic effects (eg, chemotherapy). Symptoms may be related to the excess immunoglobulin: Hyperviscosity of the blood because of the high intrinsic viscosity of the myeloma protein, insolubility in the cold (cryoglobulinemia), or formation of immunoglobulin complexes by paraprotein interactions. These lead to circulatory disturbances and microvascular occlusions. IgM production is associated with a cell type that is generally less differentiated than the plasma cell. This disease is called Waldenstrom's macroglobulinemia. The cell type is more like that seen in chronic lymphocytic leukemia.

Monoclonal gammopathies (MGs) refer to different conditions in which an increase in a monoclonal immunoglobulin is found. In 1985, a classification of four types of MG was made: (1) B-cell malignancies, (2) B-cell benign neoplasia, (3) MG in immunodeficiencies with a T/B cell imbalance, and (4) MG due to infection or antigenic stimulation. By following patients in these different categories and relating the course of the related disease to animal models, it has been tentatively concluded that MG may arise as a result of four interacting mechanisms: (1) Genetic instability of B cell leading to selected oncogene activation, (2) chronic antigen stimulation with resulting cytokine stimulation of B cells, (3) restricted clonality of the B cells in certain individuals producing oligoclonal dominance of stimulated B-cell populations, and (4) defective T-cell control. The development of the malignant B cell appears to be related to gene instability in certain individuals.

Ig Idiotypes and Therapy. The myeloma immunoglobulin idiotype not only serves as a marker for all cells in the myeloma but also may be used as a target for specific immunotherapy. In experimental models, immunization of mice with a myeloma idiotype can produce resistance to transplanted myeloma cells bearing the idiotype. There appears to be more than one mechanism for control of myeloma cell growth. The resistance may be mediated by antibodies to the idiotype (antibody-directed complement-dependent killing, opsonization, or antibody-dependent cell-mediated immunity); or by T cells (specific T-suppressor cells for the idiotype or T_{CTL} cells directed to the idiotype). In human clinical trials, mouse monoclonal anti-idiotypic infusion has had limited success. Most recipients demonstrated no effect, whereas approximately 20% have a definite antibody-related remission. Clinical trials using drug conjugated anti-idiotypic antibodies are now underway. Biologic problems in anti-idiotypic therapy include: the ability of some tumors to switch idiotype expression and escape idiotype-directed control mechanisms; the ability of tumor cells to modulate cell surface expression of antigenic molecules; and, if mouse monoclonal antihuman idiotypic antibodies are used, a host response resulting in neutralizing human antimouse immunoglobulin.

Chronic Lymphocytic Leukemia (CLL). CLL is a protracted disease consisting of a marked increase in small lymphocytes in the bone marrow and blood. Lymph node and spleen involvement may occur late in the disease, with diffuse infiltration of small lymphocytes. The tumor cells express monoclonal surface immunoglobulin or rearranged Ig gene in 90% of cases, but also express a T-cell marker, CD5. These cells are referred to as CD5+ B cells. The disease most likely starts in the bone marrow. Later in the course of disease, large numbers of mature lymphocytes extend from the bone marrow to the blood and visceral organs to give the appearance of diffuse lymphocytic lymphoma. The course of the disease is relatively long and patients with this disease often die of infection or from some unrelated disease.

Normally CD5+ B lymphocytes appear early in development and are believed to arise from a separate lineage during development than do other B cells. CD5+ B cells represent a high proportion of fetal and neonatal B cells. They are not found in the normal adult bone marrow but represent about 20% of circulating lymphocytes in adults. Nonmalignant CD5+ B cells belong to a special category of cells that spontaneously secrete IgM autoantibodies. CD5+ B cells are believed to play a role in the first-line defense against infection, as well as in many autoimmune diseases. Leukemic CD5+ B cells also express the α chain of the C3bi receptor, and many of these CLLs possess "cross-reactive" idiotypes, ie, immunoglobulin epitopes shared by different tumors. In contrast, the idiotypes of human myelomas are not shared, ie, are unique for each tumor. Thus, 20% to 30% of CLLs from different patients may express the same idiotype. This raises the possibility of anti-idiotypic–directed passive immunotherapy in which one monoclonal antibody reagent could be used for many different tumors.

Burkitt's Lymphoma. This disease features the presence of cytoplasmic and surface Ig, receptors for C3, and surface viral antigens of the Epstein–Barr (EB) virus. Burkitt's lymphoma was first identified in African children residing in high rainfall areas of Africa where mosquitos are abundant. Cases of Burkitt's lymphoma have now been identified throughout the world, and the relationship to the self-limiting disease, infectious mononucleosis, which is common in western nations, has attracted considerable attention. In African patients, the jaw is involved with a diffuse rapidly growing lymphoid tumor composed of blast cells. In Americans, abdominal, pelvic, and bone marrow involvement is more common. Chemotherapy with cyclophosphamide can produce sustained remissions in 80% of patients with African Burkitt's lymphoma. These tumors are also very responsive to radiotherapy and may undergo spontaneous remission. This supports the concept of a viral etiology, because virus-induced tumors of animals are often self-limiting or responsive to therapy in adults but grow progressively in newborns.

The presence of EB viral antigens on the cell surface provides a relatively strong potential tumor antigen to which the human host may respond. Both cell-mediated and humoral antibody responses may occur to EB viral antigens in patients with Burkitt's lymphoma. Some antigens are found on Burkitt's lymphoma cells that are not viral antigens but are new antigenic specificities unique to early EBV-transformed cells. Since antibodies to these antigens are found before antibodies to viral antigens, they have been termed early EB antigens. Antibody responses are complicated in that high antibody titers to "early antigen" expressed on Burkitt's lymphoma cells are associated with relapses, whereas responses to viral capsid antigens may be protective. Antibodies to capsid antigens are found in tumor-free relatives of patients with Burkitt's lymphoma. A reduction of antibody to early antigens is associated with the development of delayed hypersensitivity to early antigens. The relationship of antibody against capsid antigens or appearance of delayed hypersensitivity in the course of the disease remains uncertain but is believed to be protective (see infectious mononucleosis).

Transplantation-associated Lymphoproliferation. Patients who are heavily immunosuppressed, particularly recipients of cardiac or hepatic grafts, are at risk for developing an unusual lymphoproliferation lesion. The cells resemble those of large-cell lymphoma, often occur outside of lymphoid organs (muscle and fat), and may progress rapidly. Although the disease progresses with the features of a true malignancy, marker studies demonstrate a polyclonal B-cell proliferation which frequently contain EB virus. Studies on the immunoglobulin gene arrangements in these lesions often indicates a spectrum of proliferation ranging from polymorphic polyclonal proliferations with the features of a virus infection to monomorphic and monoclonal, with all the features of a non-Hodgkin's lymphoma.

Hairy Cell Leukemia (Leukemic Reticuloendotheliosis). This is a disease characterized by the appearance of an unusual mononuclear cell in the peripheral blood, associated with splenomegaly and a decrease in other cellular elements of the blood. The disease progresses slowly, and severe infections appear to be related to the decreased number of normally functioning monocytes in the blood. The hairy cell is of the size of normal nonlymphocytic mononuclear cells, has a markedly convoluted cytoplasm (hairy by scanning electron microscopy), has monoclonal cytoplasmic and surface Ig, and is capable of phagocytosis. Thus, it is a B cell with some features of macrophages and most likely represents an immature B-cell type. T-cell variants of hairy cell leukemia have also been reported, but rearrangements of Ig genes have been found in all cases so far studied in this manner. Hairy cell leukemia is particularly susceptible to treatment with interferon-α.

In summary, B-cell tumors may be considered as occurring at various stages of B-cell development, from small lymphocytes to large "blast" cells to well-differentiated plasma cells with multiple myeloma representing the most differentiated stage. Although the most impressive cellular component of multiple myeloma is the differentiated plasma cell, clearly tumor cells in different stages of the cell cycle and at different levels of differentiation must be present in the malignant population, including dividing less differentiated plasma cells. The cells in myelomas, like B-cell tumors, have surface immunoglobulin. Since the immunoglobulin produced by these cells is monoclonal, each SIg-bearing cell will contain immunoglobulin with antigens specific for that molecule (idiotype). CD5+ B cells that give rise to CLL most likely represent a separate lineage of B cells.

T-cell Tumors

These include thymoma, lymphoblastic lymphoma, acute lymphoblastic leukemia (20% to 30%), mycosis fungoides (Sezary's syndrome), and rare diffuse non-Hodgkin's lymphomas.

T-cell Markers. Monoclonal antibodies to T-cell populations are now being applied to define T-cell tumors (Fig. 24–9). These monoclonal antibodies identify T-cell differentiation markers. Previously, phenotypic markers, such as E rosette formation, lack of surface Ig, presence of terminal deoxytransferase (TdT), lack of surface HLA-D antigens, and reactivity with heteroantisera to T cells, were used. Of these, E rosettes and TdT remain the most useful markers. In addition, T-cell malignancies may be phenotyped by monoclonal antibodies (see Appendix C). Many of these, such as CD1; CD5; CD10; transferrin receptor; HLA-A, -B, and -C; and HLA-Dr are not particularly useful for delineation of T-cell lineage since they also appear on non–T-cell tissue. Others, such as E rosette receptor and antigens defined by CD3, CD4, CD7, and CD8 are essentially T-cell specific. These markers define T-cell lineage and stage of maturation arrest areas (see Fig. 24–9). However, as yet, the clinical relevance of the phenotypic identification of T-cell tumors is not clear. On the other hand, some adults with acute myelogenous leukemia (AML) have blasts that express T-cell marker CD2 or B-cell marker CD19; these patients have a more favorable prognosis than patients with AML that does not express these markers. A summary of the phenotypic characterization of some clinical types of T-cell malignancies is presented in Table 24–2 and Figure 24–9. Again the major feature of malignancies is the mono-

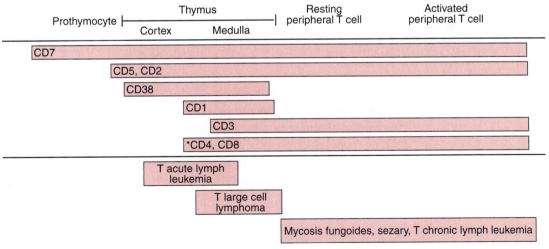

* CD4 and CD8 are present on the same cells in the thymus, but on different T cell subpopulations in blood and peripheral lymphoid organs.

Figure 24–9. T-cell differentiation markers and T-cell lymphomas. The boxes in the top half of the figure indicate the appearance of T-CLL markers detected by monoclonal antibodies at the stages of normal T-cell development. The boxes on the bottom half of the figure indicate the expression of these markers on T-cell tumors.

TABLE 24–2. PHENOTYPIC CHARACTERIZATION OF SOME CLINICAL TYPES OF T CELL MALIGNANCIES[a]

Clinical or Histologic Diagnosis	Phenotypic Characterization
T acute lymphoblastic leukemia	Heterogeneous antigen profile; most express immature T cell phenotype
T chronic lymphocytic leukemia	Mature T cell phenotype (CD4+ or CD8+), CD5+, sIg+
T lymphoblastic lymphoma	Heterogeneous antigen profile; most express immature T cell phenotypes
IgG Fc receptor positive (T_G) lymphoproliferative disease	Mature T cell phenotype CD9−, CD4−, CD1−
Cutaneous T cell lymphoma	PBL[b]: mature helper phenotype (CD9−, CD4+, CD8−, CD1−)
Mycosis fungoides/Sezary's syndrome	Skin: mature helper phenotype type (CD9+, CD4+, CD8−, CD1−)
T cell type of hairy cell leukemia	CD4+, CD8−, mature T cell phenotype
HTLV-associated Japanese, Caribbean and American adult T cell leukemia/lymphoma	Skin and PBL: mature helper phenotype (CD9−, CD4+, CD8−, CD1−)
T cell non-Hodgkin's lymphoma	Mature T cell phenotype

[a] Phenotypes in this table, when given, are the usual phenotypes for the clinical/histologic syndrome. In most cases, minor variations or alternative phenotypes have been reported.

[b] PBL, peripheral blood lymphocytes.

Modified from Harden EA, Polker TJ, Haynes BF: Monoclonal antibodies: Probes for the study of malignant T cells. In *Monoclonal Antibodies in Cancer*. Sell S, Reisfeld R (eds.). Creascent Manor, NJ, Humana Press, 1985.

clonal nature of the malignant cells (all have the same markers) as compared to normal nonmalignant polyclonal T-cell populations. Phenotypic characterization may be carried out on cell suspensions, such as from leukemic blood or effusions, as well as on frozen tissue sections. The future application of such analysis depends on clinical correlations yet to be made.

Thymoma. Tumors of the thymus are extremely rare and may be classified into three major types: Lymphoid, epithelial, and mixed. Most tumors are mixed, and it is believed that the lymphoid cell component is a nonmalignant proliferative of lymphocytes accompanying the malignant epithelial cells. Tumors of the epithelial cells of the thymus are usually composed of spindle or cuboidal epithelial cells, and mixed tumors contain elements of both. Thymic tumors present as masses in the anterior mediastinum and may be associated with a number of systemic autoimmune diseases, including myasthenia gravis, pancytopenia, multiple myeloma, thyroiditis, and dermatomyositis. In most cases, with or without systemic manifestations, the tumor is limited to the thymus; metastatic extension of thymomas (malignant thymoma) is extremely rare. Most T cells in thymomas have the phenotype of cortical (immature) thymocytes (CD1+, CD4–, CD8–). The term lymphocytic lymphoma of the thymus may be used in the rare instances when invasion of the capsule or widespread disease consisting of mainly small lymphocytes indicates malignancy. This may be a true thymic T-cell tumor.

Acute Lymphoblastic Leukemia. T-cell acute lymphoblastic leukemia begins in the bone marrow, has a rapid course, and involves the peripheral blood and lymphatics extensively. Approximately 15% to 25% of the tumors bear T-cell markers; others bear B-cell markers or no markers. Those patients with T-cell acute leukemia have a poor prognosis and respond poorly to chemotherapy, compared to patients with non–T-cell acute leukemia. T-cell leukemias are usually TdT-positive and acid phosphatase-positive. T-cell differentiation markers are heterogenous, but are generally that of immature T cells and thymocytes.

Lymphoblastic Lymphoma. This is a rare T-cell tumor, usually occurring in children, that mimics the virus-induced T-cell tumors of mice. It begins in the thymus and rapidly extends and infiltrates diffusely (T zones) into lymph node, spleen, bone marrow, and other organs and may have a terminal leukemic phase. In humans, this tumor may resemble diffuse B-cell lymphoma morphologically, but can be identified by the presence of T-cell markers. This tumor has also been termed lymphoblastic sarcoma when extensive involvement with immature lymphocytes occurs. T-cell lymphoblastic lymphomas are E rosette-positive and SIg- and Ia-negative. T-cell differentiation markers are usually of thymocyte type, but some tumors express a more differentiated phenotype.

Mycosis Fungoides and Sezary's Syndrome. These are both tumors of T cells. Mycosis fungoides begins in the skin. The disease may be grouped into three stages: (1) Skin involvement as an inflammatory-like condition that presents as dermatitis, parapsoriasis, or erythroderma; (2) infiltrated dermal plaques; and (3) gross tumors. The length of survival depends on the stage of the disease: 8 to 12 years for stage 1, 3 to 5 years for stage 2, and 1 to 3 years for stage 3. Tumors in the skin appear as solid masses with terminal extensions into visceral organs. Sezary's syndrome is a leukemic variant. The same cutaneous features as seen in mycosis fungoides are present, but tumor cells are also present in blood (leukemia). Most often, these cells have T-cell properties and may be able to function as helper cells and stimulate immunoglobulin production by B cells. The cells also bear the helper phenotype: CD4+,CD8−. The dermal lesions contain large numbers of dendritic macrophages, and it has been proposed that antigen persistence on the dendritic cells (Langerhans' cells), may result in chronic exposure to contact antigens, leading to excess intraepithelial stimulation, as well as involvement of the dermis and draining lymph nodes.

T-cell Chronic Lymphocytic Leukemia (T-cell CLL). Most CLL cells express B-cell phenotypes but, as mentioned above, may also react with a monoclonal antibody for T cells (CD5), and form E rosettes (CD5+ B cells). Approximately 2% of CLL cells are restricted to T cells as defined by E rosette formation, lack of SIg, and mature T-cell phenotype as defined by monoclonal antibodies (TdT−, CD1−, CD3+). Most T-cell CLL cells express the CD4 (helper cell) phenotype.

HTLV-associated Adult T-cell Leukemia/lymphoma. In 1980, the association of a human retrovirus with human T-cell tumors was described—human T-cell leukemia/lymphoma virus (HTLV-1). This tumor appears in high frequency in Japan, the Caribbean basin, and the southern United States. The virus infects CD4+ cells and produces a highly malignant tumor that is CD4+,CD8−. Although these cells bear the helper (CD4) phenotype, they function as suppressor cells for B-cell function in vitro. These tumors also bear HLA-B5 antigens simultaneously, presumably due to shared antigens between HLA-B5 and HTLV-1.

Lymphoproliferative Disease of Granular Lymphocytes (LDGLs). Large granular lymphocytes (LGL) contain azurophilic (blue) granules and are known for their cytotoxic activity to tissue culture cells. Three distinct, rare clinical syndromes resulting from increased numbers of circulating LGLs have been recognized. T-cell LGL leukemia (CD3+), NK-cell LGL leukemia (CD3−) and polyclonal LGL lymphocytosis.

LGLs normally exist in two major subsets: CD3– and CD3+. Clonal proliferations of either of these populations results in LGL leukemia. CD3+ LGL leukemia is associated with bacterial infections and rheumatoid arthritis and has a relative benign course. CD– LGL lymphoma has an acute clinical course with profound anemia and thrombocytopenia and is not associated with rheumatoid arthritis. Polyclonal LGL lymphocytosis may be a variant of CD3+ LGL leukemia in which it is impossible to prove clonality using TCR rearrangements. This disorder also has a benign course.

Diffuse Lymphomas. Most diffuse lymphomas are of B-cell type but a small percentage, usually of a large-cell type, are SIg negative and may express CD4 or CD8 phenotype.

Treatment of Leukemia and Lymphomas

Treatment of leukemia and lymphomas is accomplished by administration of selected antimetabolic or cytotoxic drugs. In many instances, complete cures can be effected by the proper choice of drug, dosage, and timing. Other modes of therapy include irradiation, irradiation with bone marrow transfer (see Chapter 23), or monoclonal antibodies (see Chapter 30). It is not in the scope of this text to present this subject in more detail.

MACROPHAGE TUMORS

Malignant histiocytosis or histiocytosis X are terms used for tumors of macrophages. Malignant histiocytosis is a family of diseases, including Letterer–Siwe disease, Hand–Schuller–Christian disease, and eosinophilic granuloma of bone (Table 24–3). These tumors consist of

TABLE 24–3. CLASSIFICATION OF MACROPHAGE–HISTIOCYTE DERIVED TUMORS

Histiocyte Type	Normal Tissue Distribution	Putative Malignant Tumor
Free histiocytes	Circulating monocytes	Monocytic leukemia
Fixed histiocytes	Reticuloendothelial cells	True histiocytic lymphoma
Dendritic histiocytes	Follicular zones, lymph node cortex	Hand–Schuller–Christian disease
Interdigitating reticulum cells	T-cell zone, lymph node paracortex	Hodgkin's disease
Langerhans' cells	Intraepithelial	Letterer–Siewe
Macrophage stem cell	Bone marrow	Eosinophilic granuloma

space-occupying lesions filled by mature histiocytes with abundant cytoplasm. Hand–Schuller–Christian disease and eosinophilic granuloma occur in bone, with the former also occurring predominantly in the spleen and lymph node. Letterer–Siwe disease involves the skin, lymph nodes, and spleen. The cells in these diseases contain a distinctive rod-shaped inclusion also found in intraepithelial monocytes (Langerhans' cells). Note that in the Rappaport classification, the term histiocytic lymphoma has been used for a B-cell tumor, not a true histiocytic (macrophage) tumor. True histiocytic lymphomas are believed to arise from fixed histiocytes; Letterer–Siwe disease cells may arise from Langerhans' cells.

HODGKIN'S DISEASE

Hodgkin's disease is a malignant tumor of lymphoid organs composed of mixed cell types. Hodgkin's disease has been known in some form or another for over 150 years; however, the original description by Hodgkin in 1872 of seven patients with "tumors of the absorbent glands" included lesions now known to be tuberculosis. Whereas significant advances have been made in the diagnosis and treatment of Hodgkin's disease, the etiology remains unknown. Major theories of the nature of Hodgkin's disease include that it is a form of lymphoma, an inflammatory response, or a viral infection. Until more is known about its etiology, it is best to consider Hodgkin's disease a lymphoma. As stated above, two general classifications of lymphomas are Hodgkin's and non-Hodgkin's lymphomas.

Histopathologic Classification

The major feature of Hodgkin's disease is the pleomorphism (different cell types) of the tumor lesions, in contrast to the more homogeneous cell types of the non-Hodgkin's lymphomas. Tentative agreement of the classification of Hodgkin's disease was reached at a conference in Rye, New York, in 1966. This classification scheme is important because the histologic forms of each type correlate with the clinical course (Table 24–4).

Because of the different cell types seen in Hodgkin's lymphomas, there has been controversy as to which is the cell line responsible for the tumors and which are non-neoplastic reactive cells. Monoclonal antibodies to markers of different cellular lineage have been applied to this problem. Marker studies indicate that the other cell types in Hodgkin's disease lesions are polyclonal, whereas the Reed–Sternberg cells are monoclonal. The characteristic large binuclear cell of Hodgkin's disease was described independently in the United States by Dorothy Reed, a pathology resident at Johns Hopkins University, and

TABLE 24–4. HISTOPATHOLOGIC CLASSIFICATION OF HODGKIN'S DISEASE

Type	Features	Relative Prognosis
Lymphocyte predominance	Mainly small lymphocytes Few R–S* cells	Most favorable
Modular sclerosis	Lymphoid nodules separated by fibrous bands	Favorable
Mixed cellularity	Numerous R–S cells in pleomorphic stroma	Guarded
Lymphocyte depletion	Diffuse irregular fibrosis Anaplastic R–S cells	Least favorable

* R–S, Reed–Sternberg Cells

From Lukes RJ, et al.: *Cancer Res* 26:1311, 1966.

Professor C. Sternberg, a famous German pathologist. In the United States, these cells were referred to as Reed–Sternberg cells; in Europe, Sternberg–Reed cells (Fig. 24–10).

The histopathologic classification is based on the relative proportion of lymphocytes, fibrosis, and Reed–Sternberg cells in relation to other cells (neutrophils, eosinophils, plasma cells) in the pleomorphic tumor. Reed–Sternberg cells are of particular diagnostic significance for Hodgkin's disease (Fig. 24–11).

Cellular Origin

The present evidence supports the cell of origin of Hodgkin's disease to be a particular subset of macrophages known as interdigitating reticulum cells (see Table 24–3). However, this conclusion is extremely controversial; many investigators think that the Hodgkin's tumor cells are derived from activated T or B cells. Cells in the monocyte–macrophage

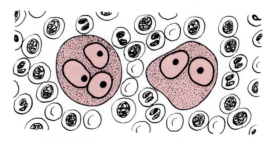

Figure 24–10. Reed–Sternberg cells are large multinucleated "giant" cells considered essential for the diagnosis of Hodgkin's disease.

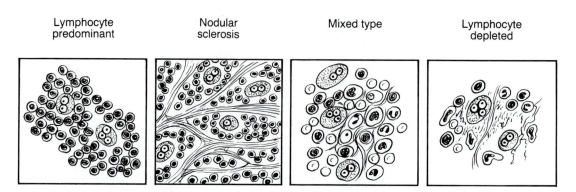

| Lymphocyte predominant | Nodular sclerosis | Mixed type | Lymphocyte depleted |

Figure 24–11. Drawing of cell types in Hodgkin's disease. Depicted is a drawing modified from a textbook by William Osler published in 1914, illustrating the different cell types seen in mixed cellularity Hodgkin's disease. The diagnosis depends on the identification of Reed–Sternberg cells in a lesion containing a mixture of other cell types. Lymphocytes and eosinophils are often prominent.

lineage exist in the body in different tissue locations and most likely have different but related functions. Reed–Sternberg cells and interdigitating cells have morphologic similarities; express similar levels of HLA-DR antigen, esterase, and acid phosphatase; and do not react with monoclonal antibodies shared by other cells in the monocyte series, but both do react with monoclonal antibody LeuM1 (CD15), which identifies an epitope on interdigitating reticulum cells. Other markers that have proven useful in the diagnosis of Hodgkin's disease are CD30 (Ki1), which also reacts with Reed–Sternberg cells and not with T cells or B cells, as well as B-cell and T-cell markers which do not label Reed–Sternberg cells, but do label other cell types in non-Hodgkin's, as well as Hodgkin's, disease lesions. As with non-Hodgkin's lymphomas, labeling with Ki67 will identify the proliferating cells and may be of some prognostic value. Double staining with CD30 and Ki67 indicates that both multinuclear and mononuclear histiocytic cells contribute to the proliferating pool of neoplastic cells.

The "non-neoplastic" component of Hodgkin's disease, the accompanying lymphocytes, and other cells may also proliferate and contribute to the cellular composition of the lesions, but are not truly malignant cells. The proliferation of these cells may be stimulated by monokines produced by the Hodgkin's (Reed–Sternberg) cells. Reed–Sternberg cells in Hodgkin's disease have been shown to secrete IL-1, IL-5, IL-6, IL-9, TNF-α, M-CSF, TGF-β, and less frequently, IL-4 and G-CSF. With some exceptions, most non-Hodgkin's disease lymphoma cells do not secrete cytokines. Exceptions are the so-called T-cell-rich B-cell lymphomas in which the tumor B cells secrete IL-4, which is responsible for the T-cell infiltrate, and angioimmunoblastic lymphadenopathy-type T-cell lymphoma in which the tumor T-cells secrete IL-6, which is responsible for the plasma cell reaction. The large number of cytokines secreted by Hodgkin's tumor cells is responsible for the varied type of nontumor cells included within the mass of the Hodgkin's lymphoma.

Staging

The clinical course of Hodgkin's disease is dependent on the extent of the disease when first diagnosed. The exact relationship between the extent of disease (stage) and prognosis is not clear, but prognosis generally becomes worse as the extent of the disease increases (Fig. 24–12).

Treatment

The treatment of Hodgkin's disease with high-dose irradiation to the total lymphoid tissue has led to substantial increases in survival times and essential cure of some patients. In addition, combined drug chemotherapy has yielded up to 80% complete remission, even in patients with far advanced disease, and has induced remission in patients who relapse after radiotherapy. Hodgkin's disease patients frequently demonstrate immunodeficiencies, particularly of the cellular immune system, and may develop infectious complications.

Angio-immunoblastic Lymph-adenopathy

This particular lesion is associated with clinical findings similar to those seen in Hodgkin's disease (fever, sweats, weight loss, skin rash, etc.). There may also be hypergammaglobulinemia (polyclonal). Histologically, there is a marked increase in small blood vessels (particularly endothelial hyperplasia) in the involved nodes, with numerous blasts and plasma cells, epithelial cells, and large numbers of dying and degenerating cells. The lesion resembles a florid proliferation of the B-cell system, although T cells may also be involved. Most patients demonstrate a rapid downhill course, with death occurring after one to two years. It is not yet clear if this condition is truly a malignant tumor. Some investigators consider this to be a non-neoplastic progressive immune reaction, but the progressive clinical course is consistent with malignancy. A variant is angioimmunoblastic lymphadenopathy with dysproteinemia. These patients usually have partial or complete displacement of lymph nodes with diffuse lymphoplasmacytic proliferation, and evidence of autoimmune or immune complex disease. As stated above, the plasma cell proliferation and differentiation in these tumors may be due to lymphokines secreted by the tumor cells.

Animal Models of Lymphoid Tumors

Animal models of lymphoma and leukemia support the concept of tissue localization of different tumor cell types. Most of the animal tumors are caused by tumor viruses. However, the tumor cells may express properties of different lymphocyte lineage and demonstrate

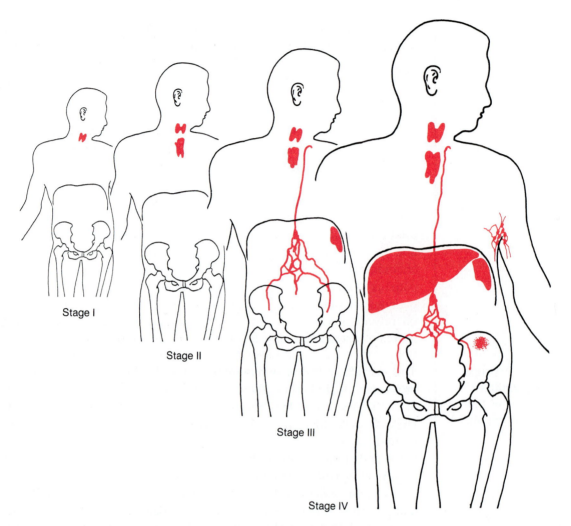

Figure 24–12. Clinical staging of Hodgkin's disease. Staging correlates well with prognosis and helps in deciding the selection of therapy. The same clinical staging is also applicable to the non-Hodgkin's lymphomas.

Stage I: Involvement of a single lymph node region.
Stage II: Involvement of two or more lymph node regions on the same side of the diaphragm.
Stage III: Involvement of lymphatic structures on both sides of the diaphragm.
Stage IV: Diffuse or disseminated involvement.

related growth patterns in vivo. Lymphoid tumors in mice, chickens, cats, and guinea pigs will be considered (Table 24–5).

MICE

Malignant tumors of both T and B cells occur in mice. A large number of transplantable T-cell tumors has been induced in mice by radiation and contain mouse leukemia virus (MuLV). These tumors almost

TABLE 24–5. ANIMAL MODELS OF LYMPHOID TUMORS

Animal	Type	Organ of Origin	Site of Proliferation	Etiology
Mouse	T cell	Thymus	Paracortex of lymph nodes	Mouse leukemia virus (MuLV)
	Null		Diffuse	MuLV
	B cell		Cortex of lymph nodes	MuLV
	Myeloma	Intraperitoneal	Intraperitoneal	Inflammatory stimulus (mineral oil)
Chicken	T cell	Thymus	Paracortex	DNA virus
	B cell	Bursa of Fabricius	Cortex	RNA virus
Cat	T cell	Thymus	Blood	FeLV
	B cell	GI tract	GI tract	FeLV
Guinea pig	B cell	Transplantable Leukemia	Blood, cortex	

always start in the thymus, bear T-cell surface markers, migrate to the proliferate in T-cell zones of lymphoid organs upon transplantation, and are similar to diffuse lymphoblastic T-cell lymphoma of man. A small number of MuLV-induced tumors do not express T-cell markers (null-cell tumors). These tumors proliferate diffusely, show no preference to T-cell zones in the lymph node, and selectively invade the red pulp of the spleen.

Malignant tumors of differentiated B cells (immunoglobulin-secreting plasma cells) occur spontaneously in C_3H mice and may be induced by injection (particularly intraperitoneally) of inflammatory agents (such as mineral oil) into BALB/c mice. In this manner, a large number of transplantable plasma-cell tumors have been produced. These tumors and their products have been used extensively to study plasma-cell tumor growth characteristics, effects of therapy, and mechanisms of immunoglobulin synthesis and assembly, and have been a major source of homogeneous immunoglobulin used for determining the structure of immunoglobulin. In addition, non-Ig–secreting myeloma cell lines are fused with spleen cells from immunized mice to produce hybridoma antibody.

The observation that plasma cell tumors may be induced in mice by inflammation suggests that such stimuli may play an etiologic role in human plasma-cell tumors (multiple myeloma). Plasma-cell tumors may be caused by chronic stimulation of the B-cell system associated with decreased T-cell control. The finding that most immunoglobulin-producing tumors produce only one class and type of immunoglobulin has been used as an argument that these tumors are in fact derived from a single clone (monoclonal). However, a number of instances of single myeloma cells of both mice and man producing more than one class of Ig have been reported.

CHICKENS

Lymphoid tumors of chickens include a DNA virus-induced tumor with T-cell markers (Marek's disease) and an RNA virus-induced lymphoma, which is most likely a B-cell tumor (lymphoid leukosis). Both of these diseases combine features of a virus infection and a lymphoid neoplasm. In Marek's disease, tumor incidence is decreased by thymectomy and increased by bursectomy. The former result is believed to be caused by a loss of T cells that can be infected by virus, and the latter effect caused by decreasing the humoral immune response to the virus infection. The tumor cells are mainly T cells. There is a multifocal diffuse lymphoid proliferation in the gonads, liver, and lymphoid organs, consisting of small and medium lymphocytes, blast cells, and other mononuclear cells. The disease may be prevented by immunization with a related nonpathogenic turkey virus. T cells may play a dual role in this disease, as cells that are infected by the virus (the predominant tumor cell) and as immunologically reactive cells that mount a cellular immune response to viral antigens. Both thymus and bursa become infected with virus, suggesting that the original target tissue is not T- or B-cell–dependent, but clearly 70% or more of the tumor cells that develop later are T cells.

In contrast, the RNA-induced tumor (lymphoid leukosis) appears to require B cells. Bursectomy results in a decrease in tumor incidence, presumably by removing B cells that become infected. This tumor usually begins in the bursa of Fabricius as a polyclonal proliferation of B cells. Eventually, one clone outgrows the rest so that at a later stage of the disease, a monoclonal B-cell tumor with surface Ig is produced. The tumor then spreads to the lymph nodes, spleen, and liver, but not to the thymus. Histologically, the tumor has the appearance of a "nodular" lymphoma (B-cell zones), and upon transplantation the cells preferentially home to B-cell zones (bursa of Fabricius) of the recipient animal.

CATS

A lymphoproliferative disease of the cat is caused by feline leukemia virus (FeLV), which shows some similarities with murine leukemia virus. The lymphoid tumors produced fall into two distinct patterns—thymic and alimentary. The thymic form is similar to the T-cell murine leukemia, with major involvement of the thymus and peripheral blood, as in acute leukemia, whereas the alimentary form occurs primarily in the gastrointestinal tract. The thymic form is of T-cell origin, and the alimentary form of B-cell origin.

GUINEA PIGS

The L_2C leukemia is an acute B-cell tumor of guinea pigs. The cells of L_2C leukemia have receptors for C_3 and express surface IgM, with a characteristic idiotype. It is different from most B-cell leukemias of man, which are chronic. This tumor is transplantable in strain 2 guinea pigs, in which it produces an acute leukemia with extension into the spleen, lymph nodes, liver, and Peyer's patches. The thymus and bone marrow are not usually involved, but the brain frequently is, and central nervous system complications are frequent. This tumor is not like most human B-cell leukemias but does have properties similar to some rare forms of human leukemias.

These animal models help to understand human lymphomas, but in fact many more different kinds of lymphoid tumors have been studied in man as the result of extensive diagnostic studies on individual tumors. Because of the nature of human immunoproliferative diseases and the necessity to classify and follow each patient individually, most of the information in the human deals with morphologic appearance, growth patterns, clinical course, response to therapy, and, more recently, immunologic markers and gene rearrangements.

Etiology of Lymphoproliferative Diseases

The etiology of cancer remains one of the major questions in medical science. A number of theories, including malignant mutations, abnormal development, and embryonic reversion, have been proposed. Three major mechanisms seem likely for lymphoid tumors—inadequately controlled responses of the immune system, viral infection, chromosomal translations or abnormal gene expressions.

LOSS OF IMMUNOREGULATION

Loss of normal immunoregulatory mechanisms has been postulated as a possible cause of lymphoid tumors. Patients who are administered drugs that depress immune responses, such as recipients of allografted organs, display an extremely high incidence of lymphoid malignancies but normal incidence of other nonlymphoid tumors. Thus, patients receiving immunosuppressive therapy may reflect loss of the ability to regulate proliferation of clones of cells that would normally be suppressed by immune regulatory (T-suppressor) cells. Further support for this concept is the observation that the incidence of many of the lymphoid tumors increases with aging. Aging is also associated with involution of the thymus, autoantibody production, and other evidence of loss of immunoregulation. In addition, the incidence of lymphoid tumors, particularly those of B-cell origin, is increased in patients with naturally occurring immune deficiency diseases such as ataxia telangiectasia. It is postulated that immune deficiencies are associated not only with losses of responding cells (T-helper cells and B cells), but also with losses of controlling cell populations (suppressor or regulatory cells). This imbalance permits inadequately controlled proliferation of the remaining lymphoid cells.

VIRAL INFECTION

Although many tumors of animals are known to be caused by viral infection, a viral etiology for most human cancers has been difficult to demonstrate. Many of the virus-induced tumors of animals are lymphoid (see above). These are usually fast-growing tumors that are more frequent in young than old animals. Virus-induced tumors of animals are similar to the acute lymphoid tumors of children, whereas the lymphoid tumors of adults are generally more chronic and may reflect loss of immune control. Adult T-cell leukemia/lymphoma caused by HTLV and Burkitt's lymphoma are two examples of viral-induced neoplasm in humans. Thus, two major etiologies of leukemia and lymphoma appear likely—virus infection and loss of immune regulation.

CHROMOSOMAL TRANS-LOCATIONS

Cells from lymphomas and leukemias demonstrate a variety of non-random chromosome translocations that may bring "promotor" areas of one gene into juxtaposition with protooncogene DNA sequences. The activation of these protooncogenes may play a key role in producing neoplastic activation of the cells. For example, in Burkitt's lymphoma, the myc oncogene in chromosome 8 is transposed to Ig heavy-chain locus on chromosome 14 resulting in activation of the oncogene. This and other such translocations are illustrated in Figure 24–13.

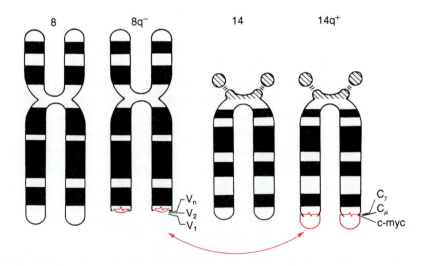

Figure 24–13. Diagram of the t(8;14) translocation in Burkitt's lymphoma cells. The *c-myc* gene on chromosome 8 translocates next to the C and Cγ genes on chromosome 14. (From Erikson J, et al.: Transcriptional activation of the translocated *c-myc* oncogene in Burkitt's lymphoma. *Proc Soc Exp Biol Med* 80:830, 1983.)

CONTROL OF DIFFERENTIA-TION

Since the basic cellular abnormality in lymphomas and leukemias is the prolonged survival of cells apparently blocked in their differentiation, molecular mechanisms responsible for the progression of normal cellular differentiation have been proposed to explain the biology of these tumors. Prolonged survival of a lymphocyte clone may be caused by viral infections (Epstein–Barr or HTLV-1), by abnormal expression of cellular genes that inhibit apoptosis (*bcl*-2) or by the mutation or deletion of cellular genes that are necessary for apoptosis.

Infection Associated with Lymphoproliferative Diseases

Patients with lymphoproliferative disease are subject to an increased incidence of clinically significant infections (see Chapter 27). This may be caused by the nature of the disease or, secondarily, by the type of treatment usually employed—chemotherapy or irradiation. Abnormalities of immune function are frequently found in patients with lymphoproliferative diseases. These include increased production of abnormal immunoglobulins, found with immunoglobulin-secreting tumors, and a variety of autoantibodies, as well as depressed immune reactivity. Some reasons for increased susceptibility to infections in these diseases are as follows: (1) Replacement of normally functioning immune cells with tumor cells that function poorly, (2) production of secreted products that inhibit inflammatory or immune reactions, (3) appearance of cells (suppressor cells) that suppress normal immune function, and (4) loss of normal homeostatic mechanisms (loss of suppressor cells), permitting overproduction of some immune products and underproduction of others.

Summary

Both benign and malignant proliferation of lymphoid cells may lead to enlargement of lymph nodes and spleen, increases in lymphoid cells in the peripheral blood, and systemic symptoms (fever, sweats, and weight loss). Benign lymphoproliferative lesions are usually made up of a heterogeneous population of lymphoid cells that may cause enlargement of lymphoid organs, but the basic structures of the organs (cortex, follicles, medulla) are usually, but not always, maintained. Malignant lymphoid tumors result from an arrest in maturation of a single cell lineage and usually consist of a homogeneous cell type that replaces or destroys the normal architecture of the organ. Strict morphologic criteria are not adequate for acceptable diagnosis of lymphoproliferative disease; immune characteristics and phenotypic markers of the cell type provide additional information in regard to diagnosis and prognosis. In many instances, the growth pattern of the tumor reflects the cell type of origin (B cells produce follicular tumors, T cells, and diffuse tumors), but considerable deviation from predicted growth patterns occurs in individual patients.

Bibliography

LYMPHOID TISSUE STRUCTURE AND LYMPHOMAS

Baird S, Raschke W: The pattern of involvement of murine lymphoid tissues by primary lymphomas of different cell lineage. *Hum Pathol* 9:47, 1978.

Lukes RJ, Collins RD: New observations in follicular lymphoma. *Gann Monogr Cancer Res* 15:209, 1973.

Mann RB, Jaffe ES, Berad CW: Malignant lymphomas: A conceptual understanding of morphologic diversity. *Am J Pathol* 94:105, 1979.

Swerdlow SH: *Biopsy Interpretation of Lymph Nodes.* New York, Raven Press, 1991.

Warnke R, Levy R: Immunopathology of follicular lymphomas: A model of B-lymphocyte homing. *N Engl J Med* 298:481, 1978.

Weissman IL, Warnke R, Butcher EC, et al.: The lymphoid system: Its normal architecture and the potential for its understanding by the study of lymphoproliferative diseases. *Hum Pathol* 9:25, 1978.

CLASSIFICATION OF LYMPHOMAS

Baird S: The usefulness of cell surface markers in predicting the prognosis of non-Hodgkin's lymphomas. *Crit Rev Clin Lab Sci* 30:1–28, 1993.

Bennett MH, Farrer-Brown J, Henry K, et al.: Classification of non-Hodgkin's lymphomas. *Lancet* 2:405–406, 1974.

Carey JL: Flow cytometric immunoanalysis of leukemia and lymphoma. *J Clin Immuno* 1:21, 1989.

Dorfman RF: Classification of non-Hodgkin's lymphomas. *Lancet* 2:961, 1974.

Ersboll J, Schultz HB: Non-Hodgkin's lymphomas: Recent concepts in classification and treatment. *Eur J Haematol* 42(suppl. 48):15, 1989.

Foon KA, Todd RF: Immunologic classification of leukemia and lymphoma. *Blood* 68:1, 1986.

Jaffe ES, Raffeld M, Medeiros LJ, et al.: An overview of the classification of non-Hodgkin's lymphomas: An integration of morphologic and phenotypic concepts. *Cancer Res* 52(suppl.):5447s, 1992.

Leong ASY: Malignant lymphoma: Nomenclature, recently recognized subtypes, and current concepts. *J Histotechnol* 15:175, 1992.

Lennert K, Mohri N, Stein H, et al.: The histopathology of malignant lymphomas. *Brit J Hematol* 31(suppl.):199, 1975.

Lukes RJ, Botler JJ: The pathology and nomenclature of Hodgkin's disease. *Cancer Res* 26:1311, 1966.

Lukes RJ, Collins RD: Immunologic characterization of human malignant lymphoma. *Cancer* 34:1488, 1974.

Lukes RS, Craver LF, Hall TC, et al.: Report of the nomenclature committee. *Cancer Res* 26:1311, 1966.

Nathwahi BN: A critical analysis of the classification of non-Hodgkin's lymphomas. *Cancer* 44:347, 1979.

O'Connor GT, Sobin LH: EORTC-CNS: International colloquium on lymphoid neoplasms. *Biomedicine* 26:385, 1977.

Rappaport H: Tumors of the hematopoietic system. In *Atlas of Tumor Pathology*, sect. 3, fascicle 8. Washington, DC, Armed Forces Institute of Pathology, 1966.

Schuurman H-K, Van Baarlen J, Muppes W, et al.: Immunophenotyping of non-Hodgkin's lymphoma: Lack of correlation between immunophenotype and cell morphology. *Am J Pathol* 129:140, 1987.

Taylor CR: Classification of lymphoma: New thinking on old thoughts. *Arch Path Lab Med* 102:549, 1978.

Weisenburger DD: Pathological classification of non-Hodgkin's lymphoma for epidemiologic studies. *Cancer Res* 52:5456s, 1992.

NONMALIGNANT LYMPHO-PROLIFERATION

Castleman B, Iverson L, Menrenden P: Localized mediastinal lymph node hyperplasia resembling cancer. *Cancer* 9:8221, 1956.

Frizzera G: Castleman's disease: More questions than answers. *Human Pathol* 16:202, 1985.

Frizerra G, Moran EM, Rappaport H: Angioimmunoblastic lymphadenopathy: Diagnosis and clinical cause. *Am J Med* 59:803, 1975.

Keller AR, Hochholzer L, Castleman B: Hyaline-vascular and plasma-cell types of giant lymph node hyperplasia of the mediastinum and other locations. *Cancer* 29:670, 1972.

Kyle RA, Bayzd ED: Benign monoclonal gammopathy: A potentially malignant condition. *Am J Med* 40:426, 1965.

Neiman RS, Dervan P, Haudenschild C, et al.: Angioimmunoblastic lymphadenopathy. *Cancer* 41:507, 1978.

Rosai J, Dorfman PF: Sinus histiocytosis with massive lymphadenopathy: A newly recognized benign clinicopathologic entity. *Arch Pathol* 87:63, 1969.

Saltzstein SL, Ackerman LV: Lymphadenopathy-induced by anticonvulsant drugs mimicking clinically and pathologically malignant lymphomas. *Cancer* 12:164, 1959.

AIDS-RELATED LYMPH-ADENOPATHY

Edelman AS, Zolla-Pazner S: AIDS: A syndrome of immune dysregulation, dysfunction, and deficiency. *Fed Aw Soc Exp Biol J* 3:22, 1989.

Ewing EP, Chandler FW, Spira TJ, et al.: Primary lymph node pathology in AIDS and AIDS-related lymphadenopathy. *Arch Pathol Lab Med* 109:977, 1985.

Ioachim HL: Pathology of AIDS. Philadelphia, JB Lippincott, 1989.

Ioachim HL, Lerner CW, Tapper ML: The lymphoid lesions associated with the acquired immune deficiency syndrome. *Am J Surg Pathol* 7:543, 1983.

Krueger GRF, Otten JK, Ortmann M, et al.: Immunopathology of AIDS: Observations in 75 patients with pre-AIDS and AIDS. *Pathol Rec Pract* 180:463, 1985.

Levine AM: Acquired immunodeficiency syndrome-related lymphoma. *Blood* 80:8, 1992.

Niedt GW, Schinella RA: Acquired immunodeficiency syndrome: Clinicopathologic study of 56 autopsies. *Arch Pathol Lab Med* 109:727, 1985.

Reichert CM, O'Leary TJ, Levens DL, et al.: Autopsy pathology in the acquired immune deficiency syndrome. *Am J Pathol* 112:357, 1983.

INFECTIOUS MONO-NUCLEOSIS

Henle G, Henle W, Diehl V: Relation of Burkitt's tumor-associated herpes-type virus to infectious mononucleosis. *Proc Natl Acad Sci USA* 59:94, 1968.

Pattengale PK, Smith RW, Perlin E: Atypical lymphocytes in acute infectious mononucleosis: Identification by multiple T and B lymphocyte markers. *N Engl J Med* 291:1145, 1974.

Purtilo DT: Lymphotropic viruses, Epstein–Barr virus (EBV and human T-cell lymphocytropic virus-I (HTLV-1)/adult T-cell leukemia virus (ATV), and HTLV-III/human immune deficiency virus (HIV) as etiologic agents of malignant lymphoma and immune deficiency AIDS research 2:S1, 1986.

Sheldon PJ, Papamichail M, Hemsted EH, et al.: Thymic origin of atypical lymphoid cells in infectious mononucleosis. *Lancet* 1:1153, 1973.

Shiftan TA, Mendelsohn J: The circulating "atypical" lymphocyte. *Hum Pathol* 9:51, 1978.

B-CELL TUMORS

Bollum FJ: Terminal deoxynucleotidyl transferase as a hematopoietic cell marker. *Blood* 54:1203, 1979.

Burke JS, Byrne GE, Rappaport H: Hairy cell leukemia (leukemic reticuloendotheliosis): A clinical pathologic study of 21 patients. *Cancer* 33:1399, 1974.

Cheson BD: *Chronic Lymphocytic Leukemia.* New York, Marcel Dekker, 1992.

Cossman J, Zehnbauer B, Garrett CT, et al.: Gene rearrangements in the diagnosis of lymphoma/leukemia. *Am J Clin Pathol* 95:347, 1991.

Dameshek W: Chronic lymphocytic leukemia: An accumulative disease of immunologically incompetent lymphocytes. *Blood* 29:566, 1967.

Fu SM, Winchester RJ, Rai KR, et al.: Hairy cell leukemia: Proliferation of a cell with phagocytic and B-lymphocyte properties. *Scand J Immunol* 3:847, 1974.

Hubbard SM, Chabner BA, DeVita VT, et al.: Histologic progression in non-Hodgkin's lymphoma. *Blood* 59:258, 1982.

Kipps TJ, Robbins BA, Kustner P, et al.: Autoantibody-associated cross-reactive idiotypes expressed at high frequency in chronic lymphocytic leukemia relative to B-cell lymphomas of follicular center cell origin. *Blood* 72:422, 1988.

Korsmeyer SJ, Hieter PA, Sharrow SO, et al.: Normal human B cells display ordered light-chain gene rearrangements and deletions. *J Exp Med* 156:975, 1983.

Levy R, Levy S, Cleary ML, et al.: Somatic mutation in human B-cell tumors. *Immunol Rev* 96:43, 1987.

Levy R, Warnke R, Dorfman R, et al.: The monoclonality of human B-cell lymphomas. *J Exp Med* 145:1014, 1977.

Pangalis GA, Boussiiotis VA, Kittas C: Malignant disorders of small lymphocytes: Small lymphocytic lymphoma, lymphoplasmacytic lymphoma, and chronic lymphocytic leukemia: Their clinical and laboratory relationship. *Am J Clin Pathol* 99:402–408, 1993.

Perry DA, Bast MA, Armitage JO, et al.: Diffuse intermediate lymphocytic lymphoma: A clinicopathologic study and comparison with small lymphocytic lymphoma and diffuse small cleaved-cell lymphoma. *Cancer* 66:1992, 1990.

Rappaport H, Winter WS, Hicks EB: Follicular lymphoma: A reevaluation of its position in the scheme of malignant lymphoma. Based on a survey of 253 cases. *Cancer* 9:792, 1956.

Salsano F, Fraland SS, Natvig JB, et al.: Some idiotypes of B-lymphocyte IgD and IgM: Formal evidence for monoclonality of chronic lymphocytic leukemia cells. *Scand J Immunol* 3:841, 1974.

Schuurman H-J, Huppes W, Verdonck LF, et al.: Immunophenotyping of non-Hodgkin's lymphoma: Correlation with relapse-free survival. *Am J Pathol* 131:102, 1988.

Schwartz BE, Pinkus G, Bacus S, et al.: Cell proliferation in non-Hodgkin's lymphomas: Digital image analysis of Ki67 antibody staining. *Am J Pathol* 134:327, 1989.

Williams ME, Lee JT, Innes DJ, et al.: Immunoglobulin gene rearrangement in abnormal lymph node hyperplasia. *Am J Clin Pathol* 96:746, 1991.

Zelenetz AD, Chen TT, Levy R: Histologic transformation of follicular lymphoma to diffuse lymphoma represents tumor progression by a single malignant B cell. *J Exp Med* 173:197, 1991.

Zukerberg LR, Medeiros LJ, Ferry JA, et al.: Diffuse low-grade B-cell lymphomas: Four clinically distinct subtypes defined by a combination of morphologic and immunophenotypic features. *Am J Clin Pathol* 100:373–385, 1993.

MULTIPLE MYELOMA

Durie BGM, Salmon SE: Cellular kinetics, staging, and immunoglobulin synthesis in multiple myeloma. *Annu Rev Med* 26:283, 1975.

Grey HM, Kohler PF: Cryoimmunoglobulins. *Semin Hematol* 10:87, 1973.

Kopp WL, Beirne GS, Borus RO: Hyperviscosity symptoms in multiple myeloma. *Am J Med* 43:141, 1967.

Kyle RA, Elveback LR: Management of prognosis of multiple myeloma. *Mayo Clin Proc* 51:751, 1976.

Lindstrom FD, Williams RC Jr: Serum anti-immunoglobulins in multiple myeloma and benign monoclonal gammopathy. *Clin Immunol Immunopathol* 3:503, 1975.

Radl J, van Camp B (eds.): Monoclonal gammapathies III: Clinical significance and basic mechanisms. *EURAGE*, 1991.

Salmon SE: Immunoglobulin synthesis and tumor kinetics of multiple myeloma. *Semin Hematol* 10:135, 1973.

Shustic C, Bergsagel DE, Pruzanski W: K and L light-chain disease: Survival rates and clinical manifestations. *Blood* 48:41, 1976.

Solomon A: Homogeneous (monoclonal) immunoglobulins in cancer. *Am J Med* 63:169, 1977.

Waldenstrom J: The occurrence of benign, essential monoclonal (M type), nonmacro-molecular hyperglobulinemia and its differential diagnosis. *Acta Med Scand* 176:345, 1964.

BURKITT'S LYMPHOMA

Burkitt DP, Wright DH: *Burkitt's lymphoma*. Edinburgh and London, Livingston, 1970.

Epstein MA, Achong BG, Barr YM: Virus particles in cultured lymphoblasts from Burkitt's lymphoma. *Lancet* 1:702, 1964.

Klein G: The biology and serology of Epstein–Barr virus (EBV) infections. *Bull Cancer* (Paris) 63:399, 1976.

Mann RB, Jaffe ES, Braylan RC, et al.: Nonendemic Burkitt's lymphoma: A B-cell tumor related to germinal centers. *N Engl J Med* 295:685, 1976.

Nkrumah F, Henle W, Henle G, et al.: Burkitt's lymphoma: Its clinical course in relation to immunologic reactivities to Epstein–Barr virus and tumor-related antigens. *J Natl Cancer Inst* 57:1051, 1976.

TRANSPLANT-ASSOCIATED LYMPHOMA

Penn I: Malignant lymphomas in transplant recipients. *Transpl Proc* 13:736, 1981.

Swennen LJ, Costanzo-Nordin MR, Fisher SG: Increased incidence of lymphoproliferative disorder after immunosuppression with the monoclonal antibody OKT3 in cardiac transplant recipients. *N Engl J Med* 323:1723, 1990.

Swerdlow AH: Posttransplant lymphoproliferative disorders: A morphologic, phenotypic and genotypic spectrum of the disease. *Histopathology* 20:373, 1992.

T-CELL TUMORS

Ball ED, Davis RB, Griffin JD, et al.: Prognostic value of lymphocyte surface markers in acute myeloid leukemia. *Blood* 77:2242, 1991.

Bani D, Moretti S, Pimpinelli N, et al.: Interdigitating reticulum cells in the dermal infiltrate of mycosis fungoides: An ultrastructural and immunohistochemical study. *Virchows Arch Pathol* 412:451, 1988.

Broder S, Edelson RL, Lutzner MA, et al.: The Sezary syndrome: A malignant proliferation of helper T cells. *J Clin Invest* 58:1297, 1976.

Castleman B: Tumors of the thymus gland. In *Atlas of Tumor Pathology*, Sect. 5, fascicle 19. Washington, DC, Armed Forces Institute of Pathology, 1955.

Guillan RA, Zelman S, Smalley RL, et al.: Malignant thymoma associated with myasthenia gravis, and evidence of extrathoracic metastases. *Cancer* 27:823, 1971.

Hinuma Y: A retrovirus associated with a human leukemia, adult T-cell leukemia. *Curr Top Microbiol Immunol* 115:127, 1985.

Kaplan J, Mastrangelo R, Peterson WD Jr: Childhood lymphoblastic lymphoma: A cancer of thymus derived lymphocytes. *Cancer Res* 34:521, 1974.

Knowles DM: Immunophenotypic and antigen receptor gene rearrangement in T-cell neoplasia. *Am J Pathol* 134:761, 1989.

Loughran TP: Clonal diseases of large granular lymphocytes. *Blood* 82:1–14, 1993.

Miller RA, Coleman CN, Fawcett HD, et al.: Sezary syndrome: A model for migration of T lymphocytes to skin. *N Engl J Med* 303:89, 1980.

Pandolfi F, Zambello R, Cafaro A, Semenzato G: Biologic and clinical heterogeneity of lymphoproliferative diseases of peripheral mature T lymphocytes. *Lab Invest* 67:264, 1992.

Reis MD, Griesser H, Mak TW: T-cell receptor and immunoglobulin gene rearrangement in lymphoproliferative disorders. *Adv Cancer Res* 52:45, 1989.

Rowden G, Lewis MG: Langerhans' cells: Involvement in the pathogenesis of mycosis fungoides. *Br J Dermatol* 95:665, 1976.

Sen L, Borella L: Clinical importance of lymphoblasts with T-cell markers in childhood acute leukemia. *N Engl J Med* 292:828, 1975.

Waldman TA: The arrangement of immunoglobulin and T-cell receptor genes in human lymphoproliferative disorders. *Adv Immunol* 40:247, 1987.

Winkelmann K (ed.): Symposium on the Sezary cell. *Mayo Clin* 49:513, 1974.

MACROPHAGE TUMORS

Anderson RC: Histiocyte medullary reticulosis with transient skin lesions. *Br Med J* 1:220, 1944.

Byrne GE, Rappaport H: Malignant histiocytosis. *Gann Monogr Cancer Res* 15:145, 1973.

Cline MJ, Golde DW: A review and reevaluation of the histiocytic disorders. *Am J Med* 55:49, 1973.

Van der Volk P, Velde J, Jansen J, et al.: Malignant lymphoma of true histiocytic origins: Histiocytic sarcoma. *Virch Arch Pathol* 391:249, 1981.

HODGKIN'S DISEASE

Aisenberg AC: Hodgkin's disease: Prognosis, treatment, etiologic, and immunologic considerations. *N Engl J Med* 270:508, 1964.

Cassazza AR, Duvall CP, Carbone PP: Summary of infectious complications occurring in patients with Hodgkin's disease. *Cancer Res* 26:1290, 1966.

Carbone PP, Kaplan HS, Musshof K, et al.: Report of the committee on Hodgkin's disease staging. *Cancer Res* 31:1860, 1971.

Chittal SM, Caveriviere P, Schwarting R, et al.: Monoclonal antibodies in the diagnosis of Hodgkin's disease: The search for a rational panel. *Am J Surg Pathol* 12:9, 1988.

Ford RJ, Metha S, Davis F, et al.: Growth factors in Hodgkin's disease. *Cancer Treat Rep* 66:663, 1982.

Gerdes J, Van Baarlen J, Pileri S, et al.: Tumor cell growth fraction in Hodgkin's disease. *Am J Pathol* 128:390, 1987.

Hodgkin T: On some morbid appearance of the absorbent glands and spleen. *Med Chir Dig* 17:68, 1832.

Hsu S-M, Hsu P-L: Aberrant expression of T cell and B cell markers in myelocyte/monocyte/histiocyte-derived lymphoma and leukemia cells. *Am J Pathol* 134:203, 1989.

Hsu S-M, Waldron JW, Hsu P-L, et al.: Cytokines in malignant lymphomas: Review and prospective evaluation. *Hum Pathol* 24:1040–1057, 1993.

Kaplan HS: Hodgkin's disease and other human malignant lymphomas: Advances and prospects—G.H.A. Clowes memorial lecture. *Cancer Res* 36:3863, 1976.

Kaplan HS: Hodgkin's disease: Biology, treatment, prognosis. *Blood* 57:813, 1981.

Kadin ME: Possible origin of the Reed–Sternberg cells from an interdigitating reticulum cell. *Cancer Treat Rep* 66:601, 1982.

Portlock CS, Robertson A, Turbow MM, et al.: MOPP chemotherapy of advanced Hodgkin's disease: Prognostic factors in 242 patients. *Proc Am Assoc Cancer Res* 17:248, 1976.

Rather LJ: Who discovered the pathognomonic giant cell of Hodgkin's disease? *Bull NY Acad Med* 48:943, 1972.

Reed DM: On the pathologic giant cell of Hodgkin's disease with special reference to its relation to tuberculosis. *Johns Hopkins Med J* 10:133, 1902.

Regula DP, Hoppe RT, Weiss LM: Nodular and diffuse types of lymphocyte predominance Hodgkin's disease. *New Engl J Med* 318:214, 1988.

Specht L, Pedersen-Bjergaard J: Hodgkin's disease: Recent concepts in classification and treatment. *Eur J Haematol* 42(suppl. 48):7, 1989.

Stein H, Schwarting R, Dallenbach F, et al.: Immunology of Hodgkin and Reed–Sternberg cells. *Rec Res Cancer Res* 117:15, 1989.

TREATMENT

DeVita VT Jr, Serpick A, Carbone PP: Combination chemotherapy in the treatment of advanced Hodgkin's disease. *Am Intern Med* 73:881, 1970.

Gale RP, Foon KA: Chronic lymphocyte leukemia: Recent advances in biology and treatment. *Am Int Med* 103:101, 1985.

Gorin NC: Autologous bone marrow transplantation: A review of recent advances in acute leukemia. *Progress in Bone Marrow Transplantation.* In Gale RP, Champlin R (eds.). New York, Liss, 1987, 723.

Kernan NA, Bartsch G, Ash RC, et al.: Analysis of 462 transplantations from unrelated donors facilitated by the national marrow donor program. *N Engl J Med* 328:593–602, 1993.

McGlave PB: The status of bone marrow transplantation for leukemia. *Hosp Pract* 20:97, 1985.

Mertelsmann R, Herrmann F: *Hematopoietic Growth Factors in Clinical Applications.* New York, Marcel Dekker, 1990.

Petz CD, Blume KG (eds.): *Clinical Bone Marrow Transplantation.* New York, Churchill Livingston, 1983.

Stevenson GT, Stevenson FK: Treatment of lymphoid tumors with anti-idiotype antibodies. *Spring Semin Immunopathol* 6:99, 1983.

Thomas ED: The role of marrow transplantation in the eradication of malignant diseases. *Cancer* 49:1963, 1982.

ANIMAL MODELS OF LYMPHOMAS

Biggs PM: A discussion of the classification of the avian leukosis complex and fowl paralysis. *Br Vet J* 117:326, 1961.

Else RN: Vaccinial immunity to Marek's disease in bursectomized chickens. *Vet Rec* 95:182, 1974.

Essex M: Immunity to leukemia, lymphoma, and fibrosarcoma in cats: A case for immune surveillance. *Contemp Top Immunobiol* 6:71, 1977.

Green I, Forni G, Konen T, et al.: Immunological studies of the guinea pig L$_2$C leukemia. *Fed Proc* 36:2264, 1977.

Hoover EA, Zeidner NS, Perigo NA, et al.: Feline leukemia virus-induced immunodeficiency syndrome in cats as a model for evaluation of antiviral therapy. *Intervirol* 30(suppl. 1):12, 1989.

Kaplan HS: On the natural history of murine leukemias: Presidential address. *Cancer Res* 27:1325, 1967.

Madel EM: History and further observations (1954–1976) of the L$_2$C leukemia in the guinea pig. *Fed Proc* 36:2249, 1977.

Payne LN, Frazier JA, Powell PC: Pathogenesis of Marek's disease. *Int Rev Exp Pathol* 16:59, 1976.

Peterson RDA, Burnmester BR, Fredrickson TN, et al.: Effect of bursectomy and thymectomy on the development of visceral lymphomatosis in the chicken. *J Natl Cancer Inst* 32:1143, 1964.

Potter M: Pathogenesis of plasmacytomas in mice. In *Cancer*, vol. 1, Becker FF (ed.). New York, Plenum Press, 1975, 161.

Puchase HG: Prevention of Marek's disease: A review. *Cancer Res* 36:696, 1976.

Rouse BT, Wells RJH, Warner NL: Proportion of T and B lymphocytes in lesions of Marek's disease: Theoretic implications for pathogenesis. *J Immunol* 110:534, 1973.

Zolla-Pazner S, Gilbert M, Fleit SA: Studies of antibody affinity in plasmacytoma-bearing mice: Evidence for a maturational defect of B lymphocytes. *Cell Immunol* 62:149, 1981.

IMMUNO-REGULATION

Gatti RA, Good RA: Occurrence of malignancy in immunodeficiency disease: A review. *Cancer* 28:89, 1971.

Jarret WF, Mackey LJ: Neoplastic diseases of the hematopoietic and lymphoid tissues. *Bull WHO* 50:21, 1974.

Kinlen L: Immunosuppressive therapy and acquired immunological disorders. *Cancer Res* 52(suppl.):5474s, 1992.

Louie S, Schwartz RS: Immunodeficiency and the pathogenesis of lymphoma and leukemia. *Semin Hematol* 15:117, 1978.

Melief CJM, Schwartz RS: Immunocompetence and malignancy. In *Cancer*, vol. 1, Becker FF (ed.). New York, Plenum Press, 1975, 121.

Yunis EJ, Ferndandes G, Greenberg LS: Tumor immunology: Autoimmunity and aging. *J Am Geriatr Soc* 24:258, 1976.

VIRUS INFECTION

Hanna MG Jr, Rapp F (eds.): Immunobiology of oncogenic viruses. *Contemp Top Immunol* 6:1, 1977.

Kaplan HS, Goodenow RS, Gartner S, et al.: Biology and virology of the human malignant lymphomas. *Cancer* 43:1, 1979.

Mueller N, Mohar A, Evans A: Viruses other than HIV and non-Hodgkin's lymphoma. *Cancer Res* 52(suppl.):5479s, 1992.

CHROMOSOMAL TRANS-LOCATIONS

Klein G: Specific chromosomal translocations and the genesis of B-cell derived tumors in mice and men. *Cell* 32:311, 1983.

Magrath I: Molecular basis of lymphomagenesis. *Cancer Res* 52(suppl.):5529s, 1992.

Nowell PC, Erickson J, Finan J, et al.: Chromosomal translocations, immunoglobulin genes, and oncogenes in human B-cell tumors. *Cancer Surv* 3:531, 1984.

Rowley J: Biological implications of consistent chromosome rearrangements in leukemia and lymphoma. *Cancer Res* 44:3159, 1984.

Temin HM: Origin of retroviruses from cellular variable genetic elements. *Cell* 21:599, 1980.

Williams DL, Look AT, Melvin SL, et al.: New chromosomal translocations correlate with specific immunophenotypes of childhood acute lymphoblastic leukemia. *Cell* 36:101, 1984.

Wolman SR, Henderson AS: Chromosomal aberrations as markers of oncogene amplification. *Human Pathol* 20: 309, 1989.

Yunis JJ, Oken MM, Theologides A, et al.: Recurrent chromosomal defects are found in most patients with non-Hodgkin's lymphoma. *Cancer Genet Cytogenet* 13:17, 1984.

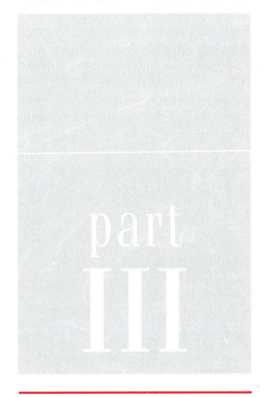

part
III

Immunity

In medical terms, immunity is protection against or exemption from a disease, usually an infectious disease. The same immune mechanisms that are responsible for the diseases discussed in the preceding section of this book (immunopathology) also mediate specific acquired resistance to infection (Table III–1). Thus immune mechanisms are "double-edged swords," protecting against infectious diseases on the one hand, and causing tissue damage and disease on the other hand. These immune mechanisms most likely evolved and were selected as a means of protection from the destructive effects of parasitic organisms and their products or as a means of resisting the growth of neoplastic cells (see Chapter 30). However, these same mechanisms may cause many of the signs and symptoms of infectious diseases. The last six chapters of this book cover immunity to infectious diseases, iatrogenic and natural modification of immunity, and tumor immunity.

TABLE III–1. IMMUNOPATHOLOGY AND IMMUNITY

Immune Effector Mechanism	Destructive Reaction "Allergy"	Protective Function "Immunity"	Protective Immunity Examples
Neutralization	Insulin resistance, pernicious anemia, myasthenia gravis, hyperthyroidism	Toxin neutralization, blockade of virus receptors	Diphtheria, tetanus, cholera, botulism, polio
Cytotoxic	Hemolysis, leukopenia, thrombocytopenia	Bacteriolysis, opsonization	Bacterial infection, staphylococci, streptococci, etc.
Immune complex	Vasculitis, glomerulonephritis, serum sickness, rheumatoid diseases	Acute inflammation, opsonization, polymorphonuclear leukocyte activation	Bacterial infections, staphylococci, streptococci, pneumococci, etc.
Anaphylactic	Asthma, urticaria, anaphylactic shock, hay fever	Focal inflammation, increased vascular permeability, increased gastrointestinal secretion and motility, expulsion of inhaled organisms by sneezing	Intestinal parasites, bacterial infections
T-cell cytotoxicity	Contact dermatitis, viral exanthems, autoimmune diseases, graft rejection	Destruction of virus-infected cells	Virus infections, tuberculosis, cancer
Delayed hypersensitivity	Autoimmune diseases, postvaccinial encephalomyelitis	Elimination of intracellular infections of macrophages	Tuberculosis, leprosy, syphilis, leishmaniasis
Granulomatous	Berylliosis, sarcoidosis	Isolation of organisms in granulomas	Tuberculosis, filariasis, schistosomiasis, leprosy, helminths, fungi

Modified from Sell S: Introduction to symposium on immunopathology: "Immune Mechanisms in Disease." *Hum Pathol* 9:24, 1978.

25

Immune Resistance to Infection

The specific immune effector mechanisms responsible for protection against infectious agents are the same as those that cause immune-mediated disease. Although it has become popular to define the immunity to infectious diseases on the basis of the type of T-helper subsets (eg, Th1 for DTH and Th2 for IgE-mediated reactions), it must be kept in mind that T-helper subsets are used for hypothetical explanations for induction of different types of immunoglobulin antibody responses based on observations on the types of lymphokines produced by different T-cell lines in vitro and do not act, as often postulated, at the level of effector mechanisms. The type of protective mechanism differs with different infectious agents (Table 25–1). With some notable exceptions, the mechanisms mediated by humoral antibody (immunoglobulin) are effective against infectious agents that exist extracellularly, such as bacteria, whereas cellular-mediated reactions (T_{CTL}, T_{DTH}, and granulomatous reactions) are effective against intracellular parasites, such as viruses and mycobacteria. T_{CTL} react with antigens on virus infected cells and kill the cells infected with virus as well as the virus. T_{DTH} activate macrophages to kill organisms that they have internalized and are most effective against parasite diseases, such as tuberculosis, leprosy, candidiasis, and leishmaniasis, in which the organisms infect macrophages. The selected infections covered in this chapter—tetanus, malaria, rheumatic fever, allergic bronchopulmonary aspergillosis, filariasis, and strongyloides—are chosen to illustrate how different immune mechanisms not only protect against infection but also cause disease (the double-edged sword of immunopathology). Immunity to smallpox, syphilis, tuberculosis, and leprosy is presented in more detail in Chapters 15–17. Finally, some other infectious dis-

TABLE 25–1. MAJOR IMMUNE DEFENSE MECHANISMS FOR INFECTIOUS DISEASES

Type of Infection	Major Immune Defense Mechanism(s)
Bacterial	Antibody
Viral	Antibody and T_{CTL}
Mycobacterial	DTH, T_{CTL} and granulomatous
Protozoal	DTH and antibody
Worms	Anaphylactic and granulomatous
Fungal	DTH and granulomatous

eases will be used to illustrate how some infectious agents avoid the attack function of specific immunity (immune evasion).

BACTERIAL INFECTIONS

Specific immunity to the destructive effects of bacteria or bacterial products is usually mediated by humoral antibody. The mechanisms of antibody-mediated and cell-mediated protection against bacterial infections are illustrated in Figure 25–1. Some bacteria produce disease not by direct effects of the organism but by the release of products called toxins, which may have severe destructive effects distant from the site of infection. Destructive bacterial toxins are rendered harmless by reaction with antibody (neutralization reaction). For instance, antitoxin antibodies inactivate toxins of diphtheria or tetanus (see below). In addition, IgA antibodies in the gastrointestinal tract may be able to block the production of watery diarrhea by *Vibrio cholerae* infection of the intestinal tract by preventing the toxin from binding to gastrointestinal lining cells (neutralization). Destruction of infecting organisms in connective tissues is accomplished by the activation of complement following the reaction of antibody with the organism. This leads to increased susceptibility of the organism to phagocytosis (toxic complex reaction) or destruction by insertion of the terminal components of complement into the bacterial cell membrane and lysis (cytotoxic reaction). Activation of mast cells by IgE-mediated reactions increases vascular permeability (endothelial cell contraction), permitting egress of blood-borne antibody or inflammatory cells into the site of infection. Specific T_{CTL} and T_{DTH} gain access to the site of infection through the contracted endothelial cells. T_{DTH} cells may also be activated by bacterial antigens and release lymphokines, which attract and activate macrophages. The activated macrophages clear the site of inflammation by phagocytosis and digestion of dead bacteria, neutrophils, and necrotic tissue, and prepare the site for healing through the release of monokines that stimulate fibroblastic proliferation and wound healing.

As an example of the role of different immune mechanisms in protection against a bacterial infection, let us assume that an anaerobic,

Immune mechanisms in bacterial skin infection

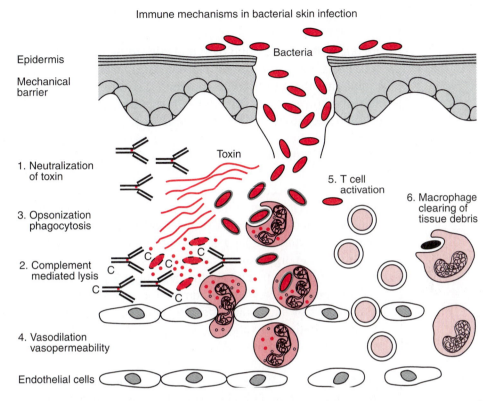

Figure 25–1. Antibody-mediated and cell-mediated mechanisms of protection against bacterial infections. Bacterial infections may be resisted by each of the antibody-mediated immune mechanisms, including: (1) Neutralization of bacterial toxins, (2) cytotoxic lysis by antibody and complement, (3) immune complex mediated acute polymorphonuclear infiltration (Arthus reaction) and opsonization of bacteria leading to increased phagocytosis, and (4) acute anaphylactic vascular events permitting exudation of inflammatory cells and fluids. During the chronic stage of the infection, cell-mediated immunity is activated: (5) T_{CTL} cells that react with antigens on the surface of virus-infected cells and cause their destruction. (6) T_{DTH} cells that react with bacterial antigens may infiltrate the site of infection, become activated, and release lymphokines that attract and activate macrophages. The activated macrophages phagocytose and degrade necrotic bacteria and tissue, preparing the lesion for healing. (7) Granulomas form when organisms cannot be destroyed by macrophages, walling off the infection from the rest of the host.

gram-negative bacillus, *Bacteroides*, which is a normal inhabitant of the intestine, gains access to the peritoneal cavity. The organism starts to multiply and the body recognizes that something is wrong. The initial host response consists of polymorphonuclear cells (PMNs), which are attracted to the site by the release of chemoattractants from the damaged tissue along with C5a, since desialyted *Bacteroides* lipopolysaccharide (LPS) endotoxin can fix complement by the alternate pathway. Another powerful PMN attractant is formylated peptides, which are the leader sequences of bacterial protein synthesis. As the PMN and resident macrophages attack the bacterial cells, antigens are released and delivered by lymphatics to lymph nodes. In the lymph nodes, macrophages present the processed antigens to T and B cells, stimulating them to become specific effector cells (T cells) or to produce specific antibody (B cells). The specific antibody reacts with antigens on the surface of the *Bacteroides* organisms and fixes complement, which may kill the cell, allow for more efficient phagocytosis, or produce inflammatory fragments (C3a, C5a), which increase circulation to the site and attract more inflammatory cells. Specific T_{CTL} or T_{DTH} cells gain access to the site due to the increased vascular permeability and also react with specific antigens. Activated T_{DTH} cells release lymphokines, which further contribute by attracting and activating macrophages. The macrophages then phagocytose and clear the site of the dead organisms, as well as the products of inflammation, and release monokines to activate the healing process.

Immune complex-mediated reactions are responsible for the boils or abscesses of cutaneous infection with *Staphylococcus aureus*. The organisms initially invade the hair follicles of the skin, causing folliculitis. This is painless and may be as far as the infection goes. However, the infection may penetrate into the subcutaneous connective tissue. The infected zone becomes filled with fibrin, polymorphonuclear cells and lymphocytes. The inflammatory reaction is driven by serum antibodies, IgG or IgM, which diffuse into the tissues and react with the staphylococcal antigens, fixing complement, and attracting more inflammatory cells. *S. aureus* produces serine proteases that cleave human immunoglobulins, thus contributing to the virulence of the infection. The infected zone becomes ringed with leukocytes and collagen, limiting the spread of infection. Necrosis of the involved tissue occurs when the PMNs release the contents of their lysosomes into the infected area. The lesions heal after they open to the surface and lose the necrotic core of tissue. The resulting defect is filled with connective tissue, leaving a scar that is usually inapparent.

VIRAL INFECTIONS

Immune resistance to viral infections is mainly by cell-mediated immunity, but humoral antibody also plays a role by preventing virus from attaching to cell receptors (Fig. 25–2). Viruses live within the host's cells and can spread from cell to cell. To be effective in attacking intracellular organisms, an immune mechanism must have the capacity to react with cells in solid tissue. This is a property of cell-mediated reactions, particularly T_{CTL}, but not of antibody-mediated reactions. Many cells infected with a virus will, at some stage of the infection, express viral antigens on the cell surface. It is at this stage that specifically sensitized T_{CTL} cells can recognize cell surface-expressed viral antigens in association with class I MHC molecules

Immune mechanisms in viral infections

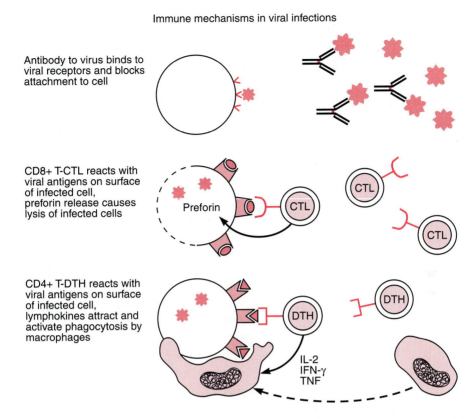

Antibody to virus binds to viral receptors and blocks attachment to cell

CD8+ T-CTL reacts with viral antigens on surface of infected cell, preforin release causes lysis of infected cells

Preforin

CD4+ T-DTH reacts with viral antigens on surface of infected cell, lymphokines attract and activate phagocytosis by macrophages

IL-2
IFN-γ
TNF

Figure 25–2. Cellular and antibody-mediated mechanisms of protection against viral infections. Circulating immunoglobulin antibody (usually IgG) or secretory antibody (usually IgA) reacts with surface antigens on the virus and prevents the virus from attaching to cells (neutralizing antibody), thereby inhibiting spread of the infection. Sensitized T_{CTL} may destroy virus-infected cells that express viral antigens associated with class I MHC molecules on the surface. T_{DTH} cells reacting with viral antigens release lymphokines that activate macrophages to eliminate intracellular viral infections of macrophages.

and destroy the virus-infected cells. Transgenic mice lacking class I MHC-restricted T cells have decreased resistance to viral infections. Adverse effects of this reaction occur if the cell expressing the viral antigens is important functionally, as is the case for certain viral infections of the central nervous system (see below). If the virus infects macrophages, lymphokines from reactive T_{DTH} cells can activate the macrophages to kill the intracellular viruses. Transgenic knockout mice lacking interferon-γ (INF-γ) receptors are susceptible to virus infections. Humoral antibody can prevent the entry of virus particles into cells by interfering with the ability of the virus to attach to a host cell, and secretory IgA can prevent the establishment of viral infections of mucous membranes. However, once the virus is within cells, it is not susceptible to the effects of antibody. Patients with deficiencies in antibody production alone usually do not have serious viral infections but develop life-threatening bacterial infections. Patients with defects in cell-mediated immunity develop serious viral infections (see Chapter 27).

MYCO-BACTERIAL INFECTIONS

Mycobacterial infections, such as tuberculosis and leprosy, are resisted by cellular mechanisms, including T_{CTL}, T_{DTH}, and granulomatous hypersensitivity (see Figure 17–4). T_{CTL} cells destroy highly infected macrophages that are unable to cleanse themselves of intracellular infections, resulting in uptake of organisms by other macrophages. T_{DTH} cells release lymphokines that activate macrophages to destroy intracellular organisms, including those released from macrophages destroyed through action of T_{CTL} cells. Interferon-γ appears to be critical for production of macrophage killing, as IFN-γ–deficient mice (IFN-γ knockout mice) are susceptible to lethal infections with *Mycobacterium bovis*. Granulomatous reactions isolate infected sites in tissues and prevent dissemination. At one time it was thought that the tissue lesions of tuberculosis required the effect of delayed hypersensitivity. The term "hypersensitivity" was coined because animals with cellular immune reactivity to tubercle bacilli developed greater tissue lesions after reinoculation of bacilli than did animals injected for the first time. The granulomatous lesions seen in tuberculosis do depend on immune mechanisms for their formation. However, these lesions are not really the cause of the disease but an unfortunate effect of the protective mechanisms; the granulomatous inflammatory reaction to the infective mycobacteria results in destruction of normal tissue. In the lung, for instance, extensive damage done by the formation of large granulomas in response to a tuberculosis infection can result in respiratory failure. The granulomatous immune response produces the lesion, but the mycobacterium causes the disease. See Chapters 16 and 17 for more details.

PROTOZOAL INFECTIONS

The mechanism of protection against protozoal infections, like viral infections, depends upon the location of the agent in the host. Protozoa are unicellular organisms that may be located intracellularly, extracellularly in the blood, both intracellularly and in the blood, or primarily in the gastrointestinal tract. Intracellular protozoans, such as *Leishmania*, are eliminated by delayed and granulomatous reactions similar to the response evoked by leprosy. In certain types of leishmaniasis, the organism is limited to focal inflamed areas of the skin. This response has histologic characteristics of a delayed hypersensitivity reaction. If this delayed hypersensitivity is lost, dissemination of the organisms may occur. Trypanosomiasis is an example of a blood-borne extracellular parasite that may also be found intracellularly; the major defense appears to be via humoral antibody as rising titers of antibody are associated with containment of symptoms. However, as discussed below, the organisms of African trypanosomiasis are able to change surface antigens in a cyclic fashion, resulting in growth of new clones in successive waves of parasitemia. Malaria protozoa multiply intracellularly but disseminate through release into the blood stream. Malarial immunity is mediated by both IgG antibody, which can effectively attack the blood-borne organism, and by T_{CTL} and T_{DTH} cells that are effective against the intracellular stage in liver cells. Therefore, humoral immunity is effective only during a short period of the malarial protozoan life cycle. Even highly immune-infected persons may be unable to clear the parasites completely because of the inability of antibody to affect the intracellular stages. The number of organisms present in the body may be controlled by antibody, and the host lives in balance with his infection. Preventive immunity to malaria may be mediated by antibodies to the sporozoite stage introduced by the mosquito vector or by preventing initial infection of hepatocytes (see below for details). *Entamoeba histolytica* is an intestinal protozoan infection of man. Although antibodies are produced, the protective effect of these antibodies remains to be demonstrated; immunity may be mediated by cell-mediated immunity or IgA antibody.

HELMINTH (WORM) INFECTIONS

The response to worm infections also depends on the location of the infestation. Worms are located in the intestinal tract and/or tissues. Tapeworms, which exist in the intestinal lumen, isolated from the tissues of the infected host, promote no protective immunologic response. On the other hand, worms with larval forms that invade tissue do stimulate an immune response. The tissue reaction to *Ascaris* and *Trichinella* consists of an intense infiltrate of polymorphonuclear leukocytes, with a predominance of eosinophils. Eosinophil granules contain basic proteins which are toxic to worms. Eosinophils are directed to attack worms by antibody-dependent cellular cytotoxicity (ADCC). Anaphylactic antibodies (IgE) are also frequently associated with helminth infections, and intradermal injection of worm extracts elicits a wheal-and-flare reaction. Children infested with *Ascaris lumbricoides* have attacks of urticaria, asthma, and other anaphylactic or atopic types of reactions presumably associated with dissemination of *Ascaris* antigens. An eosinophilic pulmonary infiltrate (pneumonia) may be found associated with migration of helminth larvae through the lung. In experimental models, expulsion of parasitic worms from the gastrointestinal tract occurs following the induction of peristalsis and diarrhea from intestinal IgE-mediated anaphylactic reactions to worms (see below). In tissues, the egg forms of schistosomes elicit a granulomatous response in which both delayed-type hypersensitivity (IL-2, TNF-γ) and anaphylactic (IL-4, IL-5, eosinophils) responses play a prominent role.

FUNGAL INFECTIONS

Cellular immunity, primarily T_{DTH}-mediated activation of macrophages, appears to be the most important immunologic factor in resistance to fungal infections, although humoral antibody certainly may play a role. The importance of cellular reactions is indicated by the intense mononuclear infiltrate and granulomatous reactions that occur in tissues infected with fungi and by the fact that fungal infections are frequently associated with depressed immune reactivity of the delayed type (opportunistic infections). Chronic mucocutaneous candidiasis refers to persistent or recurrent infection by *Candida albicans* of mucous membranes, nails, and skin. Patients with this disease generally have a form of immune deviation, ie, a depression of cellular immune reactions, with high levels of humoral antibody (see below), similar to lepromatous leprosy. Fungi appear to be resistant to the effects of antibody, so that cell-mediated immunity (CMI) is needed for effective resistance.

INSECT STINGS

Immune reactions to insect bites or stings are generally believed to be responsible for most of the irritating skin reactions that follow the bite or sting. Individuals vary markedly in their immune reactions to insect stings. Clearly, the reaction of a given person to an insect sting depends on the dominant type of immune response. Most people react to insect stings or bites, including mosquito bites, by acute cutaneous anaphylactic reactions. Systemic shock and death from wasp or bee stings, while infrequent, may develop in hyperreactive individuals. Two possible protective functions of anaphylactic reactions to insect stings are possible: (1) Immediate avoidance behavior by the recipient, which serves to reduce antigen contact, and (2) anaphylactic reactions may help prevent toxic complex reactions or delayed hypersensitivity reactions. Since potentially fatal anaphylactic reactions require much less antigen contact than other allergic reactions, the latter mechanism seems unlikely. In fact, hyposensitization via the production of blocking IgG antibodies is attempted clinically to reduce the possibility of anaphylactic reactions to insect bites (see Chapter 14). An anaphylactic reaction to insect stings may be protective in producing avoidance behavior. However, in all likelihood, anaphylactic reactions to insect bites are not protective reactions but examples of potentially protective immune reactions being applied inappropriately.

SUMMARY OF THE ROLE OF IMMUNE MECHANISMS IN PROTECTION AGAINST INFECTIONS

From the preceding discussion, it can be appreciated that each of the seven types of allergic reactions responsible for immune disease also has important functions in resistance to infection.

1. Neutralization of inactivation of biologically active toxins by antibodies is highly desirable. This is precisely what is accomplished by immunization with diphtheria toxoid.
2. Cytotoxic or cytolytic reactions directed against the infecting organisms cause their death, resulting in cure of the infection.

3. The inflammatory effect of antigen–antibody complexes in the Arthus mechanism results in chemotaxis and stickiness of leukocytes, platelets, and endothelium, and increases permeability. These effects promote defense by localization and diapedesis of leukocytes. At the dose level of a usual infection, this effect is not harmful to the host. Precipitating antibody and complement, as means of enhancing phagocytosis (opsonization), are responsible for protection against many bacterial infections.

4. The effect of histamine release (the anaphylactic mechanism) at the usual dose level results in slight vasodilation and increased capillary permeability, both effects interpreted in classic pathology as aiding defense. Eosinophilic infiltrates may be toxic to worm infestations in tissues. Smooth muscle contraction and diarrhea induced by the anaphylactic mechanism may cause expulsion of intestinal parasites.

5. T-cytotoxic reactions are protective when directed against virus-infected cells, but the loss of these cells may be the critical factor in a disease. In addition, T_{CTL} cells directed against host cells is a major mechanism for autoimmune lesions.

6. Delayed-type hypersensitivity (DTH) at the dose level occurring in infection results in local mobilization and activation of phagocytes and effective destruction of infecting agents. DTH is particularly effective against infectious agents that proliferate inside macrophages; such organisms thrive in the absence of DTH but are eliminated by DTH-activated macrophages.

7. Granulomatous hypersensitivity may serve to isolate or localize insoluble toxic materials or organisms.

Protective and Destructive Immune Effector Mechanisms to Infectious Agents

NEUTRALIZATION

Skin Tests

Schick Test. In some cases, antibody can neutralize the inflammatory activity of bacterial toxins, resulting in the absence of a reaction in immune individuals. Historically, in vivo neutralization of diphtheria toxin by antibody was determined by skin testing. A small amount of diphtheria toxin injected intradermally produces a local inflammatory reaction that is maximal at 4 to 5 hours and then fades. In an immunized individual who has antibody to diphtheria toxin, no reaction occurs; the antibody neutralizes the effect of the toxin. This test was pioneered by Bela Schick between 1910 and 1930 and is known as the Schick test. A delayed hypersensitivity reaction to diphtheria toxin may also occur. This is known as pseudoreaction and can usually be differentiated from the effects of the toxin as the delayed reaction reaches a maximum at 2 to 3 days and fades by 4 to 5 days.

Dick Test. Some human sera injected into patients with a characteristic scarlet fever rash (scarlatina) can produce a blanching of the rash at the site of injection. Not all human sera can induce this blanching. The effect is due to the presence of specific antibody to the erythrogenic toxin produced by the streptococcal organism responsible. These observations led to the development of the Dick test for scarlet fever.

The Dick test is an intradermal test for antibody to hemolytic streptococcal antigens. Filtrates of cultures of the scarlatinal strains (strains responsible for scarlet fever) of streptococci contain a toxic substance that produces a typical skin reaction in nonimmunized individuals. Individuals with neutralizing antibody do not react to this erythrogenic toxin. The reaction induced by erythrogenic toxin appears as a bright red flush within 6 to 12 hours, is maximum at 24 hours, and fades rapidly. This test only measures resistance to strains of streptococci causing scarlet fever and does not measure protection or susceptibility to streptococcal throat infection.

Tetanus. Tetanus is caused by a highly fatal endoneurotoxin (tetanospasmin) released by the anaerobic gram-negative bacillus, *Clostridium tetani.* Tetanus toxin is synthesized as a single polypeptide chain of 150,000 Da. Upon secretion, cleavage by a *C. tetani* "nickase" results in a two-chain molecule joined by a single disulfide bond, with a heavy chain of approximately 100,000 kD and a light chain of 50,000 kD. The heavy chain is able to bind to cell surface gangliosides and is taken into the cell. In the cell, the light chain is cleaved by cellular enzymes to produce a peptide fragment that blocks an elongation factor (EF2) required for protein synthesis. One activated light chain is able to block all EF2 activity in a cell. This effectively destroys, inhibits, or blocks protein synthesis and the function of the cell.

Viable tetanus organisms exist only in dead tissue and produce disease by release of toxin that diffuses into the adjacent living tissues. Spore forms of the organism are ubiquitous in soil and can infect a seemingly trivial wound. Natural defenses are essentially limited to local healing processes. The organisms multiply locally and produce endotoxin. The endotoxin is released when organisms are destroyed in the necrotic wound tissue and travels via the blood or by retrograde axonal transmission to the spinal cord. The toxin increases reflex excitability in motor neurons by blocking the function of inhibitory neurons. This results in rigidity and reflex spasms, with death most often due to respiratory failure. The incubation period is usually less than 14 days. The length of the incubation period is critical in determining the outcome (60% fatality if less than 9 days; 25% if greater than 9 days).

The major immune defense mechanism of the host is neutralization of the toxin by specific antibody, which blocks binding of the toxin to neurons (Fig. 25–3). Unfortunately, in the natural infection, the potency of the toxin is so great that even fatal doses of tetanospasmin are usually not sufficient to stimulate antibody production. However, in high incidence countries, such as Ethiopia, up to 30% of adults have

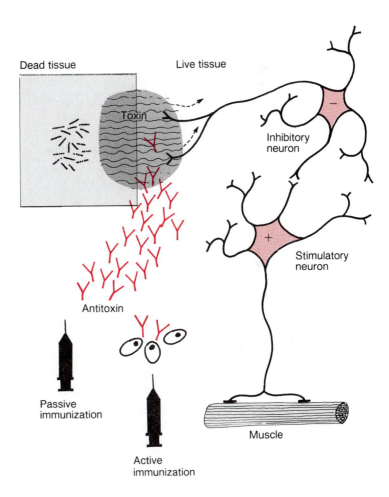

Figure 25–3. Neutralization of tetanus toxin by antitoxin. Antitoxin blocks entry of toxin into neurons. *C. tetani* release endotoxin when the organisms die in necrotic tissue. The endotoxin is taken up by axons and delivered to nerve cells, where it inactivates protein synthesis. The loss of activity of inhibitory neurons permits hyperactivity of stimulatory neurons and muscle spasm. Antitoxin provided by active or passive immunization prevents toxin from reaching inhibitory neurons.

toxin-neutralizing antibody, presumably from natural exposure. Since the organism cannot survive in living tissue because it is anaerobic, *C. tetani* benefits if the infected individual dies, at which point the entire body can be colonized. Primary therapy is directed to keeping the wound clean and debrided to avoid the anaerobic conditions favoring growth of *C. tetani*. Secondary therapy is to neutralize tetanospasmin by antibody.

In 1890, Van Behring and Kitasato demonstrated protective immunization using repeated small doses of tetanus toxin. Their report included the finding that the protection was due to a new factor present in the serum of immunized individuals (antitoxin). This classic report laid the foundation for subsequent development of immunoprophylaxis of infectious diseases using bacterial products. Antitoxin produced in horses was prepared and used to treat patients with tetanus or those with wounds that could accommodate *C. tetani*. Unfortunately, treated patients often developed another serious disease—serum sickness—caused by production of antibody to the horse antitoxin (see Chapter 13).

Active immunization with toxoid has greatly reduced the incidence of tetanus. In 1925, Ramon introduced chemically modified toxin (toxoid) for active immunization. It should be noted that antibodies directed against the *C. tetani* itself would not be useful, since the organism lives only in dead tissue, and antibody cannot reach the site of infection. In order for toxin to be active, it must be internalized into the neuron, presumably at the axon level. Antitoxin binding to toxin prevents entry of the toxin into the cell. This may be accomplished by alteration of the tertiary structure of the toxin molecule. Once the toxin is bound to the neuron or internalized, antitoxin is ineffective. Neutralization of tetanus toxin is a powerful specific and effective mechanism of protection. Artificial immunization with tetanus toxoid provides prolonged, but not permanent, protection. Antitoxin titers must be boosted by reimmunization if exposure to toxin is suspected. Reimmunization of an individual with a wound that may be infected with *C. tetani* induces a secondary antibody response that can effectively block the toxin. However, if reimmunization is delayed, elevation of the antibody titer may be too late to prevent clinical tetanus. The risk for fatal tetanus is greater in people over 60 years of age who lack protective levels of antitoxin because of a failure of booster immunizations. About 60 cases of tetanus per year are reported in the United States with a case fatality rate of 24%.

CYTOTOXICITY

Malaria

The immune response to infection by malaria includes both cellular and humoral cytotoxic effector mechanisms. Hippocrates first recognized different types of malaria by different periods of fever. During the Middle Ages, the disease was attributed to bad air "malair" (Torti, 1753). Although the role of immune mechanisms in the pathogenesis of malaria is incompletely understood, cytotoxic T cells (T_{CTL}), delayed hypersensitivity, and IgG or IgM antibodies appear to play an important role in controlling the infection through the activation of cytotoxicity directed against the infected host cells (Figs. 25–4 and 25–5). In endemic areas, natives develop resistance to malaria. Neonates in endemic areas are resistant as a result of placentally transferred maternal immunity. A peak of susceptibility occurs at about 1 year of age. However, infection at this age is less severe than in persons who first contract infection as adults.

The bite of an infected mosquito results in inoculation of hundreds to thousands of sporozoites into the bloodstream. Within minutes, the sporozoites are cleared from the bloodstream, with many going to the liver. In the liver, the sporozoites develop into merozoites within a few days or a week. Thousands of merozoites are released from infected hepatocytes and begin the blood stage of the disease. The infection can be interrupted by antibody to sporozoites if present in high titer at the time of inoculation, by antibody to merozoite antigens on the parasite surface or the newly infected blood cells, or by T_{CTL} cells that recognize antigens of the sporozoites expressed on infected liver cells and destroy the cells before merozoites are released. T_{DTH} cells may also be active, at least in some experimental models.

T_{CTL} cells are induced by endogenous presentation of sporozoite antigens in association with class I MHC antigens on infected liver cells. Upon infection of liver cells, the parasites develop within a vacuole inside the hepatocyte that prevents release of malarial antigens into the cytoplasm, thus exogenous processing of antigen cannot take place. However, the important sporozoite antigen, the circumsporate protein, is a cell surface protein that is shed into the hepatocyte during infection and appears on the surface complexed to class I MHC antigens normally expressed by the hepatocyte (see Fig. 25–5). Presentation of circumsporate antigens in the form of recombinants with intracellular bacteria, such as *Salmonella*, induces CD8+ T_{CTL} cells and may be a way to induce protective immunity to malaria.

After the hepatocyte phase, malaria organisms exist with erythrocytes during an established infection. Some of the major manifestations of malaria (anemia, fever, nephritis, and vasculitis) appear to be associated with an antibody-mediated cytotoxic reaction. The erythrocytes of patients with malaria become coated with IgG or IgM and have an increased susceptibility to phagocytosis and destruction by splenic macrophages. Epidemiologic studies indicate that the major inherited blood cell disorders, such as sickle cell anemia, have been selected for in malaria areas by conferring protection in their mild forms against *Plasmodium falciparum* malaria. This hypothesis is sup-

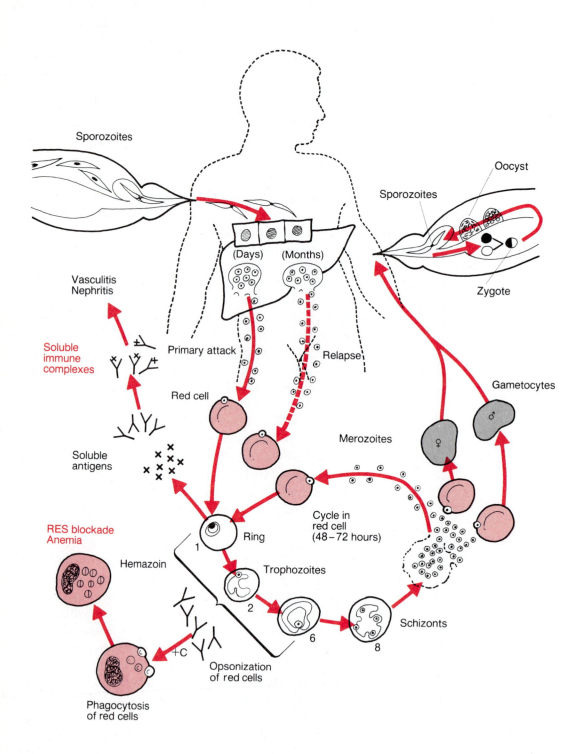

Sporozoites

Oocyst

Sporozoites

Zygote

(Days)   (Months)

Vasculitis
Nephritis

Soluble
immune
complexes

Primary attack

Relapse

Red cell

Gametocytes

Soluble
antigens

Merozoites

RES blockade
Anemia

Cycle in
red cell
(48 – 72 hours)

Hemazoin

Ring

Trophozoites

+C

Schizonts

Opsonization
of red cells

Phagocytosis
of red cells

Figure 25–4. Immune mechanisms in malaria. Malaria is transmitted from the salivary glands of mosquito to the blood of an animal by sporozoites that enter host liver cells and develop into intracellular stages. Merozoites are released into the circulation and reinfect other liver cells and red blood cells. Micro- and macrogametes are produced, which are taken up by mosquitos where they develop after fusion of micro- and microgametes and formation of an oocyst in the stomach into sporozoites. Malarial antigens are found not only in organisms but also on the surface of infected cells. Antibodies to these antigens are able to lyse organisms or infected cells, producing anemia or liver cell necrosis. Soluble antibody–antigen complexes formed may produce immune complex lesions (glomerulonephritis). The production of large numbers of opsonized red cells and particulate antigen results in accumulation of phagocytosed material in macrophages (Hemozoin pigment), reticuloendothelial blockade, and immune dysfunction. Malarial organisms are able to change antigens expressed on the cell surface, avoid destruction by antibody, and set up another cycle of infection (antigenic variation). Protective immunity may be effected by antibodies to sporozoites, which prevent infection. Protective immunity could be mediated by antibody directed to extracellular stages: (1) Sporozoites, (2) merozoites, (3) zygotes, or (4) by T-cytotoxic cells to infected hepatocytes.

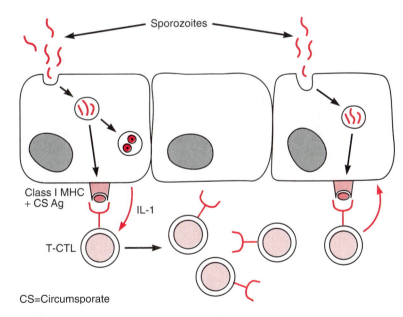

Figure 25–5. T_{CTL} immunity in malaria. Sporozoite antigen is presented to T_{CTL} precursors complexed to class I MHC cell surface markers on infected hepatocytes leading to the proliferation of a population of T_{CTL} cells that can recognize and destroy hepatocytes expressing sporozoite antigens. Since the sporozoite antigen is expressed before infective merozoites are released, preexisting specific T_{CTL} cells may be able to destroy infected cells before systemic infection is established or prevent spread of infection from liver cells to red blood cells.

ported by the finding that the red cells of the mild forms of thalassemia express higher levels of malarial antigens than do normal red cells, rendering the infected cells more susceptible to destruction by antibody, complement, and phagocytosis by neutrophils. Neutrophil killing of infected red blood cells (RBCs) is enhanced by INF-γ and other factors released from T_{DTH} cells. The destruction of infected red cells may be of such an extent that macrophages in the spleen and liver become loaded with malaria pigment (Hemozoin) from phagocytosed and degraded red blood cells. Although this reaction may help to eliminate infected cells, it also contributes to the anemia. During malarial paroxysms, parasites are released from intracellular locations in enormous numbers, resulting in the formation of immune complexes in antigen excess. Glomerulonephritis, the nephrotic syndrome (black water fever), and vasculitis are presumed to be consequences. Finally, the preoccupation of macrophages with erythrophagocytosis may contribute to the immunosuppression observed in association with malaria and production of tumor necrosis factor (cachexin), which is found in elevated levels in the serum of malaria patients, may contribute to the fever, chills, hypoglycemia, renal tubule necrosis, liver damage, pulmonary neutrophil accumulation, and other lesions seen in malaria.

The ability to produce an effective vaccine against malaria is complicated by species-specific antigens, by the stage-specific antigens that are produced during the malarial life cycle, by antigenic variation during infection, by possible genetic limitation to HLA-dependent processing of cloned peptide antigens, and by failure of a substantial proportion of immunized individuals to develop T_{CTL} cells. Vaccination against malaria may be directed to the infecting sporozoites, to the intracellular infection (merozoites, schizonts) or to the sexual stages in the mosquito (see Chapter 26 for a detailed presentation of the status of malaria vaccines).

IMMUNE COMPLEX

Rheumatic Fever

Acute rheumatic fever and chronic rheumatic heart disease are examples of the immune complex mechanism activated following an immune response to an infection. Rheumatic fever is an acute systemic inflammatory sequel to Group A β-hemolytic streptococcal pharyngitis (not to streptococcal skin infections) that can lead to chronic heart disease secondary to scarred valves. The lesions of rheumatic fever are sterile. Refinement of the diagnosis of streptococcal infection and prompt introduction of measures to eliminate the infection, usually by intensive therapy with penicillin, significantly reduce the occurrence of cardiac sequelae. The many early manifestations of this multiorgan disease often make the diagnosis difficult. To codify the diagnosis, a classification of the diagnostic criteria for rheumatic fever devised by T. Duckerr Jones in 1944 was revised in 1992 (Table 25–2). The clinical picture may be one of fleeting and transient joint pains and fever to full blown acute rheumatic fever. Acute rheumatic fever begins with abrupt fever, malaise, skin rash, and pain and swelling of the joints occurring within 4 to 5 weeks after a streptococcal throat infection. Subcutaneous nodules, Sydenham's chorea or St. Vitus' dance (involuntary and jerky movements of the extremities), and signs of acute left ventricular failure may also be seen at the beginning of the acute illness. The symptoms usually last for a month or two, although fatal heart failure can occur. After a symptomless period, the initial clinical pattern is repeated with subsequent infections of rheumatogenic strains of β-hemolytic streptococci. If the first episode has prominent cardiac symptoms and little joint inflammation, the following episodes will follow the same pattern. Thus, the occurrence of heart failure during the first episode indicates that repeated episodes will eventually lead to chronic rheumatic heart disease.

Although the incidence of acute rheumatic fever in children has decreased markedly in North America and Europe from that of 20 to 40 years ago, rheumatic heart disease still ranks as a major cause of disease in adults who contracted rheumatic fever as children. The number of admissions to the children's service at Johns Hopkins Hospital in Baltimore declined from 25 to 30 per year from 1952 to 1961 to less than 3 per year from 1976 to 1981. The decrease in the number of new cases may be due to the widespread, and often indiscriminate, use of antibiotics effective against streptococci, better general living condi-

TABLE 25–2. REVISED CRITERIA FOR THE DIAGNOSIS OF RHEUMATIC FEVER (UPDATED 1992)

Major Manifestations	Minor Manifestations	Supporting Evidence of Previous Group A Streptococcal Infection
	Clinical findings	Positive throat culture
Carditis	Fever	or rapid streptococcal
Polyarthritis	Arthralgias	antigen test
Chorea	**Laboratory findings**	
Erythema marginatum	Elevated ESR or	Elevated or rising
Subcutaneous nodules	C-reactive protein	streptococcal
	Prolonged PR interval	antibody titer

ESR, erythrocyte sedimentation rate; PR interval, timing of signal on electrocardiogram consistent with myocarditis.

Modified from Dajani AD, Ayoub E, Bierman FZ, and the Special Writing Group of the Committee on Rheumatic Fever: Guidelines for the diagnosis of rheumatic fever: Jones criteria, updated 1992. *Circulation* 87:302–307, 1992.

tions with less crowding, and a decline in the prevalence of the rheumatogenic strains of β-hemolytic streptococci. However, the disease is still common in Third World countries, and occasional local resurgences of the disease have been reported in the United States. In the state of Connecticut, the number of positive throat cultures for streptococci rose from less than 5,000 in 1955 to over 250,000 in 1972. The reasons for the decline and for the resurgences in the United States remain poorly understood, but there appears to be an increase in the prevalence of "rheumatogenic" strains of β-hemolytic streptococci.

The major pathologic features of rheumatic fever are widespread inflammation and scarring in connective tissue in the heart, joints, lungs, pleura, subcutaneous tissue, and skin. Vasculitis may involve many small and medium-sized arteries. The inflammation of the heart is a "pancarditis" involving the pericardium, myocardium, and endocardium. Myocardial fibers may show dissolution associated with a diffuse mixed inflammatory infiltrate. Scarring of the endocardium leads to marked thickening and shortening of the chordae tendinea and thickening of the valve leaflets. This may produce severe insufficiency and stenosis of the cardiac valves, most commonly the mitral valve. The classic myocardial lesion, the Aschoff body, begins as a loose focal mononuclear infiltrate around small arteries and evolves to a fibrous scar. The histologic appearance of later valvular and myocardial lesions suggests that cell-mediated immunity may be active during the chronic stages of the inflammation. Lymphocytes from rheumatic fever patients react with streptococcal antigens in vitro by proliferation, and lymphocytes from animals immunized with streptococcal antigens kill myocardial cells in vitro. Patients with late effects of rheumatic endocarditis are a major source of candidates for corrective valvular surgery.

The lesions of rheumatic fever are caused by immune-mediated inflammation. As a protective response to infection, antistreptococcal antibodies neutralize toxins and opsonize organisms. However, destructive lesions are caused by the formation of immune complexes and of antibodies to streptococcal antigens that cross-react with antigens present in the tissues of the host (molecular mimicry) (Fig. 25–6). Antibodies to a number of streptococcal antigens as well as to host proteins are found in the serum. Antibodies to streptococcal M protein cross-react with heart muscle and are believed to be responsible for inflammation of the heart (pancarditis). Monoclonal antibodies produced to group A streptococci have identified cross-reacting antigens on cardiac myocytes, smooth muscle cells, cell surface and cytoplasm of endothelial lining cells, and valvular interstitial cells. Antibodies to group A streptococcal carbohydrate correlate with the development of valvular heart disease. The chorea of rheumatic fever has been associated with autoantibodies to basal ganglia. These antibodies can be absorbed with streptococcal cell walls. Other lesions of rheumatic

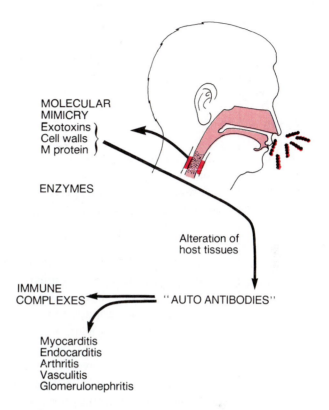

MOLECULAR
MIMICRY
Exotoxins ⎫
Cell walls ⎬
M protein ⎭

ENZYMES

Alteration of
host tissues

IMMUNE
COMPLEXES ← "AUTO ANTIBODIES"

Myocarditis
Endocarditis
Arthritis
Vasculitis
Glomerulonephritis

Figure 25–6. The immune response to streptococcal Group A antigens and rheumatic fever. Antibodies produced to streptococcal antigens cross-react with host tissue antigens. These "autoantibodies," as well as soluble immune complexes, are responsible for the lesions of rheumatic fever (myocarditis, endocarditis, arthritis, vasculitis, and glomerulonephritis).

fever are most likely the result of immune complex formation, particularly erythema marginatum (vasculitis in the dermis) and glomerulonephritis. Rheumatic nodules are small, rubbery granulomas, and most likely the end result of vasculitis caused by the deposition of immune complexes containing antigens resistant to degradation, leading to accumulation of macrophages and the formation of granulomas. In addition, streptococcal M protein can act as a superantigen, activating T cells, and stimulating subsets of T cells that react with self antigens. Although there is no clear association of rheumatic disease with HLA phenotype, the B-cell alloantigen 833 is significantly more common in rheumatic fever patients than in controls.

In summary, antibodies to streptococcal products serve to inactivate streptococcal organisms and products, as well as to initiate acute inflammatory reactions (immune complex mechanism). Cross-reaction of antistreptococcal antibodies with host tissues and formation of soluble complexes of antibodies and streptococcal antigens may cause immune complex-mediated inflammatory reactions distant from site of infection.

ANAPHYLAXIS

Allergic Broncho-pulmonary Aspergillosis

Anaphylactic reactions to fungal or bacterial antigens are not uncommon and may be responsible for some acute asthmatic attacks and dermal reactions. A serious problem is allergic reaction to fungi in the tracheobronchial flora (eg, *Aspergillus fumigatus*). "Aspergillus" comes from the Latin word aspere (to scatter). An aspergill is a brush used to sprinkle (scatter) holy water during the asperges, a short service in the Roman Catholic Church before a High Mass during which holy water is sprinkled. The name is applied to the *Aspergillus* fungus because of the resemblance of the conidiospores to the aspergill. The term aspergillus is also applied to a medieval weapon consisting of a spiked ball on the end of a chain.

The syndrome of allergic bronchopulmonary aspergillosis includes wheezing, fever, occasional expectoration of golden brown plugs that contain mycelia, systemic eosinophilia, elevated serum IgE concentrations, and the presence of antibodies to *Aspergillus* spp. in the serum. The syndrome is caused by prolonged anaphylactic reactions to aspergillus antigens (Fig. 25–7). Allergic aspergillosis most likely begins with the inhalation and trapping of aspergillial conidia in the viscous secretions present in the bronchi of an asthmatic. The spores germinate and form mycelia; antigens released from mycelia react with IgE on mast cells in the bronchial walls, resulting in greatly increased mucous secretion and bronchospasm. Allergic bronchopulmonary aspergillosis differs from most other forms of asthma in that the supply of inciting antigen is continuously replenished by replication within the bronchi and bronchioles. The anaphylactic reaction to aspergillus in bronchi may lead to formation of mucous plugs containing fungi, produce protracted construction of bronchial smooth muscle, and cause death by asphyxiation.

Almost all affected patients will react with a wheal-and-flare skin response to dermal injection of *Aspergillus* antigens (IgE). Many patients also have precipitating IgG antibodies and may have pulmonary vasculitis presumably due to immune complexes. Nonallergic patients may develop *Aspergillus* infections, which usually present as single lesions (fungus ball) in areas of previously damaged lung tissue. Invasive *Aspergillus*, in which mycelia actually extend into tissue, is different from allergic bronchopulmonary aspergillosis and is seen in patients with immune deficiency diseases.

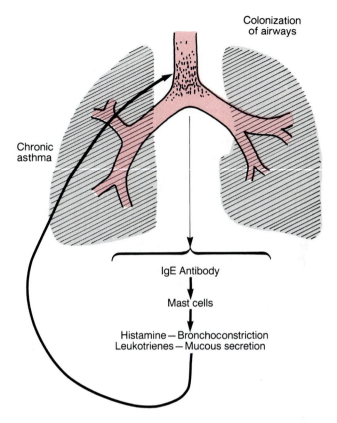

Figure 25–7. Allergic bronchopulmonary aspergillosis. Anaphylactic reaction to aspergillus infection in the bronchi cause secondary pathologic effects, leading to repeated asthmatic attacks and plugging of airways with thick mucous plugs.

Intestinal Worms

The protective action of an individual with a parasitic gastrointestinal worm infestation is to expel the worms from the gastrointestinal tract. Our understanding of how this is accomplished is based largely on studies in rodents and is still incomplete. In the human disease trichinosis, cysts of *Trichinella* are digested in the gastrointestinal tract, liberating larvae that mature into adult worms. Female adult worms release larvae that penetrate the intestinal wall and lodge in muscle tissue where they encyst. The invasion of the muscle is associated with an intense inflammatory reaction, causing fever, muscle pain, and swelling, but some larvae survive this attack and encyst. These cysts are protected niches where the encysted larvae may remain viable for many years. When uncooked meat containing these cysts is eaten, the infection is repeated.

It is believed that intestinal larvae or worms are eliminated as their microenvironment deteriorates as a consequence of immune-mediated inflammation. Mast cell mediators are involved in elimination of larval forms by producing effects such as local acidosis, mucous hyperplasia, hypermotility, and epithelial cell changes, as well as increased blood flow, edema, and attraction of other inflammatory cells, particularly eosinophils. Eosinophils contain major basic protein (MBP) that is not only toxic for worms but also attracts more mast cells. In addition, eosinophils may release leukotrienes, platelet-activating factor, and oxygen radicals that kill adult worms. Dead organisms in tissue are usually surrounded by large numbers of eosinophils. Increased mucin production by hyperplastic goblet cells may produce dislodgement of established worms or prevent attachment of larvae. Antibody and complement in mucous may increase this effect.

The ability of previously infected individuals to resist reinfection indicates that effective immunity to reinfection can be induced and that immunization with worm products might prevent primary infection through rapid expulsion of larvae. However, immunization with dead organisms or extracts have failed to induce immunity. Thus, biological interactions between the living parasite and the host appear to be required to induce effective immunity, perhaps by expression of antigens specific for developmental stages in vivo. Effective vaccines for veterinary use have been produced using irradiated larvae, and studies are underway in an attempt to produce vaccines for human nematodes.

CELL-MEDIATED IMMUNITY

Smallpox, Syphilis, and Tuberculosis

Cell-mediated immunity (CMI) to smallpox, syphilis, leprosy, and tuberculosis is presented in Chapters 16 and 17. T_{CTL}-mediated killing is responsible for destroying infected cells, as in viral exanthems (see Fig. 15–6). T_{DTH} activation of macrophage digestion and killing is the major clearing mechanism for infection with *Treponema pallidum* (syphilis) (see Fig. 16–4). T_{DTH} activation of the killing mechanisms in infected macrophages is effective in eliminating intracellular infections, such as malaria, tuberculosis, leishmaniasis, and leprosy. Effective immunity to organisms that infect macrophages depends on activating the macrophages to kill the organism they contain. If macrophages are unable to be activated, T_{CTL} may be able to lyse the infected cells, allowing activated macrophages to phagocytize them and then destroy them (see Fig. 17–4). The critical determinant of the outcome of the infection is the preferential selection of cellular immunity over antibody production, as antibody-mediated opsonization is essentially ineffective against parasites that infect macrophages. If virus-infected cells, such as neurons, perform a vital irreplaceable function, their loss results in manifestations of the disease. This loss may be caused directly by the virus itself or be secondary to the destruction of the infected cells by T_{CTL} or T_{DTH} cells.

Viral Infections

Viral Encephalitides of Animals. Animal models of virus-induced inflammation of the central nervous system (encephalomyelitis) illustrate important differences in pathogenesis involving immune mechanisms (Table 25–3).

Lymphocytic choriomeningitis (LCM). The role of CMI in producing the lesions of some infectious diseases is exemplified by lymphocytic choriomeningitis, a viral disease of mice and humans. Certain features of the experimental disease suggest that the brain lesions are due not just to the presence of the virus itself but to a CMI reaction to the viral antigens located in the brain. Systemic infection may produce immunity that prevents infection of the brain. Intracranial injection of the virus results in much more severe disease than does intracutaneous injections. If a sublethal intracutaneous injection is followed by a lethal intracranial injection, the eventual outcome depends upon the interval between the cutaneous and cranial injections. If the cranial injection follows the cutaneous injection by fewer than four days, the outcome is invariably fatal, and the course of the disease is more rapid than when the virus is given only intracranially. If seven days intervene between the cranial and cutaneous injections, the animals survive. The interpretation is that the sublethal cutaneous injection produces an immune response to the virus. If immunity is developed (seven-day interval) when the cranial injection is administered, specific CMI prevents dissemination and growth of virus. However, if the virus is already distributed before the delayed reaction develops, the reaction

TABLE 25–3. PATHOGENESIS OF SOME VIRUS-RELATED ENCEPHALITIDES OF ANIMALS

Disease	Species	Suspected Mechanism
Lymphocytic choriomeningitis	Mouse	Cellular reaction to virus antigens on neurons
Mouse hepatitis virus encephalitis	Mouse	Viral destruction of myelin
Canine distemper	Dog	Postinfectious autoimmunity to myelin or slowly progressing virus demyelination
Theiler's virus myelitis	Mouse	Postinfectious autoimmunity to myelin
Marek's disease	Chicken	Postinfectious autoimmunity to myelin
Visna	Sheep	Primary infection of monocytes; T_{CTL} and T_{DTH} destruction of myelin

of the specifically sensitized cells with the localized virus produces the lesions. In the four-day interval situation, the cutaneous injection initiates the development of CMI so that it is partially developed but not active (in the induction period) when the cranial injection is given. Since CMI, primarily T-cytotoxicity, is already partially developed, the onset of symptoms caused by reaction of T_{CTL} cells with viral antigens on infected cells occurs earlier than when the induction of CMI and the cranial injection of the virus occur at the same time. Further evidence that T_{CTL} is the mechanism responsible for the actual production of lesions is that procedures that suppress CMI (administration of immunosuppressive drugs, irradiation, thymectomy at birth, or anti-lymphocyte serum) markedly suppress the development of the symptoms of lymphocytic choriomeningitis. Some of the mice so treated may remain completely asymptomatic, even though viable virus can be isolated from brain tissue. However, these mice may develop immune complex-mediated disease because of the production of humoral antibody to LCM virus and the formation of circulating antibody–antigen complexes.

The role of histocompatibility (MHC) restriction in killing of virus-infected target cells was worked out by Peter Doherty and Rolf Zinkernagle using the LCM model. Specifically sensitized T_{CTL} cells will not lyse LCM virus-infected target cells unless the T_{CTL} cells can also recognize class I MHC antigens on the target cells. Adoptive immunization (passive transfer) of T_{CTL} cells sensitized to LCM or to immunosuppressed LCM-infected mice causes a fatal reaction within two to four days. The fatal disease only occurs when the T_{CTL} cells can recognize both viral antigens and MHC antigens on the target cells. Thus, cell injury in LCM is mediated by class I MHC-restricted T_{CTL} cells.

Mouse hepatitis virus encephalitis. Virus-induced demyelination that does not depend on an immune response is exemplified by mouse hepatitis virus. Mouse hepatitis virus infects oligodendrocytes and produces plaques of demyelination. Viral antigens are detectable in glial cells, which are intimately associated with myelin. Demyelination is believed to be caused by virus infection. In contrast to LCM, immunosuppressive treatment increases the rate of mortality in infected mice. Demyelination occurs randomly with no relation to blood vessels, in contrast to what is observed in experimental allergic encephalomyelitis. Lymphocyte infiltration is scanty and rarely detected prior to demyelination. Thus, this infection illustrates that some virus infections may cause demyelination directly without the action of immune cells.

Canine distemper. The relationship of an inadequate or inappropriate immune response to a virus-induced disease is seen in canine distemper, a naturally occurring infectious disease of dogs. The canine distemper paramyxovirus is closely related to human measles virus and produces a disease in dogs similar to human measles and the related neurologic diseases—acute encephalitis, postinfectious encephalitis, and subacute sclerosing panencephalitis (SSPE) (see below). Canine distemper produces an acute systemic disease from which most animals recover. Following this disease, however, a certain proportion of the affected animals go on to develop a demyelinating postinfectious encephalomyelitis, the pathology of which is similar to experimental allergic encephalomyelitis. The chronic phase of distemper is called "old dog encephalitis" and bears similarities to human SSPE. The distemper virus enters the brain during the acute systemic viremia, and viral inclusions can be found in glial cells. The postinfectious disease develops suddenly after a latent period of several weeks, even though it can be assumed that the virus particles are in the brain throughout the latent period. Although the role of immunopathologic mechanisms in the disease remains unclear, antibodies to viral antigens and to myelin appear in high titers in the sera of affected dogs. Since the virus does not appear to cause tissue destruction, it is likely that the demyelination is due to sensitized lymphocytes reacting to either viral antigens present in myelinated tissue or to myelin antigens rendered immunogenic from the viral infection. Humoral antibody may play a role in initiating vascular reactions or may actually be protective (eg, blocking antibody).

Theiler's myelitis. This is an inflammatory demyelination of the spinal cord of mice, occurring one to three months following infection of Theiler's mouse encephalitis virus. After initial involvement of the gray matter, patchy demyelination occurs. The pathologic picture is similar to experimental allergic encephalomyelitis (EAE) (see Autoimmunity). Immunosuppression increases the virus particles, but they are not present in the areas of demyelination. This demyelination is believed to be caused by a postinfectious autosensitization to myelin.

Marek's disease. Marek's disease is a herpesvirus-induced lymphoproliferative disease of chickens that also induces paralysis associated with perivascular infiltration of mononuclear cells and demyelination. It is postulated that there is an autosensitization to myelin, and a number of observations indicate that the demyelination is T-cell dependent. The mechanism of autosensitization in this disease is not known, but the lesions are similar to those of EAE of animals and the Guillain–Barré syndrome of humans.

Visna. Visna is a primary infection of macrophages and lymphocytes with a lentivirus with properties similar to human immunodeficiency virus (HIV). In contrast to HIV, however, there is little evidence of immune suppression. Usually, the infected sheep mount a strong immunoprotective response. However, in some cases there is a progressive meningitis and periventricular inflammation associated with perivascular mononuclear cell infiltration and demyelination. CD4+ cells predominate immediately perivascularly, but CD8+ cells are seen infiltrating the parenchyma, suggesting that T_{CTL} cells are the main effector cells.

Viral Encephalitides of Humans. The viral encephalitides of humans occur in a variety of forms, depending on the nature of the infecting agent and the type and intensity of the immune response. The disorders are classified as acute, postinfectious, latent, chronic, and slow (Table 25–4).

In the acute encephalitides (poliomyelitis, rabies, herpes simplex), the virus destroys nerve cells directly in a predictable fashion. The immune response is protective in the sense that it blocks the destructive aspects of the disease by elimination of the virus.

Postinfectious encephalomyelitis follows a mild virus infection and is caused by an autoimmune reaction of sensitized cells with myelin, presumably due to the presence of altered host antigen or virus antigen–host myelin combinations (see Chapter 21). The virus alone does not produce significant destruction. Such reactions may follow infections such as mumps, measles, distemper, or vaccination with rabies or vaccinia virus.

TABLE 25–4. VIRAL ENCEPHALITIDES OF HUMANS

Type	Examples	Mechanism
Acute	Polio, rabies, herpes	Virus destruction of cells, immune-response protective
Postinfectious	Postvaccinial Postvirus infection	Lymphocyte-mediated destruction (?autoimmune) (mumps, measles, ?multiple sclerosis)
Latent	Progressive multifocal leukoencephalopathy	Inadequate protective immunity because of secondary immune deficiency (leukemia, lymphoma) T_{CTL}-mediated attack of virus-infected cells
Chronic or slow	Subacute sclerosing panencephalitis	Persistent infection because of lack of protective response, alteration of specialized function of infected cells
	Kuru, Creutzfeldt–Jakob syndrome (?amyotrophic lateral sclerosis)	

Latent viral infections are caused by a change in the relation of the host's immune response to a virus infection that has not produced clinical manifestations, so that clinical symptoms become manifest. This may occur because of an increase or a decrease in the host's immune state. Progressive multifocal leukoencephalopathy occurs in patients whose immune state is lowered (leukemia, lymphoma). Destruction of brain cells occurs in the absence of significant inflammation. Cytomegalic inclusion disease, a systemic virus infection, also occurs in patients with depressed ability to mount an immune response (eg, AIDS, kidney transplant recipients undergoing immunosuppression with drugs). On the other hand, symptoms related to lymphocytic choriomeningitis may be produced in experimental animals with latent infections by increasing their immune response to lymphocytic choriomeningitis virus. The lesions contain numerous mononuclear inflammatory cells. Because of an immune response to the virus, not only virus-infected but also uninfected cells in the areas of inflammation may be destroyed (innocent bystander reaction). HTLV-1 encephalitis also is believed to be caused by immune destruction of infected cells. HTLV-1–associated demyelination mimics the progressive form of multiple sclerosis. The blood and spinal fluid contain antibodies to HTLV-1 and high precursor frequencies of CD8+, MHC class I-restricted T_{CTL} cells specific for HTLV-1 proteins that correlate with the degree of disease. The major pathologic findings are chronic meningitis and perivascular mononuclear cell infiltrates. The most likely pathogenesis is destruction of HTLV-1–infected cells by specific T_{CTL} cells. HIV encephalopathy often has histopathologic features typical of viral inflammation, including perivascular round cell infiltrate and glial nodules containing virus, but it may also be associated with neuronal loss or no change (see Chapter 29).

Chronic encephalomyelitis features an irregular protracted course with variation in immune reactivity and brain cell destruction by virus. The condition of subacute sclerosing panencephalitis is believed to be a later manifestation in adults following measles infection in childhood. Affected patients have brain cell inclusions and high antibody titers to measles virus. Some change in the relation between protective immunity and virus infection is believed to occur, but it is not clear whether the allergic reaction or the virus itself is the cause of the destruction. Multiple sclerosis (MS) is a chronic remitting disease with the occurrence of repeated attacks, whereas subacute sclerosing panencephalitis (SSPE) is an unremitting progressive disease caused by the dissemination of a defective yet replicating virus. SSPE is probably caused by an inadequate protective immune response to the virus, whereas MS may be caused by a delayed hypersensitivity response to myelin (see Chapter 16).

Slow virus infections, represented by kuru and Creutzfeldt–Jakob disease, have a regular, protracted, fatal course following a long latent period. These diseases are characterized by abnormal membrane accumulations. The responsible agents have not been characterized but appear to consist of "prion protein" with characteristic of membrane proteins with no RNA or DNA component. No inflammatory response or immune reactivity of the host can be demonstrated; the course of the disease is determined by characteristics of the agent. Kuru occurs in certain native tribes of New Guinea. Its incidence has decreased sharply since the ritual cannibalism involving removal of the brain and widespread contamination of those preparing the brain for consumption with tissue containing millions of infective doses of kuru has been discontinued. Kuru is caused by the progressive proliferation and dissemination of an agent that provokes no immune response and is normally not infective but becomes so if large amounts of the agent are introduced through the skin, such as occurs during preparation of brains for ritual eating.

Amyotrophic lateral sclerosis is a disease of unknown origin associated with destruction or injury of anterior cells in the spinal cord and pyramidal cells in the cerebral cortex. It has been shown that persistent infection with virus, such as LCM virus, can alter luxury functions of certain cells without affecting vital functions. Viral infections of neural cells may not actually destroy the cells but can alter their neurotransmitter function. Thus, although the function of these cells is lost, the infected cells are not destroyed by either virus or immune response to the virus. Patients with amyotrophic lateral sclerosis often have circulating immune complexes. Identification of the antigen in these complexes may give an important clue to the etiologic agent.

Viral hepatitis. Viral hepatitis (inflammation of the liver) is caused by at least five viruses: Hepatitis A virus (HAV) (infectious hepatitis); hepatitis B virus (HBV) (serum hepatitis); and hepatitis C, D, and E (Table 25–5). The first association of a specific virus with hepatitis was made possible by the study of Australia antigen, now known as hepatitis B surface antigen (HBsAg). HBsAg is the coat or surface antigen of hepatitis B virus. The core antigen (HBcAg) contains double-stranded circular DNA with DNA polymerase activity, and is antigenically distinct from HBsAg. The core virus infects and replicates within the hepatocyte nucleus. It then migrates to the cytoplasm, where it is ensheathed in a coat made by the liver cell under the direction of the viral genome.

The time of appearance of hepatitis B viral antigens and the immune response is exemplified in Figure 25–8. The viral surface antigen, HBsAg, is detected in the serum of hepatitis patients or antigen carriers by reaction with anti-HBsAg. The association with hepatitis was first made when a patient previously found to be lacking the

TABLE 25–5. HEPATITIS VIRUSES

Name	Transmission	Discovery	Disease	Genome	Family
HAV	Enteric	1979	Infectious hepatitis, self resolving	SS linear RNA	Picornaviridae
HBV	Parenteral	1968	Serum hepatitis most serious world-wide infectious agent	DS circular DNA	Hepadnaviridae
HCV	Parenteral	1988	NANB hepatitis transfusion associated	SS linear RNA	?Flaviviruslike
HDV	Parenteral	1977	Increases severity of HBV disease	SS circular RNA	Defective virus
HEV	Enteric	1990	NANB hepatitis	SS linear RNA	?Calciviridae

SS, single-stranded; DS, double-stranded; NANB, non-A, non-B hepatitis.

Modified from Dock NL: The ABC's of viral hepatitis. *Clin Micro Newsletter* 13:17, 1991.

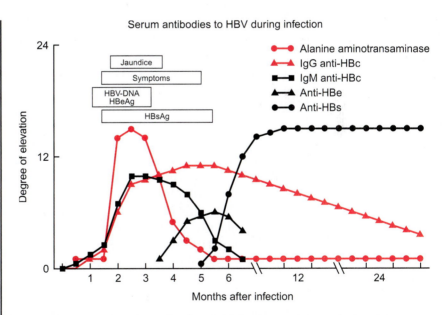

Figure 25–8. Antigen, antibody, and immune response during the course of hepatitis B infection. Within two months after infection, systemic symptoms and jaundice are associated with the presence of HBV DNA and HBV antigens in the blood and elevations of alanine aminotransaminase, which is an indicator of liver cell injury. Antibodies to HBc (core) antigens appear at about the same time. Anti-HBsAg may not become elevated until six months after the initial infection. Failure to produce anti-HBsAg is associated with a prolonged carrier state and continued production of infectious virus.

HBsAg antigen was found to possess the Australia antigen at the time of development of hepatitis. A systemic survey then demonstrated a high incidence of HBsAg antigen among patients with acute viral hepatitis and disappearance of the antigen upon their clinical recovery. Viral antigen may be identified within the liver cells of infected individuals using immunofluorescence, and viral particles may be obtained from the blood of some patients during active stages of the disease. The blood-borne particles consist mainly of viral coat particles, whereas whole viral particles (coat and nucleoprotein core) are rarely found. The detection of HBsAg antigen is now used to confirm the clinical diagnosis of hepatitis. A third antigen, the e antigen, which is distinct from HBsAg and HBcAg, may be present in long-term carriers. The presence of the e antigen is associated with chronic active hepatitis, cirrhosis, and with an infectious carrier state.

T_{CTL} CMI to viral antigens expressed on the surface of infected liver cells or to liver cell antigens rendered immunogenic by association with viral particles occurs five months to a year following infection and may be one of the mechanisms of liver cell destruction leading to elimination of virus-infected cells. In the infected cells, the capsular antigen is found in the cytoplasm and the core antigen in the nucleus. The acute lesion is destruction of hepatocytes (liver cell necrosis), most likely directly produced by virus infection; later lesions are associated with a marked infiltration of mononuclear cells. Chronic hepatitis may evolve from acute hepatitis or may arise without an obvious acute phase; is most likely due to immune lymphocytes (T_{CTL}) attacking virus-infected liver cells.

Antibodies to core antigens (anti-HBc) appear earlier in the disease than anti-surface (anti-HBsAg) antibodies. Humoral antibody and HBsAg–antibody complexes are present in the sera of patients during or recovering from the disease. Whereas humoral antibody may act to neutralize the virus, the presence of HBsAg–Ab complexes may lead to systemic toxic complex disease; polyarteritis has been found in patients with HBsAg–Ab complexes in their sera (see Chapter 13). The passive transfer of antibody to HBsAg has been used not only for prevention of disease in exposed individuals but also for therapy for patients with active viral hepatitis. A pregnant patient with fulminant HBsAg-positive hepatitis was treated successfully with plasmapheresis and anti-HBsAg plasma.

In summary, the acute destructive lesions of viral hepatitis are most likely due to direct destruction of liver cells by the virus, whereas chronic destruction is caused by a cellular reaction to the virus, killing virus-infected cells. Protection may be effected by humoral antibody, which probably acts to prevent spread of the infection from cell to cell. However, circulating HBsAg–Ab complexes may cause systemic immune complex disease.

Warts. Warts in humans are caused by a human papillomavirus and, like animal papillomavirus, more commonly causes lesions in young individuals. Spontaneous regression frequently occurs and is associated with the appearance of IgG serum antibodies, or specific cellular immunity. Patients with recurring warts are characterized by a weak or nonexistent specific immune response. Thus, a wart is a virus infestation that is effectively controlled by an immune response and only occurs persistently in individuals with an inadequate immune response to the virus.

GRANULO-MATOUS HYPER-SENSITIVITY

Granulomatous reactions occur to mycobacterial, fungal, helminth, and treponemal infections as a result of accumulation of altered macrophages that have accumulated material from phagocytosis that is difficult to break down (digest). As discussed in more detail in Chapter 17, this has a mixed effect. The granuloma can form a barrier of cells (epithelioid macrophages and reactive fibroblasts) that wall off the infectious agent from the host, but at the same time, organisms may survive within the center of the granuloma and be released with depression of the immune response due to aging, disease, or immunosuppressive treatment. When the immune response works effectively, the organisms are destroyed. However, when the immune response is unable to destroy the infecting organisms, a granuloma appears to be a "stopgap" measure to hold the organisms in check until an effective cell-mediated immune response can be developed. If the cellular response does not develop, the granulomatous reaction may not be effective. An illustrative example of this is the immune response to leprosy and syphilis (see Immune Deviation, below).

MIXED MECHANISMS

Lyme Disease

Lyme disease is manifested by stages of inflammation in which the immune response to the infecting organism is believed to be responsible for the lesions. The nature of the lesions seen resemble other immunopathologic diseases. There is demyelination similar to post-vaccinial encephalomyelitis; inflammation of the heart and heart block, similar to rheumatic fever; arthritis, similar to rheumatoid arthritis; and vasculitis, consistent with immune complex disease. The name "Lyme disease" comes from the recognition of a geographic clustering of children with what was thought to be a peculiar form of juvenile arthritis in Lyme, Connecticut, in 1977. The responsible organism, *Borrelia burgdorferi*, is a spirochete related to *T. pallidum*, the causative agent of syphilis. It is transmitted to humans through the bite of certain species of ticks. Following infection, there may be an inapparent infection or development of a complex series of lesions first involving the skin and then extending to a systemic disease (Table 25–6). The disease begins with the appearance of a pathognomonic skin lesion (stage 1), **erythema chronicum migrans**, first described in 1909 by Dr. Arvid Afselius in Sweden. It was not until 1982 that the spirochete, *B. burgdorferi*, was isolated from these skin lesions. Erythema migrans begins as a red macule or papule that expands to form a large ring of erythema with a bright red outer border and partial central clearing. This is sometimes accompanied by fever, minor constitutional symptoms, and regional swelling in the lymph nodes (lymphadenopathy). Without this characteristic lesion, the diagnosis may be very difficult.

The next stage of the disease, early infection (stage 2), evolves after spread of the Lyme disease spirochete through the blood to other organs. The major characteristics of the second stage are skin rashes, migratory joint pains, meningitis, lymphadenopathy, and severe malaise and fatigue. By this time, serum IgM antibody has usually appeared and its detection may be used to aid in the diagnosis. In addition, lymphocytes respond to *B. burgdorferi* antigens by blastogenesis, and IL-1 and TNF levels increase.

Late infection (stage 3), usually during the second or third year after infection, features prolonged episodes of arthritis, similar to rheumatoid arthritis. Synovial lesions show hypertrophy with increases in mononuclear cells and plasma cells. In a few cases, Lyme disease spirochetes have been isolated from synovial fluid, and IL-1 is elevated. At this stage, a few spirochetes may be found around lesions of obliterative endarteritis (chronic immune complex vasculitis). Thus, although the exact pathogenesis of Lyme disease is not clear, there appear to be many similarities to other immune-mediated diseases involving both antibody and cell-mediated mechanisms. Cross-reactivity (molecular mimicry) between *B. Burgdorferi* antigens and host tissues may be responsible for many of the lesions (CNS, heart, joint) that are similar to other presumed autoimmune diseases.

The diverse manifestations can make the diagnosis of Lyme disease very difficult. In the United States, Lyme disease is seen in the summer with the appearance of erythema marginatum, accompanied by flulike or meningitislike symptoms. Weeks or months later, neurologic or heart problems, migratory arthritis, or musculoskeletal pain may occur; and more than a year after onset, some patient have chronic joint, skin, or neurologic abnormalities. However, the course of the disease may vary greatly in different patients. In particular, the late neurologic symptoms are not completely codified but are different from multiple sclerosis, amyotrophic lateral sclerosis, or Alzheimer's disease. The more vague constitutional symptoms may be confused with chronic fatigue syndrome, but careful analysis can lead to the correct differential diagnosis in most cases. After the first several weeks, almost all patients develop specific antibody. However, serologic test-

TABLE 25–6. CLINICAL MANIFESTATIONS OF LYME DISEASE

System	Localized (Stage 1)	Disseminated (Stage 2)	Persistent (Stage 3)
Skin	Erythema migrans	Annular lesions, malar rash, diffuse erythema or urticaria	Acrodermatitis chronica atropicans, localized sclerodermalike lesions
Musculoskeletal		Migratory joint and bone pain, transient arthritis, myositis	Prolonged arthritis
Neurologic		Meningitis, cranial neuritis, Bell's palsy, myelitis, chorea	Chronic encephalomyelitis, spastic paraparesis, ataxia, dementia, etc.
Lymph	Lymphadenopathy	Lymphadenopathy, splenomegaly	Lymphoma
Heart		Nodal block, pancarditis	
Eyes		Conjunctivitis, iritis, choroiditis, retinal detachment, ophthalmitis	Keratitis
Liver		Mild or recurrent hepatitis	
Respiratory		Sore throat, nonproductive cough, adult respiratory distress syndrome	
Kidney		Mild hematuria or proteinuria	
Genitourinary		Orchitis	
Constitutional	Minor	Severe malaise and fatigue	Fatigue

Modified from Steere AC: Lyme disease. *N Engl J Med* 321:586–596, 1989.

ing is complicated by the fact that the tests for antibody are not yet fully standardized and differ from laboratory to laboratory. Thus, serologic testing, such as enzyme-linked immunosorbent assay (ELISA) for specific antibody, is the most practical laboratory aid in diagnosis, but results must be interpreted with caution. Diagnosis is important because *B. burgdorferi* is highly sensitive to tetracyclines, and oral treatment is effective in stage 1 or 2; treatment of stage 3 is unsettled.

The life cycle of *B. burgdorferi* depends upon ticks, which in turn depend upon certain types of mice. In the United States, the primary host for the ticks is the white-footed mouse. The mouse is tolerant of the infection and supports large numbers of *B. burgdorferi* without apparent untoward effects. The ticks can also feed on a number of other wild animals and birds without causing disease. However, humans and domestic animals, such as dogs and cattle, are not natural hosts and develop disease. Lyme disease is worldwide but has a particularly high incidence in New England and Europe. The marked increase seen during the last fifteen years in New England is explained by the conversion of farmland to woodland with measures to protect deer, which also protect deer mice, and the expansion of suburban populations into these woodland areas.

Filariasis

Host reactions to filarial infections determine the type of lesions seen. *Filaria* are roundworms with complex life cycles that live in the subcutaneous or lymphoreticular tissues and have been called connective tissue parasites. These are highly specialized parasites that are narrowly restricted regarding their sites of infection and reproduction. As higher order parasites, they have traded in fast reproductive rates and genetic modulation, which are characteristic of viruses and trypanosomes, for greater individual longevity and reproductive complexity. Filariform larvae are transmitted to man by a biting insect that serves as the intermediate host. The larvae penetrate the skin and may pass into the lymphatic system. All of the seven filariids known to infect humans may evoke allergic reactions (Table 25–7); however, only three cause serious disease: *Wuchereria bancrofti*, *Brugia malayi*, and *Onchocerca volvulus*.

The manifestations of filariasis clearly reflect the state of immune responsiveness of the host (Table 25–8). Chronic, asymptomatic filaremia is associated with specific hyporesponsiveness to filarial antigens. It is a host–parasite relationship that permits prolonged production of microfilaria, which are cleared from the circulation by the lungs, liver, and spleen without evoking symptoms. The lack of an immune response in asymptomatic microfilaremia may be due to specific tolerance, MHC-linked unresponsiveness, or to suppressive mechanisms. Although the mechanism is still in doubt, evidence has been presented favoring the presence of some suppressive mechanism, but specific tolerance based on anergy is considered possible in some cases.

Endemic normals are individuals with no signs of infection but who have IgG antibody and T-cell blastogenic responses to filarial antigens. The existence of such individuals argues that immunization resulting in a high T-cell sensitivity could provide effective protection against infection. In occult filariasis, there are neither symptoms nor microfilaria in the blood. Such individuals may be very difficult to differentiate from endemic normals, but some individuals have minimal evidence of infection, such as subconjunctival adult worms in *Loa loa* and symptomatic episodes of lymph node enlargement and respiratory

TABLE 25–7. HUMAN FILARIAL INFECTIONS

Species	Site of Infection	Immune Effector Mechanism	Distribution
Wuchereria bancrofti	Lymphatic	Multiple	Tropics
Brugia malayi	Lymphatic	Multiple	Southeast Africa
Onchocerca volvulus	Subcutaneous	Cellular	Africa, South and Central America
Loa loa	Subcutaneous	Anaphylactic	Africa
Dipetalonema perstans	Subcutaneous	Anaphylactic	Africa, South America
Dracunculus medinensis (nonfilarial)	Connective tissue	Anaphylactic	Tropics

TABLE 25–8. CLASSIFICATION AND IMMUNOPATHOLOGIC MECHANISMS IN FILARIASIS

Disease State	Age of Infection	Immune Mechanism
Asymptomatic microfilaremia	Infants	Tolerance
Endemic normal	Infants	IgG antibody and T cells
Occult filariasis	Infants	IgG antibody
Tropical eosinophilia	Adult, acute	Anaphylactic
Lymphadenitis	Adult, chronic	Delayed hypersensitivity
Lymphatic obstruction	Adult, chronic	Granulomatous

complaints in *W. bancrofti* and *B. malayi*. IgG antibodies may be responsible for the rapid, apparently complete clearance of organisms from the blood, and an asymptomatic latency is established. The comparison of endemic normals and occult filariasis to other forms of the disease indicate that both antibody and cellular immunity are important for complete control of the infection.

However, immune responses that apparently cure the infection may actually lead to disease. Thus, filarial fevers are an indication that an immune response has been activated, most likely involving immune complexes. The manifestations of tropical eosinophilia (attacks of bronchial asthma with interstitial inflammation of the lungs) are consistent with an IgE response and the formation of immune complexes. A cellular (granulomatous) response is implicated in the pathogenesis of lymphadenitis and lymphatic obstruction leading to massive edema (elephantiasis).

The development of the different, more benign host–parasite relationships is related to the age when exposure to the parasite occurs. When previously unexposed adults are infected, there is a tendency to develop acute inflammation with pain, urticaria, angioedema, and marked lymphangitis, which disappear without sequelae if exposure is terminated. However, if exposure continues, the disease progresses rapidly from temporary to permanent lymphatic obstruction. Thus, continued exposure to the organism in sensitized individuals is associated with the development of lymphatic obstruction by granulomas formed around killed microfilaria. In contrast, residents of endemic regions who contact filaria early in life may develop less frequent and less severe manifestations of the disease. In some as yet unknown way, the immune response of such persons is either specifically suppressed or is restricted to IgG antibody production, resulting in an asymptomatic carrier state or occult filariasis. Adults from outside the endemic area tend to produce IgE antibody or cellular hypersensitivity when infected. This intriguing host–parasite relationship clearly deserves further study.

Strongyloides Hyperinfection

An example of the role of delayed hypersensitivity (granulomatous reactivity) and anaphylactic mechanisms in controlling intestinal nematode infection is the occurrence of "hyperinfection" by *Strongyloides stercoralis* in immune-suppressed individuals. Infestations with *S. stercoralis* were first noted in French soldiers returning from Vietnam in 1876. It is estimated that 100 to 200 million people in the tropics and subtropics have *S. stercoralis* infections. *S. stercoralis* is also found in the southeastern United States. In one study, 4% of patients in a New Orleans Hospital were found to contain eggs or larvae in their stools.

Unique among the intestinal nematodes of humans is the ability of invasive larvae of *S. stercoralis* to mature within the gastrointestinal tract (Fig. 25–9). This allows autoinfection. Infected individuals with normal immune function remain essentially asymptomatic; the immune system provides a barrier to autoinfection. However, in immunosuppressed individuals, hyperinfection occurs.

Hyperinfected individuals are most likely asymptomatic bearers of *S. stercoralis* until a natural disease (Hodgkin's disease, lymphoma, debilitation, leprosy, etc.) or immunosuppressive therapy, such as steroids or cytotoxic drugs for graft recipients, results in depressed immunity. It is believed that anaphylactic and delayed hypersensitivity mechanisms are primarily responsible for maintenance of the asymptomatic state. Evidence for this is the association of poor prognosis with a lack of eosinophilia and the finding of hyperinfection in patients with lepromatous leprosy who have a selective deficiency in delayed hypersensitivity. In hyperinfected patients, there is a failure to develop granulomas in infected organs; such granulomas are characteristic of lesions in infected individuals with normal immune function.

The apparent pathogenesis of hyperinfection is loss of intestinal barriers to invasion of filiform larvae secondary to immunodeficiency and decreased intestinal motility, allowing more time for filiform larvae to develop from eggs and rhabdiform larvae. Patients with *Strongyloides* hyperinfection develop inflammatory changes in the intestine associated with diarrhea and ileus. Massive infiltration leads to severe inflammation in the lung, and larvae may be seen in the liver, lung, brain, and meninges. Also associated is sepsis by enteric organisms, leading to fatal meningitis. Invasion of the *Strongyloides* larvae opens the way for organisms in the gut to enter the body of an already immunosuppressed individual.

Evasion of Immune Defenses

Infectious organisms have evolved "ingenious" ways to avoid immune defense mechanisms (Table 25–9). Organisms may locate in niches not accessible to immune effector mechanisms or mask themselves by acquiring host molecules. They may change their surface antigens, hide within cells, produce factors that inhibit the immune response or fool the immune system into responding with an ineffective effector mechanism. The ultimate endpoint of coevolution of the human host and its infectious organisms results in an eventual mutual coexistence. There is no better evidence of this than the loss of this coexistence when the immune mechanisms do not function properly. Then organisms that do not normally cause disease become virulent. These are known as opportunistic infections (see Chapter 27). One of the many lessons of AIDS is that new infectious organisms will become dominant when introduced into a previously unexposed population. Previous examples of this are the devastating effects of tuberculosis and smallpox introduced to previously unexposed American Indians and of syphilis introduced into Europe in the 1490s. The genetic diversity of immune responsiveness in populations is responsible for both the inability of some individuals to develop an immune response to a new infectious agent and the ability of other individuals to make a protective response and survive. If genetic diversity in immune responsiveness is not present, a new infectious agent can annihilate a genetically unresponsive population. In a fully evolved, mature relationship, host and infectious agent coexist without detrimental effects. Thus, the ultimate evolution of the host parasite relationship is not "cure" of an infection by complete elimination of the parasite but is mutual coexistence without deleterious effects of the parasite on the host. In fact, in many human infections, the infectious agent is never fully destroyed and the disease enters a latent state that can be reactivated under different conditions, such as decreased immunity with aging or the effect of superinfection with another agent.

To illustrate some examples of how the host's immunity is avoided during an infection, the following will be briefly presented: Echinococcus, HIV, schistosomiasis, vaccinia, trypanosomiasis, measles, influenza virus, herpesvirus, ascaris, leprosy, poxviruses, Epstein–Barr virus, and leishmaniasis.

ECHINO-COCCOSIS (PROTECTED NICHE)

Echinococcosis is initiated by ingestion of eggs of the dog tapeworm *Echinococcus granulosis*. The eggs hatch in the human intestine and release embryos (oncospheres) that penetrate the gut wall, enter the bloodstream, and disseminate to deep organs, such as liver, kidney, and lung, where the larvae mature and produce cysts called hydatid cysts. Cystic hydatid disease of humans consists of multiple, unilocular, fluid-filled cysts containing viable larvae. The mature larvae (metacestodes) may survive for many years in the cyst, even though the infected individual is resistant to reinfection (concomitant immunity). The larvae are protected from immune attack by an acellular, laminated, external layer or cuticle, as well as by a thick capsule of connective tissue that walls off the site of infection similar to what occurs in the granulomas of chronic tuberculosis. Thus, the organisms survive in a pro-

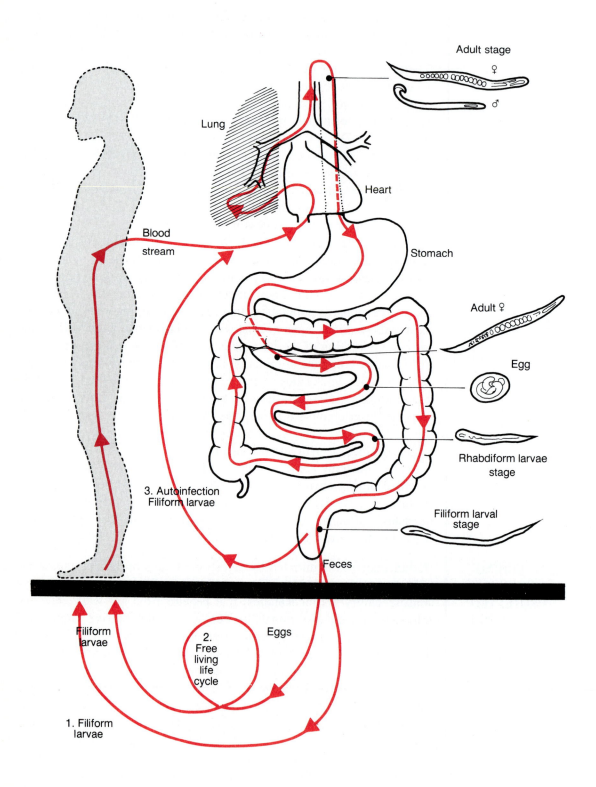

Adult stage ♀

♂

Lung

Heart

Blood
stream

Stomach

Adult ♀

Egg

Rhabdiform larvae
stage

3. Autoinfection
Filiform larvae

Filiform larval
stage

Feces

Filiform
larvae

2.
Free
living
life
cycle

Eggs

1. Filiform
larvae

TABLE 25–9. SOME MECHANISMS OF EVASION OF IMMUNE DEFENSES BY INFECTIOUS AGENTS

Mechanism	Examples
Localization in protective niches	Latent syphilis, herpes simplex, tapeworm (*Echinococcus*)
Intracellular location	Histoplasmosis, viruses (HIV), chlamydia
Resistance to phagocytosis	*S. pneumoniae*
Complement Misdirection	Schistosomiasis, vaccinia virus
Loss of cell surface antigens	Schistosomiasis
Antigenic modulation	Malaria, trypanosomiasis
Steric hindrance of receptor sites (the canyon hypothesis)	Influenza virus, rhinoviruses, ?HIV
Fc receptor induction (bipolar bridging)	Herpes simplex, cytomegalovirus, *Staphylococcus*
Immunosuppression	Malaria, measles, HIV, tuberculosis (anergy)
Extracorporal location	*Clostridium tetani, Ascaris lumbricoides*
MHC-restricted recognition of antigens	*Ascaris lumbricoides*, malaria
Downregulation of class I MHC	Adenovirus
Inappropriate immune response (immune deviation)	Lepromatous leprosy, chronic mucocutaneous candidiasis
Competing soluble cytokine receptors	Poxviruses (IL-1R, TNFR)
Suppressive lymphokines	Epstein–Barr virus (IL-10)
Multiple mechanisms (complement-mediated endocytosis, inhibition of macrophage killing, modulation of T-cell immunity)	Leishmaniasis

Figure 25–9. The life cycle of *Strongyloides stercoralis* provides three routes of human infection: (1) Infection by invasive filiform larvae excreted into the soil, (2) maturation of invasive filiform larvae from free-living organisms in the soil, and (3) autoinfection from filiform larvae that mature in the gastrointestinal tract of the host. Filiform larvae invade skin, enter the venous circulation, and pass to the alveolar capillaries. In the lung, the adolescent worms mature to adult male and female worms. The adult worms pass to the gastrointestinal tract presumably by being coughed up and swallowed. The females lodge in the mucosa of the gastrointestinal tract, set up housekeeping, and lay many eggs; the male is no longer needed and most likely is passed out in the feces. In the GI tract, eggs may mature to rhabdiform larvae and to filiform larvae. All of these forms may be passed into the soil. In addition, filiform larvae may invade the intestinal mucosa, particularly at the anal canal, permitting autoinfection.

tected niche, while the infected individual has a high titer of circulating antibody and is protected from newly acquired infection.

HUMAN IMMUNO-DEFICIENCY VIRUS (HIV) (INTRA-CELLULAR LOCATION, IMMUNO-SUPPRESSION)

The pathogenesis of AIDS and HIV infection is covered in detail in Chapter 29. HIV is carried inside monocytes and lymphocytes in the form of integrated DNA, where it is hidden from immune attack for long periods of time during latent infection. Transmission of infection from one individual to another is mediated by passage of living infected cells during intimate body contact through open lesions in the skin or mucous membranes. Even if circulating antibody to HIV antigens is present in the recipient of the infected cells, no HIV antigens are on the infected cells to which the antibody can react. The immune response does appear to be able to hold in check manifestations of the infection, but since one of the most important cells of the immune system, the CD4+ T cell, is also the prime target for HIV infection, eventually the cytolytic HIV virus destroys enough of the CD4+ T cells to produce a severe immunodeficiency. This not only allows expansion of the HIV infection but also opportunistic infections by other organisms.

CHLAMYDIA TRACHOMATIS (ENDOSOMES)

Chlamydia trachomatis is a prokaryotic obligate intracellular parasite (bacterium) that causes keratoconjunctivitis and pelvic inflammatory disease. The organisms are taken into epithelial cells by receptor-mediated endocytosis and multiply within the host cell in membrane-delimited endosomes. Within the host cell, the organisms are protected from host immune defenses. Large numbers of infective particles are released when the host cell dies.

STREPTO-COCCUS PNEUMONIAE (RESISTANCE TO PHAGOCYTOSIS)

S. pneumoniae has a thick capsule of polysaccharide that enables the bacteria to resist phagocytosis either by resident pulmonary macrophages or recruited neutrophils. Inhaled organisms are cleared by the microvilli of the respiratory epithelium. The incidence of infection is greatly increased in individuals who have defective clearing mechanisms (smokers, chronic bronchitis, asthma, etc.). In such individuals, organisms are able to colonize the nasopharynx and spread to the pulmonary alveoli. Reaction of antibodies to antigens of the cell wall activates complement, but because of the capsule, neither the Fc of IgG nor the C3b on the cell surface is able to interact with receptors of phagocytic cells. In the absence of antibody to the capsular polysaccharide, phagocytosis and killing do not occur. Activation of the inflammatory peptides of complement, particularly C5a, causes an intense polymorphonuclear reaction and, along with other mediators, such as IL-1, endogenous pyrogens, and pneumolysin (a toxin produced by pneumococci), cause a self-perpetuating inflammatory reaction that is largely responsible for symptoms and signs of the disease. In contrast to antibodies to the cell wall, antibodies to the capsular polysaccharides are extremely effective in opsonizing the organisms. Immunization with capsular polysaccharides stimulates antibodies that cause agglutination and a marked swelling of the capsule (the Quelling reaction) and protect against challenge in experimental animals. Pneumococcal vaccination is recommended for individuals at risk for infection and is likely to offer a substantial degree of protection.

SCHISTO-SOMIASIS (COMPLEMENT MISDIRECTION)

The life cycle of the *Schistosoma* spp. that infect man provides stages which express little if any antigens recognizable by infected individuals and stages that are highly immunogenic. Infection begins when motile aquatic cercariae released from the snail intermediate invade the skin of a human host. These larvae penetrate blood vessels, pass through the lung, and circulate selectively to the venous sinusoids of the gastrointestinal (*S. japonicum* and *S. mansoni*) or bladder wall (*S. haematobium*), where maturation to adult worms occurs in the venous sinuses. The adults may live for over a decade in this location. The female releases eggs, which pass through the gastrointestinal wall or bladder, where they are excreted into fresh water to infect the intermediate snail host.

The adult worms survive in the circulation of the host in the face of high titers of circulating antibodies to schistosomal antigens. This paradox has been attributed to several possible mechanisms, including very low surface antigen expression on the adult so that IgG antibody is unable to form aggregates to fix complement; absorption of host molecules such as blood group glycolipids, MHC-glycoproteins, fibronectin, and immunoglobulin bound through the Fc regions that disguise schistosomal antigens; shedding or endocytosis of surface antigens without destruction of the organisms; or membrane pumps that compensate for the ion imbalance that might be produced by immune attack. A more recent explanation is that schistosomula acquire resistance to alternate pathway-mediated complement killing by shedding glycoproteins that activate complement. This not only protects the organisms directly but also indirectly. The released glycoproteins bind to the C3 receptors on effector cells, such as eosinophils or neutrophils, damage the effector cells, and further protect the organisms. Regardless of the mechanisms, the adult organisms develop a tegument resistant to immune attack, which is not the case for the egg or larval forms.

Individuals who are infected are resistant to reinfection even though they carry live adults in their veins (concomitant immunity). There is a strong cellular immune response to antigens on the eggs that is shared with the invading larvae. This immunity prevents reinfection but also induces extensive granulomatous inflammation in the liver or bladder wall to eggs that are deposited there. Thus, the immune response that protects against reinfection is responsible for the inflammatory lesions of the disease schistosomiasis. There is also evidence that some of the cytokines released from reacting T cells, such as IL-10, IL-4, and TGF-β, may actually inhibit destruction of parasites by blocking nitric oxide metabolism of macrophages. The presence of concomitant immunity indicates that appropriate immunization of uninfected individuals with egg antigens should produce immunity to primary infection.

VACCINIA VIRUS (CONTROL OF COMPLEMENT ACTIVATION)

Vaccinia virus secretes a complement control protein (VCP), which has homology to eukaryotic regulators of complement. VCP can inhibit both classical and alternative pathways of complement activation. VCP binds to both C4b and C3b and accelerates the decay of complement convertases. Although the lesion of vaccinia is clearly cell-mediated, complement-mediated neutralization decreases the pathogenic effects of the virus, presumably by limiting spread of infection. In rabbits, lesions caused by wild-type and mutant viruses lacking the gene for VCP are similar for the first five days, but after that the lesions of the mutant virus decreased in size, whereas that of the wild type did not. Antibody to virus appears about day 5. Thus, wild-type virus is able to avoid antibody mediated attack, whereas virus lacking VCP is not.

TRYPANO-SOMIASIS (ANTIGENIC MODULATION)

Trypanosoma spp. avoid immune attack by changing the antigens that they express (antigenic variation). This mechanism is also used by other organisms, but trypanosomes have the most sophisticated system of antigenic variation now known. A relatively large portion of the trypanosome genome (approximately 2%) is devoted to antigenic variation. *Trypanosoma b. brucei* has been estimated to have 1,000 different antigen genes. The maximum number of antigen types actually identified in one clone of *Trypanosoma* is 101. Thus, when an infected individual produces an antibody to one antigen, the organism shifts to expression of a new antigen and avoids immune attack.

The genetic mechanisms for antigen switching include: (1) Gene conversion, by which the activated gene is replaced by a copy of another gene, so that the original gene activation site acts on a different gene; (2) differential activation, in which an activation factor binds to a different controlling region, activating another gene; (3) partial gene conversion, in which part of an inactive gene replaces part of an active gene; (4) reciprocal recombination, by which an inactive gene gains access to an active controlling site by unequal crossing over; and finally, (5) point mutation. Many of the variable surface glycoprotein antigen genes are found in repeat sequences at chromosomes ends (telomeres). Telomeres with extensive regions of repeated sequences are recombination "hot spots." In addition, a telomeric transcription site allows activation of a series of alternative telomeres on different chromosomes.

In the blood, antigen types succeed each other in different parasitemic waves (Fig. 25–10). Analysis of clones reveals the presence of different DNA rearrangements within a clone, suggesting a high rate of recombination or polyclonal activation. The timing of antigenic variation is important for long-term survival of the organism, since otherwise it would be possible to exhaust the antigenic repertoire and eliminate the infection. The succession of antigen types appears to be conserved in a given strain, but the mechanism controlling the sequence of antigen expression is not known.

MEASLES (IMMUNO-SUPPRESSION)

Measles was the first virus infection shown to cause a generalized immune deficiency; HIV (see Chapter 29) produces even more profound effects. Measles was first described in Baghdad by Rhazes in the 6th century A.D. It is believed to have evolved in Africa from an animal virus. It was spread into Europe in the 8th century by the Saracen invasion, where it produced vast numbers of fatalities from opportunistic infections, as well as by activation of latent tuberculosis or superinfection with tuberculosis. In 1908, von Pirquet first noted a loss of cutaneous tuberculin reactions in children who had the measles rash. Like many other infectious agents, measles produces high death rates in virgin populations but is much less virulent in exposed populations.

Measles infection is associated with depressed cellular immunity. This is not specific for measles as there is depression of skin test reactivity to other test antigens and depressed lymphoproliferative responses to antigens and mitogens in individuals with more severe

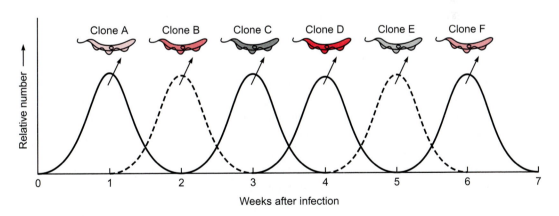

Figure 25–10. Antigenic variation during trypanosomiasis infection. Successive waves of different clones expressing different surface glycoprotein (VSG, variable surface glycoproteins) of the parasite is characteristic of trypanosomiasis. After infection, one clone of parasites, most of which carry a particular VSG, proliferates in the bloodstream. Antibody is produced to this VSG and kills most of the parasites. A few individuals survive by expressing a new VSG. This clone then expands until antibody to the new VSG is produced and kills most of the second wave. This process is repeated over and over again as new clones are produced. From Donelson JE and Turner MJ, *Scientific American* 252:44, 1985.

716 IMMUNOLOGY/IMMUNOPATHOLOGY AND IMMUNITY

manifestations, such as measles pneumonia. In vitro, the virus will infect T cells of both CD4 and CD8 subsets, as well as B cells and macrophages. However, the exact nature of the immunosuppression in vivo is not well understood. There appears to be decreased production of IL-1 and IL-2 by macrophages of lymphocytes, elevation of IgE and evidence for spontaneous suppressor cell activity. Thus, even with major advances in analyzing immune functions, the pathogenesis of measles immunodeficiency remains unclear.

INFLUENZA VIRUS (STERIC HINDRANCE)

Influenza virus has conserved structures required for infectivity, as well as rapidly modulating structures that are recognized by antibodies produced by the infected host. In order to survive in face of development of immunity in a population, the virus is able to undergo modification of those structures that are recognized by antibody without changing the structure required to bind to the specific cell receptor. Influenza virus, as well as most other animal viruses, initiates infection by specific binding of a receptor to a site on the host cell. For influenza virus, the binding site is sialyl-lactose. The virus-binding site is located in a depression in the hemagglutinin spike on the surface of the virus that is too narrow for antibody binding to occur. Thus, neutralizing antibodies react with determinants on the surface of the spike and not with the specific cell-binding domain. Human flu epidemics occur because of the appearance of new strains of influenza virus that have different surface epitopes, whereas the cell-binding structure remains unmodified (Fig. 25–11). This is known as the canyon hypothesis.

HERPESVIRUS (INTRA-CELLULAR LOCATION, BIPOLAR BRIDGING)

Although the precise role of cellular and humoral immunity in protection and pathogenesis of herpesvirus infection has not been clearly established, the intracellular location and the ability of herpes simplex virus to induce Fc receptors (FcR) on infected cells provides protection against lysis by IgG antibody and complement. Binding of the Fab domains of IgG antibodies to virus antigens expressed on the surface of infected cells has the potential to fix complement through binding of C_1 to aggregated Fcs of the bound antibodies. However, infection of human cells with herpes simplex is associated with the appearance of a novel FcR so that the Fc portion of IgG antibodies that react with the infected cells is bound to this receptor and not available to react with C_1. This is termed "bipolar bridging" (Fig. 25–12). FcR expression is also associated with other infectious agents, including cytomegalovirus, *S. aureus*, *Trypanosoma, Leishmania,* and *S. mansoni.* Staphylococcal protein A binds the $C_{\gamma2}$ and $C_{\gamma3}$ domains of IgG and impairs antibody-dependent complement-mediated killing. Induction of FcR by cytomegalovirus renders cells susceptible to infection by HIV bound to antibody.

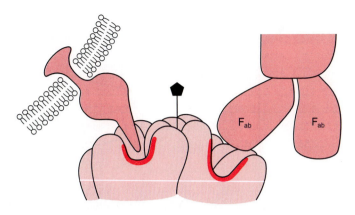

Figure 25–11. The canyon hypothesis. This hypothesis states that the virus-binding site for a cell surface receptor for the virus is located in a depression of the viral spikes on the surface of the virus particles and that this location, while able to receive the cell surface receptor (R), sterically prevents larger antibody paratopes (P) from reacting. This allows for conservation of the virus-binding site while at the same time permitting evolution of new serotypes by mutating epitopes about the rim of the canyon. Modified from Luo M, Vriend G, Kramer G et al: The atomic Structure of the Mengo Virus at 3.0A° resolution: *Science* 235:182–191, 1987.

ASCARIS LUMBRICOIDES (EXTRA-CORPORAL LOCATION, MHC-RESTRICTED RECOGNITION)

In addition to the location of the adult worms within the gastrointestinal tract lumen, where it essentially does not come into contact with the host's immune system, there is MHC-related restriction of recognition of the antigens of the tissue-invading larval stages of *Ascaris*. In mice, the ability to recognize and produce antibody to the external excretory/secretory material (ES) of the larvae is under the control of H_2 loci, not only in regard to the epitopes recognized, but also in the class of antibody produced. For instance, mouse strains differ markedly in the level of IgE production, eosinophilia, and the capacity of the immune response to inhibit migration of the larvae to the lungs, a necessary stage of the life cycle of *Ascaris*. MHC-controlled heterogeneity in the immune response explains, at least in part, the variation in disease patterns produced by infection of humans by a number of infectious agents.

LEPROSY AND SYPHILIS (IMMUNE DEVIATION)

Immune deviation or split tolerance is defined as the dominance of one immune response mechanism over another for a specific antigen and has been implicated in the tendency for certain individuals to develop IgE (allergy) antibodies rather than IgG antibodies. In addition, for reasons that are unclear but may be genetically determined, some individuals tend to make strong cellular immune responses but weak antibody response to certain antigens, whereas other individuals will have the

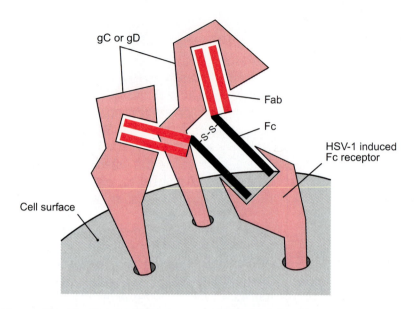

Figure 25–12. Bipolar bridging prevents complement activation. HSV infection induces Fc receptors on the surface of infected cells that tie up the Fc domain of antibody that binds to either of the dominant antigens of HSV-1, gC, or gD, through the antigen-binding site (paratope) on the Fab domain. This prevents aggregation of the Fc regions of antibodies on the surface of the cell and prevents binding of C_1 of complement. Modified from Frank I, Friedman HM: *J Virol* 63:4479, 1989.

opposite response. The course of leprosy depends upon the immune reaction of the patient (see Chapter 17). Leprosy may be classified into three overlapping groups—tuberculoid, borderline and lepromatous. In tuberculoid leprosy, there are prominent well-formed granulomatous lesions, many lymphocytes and few if any organisms. Delayed hypersensitivity skin tests are intact and there is predominant hyperplasia of the diffuse cortex (T-cell zone) of the lymph nodes. The level of antibodies is low. In lepromatous leprosy, granulomas are not formed, there are few or no lymphocytes, and lesions consist of large macrophages filled with viable organisms. Delayed hypersensitivity skin tests are depressed, and there is marked follicular hyperplasia in the lymph nodes with little or no diffuse cortex. The levels of antibodies are high, and vascular lesions due to immune complexes are seen (erythema nodosum leprosum). Borderline leprosy has intermediate findings. The prognosis in tuberculoid leprosy is good, and the response to chemotherapy is excellent. In borderline leprosy, a good response to therapy is associated with a conversion to the tuberculoid form. The prognosis in lepromatous leprosy and the response to chemotherapy is poor. The example of the forms of leprosy illustrates the role of cellular immunity (delayed hypersensitivity) in controlling the infection and the lack of protective response provided by humoral antibodies. This concept is also considered valid for immunity to *Candida albicans*. Depressed cellular immunity is associated with chronic mucocutaneous candidiasis, a condition in which the infected individual is unable to clear *Candida* infections. It is now proposed that the same holds for the clinical stages of syphilis.

A diagram illustrating the relationship of the degree of cellular and humoral immune response to the stages of syphilis and leprosy is shown below (Fig. 25–13). In this model, the primary chancre of syphilis is considered to be a delayed hypersensitivity reaction that essentially clears the site of infectious organisms. If the cellular immune mechanism is dominant, the infection will be cured. If the cellular immune mechanism is not able to clear the infection, replication of the organisms in multiple sites will stimulate secondary reactions, which again are manifestations of delayed hypersensitivity. Because of the large number of organisms now present, it may take weeks to clear the lesions, and many organisms will remain in protected niches.

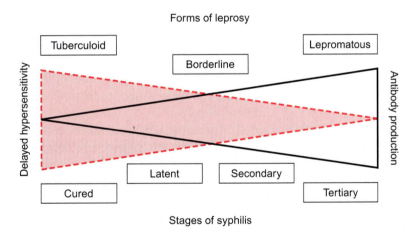

Figure 25–13. A comparison of the association of delayed hypersensitivity and antibody production in the clinical forms of leprosy and in the clinical stages of syphilis. The overlapping triangles indicate the relative strength of delayed hypersensitivity and antibody production. The cross-hatched triangle indicates delayed hypersensitivity; the open triangle, antibody production. High levels of delayed-type hypersensitivity (DTH) are associated with cure; weak DTH is associated with progressive disease; balanced DTH and antibody production are associated with borderline leprosy and latent syphilis. Progression of syphilis to the tertiary stage is most likely more related to depressed T-cell immunity, with or without high levels of antibody. The nature of the antigen-presenting cell may determine if Th1 cells are activated to help in antibody production or in development of DTH. Antibody production is stimulated by antigens processed by dendritic follicular cells; DTH is stimulated by antigens processed by interdigitating reticulum cells.

However, if cellular immunity remains strong, no further lesion development will occur, and latent infection will be maintained. If the cellular immune response declines, organisms will increase, and lesions of tertiary syphilis will appear, even in the face of high antibody titers in the serum or in the cerebrospinal fluid. In the experimental model in the rabbit, cellular immunity is able to clear dermal or testicular infection, and lesions of secondary and tertiary syphilis do not occur. Penicillin treatment of secondary or tertiary syphilis is able to reduce the number of organisms so that the low level of cellular immunity present is able to reestablish control of the infection. However, if suppression of the cellular immune response is induced by immunosuppression or AIDS, latency may be terminated more rapidly and produce a systemic infection requiring high doses of penicillin treatment.

POXVIRUSES (EFFECTOR MODULATION-SOLUBLE RECEPTORS)

Poxviruses, such as cowpox virus and vaccinia, produce soluble receptors for IL-1; and Shope fibroma/myxoma virus, which produces tumorlike lesions in rabbits, produce soluble forms of receptors for TNF and INF-γ. These receptors intercept their respective cytokines and prevent reaction with the cell surface receptor, thus preventing the decoyed mediator from binding to its cellular receptor and destroying virus-infected cells.

EPSTEIN–BARR VIRUS (EBV) (IL-10)

EBV produces a homologue of IL-10, which normally downregulates the antiviral T-cell response and also stimulate B cells that EBV infects. In this way, IL-10 production by EBV-infected B cells not only "auto-upregulates" virus production, but also blocks T_{CTL} response to infected B cells.

LEISHMANIASIS (COMPLEMENT-MEDIATED ENDOCYTOSIS, INHIBITION OF MACROPHAGE KILLING, MODULATION OF T-CELL IMMUNITY, IMMUNE DEVIATION)

Perhaps no other organism exemplifies the multiple ways that parasites can evade or even use the host immune system to its advantage than *Leishmania donovani*. Other species of *Leishmania*, such as *L. major*, *L. aethiopica*, and *L. mexicana* do not have these evasive mechanisms and usually cause only local cutaneous lesions that are controlled by delayed hypersensitivity reactions with destruction by phagocytosis and digestion by macrophages. However, infection with *L. donovani* leads to a systemic, eventually lethal, disease known as kala-azar because of its ability to evade macrophage-mediated killing. The three major evasion mechanisms used by *L. donovani* are: (1) Use of complement receptors on macrophages for endocytosis, (2) inhibition of intracellular killing by macrophages, and (3) modulation of T-cell immunity (immune deviation) (Fig. 25–14). The major pathologic features of kala-azar are intracellular accumulation of organisms in macrophages, leading to massive hepatosplenomegaly, and stimulation of monocyte hyperplasia in the bone marrow.

In pathogenic leishmaniasis, the surface lipophosphoglycan (LPG) is able to serve as an acceptor for the third component of complement. After binding to the acceptor, C_3 is converted to C_3b and the

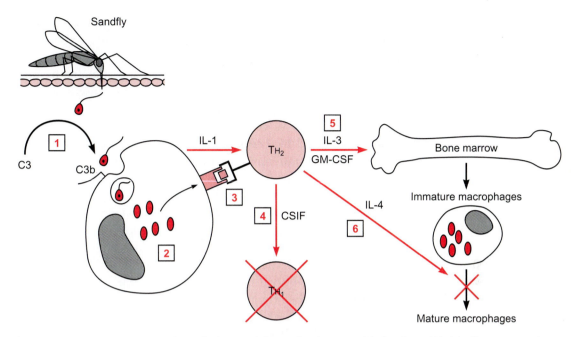

Figure 25–14. Immune evasion during *Leishmania donovani* infection. (1) Motile promastigotes injected by the bite of the infected sandfly are able to activate C_3 to C_3b, bind to macrophages through C_3b and CR1/CR3, and are endocytosed without a fatal oxygen burst. (2) Inside the cell, the promastigotes transform into amastigotes that are resistant to the oxygen-dependent and enzymatic killing process of the phagocyte. (3) Infected macrophages in T-cell zones of lymph nodes present antigens preferentially to Th2 helper cells, which release CSIF, IL-3, GM-CSF, and IL-4. (4) CSIF inhibits activation of Th1 helper cells and prevents development of T_{DTH} cells and delayed hypersensitivity. (5) IL-3 and GM-CSF stimulate the bone marrow to produce immature monocytes, which are permissive for parasite replication. (6) IL-4 inhibits maturation of monocytes to a state of being able to resist parasite infestation.

"opsonized" parasites bind to the CR1 or CR3 of the host's macrophages, which then endocytose the parasite. The effect of this is not only to protect the organism from lysis by antibody and complement activated in the classical pathway but also to facilitate the entry of the parasite into their permissive host cells.

In progressive leishmaniasis, the infecting organisms are able to survive within macrophages by the ability of the parasite to avoid the oxidative and enzymatic destructive mechanisms of the macrophage. Binding to CR1/CR3 inhibits the oxidative burst usually associated with phagocytosis. Once inside the cell, the acid phosphatase on the surface of the parasite downregulates oxygen-dependent killing, and other enzymes, as well as the surface LPG, are able to scavenge toxic oxygen metabolites. In addition, LPG and other surface molecules inhibit digestive enzymes of phagolysosomes, and the pathogenic organisms are able to maintain a neutral intercellular milieu despite the acidic environment inside the phagolysosome. Through these mechanisms, the parasite is able to convert the macrophage into a permissive cell for its survival and propagation.

Finally, in progressive disease, *Leishmania* spp. are able to modulate the T-cell immune response so that T_{DTH} cells are not induced to activate the macrophages (immune deviation), similar to what occurs in lepromatous leprosy. It appears that antigen presentation by macrophages infected by *Leishmania* somehow is directed to activation of Th2 cells in preference to Th1 cells. Epidermal Langerhans' cells internalize *L. major* and deliver processed antigens to the T-cell zones of draining lymph nodes. In mice, proliferation of organisms in dendritic macrophages in the lymph nodes correlates with the induction of Th2 cells, whereas resistance correlates with the induction of Th1 cells. The release of IL-3, IL-4, and GM-CSF by Th2 cells stimulates bone marrow hyperplasia and the release of immature macrophages from the bone marrow that are unable to destroy endocytosed organisms, providing more permissive cells for infection. In addition, factors from Th2 cells (colony-stimulating inhibitory factor [CSIF]) further inhibit Th1 cells. The inhibition of IL-2 and interferon-γ release from Th1 cells prevents not only induction of T_{DTH} cells but also macrophage activation, resulting in immunosuppression, as well as inhibition of the killing potential of macrophages.

In conclusion, the host–parasite relationship between infectious agents and their supportive hosts has evolved to allow ways for the infecting parasite to avoid immune attack of the host. There are three general ways that this is accomplished: (1) Anatomic (protective niches, intracellular location of the infection, and extracorporal location); (2) antigenic change or masking of the infectious agent (antigenic modulation, absorption of host molecules, formation of external cuticles or coats with low antigenicity and location of important surface structures in "canyons" inaccessible to antibodies); and (3) variations of the host's immune response (immune suppression, immune deviation, MHC-controlled epitope recognition, and production of competitive inhibitors of cytokines). Each of these approaches is used effectively with incredible variations to suit the characteristics and life cycles of the infecting organisms.

Summary

The double-edged sword of immune reactivity is illustrated by the role of immune effector mechanisms in resistance to infectious agents and the contribution of immune mechanisms to tissue lesions and disease. Each immune effector mechanism has a defensive function for the host. Antibody-mediated effector mechanisms generally operate against bacteria or bacterial products; cellular effector mechanisms protect against viral, mycobacterial, or fungal diseases. Neutralization or inactivation of biologically active bacterial toxins is clearly protective. This is what is accomplished by active immunization with diphtheria or tetanus toxoids. Antibody-mediated cytotoxic reactions are effective in killing bacteria or preparing bacteria for phagocytosis by opsonization. The inflammatory effect of immune complexes produces stickiness of leukocytes and platelets to vascular endothelium and increased permeability. These reactions promote defense by localization, diapedesis, and activation of polymorphonuclear leukocytes. Anaphylactic mechanisms serve to open up capillaries, permitting extravasation of blood/bone components into tissues, thus permitting delivery of inflammatory cells or antibodies to sites of infection. Spasmatic and massive diarrhea (gastrointestinal anaphylaxis) may effect expulsion of intestinal parasites. T-cytotoxic cells are effective in eliminating virus-infected cells, but deleterious effects may occur if cells with vital functions, such as neurons, are destroyed. Delayed hypersensitivity reactions result in local mobilization of lymphocytes and alteration and activation of macrophages, effects clearly necessary for defense against viral, fungal, and mycobacterial infections. Granulomatous hypersensitivity functions to isolate insoluble toxic material or microorganisms. A list of postulated specific-effector mechanisms for selected infectious diseases is given in Table 25–10. In many infectious diseases, more than one mechanism may be active, particularly if the organism exists in different stages.

TABLE 25–10. POSTULATED SPECIFIC IMMUNE DEFENSE MECHANISMS IN SOME INFECTIOUS DISEASES

Disease	Agent	Site of Infection	Defense Mechanism
Viruses (RNA)			
Influenza	Paramyxovirus	Lung	Antibody blocks cell attachment
Mumps	Paramyxovirus	Parotid gland	T_{CTL} kills infected cells
Measles (Rubeola)	Paramyxovirus	Skin systemic	T_{CTL} kills infected cells
Rabies	Rhabdovirus	Brain cells	T_{CTL} kills infected cells
Polio	Picornavirus	Systemic, neurons	Antibody blocks cell attachment
Yellow fever	Flavivirus	Viscera	Antibody blocks cell attachment
Viruses (DNA)			
Herpes	Herpesvirus	Skin, mucous membranes	T_{CTL} kills infected cells
Smallpox	Poxviridae	Skin	T_{CTL} kills infected cells
Hepatitis B	Hepatitis B virus	Liver	Antibody blocks cell attachment
Rickettsia			
Rocky Mountain spotted fever	Rickettsia rickettsii	Vascular endothelium	T_{CTL} kills infected cells
Typhus	Rickettsia prowazekii	Vascular endothelium	T_{CTL} kills infected cells
Bacteria			
Botulism	Clostridium botulinum	Exotoxin	Neutralization by antibody
Tetanus	Clostridium tetani	Exotoxin	Neutralization by antibody
Diphtheria	Corynebacterium diphtheriae	Exotoxin	Neutralization by antibody
Pertussus	Bordetella pertussis	Endo- and exotoxin	Neutralization, opsonization
Cholera	Vibrio cholerae	Enterotoxin	IgA neutralization of toxin

TABLE 25–10. POSTULATED SPECIFIC IMMUNE DEFENSE MECHANISMS IN SOME INFECTIOUS DISEASES (continued)

Disease	Agent	Site of Infection	Defense Mechanism
Staphylococcus	*Staphylococcus aureus*	Connective tissue Pyogenic abcess	Antibody neutralization of toxin, opsonization
Streptococcus	*Streptococcus β-hemolytic*	Connective tissue Cellulitis	Antibody neutralization of toxins, opsonization
Pneumonia	*Streptococcus pneumoniae*	Pneumonia	Antibody opsonization, cytotoxicity
Meningitis	*Neisseria meningitidis*	Meninges, IgA protease	Antibody opsonization, protease neutralization
Gonorrhea	*Neisseria gonorrhoeae*	Mucous surface	Antibody, opsonization, protease neutralization
Influenza	*Hemophilus influenza*	Lung, endotoxin	Antibody, opsonization, neutralization
Infantile diarrhea	*Escherichia coli*	G.I. tract, endotoxin	Antibody blocks cell attachment, neutralization, opsonization
Typhoid fever	*Salmonella typhi*	G.I. tract, systemic endotoxin	Antibody neutralization, DTH macrophage activation
Mycobacteria			
Tuberculosis	*Mycobacterium tuberculosis*	Lung	Granulomatous, DTH
Leprosy	*Mycobacterium leprae*	Dermis	Granulomatous, DTH
Spirochetes			
Syphilis	*Treponema pallidum*	Connective Tissue	DTH, ?Antibody opsonization
Lyme disease	*Borrelia burgdorferi*	Skin, systemic	Antibody, immune complex, DTH
Fungi			
Actinomycosis	*Actinomyces* spp.	Connective tissue	Immune complex opsonization granulomatous
Aspergillosis	*Aspergillus* spp.	Lung	Immune complex, granulomatous
Candidiasis	*Candida albicans*	Skin, mucous membranes	DTH, granuloma
Coccidioidomycosis	*Coccidioides immitis*	Lung	DTH, Granulomatous
Cryptococcus	*Cryptococcus neoformans*	Lung	Granulomatous
Histoplasmosis	*Histoplasma capsulatum*	Inside macrophages	DTH, macrophage activation
Protozoa			
Amebiasis	*Entamoeba histolytica*	GI mucosa	Immune complex, inflammation
Malaria	*Plasmodium* spp.	Inside cells, free in blood	Cytotoxic, immune complex opsonization T_{CTL} kills infected cells
Leishmaniasis	*Leishmania* spp.	Inside macrophages	DTH, activated macrophages
Toxoplasmosis	*Toxoplasma gondii*	Intracellular	Immune complex opsonization
Chagas' disease	*Trypanosoma cruzi*	Free in blood, intracellular	Cytotoxic, immune complex opsonization
Sleeping sickness	*Trypanosoma rhodesiense Trypanosoma gambiense*	Free in blood	Cytotoxic, immune complex opsonization
Giardiasis	*Giardia lamblia*	GI tract	IgA antibody
Helminths			
Schistosomiasis	*Schistosoma* spp.	Veins	Eosinophil ADCC
Fascioliasis	*Fasciola*	Biliary ducts	Eosinophil ADCC, granulomatous
Trichinosis	*Trichinella spiralis*	In muscle	Eosinophil ADCC, DTH
Strongyloidiasis	*Strongyloides stercoralis*	GI tract	Eosinophil ADCC, DTH
Filariasis	*Wuchereria bancroft*	Lymphatics	Eosinophil ADCC, granulomatous
	Onchocerca volvulus	Dermis	Immune complex, granulomatous
Taeniasis	*Taenia*	GI tract	Eosinophil ADCC, GI motility

Examples of the destructive capacity of immune responses to some selected infectious agents have also been presented. Tissue lesions caused by immune reactions to infectious agents usually occur when an inappropriate mechanism is activated. Thus, in leprosy, antibody causes problems due to immune complex formation but has no protective effect against the intracellular bacilli; granulomatous reactivity is protective but may cause tissue damage if activated after large numbers of organisms have already been disseminated. The relative contribution of different immune mechanisms to the pathogenesis of other infectious diseases reflects even more variations in the interplay between immune effector mechanisms in protection and pathogenesis. The ability of many organisms to cause disease depends on their ability to evade the immune defenses. For as many different immune defense mechanisms that can be recognized, infectious agents have been able to evolve ways to avoid the defenses and even ways to use the immune system to their advantage.

Bibliography

GENERAL

Braude AI: *Infection and Immunity in Clinical Physiology*. Giallium A (ed.). New York, McGraw Hill, 1957, 773.

Capron A, Dessaint JP: Effector and regulatory mechanisms in immunity to schistosomes: A hieratic view. *Ann Rev Immunol* 3:455, 1985.

Dalton DK, Pitts-Meek S, Keshav S, et al.: Multiple defects of immune cell function in mice with disrupted interferon-γ genes. *Science* 259:1739–1742, 1993.

Ellner JJ, Mahmond AAF: Phagocytes and worms: David and Goliath revisited. *Rev Inf Dis* 4:698, 1982.

Gillis HM: Selective primary health care: Strategies for control of disease in the developing world. XVII. Hookworm infection and anemia. *Rev Inf Dis* 7:111, 1985.

Keusch GT: Immune responses in parasitic diseases. *Rev Infect Dis* 4:751, 1982.

Mendes E: *Immunopathology of Tropical Diseases*, San Paulo, Brazil, Sawyer, 1982.

Prokesova L, Potuznikova B, Potempa J, et al.: Cleavage of human immunoglobulins by serine proteinase from *Staphylococcus aureus. Immunol Lett* 31:259, 1992.

Salata RA, Ravdin JI: Review of the human immune mechanisms directed against *Entamoeba histolytica. Rev Infect Dis* 8:261–272, 1986.

Sissons JGP, Oldstone MBA: Killing of virus-infected cells by cytotoxic lymphocytes. *J Inf Dis* 142:114, 1980.

Von Lichtenberg F: *Pathology of Infectious Diseases*. Boca Raton, FL, Raven, 1991.

NEUTRALIZING SKIN TESTS

Dochez AR: Etiology of scarlet fever. *Medicine* 4:251, 1925.

Dick GF, Dick GH: A skin test for susceptibility to scarlet fever. *JAMA* 82:265, 1924.

Dick GF, Dick GH: Results with the skin test for susceptibility to scarlet fever: Preventive immunization with scarlet fever toxin. *JAMA* 84:1477, 1925.

Romer PH: Veber Den Nachwis Sehr Kleiner Mengen des Diphtheriegiftes. *Z Immunitaetsforsch* 3:208, 1909.

Schick B: Die Diphtherietoxin-Hautreaktion des Menschen Als Vorprobe Der Prophylaktischen Diphtherieheilserum Injection. *Munch Med Wochenschr* 60:2608, 1913.

Schultz W, Charlton W: Serologische Beobactungen Am Scharlachexanthum. *Z Kinderheikd* 17:328, 1917.

Schwentker FF, Hodes HL, Kingland LC, et al.: Streptococcal infections in a naval training station. *Am J Public Health* 33:1455, 1943.

TETANUS

Blake PA, Feldman RA, et al.: Serologic therapy of tetanus in the United States, 1965, 1971. *JAMA* 235:42, 1976.

Brooks VB, Curtis DR, Eccles JC: Mode of action of tetanus toxin. *Nature* 175:120, 1955.

Fraser DW: Preventing tetanus in patients with wounds. *Ann Intern Med* 84:95, 1976.

LaForce FM, Young LS, Bennett JV: Tetanus in the United States: Epidermiologic and clinical features. *N Engl J Med* 280:569, 1969.

Nielsen PA, Ablondi FB, Querry MV, et al.: Antigenic and immunogenic studies on purified tetanus toxoid. *J Immunol* 98:1248, 1967.

Prevots R, Sutter RW, Strebel PM, et al.: Tetanus surveillance—United States, 1989–1990. *MMWR* 41 (no. SS-8):1, 1992.

Donelson JE and Turner MJ, *Scientific American* 252:44, 1985.

Proceedings of the 4th International Conference on Tetanus: Dakar, Senegal, April 6–12, 1975. Lyon, France, Foundation Merieux, 1975.

Rubbo SD: A reevaluation of tetanus prophylaxis in civilian practice. *Med J Aust* 2:105, 1965.

MALARIA

Aggarwal A, Kumar S, Jaffe R, et al.: Oral *Salmonella*: Malaria circumsporate recombinants induce specific CD8+ cytotoxic T cells. *J Exp Med* 172:1083, 1990.

Boyd MF (ed.): *Malariology*. Philadelphia, Saunders, 1949.

Cruz Cuhas AB, Gentilini M, Monjour L: Cytokines and T-cell response in malaria. *Biomed & Pharmacother* 48:27–33, 1994.

Hollingdale MR: Biology and immunology of sporozoite invasion of liver cells and exoerythrocytic development of malaria parasites. *Prog Allergy* 41:15–48, 1988.

Kumaratilake LM, Ferrante A, Rzepczyk C: The role of T lymphocytes in immunity to *Plasmodium falciparum*. Enhancement of neutrophil-mediated parasite killing by lymphotoxin and IFN-γ: Comparisons with tumor necrosis factor effects. *J Immunol* 146:762, 1991.

Luzzi GA, Merry AH, Newbold CI, et al.: Surface antigen expression on *Plasmodium falciparum*-infected erythrocytes is modified in α- and β-thalassemia. *J Exp Med* 173:785, 1991.

Miller LH, Good MF, Milon G: Malaria pathogenesis. *Science* 264:1878–1883, 1994.

Rener J, Carter R, Rosenberg Y, et al.: Antigamete hybridoma antibodies synergistically block transmission of malaria. *Proc Natl Acad Sci USA* 77:6797, 1980.

Riley EM, Olerup O, Troye-Blonberg M: The immune recognition of malaria antigens. *Parasitol Today* 7:6, 1991.

Rodrigues RS, Nussenzweig RS, Zavala F: The relative contribution of antibodies, CD4+, and CD8+ T cells to sporozoite-induced protection against malaria. *Immunol* 80:1–5, 1993.

Troye-Blumberg M, Perlmann P: T-cell functions in *Plasmodium falciparum* and other malarias. *Prog Allergy* 41:253, 1988.

Weidanz WP, Long CA: The role of T cells in immunity to malaria. *Prog Allergy* 41:215, 1988.

RHEUMATIC FEVER

Agarwal BI: Rheumatic heart disease unabated in developing countries. *Lancet* 2:910, 1981.

Bisno AL: The resurgence of acute rheumatic fever. *Ann Rev Med* 41:319, 1990.

Cheadle WB: Harvarian lectures on the various manifestations of the rheumatic state as exemplified in childhood and early life. *Lancet* 1:821, 871, 921, 1889.

Dajani AS, Bisno AL, Chung KJ, et al.: Prevention of rheumatic fever. *Circulation* 78:1082, 1988.

Froude J, Gibofsky A, Buskirk, et al.: Cross-reactivity between *Streptococcus* and human tissue: A model of molecular mimicry and autoimmunity. *Curr Top Microbiol Immunol* 145:5, 1989.

Gillum RF: Trends in acute rheumatic fever and chronic rheumatic heart disease: A national perspective. *Am Heart J* 111:A430, 1986.

Ginsburg I: Mechanisms of cell and tissue injury induced by group A streptococci: Relation to poststreptococcal sequelae. *J Infect Dis* 126:294–340, 419–456, 1972.

Gross L, Ehrlich JC: Studies on the myocardial Aschoff body. I. Descriptive classification of the lesions. *Am J Pathol* 10:467, 1934.

Gulizia JM, Cunningham MW, McManus BM: Immunoreactivity of antistreptococcal monoclonal antibodies to human heart valves: Evidence for multiple cross-reactive epitopes. *Am J Pathol* 138:285, 1991.

Haverkorn MJ (ed.): *Streptococcal Disease and Immunity.* New York, American Elsevier, 1974.

Husby G, van de Rijn I, Zabriskie JB, et al.: Antibodies reacting with cytoplasm of subthalamic and caudate nuclei neurons in chorea and acute rheumatic fever. *J Exp Med* 144:1094, 1976.

Kaplan El, Markowitz M: The fall and rise of rheumatic fever in the United States: A commentary. *Int J Cardiol* 21:3, 1988.

Kaplan MH, Suchy ML: Immunologic relation of streptococcal and tissue antigens. II. Cross-reaction of antisera to mammalian heart tissue with a cell wall constituent of certain strains of group A streptococci. *J Exp Med* 119:643, 1964.

Leirisalo M: Rheumatic fever: Clinical picture, differential diagnosis, and sequels. *Ann Clin Res* 9(supp. 20):1, 1977.

Markowitz M: Rheumatic fever in the eighties. *Ped Clin N Am* 33:1141, 1986.

Massell BF, Chute CG, Walker AM, et al.: Penicillin and the marked decrease in morbility and mortality from rheumatic fever in the United States. *N Engl J Med* 318:280, 1988.

Martin DR, Kick KJ: M-associated antibodies in patients with rheumatic fever. *J Med Microbiol* 17:189, 1984.

McCarty M: Lewis W. Waunamaker in the campaign against rheumatic fever. *Zbl Bakt Hyg* A260:151, 1985.

Rammelkamp CH Jr: Epidemiology of streptococcal infections. *Harvey Lect* 51:113–142, 1955, 1956.

Rijn I, Zabriske JB, McCarty M: Group A streptococcal antigens cross-reactive with myocardium: Purification of heart-reactive antibody and isolation and characterization of the streptococcal antigen. *J Exp Med* 146:579, 1977.

Stollerman GH: *Rheumatic Fever and Streptococcal Infections.* New York, Grune & Stratton, 1975.

Stollerman GH: Rheumatogenic streptococci and autoimmunity. *Clin Immunol Immunopathol* 61:131, 1991.

Tomai M, Kotb M, Majumdar G, et al.: Superantigenicity of streptococcal M protein. *J Exp Med* 172:359, 1990.

Veasy LG, Wiedmeier SE, Orsmond GS, et al.: Resurgence of acute rheumatic fever in the intermountain area of the United States. *N Engl J Med* 316:421, 1987.

Yang LC, Soprey PR, Wittner MK, et al.: Streptococcal-induced cell-mediated immune destruction of cardiac myofibrils in vitro. *J Exp Med* 146:344, 1977.

Zabriskie JB: Mimetic relationships between group A streptococci and mammalian tissues. *Adv Immunol* 7:147, 1967.

Zabriskie JB: Rheumatic fever: The interplay between host, genetics, and microbe. *Circulation* 6:1077, 1985.

ASPERGILLUS

Aisner J, Schimpff SC, Wiernick PH: Treatment of invasive aspergillosis: Relation of early diagnosis and treatment to response. *Annu Intern Med* 86:539–543, 1977.

Carbone PP, Seymour MS, Sidransky H, et al.: Secondary aspergillosis. *Annu Intern Med* 60:556–567, 1964.

English MP, Henderson AH: Significance and interpretation of laboratory tests in pulmonary aspergillosis. *J Clin Pathol* 20:832–834, 1967.

Imbeau SA, Nichols D, Flaherty D, et al.: Allergic bronchopulmonary aspergillosis. *J Allergy Clin Immunol* 62:243, 1978.

Patterson R, Greenberger PA, Radin RC, et al.: Allergic bronchopulmonary aspergillosis: Staging as an aid to management. *Am Int Med* 96:286, 1982.

Young RC, Bennett JE, Vogel CL, et al.: Aspergillosis: The spectrum of disease in 98 patients. *Medicine* 49:147, 1970.

WORMS

Maizels RM, Bundy DAP, Selkirk ME, et al.: Immunologic modulation and evasion by helminth parasites in human populations. *Nature* 365:797–805, 1993.

Maizels RM, Selkirk ME: Immunobiology of nematode antigens. In *The Biology of Parasitism*. Liss, 1988, 99285–308.

Rothwell TLW: Immune expulsion of parasitic nematodes from the alimentary tract. *Int J Patasitol* 19:139–168, 1989.

SMALLPOX, SYPHILIS, LEPROSY, TUBERCULOSIS

Orme IM, Andersen P, Boom WH: T-cell response to *Mycobacterium tuberculosis*. *J Infect Dis* 167:1481–1497, 1993.

VIRUSES

Bender BS, Croghan T, Zhang L, et al.: Transgenic mice lacking class I major histocompatibility complex-restricted T cells have delayed viral clearance and increased mortality after influenza virus challenge. *J Exp Med* 175:1143, 1992.

Kaarianen L, Ranki M: Inhibition of cell functions by RNA virus infections. *Ann Rev Microbiol* 38:91, 1984.

Mims CA: Immonopathology in virus disease. *Phil Trans R Soc Lond B* 303:189, 1983.

Russell WO: Viruses and autoimmune disease. Fifth Annual ASCP Research Symposium. *Am J Clin Pathol* 56:259, 1971.

von Pirquet CF: *Klinische Studien uber Vakzination und Vakzinal Allergie*. Leipzig, Deutickie, 1907.

VIRAL ENCEPHALITIDES OF ANIMALS

Appel MGJ, Gillespie JH: Canine distemper virus. *Virology* 11:1, 1972.

Daniels JB, Pappenheimer AM, Richardson S: Observations on encephalomyelitis of mice (D4 strain). *J Exp Med* 96:S17, 1952.

Doherty PC, Zinkernagel RM: Capacity of sensitized thymus-derived lymphocytes to induce fatal lymphocyte choriomeningitis is restricted by the H_2 gene complex. *J Immunol* 114:30, 1975.

Georgsson G, Torsteinsdottir S, Petursson G, et al.: Role of immune response in visna, a lentiviral central nervous system disease of sheep. In *Animal Models of HIV and Other Retroviral Infections*. Racs P, Letvin NL, Gluckman JC (eds.). Basel, Karger, 1993, 183–195.

Koestner A, McCullough B, Drakowka GS, et al.: Canine distemper: A virus-induced demyelinating encephalomyelitis. In *Slow Virus Diseases*. Zeman W, Lennette EH (eds.). Baltimore, Williams & Wilkins, 1974, 86.

Hotchin JE: The biology of lymphocytic choriomeningitis infection: Virus-induced immune disease. *Cold Spring Harbor Symp Quant Biol* 14:479, 1962.

Lampert PW, Garrett R, Powell H: Demyelination in allergic and Marek's disease virus-induced neuritis: Comparative electron microscopic studies. *Acta Neuropathol* (Berlin) 40:103, 1977.

Lampert PW, Sims JK, Kniazeff AJ: Mechanism of demyelination in JHM virus encephalomyelitis: Electron microscopic studies. *Acta Neuropathol* (Berlin) 24:76, 1973.

Payne LN, Frazier JA, Powell PC: Pathogenesis of Marek's disease. *Int Rev Exp Pathol* 16:59, 1976.

Stroop WG, Baringer JR: Persistent, slow, and latent viral infections. *Prog Med Virol* 28:1, 1982.

Weiner LP: Pathogenesis of demyelination induced by mouse hepatitis virus (JHM virus). *Arch Neurol* 28:298, 1973.

VIRAL ENCEPHALI-TIDES OF HUMANS

Budka H, Lassman H, Popow-Krupp T: Measles virus antigen in panencephalitis: An immunohistologic study stressing involvement in SSPE. *Acta Neuropathol* (Berlin) 56:52, 1982.

Diener TO: PrP and the nature of the scrapie agent. *Cell* 49:719, 1987.

Gajdusek DC: Unconventional viruses and the origin and disappearance of kuru. *Science* 197:943–960, 1977.

Haase AT: Pathogenesis of lentivirus infections. *Nature* 322:130, 1986.

Jacobson S, Gupta A, Mattson DH, et al.: Immunologic studies in tropical spastic paraparesis. *Ann Neurol* 27:149, 1990.

Jacobson S, Shida H, McFarlin DE, et al.: Circulating CD8+ cytotoxic T lymphocytes specific for HTLV-1 pX in patients with HTLV-1–associated neurologic disease. *Nature* 348:245, 1990.

Lampert PW: Autoimmune and virus-induced demyelinating diseases. *Am J Pathol* 91:176, 1978.

Manvelidis EE: Creutzfeldt–Jakob disease. *J Neuropathol Exp Neurol* 44:1, 1985.

Meulen V, Hall WW: Slow virus infections of the nervous system: Virologic, immunologic, and pathogenic manifestations. *J Gen Virol* 41:1, 1978.

Robertson HD, Branch AD, Dahlberg JE: Focusing on the nature of the scrapie agent. *Cell* 40:725, 1985.

Waksman B: Mechanisms in multiple sclerosis. *Nature* 318:104, 1985.

VIRAL HEPATITIS

Blumberg BS: Australia antigen and the biology of hepatitis B. *Science* 197:17, 1977.

Craske J: Hepatitis C and non-A non-B hepatitis revisited: Hepatitis E, F, and G. *J Infection* 25:243, 1992.

Deinhardt F, Jilg W: Vaccines against hepatitis. *Ann Inst Pasteur/Virol* 137E:79, 1986.

Dienstag JL: Immunopathogenesis of the extrahepatic manifestations of hepatitis infection. *Spring Immunopathol* 3:461, 1981.

Dmochowski L: Viral type A and type B hepatitis: Morphology, biology, immunology, and epidemiology. *Am J Clin Pathol* 65:741–786, 1976.

Edgington TS, Chisari FV: Immunological aspects of hepatitis B virus infection. *Am J Med Sci* 270:213, 1975.

Storch W: Immunopathology and humoral antoimmunity in chronic active hepatitis. *Scand J Gastroenterol* 23:513, 1988.

WARTS

Howley PM: The molecular biology of papillomavirus transformation. *Am J Pathol* 113:414, 1983.

Kirchner H: Immunologic surveillance and human papillomavirus. *Immunol Today* 5:272, 1984.

Lee AKY, Eisinger M: Cell-mediated (CMI) to human wart virus and wart-associated tissue antigens. *Clin Exp Immunol* 26:419, 1976.

Matthews RS, Shirodaria PV: Study of regressing warts by immunofluorescence. *Lancet* 1:689, 1973.

Morrison WL: In vitro assay of cell-mediated immunity to human wart antigen. *Br J Dermatol* 90:531, 1974.

Ogilvie MM: Serologic studies with human papova (wart) virus. *J Hyg* (Camb) 68:479, 1970.

Viac J, Thivolet J, Chardonnet Y: Specific immunity in patients suffering from recurring warts before and after repetitive intradermal tests with human papilloma virus. *Br J Dermatol* 97:365, 1977.

LYME DISEASE

Burgdorfer W: Discovery of Lyme disease spirochete: A historical review. *Zbl Bakt Hyg* A263:7–10, 1986.

Burgdorfer W, Barbour AG, Hayer SF, et al.: Lyme disease: A tick-borne spirochetosis? *Science* 216:1317–1319, 1982.

Duray PH: The surgical pathology of human Lyme disease. *Am J Surg Pathol* 11(suppl. 1):47–60, 1987.

Johnson RC, Schmid GP, Hyde FW, et al.: *Borrelia burgdorferi* sp. nov.: Etiologic agent of Lyme disease. *Int J Ays Bacteriol* 34:496–497, 1984.

Rahn DW, Malawista SE: Lyme disease: Recommendations for diagnosis and treatment. *Ann Int Med* 114:472–481, 1991.

Steere AC: Lyme disease. *N Engl J Med* 321:586–596, 1989.

Steere AC, Malawista SE, Syndman DR, et al.: Lyme arthritis: An epidemic of oligoarticular arthritis in children and adults in three Connecticut communities. *Arth Rheum* 20:7–17, 1977.

FILARIASIS

Conner DH, Palmieri JR, Gibson DW: Pathogenesis of lymphatic filariasis in man. *Parasitenkinde* 72:13, 1986.

Galindo L, Von Lichtenberg F, Baldison C: Bancroftian filariasis in Puerto Rico: Infection pattern and tissue lesions. *Am J Trop Med* 11:739, 1962.

King CL, Kumaraswami V, Poindexter RW, et al.: Immunologic tolerance in lymphatic filariasis. Diminished parasite-specific T and B lymphocyte precursor frequency in the microfilaremic state. *J Clin Invest* 89:1403, 1992.

Lie KJ: Occult filariasis and its relationship to pulmonary tropical eosinophilia. *Am J Trop Med* 11:646, 1962.

Maizels RM, Lawrence RA: Immunological tolerance: The key feature in human filariasis? *Parasitol Today* 7:271, 1991.

Nelson GS: The pathology of filarial infections. *Helminth* 35:355, 1966.

Nutman, TB: Protective immunity in lymphatic filariasis. *Exp Parasitol* 68:248–252, 1989.

Ottesen EA: Immunopathology of lymphatic filariasis in man. *Immunopathology* 2:373, 1980.

Philipp M, Davis TB, Storey N, et al.: Immunity in filariasis: Prospectives for vaccine development. *Ann Rev Microbiol* 42:685–716, 1988.

Pinder M: Loa loa: A neglected filaria. *Parasitol Today* 4:279–284, 1988.

Turner JH: Studies in filariasis in Malaya: The clinical features of filariasis due to *Wuchereria malayi*. *Trans R Soc Trop Med Hyg* 55:107, 1961.

Von Lichtenberg F: Inflammatory responses to filarial connective tissue parasites. *Parasitology* 94:S101–S122, 1987.

STRONGY-LOIDES

Cruz T, Rebokas C, Rochas H: Fatal strongyloidiosis in patients receiving corticosteroids. *N Engl J Med* 27:1093, 1966.

Gill CV, Bell DR: *Strongyloides stercoralis* infection in Far East prisoners of war. *Br Med J* 2:572, 1979.

Haque AK, Schnadig V, Rubin SA, Smith JH: Pathogenesis of human strongyloidiosis: autopsy and quantitative parasitological analysis. *Modern Pathol* 7:276–288, 1994.

Poltera AA: Fatal strongyloidiosis in Uganda. *Ann Trop Med Parasitol* 68:81, 1974.

Purtillo DT, Meyers WM, Conner DH: Fatal strongyloidiosis in immunosuppressed patients. *Am J Med* 56:488, 1974.

Rivera E, Maldonado N, Velez-Garcia E, et al.: Hyperinfection syndrome with *Strongyloides stercoralis*. *Ann Int Med* 72:199, 1970.

**IMMUNE
EVASION**

Arnon R: Immunoparasitologic parameters in schistosomiasis: A perspective view of a vaccine-orientated immunochemist. *Vaccine* 9:379, 1991.

Bernards A: Antigenic variation of trypanosomes. *Biochem Biophys Acta* 824:1, 1984.

Bloom BR: Games parasites play: How parasites evade immune surveillance. *Nature* 279:21, 1979.

Bogdan C, Rollinghoff M, Solbach W: Evasion strategies of *Leishmania* parasites. *Parasitol Today* 6:183–187, 1990.

Capron A, Dessaint J-P: Survival strategies of parasites in their immunocompetent hosts. *Adv Neuroimmunol* 2:181, 1992.

Craig PS: Immunology of human hydatid disease. *ISI Atlas Sci: Immunology* 95–100, 1988.

Cruse JM, Lewis RE: Contemporary concepts of antigenic variation. *Contr Microbiol Immunol* 8:1–19, 1987.

Davidson RA: Immunology of parasitic infections. *Med Clin N Amer* 69:751, 1985.

Donelson JE, Turner MJ: How the trypanosome changes its coat. *Scientific Am* 252:44, 1985.

Frank I, Friedman HM: A novel function of the herpes simplex virus type 1 Fc receptor: Participation in bipolar bridging of antiviral immunoglobulin. *G J Virol* 63:4479–4488, 1989.

Gooding LR: Viruses that counteract host immune defenses. *Cell* 71:5, 1992.

Halsted SB: Immune enhancement of viral infection. *Prog Allergy* 31:301, 1982.

Isaacs SN, Kotwal GJ, Moss B: Vaccinia virus complement-control protein prevents antibody-dependent complement-enhanced neutralization of infectivity and contributes to virulence. *Proc Natl Acad Sci USA* 89:628, 1992.

Johnson RT, Griffin DE, Moench TR: Pathogenesis of measles immunodeficiency and encephalomyelitis: Parallels to AIDS. *Microbiol Pathogen* 4:169–174, 1988.

Kennedy MW: Genetic control of the immune repertoire in nematode infections. *Parasitol Today* 5:316–324, 1989.

Medici MA: The immunoprotective niche: A new pathogenic mechanism for syphilis, the systemic mycoses, and other infectious diseases. *J Theor Biol* 36:617, 1972.

Moll H, Fucks H, Blank C, et al.: Langerhans' cells transport *Leishmania major* from the infected skin to the draining lymph node for presentation to antigen-specific T cells. *Eur J Immunol* 23:1595–1601, 1993.

Musher DM: Infections caused by *Streptococcus pneumoniae*: Clinical spectrum, pathogenesis, immunity, and treatment. *Clin Inf Dis* 14:801, 1992.

Pays R, Steinert M: Control of antigen gene expression in African trypanosomes. *Annu Rev Genet* 22:107–126, 1988.

Pearce EJ, Sher A: Mechanisms of immune evasion in schistosomiasis. *Contr Microbiol Immunol* 8:219–232, 1987.

Reed SG, Scott P: T-cell and cytokine responses in leismaniasis. *Curr Opin Immunol* 5:524–531, 1993.

Rinaldo CR Jr: Modulation of major histocompatibility complex antigen expression by viral infection. *Am J Pathol* 144:637–650, 1994.

Rossman MG: The canyon hypothesis. *Viral Immunol* 2:143–161, 1989.

Scott P, Pearce E, Cheever AW, et al.: Role of cytokines and CD4+ T-cell subsets in the regulation of parasite immunity and disease. *Immunol Rev* 112:161, 1989.

Smith GL: Vaccinia virus glycoproteins and immune evasion. *J Gen Virol* 74:1725–1740, 1993.

Upton C, Mossman K, McFadden G: Encoding of a homologue of the INF-γ receptor by myxoma virus. *Science* 258:1369, 1992.

Warren S: The present impossibility of eradicating the ever-present worm. *Rev Inf Dis* 4:955, 1982.

26

Immunization

Since prehistoric times, it has been observed that a previous natural exposure to an infectious agent would produce a state of specific resistance to reinfection (**active immunity**). Many procedures for intentionally inducing immunity (**immunization**) have been developed and are used prophylactically, while others are in the process of being made available for general or specific use. Because of active immunization, many infections that were considered part of growing up in the Western world 30 or 40 years ago have become so infrequent that physicians trained in the last few years have had no experience with these natural infections personally or professionally, and some major infectious diseases, such as smallpox, have been eliminated entirely. In addition, passive transfer of immunity has been applied successfully in more limited situations (**passive immunity**). On the other hand, some diseases, such as tuberculosis and syphilis, which were thought to be under control, are increasing in incidence. Further development of vaccines for such diseases should have a high priority. The application of molecular engineering to construction of vaccines has great promise in this regard.

Passive Immunity

The transfer of immune products (humoral or cellular) from a sensitized person to a nonimmunized person produces a temporary passive state of specific immunity in the recipient. Passive immunity occurs naturally in fetal life. Maternal antibodies cross the placenta and provide specific immunity for the newborn until about 3 to 4 months of age, when the infant begins to produce its own antibody (see Chapter 27). Historically, one of the first methods to attempt to produce specific immunity in humans was by the passive transfer of antiserum from other species.

HUMORAL ANTIBODY

Polyclonal Antibodies

Two forms of passive transfer of conventional humoral antibodies are used–pooled human immunoglobulin in which specific antibody is present (Table 26–1) and immunoglobulins from serum of immunized animals. There are three designated uses for intravenous administration of pooled human immunoglobulin (IVIG): (1) Replacement therapy for primary and secondary immunodeficiency diseases; (2) specific passive immunotherapy for infectious diseases; and (3) management of inflammatory or autoimmune diseases, such as Kawasaki syndrome and idiopathic thrombocytopenic purpura. IVIG has also been shown to be effective in reducing infections in high-risk neonates and in preventing postoperative infections. The use of passive immunoglobulin preparations for treatment of humoral immune deficiency diseases is discussed in Chapter 27, Immune Deficiency Diseases (see Table 27–12 for a listing of commercial immunoglobulin preparations).

For transfer of antibodies against specific infectious diseases, horse antiserum was first used after exposure to toxins of botulism, diphtheria, and tetanus. Although horse antitoxin neutralizes the toxins or the infectious agent because the host responds to the horse serum proteins by forming precipitating antibody, it also causes serum sickness (see Chapter 13). The incidence and severity of the serum sickness reaction has been reduced somewhat by using fractionated horse serum, thus eliminating many of the immunogenic serum proteins. However, horse immunoglobulin preparations are still strongly immunogenic, and should be used only in life-threatening circumstances and only after careful testing fails to detect a preexisting allergy to horse serum.

Passive serotherapy for snake bites began in the late 1800s, when Calmette produced antivenom against *Naja*. In 1899, commercial

TABLE 26–1. IMMUNE GLOBULIN PREPARATIONS AVAILABLE FOR PASSIVE IMMUNIZATION AND INDICATIONS FOR USE*

Pooled Human Immune Globulin	Specific Human Immune Globulin	Specific Equine Immune Globulin
Humoral immune deficiency	Hepatitis B	Black widow spider venom
Hepatitis A	Pertussis	Botulism toxin
Measles	Rabies	Diphtheria toxin
	Rh isoimmunization	Snake venoms
	Tetanus	
	Vaccinia	
	Varicella-zoster	

*For emergencies, call Centers for Disease Control, 404-329-3311 (day) or 404-329-3644 (night).

antivenoms were produced in the United States by the H. K. Muflord company. This was followed by a wider program for production of antiserum for therapeutic use in the early 1900s by Vita Brazil at the Institute Butantan in Sao Paulo, Brazil, where there were nearly 3,000 deaths per year from crotaline snake bites. Specific antisera proved to be effective in alleviating the symptoms of bites of snakes native to Brazil. These antisera served as the model for passive antibody treatment. Of the 26,786 snake bites reported to the Brazilian Ministry of Health between June 1986 and December 1987, only 181 deaths were reported.

Since the early 1950s, specific passive immunity is transferred using immunoglobulin preparations (eg, cold ethanol fractionation) from human plasma pools with high titers of specific antibody. For instance, death from cytomegalovirus (CMV) infection in immunosuppressed kidney transplant patients can be prevented by passive transfer of anti-CMV immunoglobulin. Pooled human immunoglobulin is effective after exposure to hepatitis, measles, or rubella (German measles) during the first trimester of pregnancy. Although cellular immunity may be required to eliminate virus-infected cells, passively transferred antibody is effective if administered shortly after exposure to hepatitis virus, and for measles, polio, rabies, smallpox, and varicella.

Monoclonal Antibodies. With the development of human monoclonal antibodies to infectious agents and their products, it can be predicted that specific passive transfer of monoclonal antibodies will not only replace the pooled immunoglobulin preparations now being used but will also be applied to treat a variety of human diseases not now treated by passive antibody transfer. Thus, human monoclonal antibodies could be used for treatment of tetanus, diphtheria, etc., as well as for other infectious diseases.

One new approach is the use of monoclonal antibodies to treat endotoxin (lipopolysaccharide [LPS]) shock that is responsible for deaths from infections with gram negative bacteria. Human monoclonal antibodies to gram-negative endotoxins have been produced that react with the core lipid A component of the toxin. These antibodies are able to block reaction of LPS with the complement and coagulation systems, as well as inhibit LPS-induced release of cytokines (tumor necrosis factor [TNF]) in vitro. However, clinical trials of two commercially produced antibodies have given inconsistent results, and have been discontinued. Monoclonal antibodies to TNF have been used in animal studies and may be available for clinical trials soon.

Other human monoclonal antibodies to *Haemophilus influenzae* type B capsular polysaccharide, pneumococcal polysaccharide, *Mycobacterium leprae*, hepatitis A and B viruses, *herpes simplex*, measles, chlamydia, malaria, HTLV, HIV, etc., are being developed for therapeutic use. The function of such antibodies is being enhanced by genetic engineering to produce hybrid antibodies, toxin and drug-linked antibodies, bispecific antibodies, anti-idiotypic antibodies and antibodies with enzyme activity (abzymes).

With advances in molecular engineering, methods are being devised to create antibodies in vitro using synthetic nucleic acids cloned into bacteriophages that code for sequences of antibody-hypervariable polypeptide chains. By mutation and selection of the bacteriophages, it may be possible to obtain combinations of genes that provide different antigen-binding specificities and produce a library of "antibodies" without immunization of animals. Such procedures could generate an endless variety of engineered antibodies for clinical use.

CELLULAR IMMUNITY

The passive transfer of cellular immune reactions using living cells is generally not satisfactory in humans because of immune rejection of the transferred cells. Passive transfer of cellular sensitivity may be accomplished if the recipient is unable to reject transferred living lymphoid cells or through use of a product of sensitized cells known as transfer factor. The former is possible with transfers between identical twins. Cellular reactivity may also be transferred if lymphoid cells are given to a recipient who is incapable of reacting because of an immunologic deficiency. However, the transferred cells may react to the recipient's tissues (graft-versus-host reaction) (see Chapter 23). Successful cell transfer depends on histocompatibility matching of donor and recipient. Transfer factor has been used with limited success in some human diseases, such as chronic mucocutaneous candidiasis. A recent development is the ability to transfer persistent immunity to immunodeficient humans using CD8+ T-cell clones specific for CMV isolated from allogeneic bone marrow donors. The use of clones of specifically reactive T cells cultivated in vitro and then transferred to immune deficient patients has promise for a wide application. (For a further discussion of the use of lymphoid cells or cell products as therapy for immune deficiencies, see Chapter 27; for cancer therapy, see Chapter 30; for bone marrow transplantation, see Chapter 23).

Active Immunity

Active immunity occurs upon recovery from a naturally acquired infection. Active immunity may be induced intentionally by inoculation, ingestion, or inhalation of a modified form of an infectious organism or a product of an organism so that the immunizing material retains the antigenicity of the intact organism but does not have the capacity to cause disease. The types of artificial immunogens that have been used in the past include low doses of a product of the organism; altered products, such as chemically modified toxins (toxoid); antibody-neutralized toxin; killed organisms; low doses of virulent organisms given by nonpathogenic or relatively innocuous routes; living attenuated (avirulent) strains; and organisms altered in such a way that they can infect but cannot complete a complex life cycle (eg, immunization of cattle against lungworm). Attenuated strains are produced by culturing virulent organisms in vitro or in unnatural hosts so that the organisms are no longer pathogenic for the natural host but retain the antigenic specificity of the virulent strains. More recently, genetically altered organisms, such as viruses lacking genes required for optimal replication, have been used experimentally to induce immunity to the native virus (see HIV vaccines, Chapter 29). The use of adjuvants to enhance specific active immunization and to direct antigen processing to preferentially induce antibody or cell-mediated immunity is discussed in Chapter 28. Recent developments in molecular biology and immunology have added new approaches to vaccine development, such as genetically engineered products, recombinant or idiotype vaccines, and direct innoculation of DNA (see below).

PROPHY-LACTIC IMMUNIZATION

The Classic Vaccine: Smallpox Variolation and Vaccination

Vaccination against smallpox (variola) is historically one of the first active immunization approaches used and represents one of the most spectacular successes in control of an infectious disease. Smallpox was once one of the most lethal and disfiguring diseases of humans. In ancient China, names were not given to infants until they had survived smallpox; so many children died from smallpox that families would run out of favorite names. The Chinese noted that milder forms of smallpox could be induced using infected tissue from people with a relatively benign course of the disease. From this observation, they developed the first method of artificial active immunization. A powder from smallpox crusts was made into a snuff that was inhaled into the nose. Although this produced fatal smallpox in up to 1 out of 50 exposed individuals, the course of the disease induced in most individuals was generally much milder than that in the naturally acquired disease. Although this would be an unacceptable result by present-day standards, it was a great improvement over the fatality rate of the natural infection. In the Western world, this process became known as **variolation.**

The introduction of variolation in the Western world is largely attributed to the efforts of Lady Mary Worthy Montague, who was the wife of the British Ambassador to Turkey. She learned of the practice of variolation in Constantinople. Infected tissue from individuals with mild forms of smallpox was injected into young uninfected people. The inoculated individuals developed "mild" disease and recovered. She returned to England and persuaded King George I to conduct "clinical trials" on prisoners at Newgate Prison. The trials were successful and variolation become a regular practice in England. In the United States, variolation was introduced by Zabdiel Boylston in Boston in 1721 at the urging of Cotton Mather. During the Revolutionary War, smallpox broke out among the American army late in 1775. However, the disease was controlled by variolation, and by September 1776, the army was again prepared to take the field free of smallpox.

In 1770, Edward Jenner noted that milkmaids, who contracted cowpox, had a mild smallpoxlike disease, but never developed any of the serious manifestations of smallpox. In 1796, he inoculated a healthy young boy with cowpox (**vaccinia**) from the sore of a dairy maid. The boy developed cowpox, which healed and was subsequently found to be resistant to challenge with smallpox. In 1807, a National Vaccine Establishment was set up in London to evaluate and compare the results of vaccination with those of variolation. By 1840, compulsory vaccination was established by law, and variolation was made illegal.

Vaccinia virus has low pathogenicity for humans and contains antigens that cross-react with smallpox virus. Dermal inoculation induces cell-mediated immunity (TCTL) that results in a cytotoxic skin reaction at the site of inoculation approximately eight days after application (see Fig. 15–6). This long-lasting cellular sensitivity protects the vaccinated person against smallpox. The term **vaccination**, now used to cover all kinds of protective immunization, is derived from the use of the vaccinia virus.

Through the application of worldwide vaccination programs monitored by the World Health Organization, the once great killer disease of smallpox has been eliminated. A few cases of smallpox were reported in Somalia in 1976, and the last known case was diagnosed in October 1977. In December 1979, an independent scientific commission certified global eradication of smallpox. The WHO continues to monitor rumors and coordinate the investigation of suspected cases, but during the last twelve years, all suspected cases turned out to be chickenpox, some skin disease other than smallpox, or a mistake in reporting. Inoculation with vaccinia virus sometimes leads to complications, such as postvaccinial encephalitis or disseminated vaccinia in a small but significant number of vaccinated individuals. Because the untoward consequences of vaccination are now more significant than the naturally occurring disease, vaccination against smallpox has been discontinued. By 1984, all countries had ceased smallpox vaccination of the general public. Until 1987, the WHO maintained a stock of vaccine sufficient to immunize 300 million people, but this reserve is no longer maintained. Since the virus gene pool has been cloned in bacterial plasmids, which provide sufficient material to solve future research

TABLE 26–2. PROPHYLACTIC IMMUNIZATION FOR HUMAN INFECTIOUS DISEASES

Disease/Organisms	Antigen Preparation	Indication	Immunization Route	Results
TOXOIDS				
Diphtheria	Formaldehyde-treated toxin	All children All adults	Intramuscular	Satisfactory
Botulism	Formaldehyde-treated toxin	On exposure	Intramuscular	Needs improvement
Tetanus	Formaldehyde-treated toxin	All children All adults	Intramuscular	Satisfactory
KILLED ORGANISMS				
Pertussis	Thiomersalate-treated	All children	Intramuscular	Needs improvement
Typhoid[a]	Phenol inactivated	Travelers[a] on exposure	Subcutaneous, intramuscular, oral	Needs improvement
Cholera	Phenol-treated	Travelers	Subcutaneous	Needs improvement
Plague	Formalin-killed	High risk groups	Intramuscular	Needs improvement
Anthrax	Phenol-treated	On exposure High risk group	Subcutaneous	Needs improvement
POLYSACCHARIDES				
Meningococcus	Quadrivalent Polysaccharide	Endemic areas (Africa) travelers	Subcutaneous	Needs improvement/short duration of protection in infants
Pneumococcus	Polysaccharide (23 types)	Susceptible individuals Elderly (>65 years)	Intramuscular	Needs improvement/ antigenicity variable
Haemophilus influenzae	Polysaccharide Protein Conjugates (DTP-Hib)	Infants and children	Intramuscular	Needs improvement

ATTENUATED ORGANISMS

Poliomyelitis[b]	Monkey tissue culture (live)	All children	Oral	Satisfactory
Measles (rubeola)	Chicken tissue culture (live)	All children; Adults born after 1956	Subcutaneous	Satisfactory
Mumps	Chicken tissue culture (live)	All children; Adults born after 1957	Subcutaneous	Satisfactory
Rubella	Human tissue culture (live)	All children	Subcutaneous	
Yellow fever[c]	Egg tissue culture (live 7D Strain)	Travelers (endemic area)	Subcutaneous	
Influenza	Egg tissue culture (4 strains) purified antigens	High-risk groups; Elderly	Subcutaneous	Satisfactory
Varicella	Tissue culture/attenuated strain	Children with leukemia	Subcutaneous	Satisfactory
Adenovirus	Live virus/enteric capsules	Military	Oral	Satisfactory
Smallpox	Vaccinia (cowpox) virus	Laboratory markers	Intradermal or subcutaneous	Needs improvement
Tuberculosis	Bacillus Calmette—Guérin	High-risk groups	Intradermal	Needs improvement

KILLED PARTIALLY ATTENUATED ORGANISMS

Typhus	Chick embryo culture	Travelers[a]	Subcutaneous	Satisfactory
Rabies	Rhesus lung tissue culture/inactivated with β-propiolactone	On exposure, high-risk groups	Intramuscular/subcutaneous	Needs improvement
Cutaneous leishmaniasis	Controlled route and dose	Virulent organisms, exposed children	Intradermal	Needs improvement
Hepatitis B	Recombinant protein hepatitis B[a], HB_sAg	High-risk groups; All children	Intramuscular	Needs improvement

a Live alternated oral vaccine also available.

b Inactivated vaccine (el PV) recommended for primary vaccination.

c Yellow fever vaccines must be approved by WHO.

d Formaldehyde-infective virus is also licensed, but is no longer produced in USA.

and diagnostic problems, it was decided that there is no need to maintain stocks of viable virus. Vaccinia virus is available for experimental use and for production of vaccinia vectors for carrying the DNA of other organisms (recombinant vaccines). Smallpox virus is now maintained in only two WHO-supervised laboratories under high security. However, the possibility that smallpox could be used for biological warfare has led to recommendations that military personnel continue to be vaccinated. There is an ongoing debate as to whether or not all remaining repositories of smallpox virus should be destroyed. At the time of this writing, the final decision has been postponed.

STANDARD IMMUNIZATION SCHEDULES

Some diseases for which active prophylactic immunization is available are listed in Table 26–2. Widely employed vaccines include those against diphtheria, whooping cough (pertussis), tetanus, measles (rubeola), poliomyelitis, rubella, and mumps. Immunizations in clinical practice are scheduled as a compromise between immunization efficiency and convenience of administration, that is, to obtain safe, adequate protection with a minimum number of visits to the doctor. Most immunizations usually require two to three applications and occasional booster injections.

Childhood Immunization

Children are usually immunized with diphtheria toxoid, killed pertussis organisms, and tetanus toxoid by three injections of the combined antigens (DPT) between 2 and 6 months of age, with another booster at 18 to 24 months. Infants younger than 2 months of age develop poor immune responses. Oral polio vaccine (OPV) is given at 2, 4, and 18 months. One inoculation with attenuated measles, mumps, and rubella virus (MMR) and *H. influenzae* polysaccharide protein conjugates[1] (HIG) given at 15 months. For more detailed immunization recommendations, see Tables 26–3 and 26–4.

TABLE 26–3. CHILDHOOD IMMUNIZATION SCHEDULE RECOMMENDED BY U.S. PUBLIC HEALTH SERVICE JANUARY 1995

Vaccine	Birth	2 months	4 months	6 months	12[†] months	15 months	18 months	4–6 years	11–12 years	14–16 years
Hepatitis B[§]	HB-1	HB-2		HB-3						
Diphtheria, Tetanus, Pertussis[¶]		DTP	DTP	DTP	DTP or DTaP at ≥ 15 months			DTP or DTaP	Td	
H. influenzae type b[**]		Hib	Hib	Hib	Hib					
Poliovirus		OPV	OPV	OPV				OPV		
Measles, Mumps, Rubella[††]					MMR			MMR or MMR		

There is some variation in recommendations. For example, the third *Haemophilus* B vaccination may be given as a four-dose schedule or a three-dose schedule. Hepatitis B vaccination may be given at birth in endemic areas. DTP = diphtheria, tetanus, pertussis; aP = acellular pertussis; Td = Tetanus and diphtheria; OPV = oral polio vaccine

From CDC MMWR 43960, 1995.

TABLE 26–4. RECOMMENDED IMMUNIZATION SCHEDULES FOR PERSONS > 7
YEARS OF AGE NOT IMMUNIZED AT THE RECOMMENDED TIME IN EARLY INFANCY

Timing	Vaccines	Comments
First visit	Td#1, OPV#1, MMR, HBV	OPV not recommended for persons > 18 years of age
2 months later	Td#2, OPV#2, HBV	OPV#2 may be given as early as 6 weeks after OPV#1
8–14 months	Td#3, OPV#3, HBV	OPV#3 may be given as early as 6 weeks after OPV#2
10 years after	Td	Repeat every 10 years Td#3

Td, tetanus, and diphtheria toxoids absorbed for adults; OPV, oral polio vaccine; MMR, measles, mumps, and rubella live vaccine; HBV, recombinant hepatitis B surface antigen.

It is difficult to overestimate the effect that childhood immunizations have had on the general health of immunized populations. For example, in the United States, only 11 cases of diphtheria were reported in the period 1985–89, and these were in unvaccinated individuals. Worldwide, the number of cases of tetanus has decreased dramatically. An example of the consequences of a breakdown in childhood vaccination is the increase in the reported number of cases of diphtheria in the new independent states of the former Soviet Union from 839 in 1989 to 47,802 in 1994 mostly in children aged 4 to 10 years. In the United States, there were 250,000 cases of measles each year prior to introduction of vaccination for measles in 1963. In 1990, even though immunization coverage was not complete, the number of cases was 22,000. It is estimated that from 1963 to 1981, the number of deaths prevented from measles was almost 5,000 and the savings in health care costs and lost work days was $4.5 million.

Adult Immunization

Vaccine-preventable diseases occur in adults who have not been immunized as children. Unless there is some contraindication, such as immunosuppressive therapy or immune deficiency disease, adults should be immunized with at least seven vaccines–especially those at high risk, such as the elderly (Table 26–5). Of particular importance is the fact that 50% to 75% of persons at high risk for influenza or who die from influenza, and who have been cared for in a healthcare institution or as an outpatient, did not receive vaccination against influenza. These clearly represent a "missed opportunity" for simple and inexpensive preventive medicine.

IMMUNIZATION FOR OTHER INFECTIOUS DISEASES

Immunization for diseases such as cholera, typhoid, typhus, and yellow fever is not done routinely but is indicated for a person traveling to areas where the disease is endemic or for high-risk groups. For example, use of acetone-treated or heat-killed organisms for typhoid vaccination has

TABLE 26–5. IMMUNOLOGIC RECOMMENDATIONS FOR ADULTS 18 YEARS OF AGE AND OLDER

Vaccine	Major Indications*	Major Precautions*
Influenza vaccine	Adults with high-risk conditions, residents of nursing homes or other chronic care facilities, medical care personnel, healthy persons age 65 years or older	History of anaphylactic hypersensitivity to egg ingestion
Pneumococcal polysaccharide vaccine (23-valent)	Adults who are at increased risk of pneumococcal disease and its complications because of underlying health conditions; healthy older adults, especially those age 65 years or older	Vaccine safety in pregnant women has not been evaluated; revaccination is not recommended
Hepatitis B vaccine	Adults at increased risk of occupational, environmental, social, or family exposure to hepatitis B	Pregnancy should not be considered a contraindication if the woman is otherwise eligible
Tetanus–diphtheria toxoid	All adults at mid-decade ages	History of a neurologic or hypersensitivity reaction after a previous dose
Measles vaccine	Adults born after 1956 without verification of live measles vaccine on or after first birthday, physician-diagnosed measles, or laboratory evidence of immunity; susceptible travelers to foreign countries	Pregnancy; history of anaphylactic reaction following egg ingestion or receipt of neomycin; immuno-suppression
Rubella vaccine	Adults without verification of live vaccine on or after first birthday or laboratory evidence of immunity; susceptible travelers to foreign countries	Pregnancy; history of anaphylactic reaction following receipt of neomycin; immunosuppression

*Refer to appropriate recommendations for more details.

From Williams WW, et al.: Immunization policies and vaccine coverage among adults. *Ann Intern Med* 108:616, 1988.

resulted in great reduction of cases in the military but induces marked local inflammation and febrile reactions. Attempts are being made to improve this vaccine through the use of attenuated organisms. Work is also underway to produce and evaluate immunogens for essentially every known infectious disease including, but not limited to, gonorrhea; syphilis; hepatitis A, C, and E; mycoplasma; rotaviruses; streptococci; respiratory syncytial virus; cytomegalovirus; and, of course, HIV and HTLV. Attempts have been made to immunize patients with treated organisms grown from cultures of the patient's own tissues (autogenous vaccines), but such procedures have not been clinically rewarding. Critically important in vaccine development is the availability of *in vitro* culture methods to produce an attenuated strain or enough of the agent for chemical modification. The breakthrough in the production of both attenuated and killed poliomyelitis vaccines was the development of *in vitro* conditions for culture of the virus. Regardless of the care taken to produce specific antigens for immunizations, it is virtually impossible to rule out dangerous contaminating materials if tissue culture methods are used. For instance, although it was impossible to know at the time, the original Salk polio vaccine was contaminated with SV40 virus, which could be responsible for the production of slow virus infections. However, there is no evidence that this contaminant produced any untoward effects. The application of modern techniques of immunology and molecular engineering now allows development of a "second generation" of vaccines with seemingly unlimited potential (see below). It is not possible to cover all of the recent progress made in vaccine development in this text. Some examples of the present state of the art for different vaccines will be presented after briefly reviewing the new approaches to vaccine production.

New Approaches to Vaccine Production

Four new approaches now being used for vaccine development are: (1) In vitro synthesis of immunogenic peptides, (2) cloning of DNA for recombinant immunogens, (3) linking of B-cell epitopes to highly immunogenic carriers (conjugates), and (4) use of anti-idiotypes as immunogens. The use of adjuvants to increase or modify the specific immune response is covered in Chapter 28.

SYNTHETIC VACCINES

In order to synthesize antigenic peptides, the amino acid sequences of the epitope recognized by the immune system must be identified, and the peptide synthesized and administered to the responding animal in an immunogenic form. The identification of epitope peptides can be accomplished by direct analysis of the amino acid sequence of the protein or deduced from the cDNA sequence for the protein. For instance, the 220 amino acid primary structure of hepatitis B surface antigen was determined from the sequence of bases in the cDNA for HBsAg. The tertiary structure was deduced, and candidate peptides for epitopes for immunization selected. The selection process includes:

1. The presence of charged amino acids that permit solubility.
2. Predicted presence of sequences on the surface of the antigenic molecule.
3. Peptides larger than 10 amino acid residue in length (small peptides tend to be poorly immunogenic).
4. The presence of a proline residue (usually present at bends in the mature polypeptide chain and important for the tertiary conformation.
5. The presence of an amino acid residue that will allow coupling to a carrier, such as cysteine.

The selected peptides are synthesized by automated methods. The peptides are then tested for immunogenicity by immunization of rabbits or other experimental animals with or without coupling to carriers. In this manner, immunogenic peptides of HBsAg, foot and mouth disease virus, and the hemagglutinin antigen of influenza A virus have been identified and tested in animals. So far, the results are encouraging but application to man requires considerably more development. In the case of influenza A hemagglutinin, antibodies to common peptides not in the four dominant strain-specific antigenic domains have been produced. This observation suggests that immunization to a common sequence conserved among different virus strains might be impossible. Some bacterial antigens that are under development are *Streptococcus pyogenes* M protein, diphtheria toxin, *Vibrio cholerae* toxin β-subunit, the heat-labile toxin of *Escherichia coli, Shigella* toxin β-subunit, as well as peptides of HIV (see Chapter 32). A major theoretical problem is the ability of these engineered antigens to mimic the conformation of the naturally produced antigenic proteins. Thus, it may be critical to construct peptides that reflect the conformational-dependent determinants, not just sequential determinants.

RECOMBINANT VACCINES

Expression of cloned DNA for immunogenic molecules in bacterial, viral, or other vectors offers unlimited potential for vaccine production. Recombinant subunit vaccines may be produced by cloning portions of the genes of pathogens that encode critical antigens into plasmids and then producing large amounts of the noninfectious antigen in the appropriate bacteria or yeast. Recombinant plasmids grown in tissue culture cells have been used to produce large amounts of the envelope glycoprotein of HIV. A subunit vaccine for hepatitis B has been produced from a purified recombinant HBsAg expressed in yeast or Chinese hamster ovary cells. The antigen forms particles that can be absorbed onto aluminum hydroxide to make a potent vaccine.

The combined use of cloned genes for selected antigens of pathogens and special delivery methods may allow induction of cellular immunity in such diseases as leprosy, syphilis, and AIDS, for which cell-mediated immunity (CMI) is believed to be the effective immune mechanism. For example, it may be possible to induce T_{CTL} cells by direct transfection of animals with DNA coding a viral protein. Plasmid DNA-encoding influenza A nucleoprotein produced T_{CTL} cells when injected into the quadriceps muscle of mice, and the mice were protected against challenge with influenza A. In addition, vaccinia virus vectors may preferentially induce T_{CTL} cells, whereas BCG vectors may direct antigen to processing cells for T_{DTH}. (See Chapter 28 for more details on vaccinia and bacillus Calmette–Guérin [BCG] vectors). Vaccinia and other viruses (adenoviruses, herpesviruses) offer genomes that can be easily manipulated through the use of restriction enzymes to construct recombinants that will synthesize the desired polypeptide product and at the same time provide a highly immunogenic, nonpathologic carrier that can amplify the foreign gene product by limited viral replication in vivo. Vaccinia virus-vectored vaccine candidates include genital herpes; infectious mononucleosis; CMV; hepatitis A, B, C, and E; AIDS; respiratory syncytial disease; influenza; rabies; Lassa fever; dengue fever; malaria; schistosomiasis;

HIV; and others. Enthusiasm for the use of vaccinia vectors in man has been tempered because of possible complications. However, inactivation of the thymidine kinase gene of the virus markedly decreases neurovirulence, thus rendering recombinants much less hazardous than the wild-type virus. A recombinant vaccinia virus–rabies vaccine that expresses the rabies G glycoprotein has been effective in producing protective immunity after a single oral immunization. Field trials are now underway using this vaccine in bats for the vaccination of animals, such as foxes, skunks, or raccoons, that propagate rabies and spread the virus in the wild. BCG, a living attenuated tubercle bacillus, may also be used as a vaccine vehicle delivering protective antigens of multiple pathogens, and may preferentially induce T_{DTH}-mediated delayed hypersensitivity (see Chapter 28). Expression vectors carrying the regulatory sequences for the major heat-shock proteins of BCG have been developed and allow the construction of recombinant BCG strains that can elicit long-lasting humoral and cellular immunity in mice.

CONJUGATE VACCINES

Conjugate vaccines are based on the covalent attachment of bacterial carbohydrate antigens or peptide haptens to selected carrier proteins. In addition, several proteins may be conjugated together to increase immunogenicity through carrier effects and to produce polyvalent vaccines. Polysaccharide antigens of *Streptococcus pneumoniae, Neisseria meningitidis, Escherichia coli, Pseudomonas aeruginosa*, and *Haemophilus influenzae* are generally considered as T-independent antigens. However, complexing these antigens with carrier proteins recognized by helper T cells may significantly increase their immunogenicity. For instance, acidic hydrazine derivatives of various proteins have been conjugated to the *H.influenzae* type b polysaccharides and tested by immunization of animals. The carrier protein increases the immune response to the carbohydrate antigen and a booster response is obtained upon reinjection. One of the carriers tested was diphtheria toxoid, and the results were such that this is now the preferred immunogen for vaccination against *H. influenzae*. Conjugate vaccines of groups A, B, and C meningococcal polysaccharides and tetanus toxoid are also under development. Such conjugates stimulate high titers of IgG antibody, whereas the polysaccharide alone tends to stimulate IgM antibodies, and are much more immunogenic in young infants and immunosuppressed individuals.

IDIOTYPE VACCINES

Antiidiotypic antibodies that react with the paratope of an antibody to an infectious organism may be used to immunize animals to produce an anti-antiidiotype that reproduces the paratope of the original antibody. By such immunization the anti-antiidiotype will have paratope specificity for the epitope on the original infectious agent. In experimental systems, antiidiotypic antibodies were the first to induce protective antibodies to *Trypanosoma rhodesiense* in mice, and antiidiotypic antibodies against antiphosphorylcholine known to protect against lethal streptococcal pneumonia infection have been successful in immunizing mice to resist infection. Delayed hypersensitivity to herpes simplex has been induced in mice using rabbit antimouse idiotype sera. The list of experimental infections for which antiidiotypic immunization has proved to be effective now includes hepatitis B, poliovirus, rabies, *Listeria monocytogenes, E. coli, S. pneumoniae, Schistosoma mansoni, T. rhodesiense*, and others. Finally, monoclonal antibodies to specific epitopes of infectious agents have been shown to be effective in producing temporary protection by passive transfer. Each of these approaches offer great expectations for future development of artificial immunization against infectious diseases.

Development of New Vaccines

Active development programs are underway applying new technologies for vaccines against essentially every infectious disease of man and animals. Each infectious disease has its individual host–parasite interaction that must be understood in order to begin to produce an effective vaccine. Some of the problems in developing vaccines and approaches to solving them will now be presented by a few illustrative examples.

BACTERIAL

Pertussis

There has been some controversy over the use of the pertussis component of the DPT vaccine. Pertussis (whooping cough) is a devastating respiratory disease in young children, and pertussis vaccination has been associated with a substantial decline in the prevalence of whooping cough. In the United States, the incidence of whooping cough dropped from a reported high of 157 cases per 100,000 in the 1930's to 1.4 per 100,000 in 1988. However, a clear decline in the prevalence of the disease had occurred prior to the introduction of pertussis vaccination in the 1940s, raising some doubts as to the role of the vaccine in the decrease in incidence. Pertussis vaccination was discontinued in Japan when two children died within 24 hours of receiving DPT, and the incidence of pertussis rose from fewer than 1,000 reported cases per year to 13,105, with 41 deaths. There is encephalopathy in 1 per 100,000 vaccine doses and permanent brain damage associated with approximately 1 in 300,000 injections. However, the rates are such that these effects could be contributed to coincidental events. In the British courts, the chief justice ruled that there was no evidence that brain damage is caused by the pertussis vaccine. Even if use of the vaccine is related to the brain damage, the continued use of pertussis vaccination is recommended as it is projected that far more children would suffer serious complications from pertussis infection if pertussis vaccinations were not done.

Although complications appear to be exceedingly rare following pertussis vaccination, there is an ongoing effort to produce a better vaccine that would eliminate the possibility for these complications. Clinical trials of "acellular" pertussis vaccines demonstrated that the major protective antigen is the protein exotoxin, called the pertussis toxin (PTX). PTX is composed of five distinct subunits (S1, S2, S3, S4, and S5); the catalytic (toxic) and dominant protective epitope is located in the S1 subunit. In this subunit, the domain bounded by tyrosine-8 and proline-15 is crucial for toxic activity. Using site-specific mutation, a substitution of lysine for arginine at position 9 produced a polypeptide that retained antigenic activity but had lost toxic activity. Using recombinant proteins, it has been possible to reconstruct the five-unit hexameric quaternary structure using recombinant mutated S1 with native S2, S3, S4, and S5 to produce a **holotoxoid**. This holotoxid may now be used for the fourth or later (booster) immunizations against pertussis (*MMWR*, October 9, 1992).

Tuberculosis and Leprosy

Tuberculosis was once one of the most prevalent and costly human plagues. During the 20th century, improved living conditions and chemotherapy greatly reduced the incidence of tuberculosis and leprosy infection. Because of the worldwide impact of tuberculosis, many countries introduced mandatory immunization with BCG. Today, BCG holds the interesting position of being one of the most widely used, poorly understood, and most controversial vaccines. BCG stands for **bacillus Calmette–Guérin**, a strain of *Mycobacterium bovis*, attenuated between the years of 1906 and 1919 by Calmette and Guérin. The use of BCG had a shaky start. M. Calmette was an abrasive French nationalist who disliked Germans and was uneasy with English. In addition, he greatly exaggerated his early results. On the other hand, M. Guérin, who lived much longer than Calmette, appears to have been much more tolerant but an ineffectual promoter of the vaccine. After years of animal experiments, human trials were carried out in 1921, and by 1924 the French government adopted the vaccine for mass use. In the 1950s, BCG vaccination against tuberculosis came into widespread use throughout the world, except for the United States and Holland, through the sponsorship of the World Health Organization. In 1939, it was shown that BCG inoculation also induced a positive Mitsuda reaction (skin reaction to leprosy antigens). The efficacy of BCG immunization has been found to vary in different studies from 0% to 80% for tuberculosis, and from 20% to 80% for leprosy. Explanations for variation in efficacy include:

1. Infection with other atypical mycobacteria that impart some protection against tuberculosis in control groups.
2. Differences in immunogenicity among BCG preparations.

3. Differences in the natural history of the disease in different populations.
4. Methodologic differences in the trials.
5. Nutritional or other environmental effects, such as incidence of infections with other agents.

These problems led 14 of the 32 countries to discontinue BCG immunization programs. In England and Wales, BCG inoculation is not required but offered to high-risk children in most districts. Now, the incidence of tuberculosis is again on the rise. The most likely reason for this rise is the increasing reservoir of infection in AIDS patients in large cities and increased exposure of a high-risk population. Thus, after a hiatus lasting a full generation, tuberculosis is coming back, and antituberculosis immunization is being reexamined.

The protective epitopes of BCG are poorly understood, but older studies suggested that the most important immunogens are polysaccharides. Thus, recombinant techniques will most likely not work, but the immunizing polysaccharide epitope can be synthesized and conjugate methodology used to produce an effective acellular vaccine. Using reactive cloned T-cell lines, which do not necessarily identify a protective immunogen, it appears that the most likely candidate is a 65 kDa antigen, but other evidence implicates larger proteoglycans.

Haemophilus influenzae

Two *H. influenzae* type b (Hib)-conjugate vaccines were licensed in the latter part of 1989 and by 1990 were approved for use in children as young as 2 years old. Following the introduction of these vaccines, the incidence of all Hib invasive infections has declined by almost 90%. The vaccine also appears to decrease transmission of infection from person to person by infected respiratory drippings. Thus, the vaccination program also protects nonimmunized children. In addition, a monoclonal antiidiotype against monoclonal antibodies to a highly conserved epitope of the outer membrane porin molecule from *H. influenzae*, are able to stimulate specific antibody to the porin epitope after immunization. This remains an interesting alternative if problems should arise with the conjugate vaccine.

Typhoid Fever

Killed typhoid vaccines have been used since the late 1890s. Three typical vaccines are now available in the United States: an oral live attenuated strain (Ty21a), a heat-phenol killed vaccine widely used for many years, and a newly licensed capsular polysaccharide (Typhium Vi/VICS). The older heat-phenol inactivated vaccine was 51% to 77% effective in preventing typhoid fever but frequently produced local pain and swelling, fever, headache, and malaise. The new, attenuated strain is administered orally. It and the VICS vaccine are as effective as the previously used killed vaccine, and appear to have a lower incidence of side effects. The live attenuated vaccine is easier to administer but should not be used for immunocompromised individuals. Routine typhoid vaccination is not recommended in the United States, but should be given to travelers to endemic areas.

Pneumococcal Pneumonia

From the end of the 1940s, the introduction of penicillin caused a temporary decline in pneumococcal infections. However, since the 1960s, the continuing high morbidity and mortality of pneumococcal pneumonia in the elderly and immunosuppressed resulted in a renewed interest in pneumococcal vaccines. Pneumococcal polysaccharide vaccine (23 valent) has been shown to reduce the risk of infection by two-thirds (60% to 70% efficiency) in high-risk groups (immunosuppressed cancer patients, elderly, etc.) and is recommended for those over 50 years of age.

Problems with the present vaccine are that it does not reliably induce immunity in children younger than 2 years, the age group that has the highest incidence of invasive pneumococcal infection and meningitis, and it has limited protective effects in immunosuppressed individuals susceptible to pneumococcal infections. Since polysaccharide antigens are T-independent, the pneumococcal vaccine does not effectively induce high-affinity antibodies or T-cell responses. Thus, conjugate vaccines with the polysaccharide coupled to carrier proteins might recruit T-cell help, isotype switching of reactive B cells and production of high-affinity IgG antibodies. The difficulty with this approach is the large number of specific pneumococcal polysaccharides and lack of knowledge of the best carrier to use. Currently manufacturers are concentrating on the six or seven most common pneumococcal types, but this requires manufacture and testing of seven different vaccines. Carrier proteins now being examined include a nontoxic variant of diphtheria toxin, tetanus toxoid, diphtheria toxoid, and meningococcal outer membrane protein. Immunization with noncapsular antigens is also under examination.

Cholera

Cholera is a potentially lethal diarrheal disease caused by the Gram-negative bacterium *Vibrio cholerae*. Of critical importance in a vaccine is the production of mucosal immunity, since the organism exerts its effect on the gastrointestinal mucosa. One of the primary protective antigens is a lipopolysaccharide O antigen, but this is now known to exist in at least two different serotypes, O1 and O139, that do not confer effective cross-immunity. Whole-killed lipopolysaccharide and toxoid antigens have been tested by parenteral injection and found to induce only weak or short-term immunity, due to their inability to induce mucosal immunity. Natural infection provides direct exposure of intestinal epithelium to *V. cholerae* and survivors develop strong mucosal immunity. Two oral vaccines designed to induce mucosal immunity are now being studied: a mixture of the nontoxic B subunit of cholera toxin and killed whole bacterial cells (RW-WC), and live attenuated organisms. The RW-WC vaccine has been tested in a field trial confers only short-term protection. However it also confers protection against diarrhea caused by pathogenic *E. coli*, which produce an enterotoxin immunologically cross-reactive with cholera B subunit. The attenuated strain *V. cholerae* vaccines have also been shown to be effective, but produce side effects (diarrhea, vomiting, intestinal cramps, etc). Currently only the live attenuated O1 vaccine CVD103-HgR has advanced beyond phase II clinical studies. A single oral dose of CVD103-HgR conferred 82–87% protection in volunteers challenged one month after vaccination. A disquieting feature is the ability of this strain to reacquire virulence by recombination with a strain possessing a conjugate sex factor. It is anticipated that ongoing work will soon provide a useful cholera vaccine.

VIRUSES

For AIDS vaccine development, see Chapter 29.

Poliomyelitis

Formalin-killed (Salk) and attenuated (Sabin) vaccines are available for immunization against polio. Surprisingly, few mutations in the Sabin vaccine strains are required to acquire attenuation. The attenuated viruses grow successfully, yet cause almost no disease. In evaluation of immunization to polio, factors in addition to protection of the immunized individual must be considered. Oral immunization by ingestion of attenuated virus induces local immunity in the gastrointestinal tract and may prevent passage of the virus through elimination of fecal contamination, while injection of killed virus is relatively ineffective in this regard. Polio infections are contracted naturally by swallowing of virus-contaminated materials. In an unprotected person, the virus passes into the bloodstream, leading to a systemic infection. Disease occurs when the virus attacks the anterior horn cells of the medulla and spinal cord. Antibody induced by injection prevents the systemic spread of the virus, but the gastrointestinal phase may still occur. On the other hand, oral immunization leads to local immunity in the gastrointestinal tract, presumably due to production of secretory antibody. This reduces the gastrointestinal phase of infection and limits spread of the virus. Persons inoculated with the killed virus may be protected from disease but can still serve as carriers. If a substantial portion of a population has received the oral vaccine, even the nonimmunized portion of the population is protected from epidemic disease. The incidence of paralytic poliomyelitis in the United States from 1951 to 1978 is given in Table 26–6. Although some controversy exists in regard to the efficiency of intramuscular injections of killed polio vaccine and of oral administration of attenuated poliovirus, oral vaccine is recommended by most authorities at this time, administered for the first time between 2 months of age and the preschool period.

TABLE 26–6. CORRELATION OF PARALYTIC POLIOMYELITIS AND VACCINE USE IN THE UNITED STATES 1951–1978

Period	Vaccine	Total Number	Average Number/ Year	Average Number/ Million/ Year
1951–1955	None	111,040	22,208	135
1956–1960	IPV only	22,970	4,594	26
1961–1965	IPV and OPV	2,341	468	2.4
1973–1978	OPV only	55	9	0.004

IPV, formalin inactivated polio vaccine.

OPV, oral (attenuated) line polio vaccine.

Modified from Sabin, AE: Paralytic poliomyelitis: Old dogmas and new perspectives. *Rev Infect Dis* 3:543–564, 1981.

Recently, largely driven by lawsuits, there has been reconsideration of reintroduction of inactivated polio vaccine. Rare cases of polio in the United States are associated with live virus in recent vaccine recipients or by transmission to contacts who were not immunized. One hundred five cases have been verified by the CDC in a 12-year period; 35 were vaccinees, and 50 were in contacts of vaccinees. A National Academy of Sciences committee has recommended that inactivated polio virus (IPV) immunization be combined with oral live virus (OPV) immunization, with two injections of IPV preceding OPV. However, this schedule would make immunization much more complicated and less accessible to many children, as well as increase costs. As yet, the recommendation for a combined polio vaccination has not been accepted.

Since 1985, through the wide use and surveillance of all cases of polio in the Americas, poliomyelitis is on the verge of being eradicated from the western hemisphere. During 1991, only nine cases of acute flaccid paralysis were confirmed to have been caused by wild-type poliovirus, and none were in the United States or Canada. This result may be attributed to the efforts of thousands of health workers and civil servants who have contributed. However, even tighter surveillance is needed to eliminate the disease entirely.

Hepatitis

Vaccines against hepatitis viruses, Epstein–Barr virus (EBV), and papillomavirus, if successful, would be the first vaccines for the prevention of cancer in humans.

Hepatitis B. Two types of vaccines are now available for immunization: Hepatitis B surface antigen (HBsAg) subviral particles purified from the serum of asymptomatic carriers and subunit HBsAg particles produced by genetic engineering in common baker's yeast (Saccharomyces cerevisiae) or in Chinese hamster ovary cells. The *env* gene of the virus (Figure 26–1) was cloned, inserted into a vector, and transfected into the productive cells. Translation products of each of the small (S), medium (M), and large (L) mRNAs of the *env* region were identified and subviral particles obtained in large amounts after lysis of the yeast cells. In animal studies direct gene transfer into skeletal muscle using plasmid DNA encoding HBsAg DNA has been effective in stimulating antibody formation, but application of the approach to humans will require much more testing.

There is a good correlation between the presence of antibodies to the *env* gene product and protection for infection. Clinical trials have shown that there is little difference between the plasma derived or the recombinant product regarding antibody response or protection against infection. However, cell-mediated immunity to HBV protein is significantly higher after recovery from natural infection than after immunization. There remains a small proportion of nonresponders to the vaccines and marked individual variation in the levels of antibodies obtained. In addition, nonresponders who subsequently become infected and recover develop a high titer of antibodies to the HBV *env* proteins. Thus, improvement is needed in the hepatitis B vaccines. One approach would be to produce a vaccine that includes additional epitopes of HBV, such as the core antigen or pre-S1 and pre-S2 epitopes not present in the *env* gene product. Pre-S1 and pre-S2 are expressed on the surface of HBV and appear to play an important role both in immunologic recognition and in reactions with cell receptors. Originally recommended for high-risk populations (neonates born to HBsAg carrier mothers, recently arrived immigrants from southeast Asia or southern Africa, etc.), HBsAg immunization is now included in recommended childhood immunizations. Despite the availability of a safe and effective vaccine, the incidence of HBV infection has increased since 1981, especially in high-risk groups, (eg, drug users). A cost-effective strategy proposed is to treat and vaccinate newborns of mothers who test positive for active infection, and then vaccinate all children at 10 years of age.

The high association of development of hepatocellular carcinomas in areas of the world with endemic hepatitis B has led to clinical trials with the intention of preventing hepatitis in children and thus also preventing hepatocellular carcinoma. Present recommendations are that babies born to HBsAg-positive mothers should receive immunoprophylaxis with hepatitis B immune globulin within 12 hours of birth along with HBV vaccine, a second HBV vaccination at one month, and a third at six months. If the level of antibody produced by such immunization is an indication, reductions in carcinomas can be expected.

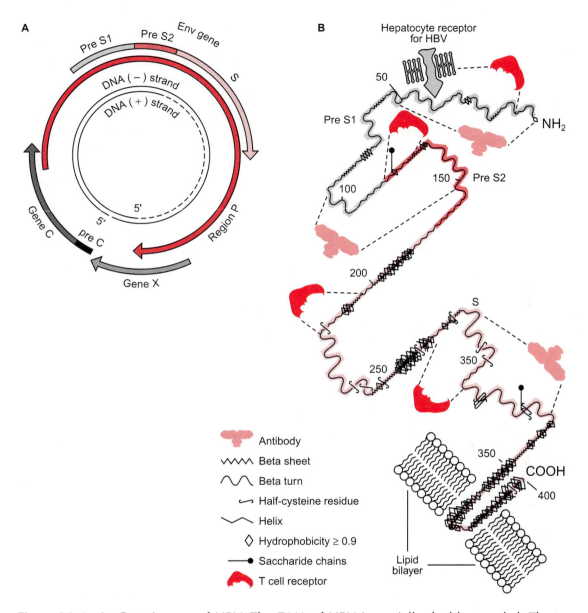

Figure 26–1. **A.** Genetic map of HBV. The DNA of HBV is partially double-stranded. The two strands (+ and -) are also called large (-) and small (+) because of the different sizes. The deleted region of the + strand is indicated with a dashed line (- - - - - -). The large open reading frame for the HBsAg (hepatitis B surface antigen), the *env* region, has been cloned, and peptides representing the B- and T-cell epitopes identified. **B.** Secondary structure of the HBsAg as predicted from the HBV *env* gene product. The large surface protein contains pre-S1, pre-S2, and S; the middle protein, pre-S2 and S; and the small protein, S only. The pre-S1 region contains the binding region for the hepatocyte receptor for HBV; the S region contains the hydrophobic membrane region inserted into the HBV lipid bilayer. (Modified from Neurath AR, Jameson BA, Huima T: Hepatitis B virus proteins eliciting protective immunity. *Microbiol Sciences* 4:45–51, 1987.)

Hepatitis A. During the past fifteen years, the virus causing hepatitis A has been isolated and identified and a formalin-inactivated vaccine produced. Hepatitis A is caused by a picornavirus that appears to have properties unique from any other RNA viruses. As with many other infectious diseases, the incidence of the disease actually increased with improving hygienic living conditions. Thus, it is an example of an infectious agent that previously infected essentially all infants at an age when infection was asymptomatic or produced only mild symptoms indistinguishable as a specific disease. Although the incidence of hepatitis is declining in general, the majority of civilian cases in European and North American populations are acquired while traveling in developing countries, and thousands of soldiers in World Wars I and II most likely had hepatitis A. Four approaches to production of a vaccine have included production of attenuated viruses in cell culture, genetically engineered capsid vaccines, synthetic peptide vaccines, and formalin-killed cell-cultured viruses. Of these, the formalin-killed virus is now available and has been effective in inducing antibody in normal volunteers. It is not known how long lasting immunity to hepatitis A will last following killed-virus vaccination. In developing countries, where a vaccine to hepatitis A would be most useful, it is very desirable to have a vaccine that is effective in producing lifelong immunity. This objective may require an attenuated virus vaccine.

Hepatitis C and E. The RNA genome of hepatitis C virus has been cloned and consists of about 1,000 nucleotides. A gene encoding an envelope protein of hepatitis C has possibilities of being used to develop a vaccine. Hepatitis E has also been cloned and may be used to develop a vaccine against this virus. Hepatitis E produces a significant mortality in pregnant women, particularly in India.

Epstein–Barr
Virus

EBV is the causative agent of infectious mononucleosis, as well as Burkitt's lymphoma in Africa and nasopharyngeal carcinoma in China. In Western countries, about 85% to 90% of all adults carry the virus; in developing countries, 100%. EBV infection is lifelong, and at any given time, about 20% of virus-positive individuals shed virus in saliva. Proposed vaccines cover about every approach possible, including attenuated virus (P3HR-1 strain), inactivated virus EBV membrane antigen, a subunit vaccine (gp340/220), and recombinant gp340. Proposed adjuvants include alum, immunostimulating complexes (ISCOMs), and muramyl dipeptide, and vectors include vaccinia and BCG (see Chapter 28). The immediate prospects all utilize the major membrane glycoprotein and a variety of delivery systems. A major problem is the lack of a good animal model system to test vaccines. It has been shown that children in Africa that are most likely to get Burkitt's lymphoma have high antibody titers. Thus, an effective EBV vaccine almost certainly should preferentially induce cell-mediated immunity. A discussion of approaches used to produce cell-mediated immunity is included in Chapter 28. These methods include identification of amphipathic peptides that represent epitopes recognized by T cells; isolation of peptides that bind to class I MHC grooves; the use of adjuvants, such as ISCOMs, that direct antigens to exogenous processing and of vectors, such as vaccinia for T_{CTL} and BCG for T_{DTH} cells.

Papilloma
Viruses

The role of antibody and CMI in protection against virus-induced tumors is also illustrated in approaches to producing a vaccine for papillomaviruses (PVs). PVs are the causative agent for up to 90% of cervical cancers. Although there are 68 different types of human papillomaviruses (HPVs), there are two types–HPV-16 and HPV-18–which are believed to be responsible for most cases. It should be possible to develop prophylactic vaccines using the L1 and L2 capsular proteins or therapeutic vaccines using the E6 or E7 onco proteins. In animal models of similar viruses it has been shown that antibody to capsular proteins of PVs reduce risk of infection but have little or no effect after infection is established. On the other hand, cell-mediated immunity (particularly T_{CTL}-mediated immunity), can induce regression of established hyperplastic lesions. Therefore, vaccination is directed to two effects—production of neutralizing antibody against capsular proteins for protection (specifically secretory IgA in the vagina) and of T_{CTL} cells to viral transforming proteins (E6 and E7), which are expressed on the surface of infected cells, for regression. A number of viral preparations, adjuvants, and vectors have been shown to be partially effective in bovine models using bovine papilloma virus-2 and clinical trials in humans using protein vaccines or vaccinia vectors will almost certainly be underway by the time this book is published.

Measles

Measles and other diseases, such as rubella and mumps, could theoretically be eliminated by effective global vaccination programs. Attenuated measles vaccines have been effective in reducing not only active measles infections but also the incidence of late-occurring disease manifestation believed to be related to measles. After its introduction in 1963 in the United States, the incidence of measles dropped 95%. In addition, the incidence of subacute sclerosing panencephalitis dropped dramatically after institution of measles vaccination. However, in 1989 and 1990, the incidence of measles increased dramatically among preschool children in inner cities, as well as in school children and in college students with high vaccination rates. The main reason for the outbreaks in preschool children was nonvaccination, either because the children were too young or from neglect. In the older children, measles occurred even though they had received the proscribed vaccinations. It had been assumed that a single vaccination would produce long-lasting immunity. Because of these outbreaks of measles, the CDC has begun an infant immunization initiative and the recommended schedule for measles vaccination has been changed to administer a second measles, mumps, and rubella vaccine (MMR) at 11 or 12 years of age, following initial immunization at 15 months. Corresponding with these new recommendations, the incidence of measles dropped markedly in 1992 and in 1993 appeared to be below pre-epidemic levels.

One problem with the original measles vaccine was that it increased the chances of getting a severe form of "atypical measles." In 1967, the Edmonston strain of attenuated live measles was developed, and in 1968, use of the inactivated vaccine was discontinued. At first, this vaccine was given with immune globulin. Ultimately, the Moraten line of a more attenuated strain was made available, that did not require coadministration of immune globulin (licensed in 1968), replaced the killed vaccine. This vaccine was found to be ineffective in the presence of maternal antibodies, which remain in the blood for about nine months after birth. This was not a major problem in the United States, where measles generally does not occur until after nine months of age, but it was a problem for developing countries where the disease attacks younger children. To address this problem, a more efficient attenuated strain that could be given at higher doses was introduced—the Edmonston–Zagred (EG) strain. In 1990, the WHO recommended that this strain be used in areas where measles in young infants remained a major health problem. However, it was soon discovered that children who had been inoculated with the EG strain were dying at higher rates from other diseases endemic in the areas of use, such as pneumonia, diarrhea, and parasitic diseases, presumably because of immunosuppressive effects of the EG-strain immunization. In October 1992, the use of this vaccine was discontinued, and the WHO measles eradication program is on hold.

Respiratory Disease Viruses/Influenza

Immunization to acute virus-induced respiratory diseases, including the common cold, remains an as yet unattained goal. The status of vaccines for respiratory disease viruses of humans is given in Table 26–7. The difficulties in developing such vaccines are exemplified by influenza, for which the most data are available.

Influenza Virus. Immunization against influenza viruses is complicated because different strains show antigenic variations. When the influenza vaccine used contains the prevalent strain of virus, the incidence of influenza in immunized individuals is reduced 75% to 90%. Influenza vaccine immunity is short-lived, and yearly boosters must be given to maintain protection. Yearly immunization for elderly and

TABLE 26–7. STATUS OF VACCINES FOR RESPIRATORY TRACT VIRUSES OF MAN

Family	Genes	Clinical Effects	Vaccine	Status	Problem
Orthomyoviridae	Influenza virus (A, B, and C)	Acute respiratory diseases (adults and children)	Formalin-killed virus	Needs improvement	Antigenic drift, expensive
Paramyxoviridae	Paramyxovirus (types 1–4)	Group, VRF, pneumonia (infants and children)	Formalin-killed virus	Unsatisfactory	No protective effect
	Pneumovirus (respiratory syncytial virus)	Pneumonia (infants)	Formalin-killed virus	Unsatisfactory	Lacks protective effect, intensifies infection
Picornaviridae	Rhinovirus (111 serotypes)	Common cold	Monovalent killed virus	Unsatisfactory	Many serotypes
	Enterovirus (70 serotypes)	Common cold, pneumonia, others	None available		Heterogeneity of genus
Cornaviridae	Coronavirus (3 types)	Coldlike illness	None available		Very great technical difficulties
Adenoviridae	Mastadenovirus (36 serotypes)	Pneumonia, URI, acute respiratory disease, cystitis, keratoconjunctivitis	Formalin-killed	Needs improvement effective for types 4 and 7	Multiple serotypes

other high-risk groups is recommended. Now each year's vaccine produced for the United States contains three virus strains (usually two type A and one type B) believed likely to circulate in the United States in the upcoming winter. The trivalent influenza vaccine prepared for the 1991–92 season, for instance, included A/Taiwan/1/86-like(H1N1), A/Beijing/353/89-like(H3N2), and B/Panama/45/90-like hemagglutinin antigens. For the trivalent vaccine for the 1992–93 and 1993–94 seasons, A/Texas/36/91-like(H1N1) replaced the A/Taiwan/1/86-like hemagglutinin antigen. Influenza vaccine is made from highly-purified egg-grown viruses that are inactivated. Its use is contraindicated in individuals with a history of allergic reactions to egg proteins. Influenza vaccination is highly recommended for any person above the age of six months who is at increased risk for complications of influenza.

Extraordinary vaccines may have to be produced to influenza variants that cause epidemics. This was the case for "swine flu" and "Russian flu" in the 1970s. These strains contained antigens not included in the available vaccines. A crash program was set up to produce a vaccine that would be effective against the new antigenic variation occurring in the swine flu virus. This required the cultivation of a large number of virus particles. A recombinant virus (X-53) was made up of the swine flu, a low-yield virus, and a high-yield laboratory virus (PR8G) by co-culturing the two viruses in chick embryos. Isolates of viral particles containing most of the core RNA of the high-yield laboratory virus and the surface antigens (and the RNA coding for the surface antigens) of the swine flu virus were made. This permitted rapid production of the large number of viruses needed for the immunization program.

Although the necessary number of doses of the vaccine were prepared in time, two factors led to discontinuation of its use. First, the expected pandemic of swine flu never really materialized, and, second, the number of complications at least partially attributed to the vaccine was not acceptable. These included unexplained sudden death in the elderly (perhaps not statistically significant from the expected death rate) and the development of the Guillain–Barré syndrome (see Chapter 21) in a small number of recipients (approximately 10 cases per million doses). The use of newly formulated swine flu vaccines between 1978 and 1981 was not associated with an increased incidence of Guillain–Barré syndrome above that seen in a nonimmunized population.

The concept of artificially providing partial protection to an infection that will limit the extent but not prevent an infection is illustrated by influenza vaccines. Influenza NA glycoprotein (NA) and hemagglutination (HA) antigens have been compared for protective effects. Both induce neutralizing antibody. Anti-HA prevents infection by blocking the ability of virus to bind to cells. Anti-NA is neutralizing in only high doses, does not prevent disease, but limits cyclic infection in vivo. Thus, influenza vaccination that produces anti-HA may prevent infection temporarily when active, whereas anti-NA will not prevent infection but will limit infection, prevent serious illness, and allow longer lasting active immunity of infection to be established. In the long run, it is possible that the partial protection provided by anti-NA may be more effective than the temporary "full protection" provided by anti-HA, since the full immunity provided by immunization to HA will decrease more rapidly than the full immunity established with immunity of infection.

A possible breakthrough in the design of influenza vaccines involves the recent finding that injection of plasmid DNA-encoding influenza protein into mice resulted in generation of nucleoprotein-specific T_{CTL} cells and protection from subsequent challenge with a heterologous strain of influenza A virus. In contrast to antibodies induced by the conventional vaccines that are strain-specific, T_{CTL} cells can respond to conserved viral antigens on different strains. If applicable to humans, this could greatly simplify influenza virus vaccination.

Respiratory Syncytial Virus (RSV). RSV causes an estimated 91,000 hospitalizations and 4,500 deaths in the United States yearly. Early attempts to product immunity using a formalin-inactivated whole virus vaccine actually resulted in more severe disease in immunized children. More recent experimental studies have shown that this vaccine induces Th2 type CD4+ cells (IL-4), whereas active infection resulting in immunity induces Th1 type cells (INF-γ). This "inappropriate" T-cell response may have prevented the development of neutralizing antibody response required for protective immunity. The IL-4 associated Th2 response favors IgE production and is also seen in progressive disease. Attention is now focused in development of RSV mutants that will not be pathogenic and will induce the "appropriate" type of immune response.

Rabies

Since the development of the first rabies vaccine by Louis Pasteur in 1885, there have been serious problems in effectiveness and dangerous complications. Rabies virus vaccines had been prepared from viruses cultured on chick embryo cultures that are then inactivated. Although the neurologic complications (autoimmune encephalomyelitis) are rare compared to the use of viruses obtained from the nervous system of infected animals, the potency of the chick embryo vaccine is not satisfactory.

In 1980, a new rabies vaccine produced in human diploid-cultured cells became available that induces antibody titers 10 to 20 times higher than the chick embryo vaccine. Two inactivated rabies vaccines are currently licensed for use in the United States. Only five injections of the cultured vaccine (in contrast to 14 to 21 injections of the duck vaccine) are required, and the frequency of allergic reactions is far lower. Use of the duck vaccine has been discontinued. Exposed individuals are given passive immunization with human rabies immune globulin on day 0 followed by the new vaccine on days 0, 3, 7, 14, and 28. Preexposure prophylaxis for animal handlers and laboratory personnel consists of three intramuscular injections on days 0, 7, and 28.

Efforts to improve the rabies vaccine have focused on the viral surface glycoprotein (protein G). Neutralizing antibody to rabies virus shows exclusive specificity for protein G, and protein G or vaccinia–rabies G gene recombinant virus has been shown to produce effective immunity experimentally. However, there is considerable antigenic variation among the G proteins isolated from different strains of infective rabies virus. Rabies ribonucleoprotein (RNP) does not show strain variation, and immunization with liposomes containing rabies RNP from one strain has conferred protection to lethal infection with another strain.

Recent efforts have been directed to inducing immunity in wild animals, particularly foxes, which serve as a reservoir for rabies in Europe. Recombinant vaccinia virus–rabies vaccines have been produced that contain the gene for the G protein and have been shown experimentally to produce effective immunity when ingested orally by foxes. Field trials in France and Belgium have demonstrated that baited vaccine is effective in immunizing feral foxes. A campaign is now underway that could lead to disruption of the viral infection and local eradication of fox rabies.

Varicella (Chickenpox)

A live, attenuated strain of varicella zoster was developed in Japan in the early 1970s (Oka strain) and has been shown to be safe, immunogenic, and highly protective, both in normal and immunocompromised children. This is available in the United States under the trade name of "Varivax-R". The Oka strain is licensed for use in Japan and has been administered to over 2 million children. It is used on a limited scale for immunosuppressed children in the United States. Trials have shown that the vaccine induces antibodies and T_{CTL}, although 98% of vaccinated children will be protected from severe disease only 70 to 85% will be completely protected from mild illness. There is still a difference of opinion, but several advisory committees have recommended routine vaccination if the vaccine is licensed in the United States. Chickenpox is usually thought of as a benign disease of childhood, but rare complications, such as bacterial superinfection, Reye's syndrome, or other encephalopathies, might be prevented by an immunization program. In addition, the vaccine has been found to be very effective in preventing varicella in high-risk groups, such as children with leukemia. Varicella vaccination has recently been recommended for healthy children, combined with MMR to be given as MMRV at 15 months of age and later at age 11 or 12.

Herpes Simplex

Herpes simplex virus (HSV) is estimated to affect over 10 million people who have recurring genital infections and about 500,000 with episodes of herpes keratoconjunctivitis. Up to 1 million Caesarian deliveries to prevent congenital infection. Vaccination for HSV is directed toward prevention of infection, as well as suppression of recurrent disease. Once the virus infects cells at the portal of entry, a latent infection is established in sensory neurons that innervate the cell. As with other viral infections, antibodies are able to prevent infection, but will have no effect on established infection; T_{CTL}-mediated cytotoxicity may help to control exacerbations of the recurrent lesions. Once HSV enters the sensory neuron, it is sequestered from the immune system until it is reactivated. The axon serves as a conduit to epithelial cells, where viral replication can take place. Over fifty vaccines have been tested since 1924, and all failed to provide protection or reduce recurrence. The most recent approach is to attempt to provide mucosal immunity in order to reduce the growth of the initial inoculum of HSV and thus the amount of virus that eventually reaches the sensory axons. The development of such a vaccine is not expected in the near future.

Rotavirus

Rotavirus is one of the most common causes for debilitating diarrhea in infants. It is an RNA virus that contains two outer capsid proteins important for vaccine development: VP7, a surface glycoprotein (four serotypes), and VP4, a protease-cleaved hemagglutinin (two serotypes). The first field trial of a rotavirus vaccine conducted in 1983 using a live, attenuated bovine strain (RIT) reduced the incidence of rotavirus diarrhea by 83%. However, the efficacy of the RIT strain could not be reproduced in later trials. Difficulties with rotavirus vaccine development are that the rabbit model of the disease is not closely predictive of results in humans and the immune mechanism responsible for defense is not well understood. Presumably mucosal defenses are paramount, but it is not easy to measure antibodies or cells in this system. Two live oral candidate vaccines are now being tested in field trials, the rhesus rotavirus tetravalent vaccine (RRV-TV) which contains viruses with the three most common V7 serotypes, and W179-9, which is derived from the bovine strain and contains the human strain VP7 gene. These vaccines have 50 to 65% efficiency. New vaccines design includes the use of reassortment vaccines incorporating more VP7 and VP4 serotypes and the use of microencapsulated viruses which persist longer in the GALT and increase the immune response.

Complications of Virus Vaccination

Vaccines prepared from live, attenuated viruses, such as for measles, mumps, rubella, and trivalent oral poliomyelitis, may cause symptomatic infection in the nervous system in 1:10,000 to 1,300,000 vaccine recipients. Vaccines prepared from killed whole organisms may cause demyelinating disease in approximately 1:100,000 recipients. Vaccines containing DNA from an oncogenic or immunosuppressive virus may produce an oncogenic or immunosuppressive effect even if the whole virus is not present in the vaccine. Recombinant vaccines, including segments of DNA that may cause transformation of cells or transactivation of other cells, could produce a variety of untoward effects.

An additional complication of vaccination is an allergic reaction to a component of the vaccine. For instance, yellow fever vaccine was once prepared in embryonated chicken eggs. Because of the possibility of anaphylactic shock, this yellow fever vaccine had to be carefully administered in patients who are allergic to eggs or chicken feathers. Influenza vaccine was also produced in eggs but was highly purified prior to use. Anaphylactic reactions have rarely been traced to trace amounts of calf serum proteins in measles vaccines.

As mentioned in several examples above, a vaccine may induce the wrong type of immune response. This problem is magnified in such infections as HIV (see Chapter 29) in which activation of the immune system may also serve to activate production of the virus.

OTHER VACCINES

Fungi

The success of vaccines against bacterial and viral infections has not extended to fungal infections. A ribosomal vaccine for *Candida albicans* protects against infection in experimental animals and could be useful in high-risk patients. A similar vaccine against *Histoplasma capsulatum* has been shown to produce effective cell-mediated immunity in animals. A killed spherule vaccine for *Coccidioides* is effective in animals and is undergoing clinical trials. Vaccines against other fungal infections, such as *Blastomyces*, *Aspergillum*, *Zygomycetes*, etc., have had very limited development.

Protozoa/Malaria

The pathogenesis and immunopathology of malaria is presented in Chapter 25. The complex life cycle of malaria places limitations on approaches to preparation of a vaccine because of antigenic variation during infection, stage specific antigens of the organisms at different points in the life cycle, and strain differences in antigenicity. Theoretically, vaccine development could be directed to prevent infection (sporozoite), to decrease the production of parasites in the infected blood (merozoite) or liver (schizont), or to the sexual stage in the mosquito (gametocyte).

Sporozoite. In the late 1960s, it was shown that vaccination with gamma-irradiated sporozoites could protect against different malaria strains. However, it was only possible to obtain enough sporozoites for limited experimental study. There is as yet no satisfactory method to cultivate the sporozoites. They must be isolated from salivary glands of infected mosquitos. This method does not yield adequate quantities for producing a vaccine for widespread human use. Because of this, vaccine efforts then focused on isolating and cloning the gene for the circumsporate (CS) protein.

The CS protein is an antigen highly represented on the surface of the infectious sporozoite stage injected by infecting mosquitos, and CS proteins contain repetitive amino acid sequences shared by different *Plasmodium* strains (Fig. 26–2). Since nearly all identified anti-CS react with the repeat amino acid sequences, the first vaccine tested was directed against these epitopes. Human volunteers vaccinated with the tetramer linked to tetanus toxoid (Asn-Ala-Asn-Pro) pro-

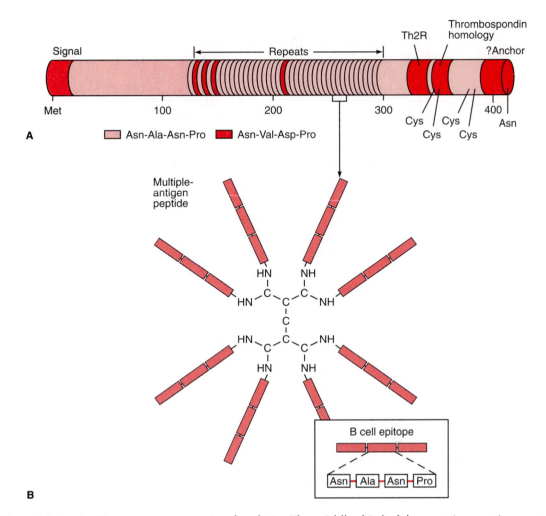

Figure 26–2. **A.** Circumsporate protein of malaria. The middle third of the protein contains a set of repetitions of two short sequences of amino acids (Asn-Ala-Asn-Pro or Asn-Val-Asp-Pro), as well as a polymorphic region (Th2R) and two pairs of cysteine residues. Hydrophobic regions at the C terminal may anchor the protein in the plasma membrane of the sporozoite. The repetitive sequences constitute epitopes that are recognized by all known antibodies against *Plasmodium* strains. **B.** Multiple-antigen peptide is a synthetic molecule in which a lysine core provides "mooring posts" for B-cell epitopes that can be processed by macrophages for presentation to T cells. In this example, all eight arms of the lysine core hold the same B cell epitope (Asn-Ala-Asn-Pro). (Modified from Nussenzweig V, Nussenzweig RS: Progress toward a malaria vaccine. *Hosp Pract* 25:41, 1990.)

duced only low titers of antibody. To increase immunogenicity of the peptide antigen it was complexed with epitopes that would be bound to class II MHC molecules and processed by T cells. In this way the poorly immunogenic peptides would be provided with a "carrier" for T-cell help. This has been accomplished using "multiple-antigen peptides" (MAPs) (see Fig. 26–2). MAPs have been shown to induce higher titers of anti-CS in experimental animals and are now being tested in humans.

Merozoite/schizont. In 1987 Manuel Patarroyo demonstrated that combinations of synthetic peptides from merozoite blood stage parasites were immunogenic and protective in monkeys. One of these peptides, SPf66, was shown to produce a 39% reduction in clinical episodes of malaria in clinical trials in Columbia, but later trials were less convincing. A more recent trial in Africa, completed in August of 1994, resulted in a 31% efficiency in preventing disease, although both vaccinated and placebo groups had a similar incidence of parasitemia. Thus, immunization with blood stage antigens may decrease clinical evidence of infection, but not prevent it. Clearly SPf66 is unlikely to be the final definitive malaria vaccine, but may find application until a better vaccine is developed.

A second approach to suppress the effects of infection is inducing CD8+ T_{CTL} cells to malaria antigens expressed on infected blood or liver cells (see Chapter 25), and by so doing decreasing the production of organisms in the infected cells. Several different ways to this approach are under study:

1. A T_{CTL} epitope appears to be shared by the C terminal CS protein and schizonts in liver cells. T cell clones that recognize this epitope in association with class I MHC have been derived in mice, and passive transfer of these cells protects against challenge with malarial sporozoites. Vaccination with this peptide conjugated to ISCOMS (see Chapter 28) or to liposomes may selectively allow presentation through class I MHC.
2. A recombinant protein form, the p190 antigen (p190-3) of *Plasmodium falciparum* merozoites, has been found that will selectively induce CD4+ and CD8+ T cells when administered in Freund's adjuvant.
3. In further studies, ampipathic analysis has been used to identify twenty two putative T_{CTL} epitopes from conserved regions of ten *P. falciparum* asexual stage proteins that are candidates for vaccine development. Peptides containing these epitopes have been further analyzed for their ability to stimulate T cells from malaria patients.

Gamete. The rationale for vaccines to the gametocytes is to produce antibodies in humans that will be ingested by the mosquitoes that are responsible for transmission of the infection and block or impair the sexual development of the malaria parasite in the mosquito. This approach has been attained in laboratory studies but has not yet been demonstrated in field trials.

Helminths

Schistosomiasis. Helminths (worms) are among the most prevalent infectious agents of humans. Programs aimed at eliminating schistosomiasis have been only partially successful. The problem may be addressed at three points in the life cycle of the organisms: (1) Preventing parasite contact between the intermediate host (snail) and definitive host (human) in the water, by sanitation and protected water supplies; (2) destruction of the intermediate host (snail); and (3) suppression of infection in the human host by vaccination or chemotherapy. Attack at all three levels may be required in order to eradicate this disease. Control of the intermediate host (snail) has proven feasible by itself in selected areas but treatment of water supplies remains costly and not possible at this time in all infected areas. Chemotherapy, particularly of infected children, who may pass thousands of schistosome eggs in their stools per day, could drastically reduce transmission of the disease since the drug of choice, praziquantel, kills adult worms and provides an over 90% reduction in worm burdens. This greatly reduces the chances of spreading infections. Unfortunately, treated people are reinfected from larvae that multiply in water snails; praziquantel treatment must be given at least once a year to maintain surveillance of infection. Even with a vigorous program monitored by the World Health Organization, the disease continues to spread. Developing countries cannot afford to give yearly doses of praziquantel; it is estimated that only 5% to 10% of infected individuals are now being adequately treated, compared to 70% to 80% of infected children who could be vaccinated.

Genetic engineering has provided at least four candidate vaccines. The most promising appears to be a protein secreted by the adult worm called p28GST, a member of the glutathione S-transferase family. In clinical trials, a single injection of p28GST has reduced the "worm burden" by up to 60% and reduced egg excretion by 65% in experimental animals. Since debilitating symptoms of the disease generally appear only in people who harbor very large numbers of organisms, a reduction of 50% or more can drastically reduce the number of infected people with clinical disease and greatly reduce transmission. Other candidate vaccines include: (1) A genetically engineered form of BCG incorporating paramyosin, a worm protein coded by a gene called Sm97; (2) a triose phosphate isomerase (TPI); and (3) another glutathione S-transferase isolated from *Schistosoma japonicum*. At the time of this writing, all four candidates were still in the running.

Theoretical approaches to schistosomal vaccine development are currently directed at the relative role of Th1- and Th2-type responses in schistosomal immunity. Th1-type responses (IgG antibody, DTH) are downregulated during Th2-type responses (IgE antibody) to schistosoma egg antigens. Both the pathology and the protection may be Th2 cytokine-dependent. It is possible that modulation to a predominant Th1 cytokine pattern, particularly IFN-γ, might be more protective and less pathogenic.

Onchocerciasis. Onchocerciasis is endemic in 34 countries in Africa, Latin America, and the Middle East, where it is estimated that over 17 million people are infected and 336,000 are blind as a result of infection. Approaches to vaccine production have followed two pathways: (1) Inoculation of parasite homogenates, extracts, dead organisms, or live attenuated organisms; and (2) attempts to identify specific antigens that are expressed at different stages of the infection. The first approach has not been successful for human filarial parasites. For the second approach, filarial antigens are divided into three groups—surface, circulating, and excretory/secretory. In experimental models, ADCC to surface antigens involving eosinophils, neutrophils, and macrophages have been shown to be effective in experimental models. Characterization of antigens using human postinfection sera and monoclonal antibodies is now underway to identify different antigens. Putative protective antigens will be cloned and used for further experimental study.

Insects/Ticks

Ticks are responsible for tremendous livestock losses, as well as for transmission of human diseases, such as Lyme disease. Animals develop a natural resistance to ticks after repeated exposure to the same tick species. However, this naturally acquired immunity, mediated by anaphylactic reactivity to larvae, is not very effective. On the other hand, vaccination-induced immunity to tick gut antigens may be much more effective in reducing numbers of adult ticks. The mechanism involves production of antibodies to gastrointestinal cells of the adult ticks. Upon ingestion of blood from immunized animals, these antibodies appear to inhibit endocytosis by gut cells and their eventual death, as well as the death of the tick. Since these gut antigens are not normally seen by the host, natural immunity does not develop to them (**concealed antigens**).

ORAL VACCINES

Oral or inhalation administration of vaccines has been proposed to deliver antigens in order to induce effective local immunity in the gastrointestinal tract, such as is done with the oral polio vaccine. Over 100 years ago, based on immunization against chicken cholera, Louis Pasteur suggested that vaccination by the oral route might be more effective against enteropathogenic bacteria than vaccination by intramuscular or subcutaneous inoculation. Such an approach has been attempted for vaccination against *Vibrio cholera*, typhoid, and dysentery. Local protection may be due to production of mucosal IgA antibody or sensitized cells and may not be reflected in titers of serum antibodies. As discussed in Chapter 3, there is an extensive gastrointestinal and bronchoalveolar-associated lymphoid system in all mammalian species that responds vigorously to antigens and produces effective antibody and cell mediated immunity. The results of limited trials of oral vaccination against adenovirus type 4, cholera, dysentery, and herpes simplex have suggested that mucosal immunity may be enhanced by oral challenge. Inhalation of influenza vaccine has been associated with production of IgA mucosal antibody, but a definite increased protective effect using this route has not been demonstrated. It has been shown in experimental studies that the most effective oral antigens are those that have lectin or lectinlike activity, such as *E. coli* pili or labile toxin β-subunit, viral hemagglutinins, and lectins. These are all believed to bind to glycolipids or glycoproteins on the intestinal mucosa (M cells) and be transported to the underlying lymphoid tissue.

ANTIFERTILITY VACCINES

Control of population growth is the major problem in large areas of the world, particularly India and China. Conventional birth control methods are difficult to apply to many of the people who most need them. Conceptually, it is possible to immunize against an antigen that is unique to a reproductive organ and has a fertility-related function that could be blocked by antibody. Potential antigens include reproductive hormones, sperm, embryonic tissue, and/or egg antigens.

Chorionic Gonadotropin

Successful trials in baboons and women have demonstrated that immunization to human chorionic gonadotropin (hCG) can effectively decrease fertility without producing side effects, either in the women immunized or in infants that are born to hCG-immunized mothers. However, the immunogenicity is not uniform; many women do not develop effective antibody titers. Peptides containing hormone-specific epitopes have been developed that may provide cheaper and more effective vaccines. A problem is the relatively low immunogenicity of proteins and peptides. This may be overcome with the appropriate selection of an adjuvant for delivery.

Sperm Antigen

A more consistent immunizing protocol or antigenic preparation is lactic dehydrogenase—C4 (LDH-C4)—an isozyme of LDH found only in male germinal cells. This enzyme may be purified to crystalline homogeneity. Female rabbits and mice immunized with LDH-C4 have significantly reduced pregnancies. This effect is reversible when serum antibody levels fall after immunization. Other potential sperm antigens are being studied at this time.

Luteinizing
Hormone-
releasing
Hormone (LHRH)

Immunization against LHRH may provide a means of controlling spermatogenesis. Luteinizing hormone (LH) regulates steroidogenesis in
Leydig cells in the testes. Effective suppression of spermatogenesis is
accomplished in mice immunized with LHRH–carrier conjugates, such
as LHRH–tetanus toxoid. The effect is reversible, as spermatogenesis
will reappear as the titers of antibody decrease with time. Clinical trials are now proposed not only for fertility control but also for treatment
of prostate cancer.

Egg Antigens

Although little is known about egg antigens, at least three unique glycoproteins are found in the zona pellucida, the noncellular gelatinous
layer surrounding the mature oocyte. Antibodies to these glycoproteins
are able to block fertilization in vitro, and passive immunization has
been effective in decreasing pregnancies in experimental animals.
Treatment of isolated ova with antizona antibodies produces an antibody–antigen layer on the zona surface that inhibits sperm attachment
and penetration through the zona. In monkeys, immunization with
porcine zona antigen preparations resulted in a reversible infertility
that lasted for about one year, indicating no permanent damage to the
ovary. Efforts are now underway to identify the smallest and most
effective zona antigen, as well as acceptable and effective immunization vectors and dosage.

Embryonic
Antigen

Antibodies to embryonic antigens, such as the F9 antigen found on the
blastocyst of mouse embryos, may also reduce fertility, but little is
known of human embryonic antigens that could provide effective
antifertility immunogens. The use of antifertility vaccines is clearly at
an early developmental stage and not yet practical as an effective
means of birth control.

Implementation of Vaccination

TESTING AND CLINICAL TRIALS

Evaluation of the effectiveness of a vaccine poses considerable problems. If an experimental animal is available, the vaccine can be tested
for its ability to protect the infected animal. In many cases, either an
animal model is not available or the experimental disease does not
resemble the human disease. The ability of the vaccine to induce antibody formation or delayed hypersensitivity in humans can be tested,
but the presence of antibody or cellular sensitivity may not necessarily be correlated with resistance to disease. This has been a major
problem with development of vaccines for HIV infection. The only
valid method is to test the ability of the vaccine to reduce the incidence or severity of disease in human clinical trials. This requires

painstaking planning and evaluation. Protection of the immunized individual may not be the sole criterion of effectiveness; the effect of immunization on populations ("herd immunity") must also be considered. It is not sufficient just to compare exposure of vaccinated and unvaccinated groups to infection. The protective effect of a vaccine should be related to a specific amount of exposure to infection, not just comparable exposure.

RELATIVE STATE OF IMMUNITY

Specific or nonspecific resistance to infection is a relative state. The effect of different doses of infectious agents or their products on experimental animals clearly demonstrates that administration of sufficiently large numbers of organisms can overcome the resistance of a highly immune animal. High doses of toxins can be given that will kill animals with high titers of neutralizing antibody. Thus, immunity to infection is not an absolute condition but depends on a large number of complex variables, including not only the resistance of the host but also the dose, route of contact, and virulence of the infecting agent. In leprosy, chemotherapy may reduce the organism load in a given person, permitting immune defense mechanisms to achieve the upper hand. In an extensive chemotherapeutic eradication program in Malta, there has been a marked reduction in the incidence of the leprosy.

LIABILITY FOR VACCINE MANUFACTURE

Vaccine production has become complicated by financial liability of manufacturers for untoward effects of vaccine administration. Large financial payments have been awarded to claimants under the tort legal system. Because of this, many manufacturers have decided not to continue producing proven vaccines. Yet there is a great worldwide need to develop and test new vaccines. The American Academy of Pediatrics has recommended that a manufacturer not be held liable if its product is listed in the Vaccine Compensation Table and if the vaccine has been tested, manufactured, distributed, and labeled in accordance with the requirements of the Food and Drug Administration and that all claimants file for compensation via a federal no-fault system. The Vaccine Injury Compensations Program, created by the National Childhood Vaccine Injury Act of 1986, provides a no-fault system of compensation for individuals of families whose members are injured by mandated childhood vaccines, including DPT, DT, measles, mumps, rubella (MMR), and polio vaccines. This has resulted in a tenfold drop in suits against manufacturers of DPT and a standardized review process that greatly reduces legal costs. The basis for the program is the use of a vaccine injury table, which lists specific conditions and time frame in which claims may be made. However, some leeway must be given for development and testing of new vaccines, particularly those that are urgently needed in developing countries.

Vaccination in Developing Countries

A major effort to make available existing vaccines, as well as developing new vaccines for use in the Third World has been the goal of the Expanded Program on Immunization adopted by the World Health Assembly in 1977. A listing by the Institute of Medicine of the National Academy of Sciences of the U.S.A. of the pathogens for which new or improved vaccines are needed in the Third World is given in Table 26–8. To this list must be added diseases such as AIDS, gonorrhea, and syphilis, which are considered sexually transmitted diseases, that are also needed for the developed countries, as well as HTLV. The difficulty of implementing other methods for reducing infectious diseases in the Third World, such as vector control, sanitation, housing, and treatment, makes vaccination a particularly attractive means of controlling infectious diseases. The first goal of the WHO was to make available vaccines against six infectious diseases already proven to be effective in developed countries: Measles, tetanus, pertussis, tuberculosis, diphtheria, and poliomyelitis. In 1974, it was estimated that only 5% of children in the developing world were immunized against these diseases; by the late 1980s, this percentage had been increased to 50%; and the goal of the 1990s is to reach every child.

The major obstacles to testing, mass production, and distribution of the needed vaccines are economic and political. The conjoined efforts of such organizations as the WHO, the United Nations Children's Fund, the World Bank, the UN Development Program, and the Rockefeller Foundation were formalized by formation of the Task Force for Child Survival in 1984. Implementation of a bidding system to purchase vaccines from manufacturers has resulted in very low prices, such as 50 cents for all six vaccines listed above and $1.00 for hepatitis B vaccine. In addition, the mass production of new vaccines is being encouraged by the willingness of manufacturers to undertake the development and production of new vaccines at close to cost under contractual agreements.

TABLE 26–8. PATHOGENS IDENTIFIED BY THE IOM OF THE U.S. NATIONAL ACADEMY OF SCIENCES AS TARGETS FOR NEW OR IMPROVED VACCINES NEEDED FOR THIRD WORLD COUNTRIES

Pathogen	Potential Effects	Cases Per Year (and Deaths)	Industrial Demand
Dengue virus	Fever, shock, internal bleeding	35,000,000 (15,000*)	Small (travelers to endemic areas)
Intestinal-toxin-producing *Escherichia coli* bacteria	Watery diarrhea, dehydration	630,000,000 (775,000*)	Small

Haemophilus influenzae type b bacterium	Meningitis, epiglottal swelling, pneumonia	800,000 (145,000*)	Great
Hepatitis A virus	Malaise, anorexia, vomiting, jaundice	5,000,000 (14,000)	Small
Hepatitis B virus	Same as hepatitis A; Chronic cirrhosis or cancer of liver	5,000,000 (822,000)	Moderate
Japanese encephalitis virus	Encephalitis, meningitis	42,000 (7,000*)	Small (travelers)
Mycobacterium leprae	Leprosy	1,000,000 (1,000)	None
Neisseria meningitidis bacterium	Meningitis	310,000 (35,000*)	Some (during epidemics)
Parainfluenza viruses	Bronchitis, pneumonia	75,000,000 (125,000*)	Great
Plasmodium protozoa	Malaria (with anemia, systemic inflammation)	150,000,000 (1,500,000*)	Moderate (travelers)
Rabies virus	Always-fatal meningitis and encephalitis	35,000 (35,000*)	Small
Respiratory syncytial virus	Repeated respiratory infections, pneumonia	65,000,000 (160,000*)	Great
Rotavirus	Diarrhea, dehydration	140,000,000 (873,000*)	Great
Salmonella typhi bacterium	Typhoid fever (with platelet and intestinal damage possible)	30,000,000 (581,000*)	Small (travelers)
Shigella bacteria	Diarrhea, dysentery, chronic infections	250,000,000 (654,000*)	None
Streptococcus Group A bacterium	Throat infection, then rheumatic fever, kidney disease	3,000,000 (52,000*)	Small
Streptococcus pneumoniae bacterium	Pneumonia, meningitis, serious inflammation of middle ear	100,000,000 (10,000,000*)	Small to moderate
Vibrio cholerae bacterium	Cholera (with diarrhea, dehydration)	7,000,000 (122,000*)	Small (travelers)
Yellow fever	Fever, jaundice, kidney damage, bleeding)	85,000 (9,000*)	Small (travelers)

PATHOGENS listed here were identified by the Institute of Medicine of the U.S. National Academy of Sciences as ones for which new or greatly improved vaccines are needed in the Third World and could feasibly be developed and licensed by 1996. Many manufacturers, however, are reluctant to invest in vaccine development for the Third World because the process is costly and the prospect is poor for recouping such expenses from sales there. The number of cases and deaths due to each pathogen are estimated based on the institute's 1986 report, *New Vaccine Development, Establishing Priorities*. The asterisk indicates diseases for which children account for roughly half of the deaths or more. Virtually all deaths from dengue fever, parainfluenza, respiratory syncytial virus, rotavirus, and pneumococcal meningitis occur in children. Two kinds of vaccines are already being made for hepatitis B.

From Robbins A, Freeman P: Obstacles to developing vaccines for the Third World. *Sci Am* 256:126, 1988.

Summary

Specific immunity may be conferred passively by transfer of immune serum or cells to a naive recipient or by active immunization. Passive immunity by transfer of antibody is effective if immediate neutralization of toxin or other agents is needed. Passive transfer of specific cellular immunity has been generally unsuccessful in humans except in anecdotal cases where transfer factor has been beneficial in selected diseases such as chronic mucocutaneous candidiasis.

Active immunization has changed the history of mankind in that a number of previously uncontrolled infectious diseases are now rarely seen or even eliminated. Vaccinations against smallpox has eliminated one of history's greatest scourges. Some other diseases now essentially under control by active immunization include tetanus, diphtheria, poliomyelitis, measles, and mumps.

New approaches to production of vaccines using synthetic antigens, antigens produced by gene cloning, conjugation techniques, and antiidiotypic immunogens give promise that improved vaccination methods will lead to control of additional infectious diseases in the future. Vaccines to *Haemophilus influenzae* type b and hepatitis B are now available and others, such as vaccines against schistosomiasis, malaria, and some other pathogens, have reached the level of clinical trials. Unless politics or economic problems interfere, control of many of mankind's worst diseases may be at hand.

Bibliography

PASSIVE IMMUNITY

Baker CJ, Melish ME, Hall RT, et al.: Intravenous immune globulin for the prevention of nosocomial infection of low-birth-weight neonates. *N Engl J Med* 327:213–219, 1992.

The intravenous immunoglobulin collaborative study group: Prophylactic intravenous administration of standard immune globulin as compared with core liposaccharide immune globulin in patients at high risk of postsurgical infection. *N Engl J Med* 327:234–240, 1992.

Hawgood BJ: Pioneers of antivenomous serotherapy: Dr. Vital Brazil (1865–1950). *Toxicon* 30:573, 1992.

Larrick JW: Potential of monoclonal antibodies as pharmocologic agents. *Pharmacol Rev* 41:539, 1989.

Lerner RA, Kang AS, Bain SJ, et al.: Antibodies without immunization. *Science* 258:1313, 1992.

Lipsky PE; NIH Concensus Development Panel: Intravenous immunoglobulin. *NIH Consensus Statement* 8:1, 1990.

Metselaar HJ, Rothbarth PH, Brouwer RML, et al.: Prevention of cytomegalovirus-related death by passive immunization. *Transplant* 48:264, 1989.

Riddell SR, Watanabe KS, Goodrich JM, et al.: Restoration of viral immunity in immunodeficient humans by the adoptive transfer of T-cell clones. *Science* 257:238, 1992.

Shackleford PG, Strauss AW: Kawasaki syndrome. *N Engl J Med* 324:1664, 1991.

Steim ER: Standard and special human immune globulins as therapeutic agents. *Pediatrics* 63:301, 1979.

Theakston RDG, Warrell DA: Antivenoms: A list of hyperimmune sera currently available for the treatment of envenoming by bites and stings. *Toxicon* 29:1419–1470.

Ziegler EJ, McCutchan JA, Fierer J, et al.: Treatment of gram-negative bacteremia and shock with HA-iA human monoclonal antibody against endotoxin. *N Engl J Med* 324:429, 1991.

SMALL POX

Behbehani, AM: The smallpox story: Life and death of an old disease. *Microbiol Rev* 47:455, 1983.

Bloch H: Edward Jenner (1749–1823): The history and effects of smallpox, inoculation, and vaccination. *Am J Diseases of Children* 147:772–774, 1993.

Henderson DA: Smallpox eradication. *Proc Soc Lond (Biol)* 199:83, 1977.

Jenner E: *Inquiry into the Cause and Effects of the Variolae Vacciniae*. London, Low 1798; republished in 1896 by Cassell.

Jezek Z, Khodakevich LN, Wickett JF: Smallpox and its posteradication surveillance. *Bull WHO* 65:425, 1987.

Sabin, AB: Eradication of smallpox and elimination of poliomyelitis: Contrast in strategy. *Jap J Med Sci Biol* 34:109, 1981.

von Pirquet CF: Klinische Studien uber Vakzination and Vakzinale Allergie. Leipzig, Deuticke, 1907.

PROPHYLACTIC IMMUNIZATION

Baker CJ, Kasper DL: Group B streptococcal vaccines. *Rev Inf Dis* 7:458, 1985.

Belanti J: Pediatric vaccinations: Update 1990. *Pediatr Clin N Am* 37:513, 1990.

Beneson AS: Immunization and military medicine *Rev Inf Dis* 6:1, 1984.

Bernier RH; Ad Hoc Working Group for the Development of the Standards for Pediatric Immunization Practices: Standards for pediatric immunization practices. *MMWR* 42(RR5):1–13, 1993.

Burnett WN: Vaccine development: Necessity as the mother of invention. *New Biologist* 4:269–273, 1992.

Centers for Disease Control (MMWR): Update on Adult Immunization: Recommendations of the immunization practices advisory committee (ACIP). *MMRP Atlanta, GA* 40:1, Nov. 15, 1992.

Cryz SJ (ed.): *Vaccines and Immunotherapy*. New York, Pergamon Press, 1991.

Cvjetanovic B: Immunization programmes. *WHO Chron* 27:66, 1973.

Dudgeon JA: Immunization in times ancient and modern. *J Royal Sci Med* 73:581, 1980.

Eickhoff TC: Immunization. The adult thing to do. *J Inf Dis* 152:1, 1985.

Glenny AT, Hopkins BE: Diphtheria toxoid as an immunizing agent. *Br J Exp Pathol* 4:823, 1923.

Heggie AD: Immunization against infectious disease. *Med Clin N Am* 67:17, 1983.

Hill DR: Immunizations for foreign travel. *Yale J Biol Med* 65:293, 1992.

Holt LB: *Developments in Diphtheria Prophylaxis*. London, Heinemann, 1950.

Krugman S, Katz SL: Childhood immunization procedures. *JAMA* 237:2228, 1977.

Potkin SA, Mortimer, EA (eds.): *Vaccines*. Philadelphia, WB Saunders, 1988.

National Vaccine Advisory Committee: Adult Immunization, National Vaccine Program. DHHS, Washington DC 1994.

Smith DT: Autogenous vaccines in theory and practice. *Arch Intern Med* 125:344, 1970.

Velimirovic B: Social, economic, and psychological impacts of childhood diseases subject to immunization. *Infection* 19:237, 1991.

Williams WW, Hickson MA, Kane MA, et al.: Immunization policies and vaccine coverage among adults: The risk for missed opportunities. *Ann Int Med* 108:616, 1988.

NEW APPROACHES TO VACCINE DEVELOPMENT

Dorner F, McDonel JL: Bacterial toxin vaccines. *Vaccine* 3:94, 1985.

Girand M: Vaccines. In *Human Gene Transfer. INSERM* 219:33, 1991.

Koff WC, Six HR (eds.): *Vaccine Research and Developments*, vol 1. New York, Marcel Dekker, 1992.

Liew FY: New aspects of vaccine development. *Clin Exp Immunol* 62:225, 1985.

Mizrahi A, Hertman I, Klingberg MA, et al.: New developments with human and veterinary vaccines. New York, Liss, 1980.

Morin B, Simons K: Subunit vaccines against developed viruses: Virosomes, micelles, and other protein complexes. *Vaccine* 3:83, 1985.

Stover CD, de la Cruz VF, Fuerst TR, et al.: New use of BCG for recombinant vaccines. *Nature* 351:456, 1991.

Woodrow GC, Levine MM: *New Generation Vaccines*. New York, Marcel Dekker, 1990.

SYNTHETIC VACCINES

Arnon R: Synthetic peptides as the basis for vaccine design. *Molec Immunol* 28:209, 1991.

Brown F: Synthetic viral vaccines. *Ann Rev Microbiol* 3:221, 1984.

RECOMBINANT VACCINES

Brown F, Schild GC, Ada GL: Recombinant vaccinia viruses as vaccines. *Nature* 319:549, 1986.

Esposito JJ, Murphy FA: Infectious recombinant vectored virus vaccines. *Adv Vetern Sci Comp Med* 33:195, 1989.

Macrina FL: Molecular cloning of bacterial antigens and virulence determinants. *Ann Rev Microbiol* 38:193, 1984.

Pastoret PP, Brochier B: Development of a recombinant vaccinia–rabies vaccine for oral immunization of foxes against rabies. *Develop Biol Stand* 79:105, 1992.

Tartaglia J, Paoletti E: Live recombinant viral vaccines. In *Immunochemistry of viruses. II. The basis for serodiagnosis and vaccines*. New York, Elseiver, 1990.

Ulmer JB, Donnelly JJ, Parker SE, et al.: Heterologous protection against influenza by injection of DNA encoding a viral protein. *Science* 259:1745, 1993.

CONJUGATE VACCINES

Borras-Cuesta F, Petit-Camurdan A, Fedon Y: Engineering of immunogenic peptides by co-linear synthesis of determinants recognized by B and T cells. *Eur J Immunol* 17:1213, 1987.

Cruse JM, Lewis RE: *Conjugate Vaccines*. Farmington, CT, S Karger, 1989.

Garner CV, Pier GB: Immunologic considerations for the development of conjugate vaccines. *Contrib Microbiol Immunol* 10:11, 1989.

IDIOTYPE VACCINES

Bona C, Moran T: Idiotype vaccines. *Ann Inst Pasteur* 136:21, 1985.

McNamara MK, Ward RE, Kohler H: Monoclonal idiotope vaccine against streptococcal pneumonia infection. *Science* 226:1325, 1984.

Hiernaux JR: Idiotypic vaccines and infectious diseases. *Infect Immun* 56:1407, 1988.

Sacks DL, Kelsoe GH, Sacks DH: Induction of immune responses with antiidiotypic antibodies: Implications for the induction of protective immunity. *Springer Semin Immunopath* 6:79, 1983.

UytdeHaag FGCM, Bunschoten H, Weijer K, et al.: From Jenner to Jerne: Towards idiotype vaccines. *Immunol Rev* 90:93, 1986.

Zhou E-M, Dreesman GR, Kennedy RC: Antiidiotypic antibodies: A new generation of vaccines against infectious agents. *Microbiol Sci* 4:36, 1987.

ACTIVE IMMUNIZATION —OTHERS

Germanier R (ed.): *Bacterial Vaccines*. Orlando, FL, Academic Press, 1984.

PERTUSSIS

Burnette, WN: The advent of recombinant pertussis vaccines. *Biotechnology* 8:1002, 1990.

Pittman M: History and the development of pertussis vaccine. *Develop Biol Standard* 73:13, 1991.

TUBERCULOSIS AND LEPROSY

Clemens JD, Chuong JJH, Feinstein AR: The BCG controversy: A methodologic and statistical reappraisal. *JAMA* 249:2362, 1983.

Crowle AJ: Immunization against tuberculosis: What kind of vaccine? *Infect Immun* 56:2769, 1988.

Ellner JJ: Immunology of human tuberculosis: Perspectives for vaccine development. *Chest* 95:237S, 1989.

Fine PEM: BCG vaccination against tuberculosis and leprosy. *Br Med Bull* 44:691, 1988.

Freerksen E, Rosenfeld M: Leprosy eradication project of Malta: First published report after 5 years running. *Chemotherapy* 23:356, 1977.

Joseph CA, Watson JM, Fern KJ: BCG immunisation in England and Wales: A survey of policy and practice in schoolchildren and neonates. *Br Med J* 305:495, 1992.

Smith FB: Tuberculosis and bureaucracy: Bacille Calmette et Guérin: Its troubled path to acceptance in Britain and Australia. *Med J Aust* 159:408–411, 1993.

Turk JL, Bryceson ADM: Immunologic phenomena in leprosy and related diseases. *Adv Immunol* 13:209, 1971.

HAEMOPHILUS INFLUENZA

Cochi SL, Biloome CV, Hightower J: Immunization of U.S. children with *haemophilus influenzae* type B polysaccharide vaccine. *JAMA* 253:521, 1985.

Eskola J, Kayhty H, Takala AK, et al.: A randomized, prospective field trial of a conjugate vaccine in the protection of infants and young children against invasive *Haemophilus influenzae* type b disease. *N Engl J Med* 323:1381, 1990.

Hamel J, Broder BR: Induction of an immune response to the porin of *Haemophilus influenzae* type b by monoclonal antiidiotypic antibodies. *Microbiol Pathogen* 9:81, 1990.

TYPHOID

Centers for Disease Control MMWR: Typhoid Immunization 43:1–7, 1994.

Woodruff BA, Pavia AT, Blake PA: A new look at typhoid vaccination. *JAMA* 265:756, 1991.

PNEUMO-COCCAL DISEASE

Gable CB, Holzer SS, Engelhart L, et al.: Pneumococcal vaccine: Efficacy and associated cost savings. *JAMA* 264:2910, 1990.

Heilmann C: Human B- and T-lymphocyte responses to vaccination with pneumococcal polysaccharides. *Acta Pathol Microbiol Immunol Scand* 98(suppl. 15):5, 1990.

Shapiro ED, Berg AT, Austrian R, et al.: The protective efficacy of polyvalent pneumococcal polysaccharide vaccine. *N Engl J Med* 325:1453, 1991.

Siber GR: Pneumococcal disease: prospects for a new generation of vaccines. *Science* 265:1385–1386, 1994.

CHOLERA

Mekalanos JJ, Sadoff JC: Cholera vaccines: fighting an ancient scourge. *Science* 265:1387–1389, 1994.

VIRUSES—GENERAL

Jordan WS: Program for accelerated development of new viral vaccines. *Prog Med Virol* 35:1, 1988.

Melnick JL: Virus vaccines: 1986 update. *Prog Med Virol* 33:134, 1986.

POLIO

Andrus JK, de Quadros CA, Olive J-M: The surveillance challenge: Final stages of eradication of poliomyelitis in the Americas. *MMWR* 41(SS-1):21, 1992.

Baguley DM, Glasgow GL: Subacute sclerosing panencephalitis and the Salk vaccine. *Lancet* 2:763, 1973.

Enders JF, Weller TH, Robbins FC: Cultivation of the Lansing strain of poliomyelitis virus in cultures of various human embryonic tissue. *Science* 109:85, 1949.

Minor PD: The molecular biology of poliovaccines. *J Gen Virol* 73:3065–3077, 1992.

Sabin AB: Paralytic poliomyelitis: Old dogmas and new perspectives. *Rev Infect Div* 3:543, 1981.

Sabin AB: Present position of immunization against poliomyelitis virus with live virus vaccines. *Br Med J* 1:663, 1959.

Salk J, Salk D: Control of influenza and poliomyelitis with killed-virus vaccines. *Science* 195:834, 1977.

HEPATITIS B

Bloom BS, Hollman AL, Fendrick AM, et al.: A reappraisal of hepatitis B virus vaccination strategies using cost-effectiveness analysis. *Ann Int Med* 118:298–306, 1993.

Da Villa G, Piazza M, Iorio R, et al.: A pilot model of vaccination against hepatitis B virus suitable for mass vaccination campaigns in hyperendemic areas. *J Med Virol* 36:274, 1992.

Davis HL, Michel M-L, Mancini M, et al.: Direct gene transfer in skeletal muscle: plasmid DNA-based immunization against hepatitis B virus surface antigen. *Vaccine* 12:1503–1509, 1994.

Ellis RW: *Hepatitis B vaccines in clinical practice.* New York, Marcel Dekker, 1992.

Neurath AR, Jameson BA, Huima T: Hepatitis B virus proteins eliciting protective immunity. *Microbiol Sci* 4:45, 1987.

Stephenne J: Recombinant versus plasma-derived hepatitis B vaccines: Issues of safety, immunogenicity, and cost effectiveness. *Vaccine* 6:299, 1988.

Sylvan SPE: Cellular immune responses to hepatitis B virus antigens in man. *Liver* 11:1, 1991.

Whittle HC, Inskip H, Hall AJ, et al.: Vaccination against hepatitis B and protection against chronic viral carriage in the Gambia. *Lancet* 337:747, 1991.

HEPATITIS A

Flehmig B, Heinricy U, Pfisterer M: Prospects for a hepatitis A virus vaccine. *Prog Med Virol* 37:56, 1990.

Siegl G, Lemon SM: Recent advances in hepatitis A vaccine development. *Virus Res* 17:75, 1990.

EPSTEIN–BARR VIRUS

Arrand JR: Prospects for a vaccine against Epstein–Barr virus. *Cancer J* 5:188, 1992.

Morgan B, Finerty S, Lovgren K, et al.: Prevention of Epstein–Barr (EB) virus-induced lymphoma in cottontop tamarins by vaccination with the EB virus envelope glycoprotein gp340 incorporated into immune-stimulating complexes. *J Gen Virol* 69:2093, 1988.

Epstein MA: Epstein–Barr virus: Is it time to develop a vaccine program? *J Natl Cancer Inst* 56:697, 1976.

PAPILLOMA VIRUSES

Crawford L: Prospects for cervical cancer vaccines. *Cancer Surveys* 16:215–229, 1993.

Dillner J: Immunobiology of papillomavirus: Prospects for vaccination. *Cancer J* 5:181, 1992.

Galloway DA: Human papilloma vaccines: a warty problem. *Infect Agents DIS* 3:187–193, 1994.

Kirchner H: Immunobiology of human papillomavirus infection. *Prog Med Virol* 33:1, 1986.

zur Hausen H: Viruses in human cancers. *Science* 254:1167, 1991.

MEASLES

Centers for Disease Control: Rubella prevention: Recommendations of the immunization practices advisory committee (ACIP). *MMWR* 39:1, 1990.

Centers for Disease Control: Measles vaccination levels among selected groups of preschool-aged children—United States. *MMWR* 40:36, 1991.

Hilleman MR: Past, present, and future of measles, mumps, and rubella virus vaccines. *Pediatrics* 90:149, 1992.

INFLUENZA

Centers for Disease Control: Prevention and control of influenza: Recommendation of the immunization practices advisory committee (ACIP). *MMWR* 40:RR-6, 1, 1991; *MMWR* 41:RR-9,1, 1992; *MMWR* 42:RR-6, 1993.

Fazekas de St. Groth S: Evolution and hierarchy of influenza viruses. *Arch Environ Health* 21:293, 1970.

Killbourne ED: Influenza as a problem in immunology. *J Immunol* 120:1447, 1978.

Lennette EH: Viral respiratory diseases and antivirals. *Bull WHO* 59:305, 1981.

Ulmer JB, Donnelly JJ, Parker SE, et al.: Heterologous protection against influenza by injection of DNA encoding a viral protein. *Science* 259:1745–1749, 1993.

RESPIRATORY SYNCYTIAL VIRUS

Hall CB: Prospects for a respiratory syncytial virus vaccine. *Science* 265:1393–1394, 1994.

VARICELLA

Gershon AA: Varicella vaccine: Still at the crossroads. *Pediatrics* 90:144, 1992.

Gershon AA, Steinberg SP, NIAID Collaborative Varicella Vaccine Study Group: Live attenuated varicella vaccine: Protection in healthy adults in comparison to leukemic children. *J Infect Dis* 161:661, 1990.

Plotkin SA: Vaccines for varicella-zoster virus and cytomegalovirus: Recent progress. *Science* 265:1383–1384, 1994.

Roizman B: Introduction: Objectives of herpes simplex virus vaccines seen from a historical perspective. *Rev Infect Dis* 13 (suppl. 11):S892, 1991.

RABIES

Dietzschold B, Wang H, Rupprecht CE, et al.: Induction of protective immunity against rabies immunization with rabies virus ribonucleoprotein. *Proc Natl Acad Sci USA* 84:9165, 1987.

Hennessen W, Regamey RH (eds.): Joint WHO/IABS symposium on the standardization of rabies vaccines for human use produced in tissue culture (Rabies III). Basel, S Karger, 1978.

Pastoret P-P, Brochier B, Blancou J, et al.: Development and deliberate release of a vaccinia–rabies recombinant virus for the oral vaccination of foxes against rabies. In *Recombinant Poxviruses*. Binns MM, Smith GL (eds.). Boca Raton, FL, CRC Press, 1992, 163–206.

Suss J, Sinnecker H: Immune reactions against rabies virus: Infection and vaccination. *Exp Pathol* 42:1, 1991.

Wiktor TJ: Historical aspects of rabies treatment. In *World's Debt to Pasteur*. New York, Liss, 1985.

ROTAVIRUS

Glass RI, Geutsch J, Smith JC: Rotavirus vaccines: Success by reassortment. *Science* 265:1389–1391, 1994.

FUNGI

Segal E: Vaccines against fungal infections. CRC Critical Reviews in Microbiology. 14:229–271, 1987.

MALARIA

Brown IN: Immunologic aspects of malaria infection. *Adv Immunol* 11:268, 1969.

Good MF, Berzofsky JA, Miller LH: The T-cell response to the malaria circumsporozoite protein. *Annu Rev Immunol* 6:663, 1988.

Hommel M: Steps toward a malaria vaccine. *Res Immunol* 142:618, 1991.

Nussenzweig V, Nussenzweig RV: Rationale for the development of an engineered sporozoite malaria vaccine. *Adv Immunol* 45:283, 1989.

Nussenzweig RS, Long CA: Malaria vaccines: multiple targets. *Science* 265:1381–1383, 1994.

Playfair JHL, Taverne J, Bate CAW, et al.: The malaria vaccine: Antiparasite or antidisease? *Immunol Today* 11:25, 1990.

Quakyi IA, Taylor DW, Johnson AH, et al.: Development of a malaria T-cell vaccine for blood stage immunity. *Scand J Immunol* 36(suppl. 11):9, 1992.

Suss G, Pink JRL: A recombinant malaria protein that can induce Th1 and CD8+ T-cell responses without antibody formation. *J Immunol* 149:1334, 1992.

Tanner M, Teuscher T, Alonso PL: SPf66–The first malaria vaccine. *Parasitol Today* 11:10–13, 1995.

SCHISTO-SOMIASIS

Capron A, Dessaint JP, Capron M: Immunoregulation of parasites. *J Allerg Clin Immunol* 66:91, 1980.

Capron A, Dessaint JP: Vaccination against parasitic diseases: Some alternative concepts for the definition of protective antigens. *Ann Inst Pasteur/Immunol* 139:109, 1988.

Pearce EJ: Proselytizing with immunity. *Nature* 363:19–20, 1993.

Wakelin D: Immunity to intestinal parasites. *Nature* 273:617, 1978.

ONCHO-CERCIASIS

Braun G, Engelbrecht F, Taylor DW: Molecular biology of *Onchocerca volvulus* and development of experimental vaccines. In *Basic Research in Helminthiases*. Ehrlich R, Neito A, Yazabal L (eds.). Montevideo, Deiciones LOGOS, 1990, 145.

INSECTS/TICKS

Shulman S: Allergic responses to insects. *Annu Rev Entomol* 12:323, 1967.

Stebbings JH: Immediate hypersensitivity: A defense against arthropods. *Perspect Biol Med* 17:233, 1974.

Willadsen P, Kemp DH: Vaccination with "concealed" antigens for tick control. *Parasitol Today* 4:196, 1988.

ANTIFERTILITY VACCINES

Alexander NJ, Bialy G: Contraceptive vaccine development. *Reprod Fertil Dev* 6:273–280, 1994.

Ladd A: Progress in the development of anti-LHRH vaccine. *AJRI* 29:189–194, 1993.

Murdoch WJ: Immunoregulation of mammalian fertility. *Life Sciences* 55:1871–1886, 1994.

Sacco AG: Zona pellucida: Current status as a candidate antigen for contraceptive vaccine development. *Am J Repro Immunol* 15:122, 1987.

Stevens VC: Future perspectives for vaccine development. *Scand J Immunol* 36 (suppl. 11):137, 1992.

Stevens V: Vaccine delivery systems: Potential methods for use in antifertility vaccines. *AJRI* 29:176–188, 1993.

Talwar GP, Hingorani V, Kumar S, et al.: Phase I clinical trials with three formulations of antihuman chorionic gonadotropin vaccine. *Contraception* 41:301, 1990.

ORAL VACCINATION

Bienenstock J, Befus AD: Mucosal immunity. *Immunology* 41:249, 1980.

de Aizpurua HJ, Russel-Jones GJ: Oral vaccination: Identification of classes of proteins that provoke an immune response upon oral feeding. *J Exp Med* 167:440, 1988.

Clements JD, Lyon FL, Garry RF: Immunological protection against mucosal pathogens by direct stimulation of antibody-forming cells in the gut-associated lymphoid tissues. In *Immunopharmacology of Infectious Diseases*. New York, Liss, 1987.

Soulsby EJL: The mechanism of immunity to gastrointestinal nematodes. In *Biology of Parasites*. New York, Academic Press, 1966.

EVALUATION

Creese AL, Henderson RH: Cost-effectiveness appraisal of immunization programmes. *Bull WHO* 60:621, 1982.

D'Archy Hart P: Efficacy and applicability of mass BCG vaccination in tuberculosis control. *Br Med J* 1:587, 1967.

Frenkel JK: Models for infectious disease. *Fed Proc* 28:179, 1969.

Fulginiti VA: Immunizations: Current controversies. *J Pediatr* 101:487, 1982.

Greenwood M, Yule UG: The statistics of antithyphoid and anticholera inoculations, and the interpretation of such statistics in general. *Proc R Soc Med* 8(pt. 2):113, 1915.

Halloran ME, Haber M, Longini IM, et al.: Direct and indirect effects in vaccine efficiency and effectiveness. *Am J Epidemiol* 133:323, 1991.

Nokes DJ, Anderson RM: Vaccine safety versus vaccine efficacy in mass immunization programmes. *Lancet* 338:1309, 1991.

Sisk JE, Riegelman RK: Cost effectiveness of vaccination against pneumococcal pneumonia: An update. *Ann Int Med* 104:79, 1986.

LIABILITY

Aukrust L, Almeland TL, Refsum D, et al.: Severe hypersensitivity or intolerance reactions to measles vaccine in six children. *Allergy* 35:581, 1980.

Fenichel GM: Neurological complications of immunization. *Ann Neurol* 12:119, 1982.

Leinikki PO: Vaccination policies for the 1980s. *Am Clin Res* 14:195, 1982.

Mason JO: Protecting physicians from vaccine liability. *JAMA* 266:2951, 1991.

Peter G. Vaccine crisis: An emerging social problem. *J Infect Dis* 151:981, 1985.

IMMUNIZATION IN DEVELOPING COUNTRIES

Bres P: Immunization in developing countries. *Ann Inst Pasteur/Immunol* 136D:293, 1985.

Poore P: Vaccination strategies in developing countries. *Vaccine* 6:393, 1988.

Robbins A, Freeman P: Obstacles to developing vaccines for the Third World. *Sci Am* 256:126, 1988.

Walsh J: Establishing health priorities in the developing world. *United Nations Development Program*. Adams Pub Group, 1988.

27

Immunodeficiency Diseases

The occurrence of repeated or unusual infections in an individual may reflect a deficiency in defense mechanisms against infection (Table 27–1). Such deficiencies must be especially considered if the infecting organism is one that is not usually responsible for human diseases (opportunistic infection). The type of infection observed is determined by the kind of immune abnormality present. Antibody deficiencies are associated with bacterial infections; cell-mediated immunity deficiencies are associated with viral, fungal, protozoal, and mycobacterial infections. Immunodeficiency diseases are classified as primary or secondary. Primary immunodeficiencies result from genetic or developmental abnormalities in the acquisition of immune maturity. Secondary deficiencies are caused by diseases that interfere with the expression of a mature immune system.

Both immune and nonimmune specific levels of defensive reactions must be considered in evaluating resistance to infection. Since the major role of inflammation is defense against infection and repair of injury, any alteration in the inflammatory response or defect in the natural barriers to infectious organisms may lead to an increase in infections. For instance, infections are a major complication of burn patients who have lost their external barrier to infection. The depression of pulmonary-clearing mechanisms due to the loss of the ciliary activity of bronchial lining cells associated with exposure to cigarette smoke is another example. In addition, there is a genetic disorder resulting in a microtubule defect that affects the mobility of cilia (**immotile cilia syndrome**). Affected male patients also have immobile sperm and chronic respiratory infections, frequent *Hemophilus influenza* infection, and abundant mucous secretions. Because of the complexity of

TABLE 27–1. CHARACTERISTICS OF INFECTIONS ASSOCIATED WITH IMMUNODEFICIENCY DISEASES

Increased frequency
Increased severity
Prolonged duration
Unexpected complications and unusual manifestations
Infection with agents with low infectivity

immune deficiencies and the diverse clinical presentation of deficiency states, a careful systematic diagnostic work-up must be carried out in order to select appropriate therapy.

There are more than seventy different kinds of primary immunodeficiencies involving B cells (antibodies), T cells (cell-mediated immunity), phagocytic cells, and complement proteins. Although the incidence of a selective IgA deficiency is the most common (1:500), it is not usually associated with any clinical manifestations. Approximately 370 infants are born annually with a clinically significant primary immunodeficiency, distributed as follows:

Antibody (B-cell) immunodeficiencies	50%
Cellular (T-cell) immunodeficiencies	40%
Combined with antibody deficiency	30%
T cell only	10%
Phagocytic deficiencies	6%
Complement deficiencies	4%

Maturation of Immunity

DEVELOPMENT OF THE IMMUNE SYSTEM

Much of our understanding of the relationship of the developing immune system to immunodeficiencies stems from the brilliant insight of Robert A. Good in his study of naturally occurring immunodeficiency diseases of man ("experiments of nature") and the phylogeny of immunity in experimental animals. All white blood cells, including immune cells, arise from a common ancestral cell in the blood-forming organs (fetal liver, yolk sac, and bone marrow). In order for potentially immunologically competent cells to mature and obtain the capacity to recognize antigen, they must come in contact with, or be affected by, products of endodermal tissue. The embryonal endodermal-associated lymphoid tissue, termed the central lymphoid tissue, consists of the thymus, tonsils, appendix, Peyer's patches, liver, and, in fowl, the bursa of Fabricius. The peripheral lymphoid tissue is the remaining lymphoid tissue, including lymph nodes and spleen. If needed, the reader should refer to Chapter 3 for a more detailed exposition of lymphoid organs. The major sites of hereditary immunodeficiencies in maturation are at the stem cell (combined immune deficiency), T cell (deficiencies in cell-mediated immunity) or B cell (antibody deficiencies). T-cell defects may occur at the level of the precursor in the bone marrow, at the level of the thymus, or at the level of the thymus-derived peripheral T cell. Similarly, B-cell deficiencies may arise at the level of the bone marrow precursor or during maturation of B cells. With increasing understanding of the immune system, a number of more specific defects in immunoglobulin isotype switching, cell receptors, adhesion molecules, and lymphokines have now been recognized. For example, severe immunodeficiency in children with a defect in T-cell activation at the level of interaction between the T-cell receptor and G proteins has recently been reported.

IMMUNE RESPONSE OF IMMATURE ANIMALS

Fetal and neonatal animals may be induced to form antibody or develop high levels of immunoglobulins if given strong antigenic stimuli but often have a delayed or blunted response to T-dependent antigens. Neonatal animals normally are protected by maternal antibody received by placental transfer or by absorption of colostral antibodies shortly after birth (Fig. 27–1). The newborn animal begins to produce its own antibodies due to natural stimulation within the first three months after birth. The development of "normal" lymphoid tissue and "normal" immunoglobulin levels depends upon contact with antigen; germ-free animals that have a markedly reduced antigenic load maintain very low levels of serum immunoglobulins and have undeveloped, immature lymphoid tissue. However, germ-free animals have genetically normal immune systems and can respond to appropriate antigenic stimuli. In contrast, children with severe congenital immunodeficiencies, who have been maintained in germ-free isolators with the hope of acquiring immune maturity later in life, have died from infection or complications of bone marrow transplantation when removed from the germ-free environment.

HYPOGAMMA-GLOBULINEMIA OF INFANCY

A temporary functional delay in the production of immunoglobulins by a newborn may cause a transient hypogammaglobulinemia of infancy. Hypogammaglobulinemia occurs when the normal catabolism of placentally transferred maternal IgG commencing after birth is associated with an abnormal delay in the onset of the immunoglobulin synthetic capacity by the infant. This temporary immunoglobulin deficiency usually terminates between 9 and 18 months of age. Since it is only temporary, hypogammaglobulinemia of infancy is not considered a primary immune deficiency disease. If it continues, a true permanent immune deficiency disease must be considered.

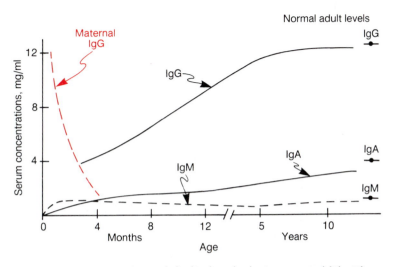

Figure 27–1. Serum immunoglobulin levels during normal life. The new-born human has high levels of serum IgG because of maternal transfer of IgG across the placenta. Colostrum provides additional immunoglobulin, particularly gastrointestinal IgA. During infancy, serum IgM becomes elevated within one month; serum IgG, between 4 and 8 months; and serum IgA rises gradually over the first 10 years of life because of synthesis by the child. Neonates also have decreased cellular immune responses, even though the CD4+ T-cell count may be >1,500/mm^3, most likely due to immature immune regulation.

NEONATAL WASTING SYNDROME (TORCH)

"Wasting" of newborn infants is seen following infection in utero with a number of organisms that are able to cross the placenta from the mother to the fetus (ie, rubella) or with infection at birth because of organisms in the birth canal (herpes). A newborn infant with low birth weight, microencephaly, eye abnormalities, and liver and other visceral abnormalities may reflect the effects of congenital infection with a number of otherwise unrelated agents given the term TORCH. TORCH refers to toxoplasmosis, rubella, cytomegalovirus, and herpes simplex, in recognition of the infectious organisms most frequently recognized as the causative agents. Other infectious agents, such as *Treponema pallidum* (congenital syphilis) and *Listeria*, may produce similar findings, so that the O in TORCH may be considered to stand for "other" infectious agents. In addition, congenital infection with HIV can cause congenital AIDS so that the H may be for HIV, as well as herpes. The chronic infectious state is the result of immaturity of the infant's immune system at the time of infection. Such infections are not able to be controlled by the infant's immune system or by passively transferred immunity from the mother, resulting in chronic wasting disease. In addition to immunodeficiencies, congenitally infected infants frequently also have other developmental abnormalities, ie, blindness, mental retardation, and heart defects.

Primary Immuno-deficiencies

Developmental abnormalities may result in a permanent loss of immune cells at specific anatomic sites. Such abnormalities may occur at one of the major sites of immune development mentioned above—the ancestral anlage, the thymus-dependent system, or the humoral antibody/immunoglobulin-producing system. These levels of development where immunodeficiencies may occur are illustrated in Figure 27–2. Essentially, three major primary immune deficits occur—combined antibody and cellular, antibody alone, and cellular alone.

MOUSE MODELS OF PRIMARY IMMUNO-DEFICIENCIES

Understanding of heritable human immunodeficiency diseases has been aided by a number of genetic defects in the mouse that produce effects similar to human immunodeficiencies (Table 27–2).

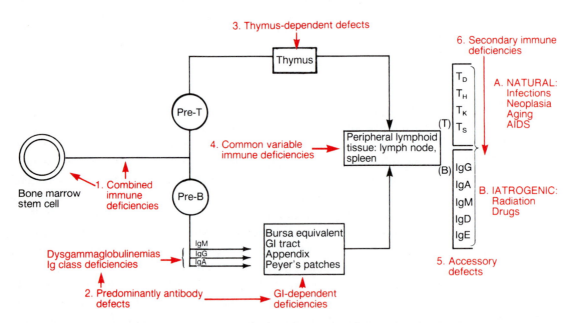

Figure 27–2. Postulated sites of defects in immune diseases. The type and severity of infections seen are related to the deficiency type and the level of development affected. Numbers 1–5 indicate the possible sites of developmental defects in primary immunodeficiencies: (1) Combined immunodeficiencies, (2) predominantly antibody defects (dysgammaglobulinemias), (3) thymus-dependent defects, (4) common variable deficiencies, and (5) defects in accessory systems, such as complement or phagocytic capacity. Number (6) marks secondary immunodeficiencies that affect an already developed immune system and occur due to other disease states or because of treatment for other diseases.

TABLE 27–2. SOME IMMUNODEFICIENCY MUTATIONS IN MICE

Gene Name	Gene Symbol	Chromosome	Major Manifestations
Nude	*nu*	11	Thymic aplasia, hairless, T-cell deficiency, increased NK and macrophage activity
SCID	*scid*	16	Absence of T and B cells, defect in antigen receptor gene rearrangement, normal myeloid, NK and macrophage function
Motheaten	*me*	6	Decreased T-cell, B-cell, and NK activity, increased macrophage proliferation, granulo-cytic skin lesions, and pneumonitis
Dominant hemimelia	*Dh*	1	Absence of spleen, decreased IgM, IgG_2, antibody responses
X-linked	*xid*	X	B-cell dysfunction, reduced IgM, IgG_3, defective antibody responses
Hemolytic complement	*Hc*	2	Homozygotes lack C5, impaired neutrophil chemotaxis, increased infections
Beige	*bg*	13	Decreased NK, T_{CTL}, lysosomal membrane defect, decreased granulocyte chemotaxis
Steel	*Sl*	10	Loss of stem cell growth factor (c-kit ligand), mast-cell defect, impaired resistance to parasitic infections
Hairless	hr^{rh}	14	Decreased T-cell response to mitogens, reduced antibody formation, thymic lymphomas
Dwarf	*dw*	11	Decreased cortical thymocytes, primary defect in anterior pituitary

COMBINED IMMUNO-DEFICIENCIES (TABLE 27–3)

Anlage Defects (Reticular Dysgenesis). The failure of development of all blood cell lines, presumably because no hematopoietic stem cells are present, is known as reticular dysgenesis. Affected fetuses lack all types of white blood cells and at autopsy have no lymphoid tissue. All have been stillbirths. The genetic defect is unknown.

Severe Combined Immuno-deficiencies (SCIDs)

SCIDs has an incidence of 1:100,000 births and may have several etiologies, including a failure in development of stem cells; a failure in thymic function, because of inborn errors of metabolism in which purine synthesizing enzymes are inactive or defective (see below); or because of a lack of cell receptors, such as IL-2R. In SCID, mice precursor lymphocytes have active, but defective, VDJ recombinase activity. They are able to cleave the immunoglobulin genes at the appropriate sequences but are unable to join the cleaved ends of the coding strands of the variable region gene segments correctly. The molecular basis for the X-linked human immune disorders is shown in Table 27–4. Severe combined immunodeficiencies include autosomal recessive and X-linked SCID (XSCID), Wiskott–Aldrich syndrome, and ataxiatelangiectasia.

TABLE 27–3. COMBINED IMMUNODEFICIENCY DISEASES

	Usual Phenotypic Expression						
Designation	Serum Ig	Serum Antibodies	Circulating B Cells	Circulating T Cells	CMI	Presumed Nature of Basic Defect	Inheritance
1. Reticular dysgenesis	None	None	None	None	None	No anlage	?
2. Swiss type agamma-globulinemia	Decreased or absent	Absent	Decreased or absent	Decreased or absent	Absent	No lymphoid stem cell	AR
3. Thymic alymphoplasia	Decreased or absent	Absent	Decreased or absent	Decreased or absent	Absent	No lymphoid stem cell	X-linked
4. Wiskott–Aldrich syndrome[a]	Increased IgA, IgE; decreased IgM	Decreased	Normal	Progressive decrease	Progressive decrease	Cell membrane defect affecting all hematopoietic stem cell derivatives	X-linked
5. Ataxia-telangiectasia[a]	Often decreased IgA, IgE, and IgG; increased IgM (monomers)	Variably decreased	Normal	Decreased	Decreased	Unknown: defective T cell maturation	AR

[a]Characteristic associated features: Wiskott–Aldrich syndrome—thrombocytopenia, eczema; ataxia–telangiectasia—cerebellar ataxia, telangiectasia, ovarian dysgenesis, chromosomal instability, decreased α-fetoprotein.

TABLE 27-4. DISEASE GENES FOR THREE X-LINKED IMMUNE DISORDERS

Clinical Disease (Abbreviation)	Genetic Locus	Protein Name (Abbreviation)	Gene Family	Genomic Span	cDNA Size	Amino Acids	Gene Alterations in Unrelated Patients
X-linked severe combined immunodeficiency (SCID)	Xq13.1	IL-2R receptor γ chain	Cytokine receptor	4.2 kb	1.8 kb	369	Single base changes forming a premature stop codon, single base changes substituting an amino acid, single base changes eradicating a splice donor site, microdeletions, microinsertions, decreased mRNA in half of cases
X-linked agammaglobulinemia (XLA) (Brutons)	Xq22	B-cell tyrosine kinase	Non-receptor tyrosine kinase	20 kb	2.6–3 kb	659	Intragenic deletions, single base changes substituting an amino acid, decreased mRNA
X-linked immunodeficiency with hyper-IgM (HIGM)	Xq26	CD40 ligand, glycoprotein 39	Type II trans-membrane glyco-protein, related to TNFα,β	15 kb	1.5–1.8 kb	260	Microdeletions, single base changes substituting an amino acid, single base changes forming a premature stop codon, normal mRNA levels

Modified from Puck JM: Molecular basis for three X-linked immune disorders. *Human Mole Genetics* 3:1457–1461, 1994.

Swiss-type Agammaglobulinemia and Thymic Alymphoplasia. His-torically, the term "Swiss-type agammaglobulinemia" was used for the autosomal recessive form and "thymic alymphoplasia" for the X-linked form (XSCID) of SCID. Infants with SCID fail to grow nor-mally and have severe infections. Symptoms may appear within the first few days of life, but in most cases, infectious complications do not appear until 4 to 6 months of age. Early clinical developments are per-sistent oral candidiasis (thrush), chronic diarrhea, pneumonia otitis media, and recurrent sepsis, associated with failure to thrive (wasting). Patients with SCID are susceptible to a wide variety of infections and developed progressive vaccinia when smallpox immunizations were done, or BCGosis if immunized with BCG.

Maternal transfer of some cellular immune function, as well as immunoglobulin, may partially protect the infant or contribute to wast-ing. Children with SCIDs frequently develop a skin rash, consistent with that of a graft-versus-host reaction, believed to be caused by maternal lymphoid cells. Maternal lymphocytes may cross the placenta during gestation. Normally such placentally transferred cells are rejected by the immune system of the fetus. However, if the fetus is unable to react to them, the foreign cells may proliferate in the immune-deficient child and produce a graft-versus-host reaction. Such cells may also provide some cellular immunity and protect the child from fulminant viral infections during the first 4 to 6 months of life.

All major immunoglobulin groups (IgG, IgA, and IgM) are severely depressed (total <0.25 mg/mL) and there is a striking defi-ciency of lymphocytes in the blood (<1,000/mL). At autopsy, only a few plasma cells and lymphocytes are found, and the thymus is atrophic and lacks Hassall's corpuscles. A deficiency in the reactivity of lymphocytes from patients with SCID can be demonstrated by the lack of in vitro stimulation by phytohemagglutinin. XSCID has been shown to be due to a lack of the γ chain for the IL-2 receptor. This chain is also shared by the IL-4 and IL-7 receptor, so that multiple stages in growth of T and B cells are affected. The presence of epithe-lial remnants in the thymus associated with an absence of lymphocytes suggests a defect in the production of prothymocytes, as well as of B stem cells (ie, a defect at the level of the lymphoid stem cell that gives rise to both T- and B-cell lineages).

Wiskott–Aldrich Syndrome. This syndrome is an x-linked recessive combined immunodeficiency with a marked deficiency in IgM and usually depressed cellular immunity resulting in death in early infancy from infections. Serum IgA and IgG levels are usually normal, but affected males have defects in T-cell functions. There is also eczema and thrombocytopenia (low blood platelets), and bleeding may be the first manifestation of the disease. A glycoprotein (glycophorin, CD43) common to T cells and platelets, is reduced in these patients. CD43 enhances the antigen-specific activation of T cells and its deficiency possibly contributes to the pathogenesis of this disease. CD43 binds to intercellular adhesion molecule-1 (ICAM-1), and loss of this binding would be expected to reduce cell signaling. Inactive CD43 may result from increased activity of calpein, which cleaves CD43. It has been proposed that calpein inhibitors might be used for therapy.

Ataxia Telangiectasia. Ataxia telangiectasia is an autosomal recessive combined immune deficiency disease. The serum IgA is very low, IgG is low or normal, and IgM is usually normal; the lymphoid organs are atrophic or absent. There is also oculocutaneous telangiectasia (dilated and redundant vessels), progressive cerebellar ataxia, and increased lymphoreticular malignancies.

Purine Metabolism and Primary Immunodeficiencies. A number of children with SCID have enzymatic defects in the purine biosynthesis pathways. Purine interconversions are required for normal maturation of the rapidly dividing cells of the lymphoid system. Blocks in purine biosynthesis may lead to accumulation of deoxynucleosides that are toxic to lymphocytes (Fig. 27–3). These include a T-cell deficiency, a B-cell deficiency, and a combined deficiency (Table 27–5).

Bare Lymphocyte Syndrome. Rare patients with combined immunodeficiencies have decreased expression of class I and less frequently class II MHC determinants on blood mononuclear cells due to a defect of gene transcription. This defect in MHC expression on lymphocytes apparently interferes with the self-recognition mechanisms required for induction of effective immune responses. These individuals may have normal or decreased serum Ig and antibodies and/or normal or decreased CMI. Severely affected individuals develop oral candidiasis, *Pneumocystis carinii* pneumonia, bacterial pneumonia, herpes, diarrhea, and wasting. Although B-cell numbers are normal, there are very few plasma cells and very low serum immunoglobulin levels in patients with clinical manifestations.

A defect in T-helper cell–B-cell communication also has been reported in **hypogammaglobulinemia with partial albinism**, a very rare syndrome (two cases reported) associated with an absence of Langerhans' cells in the skin and repeated upper and lower respiratory infections. Finally, the T cells of a child with SCID and graft-versus-hostlike lesions were found to have TCR α/β but were "double negative" for CD4 and CD8. As more analysis of the cell surface phenotype of T and B cells from patients with immunodeficiency diseases are done, it is likely that a number of different abnormalities will be discovered.

Common Variable Immunodeficiencies. Common variable immunodeficiencies (CVIs) are listed in Table 27–6. They are late onset immune deficiencies (after 4 to 5 years of age and usually later) with

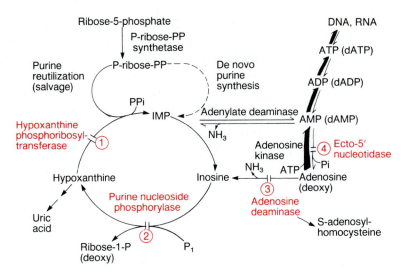

Figure 27–3. Purine metabolism and immunodeficiencies.

TABLE 27–5. CLINICAL SYMPTOMS AND EXPRESSION OF DISEASES ASSOCIATED
WITH DEFECTS IN PURINE METABOLISM

1. *Hypoxanthine guanine phosphoribosyltransferase (Lesch–Nyhan syndrome).*

(Possible B Cell Immunodeficiency.) There is a marked overproduction of purines and
overexcretion of uric acid. These children have severe neurological impairment and self-
destructive behavior. Their lymphocytes respond poorly to stimulation with pokeweed
mitogen.

2. *Purine nucleotide phosphorylase (PNP) deficiency (T-cell immunodeficiency).*

Features large quantities of ribonucleosides (inosine and guanosine), as well as 2'-
deoxyribonucleosides (2'-deoxyinosine and 2'-deoxyguanosine) in urine, in red cells, and
in lymphocytes; a loss of purines that are necessary for lymphocyte proliferation, and
severe impairment of DNA synthesis. There is recurrent infection and anemia, severe
lymphopenia, pronounced depression of lymphocytes responses to mitogenic and allogeneic cell stimuli and decreased T-cell rosette formation.

3. *Adenosinedeaminase (ADA) deficiency (T and B cell immunodeficiency).*

Children have high concentrations of AMP and dAMP in erythrocytes and lymphocytes (2
to 10 times normal) and large amounts of 2'-deoxyadenosine are excreted in urine. They
have respiratory infections, lymphopenia, and no delayed hypersensitivity response to
Candida, mumps, and streptokinase–streptodornase. Their lymphocytes respond poorly to
phytohemagglutinin, pokeweed mitogen, and allogeneic cells, and they fail to develop
isohemagglutinins.

4. *Ecto 5'-nucleotidase deficiency (B-cell immunodeficiency).*

Children have increased concentrations of toxic deoxyribonucleotides in lymphocyte
subpopulations and agammaglobulinemia.

TABLE 27–6. COMMON VARIABLE IMMUNODEFICIENCY

Designation	Usual Phenotypic Expression					Presumed Nature of Basic Defect	Inheritance
	Serum Ig	Serum Antibodies	Circulating B Cells	Circulating T Cells	CMI		
1. Common variable immunodeficiency with predominant B-cell defect	Decreased	Decreased	Near normal numbers but abnormal proportions of subtypes	Variable	Variable	Intrinsic defect in cells differentiation of immature to mature B cells	Unknown AR, AD
2. Common variable immunodeficiency with predominant immunoregulatory T-cell disorder							
(A) Deficiency of T-helper cells	Decreased	Decreased	Normal	Variable	Variable	Immunoregulatory T-cell disorder: defect in thymocyte to T-helper cell differentiation	Unknown
(B) Presence of activated T-suppressor cells	Decreased	Decreased	Normal	Variable	Variable	Immunoregulatory T-cell disorder—cause unknown	Unknown
3. Common variable immunodeficiency with autoantibodies to B or T cells	Decreased	Decreased	Decreased	Decreased	Variable	Variable; no differentiation defect known	Unknown

CMI, cell-mediated immunity; AR, autosomal recessive; AD, autosomal dominant.

different immune defects not associated with an identifiable cause (ie, not related to drugs, etc.). Clinically, the immune defects may be predominantly in antibody, due to (1) abnormalities in B-cell numbers or maturation, (2) defects in T-helper cells or increased activity of T-suppressor cells, or (3) autoantibodies to T or B cells. In all cases, there is a decrease in one or more immunoglobulin class associated with variable defects in cellular immunity. These defects appear to be abnormalities in control of the immune response, a maturation arrest at the level of the germinal center B cells, or defects in transmembrane signaling. For more information on testing for defects in CVI, see Figure 27–8.

PREDOMINANTLY ANTIBODY DEFECTS (DYSGAMMA-GLOBULINEMIAS)

A listing of immune deficiencies with diminished production of humoral antibody is given in Table 27–7. The dysgammaglobulinemias include all of the six possible combinations of depressed levels of a major immunoglobulin group or groups associated with normal or elevated levels of the other immunoglobulins: Selective IgA or IgG deficiency; selective IgM deficiency; deficiencies of IgG and IgA with normal IgM (type I dysgammaglobulinemia, usually associated with cellular immunodeficiency); deficiencies of IgM and IgA with normal IgG (type II dysgammaglobulinemia); and deficiency of IgG and IgM associated with normal or elevated levels of IgA. Some of these are considered to be late-appearing, genetically controlled developmental or isotype switch defects, whereas others may be acquired abnormalities of control of the immune response. The classic example, the first recognized immunodeficiency, is Bruton's disease.

Bruton's Congenital Sex-linked Agamma-globulinemia (Infantile Sex-linked Agamma-globulinemia)

This disease has an incidence of 1:50,000 births. Symptoms appear when transplacentally acquired maternal antibodies disappear from the circulation at the age of 5 to 6 months. Affected infants lack all three types of the major immunoglobulins but can develop reactions of the delayed type. The structure of the thymus is normal. There is a striking lack of tonsillar, appendiceal, and Peyer's patch lymphoid tissue, and plasma cells are absent. However, there are near normal numbers of pre-B cells expressing Ig-heavy chains in the bone marrow, indicating a block in the transition of pre-B-cells to B cells, not a lack of B-cell precursors. The B cells do not respond to lymphokines that usually drive B-cell maturation. The missing gene encodes for B cell tyrosine kinase that is required for B-cell maturation. This disease may be treated with antibiotics or gamma globulins. Treatment prolongs duration and quality of life, but early death is usual without treatment. In the future, these patients may be treated by gene transfer therapy using their own bone marrow stem cells containing good copies of the defective gene.

TABLE 27–7. PREDOMINANTLY ANTIBODY DEFECTS

Designation	Usual Phenotypic Expression					Presumed Pathogenesis/ Differentiation Defect	Inheritance
	Serum Ig	Serum Antibodies	Circulating B Cells	Circulating T Cells	CMI		
1. Bruton's X-linked agammaglobulinemia	All isotypes decreased	Decreased	Usually absent	Normal	Normal	Intrinsic defect in pre-B to B-cell differentiation	X-linked
2. Autosomal recessive agammaglobulinemia	All isotypes decreased	Decreased	Decreased	Normal	Normal	Intrinsic defect in pre-B to B-cell differentiation	AR
3. Ig deficiency with increased IgM (and IgD)	IgM and IgD increased, IgG and IgA decreased	IgM increased, IgG + IgA decreased	Normal IgM- and IgD-bearing cells, no IgG- or IgA-bearing cells	Normal	Normal	Intrinsic isotype switch defect: failure of IgM^+, IgD^+ B-cell maturation to IgG^+, IgA^+, IgE^+ B cells	X-linked or AR or AD or unknown
4. IgA deficiency	IgA decreased	IgA decreased	Immature serum IgA B cells	Usually normal	Usually normal	Defective IgA ($\pm$ IgG subclass) B-cell maturation	Unknown: some AR
5. Selective deficiency of other Ig isotypes IgD	Decrease in IgM, IgE, or IgD	Decrease of the deficient isotype	Normal	Normal	Normal	Differentiation defect of IgM B cell to isotype-specific plasma cell	Unknown
6. κ chain deficiency	Ig (κ) decrease	Decreased	Normal or decreased κ^+ B cells	Normal	Normal	Unknown	Unknown
7. Antibody deficiency with normal or hypergammaglobulinemia	Normal	Decreased	Near normal	Normal	Variable	B-cell differentiation defect: defective T-cell help	Unknown
8. Immune deficiency with thymoma	All isotypes decreased	Decreased	Absent or very low	Variable	Variably decreased	Unknown defect in pre-B cell maturation	None
9. Transcobalamin 2 deficiency	All isotypes decreased	Decreased	Normal	Normal	Normal	Defect in B_{12} transport resulting in defective cell proliferation; B cell to plasma cell differentiation	AR
10. Transient hypogammaglobulinemia of infancy	IgG and IgA decreased	Decreased	Normal	Decreased T-cell help	Variable	IgG/IgA B cell to IgG/IgA plasma cell differentiation defect: delayed maturation of T cell help; ? other	Unknown (frequent in heterozygous individuals in families with SCID)

CMI, cell-mediated immunity; AR, autosomal recessive; AD, autosomal dominant; SCID, severe combined immune deficiencies.

Modified from WHO Meeting Report: *Clin Immunol Immunopathol* 28:450–475, 1983.

Dysgamma-
globulinemias

Findings in other dysgammaglobulinemias are listed in Table 27–7. Single deficiencies of an immunoglobulin class are often associated with no clinical problems. Selective IgM deficiencies are rare and are associated with autoimmune disease and increased incidence of pneumococcal pneumonia. IgA deficiencies $<5\mu g/dL$ are associated with autoantibodies to IgA, allergies, recurrent sinopulmonary infections, and autoimmune diseases. It is postulated that IgA deficiency allows intestinal transfer of environmental antigens that induce antibodies that cross-react with host antigens or that there is a common genetic defect in IgA-deficient and autoimmune individuals. It is the most common immune deficiency (1:500), but most IgA deficient individuals are asymptomatic. Symptomatic IgA deficiencies may be those with associated IgG subclass deficiencies. Immunoglobulin subclass deficiencies sometimes occur in pairs, such as IgG_2 and IgG_4 together. In addition, IgG subclass deficiencies are not stable; a patient presenting with one subclass deficiency may develop additional deficiencies or switch to a different subclass deficiency. Selective deficiencies of IgG are usually asymptomatic but may be associated with increased infection with pneumococci, *Hemophilus influenza* and *Staphylococcus aureus*.

Hyper-IgM Syndrome. The hyper-IgM syndrome is an X-linked disorder expressed by increased levels of IgM but depressed IgA and IgG. It is due to a defect in isotype switching from IgM to other classes. This is associated with recurrent pyogenic infections but, fortunately, is very rare. The defect is not in the B-cell immunoglobulin genes but in signaling through CD40 on IgM-expressing B cells and the CD40 ligand on activated T cells (Table 27–4). The CD40 ligand gene is located on the X chromosome and is defective in hyper-IgM patients. Without the CD40 signaling pathway, activated B cells continue to produce IgM and do not switch to other Ig classes. Eventually, it may be possible to replace the gene responsible by giving these patients a functioning copy of the gene.

Hyper-IgE Syndrome. This syndrome features very high serum levels of IgE (>3,000 IU/mL), diminished antibody responses to specific immunizations, and pulmonary and upper respiratory infections, predominantly *S. aureus*. Also found is a high eosinophil count, a pruritic dermatitis, and growth retardation. It is suspected that there may be defective IFN-γ production since IFN-γ turns off IgE production. Clinical trials using IFN-γ treatment are now underway.

Hypercatabolic
Disgammaglob-
ulinemias

Most of the hereditary dysgammaglobulinemias are caused by a decreased synthesis of immunoglobulins, but low immunoglobulins may also be caused by increased catabolism. Increased catabolism of all immunoglobulin classes is found in **familial hypercatabolic hypoproteinemia**, of IgG in **myotonic dystrophy**, and of both immunoglobulin and lymphocytes in **intestinal lymphangiectasia**. Although these patients may have very abnormal laboratory tests, they usually do not have increased infections.

PREDOMINANTLY DEFECTS IN CELL-MEDIATED IMMUNITY (THYMUS-DEPENDENT DEFECTS)

Defects in T-cell function, with relatively normal B cells, are usually caused by failure of the thymus to develop normally.

Thymic Aplasia (DiGeorge Syndrome)

In this syndrome, there is absence of the thymus, deficiency of cellular reactions, and a normal immunoglobulin-producing system. The third and fourth pharyngeal pouches fail to develop, resulting in an absent or rudimentary thymus, absent parathyroids, and aortic arch defects. Neonatal tetany occurs due to a lack of parathyroid hormone. In complete DiGeorge syndrome, T-cell levels are markedly depressed, and responses to T-cell mitogens (phytohemagglutinin [PHA]) are absent. In patients with partial DiGeorge syndrome, which is more prevalent, there are intermediate peripheral blood lymphocyte counts and T-cell responses. Serum immunoglobulin levels are often normal. These patients are susceptible to viral and fungal infections.

Thymic Dysplasia

(Nezelof's Syndrome, Autosomal Recessive Lymphopenia with Normal or Abnormal Immunoglobulins). These patients have a vestigial embryonic thymus associated with diminished cellular immunity, and normal immunoglobulins. No lymphocytes are evident in the lymphoid tissues, although plasma cells are normal. Parathyroid tissue is normal. Wasting disease similar to that observed in neonatally thymectomized mice may be the terminal event. It is possible that a prethymic lymphocyte defect (prothymocyte) is responsible for the deficiency.

Down Syndrome

Patients with Down syndrome (mental retardation, abnormal brain development, and "mongoloid faces" associated with trisomy of chromosome 21) have up to a hundredfold higher mortality from respiratory infections than normal. They have smaller than normal thymi with large Hassal's corpuscles and marked depletion of thymocytes. There is also hypoplasia of the thymus-dependent zones of the spleen and lymph nodes, and a selective deficiency in the response of blood T cells to bacterial and fungal antigens, although not to T-cell mitogens. There are also varied abnormalities in phagocytosis, but B-cell function is usually normal. The relationship of the thymic abnormalities to the increased mortality from respiratory infection is not clear. The pathogenesis of the immunosuppression and its relationship to the inheritance of the other abnormalities is not known. It may be a secondary immunodeficiency.

Omenn's Syndrome	This syndrome is characterized by eosinophilia and infiltration of the skin and gastrointestinal mucosa with CD25+-activated T cells. There is an increased proportion of $T_{\gamma\delta}$ cells and the $T_{\alpha\beta}$ cells have restricted heterogeneity. Although T cells are present in large numbers in the skin and gastrointestinal tract, the T cells in the thymus and lymphoid organs are reduced.
T-cell Receptor Gene Mutations	These mutations may result in lack of expression of γ chain or lack of γ, δ, and ϵ subunits, most likely due to deletions of the exons that encode the transmembrane domain of the protein and produce functional signaling defects. One child of a pair of siblings who inherited mutations in the CD3-γ gene from both parents, died at the age of 31 months with severe combined deficiency and features of autoimmunity, whereas the brother was alive and healthy at 10 years of age. Two independent point mutations were identified in both the genes coding for the CD3-γ protein subunit of the T-cell receptor–CD3 complex, which hindered but did not abolish the expression of the T-cell receptor–CD3 complex on the surface of T cells. About half of the complexes that lacked the CD3-γ chain reached the cell surface, indicating that the CD3-γ protein is not essential for expression of about half of the TCR–CD3 complexes. The expressed TCRs contained α, β, CD3-δ and CD3-ϵ, and CD3-ζ subunits. The reason why one sibling had severe disease and the other, with the same genetic defect, did not, is not clear. An abnormality in nuclear factor of activated T cells (NF-AT) has been reported to result in defective production of IL-2, -3, -4, and -5 as a result of decreased transcription of the cytokine genes. This resulted in a clinical presentation of SCID.
Idiopathic CD4+ Lymphocytopenia (ICL)	ICL is an abnormal laboratory finding without a disease. With the widespread determination of CD4+ T-cell levels in the blood as a test for AIDS, individuals have been identified with low CD4 counts, but without disease. ICL includes two or more counts of CD4+ T cells below 300/mm^3 of blood or a percent-

age of less than 20 of CD4+ lymphocytes, with no evidence of HIV-1 or HIV-2 infection and no defined cause that accounts for the low level of CD4+ cells.

INFLAMMATORY DEFECTS

Defects in Inflammatory Mechanisms

Immunologically mediated defense against bacterial infections involves: (1) The reactions of specific antibody with the bacteria, (2) the activation of complement components resulting in chemotaxis and immune phagocytosis, (3) the ingestion of the bacteria by phagocytic cells (polymorphonuclear leukocytes or macrophages), and (4) the destruction of the ingested bacterial by products of the phagocytic cells. Therefore, increased susceptibility to bacterial infections may be due to a deficiency in certain complement components or an abnormality in phagocytic cells (phagocytic dysfunction), as well as to a lack of immunoglobulin antibody.

Complement Deficiencies

A listing of complement deficiencies is given in Table 27–8. Activation of complement occurs upon reaction of antibody with antigen. If the antigen is an infectious agent, the complement system may activate phagocytosis (opsonization) or cause lysis of the offending agent. Thus, a deficiency in complement might be expected to be associated with an immune deficient state. Deficiencies in a complement component are extremely rare. Most occur as autosomal recessive inherited abnormalities. Complement deficiencies are also associated with rheumatoid diseases, primarily systemic lupus erythematosus. Chronic complement consumption may also be associated with glomerulonephritis (hypocomplementemic glomerulonephritis). A deficiency in C1 inhibitor is associated with hereditary angioedema in which massive swelling lesions of the body surface or gastrointestinal tract are believed to be caused by loss of control of early complement components C1, C4, and C2 and increased formation of anaphylatoxin resulting in increased vascular permeability and edema. C1-inhibitor deficiency is the most commonly identified complement disorder and may be caused by insufficient production or an abnormal protein. The increased availability of reliable assays for complement components allows for screening for complement deficiencies (see below) and has made recognition of deficiencies in complement more frequent.

Phagocytic Dysfunction

Disorders of neutrophil or macrophage function include a lack of production (congenital neutropenia, leukemia), accessory deficiencies (complement), membrane receptor abnormalities (bare leukocyte syndrome), activation defects (Job's syndrome), phagocytic dysfunction, and extrinsic factors, such as drug effects (steroids) or immunoglobu-

TABLE 27–8. COMPLEMENT DEFICIENCIES

Component	Chromosomal Location	Inheritance of Deficiency	Approximate Number Kindreds/Patients	Clinical Manifestations
C1q	1p	Autosomal recessive	14/24	Rheumatic diseases and pyogenic infections
C1r/s	12p/12p	Autosomal recessive	7/11	Rheumatic diseases
C4	6p	Autosomal recessive	17/21	Rheumatic diseases and pyogenic infections
C2	6p	Autosomal recessive	79/109	Rheumatic diseases and pyogenic infections
C3	19q13	Autosomal recessive	14/19	Pyogenic infections and rheumatic diseases
C5	9q	Autosomal recessive	17/27	Meningococcal sepsis and meningitis
C6	5q	Autosomal recessive	49/77	Meningococcal sepsis and meningitis
C7	5q	Autosomal recessive	50/73	Meningococcal sepsis and meningitis
C8	1p A,B 9q G	Autosomal recessive	52/73	Meningococcal sepsis and meningitis
C9	5p	Autosomal recessive	15/18	Meningococcal sepsis and meningitis
Factor D	?	Unknown	2/3	Meningococcal sepsis and meningitis/sinopulmonary infections
C1 inhibitor	11q	Autosomal dominant	100s/100s	Angioedema
C4-binding protein	1q	Unknown	1/1	Behcet's disease and angioedema
DAF	1q	Unknown	2/2	Inab phenotype
Factor I	4q	Autosomal recessive	12/14	Pyogenic infections
Factor H	1q	Autosomal recessive	8/13	Hemolytic uremic syndrome
Properdin	Xp	X-linked recessive	23/70	Meningococcal sepsis and meningitis
CD59	11p	Unknown	1/1	Paroxysmal nocturnal hemoglobinuria

Modified from Frank M: *New Engl J Med* 316:152S, 1987.

lin abnormalities (rheumatoid factor, IgA, IgE). Phagocytic dysfunction occurs when phagocytic cells cannot ingest bacteria normally or can ingest but cannot kill. Such dysfunctions may be due to an abnormality in the digestive vacuole (lysosome) or to a lack of digestive enzymes in the vacuole. A summary of the steps in phagocytosis and the postulated level of phagocytic defects is illustrated in Figure 27–4. These disorders are characterized by increased susceptibility to bacterial infections associated with the accumulation of lipochrome-laden macrophages and granulomas in the affected tissues. The granulomas are caused by a reaction to bacterial products and the debris of the dead

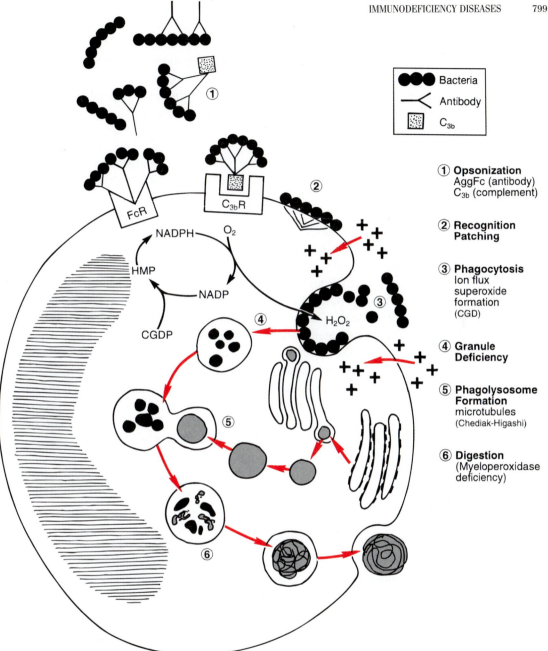

Figure 27–4. Schematic drawing of steps in phagocytosis and postulated levels of defects in phagocytic disorders:

1. Opsonization—aggregated Fc, C_3b (defects in antibody or complement).
2. Recognition through receptors and patching (defect in adhesion molecules).
3. Ingestion—cation influx stimulates transduction of hexose monophosphate shunt and conversion of O_2 to H_2O_2 (defect in chronic granulomatous disease).
4. Specific granule formation—congenital lack of granules precludes intracellular digestion.
5. Fusion of lysosome and phagosome to form phagolysosome (defect in Chediak–Higashi)—microtubule defect.
6. Digestion of bacteria in phagolysosome (defect in myeloperoxidase deficiency).

and dying phagocytic cells. Macrophages stuffed with material that they are unable to digest accumulate in tissues. Such macrophages are able to phagocytose normally but process ingested materials less rapidly or efficiently. The following are examples of phagocytic deficiencies.

Deficiency of Opsonization. This is not a defect in the phagocytic cell itself, but in opsonizing molecules, antibody, and complement.

Deficiencies of Receptor Molecules. Some individuals have a lack of surface adherence glycoproteins on their phagocytic cells. These include LFA-1, the iC3b receptor and p150,95. Each of these has a distinct α-subunit but a common 95,000 dalton β-subunit. LFA-1 is present on lymphocytes, monocytes, and neutrophils and is critical for cell adherence-related functions. iC3b is the opsonic fragment of the third component of complement. The function of p150,95 is not known. There is a genetic defect in the ability to synthesize the common β-subunit so that affected patients have an absence or deficiency of these molecules on the surface of their white cells. These receptors are required for phagocytosis and chemotaxis and most of the clinical manifestations are the result of phagocytic defects. There is also a mild T-cell deficiency manifested by decreased help for B cells and lowered cytotoxic activity, presumably because of poor cell–cell adhesion. This is inherited as an autosomal recessive and exists in severe and mild forms depending on decreased or complete lack of expression of LFA-1. There is partial compensation by increased CD2-LFA-3, and LFA-1 expression may be increased by IFN-γ.

Chronic Granulomatous Disease of Children (CGD). There is a deficiency in nicotinamide-adenine dinucleotide phosphate oxidase activation, with a failure to develop superoxide and hydrogen peroxide and hydrogen radicals. It is estimated to affect about 4,000 people worldwide. It is inherited by a defect of any one of four genes. Two-thirds of cases have the sex-linked form, affecting male children. Mothers of affected children have partial defects. Neutrophils from patients with X-linked form of CGD lack the enzyme cytochrome b_{558}, whereas neutrophils from patients with the autosomal recessive forms have normal levels of this enzyme. Cytochrome b_{558} is a 22,000-dalton peptide that is tightly bound to a highly glycosylated 91,000-dalton peptide. Patients with X-linked cytochrome b_{558}-negative CGD have defects in the gene coding for the 91,000-dalton subunit of the cytochrome complex. It is believed that the 91,000-dalton subunit is required to anchor the cytochrome complex in the cell membrane. The genetic basis for the cytochrome b_{558}-positive CGD is not known, but the neutrophils of these patients fail to phosphorylate a 44,000-dalton membrane-associated protein found in activated neutrophils.

The functional problem in CGD is that the first line of bacterial killing, oxidative-dependent killing, fails. The neutrophil dies during the battle with the invading microorganism, leaving macrophages to deal with dead cells and the invading organisms. Macrophages (which also lack respiratory burst activity) ingest the debris and kill the microorganisms using nonoxidative defenses (eg, lysozyme, neutral proteases, defensins). This killing is usually successful, but prolonged, leading to the formation of granulomas after each infectious episode. Marked improvement has been noted following IFN-γ treatment.

It has been suggested that CGD might be called Jonah's syndrome. The Biblical character Jonah was phagocytized by a large multicellular organism that was unable to digest him, and he was eventually released. The enzymatic defect in CGD is tested by the inability of isolated polymorphonuclear cells from affected individuals to kill bacteria in vitro or to reduce the dye nitroblue tetrazolium, which measures superoxide formation.

Specific Granule Deficiency. This is a group of disorders in which phagocytic granules are not formed. Patients with a lack of granules have depressed inflammatory responses and recurrent severe bacterial infections of the skin and deep tissues. Specific granule markers, such as lactoferrin, vitamin B_{12} binding protein, and defensins, may be deficient.

Chediak–Higashi Syndrome. This syndrome features a microtubular defect, with a deficit in phagosome–lysosome fusion. Large abnormal lysosomes are seen in all white cells. The defect is inherited as an autosomal recessive, and there is a partial defect in heterozygotes. Affected individuals may also have albinism and lymphoproliferative diseases.

Myeloperoxidase Deficiency (MPD). Myeloperoxidase is responsible for the azurophilic granules in neutrophils, and its activity in inflammation causes the greenish color of pus. In the presence of hydrogen peroxide and halide, myeloperoxidase produces hypochlorous acid and chlorine, which is very toxic for bacterial cells. Hereditary MPD is a relatively common (1:3000) autosomal recessive disorder, with about one-third having a total absence of myeloperoxidase and the other two-thirds having a partial absence. Fortunately, increased infection in this disorder is unusual, most likely because other microbiological mechanisms compensate for the deficiency.

Interleukin Deficiencies

Deficiencies in interleukin-1 or interleukin-2 production may occur secondary to loss of function of macrophage (IL-1) or lymphocyte (IL-2) populations. However, the clinical significance of interleukin deficiencies has not been extensively documented. IL-2 production by blood lymphocytes appears to be depressed in burn patients and may be responsible for depressed cellular immunity in some burn patients. A simplistic explanation for the defects in B-cell maturation seen in common variable hypogammaglobulinemas could be a failure of production or response to B-cell differentiation factors, such as IL-4, IL-5, and IL-6. However, no convincing evidence for such a defect has been found.

Secondary Immuno-deficiencies

Secondary immunodeficiencies may result from naturally occurring disease processes or subsequent to the administration of suppressive agents. In either case, the process operates on an already developed immune system and, therefore, either destroys or interferes with the expression of established defense mechanisms. "Opportunistic" infection with organisms not usually pathogenic for normal individuals is a common terminal event in these patients.

Diseases affecting cellular immune reactions include Boeck's sarcoidosis, leprosy, tuberculosis, measles, diabetes, cancer, and now, most critically, AIDS. Each of these diseases may affect lymphoid tissue directly or secondarily alter nonspecific innate defense systems. Burn patients not only have destroyed epithelial barriers but also have a decreased ability to produce IL-2. Uremic patients have depressed cell-mediated immunity.

Multiple abnormalities have been reported in patients with diabetes. Vascular changes lead to decreased tissue perfusion resulting in increased susceptibility to tissue damage as well as an impaired ability to mount an inflammatory response. In addition, abnormalities in glycogen metabolism depress the phagocytic and digestive capacity of neutrophils and macrophages. There may be depressed numbers of T cells in the blood, decreased responsiveness to PHA, increased CD4:CD8 ratio, decreased IL-2 production, and decreased natural killer (NK) cell function, as well as decreased chemotaxis and bacterial killing by neutrophils in vitro. Some patients have low C4 levels. Although it is clear that diabetic patients have increased susceptibility to infections, there is no general agreement on why this is true.

IATROGENIC DEFICIENCIES

The mechanisms of action of the so-called immunosuppressive agents is extremely varied (Table 27–9). These agents may affect (1) the specific induction of the immune response (primary response), (2) the expression of humoral antibody formation only, (3) the expression of cellular immunity only, or (4) the expression of both humoral and cellular immunity. Each these agents have systemic effects on cells other than those of the lymphoid system. The damage caused by these agents in vivo is quite variable. In high doses, most cause derangements of any tissue that is metabolically active (eg, depression of the bone marrow with subsequent loss of peripheral blood cell elements) or denudation of the lining epithelium of the gastrointestinal tract.

TABLE 27–9. MECHANISM OF ACTION OF IMMUNOSUPPRESSIVE AGENTS

Agents	Mechanisms of Action	Examples
Irradiation	Direct destruction of lymphoid cells, toxic for proliferating cells	Whole body, localized, extracorporeal
Steroids	Multiple, direct destruction of lymphoid cells, alterations in protein synthesis and lymphocyte circulation; antiinflammatory	Hydrocortisone, prednisone
Alkylating agents	React chemically with nucleophilic centers of molecules, in particular DNA, RNA, and proteins; B cells > T cells	Nitrogen mustard, cyclophosphamide, chlorambucil, busulfan
Purine analogs	Incorporated into DNA and RNA and interfere with nucleic acid synthesis; T cells > B cells	Azathioprine, 6-mercaptopurine, thioguanine
Pyrimidine analogs	Inhibition of enzyme activity; active in RNA and DNA synthesis; B cells > T cells	5-Fluorouracil, azaribine, 5-fluoro-2-deoxyuridine, cytosine arabinoside
Folic acid antagonists	Bind to dihydrofolate reductase, thereby interfering with purine, protein, and DNA synthesis	Methotrexate, amethopterin, aminopterin
Methylhydrazines	Formation of hydroxyl radicals causes changes in DNA similar to ionizing radiation	Procarbazine
Hydroxyureas	Kills DNA synthesizing cells, blocks entry of cell into S	Hydroxyurea
Alkaloids	Blocks assembly of the mitotic spindle leading to metaphase arrest; also inhibits RNA and protein synthesis	Vinblastine, vincristine
Enzymes	Hydrolysis of L-asparagine to L-aspartate and ammonia	L-Asparaginase
Antibiotics	Multiple actions: (1) inhibits DNA-dependent RNA polymerase, (2) alkylating agent, (3) DNA binding	Mithramycin, mitomycin, actinomycin C
Antilymphocyte globulin	Alters lymphocyte circulation; lymphocytotoxic, opsonization of lymphocytes, receptor blockage	Horse, goat, rabbit, antihuman lymphocyte globulin
Cyclosporine A	Blocks T cell helper effect, other effects?	New wonder drug for organ transplantation

Modified from Gerber NL, Steinberg AD: *Drugs* 11:14–35, 1976.

The effect of various drugs on the immune response is best considered in relation to the site of action during an immune response. Immunosuppressive therapy has become of paramount importance in preventing homograft rejection, especially in regard to organ transplantation. Experimental results indicate that such agents may be effective in suppressing various autoimmune reactions. These benefits are counterbalanced by the increased incidence and severity of opportunistic infections. See Chapter 28 for a more detailed and systematic discussion of immunosuppressive agents.

INFECTIOUS DISEASES

Infectious diseases produce a generalized debilitation or may be associated with a selective "anergy" to the infectious agent. Anergy specifically refers to a loss of skin test DTH reaction to antigens of infectious organisms. This may represent lymphocyte sequestration or a disproportionate response of a nonprotective immune mechanism. For instance, in leprosy (see Chapter 17), high antibody production (lepromatous leprosy) is associated with progressive disease, whereas high DTH and granulomatous reactivity (tuberculoid leprosy) is associated with arrested disease. The "wrong" type of immune response appears to have occurred, ie, protection against leprosy requires cellular immunity—antibody alone is not effective. If the individual infected with leprosy produces antibody but not DTH, protection is not effective. The most striking association of immunodeficiency with infection is in AIDS (see Chapter 29). Selected immune responses to other infectious agents are discussed further in Chapter 25.

Chronic Mucocutaneous Candidiasis (CMC)

CMC patients have histories of *Candida* infections associated with high antibody responses to *Candida* and absent delayed skin test responses to *Candida* antigens. These patients frequently have polyendocrinopathy, suggesting autoimmune destruction of endocrine organs. As in lepromatous leprosy, these patients respond poorly to therapy unless delayed hypersensitivity can be demonstrated. CMC is another example of **immune deviation** in which the type of immune response determines the nature of the disease manifested, ie, antibody is not effective; cellular immunity (particularly delayed hypersensitivity) is.

X-linked Lymphoproliferative Syndrome (Duncan's Syndrome)

Abnormalities of B-cell differentiation and proliferation are found in patients with Epstein–Barr virus (EBV) infections (infectious mononucleosis, Burkitt's lymphoma). The name of the first patient recognized to have this syndrome was Duncan. EBV infects B cells, leading to polyclonal B-cell proliferation on the one hand and lack of differentiation and agammaglobulinemia on the other hand. These patients have variable immunodeficiencies. They generally make a poor anti-EBV response but do not have a high incidence of opportunistic infections. It is thought that there is lack of appropriate T-suppressor control of B cells or abnormal T-helper function. The syndrome usually affects males between ages 3 and 23.

The finding of a number of X-linked immunodeficiencies (Table 27–10) implies a gene complex controlling immune development or expression on the X chromosome. In Duncan's syndrome, there appears to be a mutation at Xq26–27.

TABLE 27–10. X-LINKED IMMUNODEFICIENCIES

Bruton's agammaglobulinemia
SCID (Swiss-type)
Wiskott–Aldrich syndrome
Hyper-IgM syndrome
X-Linked lymphoproliferative syndrome
Chronic granulomatous disease of children

Acquired Immunodeficiency Syndrome (AIDS)

Full blown AIDS features essentially a wasting syndrome as a result of a loss of cell-mediated immunity, permitting a variety of opportunistic infections. HIV infects CD4+ T cells. Although the pathogenesis of AIDS is not fully understood, the most likely hypothesis is that the causative virus directly inhibits functions of T-helper cells. The classic, but not invariable, presentation is of oral *Candida* infection or of enlarging perianal ulcers containing herpes simplex (genital herpes). This is often followed by a prolonged course characterized by weight loss, fever, lymphadenopathy, multiple cutaneous nodules, and evidence of other opportunistic infections, including: Cytomegalovirus, *Pneumocystis carinii, Mycobacterium avium intracellulare*, and *Candida albicans*, as well as syphilis, tuberculosis, and gonorrhea. There is a marked depression in cellular immunity and a marked decrease in CD4+ T cells in the peripheral blood (<500 cm). (See Chapter 29, Immunology of AIDS.)

CANCER

Cancer causes depressed immunity in many ways (see Chapter 30). Perhaps the most significant is the general debilitation seen in terminal cancer patients. In addition, cancer patients are often treated with drastic chemotherapy or irradiation, further compromising immunity and setting the stage for opportunistic infections. Although "immunosuppressive" factors isolated from cancer tissue have been shown to suppress immune reactivity in vitro, the role of such factors in clinical immunosuppression remains poorly defined.

Leukemias and Lymphomas

(See Chapter 24.) Selected immune effects may be seen with tumors of the white blood cells and lymphoid organs. In leukemia, the normal inflammatory function of the white blood cells is depressed because the neoplastic cells force out the normal population by occupying "living space." Neoplastic leukemia cells are unable to provide the same function as normal cells; lymphocytes of chronic lymphocyte leukemia do not function properly. However, some acute lymphocytic leukemia (ALL) cells may function as suppressor T cells. The addition of small numbers of some ALL cells to normal peripheral blood lymphocytes will inhibit lipopolysaccharide (LPS)-induced Ig synthesis. In addition, autoantibodies to lymphocytes, particularly T cells, may be associated with lymphoproliferative disease and cause abnormalities in T cell function.

Other lymphoproliferative neoplasias may affect both cellular and humoral immunity, either by occupying the bone marrow and forcing out normal products (living space) or by producing abnormalities in immune control systems. In Sezary's syndrome, there is a malignant proliferation of T-helper cells. When graded numbers of Sezary cells are added to B cells, the amount of immunoglobulin synthesized as a result of LPS stimulation increases. However, at high T:B ratios, normal T cells suppress B-cell Ig synthesis; this may occur in later stages of the disease. In addition, it is not likely that Sezary cells can provide the T-cell help that is required for a specific immune response.

Multiple Myeloma (Plasmacytoma)

A number of immune abnormalities have been found in patients with tumors of plasma cells (multiple myeloma). Most notably, these tumors produce large amounts of nonantibody monoclonal immunoglobulin. There is suppression of normal antibody responses to immunization. The primary cause of this appears to be due to "suppressor macrophages," which can inhibit the normal response of B cells. In addition, these patients have defects in complement and granulocyte function. The high levels of circulating myeloma immunoglobulin also increases the catabolic rate of normal immunoglobulin so that there is less functional antibody. In addition, there are large numbers of T cells with membrane-bound Fc receptors (FcR) for the immunoglobulin isotope of the paraprotein being secreted by the plasma cell tumor. These isotope-specific T cells have a suppressor phenotype and can inhibit normal B-cell production of immunoglobulin of the same isotope as the myeloma protein.

MALCIRCULATION OF LYMPHOCYTES

Lymphocytopenia (low numbers of blood lymphocytes), particularly of T cells, is frequently found in diseases such as Hodgkin's disease, Crohn's disease, hepatitis, rheumatoid arthritis, multiple sclerosis, and tuberculosis. The lymphopenia in these diseases may be due to sequestration of lymphocytes in tissues so that the numbers of lymphocytes in the blood is lower. In Hodgkin's disease, there also appears to be a selective sequestration of T-helper cells in the spleen. Splenectomy of patients with Hodgkin's disease may be associated with correction of the lymphopenic condition. T cells may be sequestered in the lesions of Crohn's disease, chronic hepatitis, rheumatoid arthritis, and tuberculosis. Such maldistribution of lymphocytes may lead to depressed immune responsiveness in other organ systems, such as anergy in tuberculosis and Hodgkin's disease.

TRAUMA

Bacterial sepsis is responsible for 75% of deaths following major thermal burns or traumatic injury. In thermal injury, there is a loss of host mechanical barriers to invading organisms, not only over the skin but also in the lungs due to inhalation, producing a chemical tracheobronchitis with dysfunction of ciliary and alveolar macrophage function. Although conflicting results have been reported, there appears also to be an increase in "T-suppressor activity" after burns, and abnormalities in chemotaxis and neutrophil function following major trauma.

Surgery is an immunosuppressive event that is intensified if the patient has an underlying disease, trauma, or complications that may contribute to suppression. The mere act of surgery violates the barriers of the body, and even with great attention to sterile procedures, the surgical patient is more likely to become infected. Surgery, as a function of its duration, complexity, and magnitude, directly influences immune reactions. On the other hand, resection of inflammatory or infected lesions, removal of tumors, or drainage of an abscess can return altered host defenses to normal. Attempts to identify immunopharmacologic treatments that might alleviate surgical immunosuppression have not been fruitful.

CHRONIC FATIGUE SYNDROME

Chronic fatigue syndrome (CFS) is a complex of clinical findings with no clear pathogenesis, associated with a variety of infectious agents. The major symptom is relapsing fatigue, with all other chronic clinical conditions excluded. Other symptoms include low grade fever, sore throat, lymph node pain, generalized muscle weakness, generalized headaches, arthralgias, neuropsychological symptoms, and sleep disturbances. Laboratory test abnormalities include: Elevated antibodies to viruses, abnormal gammaglobulin levels (high or low), increased serum IL-2 levels, decreased IL-2 production in vitro, increased CD4:CD8 ratio, increased or decreased NK activity, and variable antinuclear antibody levels. Infectious associations include a variety of agents. Most often implicated are Epstein–Barr virus, *Borrelia burgdorferi*, *Mycobacterium tuberculosis*, enteroviruses, and HTLV-1, but no convincing association has been established. The ability of tumor necrosis factor (TNF) or IL-2 to produce symptoms similar to CFS has suggested that they might be responsible, but clinical testing has not found increased levels of TNF or IL-2.

Opportunistic Infections

The clinical manifestation of immune deficiency diseases are due to infections, often with organisms that are not usually pathogenic in a normal individual. Because many patients have immune deficiency secondary to another disease, they are exposed to organisms in the hospital and acquire the infection in the hospital. Such infections are termed **nosocomial**. A partial listing of pathogens in the immunocompromised host and the source of infection is given in Table 27–11. Most infections are acquired from the patient's own flora, but *Aspergillus* and zygomyces infections are nosocomial. Some infections may be traced to application of devices, such as urinary catheters or endotracheal tubes, particularly *Staphylococcus epidermidis* and *Corynebacterium*. Such hospital manipulations may help establish infections with host organisms by breaching of mechanical barriers.

Evaluation of Immuno-deficiency

The primary clue to the diagnosis of an immunodeficiency disease is obtained by history and physical examination; clinical tests serve for confirmation, definition of the type and severity of the defect, and as a guide for therapy. The clues to immunodeficiency are the type, severity, cause, and frequency of infections in a patient. Also important is the presence of other factors, such as drug therapy, cancer, etc. A summary of the laboratory evaluation of immunodeficiency disease is given in Figure 27–5.

A patient with a history of recurrent infections must be critically examined for a potential defect in defense against infectious agents. The age, condition, and clinical and family history of the patient are vital in establishing the necessity for further laboratory work-up.

TABLE 27–11. SOME NOSOCOMIAL PATHOGENS
IN THE IMMUNOCOMPROMISED HOST

Source of Infection	Endogenous	Exogenous
Bacteria		
Staphylococcus aureus	++	+
Staphylococcus epidermidis	++	0
Corynebacterium	++	0
Gram-negative rods (*Escherichia Coli, Pseudomonas, Klebsiella*)	++	+
Fungi		
Candida, yeasts	++	0
Aspergillus	0	++
Zygomyces	0	++
Viruses		
Herpes simplex	++	0
Varicella-zoster	+	+
Cytomegalovirus	+	+
Parasites		
Pneumocystis carinii	++	+
Toxoplasma	++	+
Cryptosporidia	+	+

Modified from Young LS: Infection in the compromised host. *Hospital Proc* 16, 73–84, 1981.

History and Physical

	Inflammation	Phagocytosis	Humoral antibody	Cellular sensitivity
Screening tests	White blood cell count and differential C50 hemolytic complement	White blood cell count and morphology	Immunoelectrophoresis Serum Ig levels	Skin tests T_4/R_8 ratios
Diagnostic tests	Complement levels Inhibitor levels Cell adhesion molecules	Phagocytic index Bactericidal tests NBT test Cell surface glycoproteins Lymph node biopsy Cell adhesion molecules	Serum IgE Secretory IgA B cell levels Isohemagglutinins Purine metabolizing Enzymes	SRBC rosettes Mitogen responses X ray for thymus Lymph node biopsy T-cell receptors
Experimental tests	Complement fragment assays	Chemotactic assays C reactive proteins Specific phagocytic enzymes	Skin tests Responses to immunization Ig synthesizing capacity	Interleukin levels Serum inhibitors Sensitization to DNCB Skin graft rejection

Figure 27–5. Evaluation of immunodeficiency.

Because of the complexity of findings in primary or secondary immunodeficiencies, a systematic series of tests should be performed to permit adequate evaluation. Some of the tests indicated are presented below. From the type of recurrent infection, one can obtain a clue to the type of deficiency. If mainly viral or fungal, a defect in delayed hypersensitivity (T-cell function) must be suspected. Recurrent bacterial infections indicate a defect in humoral antibody production, polymorphonuclear neutrophils, or complement. Complete white blood count and differential is an obvious first-level evaluation for major abnormalities in numbers or types of white cells in the blood. Serum immunoglobulin levels will reveal major disorders in humoral defenses. The availability of a large number of monoclonal antibodies and new methods for phenotypic analysis of lymphocyte subpopulations has made this a more practical and popular early evaluation technique; of particular importance are CD3, CD4, and CD5. Various nonimmunologic factors can be tested by measuring general inflammatory indices (eg, white blood count) or serum factors (eg, complement or various inhibitors). Phagocytic capacity should be determined to rule out a phagocytic defect. Humoral antibody capacity can be measured by determining serum immunoglobulin concentrations; by the presence of preformed antibody or the number of B lymphocytes; by the response to antigens that elicit antibody, such as immunization to diphtheria, pertussis, and tetanus (DPT); or by the response to specifically selected antigens such as keyhole limpet hemocyanin (KLH). Skin tests may also demonstrate anaphylactic or Arthus reactivity. Polyclonal activation of the patient's lymphocytes with LPS or pokeweed mitogen (PWM) and the effect of cell fractionation or mixing with normal cells may be particularly revealing (Fig. 27–6). Delayed reactivity can be determined by the transformation response of blood lymphocytes to mitogens, such as phytohemagglutinin or concanavalin A, as well as to selected specific antigens. The production of lymphocytic mediators, such as macrophage inhibitory factor or IL-2, as well as the presence of serum inhibitors of transformation, can be measured. In addition, the number of blood lymphocytes that react with monoclonal antibodies to T-cell surface markers are used to phenotype T-cell subpopulations. More recent tests may determine genetic abnormalities in the T-cell receptor subunits or cell adhesion molecules. In vivo tests for delayed hypersensitivity include skin tests to antigens, such as the purified protein derivatives of tubercle bacilli, coccidioidin, etc.; the ability to induce contact reactivity to dinitrochlorobenzene (DNCB) or other haptens; skin graft rejection; x-ray examination for the thymic shadow; and, in rare cases, lymph node biopsy. From the results of a selection of these tests, one can define the nature of defect leading to recurrent or unusual infections and institute appropriate therapy.

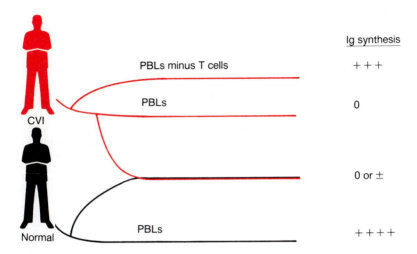

Figure 27–6. Induction of Ig synthesis by mitogens in lymphocyte cultures of some patients with common variable immunodeficiency. Peripheral blood lymphocytes (PBLs) of an immune-deficient patient will not synthesize Ig if exposed to mitogen (polyvalent stimulants). Removal of T cells from PBLs allows the patient's blood B cells to respond. If the patient's PBLs are added to cultures of PBLs from a normal person, Ig synthesis normally found is suppressed. Such an observation is consistent with T-suppressor cells in the blood of an immune-deficient patient, causing suppression of the B-cell system.

Therapy

Treatment of immunodeficiency diseases may be divided into three general approaches: (1) Treatment of the infectious agent by antibiotics; (2) treatment of the underlying disease, if present; and (3) specific replacement of the immune defect. In this chapter, only replacement will be presented (Table 27–12).

PASSIVE ANTIBODY

Since immunoglobulin deficiencies are caused by the lack of antibody, immunologically competent cells, or both, attempts have been made to correct these deficiencies by replacing the missing defense system. For many years, the antibody deficiency syndromes have been treated with partial success by injections of pooled normal immunoglobulins. Five commercially available preparations are available for intravenous administration (Table 27–13). The manufacturers recommend 100 to 200 mg/kg at monthly intervals. These preparations contain about the same spectrum of specific antibodies. Preparations with low IgA should be administered to patients with combined IgG–IgA deficiencies to prevent allergic reaction to IgA. Whereas such injections give some protection, they do not provide the high levels of specific antibody that are produced in response to an infectious organism by a normal person and do not provide any cell-mediated immunity. However,

TABLE 27–12. REPLACEMENT THERAPY FOR IMMUNE DEFECTS

1.	Immunoglobulin deficiencies:	Passive immune globulin
2.	Thymus deficiencies:	Bone marrow transplants treatment of choice; thymus transplants rarely effective
3.	Combined–Variable	
	Transfer factor:	Wiskott–Aldrich, mucocutaneous candidiasis; not used in standard treatment regimens
	Thymic Factors:	Thymosin, thymopoietin, factor thymic serique; restores E rosettes and in vitro functions but no convincing beneficial effect seen in clinical trials
	Bone marrow:	Stem cell problem—graft-versus-host reaction, HLA matching, other procedures to prevent GVH; most effective therapy
	Fetal thymus and liver:	Anecdotal reports of success difficult to evaluate

passive immunoglobulin remains the most effective maintenance procedure for patients with hypogammaglobulinemia, supplemented with antibiotics to cover specific infections.

PASSIVE CELL-MEDIATED IMMUNITY

Attempts have been made to treat immunologic deficiencies of the cellular and combined cellular and immunoglobulin types by bone marrow or thymus transplantation or transfer of cell products. Such transplants must be selected carefully to correct the specific immune deficiency with a minimum potential of unwanted effects, particularly graft-versus-host reactions. For general application, only bone marrow or stem cell transplantation has met with consistent clinical suc-

TABLE 27–13. COMMERCIALLY AVAILABLE LICENSED GAMMAGLOBULIN PREPARATIONS

Product	Manufacturer	Isolation	Comments
Gamimmune N	Cutter Biol., Berkeley, CA	Cold ethanol, ph 4.0	5% in maltose, low IgG4, delivery pH 4.0
Gammagard	Baxter Corp., Glendale, CA	Cold ethanol, DEAE	5% in glucose, low IgA, IgG4, delivery pH 6.8
IVEEGAM	Immuno-US, Rochester, MN	Cold ethanol, PEG, trypsin	5% in glucose, lyophilized
Sandoglobulin	Sandoz, East Rutherford, NJ	Cold ethanol, pepsin	3 or 6% in sucrose, lyophilized, delivery pH 6.6
Venoglobulin-I	Alpha Therapeutics, Los Angeles, CA	Cold ethanol, PEG, DEAE	5% in mannitol, delivery pH 6.8

Modified from Huston DP, et al.: *J Allerg Clin Immunol* 87:1, 1991.

cess. Patients with only cellular deficiencies, such as DiGeorge's syndrome, have rarely been successfully treated with thymus transplants. Patients with combined immunodeficiencies may be reconstituted by transfer of bone marrow cells that contain stem cells. Reconstitution of immune reactivity is due to proliferation of donor cells that repopulate the host tissue.

Thymus Transplants

Fetal thymus transplants have been reported to restore cellular immunity in a few patients with combined immunodeficiencies; these people have then been maintained with passive gammaglobulin to cover humoral antibody deficiency. The responding cells in patients treated with transplantation of the thymus are of donor origin, indicating the presence of T-cell precursors in the transplanted thymus. But B-cell precursors are not present, and humoral antibody production is not restored. The thymus must be selected from fetuses before the fourteenth week of gestation. Under these circumstances, only minimal graft-versus-host reactivity has been observed. However, thymus transplantation is not generally found to be useful in present practice.

Thymic Factors

Thymic factors are of historical interest but are not now used for therapy. The thymus produces soluble factors that induce T-cell maturation. In 1963, it was noted by two different groups that thymic tissue implanted in diffusion chambers into thymectomized mice could restore T-cell function. However, in vivo effects of injections of extracts of thymic tissue were generally ineffective in inducing T-cell function in thymectomized mice. Thymic extracts added to undifferentiated stem cells (T-cell precursors), such as lymphocytes from nude mice, which congenitally lack a thymus but produce presumptive T-cell precursors in bone marrow, induce expression of the cell surface markers of mature T cells and T-cell helper function in vitro. The thymus factor is produced by thymic epithelial cells, as demonstrated by reconstitution of thymectomized mice by implants of epithelial cells in millipore chambers. In vivo and in vitro treatment with thymosin will increase the percentage of E rosettes (presumptive T cells) in immune-deficient patients, and cases claiming clinical improvement as a result of thymosin injection have been reported. Chemically synthesized thymic humoral factor (THF-γ2) has been tested in preliminary trials. However, beneficial effects in convincing systematic clinical trials have not been found. In most patients who received thymosin, thymosin treatment was only part of rigorous therapy employing other agents, so it is impossible to judge the effect of thymosin alone. It must be stressed that thymic factors cannot be expected to have an effect on patients with severe combined immunodeficiency who lack stem cells upon which a humoral thymus factor can act, but they may be able to induce maturity in patients who lack thymus epithelial cell function. In fact, thymic humoral factors do not increase rosettes in patients with severe combined immunodeficiency; however, after bone marrow transplantation, induction of T-cell rosettes may be possible. (See Chapter 3 for more details on thymic factors.)

Transfer Factor

Transfer factor, a dialysate of an extract from peripheral blood lymphocytes, has been used to treat certain immune-deficient patients in experimental trials, but is not used generally. This factor has been applied to such diseases as Wiskott–Aldrich syndrome and mucocutaneous candidiasis, which have a variable course with temporary spontaneous improvement. Therefore, the clinical improvement noted in many cases cannot be unequivocally attributed to the effect of transfer factor. Transfer factor therapy appears to be most applicable for patients with a specific infection, such as candidiasis, coccidiomycosis, or histoplasmosis, but consistent beneficial results have not been obtained. In these cases, the administration of transfer factor obtained from the blood lymphocytes of individuals with a positive skin reaction to antigens of the infectious agent may induce a prompt reaction in infected individuals. Transfer factor is only useful in patients with a limited deficiency and not a stem cell deficiency; transfer factor may push arrested cells to limited differentiation but cannot replace an absent cell type.

Stem Cell Transplantation

(See Transplantation, Chapter 23.) In severe combined immunodeficiency, it is possible that stem cell function may be replaced by transfer of bone marrow or blood stem cells. The transplantation of living immunocompetent cells to an immunodeficient recipient is possible because the recipient is unable to reject the transplanted cells. However, the transplanted immunocompetent cells may react to the recipient tissues, and death may result from a graft-versus-host reaction. The first successful bone marrow transplant in an SCID infant was carried out in 1968. Since then a number of successful transplants of bone marrow cells have been made to immunodeficient individuals with not only some spectacular successes but also some disappointing failures. Using HLA-matched sibling donors, there is about a 75% successful long-term survival; using unrelated HLA-matched donors, there is about a 50% long-term survival. With improvement in matching tests, this figure should improve. The establishment of an international marrow donor registry has made HLA phenotypically matched marrow from unrelated donors available to patients who lack a suitable related donor. However, it costs $25,000 to screen for a donor, and there often is no insurance reimbursement. There is now the possibility of replacing the specific genes that are missing in SCIDs with adenosine deaminase deficiency by transferring back to the patient his own bone marrow stem or cord blood cells that have had the missing human gene inserted.

Bone marrow transplant recipients have cellular and humoral immunodeficiencies for months to years after transplantation. The precise reasons for this effect is not clear, but it appears that the immune system undergoes a recapitulation of ontogenesis. Immature B cells undergo differentiation processes and have low IgG levels that correlate with the incidence of pneumococcal infections after transplantation. There is also evidence of insufficient T-cell help and/or exaggerated CD8+ T-cell or NK-cell suppression. Because of the frequency of immunoglobulin deficiencies after transplantation, administration of intravenous passive immunoglobulins may have beneficial effects in individual patients, and reimmunization with childhood vaccines is often recommended.

Liver Transplants

In one case, an allograft of fetal liver to a 3-month-old boy with SCID and adenosine deaminase (ADA) deficiency restored both T- and B-cell functions, as well as ADA activity and clinical improvement. One year later, the child died with a fatal immune complex glomerulonephritis, which could have resulted from reaction to exogenous antigen or from a graft-versus-host reaction.

Summary

Primary immunodeficiency diseases are genetically controlled developmental abnormalities in the maturation of the immune system. The type of deficiency manifested depends on the level of maturational arrest that the abnormality affects. Secondary immunodeficiencies are the result of naturally occurring diseases or administration of immunosuppressive agents that operate on a mature immune system. The type of deficiency observed depends on the location of the defect for the given disease or the mechanism of action of the immunosuppressive agent. Defects may occur in antibody formation, cellular immunity, accessory systems (complement, phagocytosis), or in mechanical barriers or other nonspecific innate immune mechanisms. Patients with immune defects acquire pathogenic infections with organisms that are not usually pathogens in normal individuals (opportunistic infections). Replacement of the specific defect or therapy of the infection or an underlying disease causing the immune defects may be effective.

Bibliography

DEVELOPMENT AND MATURATION OF THE IMMUNE SYSTEM

Cooper MD, Peterson RDA, South MA, et al.: The functions of the thymus system and the bursa system in the chicken. *J Exp Med* 123:75, 1966.

Good RA, Gabrielsen AE (eds.): The thymus. In *Immunobiology*. New York, Harper & Row, 1964.

Miller JFAP, Osoba D: Current concepts of the immunological function of the thymus. *Physiol Rev* 47:437, 1967.

Parrott DM, DeSousa MAB, East J: Thymus-dependent areas in lymphoid organs of neonatally thymectomized mice. *J Exp Med* 123:191, 1966.

Smith RT, Meischer P, Good RA: *The Phylogeny of Immunity*. Gainesville, University of Florida Press, 1966.

Waksman BH, Arnason BG, Jankovic BD: Role of the thymus in immune reactions in rats. III. Changes in the lymphoid organs of thymectomized rats. *J Exp Med* 116:187, 1962.

Warner NL, Szenberg A: The immunologic function of the bursa of Fabricius in the chicken. *Annu Rev Microbiol* 18:253, 1964.

MOUSE MODELS

Bosma MJ, Carroll AM: The *scid* mouse mutant: Definition, characterization, and potential uses. *Annu Rev Immunol* 9:323-350, 1991.

Cohen PL, Eiserberg RA: Single gene models of systemic autoimmunity and lymphoproliferative disease. Ann Rev Immunol 9:243-269, 1991.

Rihova B, Vetvica V (eds.): *Immunological Disorders in Mice*. Boca Raton, FL, CRC Press, 1990.

Shultz LD: Immunologic mutants of the mouse. *Am J Anat* 191:303, 1991.

PRIMARY IMMUNO-DEFICIENCIES

Afzelius BA: The immobile cilia syndrome: A microtubule-associated defect. *CRC Crit Rev Biochem* 19:63, 1985.

Allen RC, Armitage RJ, Conley ME, et al.: CD40 ligand gene defects responsible for X-linked hyper-IgM syndrome. *Science* 259:990, 1993.

Ammann AJ: Selective IgA deficiency: Presentation of 30 cases and a review of the literature. *Medicine* (Baltimore) 50:223, 1971.

Arnaiz-Villena A, Timon M, Corell A, et al.: Brief report: Primary immunodeficiency caused by mutations in the gene encoding the CD3-γ subunit of the T-lymphocyte receptor. *N Engl J Med* 327:529, 1992.

Barton RW, Goldschneider I: Nucleotide-metabolizing enzymes and lymphocyte differentiation. *Molec Cell Biochem* 28:135, 1979.

Braun J, Galbraith L, Valles-Ayoub Y, et al.: Human immunodeficiency resulting from a maturational arrest of germinal center B cells. *Immunol Lett* 27:205, 1991.

Fundenberg HH, Good KA, Goodman HC, et al.: Primary immunodeficiencies: Report of a World Health Organization committee. *Pediatrics* 47:927, 1971.

Good RA, Bergsma D (eds.): *Immunologic Deficiency Diseases in Man*, vol. 4, no. 1. New York, National Foundation Press, 1968.

Gougeon M-L, Morelet L, Doussau M, et al.: Hyper-IgM immunodeficiency syndrome: Influence of lymphokines on in vitro maturation of peripheral B cells. *J Clin Immunol* 12:1, 1992.

Greenberg F: DiGeorge syndrome: An historical review of clinical and cytogenetic features. *J Med Genet* 30:803–806, 1993.

Hirschhorn R: Inherited enzyme deficiencies and immunodeficiency: Adenosine deaminase (ADA) and purine nucleoside phosphorylase (PNP) deficiencies. *Clin Immunol Immunopathol* 40:157, 1986.

Illum N, Ralfiaer E, Pallesen G, et al.: Phenotypical and functional characterization of double-negative (CD4-CD8-) αβ T-cell receptor positive cells from an immunodeficient patient. *Scand J Immunol* 34:635, 1991.

Kellems RE, Yeung CY, Ingolia DE: Adenosine deaminase deficiency and severe combined immunodeficiencies. *Trends Genet* 1:278, 1985.

Kondo M, Tskeshita T, Ishii N, et al.: Sharing of the interleukin-2 (IL-2) receptor γ chain between receptors for IL-2 and IL-4. *Science* 262:1874–1877, 1993.

Kondo N, Inoue R, Kasahara K, et al.: Failure of IgG production due to a defect in the opening of the chromatin structure of Ig1 region in a patient with IgG and IgA deficiency. *Clin Exp Immunol* 99:21–28, 1995.

Levin S: The immune system and susceptibility to infection in Down syndrome. In *Oncology and Immunology of Down's Syndrome* (McCoy EE, Epstein CJ, eds.) New York, Liss, 1987, 143–162.

Levitt D, Haber P, Richik, et al.: Hyper-IgM immunodeficiency: A primary dysfunction of B lymphocyte isotype switching. *J Clin Invest* 72:1650, 1983.

Liblau RS, Bach J-F: Selective IgA deficiency and autoimmunity. *Int Arch Allerg Immunol* 99:16–27, 1992.

Malynn BA, Blackwell TK, Fulop GM, et al.: The *scid* defect affects the final step of the immunoglobulin VDJ recombinase mechanism. *Cell* 54:453, 1988.

Mandell LA: Infections in the compromised host. *J Int Med Res* 18:177, 1990.

Nahmias AJ, Keyserling HL: The TORCH complex: Neonatal infections associated with toxoplasma and rubella, cytomegalovirus, and herpes simplex virus. *Pediatr Rec* 5:405, 1971.

Omenn GS: Familial reticuloendotheliosis with eosinophilia. *N Engl J Med* 273:427, 1965.

Park JK, Rosenstein YJ, Remold-O'Donnell E, et al.: Enhancement of T-cell activation by the CD43 molecule whose expression is defective in Wiskott–Aldrich syndrome. *Nature* 350:706, 1991.

Peterson RDA, Cooper MD, Good RA: The pathogenesis of immunologic deficiency diseases. *Am J Med* 38:579, 1965.

Puck JM: Molecular basis for three X-linked immune disorders. *Human Mole Genetics* 3:1457–1461, 1994.

Seggev JS, Ben-Yosef N, Meytes D: Is selective IgA deficiency associated with morbidity? Review and reevaluation. *Israel J Med Sci* 24:65, 1988.

Seligman M, Fudenberg HH, Good RA: Editorial: A proposed classification of primary immunologic deficiencies. *Am J Med* 45:817, 1968.

Sleasman JW, Harville TO, White GB, et al.: Arrested rearrangement of TCRVβ genes in thymocytes from children with X-linked severe combined immunodeficiency disease. *J Immunol* 153:442–448, 1994.

Steim ER: *Immunologic Disorders in Infants and Children.* 3rd ed., Orlando, FL, Saunders, 1990.

Touraine JL, Betuel H, Souillet G, et al.: Combined immunodeficiency disease associated with absence of cell surface HLA-A and -B antigens. *J Pediatr* 93:47, 1978.

Ugazio AG, Maccariio R, Notarangelo LD, et al.: Immunology of Down syndrome: A review. *Am J Med Genet* 7S:204, 1990.

Vetrie D, Vorechovsky I, Sideras P, et al.: The gene involved in X-linked agamma-globulinemia is a member of the *src* family of protein-tyrosine kinases. *Nature* 361:226, 1993.

Wara DW, Goldstein AL, Doyle NE, et al.: Thymosin activity in patients with cellular immunodeficiency. *N Engl J Med* 292:70–74, 1975.

Wirt DP, Brooks EG, Vaidya S, et al.: Novel T-lymphocyte population in combined immunodeficiency with features of graft-versus-host disease. *N Engl J Med* 321:370, 1989.

Wong B: Parasitic diseases in immunocompromized hosts. *Am J Med* 76:479, 1984.

PHAGOCYTIC DEFECTS

Anderson DC: Leukocyte adhesion deficiency: An inherited defect in the MAC-1, LFA-1, and p150,95 glycoproteins. In *Gene Transfer and Gene Therapy*. New York, Liss, 1989, 315–323.

Clark RA, Malech HL, Gallin JI, et al.: Genetic variants of chronic granulomatous disease: Prevalence of deficiencies of two cytosolic components of the NADPH oxidase system. *N Engl J Med* 321:647, 1989.

Crowley CA, Curnutte JT, Rosin RE, et al.: An inherited abnormality of neutrophil adhesion: Its genetic transmission and its association with a missing protein. *N Engl J Med* 302:1163, 1980.

Davis SD, Schallar S, Wedgewood RJ: Job's syndrome: Recurrent "cold" staphylococcal abscesses. *Lancet* 1:10134, 1966.

Douglas SD, Fundenberg HH: Host defense failure: The role of phagocytic dysfunction. *Hosp Pract* 4:29, 1969.

Gabign TG, Babior BM: The killing of pathogens by phagocytes. *Am Rev Med* 32:313, 1981.

Galin JI, International Chronic Granulomatous Disease Cooperative Study Group: A controlled trial of interferon-gamma to prevent infection in children with chronic granulomatous disease. *N Engl J Med* 324:509, 1991.

Good RA, Quie PG, Windhorst DB, et al.: Fatal (chronic) granulomatous disease of children: A hereditary defect of leukocyte function. *Semin Hematol* 5:215, 1968.

Kohl S, Springer TA, Schmalstieg FC, et al.: Defective natural allocytotoxicity and polymorphonuclear leukocyte antibody-dependent cellular cytotoxicity in patients with LFA-1/OKM-1 deficiency. *J Immunol* 133:2972, 1984.

Landing BH, Shirkey HS: A syndrome of recurrent infection and infiltration of viscera by pigmented lipid histiocytes. *Pediatrics* 20:431, 1957.

Yang KD, Hill HR: Neutrophil function disorders: Pathophysiology, prevention, and therapy. *J Pediatr* 119:343, 1991.

COMPLEMENT

Carreer FMJ: The C_1 inhibitor deficiency: A review. *Eur J Clin Chem Clin Biochem* 30:793, 1992.

McClean RH, Winkelstein JA: Genetically determined variation in the complement system. *J Pediatr* 105:179, 1984.

Ross SC, Densen P: Complement deficiency states and infections: Epidemiology, pathogenesis and consequences of neisserial and other infections in an immune deficiency. *Medicine* 63:243, 1984.

Schur PH: Inherited complement component abnormalities. *Annu Rev Med* 37:333, 1986.

INTERLEUKINS, LYMPHOKINES, AND MONOKINES

Friedman RM, Vogel SN: Interferons, with special emphasis on the immune system. *Adv Immunol* 34:97, 1983.

Spickett GP, Farrant J: The role of lymphokines in common variable hypogamma-globulinemia. *Immunol Today* 10:192, 1989.

Voss SD, Hong R, Sondel PM: Severe combined immunodeficiency interleukin-2 (IL-

2), and the IL-2 receptor: Experiments of nature continue to point the way. *Blood* 83:626–635, 1994.

SECONDARY IMMUNO-DEFICIENCIES

Baker CC: Immune mechanisms and host resistance in the trauma patient. *Yale J Biol Med* 59:387, 1986.

de Sousa M: Lymphocyte maldistribution and immunodeficiency. *Hosp Pract* 15:71, 1980.

Jacobson DR, Zolla-Pazner S: Immunosuppression and infection in multiple myeloma. *Semin Oncol* 13:282, 1986.

Kyle DV, deShazo RD: Chronic fatigue syndrome: A conundrum. *Am J Med Sci* 303:28, 1992.

Meakins JL: Surgeons, surgery and immunomodulation. *Arch Surg* 126:494, 1991.

Moutschen MP, Scheen AJ, Lefebvre PJ: Impaired immune responses in diabetes mellitus: Analysis of the factors and mechanisms involved; relevance to the increased susceptibility of diabetic patients to specific infections. *Diabet Metabol* 18:187, 1992.

Scharff MD, Uhr JW: Immunologic deficiency disorders associated with lymphoproliferative diseases. *Semin Hematol* 2:47, 1965.

Ward PA, Berenberg JL: Defective regulation of inflammatory mediators in Hodgkin's disease: Supernormal levels of a chematactic inhibitory factor. *N Engl J Med* 290:76, 1974.

DIAGNOSIS OF IMMUNO-DEFICIENCIES

Asherson GL, Webster ADB: Diagnosis and treatment of immunodeficiency disease. St. Louis, Mosby, 1980.

Bellanti JA, Schlegel RJ: The diagnosis of immune deficiency diseases. *Pediatr Clin North Am* 18:49, 1971.

Hong R: Evaluation of immunity. *Immunol Invest* 16:453, 1987.

Miller ME: Clinical aids in diagnosis of immunologic disease. *Clin Pediatr* 8:189, 1969.

Moore EC, Meuwissen HJ: Immunologic deficiency disease: Approach to diagnosis. *NY State J Med* 73:2437, 1973.

Schmidt, RE: Monoclonal antibodies for diagnosis of immunodeficiencies. *Blut* 59:200, 1989.

Shearer WT: Appropriate laboratory testing for immunodeficiency. *Am Assoc Clin Chem* 1:1, 1983.

Waldman TA, Broder S: Polyclonal B-cell activities in the study of the regulation of immunoglobulin synthesis in the human system. *Adv Immunol* 32:1, 1982.

THERAPY

Ammann AJ, Wara DW, Salmon S, et al.: Thymus transplantation: Permanent reconstitution of cellular immunity in a patient with sex-linked combined immunodeficiency. *N Engl J Med* 289:5, 1973.

Asanuma YA, Goldstein AL, White A, et al.: Reduction in the incidence of wasting diseases in neonatally thymectomized mice by injection of thymosin. *Endocrinology* 86:600, 1970.

Ascher MS, Gottlieb AA, Kirkpatrick CH: *Transfer Factor: Basic Properties and Clinical Application*. New York, Academic Press, 1976.

Cleveland WW, Fogel BJ, Brown WT, et al.: Foetal thymic transplant in a case of DiGeorge syndrome. *Lancet* 2:1211, 1968.

Good RA: Progress toward a cellular engineering. *JAMA* 214:1289, 1970.

Dekoning J, Van Bekkum DW, Dicke KA, et al.: Transplantation of bone marrow cells and fetal thymus in an infant with lymphopenic immunologic deficiency. *Lancet* 1:1223, 1969.

Hanszel ZT, Burstein Y, Bucher V, et al.: Immunomodulation of T-cell deficiency in humans by thymic humoral factor: From crude extract to synthetic humoral factor-γ2. *J Biol Res Modif* 9:269, 1990.

Huston DP, Kavanaugh AF, Rohane PW, et al.: Immunoglobulin deficiency syndromes and therapy. *J Allergy Clin Immunol* 87:1, 1991.

Incefy GS, Boumsell L, Touraine JL, et al.: Enhancement of T-lymphocyte differentiation in vitro by thymic extracts after bone marrow transplantation in severe combined immunodeficiencies. *Clin Immunol Immunopathol* 4:258, 1975.

Kruskal BA, Ezekowitz AB: Cytokines in the treatment of primary immunodeficiency. *Biotherapy* 7:249–259, 1994.

Lawrence HS: Transfer factor. *Adv Immunol* 11:195, 1969.

Lawrence HS: Selective immunotherapy with transfer factor. *Clin Immunobiol* 2:116, 1974.

Parkman R: The biology of bone marrow transplantation for severe combined immunodeficiency. *Adv Immunol* 49:381, 1991.

Parkman R, Gelfand EW: Severe combined immunodeficiency disease, adenosine deaminase deficiency, and gene therapy. *Curr Opin Immunol* 3:547, 1991.

Storek J, Saxon A: Reconstitution of B-cell immunity following bone marrow transplantation. *Bone Marrow Transplant* 9:395, 1992.

28

Immunomodulation

Immunomodulation is an induced alteration of immunity by synthetic chemicals, natural substances, or radiation, as well as by specific antigens or antibodies, and the actions of lymphokines, cytokines, complement, kinins, inflammatory mediators, autoacoids, and neuropeptides. The immune response may be affected at various levels by many different agents. Modulation of the immune response may involve induction, expression, amplification, or inhibition of the afferent, central, efferent, or accessory phase of the immune response (Fig. 28–1). Because immunomodulation has widespread application in many clinical and experimental models, many of the agents listed in this chapter are covered in more detail in other chapters, including desitization for allergies (Chapter 14), prevention of Rh sensitization (Chapter 12), pharmacologic intervention in accessory mechanisms of inflammation (Chapters 8 and 9), immunization for prevention of infectious diseases (Chapter 26), and immunotherapy for cancer (Chapter 30). In this chapter, modulation of the immune response will focus on specific and nonspecific effects on induction and expression of the immune system in general, rather than on accessory inflammatory mechanisms, such as mast cell degranulation (Chapter 14) or complement activation (Chapter 8).

Immunomodulation may be specific, limited to a given antigen, or nonspecific, with a general effect on immune responses (Table 28–1). Major attempts have been made to enhance or inhibit immune responses in man and experimental animals. Therapeutic stimulation of the immune response is desirable in some cases, such as patients with immunodeficiencies, whereas suppression of the immune response is sought for others, such as transplant recipients or patients with autoim-

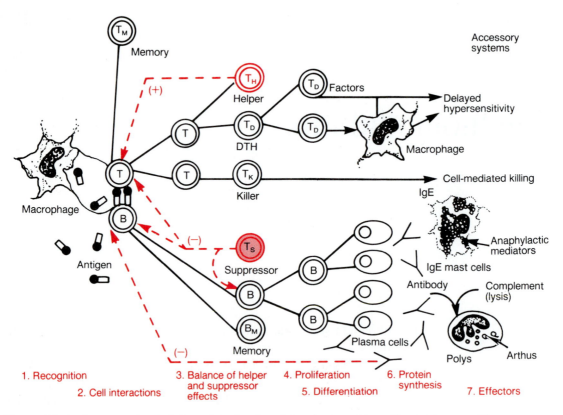

Figure 28–1. Immune modulation. Levels of activity that may be affected by specific or nonspecific agents include: *Afferent*: (1) antigen recognition and processing, (2) lymphoid cell interactions; *Central*: (3) helper and suppressor cell functions, (4) proliferation of responding cell populations, (5) differentiation of effector cells, (6) synthesis of immune products, such as lymphokines or specific antibody; and *Efferent*: (7) T cell-mediated reactions, antibody–antigen reactions, and accessory effector systems (macrophage, mast cell, and complement activity).

mune diseases. Specific immunomodulation may be actively achieved by administration of antigen in a form or by a route that suppresses induction of immunity (tolerance), or changes activity from one form to another (immune deviation). Immunization vehicles may be used to increase or modify response to a given antigen (adjuvants). In addition, specific immunomodulation may be produced passively by transfer of immune products (cells or antibody) or by factors that affect specific responsiveness (ie, transfer factor). Nonspecific immunostimulation may be achieved by administration of such agents as interferon, interleukins, or cytokines that increase some component of the immune response not involving specific antigen recognition. Such agents generally act on some accessory cell type, such as the macrophage or natural killer (NK) cells. Nonspecific suppression of the immune response

TABLE 28–1. CLASSIFICATION OF IMMUNOMODULATION

Stimulation

    Specific
        1. Active immunization (antigen, adjuvant, vectors)
        2. Passive transfer (cells, antiserum, transfer factor)

    Nonspecific (biological response modifiers)
        1. Macrophage activators (bacteria, levamisole)
        2. B-cell activators (endotoxin)
        3. T-cell activators (interleukins, interferon)
        4. NK activators (IL-2, IL-12)
        5. Nutritional (β-carotene, retinoids)

Suppression

    Specific
        1. Tolerance (suppressor cells, clonal elimination, antiidiotype suppression)
        2. Hyposensitization/desensitization (allergic immunotherapy)
        3. Passive transfer (neutralization)

    Nonspecific
        1. Depletion
        2. Irradiation
        3. Drugs
        4. Antileukocyte sera, monoclonal antibodies
        5. Suppressive factors (immunoregulatory globulin)

may be achieved by agents that interfere with the induction or expression of an immune response. Such agents include radiation, drugs (steroids, antimetabolites, cyclosporine), and immune reagents, such as antilymphocyte or antimacrophage sera or monoclonal antibodies. The effect of immune modulating agents is dependent on dose, particularly the relationship of antigen stimulation to the time of administration of the agent. For instance, radiation given before antigen may increase the magnitude of the immune response, whereas radiation given after antigen (during the proliferation of antigen-activated cells) will greatly inhibit the response. Cyclophosphamide at moderate daily doses leads to suppression of immune functions, including T- and B-cell depletion, impairment of NK activity and blocking of T- and B-cell differentiation. However, at low doses, cyclophosphamide has a selective effect on suppressor cells resulting in enhancement of antibody and effector T-cell production.

Stimulation of Immune Responses

SPECIFIC IMMUNO-STIMULATION

Active Immunization

Classically, immunologists have directed specific active immunization either for the induction of protective immunity to infectious agents (or cancer) or to produce immunologic reagents to identify, isolate, or measure a given antigen (immunoassays). For protective immunization, isolated proteins might be used, but most often the specific protective immunogens were not known and whole killed or attenuated organisms were used. (For more details on protective immunization see Chapter 26, Immunization). For molecular isolation, characterization, or assay, purified antigens are the immunogens of choice, but often mixtures of antigens produce antisera that are critical for identification of glycoproteins, lipids, or nucleic acids. These types of immunizations are almost always carried out to induce immunoglobulin antibodies.

The form of delivery of the immunogen can determine the type of immune response (Table 28–2). In the late 1950s, it was shown that immunization with very low doses of protein antigens could direct the immune response to delayed hypersensitivity rather than antibody formation, which occurred when higher doses were used. This phenomenon became known as "immune deviation." The use of complete Freund's adjuvant (see below) also enhanced DTH to low antigen doses. With the recognition of different classes of helper T cells—Th1 and Th2—as well as different pathways of antigen processing, ways are being studied that will preferentially direct a specific immune response to T_{DTH} or T_{CTL}. Recently, two developments in immunology have resulted in approaches to direct specific immunization to epitopes that will stimulate T-cytotoxic cells. The first is molecular analysis of immunogens to identify epitopes that will be recognized by class I-restricted T cells. The second is the use of ISCOMs that direct antigens to class I restricted (endogenous) processing (see below). Recombinant vaccines using vaccinia vectors will infect epidermal cells, leading to endogenous processing and stimulation of T cytotoxicity (T_{CTL}), whereas BCG vectors that infect monocytic cells may preferentially induce delayed hypersensitivity (T_{DTH}).

Antigen Form. The classic or **exogenous** processing of immunogens is accomplished by class II MHC-positive antigen-presenting macrophages or activated B cells, which deliver the processed immunogen to CD4+ T-helper cells to induce B cells to produce immunoglobulin antibody (see Chapter 7). The epitopes identified by antibodies are usually directed to conformational or topographic surface epitopes formed by folding of the antigen. Because of this, parts of the epitope may be contributed by different amino acid sequences in the unfolded molecule.

TABLE 28–2. RELATIONSHIP OF IMMUNIZATION METHODS TO TYPE OF
IMMUNE RESPONSE

Circulating antibody, exogenous processing, class II MHC-positive follicular dendritic
cells/lymph node or spleen:
    Soluble protein
    Alum

Secretory antibody (IgA), exogenous processing, class II MHC-positive follicular
dendritic cells/GALT:
    Oral route

T-cytotoxicity, endogenous processing, class I MHC-positive epithelial cells/skin:
    ISCOMs
    Vaccinia vectors
    DNA transfection

Delayed hypersensitivity, exogenous processing, class II MHC-positive interdigitating
reticulum cells/lymph node:
    Low antigen dose
    Freund's adjuvant
    Muramyl dipeptide
    BCG vectors

The **endogenous** pathway delivers peptide fragments associated with class I MHC molecules and can be accomplished by many nucleated cells. By analysis of the primary amino acid sequence of a potential immunogen, it is possible to predict peptides that will be recognized by CD8+ T cells. Such peptides are made up of seven to twelve amino acids that form amphipathic helixes. Amphipathicity refers to alternating hydrophobic and hydrophilic residues in an α-helix arranged so that hydrophobic and hydrophilic residues alternate about every three to four residues. Since there are about 3.6 residues per turn, this sequence aligns the hydrophobic residues on one side of the helix and hydrophilic residues on the other side of the helix. The hydrophobic side attaches to the cleft in the class I MHC molecule on the surface of the class I MHC+ antigen-processing cell, whereas the hydrophilic side binds to the CD8+ T-cell receptor (Fig. 28–2). Using this approach, a number of T-cell epitopes in antigens of infectious agents have been identified. Once the peptide having the putative

T-cell epitope has been identified and synthesized, it is necessary to be able to deliver it to the endogenous processing system (see ISCOMS, below).

Adjuvants. The most effective way to increase the specific immune response to a given antigen is to administer the antigen (immunogen) along with an agent that will enhance the reactivity of the reacting cells. Such agents are termed adjuvants. The mechanism of action of adjuvants is not well understood, but they are believed to attract macrophages and reactive lymphocytes to the sites of antigen deposition, to localize antigens in an inflammatory site (depot effect), to delay antigen catabolism, to activate the metabolism of antigen-processing cells, and to stimulate lymphoid cell interactions. Adjuvants will also produce a nonspecific increase in immune reactivity; much of the immunoglobulin produced by adjuvant–antigen stimulation is not specific antibody. Injection of adjuvant with or without antigen can produce a sustained hyperglobulinemia. Effective adjuvants include oils, mineral salts, double-stranded nucleic acids, products of microorganisms, and a variety of other agents.

Water–Oil Emulsions. The most widely used adjuvant for experimental immunization is Freund's adjuvant. This adjuvant consists of a water or saline in oil emulsion. Typically, soluble antigen is dissolved in

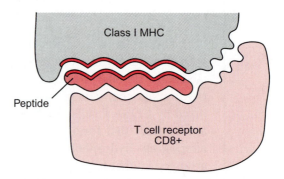

Figure 28–2. Cooperative binding of a T-cell epitope with class I MHC and CD8+ T-cell receptor. Peptides processed for T_{CTL} recognition have hydrophilic amino acids alternating with hydrophobic amino acids in a manner that aligns the hydrophilic sites on one side of an α-helix and hydrophobic sites on the other side. The hydrophilic side has affinity for the T-cell receptor, whereas the hydrophobic site binds to the class I MHC on the antigen-processing cell. Peptides which have these "amphipathic" structures are presented to reactive CD8+ T cells by the endogenous antigen-processing pathway.

saline and emulsified in equal parts of an oil, such as Bayol F (42.5% paraffin, 31.4% monocyclic naphthalene, and 26.1% polycyclic naphthalene) or Arlacel A (mannite monolate). The addition of killed mycobacteria greatly increases the adjuvant activity. Emulsions without mycobacteria are called incomplete (incomplete Freund's adjuvant) and emulsions containing mycobacteria are termed complete (complete Freund's adjuvant). The glycolipid and peptidoglycolipid portions (wax D) of the mycobacteria are responsible for the increased effect of complete Freund's adjuvant. In producing antisera in animals, it is common to use complete Freund's adjuvant for the initial immunization and incomplete Freund's adjuvant for booster immunizations. Repeated immunization with complete Freund's adjuvant can lead to severe necrotic reactions at the site of the injection because of extreme hypersensitivity to the mycobacterial component. To be fully effective, adjuvants must be injected intradermally or subcutaneously. Adjuvant immunizations are particularly effective in producing antibody responses to small doses of immunogen and in inducing primed T cells. In some instances, complete Freund's adjuvant induces extremely active delayed hypersensitivity responses. Freund's adjuvant is noted for the ability to induce cellular autoimmune reactions (see Chapter 21) and in stimulating antibody responses in low responder animals, probably through activation of T-helper cells.

Mineral Salts (Alum). Solutions of antigens precipitated with mineral salts (alum) such as calcium phosphate, silica, or alum [aluminum potassium sulfate, $[AlK(SO4)_2 12H_2 0]$ or aluminum phosphate $(AlPO_4)$], produce granulomas at the site of injection and in draining lymph nodes. The alum-induced immune granulomas function similarly to those produced by incomplete Freund's adjuvant. Alum-precipitated immunogens have been used in man to increase the extent of an immune response for prophylactic immunization to antigens such as diphtheria toxoid.

Microbial Extracts (Endotoxins). Microbial endotoxins may produce a marked increase in immune responses. The endotoxins most active are intracellular lipopolysaccharides produced by gram-negative bacteria. They can function as adjuvants when administered systemically but are more effective if injected locally along with antigens. Many of these endotoxins are capable of stimulating immunoglobulin synthesis and proliferation by B cells in vitro and of attracting and enhancing phagocytosis by macrophages. Endotoxins increase antibody production when given in vivo and have little, if any, effect on delayed hypersensitivity. Endotoxins seem to activate B cells nonspecifically (poly-clonal activation) but will enhance a specific antibody response if a given antigen is present.

Cell Wall Extracts. The cell walls of certain bacteria (mycobacteria) and fungi also serve to enhance immune reactivity. In general, the effect is less but similar to that of complete Freund's adjuvant. These agents also produce a marked nonspecific activation of the effector arm of immune responses that involve macrophages. They attract and activate macrophages, thus increasing phagocytosis at the site of antigen-induced inflammation.

Synthetic immunostimulants derived from bacterial cell walls are exemplified by peptidoglycan derivatives such as muramyl dipeptide (MDP).

MDP is a simple dipeptide derivative of muraminic acid and is the minimal molecule capable of replacing mycobacterial cell walls in complete Freund's adjuvant. However, this compound is toxic and produces fever, leukopenia, and platelet lysis in animals. Muramyl dipeptide has been combined with liposomes to stimulate the immune system of patients with cancer nonspecifically (see Chapter 33). Synthetic disaccharide peptides, such as disaccharides from lacto-bacilli coupled to the dipeptide L-alanyl-D-isoglutamine, may be even more active than MDP and less toxic. Other artificial saccharides, lipids, and peptidolipids structurally related to MDP are also being tested for possible clinical use. The primary action of adjuvants is on macrophage activation resulting in increased T- and B-cell proliferation, presumably through IL-1 production.

Mycobacteria and other organisms also produce 6,6'-diesters of trehalose called mycolic acids (or cord factors) which have various α-branched β hydroxy acids.

These and related glycolipids contain a balance of lipophilic and hydrophilic groups and interact with cell membranes. They are chemotactic for macrophages and function as adjuvants in attracting and activating macrophages. Attempts are now underway to produce derivatives of adjuvant molecules and test combinations of molecules to achieve maximum immunostimulation with minimum toxicity for use in vaccines.

Polynucleotides. Double-stranded polynucleotides, such as polyinosine–polycytidylic acid [poly-(IC)] or polyadenylic–polyuridylic acid [poly-(AU)] are also potent adjuvants and immunostimulants. They appear to act through activation of antigen-reactive T cells. Polynucleotides are not effective in T cell-depleted animals. The mechanism of action is believed to be through elevation of cyclic AMP in antigen-reactive T cells. Polynucleotides may also serve to activate macrophages nonspecifically, perhaps through stimulation of T-cell factors.

ISCOMs. Delivery of antigens to the endogenous processing pathway may be accomplished by the use of ISCOMs (Fig. 28–3). ISCOMs are glycosides that form micelles with the peptide and are able to penetrate cell membranes, as liposomes do, to introduce the antigen into the endoplasmic reticulum, allowing endogenous processing and presentation by the class I pathway. This approach is now being applied to retroviruses, such as feline leukemia virus and HIV. Such methods give promise of being able to direct vaccination to the type of cell-mediated immunity that is effective against tumor-specific antigens. However, some T-suppressor cells also belong to the CD8+ population. In view of the effect of T-suppressor cells to inhibit induction of immune effector mechanisms, it may be that the use of peptides and ISCOMs that stimulate CD8+ cells may actually enhance infection rather than inhibit it.

Vectors

Vaccinia. Vaccinia virus, the attenuated derivative of a mixture of cow, horse, and human poxvirus used for immunization against smallpox (see Chapter 26), has been used in experimental animals to deliver

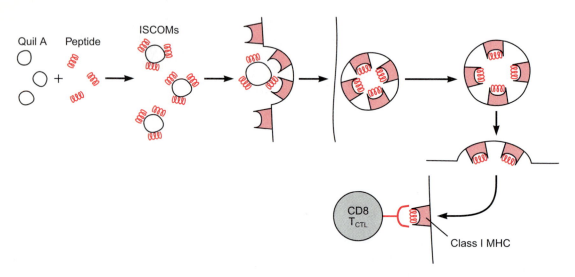

Figure 28–3. Immunostimulating complexes (ISCOMs). ISCOMs form structures with peptide antigens that direct the processing of the antigen to the endogenous pathway, presentation via class I MHC surface molecules, and induction of CD8+ T_{CTL}.

antigens for expression in epithelial cells leading to induction of antibody and/or T_{CTL}s. Vaccinia virus replicates in the cytoplasm of infected cells, and antigenic vaccinia peptides are presented in the grove of the class I MHC on the surface of the infected cell. In this form the antigenic peptides react with the T-cell receptor of CD8+ T_{CTL} precursors with eventual stimulation of T-cytotoxic immunity. Cloned complementary DNA for genes for immunogens of other infectious agents may be inserted into the nonessential regions of vaccinia DNA. Up to 25,000 bp of DNA can be introduced to the vaccinia genome without any deletions being required. The foreign gene is flanked with vaccinia virus DNA sequences and then the product, usually a plasmid, is introduced into a cell that has been infected with the whole virus. Recombination results in insertion of the foreign DNA into about 0.1% of the progeny virus. After infection of epithelial cells, expression of the foreign genes is controlled by the poxvirus promoters. The foreign genes cannot contain introns because splicing does not occur in the cytoplasm of the infected cells. Special insertion or transfer vectors are available that greatly simplify the construction and isolation of recombinant viruses. Protection against challenge with viral infections in experimental animals immunized with vaccinia recombinants is associated with neutralizing antibody for many virus infections, including influenza, parainfluenza, respiratory syncytia, measles, rabies, and Epstein–Barr viruses. In other infections, such as murine cytomegalovirus, lymphocytic choriomeningitis virus, and Friend leukemia virus, protection correlates with T_{CTL}.

Bacille Calmette–Guérin. BCG most likely specifically infects class II MHC-positive antigen-presenting macrophages and induces T_{DTH} though presentation of antigen in association with class II MHC by interdigitating reticulum cells in the paracortical regions of lymph nodes. Thus, whereas vaccinia vectors select for T_{CTL}, BCG may select for T_{DTH}. BCG is a live, attenuated bovine tubercle bacillus used to immunize against tuberculosis. It is effective in inducing activation of mycobacterial-infected macrophages, which are then able to purge themselves of the infection through activation of cellular enzymes and oxidative metabolites, so-called angry macrophages. BCG is the most widely used vaccine in the world, having been given to over 3 billion people since 1948, with a very low incidence of serious complications and a case fatality rate of $0.19/10^6$ inoculations. It can be given at any time after birth and is unaffected by maternal antibodies. It is a potent adjuvant for DTH, and after a single inoculation, BCG sensitizes to tuberculoprotein for up to 50 years. It can be administered as an oral vaccine, is heat stable and is inexpensive to produce. BCG vectors have been designed and constructed (Fig. 28–4). An expression cassette permits convenient insertion of DNA coding sequences and extra-chromosomal, and integrative expression vectors carrying the regulatory sequences for major BCG heat-shock proteins allow expression of foreign antigens.

Passive Immunization

Specific immunity may be passively transferred using antiserum, antibody preparations, or cells. The passive transfer of antibody preparations for protection against tetanus and other infectious diseases is discussed under Immunization in Chapter 26, for treatment of immunodeficiency diseases in Chapter 27 and for immunotherapy of cancer in Chapter 30. The passive transfer of immunocompetent cells in humans is limited because for MHC-related graft-versus-host disease. However, passive transfer of lymphoid cells is employed for treatment of cancer, either to replace lymphoid depletion after radiation or chemotherapy for leukemia or lymphoma (see Chapter 24) or of activated autologous cells as cancer therapy (see Chapter 30).

NONSPECIFIC IMMUNO-STIMULATION

Many of the agents mentioned above, such as oils, salts, endotoxins, mycobacterial cell walls, and polynucleotides, produce a generalized increase in immune responsiveness by nonspecifically activating the effector arm of immune responses (nonspecific immunostimulation) as well as functioning as adjuvants in the induction of antigen-specific immune responses in the presence of specific antigen. These agents may also act nonspecifically to activate T cells, B cells, macrophages, or complement. Such stimulation has been widely used in attempts to potentiate or stimulate immune responses to tumors (see Chapter 30). Agents that are most effective in this regard are BCG,

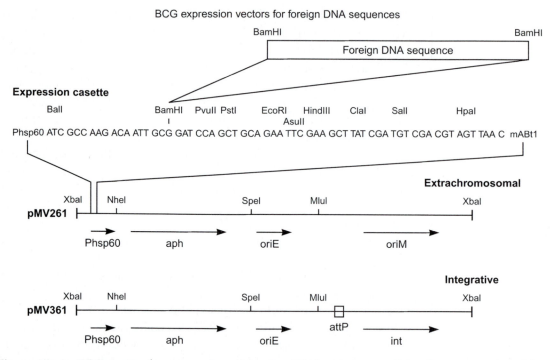

Figure 28–4. BCG vector for expression of foreign DNA sequences. Extrachromosomal and integrative BCG expression vectors are shown. Plasmids pMV261 and pMV361 share common elements, including an expression cassette that permits convenient insertion of DNA coding sequences, the Tn*903*-derived *amp* gene conferring kanamycin resistance as a marker to select recombinants and the *Escherichia coli* origin of replication (*oriM*) or the *attP* and *int* genes of mycobacteriophage L5. The expression cassette contains the regulatory sequences for major BCG heat-shock proteins which allows expression of foreign antigens and ten unique cloning sites for insertion of foreign DNA sequences.

Corynebacterium parvum, Listeria monocytogenes, and *Bordetella pertussis,* as well as polynucleotides and levamisole. Other agents include products of activated cells, such as interleukins and interferon. These are classified as biologic response modifiers, a general term used for biologic products that alter the defensive responses of an individual.

Macrophage Activators

Bacterial macrophage activators, such as BCG, *C. parvum,* and *L. monocytogenes,* act to increase phagocytosis and to activate the intracellular digestive enzymes of macrophages. Following injection of these organisms, macrophage activity is increased in the following ways: Content of lysosomal enzymes, adherence to glass, rate of phagocytosis, and bacteriocidal activity. Such macrophages are called activated, angry or armed. In general, nonspecific stimulators act by enhancing the activities of the macrophage in the effector arm of the immune response, thus increasing the magnitude of expression of delayed hypersensitivity reactions and resistance to intracellular bacterial infections. This action may be mediated through activation of T cells to release macrophage-activating factors, but there is evidence that macrophage activation need not always require T cells. BGG, *C. parvum*, or *L. monocytogenes*-treated animals demonstrate an increased resistance to antigenically unrelated organisms and an enhanced ability to reject some transplanted syngeneic tumors; BCG is being used clinically for the treatment of bladder cancer (see Chapter 30).

Levamisole is able to restore the phagocytic and T-cell responses of compromised animals but has little stimulatory effect on normal animals. Given just before tumor transplantation, levamisole decreases growth of transplantable tumors in animals, but timing of the administration is critical. Increased tumor growth may occur if levamisole is given five days before the tumor begins to grow. Clinically, levamisole has been reputed to have a beneficial effect in immune deficiency diseases, cancer, and other diseases, but the results of systematic clinical trials are not yet available. Injections of *B. pertussis* result in a marked lymphocytosis because of increased recirculating and decreased homing of small lymphocytes; pertussis-treated animals also tend to produce IgE type antibody and demonstrate an increased sensitivity to anaphylactic reactions.

Liposomes are artificial organelles, composed of phospholipids, which form a vesicular lipid bilayer structurally resembling soap bubbles. Because of their vesicular structure, drugs or other agents may be enclosed within the lipid bilayer. Liposomes are selectively taken up by cells of the reticuloendothelial system (ie, macrophages). Thus, liposomes serve as a selected drug delivery system to macrophages for exogenous processing. Liposomes have been used to deliver antifungal agents, such as amphotericin B, to infected macrophages in patients with cutaneous leishmaniasis, coccidioidomycosis, or cryptococcal meningitis. This targeted delivery allows a twentyfold increase in the effective dose of these drugs because of limiting the toxicity to other organs (ie, kidney).

B-cell Activators

The major B-cell activators are bacterial lipopolysaccharides (endotoxins). The agents nonspecifically activate proliferation and differentiation of B cells and produce marked polyclonal increases in immunoglobulin synthesis in vitro. In addition, endotoxins may act as adjuvants (see above). There is no active use for endotoxins as therapeutic agents known to the author at this time.

T-cell Activators

Lymphokines and monokines (biologic response modifiers) are products of lymphocytes or macrophages that act on other cells as effector molecules, or on other white cells to increase or decrease immune reactivity (interleukins) (see Chapter 9). These cytokines have many different effects on different cells, but at this point their effect on T cells will be emphasized. Some lymphokines or interleukins that have potential for use as modulators of immunity are listed in Table 28–3. Thymic humoral factors and transfer factor are discussed in more detail under Immune Deficiency Diseases (Chapter 27). Thymic humoral factors are able to induce T-cell differentiation in vitro and some anecdotal reports suggest a beneficial effect in treatment of patients with T-cell deficiencies. Transfer factor, a lysate of lymphocytes from patients who are highly sensitive to a given antigen, has been used to control or modify selected diseases, such as chronic mucocutaneous candidiasis. In this disease, there is preferential production of humoral antibody over development of delayed hypersensitivity (immune deviation), as is seen in lepromatous leprosy. Transfer factor appears to be able to restore delayed hypersensitivity to *Candida* in some patients and result in clinical improvement. Both of these factors give inconsistent results. The application of growth factor to stimulation of proliferation of hematopoiesis is presented in Chapter 3.

Interferons

Interferons are a family of glycoproteins produced by lymphocytes and other cells (see Chapter 9). Interferons available for clinical use include both natural products from cultured cells and interferons produced by recombinant DNA techniques. Most clinical studies have been done using α-interferon, but now highly purified α-, β- and γ-interferons are each being tested in clinical trials (Table 28–4). Alpha-interferon is produced by virus-infected lymphocytes within six hours of infection; beta by fibroblasts; and gamma by mitogen- or antigen-activated lymphocytes. Alpha-interferon exists in up to 25 different forms; β- and γ-interferon also exist in different forms, but how many is not yet known. Recombinant and natural α-interferons appear to be very similar. In clinical trials, α-interferon has had little or no effect on epithelial tumors but has been associated with remissions in about 10% of patients with lymphoma, myeloma, and melanoma. Very preliminary results with β- and γ-interferons have given similar results. Untoward side effects at high doses include fever, intolerable fatigue, weight loss, and malaise. The mechanism of action of interferons remains unclear. Interferons may have a direct cytostatic effect on some tumors and may act by this mechanism rather than by specific effects on the immune system. More promising preliminary results have been obtained in viral infections. Inhalation of interferon may

TABLE 28–3. LYMPHOKINES AND INTERLEUKINS: ACTION AND THERAPEUTIC USE

Lymphokine	Function	Possible Therapeutic Use	Clinical Status
Thymic hormones	Stimulates T-cell differentiation	Thymic deficiencies	Anecdotal, inconsistent
Transfer factor	Transfers specific T-cell sensitivity	T-cell deficiencies	Anecdotal, inconsistent
Macrophage maturing factors	Activate macrophages	Nonspecific tumor immunity	Not used
*Interferons	Inhibits proliferation, activates NK cells, increases immune response	Nonspecific tumor immunity, virus infections	Clinical trials underway, approved for chronic granulomatous disease (IFN-γ)
Lymphotoxin	Kills target cells	Tumor therapy	Not used
Suppressor factors	Inhibit T- or B-cell functions	Transplantation, autoimmunity	Not used
Interleukin-1	Activates T cells, increases IL-2R, Chemoprotective	Cancer, virus infections, neutropenia	Under study
*Interleukin-2	Activates T cells and NK cells	Cancer	Clinical trials underway
Interleukin-3	Growth factor	Bone marrow stimulation	Under study
Interleukin-4	B-cell differentiation	B-cell tumors, immuno-deficiency diseases	Clinical trials underway
Interleukin-6	Stimulates hematopoiesis	Chemoprotective	Trials to begin
Interleukin-11	Stimulates hematopoiesis	Chemoprotective	Clinical trials underway
Interleukin-12	Activates NK	Cancer	Under study
Eosinophil–chemotactic factor	Attracts eosinophils	Parasitic infection	Not used
Vascular permeability factors	Contracts endothelial cells	Cancer	Not used
Tumor migration inhibitory factor	Inhibits migration of cancer cells in vitro	Cancer	Not used
Tumor necrosis factor	Toxic or static for cancer cells in vitro	Cancer	Experimental, highly toxic
	G-CSF	Hematopoiesis	Chemoprotective FDA approved
GM-CSF	Hematopoiesis	Bone marrow transplantation	FDA approved

G-CSF, granulocyte colony-stimulating factor; GM-CSF, granulocyte–monocyte-stimulating factor (see Chapter 3).

prevent upper respiratory viral infections or modulate symptoms of colds and flulike virus infections.

Interleukin-1 (IL-1)

IL-1 is an inflammatory glycopeptide that is produced by many types of cells and has protective effects against lethal infections when administered to experimental animals. There are two structurally different IL-1 molecules—IL-1α and IL-1β—but they bind to the same receptors and have similar biologic effects. IL-1 has protected animals from a variety of infectious agents including: *Pseudomonas aeruginosa, Klebsiella pneumonia, S. typhimurium, Escherichia coli, Staphylococcus aureus, Streptococcus pneumoniae, Listeria monocytogenes,*

TABLE 28–4. INTERFERONS USED FOR CLINICAL TRIALS

Type	Source	Purity
Alpha		
Natural	Virus-activated lymphocyte cultures	Variable
Lymphoblastoid	Cultured lymphoma cells	Variable
Recombinant α2, A or D	E. coli, plasmid cDNA	Pure
Beta		
Natural	Cultured fibroblasts or SV40 transformed cells	Variable
Recombinant β1 or B	E. coli, plasmid cDNA	Pure
Gamma		
Natural	Activated lymphocytes	Variable lymphocyte lines
Recombinant 1	E. coli, plasmid cDNA	Pure

and *Candida albicans*. The mechanism of action of IL-1 in experimental infection is not clear. It may act by a direct antimicrobial effect; macrophage or neutrophil attraction and activation; stimulation of IL-6, IL-8, or TNF; induction of acute-phase proteins, etc., but experimental observations on the role of these mechanisms is conflicting. Use in humans has been limited because of toxicity.

Interleukin 2 (IL-2)

Interleukin-2 is produced by activated T lymphocytes and stimulates a number of activities in other lymphocytes, including activation of helper and cytotoxic T cells, B cells, and NK cells (see Chapter 9). Interleukin-activated NK cells demonstrate increased capability of lysing tumor cells in vitro, and such activated cells reduce tumor growth in experimental models. IL-2 administered to animals has a very short half-life in serum (approximately 2 minutes) and little or no effect on tumors. In addition, IL-2 has not been effective in treatment of immune deficiency diseases. However, clinical trials in which the blood lymphocytes from cancer patients are treated with IL-2 in vitro and then injected back into the same patient are now underway with some promising individual results. High-dose IL-2 therapy is now approved for use in the treatment of patients with metastatic renal cell carcinoma and is being considered for approval for treatment of metastatic melanoma (for more details, see Immunology of Cancer, Chapter 30).

Thymic Hormones

The thymus is believed to exert its influence over the maturation of pre-T cells, at least partially through the action of secreted effector molecules known collectively as thymic hormones. Some peptides isolated from thymic epithelium that have been shown to have effects in vitro include thymosin α-1, thymopoietin, thymic humoral factor, and thymulin. Although there have been anecdotal reports of improvement in the clinical condition of patients with immunodeficiency diseases or chronic infections after treatment with these peptides, no clear results have been obtained from controlled clinical trials.

Nutritional Stimulators (β-carotenes and Retinoids)

Carotenoids and retinoids in the diets of experimental animals stimulate T-cell maturation and activation, B cell-mediated antibody production and macrophage activities, including phagocytosis cytotoxicity and antigen presentation. Although carotenoids and retinoids have other, perhaps more direct, effects on proliferating cells, their immunologic effects may at least partially explain the observation that these dietary factors help decrease the development of cancer. Retinoids act on the differentiation process of immune cells, increasing mitogenesis and enhancing phagocytosis. Carotenoids modify the release of some cytokines after activation of lymphoid cells, increase T-helper cells, and increase the activity of NK cells, as well as decrease the immunotoxic effect of oxide radicals. These factors are recommended to supplement the diet of AIDS patients with the hope of increasing immune defenses against opportunistic infection.

Suppression of Immune Responses

SPECIFIC IMMUNO-SUPPRESSION

Tolerance

The subject of recognition of self and nonself is presented in detail in Chapter 6; tolerance and autoimmunity are presented in Chapter 21. Specific tolerance, the lack of ability to mount an immune response to a given antigen while maintaining the ability to respond to other antigens, is particularly desirable in the treatment of specific allergies or in preparation for organ transplantation. In these situations, it is the goal of therapy to eliminate or suppress the undesirable immune response to the allergen or transplantation alloantigen but not induce a general immunosuppression. Although tolerance has been demonstrated repeatedly in experimental animals, the application to humans has proved difficult, if not impossible. Hypothetically, tolerance could be induced in two ways: by blocking or eliminating the specifically reacting cells (clonal elimination), or by suppressing the reactive cells by specific immune-controlling products. This latter effect may be produced by specific suppressor cells, by products (suppressor factors) of cells, or by specific immunoglobulin antibody that provides a feedback mechanism to limit further production of antibody. Tolerance may be induced in experimental animals by either antigen exposure or by passive transfer. In some cases, specific tolerance may be induced in atopic individuals by administration of atopic antigens (see Chapter 14). In addition, tolerance may also be produced in some transplant recipients who survive for a long time. In such cases, it may be possible to withdraw nonspecific immunosuppressive therapy without serious rejection occurring. The mechanism for this phenomenon is not clear, however, and other mechanisms, such as masking of graft antigens, may be operating.

Hypo-sensitization/Desensitization

Hyposensitization (see Chapter 14) is replacement of expression of one effector mechanism by another. It is a form of immune deviation, in which the effect of the replaced effector mechanism is more detrimental than the mechanism that replaces it. For instance, in atopic individuals who have IgE antibody, this is achieved by injection immunotherapy to induce IgG antibody to the same allergen. Expression of anaphylactic or atopic reactions requires antigen reacting with IgE antibody on effector (mast) cells. If IgG antibody is also present, competition of the IgG with mast-cell-bound IgE antibody may eliminate the anaphylactic symptoms.

Desensitization is accomplished by "using up" antibody by increasing doses of antigen given under controlled conditions (see also Chapter 14). If antigen administration is discontinued, the immune state will be reestablished. Desensitization may be effective in decreasing anaphylactic and delayed hypersensitivity reactions.

Passive Transfer

Theoretically, passive transfer of antiidiotype antibodies should downregulate the production of the antibodies with which the antiidiotype serum reacts. This effect has been shown in a number of experimental models in animals but has not yet been effectively applied to human diseases, such as myasthenia gravis or Graves' disease, which are due to autoantibodies. Antibodies to idiotopes on B cells have been anecdotally successful in producing remissions in patients with B-cell lymphomas.

Passive transfer of antibodies can specifically inhibit the activity of biologically active molecules. In addition to passive immunotherapy of infectious diseases caused by toxins, such as tetanus and diphtheria, passive antibodies have been effective in treating humans for neutralization of snake venom and overdoses of drugs, such as cardiac glycoside poisoning (digitalis). The Fab fragment of IgG is often used because it diffuses more readily into tissue fluids than whole antibody or F(ab′)2 fragments, and Fab fragments joined to small molecules are readily excreted by glomerular filtration in the kidney. Using specific

Fab fragments, digitalis toxicity can be reversed within 30 minutes of administration.

NONSPECIFIC IMMUNO-SUPPRESSION

A variety of procedures, physical agents, or drugs have been used to suppress immune reactivity. The objective is to interfere with either the induction or expression of an immune response. The mechanisms include physical removal of serum or certain cell populations, killing of cells, interference with metabolism of reactive cells, blocking of cell surface receptors, or altering the tissue distribution of reactive cells. In addition, depending on the immune mechanism involved, blocking of effector mechanisms may be achieved by drugs that lower complement, interfere with mediators, depress mast cell sensitivity, block end organ responses to anaphylactic mediators (atopic reactions), or interfere with accessory cell (polymorphonuclear, macrophage) activity.

The mechanism of action of immunosuppressive agents is extremely varied (Table 28–5). These agents may affect the specific induction of both humoral and cellular immune responses (primary response), humoral antibody formation only, cellular immunity only, the expression of a given effector mechanism, or produce nonspecific depression of accessory cells involved in inflammation. They may cause the establishment of specific tolerance or the failure of expression of a primary response to a given antigen, even though memory is induced so that a secondary response occurs upon reexposure to the same antigen. The enhancement of an immune response following the administration of an "immunosuppressive" drug is believed to be caused by decreasing the number of suppressor cells so that when antigen is given, a greater than normal immune response may be observed. All these agents have systemic effects on cells other than those of the lymphoid system that seriously limit their usefulness. In high doses, most cause derangements of any tissue that is metabolically active (eg, depression of the bone marrow with subsequent loss of peripheral blood cell elements or denudation of the lining epithelium of the gastrointestinal tract).

The effect of various drugs on the immune response is best considered in relation to the stage of interference in the response (see Fig. 28–1). Immunosuppressive therapy has become of paramount importance in preventing homograft rejection, especially in regard to organ transplantation, and experimental results indicate that such agents may be effective in prevention of suppression of various autoimmune reactions, but the incidence and severity of opportunistic infections and neoplasms are substantially increased.

Clinically, various combinations of irradiation, steroids (prednisone), antimetabolites (azathioprine), alkylating agents (cyclophosphamide), cyclosporine, FK506, and antilymphocyte serum have been

TABLE 28–5. STAGES OF IMMUNE RESPONSE AND EFFECT OF IMMUNE-MODULATING AGENTS

Agent	Example	Mechanism of Action	(1) Antigen Processing	(2) Cell Interaction	(3) Suppressor/ Helper Function	(4) Proliferation	(5) Differentiation	(6) Protein Synthesis	(7) Accessory or Effector System
Irradiation	Whole body, total lymphoid, extracorporeal	Blocks proliferation, lymphocytolytic	Decreases number of macrophages	Loss of cells	Helper > suppressor	+++ T > B	May block B cell isotype switch	Indirect	Decreases T-cytotoxic cells, macrophages
Steroids	Hydrocortisone, prednisone, etc.	Alter mRNA and protein synthesis	Decrease antigen processing and binding by macrophages	Sequestration of lymphocytes	Suppressor > helper	++ T > B	May block B cell isotype switch	Decrease IL-2 and lymphokine production	Vasoconstriction, inhibits inflammatory response and PMN margination
Alkylating agents	Cyclophosphamide, nitrogen mustard, busulfan, cisplatin	React chemically with nucleophilic portions of DNA, RNA and proteins	Decrease phagocytosis, number of macrophages	Loss of cells in tissue	Suppressor ≫ helper (especially for DTH)	B > T	Block T_H and B cell differentiation	Decrease lymphokine production	Decrease NK activity, phagocytosis
ANTIMETABOLITES									
Purine analogues	Azathioprine, 6-mercaptopurine	Incorporated into DNA and RNA							
Pyrimidine analogues	5-Fluorouracil, cytosine arabinoside	Inhibit DNA and RNA synthesizing enzymes							
Folic acid antagonists	Methotrexate, aminopterin	Bind to dihydrofolate reductase, inhibit DNA synthesis	Decrease number of macrophages	Loss of cells secondary to inhibition of proliferation	Suppressor ≫ helper	+++ T > B	Block B cell differentiation, helper cells may be resistant	Indirect	Decrease numbers of inflammatory cells
Methyl-hydrazines	Procarbazine	Formation of hydroxyl radicals, radiomimetic							
Hydroxyureas	Hydroxyureas	Kills DNA synthesizing cells							

Alkaloids	Vinblastine, vincristine	Block mitotic spindle	Decrease binding by macrophages	Decrease lymphocyte-macrophage interaction	Suppressor > helper	+++ T > B	Synchronize cells, can make tolerant	Inhibit protein synthesis	Block lysis of target cells by T-cytotoxic cells
Inhibitors of protein synthesis	Antibiotics, actinomycin D, puromycin	Inhibit DNA dependent RNA polymerase, DNA binding etc.	Decrease phagocytosis and processing by macrophages		Helper > suppressor	++ B > T	Block B cell differentiation	Block antibody and lymphokine production	Decrease complement synthesis, decrease phagocytosis
T-cell blockers	Cyclosporine, FK506	Block cell activation, IL-2 receptors	?	Lymphocyte depletion in tissues	Helper ≫ suppressor	++++ T ≫ B	Block T cell effector	Decrease IL production	Decrease leukotrienes and prostaglandins
Nonsteroidal antiinflammatory agents	Indomethacin, aspirin	Inhibit prostaglandin synthesis	0	0	Block prostaglandin E inhibition of suppressor cells	Block prostaglandin inhibition of proliferation	0	Decrease IL production	Decrease DTH, NK, decrease inflammation, decrease collagenase release from macrophages
Interferon	α, β, γ	Acts on cell surface, stimulates proliferation and differentiation	Increases phagocytosis, increases binding to macrophages	Increases interactions	Increases helper activity	Increases at low doses, decreases at high doses	Increases differentiation of B cells, T effector cells	Increases antibody and lymphokine production	Synergizes with lymphokines, increases NK activity
Antilymphocyte serum	Heterologous ALG, monoclonal antibodies	Lymphocytotoxicity	"Blindfolding" of receptors	Lymphocyte depletion	May be made specific	Indirect	Decreases production of factors	0	Blocks effector cell recognition of target
Adjuvants	Mycobacterial cell walls, muramyl dipeptides, BCG	Increase numbers and metabolic activity of macrophages at site of infection	Increase antigen processing	Increase lymphocyte-macrophage interactions	Increase helper cells	Increase polyclonal B cells	Increase production of factors, IL-1	Stimulate macrophage protein synthesis	Macrophage activation

IL, interleukin; NK, natural killer; DTH, delayed-type hypersensitivity; PMN polymorphonuclear leukocytes; BCG, bacillus Calmette–Guérin; ALG, antilymphocyte globulin.

used effectively to prevent graft rejection, modify graft-versus-host disease and control autoimmune diseases. The most widely used immunosuppressive regimen for graft recipients, prednisone and aza-thioprine, was replaced with cyclosporine, and now a new drug—FK506—is under active investigation. In selected instances, total lymphoid irradiation and antilymphocyte globulin are also used. The effect of cyclophosphamide is difficult to control, and it must be used carefully and selectively. Antilymphocyte globulin (ALG) may allow reduction in dose or use of other drugs, but the clinical effectiveness of ALG has been disappointing.

Prolonged immunosuppression has two major complications—increased susceptibility to infections and increased risk of cancer. Infection with a variety of opportunistic organisms is seen in graft recipients, particularly bacterial and *Candida* infections immediately after suppression because of a loss of granulocytes; viral infections—especially cytomegalovirus—from one to three months of treatment; and *Pneumocystis carinii* and herpes zoster after three months. Increased risk of cancer may be caused by loss of immune surveillance or to loss of control of the immune system due to alterations in suppressor and inducer activity. Increases in B-cell malignancies in immunosuppressed patients may result from a loss of suppressor activity combined with increased antigenic stimulation provided by an organ graft or opportunistic infection, leading to polyclonal B-cell activation. In a number of instances, polyclonal B-cell tumors containing Epstein–Barr virus have been seen.

Depletion

Plasmapheresis. Therapeutic plasmapheresis is the process whereby plasma, containing antibodies, immune complexes, hormones, drugs, or other substances soluble in plasma, are removed from the circulation and replaced by a harmless substance. In immune-mediated diseases, this process can be used to remove circulating antibodies or antibody–antigen complexes. Plasmapheresis has been used to supplement treatment of antibody or immune complex-mediated diseases, such as systemic lupus erythematosus, antiglomerular basement membrane (anti-GBM) glomerulonephritis, factor VIII deficiency, myasthenia gravis, and pemphigus. In general, plasmapheresis is successful if the process of autoantibody or immune complex formation is self-limited, as is the case of anti-GBM glomerulonephritis. In the other diseases, removal of antibody usually produces an immediate beneficial effect. However, the short-term effects of plasmapheresis may be followed by a rebound of increased antibody formation and more severe disease manifestations. Thus, plasmapheresis may be used to control acute life-threatening situations, such as respirator-dependent myasthenia gravis, but to be effective in the long term, it must be followed by the use of immunosuppressive drugs to establish a sustained remission of disease.

Lymphocyte Depletion. Extirpation of specific lymphoid organs or removal of cells may lead to loss of immune responsiveness. Neonatal thymectomy of most mammals produces a loss of responsiveness of the T-cell system, whereas bursectomy of chickens produces a loss of B-cell function. Removal of circulating lymphocytes by chronic thoracic duct drainage has also resulted in depression of T-cell functions, mainly by removal of long-lived T cells. In animals, this technique has been used to prolong allograft survival. These procedures are not readily applicable to modulation of immune responses in humans.

Irradiation

The effects of irradiation have been studied extensively in animals. Large doses of radiation (900 to 1200 rads) destroy the host's capacity to muster an immune response by destroying both unstimulated immunologically competent cells and memory cells, so that both the primary and the secondary responses may be lost. Smaller doses (300 to 500 rads) affect primary immune responses more than secondary responses. If induction of the antibody response is carried out at a suitable time prior to sublethal irradiation, primary antibody production may actually be greatly enhanced, presumably because of the disproportionate proliferation of antigen-induced proliferating cells; depletion of other nonsensitized cells permits more living space for sensitized cells to expand into. On the other hand, low to moderate doses of irradiation affect helper activity much more than suppressor activity, so that increased T-suppressor function may result in a tolerance-like state.

The proliferative phase of the immune response is most sensitive to radiation, so that suppression by radiation will be most effective if given when antigen-induced proliferation is occurring. Both T cells and B cells are susceptible to irradiation, but phagocytic capacity is relatively radioresistant. The precursors of the effector population, such as unstimulated T or B cells, are radiosensitive, whereas effector cells are resistant. For instance, T-cell help for a primary response is extremely radiosensitive, but T-cell help of primed animals (secondary T-cell help) is radioresistant. Thus, primary responding immunocompetent cells are radiosensitive but memory cells are relatively resistant.

Although whole body irradiation has been used in the past on human transplant recipients to suppress rejection reactions, whole body irradiation is no longer given because of the many harmful effects on other cell systems. Therapy involving extracorporal irradiation of the blood is difficult to manage, the procedure is expensive and only circulating lymphocytes are exposed. Whole body irradiation has been modified to "total lymphoid irradiation" (TLI) with application to prolonging allograft survival by induction of specific tolerance. In addition, clinical trials of TLI for control of autoimmune diseases are now underway. TLI delivers high doses of radiation to lymphoid tissues while protecting radiosensitive nonlymphoid tissues. Lead shielding sharply limits the radiation to lymph nodes, thymus, and spleen, while protecting kidneys, lungs, brain, bone marrow, gastrointestinal tract, etc. This procedure was developed in the 1960s by Henry Kaplan of Stanford for the treatment of Hodgkin's disease and other lymphomas. Patients who are treated with TLI have immune suppression as effective as those treated by steroids, cytotoxic drugs, and antilymphocyte serum, with a much lower incidence of bacterial or viral infections. This is most likely due to the protection of the stem cell population in the bone marrow. In addition, there appears to be the selective generation of suppressor cells following TLI so that exposure to antigen following TLI can result in specific tolerance-like conditions, particularly in generation of cytotoxic T cells. Thus, TLI theoretically has great potential, perhaps in combination with other forms of therapy, to control graft rejection or autoimmune disease, by favoring specific control of immune reactions by T-suppressor cells.

Ultraviolet light irradiation, in experimental systems, produces depressed delayed hypersensitivity responses by two mechanisms—loss of antigen-presenting cells (class II MHC+ macrophages) and induction of specific T-suppressor cells. Clinical applications of this phenomenon have not yet been identified.

Drugs

A large number of drugs are used to modify the immune response and its effector mechanisms.

Steroids. Corticosteroids produce multiple effects in animals, and it is difficult to determine which effect may be most important for a given therapeutic result. Corticosteroids act through cytoplasmic receptors that are present in essentially all nucleated mammalian cells. Steroids are derivatives of cholesterol, are fat soluble, and pass freely through the cell membrane, combine with cytosol receptors, are transported to the nucleus. The receptor-hormone complex blocks activation of immune cells by interferating directly with activation by NF-κB or by stimulating IκBα production. IκBα directly binds and inactivates NF-κB. There two actions block activation of immune cells by NF-κB and effectively inhibit an immune response.

The major action of steroids is as an antiinflammatory agent. Careful studies indicate that steroids have little effect on the specific induction of immune responses at the central level except at very high doses. Three other major effects of steroids may be considered: leukocyte circulation, leukocyte function, and vasoconstriction. Steroids may alter the effector stage of the immune response by affecting the tissue distribution of lymphocytes and macrophages or decreasing the phagocyte capacity of macrophages. Steroids also inhibit production of interleukins (IL-1 and IL-2) and block chemotaxis of inflammatory cells. Steroids are potent vasoconstrictors and limit access of inflammatory cells to sites of inflammation in tissues. In asthma, steroids may also act as a β-agonist potentiator, contributing to bronchodilation and inhibiting the migration of eosinophils. Steroids also inhibit synthesis of prostaglandins and reduce late stages of chronic inflammation. Steroids appear to inhibit phospholipid lipase, resulting in decreased formation of arachidonic acid. Thus, beneficial effects of steroids in many immune diseases is a modulation of inflammation rather than effecting specific immunity. Man is more resistant than some experimental animals (mice, rats, and rabbits) to the effects of steroids so that close extrapolation of experimental results in these species to man is not possible. Steroids are widely used to control severe immunopathologic processes, particularly autoimmune diseases, graft rejection, and asthma, but considerable caution is needed because of the dangerous side effects. See chapter 22.

Alkylating Agents. These drugs are called radiomimetic because the effect of their administration resembles the effect of irradiation. They are generally chemically active agents that combine with DNA and interfere with cell proliferation. Included are nitrogen mustard, cyclophosphamide, tetramine, busulfan, cisplatinum, and mustard gas. The action of these drugs is only temporary, and immune reactions return when therapy is discontinued. The effects on DNA may be the most important. Alkylation of DNA of resting lymphocytes may have little or no effect until the cells are stimulated to proliferate. Lymphoid cells have the capacity to repair the lesions produced so that if the drug is given long before antigen exposure, cellular proliferation following antigen exposure will proceed normally. However, if given at the time of antigen-induced proliferation, alkylating agents can greatly reduce, and may even eliminate, the responding cells leading to tolerance by clonal elimination. High doses of alkylating agents generally suppress secondary B-cell responses more than secondary T-cell responses because of the higher metabolic activity of antibody-producing cells.

Cyclophosphamide. Cyclophosphamide is the alkylating agent most widely used. In addition to affecting DNA synthesis, cyclophosphamide and other alkylating agents can inhibit glycolysis, respiration,

RNA synthesis, protein synthesis, and a variety of enzyme functions. Cyclophosphamide appears to act principally on B cells directly and on precursors of suppressor T cells, which are more sensitive than B cells. The effect on a primary antibody response is much greater than on a secondary response. At moderate doses, cyclophosphamide may inhibit antibody responses by action on B cells. At low doses, enhancement of antibody production by action on suppressor T cells or on suppressor macrophages is observed. Augmentation of delayed hypersensitivity reactions may also be obtained. After high doses, during the recovery phase, suppressor cell activity may be increased.

The effect of cyclophosphamide in humans is obviously dose-dependent and has been difficult to evaluate. High doses result in lymphopenia and inhibition of B-cell responses that is greater than inhibition of T-cell responses. In general, established delayed hypersensitivity is resistant. Suppressor cells for delayed hypersensitivity appear to be sensitive at lower doses of cyclophosphamide than are T-helper cells for antibody production by B cells. This may explain the finding that cyclophosphamide given before antigen will enhance delayed hypersensitivity but will suppress antibody production if higher doses are given.

Antimetabolites. Antimetabolites interfere with the synthesis of RNA, DNA, or protein and prevent cell division and proliferation.

Purine Analogs. The mechanism of action of these drugs is multiple. Azathioprine inhibits RNA and DNA synthesis but also interferes with enzyme and coenzyme activity, purine conversions, and incorporation of purine into amino acids. Very large doses may not only depress bone marrow function severely but also antibody production, cellular immunity, and even secondary responses. At lower doses, the secondary response is not affected. The effects of 6-mercaptopurine or azathioprine, which is metabolized to 6-mercaptopurine, on antibody formation are determined by the timing of the drug administration with respect to antigenic stimulus, the dose of the drug, the dose of the antigen, and the nature of the antigenic challenge. By varying these parameters in experimental animals, one may obtain suppression of all classes of antibody, selective suppression of IgG antibody, enhancement of IgM synthesis, or enhancement of both IgM and IgG antibody.

The suppressive effects of azathioprine are most impressive if given 24 hours after antigen injection because of its antiproliferative effect or action on early events in the immune response. T cells appear to be the principal cells affected, because alkylating agents are particularly effective in inhibition of T rosette formation, mixed lymphocyte reactions, graft rejections, and delayed hypersensitivity reactions, including experimental autoimmune diseases, whereas specific antibody responses are relatively spared.

Pyrimidine Analogs. These agents interfere with RNA and DNA synthesis, and, experimentally, doses can be given that suppress humoral immunity while sparing T-cell reactions, such as skin graft rejection or contact sensitivity. Pyrimidine analogs are used extensively in cancer chemotherapy and may contribute significantly to the decreased resistance to bacterial infections observed in such patients.

Folic Acid Antagonists. Folic acid antagonists prevent the conversion of dihydrofolic acid to tetrahydrofolic acid by binding to the enzyme dihydrofolate reductase. This in turn blocks methylation of deoxyribonucleic acid and thymidylic acid (required for DNA synthesis) and interferes with transport of carbon fragments for purine and protein synthesis. In appropriate doses, these agents can partially suppress immune reactions without causing bone marrow suppression, but this side effect has limited the clinical usefulness of folic acid antagonists in controlling immune response. In addition, methotrexate is excreted by the kidney so that toxic levels may be achieved at low doses if given to patients with impairment of renal function, such as renal transplant recipients.

Other Antimetabolites. Other antimetabolites may affect immune responses in a variety of ways (see Table 28–4). Actinomycins inhibit RNA synthesis by combining specifically with the guanine base of the DNA molecule without markedly inhibiting DNA synthesis. This results in a reduction in RNA synthesis at the time of the primary injection of antigen. Agents that inhibit protein synthesis without preventing RNA synthesis (puromycin, streptomycin, erythromycin, chloramphenicol) have very little inhibitory effect on primary immunization unless large doses are given. With doses of chloramphenicol large enough to block protein synthesis and depress antibody formation during the primary response, the development of an anamnestic response on reexposure is not affected, indicating interference not in induction but at a later stage in antibody production. Aminoacridines intercalate between both RNA and DNA. Administration of acriflavine greatly suppresses the primary responses. No apparent interference with cell replication is observed. Dimeric alkaloids (vinblastine, vincristine) completely inhibit antibody formation and cellular reactivity when given at the same time as antigen. They also appear to inhibit proliferation of lymphoid cells. In addition, vincristine has a nonspecific antiinflammatory effect. The mechanism of action of these drugs is not well understood, although interference with gene expression is most likely.

Antibiotics. Antibiotics may cause an increase in incidence and severity of clinical infections with unusual organisms (*Candida albicans, Aspergillus*). The mechanisms by which antibiotics operate to decrease resistance to these organisms include overgrowth of organisms not susceptible to the given antibiotic because of a decrease or absence of competing susceptible organisms, inhibition of immune responses, and inhibition of phagocytosis. In large doses, the tetracyclines may have a marked effect on all types of immune reactivity.

T-cell Blockers. The primary mechanism of action of two relatively new microbial products that have had a major impact on clinical transplantation, cyclosporine and FK506, is through inhibition of T-cell activation. Although chemically different, both cyclosporine and FK506 belong to a growing class of macrocyclic immunosuppressants that affect a similar subset of calcium-associated signaling events involved in T-cell activation.

Cyclosporine (Cyclosporin A). The immunosuppressive effects of cyclosporine, a metabolite of a soil fungus, *Trichoderma polysporum Rifai* (now called *Tolycopaladium inflatum*) were first noted in 1972 as inhibition of antibody (hemagglutinin) formation following treatment of mice in vivo during immunization with sheep erythrocytes. The active compound is a cyclic polypeptide containing eleven amino acids. Cyclosporine works by binding to the cytoplasmic cyclophilin proteins and interfering with the T-cell signal-transduction cascade. Upon binding with cyclophilin, pentameric "supermolecules" are formed that associate in pairs to form a "decameric sandwich." The significance of this remarkable structure in immunosuppression is not clear, but it does result in an inhibition of the isomerase activity of cyclophilin. Cyclosporine preferentially blocks T-cell activation by mitogens and by antigens by inhibiting CA++ fluxes required for activation. There is decreased production of mRNA for early activation products, such as IL-2, IFN-γ, and c-*myc*. Cyclosporine also inhibits mixed lymphocyte reactions (proliferation) and generation of cytotoxic cells, but not the effector function of primed killer cells. NK, ADCC, nonspecific accessory cell function, neutrophil function, and wound healing are not affected, so that the immunosuppressive effect is primarily directed to T-cell activation, and the effect is reversible in most, but not all, systems. Cyclosporine is also able to block B-cell activation, but T cells are more sensitive. Cyclosporine enhances the specific peripheral elimination of reactive T cells following administrative of superantigens in animals, but, paradoxically, it abrogates the development of the specific anergy that usually occurs after superantigen injection. The success of cyclosporine in experimental organ transplantation shows that it is effective in prolonging allograft survival with a minimal number of side effects of infectious complications.

Clinical trials using cyclosporine to control allograft rejection have been highly successful. In 1981, the preliminary results of two groups suggested a marked improvement in one-year survival rate of cadaveric donor kidneys. Subsequently, a number of studies have supported these preliminary conclusions. Cyclosporine has also been effective in reducing graft-versus-host disease, as well as increasing takes and reducing infections in human bone marrow transplant recipients. In addition, cyclosporine has made orthotopic liver allografting a feasible procedure in humans, and it is also being used for pancreas and heart transplantation. Cyclosporine appears to interfere less with nonlymphoid cell function, particularly other hematopoietic bone marrow cells, and permit reduction in dose of other agents (such as steroids). This results in more specific immune control with fewer infections. Since most grafted patients actually die from infection rather than graft rejection, the ability to produce more limited immune suppression, allowing fewer infections, appears to be critical. Interestingly, systemic cyclosporine treatment is effective in reducing the lesions of severe psoriasis, but local administration is ineffective.

In human transplant recipients the major side effect of cyclosporine is nephrotoxicity. In renal transplant patients, the differentiation between an allograft rejection reaction and cyclosporine toxicity has been difficult and is controversial. Both are associated with glomerulitis and a diffuse cellular infiltrate. The fact that nephrotoxicity occurs in patients receiving cyclosporine for bone marrow or liver transplantation demonstrates that toxicity exists separate from renal graft rejection. In long-term renal transplant recipients there is no evidence of progressive loss of renal function due to cyclosporine toxicity.

FK506. FK506 is a macrolide isolated from fermentation broth of *Streptomycetes tsukubaensis* that acts in a manner similar to cyclosporine but appears to be up to 100 times more effective than cyclosporine in preventing graft rejection, with no increase in toxicity. A macrolide is a class of antibacterial antibiotics with a macrolide ring, ie, a large lactone ring containing multiple keto and hydroxyl groups, linked glycosidically to one or more sugars. These antibiotics are produced by *Streptomyces* species. FK506 binds to a family of cytoplasmic proteins, known as FKBPs (FK binding proteins or immunophilins). FKBPs have an isomerase activity similar to cyclophilin, and binding to FK506 inhibits the activity. FK506 has a marked inhibitory effect on lymphocyte activation, blocks Ca^{++} fluxes, selectively inhibits the expression of early T-cell activation genes (IL-2, IL-3, IL-4, INF-γ, TNF-α GM-CSF and C-*myc*), and increases the proportion of peripheral lymphocytes with the CD8+ (suppressor) phenotype. Although FK506 may produce vasculitis and diabetes in experimental animals, at doses used for effective prevention of graft rejection in humans, little, if any, acute toxic effects have been reported. In ongoing clinical transplantation use, FK506 is considered by some as the new "wonder drug," that will replace cyclosporine.

Rapamycin. Rapamycin is structurally related to FK506 and functions similarly in binding to and inhibiting isomerase activities of FKBPs. However, it is more effective than FK506 in inhibiting proliferation of T and B cells but less effective in inhibiting lymphokine secretion. Although both drugs bind to the same intracellular receptor (immunophilin), each of the drug–immunophilin complexes apparently interacts differently with other molecules to form functionally different complexes that ultimately mediate the specific suppressive effects peculiar to each drug. In general, both are effective in inhibiting Ca++ dependent T- and B-cell division, but rapamycin also inhibits Ca++ independent T- and B-cell division and proliferation, such as that induced by IL-2, IL-4, and IL-1. On the other hand, FK506 inhibits the nuclear factor of activated T cells (NF-AT) and the expression of the IL-2R after activation, whereas rapamycin inhibits neither. In experimental animals, rapamycin is more effective than FK506 in increasing tissue graft survival and suppressing graft-versus-host disease. Since only a small amount of drug–immunophilin complex is required for suppression, the excess immunophilin in each cell could allow the binding of low concentrations of both rapamycin and FK506. The combined use of low doses of both drugs has been shown to be highly effective in preventing graft rejection in some animal systems. Clinical trials of combination therapy are now underway.

Nonsteroidal Antiinflammatory Agents. Nonsteroidal antiinflammatory drugs (NSAIDs) act to suppress inflammation mediated by prostaglandins and leukotrienes (eicosanoids) (see Chapter 8). These drugs affect signal transduction proteins (G proteins) of inflammatory cells. Aspirin and related drugs are able to insinuate themselves into cell membranes and disrupt the response to extracellular signals. This action is very effective in blocking the ability of neutrophils to adhere to vascular endothelium. Another effect of nonsteroidal antiinflammatory drugs on immune responses is through inhibition of cyclo-oxygenase and decreased prostaglandin E production from arachidonic acid. Prostaglandin E acts as an inhibitor of cellular immune responses, so that depressed delayed hypersensitivity reactions can be restored by administration of cyclo-oxygenase inhibitors. Indomethacin increases cell-mediated immune responses in patients with decreased activity, sometimes restoring delayed hypersensitivity in anergic patients. Suppressor T cells have a high density of prostaglandin E receptors. Cyclo-oxygenase inhibitors depress immunoglobulin synthesis, presumably by reversal of prostaglandin E inhibition of suppressor cells.

Endogenous prostaglandin E_2 (PGE_2) can induce or increase autoantibody production through inhibition of suppressor cell activity. Cyclo-oxygenase inhibitors may act to decrease autoantibody production in patients with diseases such as rheumatoid arthritis by releasing prostaglandin E-induced inhibition of suppressor cells, thus damping antibody-producing B cells.

Antileukocyte Sera

Antileukocyte serum is an antiserum that contains antibody activity directed against white cells. The most widely used is antilymphocyte serum (ALS). Antileukocyte globulin is a purified fraction of antileukocyte serum containing the antibody-active immunoglobulin portion of the antiserum. Xenogeneic (heterologous) antileukocyte serum is produced by immunizing an animal of one species (rabbit) with white cells obtained from another species (thymus or spleen of mouse). With proper selection of the cell source and care in preparation, an antiserum can be obtained that reacts specifically with a white cell fraction (ie, lymphocytes) from the donor animal. The reactivity of this antiserum may be demonstrated in vitro by its ability to agglutinate the target white cells and to lyse the white cells in the presence of complement (cytotoxicity).

Antilymphocyte Serum. The effect of antilymphocyte serum on in vivo immune reactions is best understood by consideration of the role of the lymphocyte in different stages of the immune response. Antilymphocyte serum blocks cellular reactions, presumably by cytotoxic destruction of the lymphocytes (sensitized cells). This effect appears to be specific, as other tissues are not affected. Antilymphocyte serum may also prevent a primary response to antigen, presumably by an effect on precursor cells, and if administered in large enough doses, may even suppress or eliminate a second-set graft rejection or secondary antibody responses (loss of immune memory). The serum does not reduce reactions mediated by humoral antibody in animals that are already immunized (Arthus reaction) or nonimmune inflammatory reactions that are induced by cotton wool or turpentine. Antilymphocyte sera specific for different functional lymphocyte populations have been developed. Antisera to T cells generally kill T cells and inhibit T-cell functions in vitro and in vivo, whereas antisera to B cells may prevent maturation of antibody-forming cell precursors and thus inhibit antibody formation. Such antisera have been used to further define the role of different lymphoid cell populations in immune reactions.

The possible mechanisms of immunosuppression by antilymphocyte serum include direct destruction of lymphocytes (lymphocytotoxicity), resulting in lymphopenia; opsonization of lymphocytes with clearance of affected cells by the reticuloendothelial system; coating of lymphocytes with antibody so that the lymphocytes can no longer react with antigen (blindfolding); stimulation of proliferation of lymphocytes that do not have the ability to react with antigen (sterile activation); specific cytotoxic effect upon one class of lymphocytes (long-lived) with the ability to recognize antigen, with little or no effect on nonspecific short-lived lymphocytes (selective lymphocytotoxicity); inactivation of a thymic factor responsible for development of immunologically competent cells (thymus effect); direction of immunologically reactive cells toward producing an immune response to the injected serum and away from a response to other antigens (antigenic competition); or coating of the target organ (skin graft) with antibodies so that the antigens of the target organ are not recognized by the recipient (target organ coating). None of the above satisfactorily explains all the immunosuppressive effects of antilymphocyte serum. In spite of the voluminous experimental data indicating that this material may profoundly affect the immune responses of experimental animals, a statistically significant effect of antisera to human lymphocytes upon allograft survival in human recipients has been difficult to demonstrate. However, recent results indicate a prolongation of skin and kidney graft survival in some recipients treated with antilymphocytic globulin, and a higher success rate of bone marrow grafts in patients treated prior to transplantation. In these patients, antilymphocytic globulin eliminates immunocompetent cells and reduces graft-versus-host reactions.

Antipolymorphonuclear Leukocyte Serum. This serum has also been applied to experimental situations. Antineutrophil sera will reduce non-immune neutrophil-mediated inflammation induced by urate crystals, as well as antibody-induced skin reactions and glomerulonephritis. Antineutrophil sera will produce a rapid neutropenia through reticuloendothelial clearance, with subsequent reduction of cells available for inflammatory reactions. Anti-eosinophil serum has been used to inhibit passive cutaneous anaphylactic reactions in guinea pigs, suggesting that eosinophils may play a role in some anaphylactic reactions.

Antimacrophage Serum. Experimentally, xenogeneic antisera to macrophages has also been used to inhibit antibody formation, presumably by interfering with antigen processing or phagocytosis. In addition, antimacrophage sera may interfere with the effector arm of delayed hypersensitivity, exemplified by prolongation of skin allograft survival, the passive transfer of delayed hypersensitivity, and a small decrease in adjuvant-induced arthritis. Antimacrophage sera may eliminate macrophages directly by killing or through clearing by the reticuloendothelial system, resulting in a lowering of peripheral mononuclear cells. Application of antimacrophage or antipolymorphonuclear sera to human diseases has not yet been proven feasible.

Monoclonal Antibodies. The problems relating to variability in different preparations of xenogeneic ALG in immunomodulation may be circumvented by monoclonal antibodies. Monoclonal antibodies to helper/inducer T cells have been shown to reduce circulating lymphocytes in clinical trials and prolong graft survival in monkeys. Anti-CD3 (OKT3) is a potent immunosuppressive that is usually used in graft recipients who are no longer adequately controlled by ALG or steroid suppression (see Chapter 23). Recent clinical trials with anti-CDs in treatment of leukemias are discussed in Chapter 24.

Monoclonal antibodies to T cells have been used more successfully in vitro to remove functioning T cells from bone marrow cell populations. The specificities used include CDs 2, 3, 5, 6, 7, 8, and 18. Three methods have been employed to remove cells mediating graft-versus-host reactions: T-lymphocyte depletion by lectin agglutination using soybean agglutinin, by antibody and complement cytotoxicity and by antibody–toxin (ricin) conjugates. Such treatment can reduce serious graft-versus-host reactions in bone marrow recipients receiving allogenic transplants from HLA-mismatched donors from 75% to 30% and in matched donors from 45% to 10%. OKT3 treatment was first thought to have few side effects, but it has been shown to induce "cytokine-release syndrome" or CRS. CRS includes fever, headache, rigors, hypertension, diarrhea, nausea/vomiting, and a number of other symptoms. It is believed to be caused by activation of T cells to produce and release cytokines following reaction of OKT3 with the epsilon chain of the CD3/TCR complex. As discussed in Chapter 23, anti-CD34 is used to isolate stem cells from the peripheral blood after mobilization by growth factors. These stem cells are then used for gene transfer to the autologous donor.

The major limitation to the use of monoclonal antibodies at the present time is the production of antibody by the patient to the monoclonal antibodies, which are mouse immunoglobulins. This results in clearance of the monoclonal antibody and an obliteration of the beneficial effect. Effects are now underway to identify human cell lines, which could be used to generate human–antihuman monoclonal antibodies that would circumvent this problem. (See Chapter 30 for further discussion of application of monoclonal antibodies to cancer therapy.)

Clinical
Application of
Immuno-
suppressive
Agents

In practical terms, seven major immunosuppressive agents are now used clinically; steroids, alkylating agents, purine analogs, folic acid antagonists, cyclosporine, FK506, and antilymphocyte globulin. The effectiveness of these agents in immune-mediated diseases other than transplantation and immune deficiencies is shown in Table 28–6. The effectiveness of cyclosporine in the treatment of autoimmune diseases is unpredictable and that of FK506 not yet known. Immunosuppression is a well-established therapy for graft recipients and certain autoimmune or immune complex-mediated diseases. In many other diseases, immunosuppressive therapy is of questionable merit. Although individual reports may claim a beneficial effect of immunosuppressive drugs, in many situations the efficacy of such treatment has not been critically evaluated. Antimetabolites may be used to decrease the dose of steroids required for maintenance. The "steroid-saving" effect may be of great benefit in some patients. Careful monitoring of the immune reactivity of immunosuppressed patients must be performed to ensure that immune reactivity is not reduced to the point at which opportunistic infections will become manifest. Such infections were common during the first few years of renal transplantations; most transplant recipients did not die from rejection crises but from infections. With careful monitoring of recipients and titration of immunosuppressive drugs, a substantial improvement in survival of renal allograft recipients has taken place.

Immuno-
suppressive
Factors

A number of serum proteins and cellular extracts may nonspecifically suppress immune induction of expression. Although many reports have convincingly demonstrated effects in vitro, it is not clear how significant the effects of these proteins are in vivo. Theoretically, it is possible that some of these factors could be used passively to suppress immune reactivity. As a group, these proteins have been termed immunoregulatory globulins. Included are α_2 globulin (immunoregulatory α-globulin), α_2-macroglobulin, pregnancy-associated α-globulin, α-fetoprotein, very low-density lipoprotein, and C-reactive protein. Immunoregulatory α-globulin has been studied extensively. Among the reactions inhibited are mitogen and antigen proliferation responses, plaque-forming cell responses, delayed hypersensitivity skin reactions, allograft rejections, and immunity to syngeneic tumors. The effect of α_2-macroglobulin (α_2M) on immune reactivity is probably because of the ability of α_2M to inhibit the activity of proteases and inactivate inflammatory mediators, such as kallikrein and plasminogen activator. Pregnancy-associated α-macroglobulin is a serum protein that increases dramatically during pregnancy and decreases just as dramatically after birth. The addition of this protein to lymphocyte cultures in vitro markedly suppresses mitogen-induced T-cell responses. This protein appears to be different from α_2-macroglobulin, but the precise relationship is not clear, because sensi-

TABLE 28–6. CLINICAL USE OF IMMUNOSUPPRESSIVE DRUGS

Disease Treated	Steroids	Alkylating Agent (Cyclophosphamide)	Purine Analog (Azathioprine)	Folic Acid Antagonist (Methotrexate)	ALG[a]
Neutralization					
Hemophilia (anticoagulants)	+[b]	+	−	−	−
Myasthenia gravis	+	−	−	−	−
Cytotoxic					
Autoallergic hemolytic anemia	++	+	−	−	−
Idiopathic thrombocytopenic purpura	++	+	−	−	−
Toxic complex					
Nephrotic syndrome (minimal)	++	+	−	−	−
Chronic glomerulonephritis	+	+	−	−	−
Systemic lupus erythematosus	++	+	+	−	−
Rheumatoid arthritis	++	++	++	++	−
Progressive systemic sclerosis	+	−	−	−	−
Psoriasis	++	−	+	++	−
Pemphigus	++	+	+	+	−
Dermato(poly)myositis	++	+	+	+	−
Anaphylactic					
Asthma, chronic	+	−	−	−	−
Delayed hypersensitivity					
Organ transplantation	++	+	++	+	+
Bone marrow transplantation	−	−	−	−	−
Multiple sclerosis	+	−	−	−	−
Ulcerative colitis	++	+	+	+	
Regional enteritis	++	+	+	−	−
Sjögren's syndrome	+	−	−	−	−
Thyroiditis	−				
Chronic active hepatitis	+	−	−	−	−
Granulomatous					
Wegener's granulomatosis	+	++	+	−	−

[a]ALG, antilymphocyte globulin.

[b]++, effective; +, questionably effective; −, not effective.

Modified from Gerber NL, Steinberg DO: *Drugs* 11:14–112, 1976.

tive assays indicate its presence in many normal sera. Another pregnancy-associated protein, α-fetoprotein, has also been reported to have immunosuppressive properties in vitro although conflicting reports have appeared. The possible role of pregnancy-associated α-macroglobulin and α-fetoprotein in protecting the fetus from maternal immune rejection has attracted considerable attention, but has not yet been demonstrated convincingly. A species of low-density lipoprotein found in human sera suppresses lymphocyte stimulation in vitro and inhibits antibody formation in mice. C-reactive protein is a α_2-glycoprotein in serum, which increases in concentration in humans with various acute febrile illnesses. It is called C-reactive protein because of its ability to precipitate the C polysaccharide of pneumococcal cell walls and polycations (see Chapter 8). Following this reaction, C-reactive protein is able to fix complement via the classical pathway. C-reactive protein selectively binds to the T lymphocytes of humans, inhibits E-rosette formation, and suppresses the proliferation response to allogenic cells (mixed lymphocyte reaction).

In summary, several nonantigen specific immunosuppressive serum factors have been identified and partially characterized. Immunoregulatory α-globulin, α-macroglobulin, low-density lipoprotein inhibitor, and C-reactive protein may help control the extent of an inflammatory process or immune reaction. Pregnancy-associated α-globulin and α-fetoprotein could help block allorejection of the fetus. However convincing evidence for a significant therapeutic role of these proteins has yet to be reported.

Summary

Immunopharmacology is the study of naturally occurring substances and synthetic drugs that modulate immunity. Modulation of the immune response may be antigen-specific or -nonspecific. The immune response may be affected at different stages of the immune response—afferent, central, efferent, or accessory mechanisms. Stimulation of an active specific immune response may be directed by antigen selection and enhanced by a variety of adjuvants. Specific passive immunization may be accomplished by transfer of humoral antibody or specifically sensitized lymphocytes. Specific active and passive immunization have been effective in protection of normal individuals against many infectious diseases (Chapter 26). Macrophage activation, lymphokines, and interleukins can nonspecifically increase the immune response either at the level of induction or expression.

Suppression of immune responses may also be specific or nonspecific. Specific mechanisms involve tolerance, hyposensitization, or desensitization using specific antigen. Nonspecific suppression may be accomplished with a number of agents, including irradiation, steroids, alkylating agents, antimetabolic drugs, cyclosporine, FK506, antilymphocyte globulin, or monoclonal antibodies. Clinically, immune stimulation of responses is desired in patients with immune deficiency diseases or cancer. In immunodeficiency, when a specific defect can be replaced, such as immunoglobulin antibody in patients with humoral immune deficiencies or thymic grafts in patients with thymus deficiencies, specific passive immunity is effective (Chapter 27). Clinical trials for immune modifiers in cancer have been less rewarding (Chapter 30). Immune suppression is necessary for success of allografts and may be useful in control of certain autoimmune diseases.

Specific immune suppression involving antibody feedback has been spectacularly successful in preventing erythroblastosis fetalis (Chapter 12), and antigen injection therapy is often helpful in decreasing allergic symptoms in hay fever (Chapter 14). A combination of irradiation, steroids, antimetabolic agents, cyclosporine (or FK506), and antilymphocyte globulin are used to control graft rejections but frequently result in complicating opportunistic infections. Monoclonal antibodies may provide more precise and effective modulation of immune responses. Although many beneficial effects have resulted from clinical application of immune modification, many other approaches to immunotherapy, particularly in cancer treatment, have been only partially successful.

Bibliography

SPECIFIC ACTIVE IMMUNIZATION

Alving CR: Immunologic aspects of liposomes: Presentation and processing of liposomal protein and phospholipid antigens. *Biochem Biophys Acta* 1113:307–322, 1992.

Chambers DA, Cohen RL, Perlman RL: Neuroimmune modulation: Signal transduction and catecholamines. *Neurochem Int* 22:95–110, 1993.

Claassen E, deLeeuw W, deGreeve P, et al.: Freund's complete adjuvant: An effective but disagreeable formula. *Forum Immunol* 44:478–483, 1993.

Cornette JL, Margalit H, DeLisi C, et al.: Identification of T-cell epitopes and use in construction of synthetic vaccines. *Meth Enzymology* 178:611, 1989.

Freund J: The mode of action of immunological adjuvants. *Adv Tuber Res* 7:130, 1956.

Hamaoka T, Katz D: Mechanism of adjuvant activity of poly A:U on antibody responses to hapten–carrier conjugates. *Cell Immunol* 7:246, 1973.

Kersten GFA, Spiekstra A, Beuvery EC, et al.: On the structure of immune-stimulating saponin–lipid complexes (ISCOMS). *Biochem Biophys Acta* 1062:165, 1991.

Margalit H, Spouge JL, Cornette JL, et al.: Prediction of immunodominant helper T-cell antigenic sites from the primary sequence. *J Immunol* 138:2213, 1987.

Morein B, Sundquist B, Hoglund S, et al.: ISCOM, a novel structure for antigenic presentation on membrane proteins from enveloped viruses. *Nature* 308:457, 1984.

Munoz J: Effect of bacteria and bacterial products on antibody responses. *Adv Immunol* 4:397, 1964.

Persson U, Moller E: The effect of lipopolysaccharide on the primary immune response to the hapten NHP. *Scand J Immunol* 4:571, 1975.

Reed CE, Benner M, Lockey SD, et al.: On the mechanism of the adjuvant effect of *Bordetella pertussis* vaccine. *J Allergy Clin Immunol* 49:1741, 1972.

Skidmore BJ, Chiller JM, Morrison DC, et al.: Immunologic properties of bacterial lipopolysaccharide (LPS): Correlation between the mitogenic, adjuvant, and immunologic activities. *J Immunol* 114:770, 1975.

Symoens J, Rosenthal M: Levamisole in the modulation of the immune response: The current experimental and clinical state. *J Reticuloendothel Soc* 21:175, 1977.

Warren HS, Vogel FR, Chedid LA: Current states of immunologic adjuvants. *Am Rev Immunol* 4:369, 1986.

White RG: The adjuvant effect of microbial products on the immune response. *Annu Rev Microbiol* 30:579, 1976.

VACCINIA VECTORS

Mackett M, Smith GL: Vaccinia virus expression vectors. *J Gen Virol* 67:2067, 1986.

Moss B: Vaccinia virus: A tool for research and vaccine development. *Science* 252:1662, 1991.

Moss B, Flexner C: Vaccinia virus expression vectors. *Ann Rev Immunol* 5:305, 1987.

BCG VECTORS

Bloom BR: New approaches to vaccine development. *Rev Infect Dis* 11(suppl. 2):2460–2466, 1989.

Calmette A: *La Vaccination Preventive Contre la Tuberculose par BCG.* Paris, Masson, 1927.

Collins FM: Antituberculous immunity: New solutions to an old problem. *Rev Infect Dis* 13:940–950, 1991.

Stover CK, de la Cruze VF, Fuerst TR, et al.: New use of BCG for recombinant vaccines. *Nature* 351:456, 1991.

NONSPECIFIC IMMUNE STIMULATION

Bast RC Jr, Zbar B, Borsos T, et al.: Medical progress: BCG and cancer. *N Engl J Med* 29:1413, 1458, 1974.

Chirigos MA: Immunomodulators: Current and future development and application. *Thymus* 19:(suppl. 1):S7, 1992.

Christie GH, Bomford B: Mechanisms of macrophage activation by *Corynebacterium parvum.* I. In vitro experiments. II. In vivo experiments. *Cell Immunol* 17:141, 1975.

Dodet B: Cytokines in the clinics. Choose your weapon! *Eur Cytokine Netw* 5:369–377, 1994.

Douglas RM, Moore BW, Miles HB, et al.: Prophylactic efficiency of intranasal α_2 interferon against rhinovirus infections in the family setting. *N Engl J Med* 314:65, 1986.

Durum SK, Schmidt JA, Oppenheim JJ: Interleukin-1: An immunologic perspective. *Am Rev Immunol* 3:363, 1985.

Fahey JL, Sarna G, Gale RP, et al.: Immune interventions in disease. *Ann Int Med* 106:257, 1987.

Lanzavecchia A: Identifying strategies for immune intervention. *Science* 14:937–944, 1993.

Lasic DD: Liposomes. *Am Scientist* 80:20, 1992.

Mackaness GB: The immunological basis of acquired cellular resistance. *J Exp Med* 120:105, 1964.

Murahata RI, Mitchell MS: Modulation of immune response by BCG: A review. *Yale J Biol Med* 49:283, 1976.

Prabhala RH, Garewal HS, Meyskens FL, et al.: Immunomodulation in humans caused by beta-carotene and vitamin A. *Nutrit Res* 10:1473, 1990.

Rosenberg S: Lymphokine-activated killer cells: A new approach to immunotherapy of cancer. *J Natl Cancer Inst* 75:595, 1985.

Smith KA: Interleukin-2. *Ann Rev Immunol* 2:319, 1984.

Talmadge JE, Herberman RB. The preclinical screening laboratory: Evaluation of immunomodulatory and therapeutic properties of biological response modifiers. *Cancer Treat Reports* 70:171, 1986.

Vogels MTE, Van Der Meer JWM: Use of immune modulators in nonspecific therapy of bacterial infections. *Antimicrob Agents Chemother* 36:1, 1992.

SPECIFIC IMMUNO-SUPPRESSION

Ishizaka K: Regulation of IgE synthesis. *Annu Rev Immunol* 2:159, 1984.

Nossal GJV: Cellular mechanisms of immunologic tolerance. *Annu Rev Immunol* 1:33, 1983.

Scherrmann JM, Terrien N, Urtizberea M, et al.: Immunotoxicology: Present status and future trends. *Clin Toxicol* 27:1, 1989.

NONSPECIFIC IMMUNO-SUPPRESSION

Anderson RE, Warner NL: Ionizing radiation and the immune response. *Adv Immunol* 24:215, 1976.

Beard D, Mastrangelo MJ: Elimination of immune suppressor mechanisms in humans by oxazaphosphorines. *Meth Find Exptl Clin Pharmacol* 9:569, 1987.

Belzer FO: Immunosuppressive agents: A personal historic perspective. *Transp Proc* 3(suppl. 3):3, 1988.

Benjamin E, Sulka E: Antikorperbildung nach experimenteller schadigung des hamatopoetischen durch rontgenstrahlen. *Wien Klin Wochenschr* 21:10, 1908.

Bierer BE, Holländer G, Fruman D, et al.: Cyclosporin A and FK506: Molecular mechanisms of immunosuppression and probes for transplantation biology. *Current Opin Immunol* 5:763–773, 1993.

Bierer BE, Jin YJ, Fruman DA, et al.: FK506 and rapamycin: Molecular probes of T-lymphocyte activation. *Transplant Proc* 23:2850, 1991.

Boumpas DT, Chrousos GP, Wilder RL: Glucocorticoid therapy for immune-mediated diseases: Basic and clinical correlates. *Ann Int Med* 119:1198–1208, 1993.

Braun DP, Harris JE: Modulation of the immune response by chemotherapy. *Pharmac Ther* 4:89, 1981.

Claman HN: Antiinflammatory effects of corticosteroids. *Clin Allergy Immunol* 4:317, 1984.

Dyminski JW, Argyris BF: Prolongation of allograft survival with antimacrophage serum. *Transplantation* 8:595, 1969.

Fahey JL, Sarna G, Gale RP, Seeger R: Immune interventions in disease. *Ann Int Med* 106:257, 1987.

Gerber NL, Steinberg AD: Clinical use of immunosuppressive drugs, Parts I and II. *Drugs* 11:14(I)90(II), 1976.

Goodwin JS: Immunologic effects of nonstandard antiinflammatory drugs. *Am J Med* 77:7, 1985.

Hadden JW, Merriam LK: Immunopharmocologic basis of immunotherapy. *Clin Physiol Biochem* 3:111, 1985.

Halloran PF, Madrenas J: The mechanism of action of cyclosporine: A perspective for the 90s. *Clin Biochem* 24:3, 1991.

Hengst JCD, Cempe RA: Immunomodulation by cyclophosphamide. *Clin Immunol Allerg* 4:199, 1984.

Jeyarajah DR, Thistlethwaite JR: General aspects of cytokine-release syndrome: Timing and incidence of symptoms. *Transplant Proc* 25(suppl. 2):16–20, 1993.

Johansson A, Moller E: Evidence that the immunosuppressive effects of FK506 and cyclosporine are identical. *Transplant* 50:1001, 1990.

Jones JF: Plasmapheresis in the treatment of immunological diseases. *Clin Immunol Allergy* 5:13, 1985.

Kripke ML: Immunologic mechanisms in UV radiation carcinogenesis. *Adv Cancer Res* 34:69, 1981.

Lands WEM: Mechanisms of action of antiinflammatory drugs. *Adv Drug Res* 14:147, 1985.

Mevleman J, Katz P: The immunologic effects and use of glucocorticoids. *Med Clin N Amer* 69:805, 1985.

Monaco AP, Campion J-P, Kapnick SJ: Clinical use of antilymphocyte globulin. *Transplant Proc* 9:1007, 1977.

Morris RE: Rapamycin: FK506's fraternal twin or distant cousin. *Immunol Today* 12:137, 1991.

Norbury KC: Immunotoxicologic evaluation: An overview. *J Am Col Toxicol* 4:279, 1985.

Parsons WH, Sigal NH, Wyvratt MJ: FK506: A novel immunosuppressant. *Ann NY Acad Sci* 685:22–36, 1993.

Pflugl G, Kallen J, Schirmer, et al.: X-ray structure of a decameric cyclophilin–cyclosporin crystal complex. *Nature* 361:91, 1993.

Schleimer RP: The mechanism of antiinflammatory steroid action in allergic diseases. *Am Rev Pharmacol Toxicol* 25:381, 1985.

Sell S: Antilymphocytic antibody: Effects in experimental animals and problems in human use. *Ann Intern Med* 71:177, 1969.

Sigal NH, Dumont FJ: Cyclosporin A, FK506, and rapamycin: Pharmacologic probes of lymphocyte signal transduction. *Annu Rev Immunol* 10:519, 1992.

Simpson DM, Ross R: Effects of heterologous antineutrophil serum in guinea pigs: Hematologic and ultrastructural observations. *Am J Pathol* 65:79, 1971.

Slavin S: Total lymphoid irradiation. *Immunol Today* 8:3, 1987.

Taliaferro WH: Modification of the immune response by radiation and cortisone. *Ann NY Acad Sci* 69:745, 1957.

Turk JL, Parker D, Poulter LW: Functional aspects of the selective depletion of lymphoid tissue by cyclophosphamide. *Immunology* 23:493, 1972.

Vanek Z, Mateju J, Curdova E: Immunomodulators isolated from microorganisms. *Folia Microbiol* 36:99, 1991.

Vanier LE, Prud'homme GJ: Cyclosporin A markedly enhances superantigen-induced peripheral T-cell deletion and inhibits anergy induction. *J Exp Med* 176:37, 1992.

IMMUNO-SUPPRESSIVE FACTORS

Abernethy TS, Avery OT: The occurrence during acute infections of a protein not normally present in the blood. I. Distribution of the reactive protein in patients's sera and the effect of calcium on the flocculation reaction with the C polysaccharide of pneumococcus. *J Exp Med* 73:173, 1941.

Curtiss LK, DeHeer DH, Edgington TS: In vivo suppression of the primary immune response by a species of low-density serum lipoprotein. *J Immunol* 118:648, 1977.

Gallin JT, Kaplan AP: Mononuclear cell chemotacic activity of kallikrein and plasminogen activator and its inhibition by C_1 inhibitor and α_2-macroglobulin. *J Immunol* 113:1928, 1974.

Mortensen RF, Osmand AP, Gewurz H: Effects of C-reactive protein on the lymphoid system. I. Binding to thymus-dependent lymphocytes and alteration of their functions. *J Exp Med* 141:821, 1975.

Mowbray JF: Effect of large doses of an α_2-glycoprotein fraction on the survival of rat skin homografts. *Transplantation* 1:15, 1963.

Ptak W, Guminska M, Stachurska B, et al.: Inhibitory effect of α-globulins of different origin on the cell-mediated immune response in mice. *Int Arch Allergy* 53:145, 1977.

Stimson WH: Studies on the immunosuppressive properties of a pregnancy-associated α-macroglobulin. *Clin Exp Immunol* 25:199, 1976.

Immunology of AIDS

29

Human
Immuno-
deficiency
Virus

AIDS-RELATED RETROVIRUSES

The acquired immunodeficiency syndrome (AIDS) is an incurable secondary immune deficiency caused by infection with a human retrovirus called human immunodeficiency virus (HIV). HIV infects and kills CD4+ helper T cells as well as dendritic macrophages, resulting in a profound, irreversible immunosuppression that progresses to death from fatal opportunistic infections in most infected individuals.

HIV belongs to subfamily *Lentivirinae* (slow viruses) in the family of animal retroviruses (Table 29–1). In general, retroviruses either cause proliferation (transforming) or destruction (cytopathic) of the cells they infect. Human T-cell leukemia viruses—HTLV-1 and HTLV-2—are transforming viruses. Transforming viruses are also called oncoviruses because they cause cancers in a variety of animals. HIV is a cytopathic virus. The cytopathic viruses were first identified in animals where they cause "wasting" diseases after a long interval of latent or subclinical infection. Because of the chronic nature of the diseases they caused (slow diseases), this group of viruses was called "lentiviruses" or slow viruses. HIV produces a profound immunosuppression in almost every infected individual. In contrast, HTLV-1 infection produces proliferation of lymphocytes and a particular form of leukemia, adult T-cell leukemia (ATL), in a very small percentage of infected individuals. It was once proposed that HIV be called HTLV-3. However, HTLV-1 is an oncovirus, whereas HIV is a lentivirus.

There are two HIVs: HIV-1 and HIV-2; they share about 60% RNA sequence homology in some regions and 30% to 40% in other

TABLE 29–1. REPRESENTATIVE RETROVIRUSES

Group	Examples	Comments
Oncoviruses		
Avian leukosis	Rous sarcoma	Contains src
	Avian myeloblastosis	Contains myb
	Avian erythroblastosis	Contains erbA and erbB
Mammalian type C	Moloney murine leukemia	Causes T-cell lymphoma
	Harvey murine sarcoma	Contains H-ras
	Abelson murine leukemia	Contains abl
	Feline leukemia	Causes T-cell lymphoma
Mammalian type B	Mouse mammary tumor	Mammary CA, T-cell lymphoma
Mammalian type D	Mason-Pfizer monkey	Immunodeficiency (SAIDS)
HTLV-BLV	Human T-cell leukemia	Causes T-cell lymphoma
	Bovine leukemia	and neurological disease
Lentivirinae		
Lentiviruses	Human immunodeficiency	Cause of human AIDS
	Simian immunodeficiency	AIDS in monkeys
	Visna/maedi	Neurologic and lung disease in sheep
	Equine infectious anemia	
	Caprine arthritis/encephalitis	
Spumavirinae		
"Foamy" viruses	Many human and simian forms	Benign

regions. HIV-1 is by far the most common cause of AIDS in the western world. HIV-2 produces a disease similar to HIV-1 and is present in high incident in West Africa but is being found increasingly outside of Africa. HIV-2 is very closely related to simian immunodeficiency virus (SIV), which causes a form of AIDS with encephalitis in monkeys (macaques) that is very similar to AIDS in humans (SIVmac).

THE HIV GENOME

The essential features of the genome of the virus and the structure of the virus are presented in Figure 29–1. The *gag, pol* and *env* gene regions code for core structural proteins, enzymes required for virus replication, and surface (envelope) proteins, respectively. The *gag, pol* and *env* genes are common to all retroviruses, and have different levels of RNA sequence homology. The term *gag* originally referred to "group antigens"—the products of the *gag* region are recognized serologically as specific for different retrovirus groups. The *gag* and *pol* proteins are found in the core of the viral particle, whereas *env* glycoproteins are imbedded into or are on the surface of the lipid bilayer of the viral capsid.

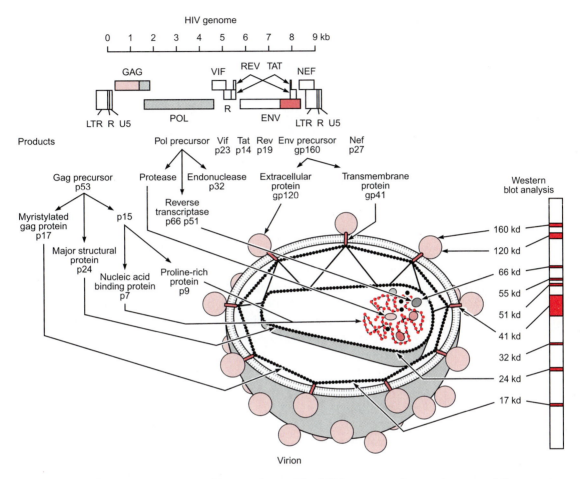

Figure 29–1. The HIV genome and its products. The HIV genome, its products, and the structure of the virion are related to the proteins identified by western blot (see Fig. 29–7). The HIV genome consists of two long terminal repeats (LTRS), structural (*gag, pol* and *env*) regions, and split segments coding for controlling factors. The *gag* region codes for internal structural proteins including nucleic acid-binding proteins (p7 and p9), the major structural protein of the nucleoid (p24) and p17, which covers the inner leaflet of the viral envelope. *Pol* codes for reverse transcriptase and other enzymes that are necessary for synthesis, processing, and assembly of virion. *Env* codes for the extracellular (gp120) and transmembrane (gp41) glycoproteins of the virion membrane. *Vif, rev, tat,* and nef code for activating and controlling factors for HIV synthesis (see text).

The *gag* gene codes for a 53 kDa precursor polypeptide that is cleaved during assembly of the virus by HIV protease to form p24, p7, p9, and p17 proteins. The most abundant *gag* protein, p24, is derived from the central portion of p53 and forms the core shell of the virus. P24 is strongly immunogenic during infection, and antibodies to p24 are usually the first seen. P7 and p9 are located in the RNA nucleoid and are derived from a p15 precursor that is cleaved from the carboxyl-terminus of p53. P17 comes from the amino terminus of p53 and lines the inner surface of the viral envelope. It appears to serve as a scaffold for the assembly of the viral envelope.

The *pol* precursor is cleaved to produce three enzymes that function at different stages of viral replication: RNA-dependent DNA polymerase (reverse transcriptase), endonuclease, and protease. The reverse transcriptase directs DNA synthesis from the genomic RNA strand during early infection. The p32 endonuclease removes the RNA in the RNA–DNA hybrid prior to the formation of DNA–DNA hybrids. The protease catalyzes processing events during the later stages of viral assembly, cleaving the protein precursors to allow formation of the virus.

The *env* gene codes for a glycosylated precursor of 160 kDa that is cleaved to yield the amino terminal gp120 and the carboxyl terminal gp41. Gp120 localizes on the external surface of the viral envelope. Gp41 has carboxyl-terminal hydrophobic amino acids, which form the transmembrane anchor that holds the gp120 external protein by noncovalent interactions. A specific portion of the extracelluar gp120 binds to the amino-terminal domains of CD4 molecules on the surface of lymphocytes and monocytes. After binding to CD4, the gp120 is cleaved off by a protease, exposing the underlying gp41. Gp41 has amino-terminal residues similar to the fusogenic domain of paramyxoviruses and initiates endocytosis of the virus by fusing to the cell membrane. Gp41 may serve to permit infection of cells not expressing CD4 by allowing the virus to fuse with CD4⁻ cells. Antibodies to gp41 can block the formation of syncytia (fused infected cells in vitro) by HIV.

HIV REPLICATION AND GENE EXPRESSION

HIV, like other retroviruses, has sets of transactivators and cis-acting factors controlling transcription (Table 29–2). The two major products which regulate viral gene expression are *tat* and *rev*.

Tat

Tat acts as a highly effective *trans*-activator of HIV LTR-dependent transcription by increasing initiation or promoting elongation of transcripts. The two *tat* coding exons are joined by RNA splicing to produce a transcript that encodes the 14-kDa *tat* protein. The *tat* protein activates transcription by binding to an RNA stem-loop structure called the trans-activating response element (TAR) that is located between sequences from +19 to +42 in the 5′ LTR. There is evidence that the trans-activating effects of *tat* may cause proliferation of other cells, leading to the lesions of lymphoma or Kaposi's sarcoma. In addition, T-cell activation factors, such as nuclear factor-κB and nuclear factor of activated Tcells (N-FAT) react with sequences in the LTR upstream from TAR after *tat* binding to form an activation complex for HIV replication (see below).

Rev | *Rev* is a 19-kDa protein that is encoded by RNA sequences which overlap those of *tat* but are in a different reading frame. *Rev* reacts with the *rev*-responsive region (RRE), which is a 204-nucleotide sequence (nt62 to nt265) in the *env* region of HIV. *Rev* acts posttranscriptionally to regulate viral mRNA transport from the nucleus and/or splicing of long HIV transcripts, which code for *gag*, *pol*, and *env* precursors.

HIV LIFE CYCLE | The HIV life cycle is depicted in Figure 29–2. The mature virion forms a sphere with 72 spikes that contain the *env* (gp120 and gp41) glycoproteins. A region on the viral envelop gp120 binds to a domain on CD4 on the lymphocyte surface. This interaction causes a conformational change in the gp120, resulting in activation of a proteolytic cleavage site on gp120, with removal of part or all of this protein. This allows interaction of the external portion of gp41 (the fusion domain) with a proposed fusion receptor on the lymphocyte surface. HIV then fuses with the cell and is internalized. The virion is uncoated in the cytoplasm and virion-associated reverse transcriptase produces hybrid RNA/DNA molecules. These are converted to double-stranded linear DNA molecules by HIV endonuclease. The linear HIV DNA is translo-

TABLE 29–2. HIV-ACTIVATING PROTEINS

Name		Size	Cellular Localization	Function
tat	Transactivator	p14	Nucleus/cytoplasm	Transactivator of all viral proteins and lymphocytes
rev	Regulator of expression	p18	Nucleus	Expression of virion proteins
vif	Virion infectivity factor	p23	Cytoplasm/inner membrane	Determine virus infectivity
nef	Negative factor	p27	Cytoplasm	? Reduces virus expression
vpu	(x)	p16	Cell membrane protein	? viral assembly
vpr	Viral protein R	p15	?	Increases viral replication

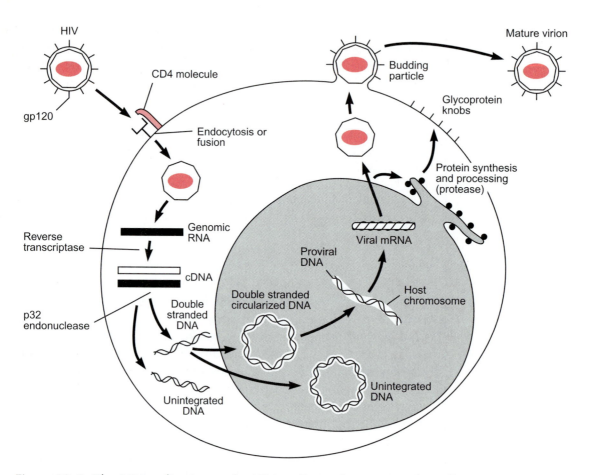

Figure 29–2. The HIV replication cycle. HIV replicates by entering the cell, using reverse tran-scriptase to synthesize complementary DNA copies of virion RNA, which insert into the host genome and then are used as templates for viral RNA synthesis. The integrated DNA may remain inactive for a long time but will be activated to synthesize viral RNA when the infected cell is stim-ulated to proliferate by mitogens, antigens, allogenic cells, or other viral infections through trans-activating factors. The newly synthesized viral RNA is then assembled into a nucleoid in the cyto-plasm and the virion formed during budding forms the cell where the external glycoproteins are added along with host-cell membrane structures, such as MHC markers. (Modified from Ho DH, Pomerantz RJ, Kaplan JC: Pathogenesis of infection with human immunodeficiency virus. *N Engl J Med* 317:278–286, 1987.)

cated to the nucleus of the infected cell where covalently closed super-coiled molecules are generated, and the viral DNA is integrated into the host DNA. In the integrated proviral form, HIV may remain latent in infected cells for months or years. Activation of infected cells causes production of host cellular transcription factors that form activation complexes with *tat*. This leads to the synthesis of *gag*, *pol* and *env* pre-cursor polypeptides, which are then assembled into viral particles together with two copies of single-stranded genomic HIV RNA. During budding from the cell, surface proteins, such as MHC molecules, are also incorporated into the viral coat. The final maturation steps, such as cleavage of the *gag* and *pol* precursor proteins and other post-translational modifications of viral proteins, occur during the budding process. Acquisition of host proteins in the viral coat produces "pseudotypes" of HIV with different host-derived surface epitopes.

AIDS

EPIDEMIOLOGY

Although there is retrospective evidence that the first case of AIDS in the United States was seen in 1968, it is generally accepted that AIDS was first recognized in the United States in June of 1981 when the Centers for Disease Control published a report of five cases of *Pneumocystis carinii* and Kaposi's sarcoma in young homosexual men. One month later, twenty-six more cases were reported from New York and Los Angeles. By February 1983, more than 1,000 cases had been reported in the United States. At first, diagnosis and recognition of the disease depended on clinical signs and symptoms. With the development of laboratory tests for HIV infection (see below), surveillance for AIDS became much more accurate. The incidence of AIDS has essentially doubled every year from 1981 to 1990. It is estimated that over one million people in the United States are infected with HIV and that about 200,000 of these will die yearly. The estimated cost of medical care for these patients is approximately $10 billion. The World Health Organization estimates that there are between eight and ten million people infected worldwide, and that eight to ten times this number will be infected by the 21st century. As the rate of infection peaks and starts to decline in Africa, it is increasing exponentially in Asia, where it is projected that there will be up to 1.5 million new adult infections per year.

The origin of AIDS is not clear. HIV appears to have surfaced in central Africa as early as 1959, but the disease was not recognized as endemic there until the late 1970s. HIV may have evolved from a monkey virus (SIV) within the last 30 to 50 years or may have existed unrecognized in isolated areas of central Africa for many years. The rapid mutation rates of the retrovirus family is consistent with either possibility. The evolutionary precursor may have been present for a long time in monkeys and HIV a recent mutation transmitted to humans. On the other hand, the virus may have been present in humans for a long time in limited populations and the present human epidemic a recent event.

A shift in circumstances may have allowed an avirulent HIV strain to mutate to a virulent strain. Opening up areas of endemic infection in Africa by war, tourism, and commercial trucking has greatly increased the spread of HIV infection. The availability of many more susceptible hosts may have allowed more virulent strains of HIV to become established. A virulent organism requires more hosts for perpetuation as infected individuals survive for relatively short times and are not able to pass the infection to as many other individuals as individuals with infections with less virulent organisms. Confined to an isolated population where no carrier has numerous sex partners, a sexually transmitted organism is better off not producing illness, allowing the host to live and be mildly infective for many years. There is evidence for a relatively avirulent strain of HIV that fits this description. A group of six individuals in Australia has been infected with the same strain of HIV-1 and has had normal CD4 counts for seven to ten years and are asymptomatic. HIV-2 is now much less virulent than HIV-1. However, if allowed to spread as HIV-1 has been, HIV-2 may mutate to more virulent strains.

HIV TRANSMISSION

HIV is transmitted by passage of viable infected blood lymphocytes or macrophages, such as by transfusion of infected blood, by sharing of contaminated needles by intravenous drug users, by passage of infected lymphocytes or macrophages in semen or cervical secretions during sexual contact through contusions or breaks in the skin or mucous membranes, or by direct passage of virus through the mucous membranes of the genital tract. Experimental studies in monkeys have suggested that vaginal immunization produce IgA and IgG antibodies in vaginal secretions that might block HIV transmission. Although infected mononuclear cells expressing viable virus can transfer HIV to epithelial cells directly, sexual transmission is increased if the act results in trauma to the skin or mucous membranes, such as is common during anal intercourse, and transmission rates are higher if there is a coexisting genital ulcer disease, such as herpes, syphilis, or chancroid. Presumably, the ulcerative lesions increase the possibility of passage of infected white blood cells. A particular HIV-I subtype, "CladeE," isolated in Thailand, appears to be much more readily transmitted by heterosexual contact than subtype B, which is found in North America and Europe. Maternal–fetal transmission most likely occurs via transplacental transfer of infected cells from the mother to the fetus, but transmission by nursing is also possible. Human hyperimmune globulin to HIV for passive immunization of pregnant women who are HIV-positive may prevent interuterine infection of their fetuses.

The first cells targeted for HIV infection are most likely monocytes, particularly the follicular dendritic cell (Fig. 29–3), but a wide range of different cell types, including many epithelial cells, are susceptible to HIV infection. During inapparent infection, cells of the monocytic series, including macrophages and astrocytes in the brain,

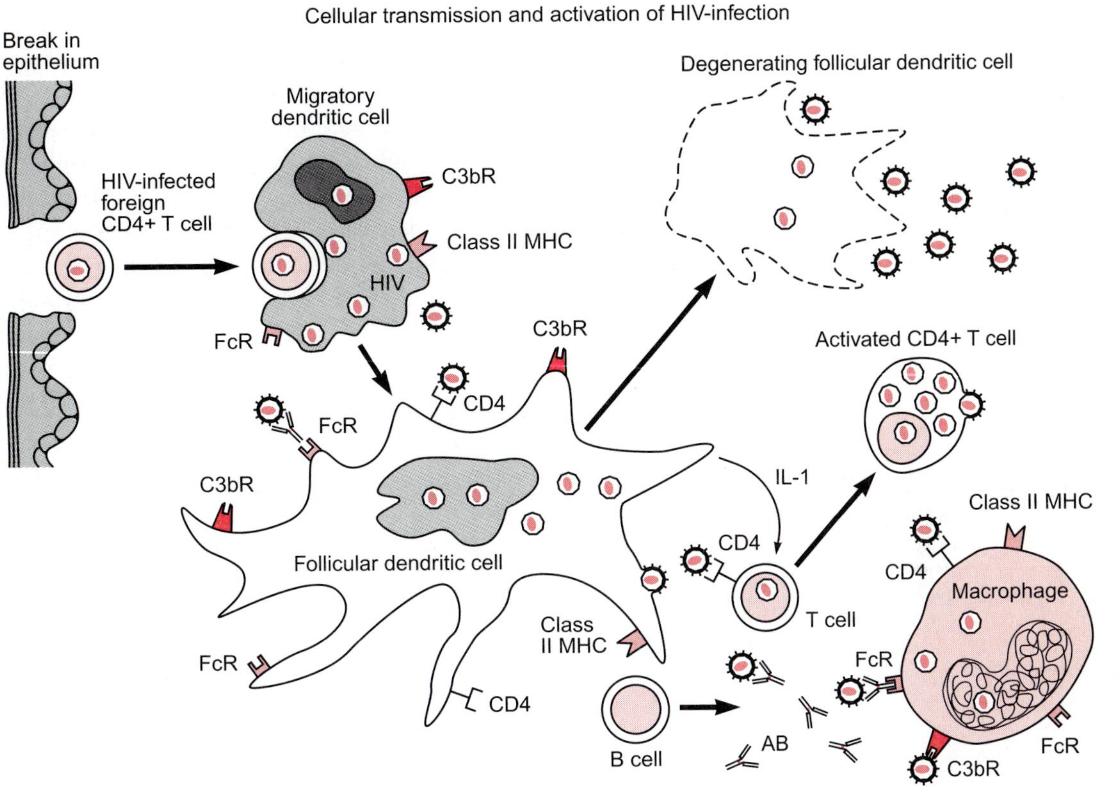

Figure 29–3. Cellular transmission of HIV infection. The most likely means of transmission of HIV infection is through HIV-infected CD4+ peripheral blood lymphocytes that enter the body through breaks in the epithelial surface. The infected CD4+ cells are phagocytosed by migratory dendritic cells, which localize in follicles in draining lymph nodes. The infection is passed from the DNA of the lymphocytes to the DNA of the migratory phagocytic cells. Infection may be increased due to the presence of FcR, C3bR, and CD4 on the macrophages. During immune activation, the infection is passed to host CD4+ T-helper cells through class II MHC–antigen receptor interactions. During this process, HIV is passed from dendritic antigen-presenting cells to CD4+ T-helper cells, and stimulation of the infected T-helper cells activates virus production (see Fig. 29–5). HIV infection eventually causes disintegration of the lymph node structure by destruction of CD4+ T cells and degeneration of follicular dendritic cells.

dendritic follicular cells in lymph nodes, and Langerhans' cells (dendritic macrophages) in the skin, contain HIV by in situ hybridization. SIV DNA sequences have been identified in the Langerhans' cells in the mucous membranes of the vagina of monkeys infected via the vaginal route. Infected monocytes may serve as "reservoirs" for HIV and deliver HIV to the brain. In addition, infection may be passed from macrophages to CD4+ lymphocytes during immune stimulation (see below) or to epithelial cells that have internalized infected monocytes. There appears to be a continuous cycle of infection from T cells to macrophages (follicular dendritic cells). Virus is passed from the infected monocytes to CD4+ lymphocytes during cell contact and activation. Infected CD4+ lymphocytes produce viruses and die. The released viruses are coated with IgG antibody and transported to the germinal centers where they are picked up by dendritic macrophages after binding to Fc receptors. The level of detection of HIV infection in blood mononuclear cells does not necessarily reflect the level of infection in the lymph nodes, where the number of viruses per CD4+ T cell may be much higher. In addition, there are many variants of HIV that

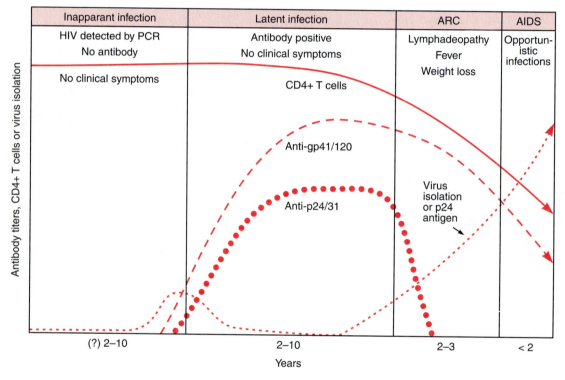

Figure 29–4. Natural history of HIV infection. The course of AIDS includes a period of inapparent infection that may be preceded by a short acute "flu-like" illness; a long latent period, followed by ARC; and then full-blown AIDS, signaled by the diagnosis of an opportunistic infection. During the period of inapparent infection, HIV sequences may be detected in cells of the macrophage series in tissues by in situ hybridization, but there is no other evidence of infection. Antibody to HIV antigens, anti-gp41 and anti-p24, may be detected during the asymptomatic latent period by western blotting. Progression to ARC is signaled by development of systematic symptoms (fever, weight loss, diarrhea, etc.), decreased numbers of CD4+ cells in the blood, lymphadenopathy, appearance of HIV antigen in the blood , and falling titers of anti-p24. Once ARC is recognized, progression to symptomatic AIDS may occur in a few months or several years. (Modified from Bolognesi DP: Natural immunity to HIV and its possible relationship to vaccine strategies. *Microbiol Sci* 5:236–241, 1988.)

that have now been identified that have different tropism for lymphocytes or macrophages. Monocytotropic HIV variants produce a higher incidence of brain infection.

NATURAL HISTORY OF HIV INFECTION

Inapparent Infection

Although there are a number of variations seen in different patients, a typical course of the natural history of HIV infection is illustrated in Figure 29–4 and features listed in Table 29–3.

A striking feature is the long time period between initial exposure and expression of manifestations of the disease that may occur in some individuals. Up to 40% of infected individuals experience an acute flu-like illness accompanied by swollen lymph nodes and a nonpruritic rash that resolves after a few days or weeks. Early on, it was reported that a few individuals survived only a few months with acute AIDS. However, it is believed that most infected individuals will not have any symptoms immediately after infection but enter a period of inapparent infection or latency. Inapparent infection has been recognized as a state with no clinical or laboratory abnormalities, except that proviral sequences may be detected in some blood or tissue cells (usually cells of the monocyte series) by extremely sensitive techniques (ie, polymerase chain reactions or in situ hybridization). The average duration of inapparent infection is not known at this time, but viral sequences have been detected by polymerase chain reactions in some individuals for up to two years prior to seroconversion. In simian AIDS (SIV), peripheral blood cells from animals previously known to be infected, but with neither laboratory tests (including PCR) nor clinical evidence of infection, are able to transfer the disease to naive animals. It has been reported that the blood lymphocytes of some individuals with no

TABLE 29–3. STAGES OF HIV INFECTION

Inapparent Infection (? up to 10 years)	HIV proviral sequences may or may not be detected by PCR Serologic tests negative No clinical signs or symptoms Blastogenic response of lymphocytes to HIV antigens may be detected	
Latent infection (2 to 10 years)	Serum antibody to HIV antigens detected No clinical signs or symptoms	
AIDS-related complex (2 to 3 years)	**Symptoms** Fever Weight loss Diarrhea Lymphadenopathy Fatigue Night sweats	**Laboratory Findings** HIV antibody Decreased CD4+ T cells Leukopenia Thrombocytopenia Anemia Hypergammaglobulinemia Low mitogen response Decreased DTH skin test
AIDS (less than 2 years)	Opportunistic infections CD4+ blood lymphocytes <200/μL	

other indications of HIV infection may be stimulated to proliferate by HIV antigens. This may indicate an early effective cellular immune response in infected individuals that precedes antibody formation.

Latent Infection (Pre-AIDS)

Latency is defined as a state in which there is no symptomatic evidence of disease, but the serologic test—antibody to HIV—is positive. The duration of inapparent infection has not yet been clearly documented, but latency may last from two to ten years before progressing to AIDS-related complex (ARC). There is evidence that those individuals who have evidence of HIV infection but respond early with antibody to p24 are less likely to progress to AIDS than those with low anti-p24.

AIDS-related Complex (ARC)

Clinical manifestations of fever, weight loss, diarrhea, enlarged lymph nodes, fatigue, and night sweats define the AIDS-related complex. Laboratory abnormalities include decreased CD4+ lymphocytes, leukopenia, thrombocytopenia, anemia, increased serum immunoglobulins, decreased response of lymphocytes to mitogen stimulation, and absence of delayed hypersensitivity skin tests. Any combination of these in the presence of a positive serologic test for HIV is considered ARC or "pre-AIDS."

AIDS

Technically, the CDC has proffered for surveillance purposes a definition of AIDS that includes all HIV-seropositive persons with a CD4+ cell count of $<200/mm^3$ within the diagnosis of AIDS. This definition affects estimates of the time from HIV infection to AIDS and survival time after diagnosis. Previously, AIDS was determined clinically as any time there was a manifestation of an opportunistic infection occurring on the background of ARC (Table 29–4). Most of these opportunistic infections are secondary to a defect in delayed hypersensitivity. Opportunistic infections of an amazing variety are, in fact, responsible for most of the clinical manifestations of AIDS. More than half of AIDS patients develop *P. carinii* pneumonia, and almost all have oral candidiasis. Cytomegalovirus infection is frequently associated with clinical deterioration, and almost all AIDS patients have rapidly deteriorating courses once opportunistic infection occurs.

The prominence of opportunistic infections with organisms that are not usually pathogenic (such as *Mycobacterium avium* and *Pneumocystis carinii*, in contrast to other organisms, such as staphylococci or streptococci, that are more common pathogens in immunologically normal individuals) is most likely due to the fact that AIDS patients will grow whatever organisms are contacted that are normally held in check by DTH. AIDS patients have a more prominent deficit in cell-mediated immunity than in antibody production and so are more susceptible to infections normally controlled by DTH or T cytotoxicity than those controlled by humoral antibody. The organisms seen in AIDS patients

TABLE 29–4. CLINICAL SYNDROMES DIAGNOSTIC OF AIDS IN
HIV-SEROPOSITIVE INDIVIDUALS

Organism	Comment
Viruses	
Cytomegalovirus	Found in almost all AIDS patients; encephalitis, pneumonia, hepatitis, colitis, disseminated
Herpes simplex	Skin ulcers, persistent and recurrent
Varicella-zoster	Local, severe, and disseminated
Epstein–Barr	Aggressive B-cell lymphomas, CNS lymphomas, intestinal lymphomas
Papilloma	Invasive cervical cancer
HIV	HIV encephalopathy
Bacteria	
Mycobacterium avium	Disseminated, GI; many acid fast organisms
Mycobacterium tuberculosis	Adenitis, pulmonary
Listeria monocytogenes	Bacteremia
Salmonella	Recurrent septicemia
Variable	Recurrent pneumonia
Parasites	
Pneumocystis carinii	Pneumonia; large numbers of organisms
Toxoplasma gondii	Encephalitis, brain abscess
Cryptosporidium sp.	Gastroenteritis, diarrhea
Fungi	
Candida sp.	Oropharyngitis, esophagitis, vaginitis
Cryptococcus neoformans	Meningitis, disseminated; pneumonia
Histoplasma capsulatum	Disseminated

Modified and updated from Armstrong D, et al.: Treatment of infections in patients with acquired immunodeficiency syndrome. *Ann Intern Med* 103:738–743, 1985.

are determined largely by their prevalence in the environment. The increase in active infections with some classic pathogens in AIDS patients has led to an increase in previously declining diseases, such as syphilis and tuberculosis, in non-AIDS contacts; children of parents with AIDS and tuberculosis are contracting tuberculosis. As a result, tuberculosis, once believed to be under control, is again threatening to become a major public health hazard in western countries.

The effect of short-term treatment of infected patients with an inhibitor of the protease of HIV-1 (ABT-538) has shown that there is an extremely rapid turn-over of virions and CD4+ lymphocytes in actively infected individuals. It appears that the immune response is actually handling large amounts of new viruses being continually produced at high rates (estimated at 10^9/day). There is rapid turnover of HIV-1 virions as new CD4+ lymphocytes are produced, infected, and killed at a high rate with a half-life of about 2 days. The vast majority of plasma virions derives from continuous rounds of infection of newly formed CD4+ lymphocytes. These infected lymphocytes appear to be located in lymphoid organs. This high turnover of virus provides ample opportunities for generation of viral diversity and escape from therapy. There is almost complete replacement of wild-type virus in the plasma by drug-resistant variants within 14 days. New assays for HIV RNA are now being used to measure viral load and direct therapy to those patients with high levels of HIV RNA in the blood.

IMMUNE STIMULATION AND ACTIVATION OF AIDS

The process of immune activation, which is critical for protection against infection, may, in the case of HIV infection, activate expression of HIV and accentuate progression of inapparent infection to AIDS (Fig. 29–5). The interaction of antigen-processing dendritic macrophages with CD4+ T-helper cells during induction of an immune response may serve to transmit virus from HIV-infected dendritic cells to CD4+ T cells through formation of cell–cell interactions. Then, activation of the CD4+ T cells by interleukins produced by macrophages, such as IL-1 and tumor necrosis factor, may stimulate HIV production by activated T cells. In addition to the viral activation factors mentioned above, several cellular transcription factors are also involved in regulation HIV gene expression. The HIV (long terminal repeat (LTR) contains binding sites for factors produced by activated T cells, such as nuclear factor of activated T cells (NF-AT-1), nuclear factor κB (NF-κB), as well as other transcription factors, and the *Tat*-binding proteins, which can cause large increases in LTR directed gene expression. These factors interact with *tat* at sites on the LTR of the HIV gene forming a "transcription complex" that stimulates high levels of transcription of the HIV gene and together can result in very high levels of viral replication (Fig. 29–6).

Thus, events which lead to activation of T cells may contribute to increased HIV production in latent individuals and to the onset of ARC or AIDS. In addition, other viruses, including herpesviruses (cytomegalovirus, Epstein–Barr virus, and herpes simplex virus), adenoviruses, hepatitis virus, and HTLV-I can transactivate the HIV LTR. Infection with these agents may not only stimulate an immune response leading to immune activation of HIV infection, but also produce cofactors that act synergistically to transactivate HIV gene transcription. The presence of these infectious agents in the patient with activated HIV destruction of CD4+ T-helper cells results in impaired ability of the immune system to combat the infection, further contributing to the pathogenesis of AIDS. Finally, AIDS patients may eventually develop autoantibodies and autoreactive T_{CTL} cells that may contribute to lesions such as orchitis, thrombocytopenic purpura, demyelinating neuritis, and graft-versus-host–like lesions. The occurrence of so many different infections and inflammatory components in the AIDS picture has led some to question whether AIDS is actually

Immune induction and cell transmission of HIV-infection

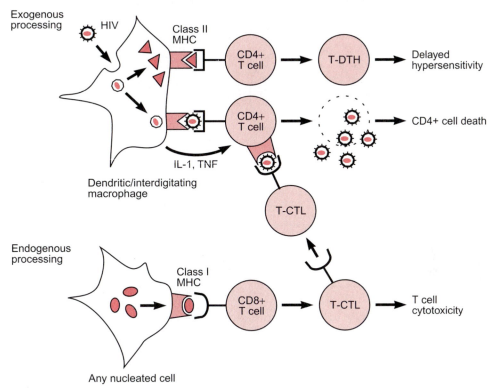

Figure 29–5. Induction of immunity and immune activation of HIV infection. HIV may be 1) processed as an exogenous antigen, 2) infect antigen presenting macrophages and 3) produce antigens that are processed by the endogenous pathway. On the one hand, antigen processing may lead to protective delayed hypersensitivity or T-cytotoxicity. On the other hand, stimulation of dendritic macrophage/CD4+ T-cell interactions by other antigens or infections may result in transfer of virus from macrophages to CD4+ T-cells and activation of HIV production in infected T-cells. Immunosuppression may be effected by CD8+ T_{CTL} reacting with HIV or cell surface antigens on CD4+ T_{DTH}.

caused by HIV or if HIV infection is secondary to immunosuppression in multiple infected patients. Similar epidemiologic and pathogenic questions could be raised about other complex diseases. For instance, the same logic that HIV does not cause AIDS has been used to argue, disingenuously, that tubercle bacillus does not cause tuberculosis.

LABORATORY DIAGNOSIS OF HIV INFECTION

The laboratory diagnosis of latent AIDS has depended on the detection of antibody to HIV in sera from infected patients, but recent advances in detecting HIV or provirus in patients may lead to more accurate and sensitive tests (Table 29–5). There are now available more than 130 tests from more than 40 commercial companies available for testing for antibodies to human retroviruses. The most widely applied screening

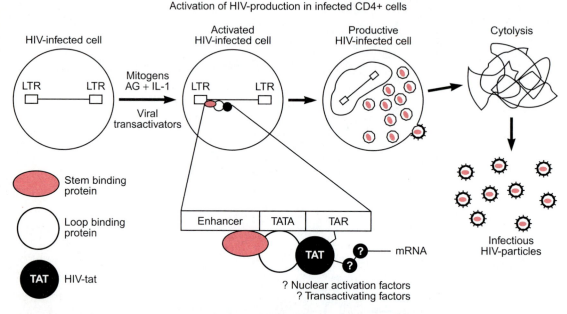

Figure 29–6. Activation of HIV in stimulated lymphocytes. Stimulation of proliferation of HIV-infected T cells activates production of HIV virions. Nuclear activation factors in stimulated lymphocytes (NF-κB, NF-AT) form an activation complex with tat that promotes HIV mRNA synthesis and virion assembly, leading to death of the HIV-infected cell. The inserts show the *tat*-binding region (TAR) and a model of the activation complex. After RNA transcripts initiate, *tat* binds to nascent transcripts at TAR. After this, cellular factors are recruited (?) that enhance transcription and/or elongation of the mRNA.

test is an enzyme-linked immunosorbent assay (ELISA). This test is very sensitive and easy to do; however, there is a problem with false positives. The initial reaction depends on antibody binding to plastic beads coated with HIV antigens. Some human sera contain immunoglobulins that bind to these beads nonspecifically or to trace contaminating materials in the beads. Because the HIV antigens are prepared from human cell lines, trace contamination of human MHC antigens may account for some false positives due to reactivity of antibodies to MHC antigens found in multiparous women or frequently transfused patients. Second generation tests using artificially derived recombinant antigens expressed in bacterial or fungal systems or chemically synthesized peptides that are now under evaluation should eliminate these problems.

A positive ELISA is confirmed first by a repeat of the ELISA on a new sample and then by western blot. Western blots detect antibodies to HIV antigens after electrophoresis of the antigens in a polyacrylamide gel (Fig. 29–7). Although this test is much more specific than

TABLE 29–5. LABORATORY TESTS FOR AIDS

Screening: ELISA for antibody
Confirmation: Western blot
Others:
p24 Antigen ELISA
Radioimmunoprecipitation (gp 120/160)
Culture in vitro: Cytopathic effect
Polymerase chain reaction
Indirect immunofluorescence
In situ hybridization
Prognosis: CD4+ blood lymphocyte count

the ELISA, there has been considerable variation in its application among different laboratories. However, it is now the accepted standard for HIV diagnosis. Positive interpretation depends on the bands that appear on the nitrocellulose membrane (Table 29–6). The most important are p24 (the major structural protein), p31 (endonuclease), and p41 (transmembrane protein) or gp120/gp160 (extracellular protein). Approximately 0.5% of individuals tested by western blotting will have indeterminant results. The reactivity is usually to only one or more of the HIV-1 core proteins (p17, p24, and p55), and therefore does not meet the definition of a positive specimen or a negative specimen. Approximately 1% to 5% of individuals with indeterminant test will seroconvert within six months. The Centers for Disease Control recommendation is: "A person whose western blot test results continue to be consistently indeterminant for at least six months—in the absence of any known risk factors, clinical symptoms, or other findings—may be considered to be negative for antibodies to HIV-1."

Some laboratories will also carry out in vitro culture assays. These are done by adding the tissue, blood, or other test material to a tissue culture line or mitogen-stimulated freshly prepared human peripheral blood mononuclear cells (PBMCs) that will support the growth of HIV. The most useful are human T-cell lines transformed by HTLV-1. After several days' incubation, the cultures as assayed for the presence of HIV-produced reverse transcriptase, or for HIV p24 antigen. Cytopathic effects (syncytia formation, cell death) may also be used to detect HIV infection but is less reliable than the other assays.

Polymerase chain reactions (PCRs) can detect extremely small amounts of HIV RNA or integrated DNA. For PCRs, oligonucleotide primers containing HIV sequences are added to RNA or DNA extracted from test cells. In the presence of a thermostable DNA polymerase, multiple cycles of replication are controlled automatically to allow rapid and exponential synthesis of new DNA sequences that depend on the presence of HIV RNA or DNA in the original sample. In this way, the RNA or DNA present can be multiplied over 10 million

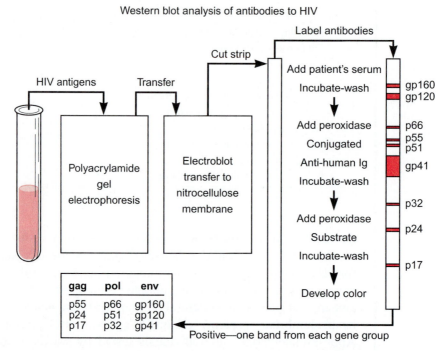

Figure 29–7. Western blot test for antibody to HIV proteins. HIV antigens are obtained from tissue culture, electrophoresed in a polyacrylamide slab gel, the separated proteins transferred to a nitrocellulose membrane, and reaction with antibody identified by a color reaction after incubation with patient's sera, followed by peroxidase labeled goat-antihuman Ig. Antibodies reacting with the individual identifiable proteins can be detected. The separated antigens are transferred to a nitrocellulose membrane by electrophoretic blotting and the blot cut into strips that are reacted with test and control sera. During incubation, antibodies to HIV antigens will react with the antigens in the blot and can be visualized by addition of peroxidase labeled antihuman Ig and enzymatic reaction with a colorless substrate that is converted to color. If antibody binds to the proteins on the nitrocellulose strip, a band of color will appear. In this way, antibodies to the different antigens of HIV can be identified.

TABLE 29-6. INTERPRETIVE CRITERIA FOR WESTERN BLOT TESTS

American Red Cross	At least one band from each gene product region *gag* AND *pol* AND *env*
ASTPHL/CDC	Any two of p24, gp41, or gp120/160
Du Pont	p24 AND p31 AND gp41 or gp120/160

gag region, p18, p24, p55.

pol region, p31, p51, p66.

env region, gp41, gp120, gp160.

times in just a few hours. The presence of the expanded nucleotide sequences can then be detected with the appropriate cDNA probe. The major problem with the clinical application of PCRs is the well-known high risk of false positives. Every laboratory with experience in PCR has had problems with false-positive results at one time or another. Strict guidelines on sample preparation, PCR conditions, and positive and negative controls need to be standardized among different laboratories. When done carefully, PCRs can detect HIV-1 proviral sequences directly from infected cells taken from the patient.

In situ hybridization using oligonucleotide probes for HIV sequences may be used to identify cells infected with HIV. Using this technique, HIV has been identified in macrophages and other cells in infected tissue, as well as in lymphocytes. The localization of HIV DNA sequences in dendritic cells in lymphoid follicles has led to the postulate that such cells may serve as a site for chronic "latent" HIV infection.

During 1992, reports appeared of rare cases of clinical AIDS in which no evidence of HIV infection could be detected. In a review by the CDC, twenty-one patients with unexplained CD4+ lymphocyte depletion below 200 cells/μL, but without HIV infection, were identified. Five patients who developed opportunistic infections were reviewed in depth. No evidence of clustering or other findings suggesting another, yet unknown virus, was found. The condition has been termed "idiopathic CD4+ T lymphocytopenia (ICL)" (see Chapter 30).

IMMUNE DYSFUNCTION IN AIDS

There are a number of possible mechanisms of immune dysfunction in AIDS that can explain the loss of defense against infections (Table 29–7). The most direct is the infection and destruction of CD4+ lymphocytes by HIV. The most consistent finding in patients with AIDS is the loss of CD4 lymphocytes. Since CD4 lymphocytes are also "helper" cells, the loss of this function may cause depressed cellular defenses, as well as impaired antibody responses. Other suggested possibilities include the decreased production of CD4+ cells, HIV-medicated dysfunction in signal transduction and in T-cell development and maturation loss of specific immune responsiveness to infectious agents reflected by the loss of specific lymphocyte proliferation responses to specific antigens of infectious agents (anergy), increased T-cell suppressor activity, blocking of T-cell receptors by HIV proteins, nonspecific activation of B cells leading to nonspecific hyperglobulinemia but also to decreased specific antibody production, decreased neutrophils and loss of acute inflammatory reactivity, and blocking or destruction of macrophages, as well as autoimmunity to lymphocyte antigens contributing to destruction of CD4+ cells. Decreased hematopoiesis may contribute not only to lymphopenia but also to granulocytopenia, thrombocytopenia, and anemia.

The immune dysfunctions seen in early ARC point to hyperacti-

TABLE 29–7. IMMUNE DYSFUNCTIONS IN AIDS

Infection and destruction of CD4+ helper cells

Interference with production of CD4+ helper cells

Loss of DTH reactivity to antigens of infectious agents

Increased T-suppressor activity

Blocking of T-cell receptors by HIV products

Nonspecific activation of B cells leading to hyperglobulinemia
and B-cell lymphomas

Decreased specific antibody formation

Decreased neutrophils

Decreased monocytes

Autoimmunity to T cells:

  Autoantibody

  Autoreactive T-killer cells to activated CD4+ lymphocytes
    in the presence of HIV gp120.

Increased expression of cell adhesion molecules (CD11/18)

vation and stimulation of autoimmune reactivity suggesting some abnormality of immune regulation rather than strictly an immune deficiency through direct destruction of CD4+ cells by HIV infection. HIV infection may alter T-cell signal transduction by gp120 binding to CD4, formation of peptides of gp120 may activate the Fas cell death pathway, production of HIV superantigens or direct interference with receptors, kinases, phosphatases, cytokines or cyclins. As a result T cells may fail to respond to foreign antigens or be directed to enter programmed cell death (apoptosis) pathways. The immune abnormalities in AIDS have been compared to the immunostimulatory phase of graft-versus-host reactions. This implicates an immunostimulatory event causing the activation of CD4 helper cells and B cells as the initiating factor in latent AIDS. Activation of CD4+ T-helper cells may increase the infection level of AIDS by activation of transcription of the HIV provirus and proliferation of CD4+ cells provides a higher number of potentially infectable cells. In addition, immune stimulation may contribute to autodestruction of activated CD4+ cells by T_{CTL} cells or autoantibodies that are stimulated by the activation process. T_{CTL} cells have been shown to be able to recognize the gp120 protein of HIV in association with class II MHC on activated CD4+ cells.

Another factor is the increased expression of CD11/18 adhesive molecules in HIV-infected lymphocytes and monocytes. The increased adhesive molecules may account for the extravascular accumulation of mononuclear cells in tissues of AIDS patient associated with lesions that are not directly related to immune deficiency such as myositis, pulmonary dysfunction, and dementia. In any case, the most important clinical manifestations are secondary to an inability to defend against a wide variety of infectious agents that are not usually pathogenic. This secondary immune deficiency is reflected primarily in a loss of delayed hypersensitivity mechanisms, but also in decreased antibody production.

PATHOLOGY AND CLINICAL STAGING
Staging

Clinical staging of AIDS using seropositivity, CD4:CD8 lymphocyte ratios, CD4 depletion and degree of lymphopenia (low white blood cell count), as well as decreasing titers of antibody to p24, loss of reactivity to delayed-type skin testing (see Fig. 29–4) and viral load in blood are useful in predicting when patients can be expected to develop opportunistic infections. The most useful indicators of progressing disease is a CD4+ lymphocyte count below 400/mm^3, falling antibody titer to p24 and appearance of HIV RNA in the blood. In one study, nearly all deaths occurred in individuals with fewer than 50 CD4+ cells/mm^3. Lymphadenopathy appearing in the context of seropositivity is critical for defining transition from latency to ARC. In fact, the term lymphadenopathy syndrome (LAS) was used to emphasize this. Loss of DTH skin reactivity to standard test antigens (purified protein derivative, mumps, *Candida*, tetanus toxoid, and trichophyton) is an independent predictor of progression to AIDS in persons with HIV infection.

Lymph Nodes

Pathologic examination of the lymph nodes reveals a progression of lesions from hyperplasia to lymphoid depletion. Early in ARC, lymph nodes show hyperplasia of both nodular and diffuse cortex. This evolves to florid nodular hyperplasia, followed by a mixed pattern of follicular hyperplasia and follicular fragmentation. Generalized lymphocyte depletion is then seen with severe follicular atrophy. HIV proviral sequences may be detected within the follicular dendritic cells using radiolabeled RNA during the hyperplastic phase, but little or no HIV RNA is seen after follicular involution with advancing disease. Thus, the follicular dendritic cell may play a critical role in the cellular interactions involved in activation of HIV infection (see Fig. 29–3). A number of other infectious agents, such as herpesvirus, cytomegalovirus, mycoplasma, etc., as well as superantigen activation of T cells, have been implicated in either activation of HIV production or induction of cell death (apoptosis) in T cells.

Kaposi's Sarcoma

The development of Kaposi's sarcoma, a vascular neoplasm, a major feature of cases described in the early 1980s, appears to be less prominent in the more recent phase of the epidemic. Kaposi's sarcoma is believed to result from transactivation by *tat* or from the action of oncostatin M, a protein produced by T cells infected by human retroviruses. Oncostatin M (30 kDa) not only stimulates Kaposi's sarcoma cells to grow but also activates them to produce IL-6, which may augment proliferation of the sarcoma cells. The identification of herpesvirus-like DNA sequences in AIDS-associated Kaposi's sarcoma (KS) raises the possibility of infection with a new human herpesvirus. However, there is as yet no evidence that this putative virus causes KS.

HIV Encephalopathy

Early in the history of the manifestations of AIDS, neurologic dysfunction (AIDS encephalitis) was reported. Clinically, the affected patients manifested cognitive changes, lethargy, social withdrawal, and psychomotor retardation, with marked dementia in the late stages of the illness. Some affected patients have severe cortical nerve cell loss associated with profound encephalopathy and encephalitis, but many symptomatic patients do not have these lesions. The now classic feature of HIV encephalitis is the development of perivascular multinucleated giant cells in the central nervous system. These cells contain virus particles and are believed to result from syncytia formation of infected monocytes similar to that seen in vitro. In addition, there are nonspecific loose collections of microglial and giant cells (microglial nodules) and diffuse leukoecephalopathy (pallor of the white matter). The only cells in the CNS that can be readily demonstrated to contain HIV-1 are monocyte derived–macrophages, microglial cells, or giant cells. The exact relationship between HIV encephalitis and dementia is not clear. Some people with typical HIV-1–associated dementia have no neuropathologic evidence of HIV-1 encephalitis. In addition, no convincing infection of neuroectodermally derived nerve or glial cells has been demonstrated in any AIDS patient. Suggested explanations are that there is sufficient involvement of the subcortex to affect the cortex indirectly, that there are toxic proteins produced by HIV (gp120), or toxic products released from HIV-infected macrophages (cytokines, TNF-α). Some patients develop spasticity and leg weakness associated with a spongioform or vacuolar change in the lateral and dorsal columns of the spinal cord (vacuolar myelopathy). AIDS patients may also exhibit a variety of central nervous symptoms as a result of opportunistic infections as well as lymphoma, vasculitis, and other lesions. Clearly, we have much to learn about the neuropathologic mechanisms in HIV infection.

Opportunistic Infections

At autopsy, the ravages of AIDS are revealed in multiple pathologic changes. Profound depletion of lymphoid organs and lesions caused by different opportunistic infections reflects the severe terminal immunosuppression characteristic of the disease. Prominent infections include necrotizing arteritis and intestinal ulcerations with cytomegalovirus inclusions, enlarged lymph nodes containing macrophages filled with *M. avium*, and pulmonary alveoli filled with many clinics. After diagnosis, therapy is started if CD4 count is less than 400/mm^3. Patients with higher CD4 counts are followed up every 3 to 6 months and treated if their CD4 count falls below 400. Treatment of asymptomatic HIV-positive patients with AZT has been reported to delay the onset of AIDS in some studies, but more recent enlarged studies indicate that this approach is not really helpful.

Virus Production and Assembly

Inhibition of virus in vitro has been obtained using four approaches: Antisense oligonucleotides, which interfere with viral RNA production; guanosine analogues, such as ribavirin, which inhibit mRNA production; protease inhibitors, which interfere with later stages of virus assembly; and agents that inhibit glycosylation of viral envelope proteins. Protease inhibitors are undergoing phase 1 trials. It is hoped that since protease inhibitors act at different stages of virus reproduction than zidovudine, they will synergize with zidovudine. Finally, if a gene coding for a toxic protein, such as diphtheria toxin, is put under control of HIV regulatory sequences, HIV-infected cells that are superinfected with the new construct in vitro will die, whereas normal cells are unaffected. By the time this book is published, clinical trials using this approach may be underway.

Immune Reconstitution

Attempts to reconstitute AIDS patients by transfer of immune competent cells or immune serum have not been successful, even when there are identical twins as donor and recipient. Biologic response modifiers, such as IL-2 and INF-γ, as well as cyclosporine, levamisole, and thymopoietin, have also not been effective.

Opportunistic Infections

Treatment of the opportunistic infections in AIDS patients may have temporary beneficial effects. For instance, acyclovir may slow the progression of cytomegalovirus, and amphotericin B is effective against cryptococcal infections. Aerosolized pentamidine has been effective in prevention of *P. carinii* pneumonia.

Passive Immunotherapy

It has been proposed to inject "cocktails" of human monoclonal antibodies to HIV virus or autologous human CD4+ T-cell lines derived from cells taken from AIDS patients in an attempt to induce remissions in AIDS patients. Since anything that might possibly work is fair game for National Institutes of Health (NIH) support, these approaches are now in clinical trials.

Trials are now underway to treat advanced AIDS patients with transfer of bone-marrow cells from other species, such as baboons or pigs, into humans on the possibility that the transferred cells may be able to replace the patient's cells and will be resistant to HIV infection. In addition, there are plans to use transferred human CD4+ T-cells and hematopoietic stem cells genetically engineered to be resistant to HIV replication, such as by introducing a mutant *rev* gene.

VACCINATION AGAINST HIV INFECTION

From what is known about animal retroviruses, such as feline leukemia virus, it may be possible to immunize individuals and provide protection against HIV infection. Some of the possible approaches to a vaccine are listed in Table 29–9. Although there are conflicting reports regarding effectiveness, a vaccine for feline leukemia virus has been prepared from polypeptides shed from FeLV-infected tumor cell lines. This vaccine contains the gp70/85 surface polypeptide of the FeLV.

Current vaccine trials are directed toward therapy, not prevention. It is hypothesized that it may not be possible to prevent HIV infection but that the immune system may be activated to hold the infection in check. Stage 1 clinical trials using recombinant gp160 (VaxSyn HIV-1) purified from cultures of lepidopteran cells infected with recombinant baculovirus have shown that the vaccine is safe and induces antibody HIV-1. After appropriation by Congress for $20 million, critical review of preliminary results by scientifically competent committees led to redirection of this approach. One direction of trials will focus on the effectiveness of active immunization on prevention of transmission of HIV from mother to child. It is predicted that at least 50% of pediatric AIDS may be prevented if this approach is successful.

Extensive experimentation has not provided evidence that vaccines made of pieces of HIV will provide protection. Vaccinia vectors containing open reading frames of the HIV genome, such as *gag* and *pol*, are able to induce antibody and CMI to HIV antigens in chimpanzees, but do not provide protection to challenge. Although there is disagreement, it is the opinion of many that such recombinant vaccines will not work. However, more careful selection of epitopes that are important for the initiation of infection, such as the V3 loop and the CD4-binding site on the gp120 molecule, may provide protective immunogens (see below). In preliminary trials, immunization with

TABLE 29–9. POSSIBLE APPROACHES TO AN AIDS VACCINE

Antigens	Carriers
Recombinant DNA Products	**For T Cytotoxicity**
gp120	ISCOMS
gp160	Vaccinia vectors
Peptides	DNA transfection
V$_3$ *loop* (gp120)	
CD4 receptor (gp120)	**For DTH**
Genetically Modified Virus	Freund's adjuvant
Avirulent deletions	Muramyl dipeptide
Whole Inactivated HIV	BCG vectors
Formalin	
Antiidiotypes	
Experimental	
Passive antibody or sensitized T cells	

recombinant vaccinia/env vector, followed by boosting with gp120, induced much higher T-cell responses in seronegative human volunteers than the response in subjects receiving either vaccine alone.

The most successful experimental vaccine is a genetically modified simian immunodeficiency virus (SIV, see below) with a deletion in the *nef* region. Monkeys vaccinated with this "weakened" form of SIV were healthy for over three years, had low virus levels and normal CD4+ lymphocyte counts. Vaccinated monkeys were resistant to challenge with high doses of fully infectious SIV that were fatal to nonvac-cinated control monkeys. Because this "immunization" is essentially inducing an infection with a low-virulence form of the virus, there are many reservations that would have to be overcome before such an approach would be applicable to humans. First, it would not seem to be a good idea to intentionally infect a human with a viable virus, and second, if an individual is already infected with a virulent form of the virus, superinfection with a less virulent form may not provide any beneficial effect.

Experimental trials with inactivated HIV have not provided convincing evidence of protection. Infection of chimpanzees with inactivated whole virus has resulted in some protective effects, but the vaccines have been shown to contain human antigens from the cell lines used to prepare the virus. Chimpanzees "vaccinated" with normal human blood cells were also resistant to challenge with HIV grown in human cells. Purified HIV grown in human cell lines contain HLA antigens. These results are interpreted to show that HIV grown in human cells will acquire human antigens in the viral envelope (pseudotypes) and that an immune response in the chimpanzees to the human antigens are responsible.

Hypervariable regions of gp120 appear to be the most likely candidates to provide immunogenic peptides (Fig. 29–8). This major surface molecule of the HIV virus contains five hypervariable regions. Of these, a segment in the third region from 315 to 329 is not only the immunodominant region with which neutralizing antibody reacts, but it also is the site of epitopes that stimulate transformation of sensitized lymphocytes, as well as an active site for CD8+ T-cytotoxic lymphocytes. In addition, amphipathicity of different regions of gp120 have been analyzed to find potential amphipathic α-helical domains that might be selectively immunogenic for CD8+ T_{CTL}. Three T-cell stimulating regions are aa residues 428 to 443, gp120 (envT1); aa residues 112 to 124, gp120 (envT2); and aa residues 834 to 848, gp160 (envT4) of the *env* region. Of particular interest is the envT1, as it contains the CD4-binding site. Immunization of healthy volunteers with these peptides in alum resulted in stronger in vitro responses of T cells, as measured by IL-2 production after exposure to antigen, than was found in T cells from infected patients. In fact, in naturally infected individuals, only 62% demonstrated T-cell recognition of p24; 18% gp160; and 23% gp120. It is possible that some of these peptides individually or in com-

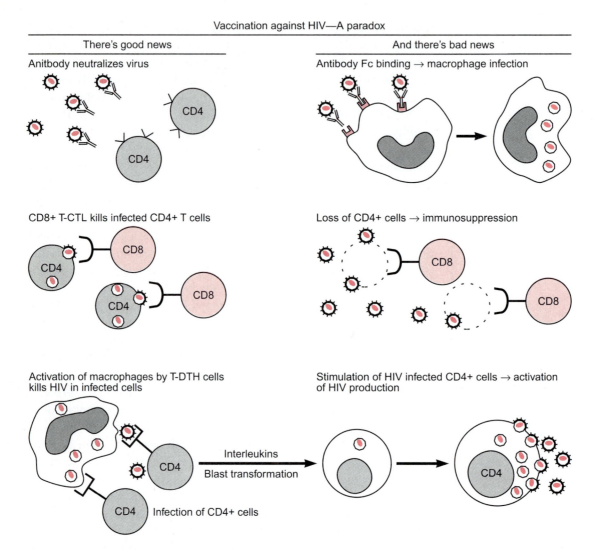

Figure 29–8. Destructive immunity in HIV infection—a paradox. Antibody to HIV may neutralize the virus (block infection) or increase infectivity by providing aggregated Fcs or binding of C_3b that increase adherence and infection of macrophages. CD8+ T_{CTL} cells limit infection by killing virus-infected cells but also reduce the number of CD4 T-helper cells and produce immunosuppression. Delayed hypersensitivity reactions can activate macrophages to kill intracellular viruses but also stimulate HIV production in infected cells.

bination might not only provide a protective vaccine but also stimulate T-cell responses in already infected individuals (vaccine therapy). In one study, immunization with a candidate gp160 vaccine resulted in new humoral (antibodies to different epitopes) and cellular (T-cell proliferation) responses in 19 of 30 HIV-infected individuals, and booster effects were noted on repeated immunizations. Thus, postinfection immunization is effective in increasing the immune response to HIV; it is not yet known if this has a beneficial effect on the course of infection.

Selection of immunization protocols for the desired type of immune response may be critical (see Chapter 26). Although there is still much to be known about the role of different immune responses in defense against AIDS, it seems likely that the most desired response is T cytotoxicity. However, there is a paradox in that immune products may increase, as well as inhibit, the progression of HIV infection (see below and Fig. 29–9). Immunization protocols that may specifically induce CD8+ T_{CTL} cells include ISCOMs, vaccinia vectors, and DNA transfection. Key to induction of T_{CTL} cells is endogenous antigen presentation by class I MHC-positive cells. Most immunization protocols involve nonliving antigens, which are processed by the endosomal system (exogenous processing). This processing usually leads to production of humoral antibodies and CD4+ MHC class II-restricted helper or cytotoxic T cells. Organisms, such as viruses or malaria protozoa, which live within epithelial cells, produce antigens that are not processed by the exogenous endosomal system (endogenous processing) and induce CD8+ class I-restricted T_{CTL}. ISCOMs, vaccinia vectors, and DNA transfection are able to deliver amphipathic peptides to class I MHC molecules for endogenous antigen processing. ISCOMs are stable matrix structures produced by incorporation of protein or

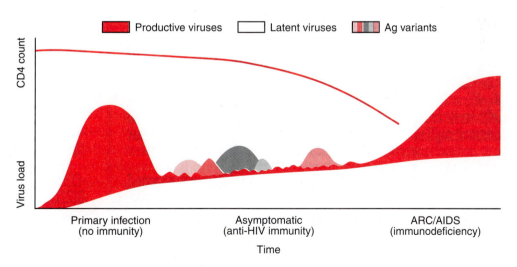

Figure 29–9. HIV vaccination and viral evolution. In natural infection, at the end of the inapparent stage, a wave of wild-type virus replication may occur in the absence of immunity, leading to the latent stage. Then, during the latent stage, specific immunity controls viral replication as new antigenic variants emerge. With development of ARC and AIDS, specific immunity is lost and the viral load increases rapidly. (From Sonigo P, Girard M, Dormont D: Design and trials of AIDS vaccines. *Immunol Today* 11:465, 1990.)

peptide antigens into an adjuvant glycoside. ICSOMs are processed during an immune response like an endogenous antigen in which the antigen is presented in association with class I MHC (see Chapter 28). Thus, ISCOMs could direct the immunodominant gp120 peptide to induction of an immune effector cell that will prove to be selectively protective rather than pathogenic. Vaccinia vectors will infect epithelial cells and present antigen endogenously, and transfection of epithelial cells with DNA that produces peptide antigens will also lead to endogenous presentation.

Major problems in inducing a protective immune response to HIV infection are: (1) The intracellular location of the viral DNA in a provirus form, (2) variations in the antigen expression of HIV, and (3) stimulation of nonprotective, immunopathologic immune responses.

Intracellular Location

Because of the intracellular location of HIV and the integration of HIV DNA into the host genome, it may not be possible to produce immunity that will prevent transmission by HIV-infected cells, as these cells may not express HIV antigens on the cell surface. Such infected cells might be able to infect the recipients cells by direct interaction and fusion with uninfected cells, even in the presence of an immune response to the virus.

Antigenic Modulation of HIV During Infection

HIV is highly mutable, most likely because of inaccuracy in reverse transcriptase. This results in a single predominant virus genotype in an infected individual with multiple, related, minor variants of the virus in the same individual. Most of the variants express minor differences in the gp120 membrane glycoprotein, which could be important immunologically or biologically. The "evolution" of variants could allow HIV to shift antigenicity and avoid attack by specific antibodies or to change the nature of the infectivity by producing variants with different trophism for lymphocytes or monocytes and different abilities to infect the brain (Fig. 29–9). Single amino acid substitutions in the V3 hypervariable region of gp120 may eliminate reactivity with specific neutralizing antibody or T_{CTL} cells. It is postulated that the slow rise in antigenic diversity of HIV during an infection results in a level of diversity that eventually cannot be controlled by the immune system. This model predicts that antigenic diversity is a major factor that drives disease progression, enabling the virus to escape from control by the immune response.

Inappropriate Immune Response

The effect of immunization may actually enhance immune defects in AIDS patients (see Fig. 29–8). On the one hand, antibody may neutralize virus in vitro but provide aggregated Fcs that facilitate binding and uptake of virus by macrophages. Cytotoxic T cells may hold the infection in check by killing HIV-infected cells. On the other hand, specific T_{CTL} may mediate depletion of CD4+ cells in AIDS patients. CD4+ T cells are killed by gp120 *env* specific killer cells in vitro that recognize class II MHC markers in the context of gp120 on activated CD4+ T cells. Thus, immunization against gp120 may actually contribute to the immune deficiency of AIDS by activating an autoimmune mechanism that selectively kills CD4+ lymphocytes. Delayed hypersensitivity to HIV may activate macrophages to destroy HIV in their cytoplasm, but coactivation of macrophages and infected CD4+ T_{DTH} may result in stimulation of virus proliferation in activated CD4+ infected cells.

ANIMAL MODELS OF CYTOLYTIC RETROVIRAL INFECTIONS

There is a critical need for the development of more useful animal models, particularly those addressing the question of therapy of—and a vaccine for—AIDS. A listing of the most relevant animal models is given in Table 29–10. Thought by many to be the most promising animal model for AIDS is that of simian immunodeficiency virus in macaques (SIVmac). SIVmac is carried without symptoms in African green monkeys (cercopithecus) and the sooty mangaby (cercocebus) but produces an AIDS-like illness in Asian macaques (rhesus). SIV does not appear to inhibit the functions of lymphocytes in African green monkeys and induces a very weak immune response. Combined HIV/SIV chimeric viruses infect macaques or cynomolgus monkeys. Immunization of macaques with gp subunits in vaccinia virus with boosting in baculovirus vectors has produced resistance to infection with SIV. Testing of an SIV vaccine in macaques using inactivated

TABLE 29–10. ANIMAL MODELS FOR AIDS

EXPERIMENTAL			
Species	Agent	Result	Use
Chimpanzee	HIV-1	Latent infection	Vaccine testing
Macaques	SIV	Wasting disease, AIDS-like	Vaccine testing, therapy pathogenesis
Rabbits	HIV	Defective infection	Latent infection
Mice	Transgenic (complete)	AIDS-like disease	
	Transgenic (tat)	Kaposi's sarcoma	Pathogenesis
	SCID-human	AIDS-like disease	Therapy
	Lymphoid cell chimera		
NATURALLY OCCURRING			
Sheep	Visna	Chronic neurodegeneration	Pathogenesis
Goats	Caprine	Chronic arthritis	Pathogenesis
Horses	EIAV	Hemolytic anemia	Pathogenesis

human cells infected with SIV has produced the unexpected result that uninfected human cells (the control vaccine) produced protection against SIV infection, as did SIV-infected cells.

The course of infection with HIV in chimpanzees appears to be similar to latent AIDS in humans and inapparent infections in rabbits. Chimpanzees have humoral and cellular responses similar to those of humans and contain CD4+ T cells but do not manifest AIDS-like symptoms when infected with HIV. The chimp model may be used for vaccination trials to determine if a vaccine can prevent infection but not for pathogenesis or therapy. So far, chimps have been immunized with synthetic peptides, recombinant vaccinia vectors containing HIV DNA, or gp120, and have had mixed responses to HIV infection. Although most studies have not shown resistance to HIV infection after immunization, chimps immunized with a combination of immunogens including the V_3 peptide or with formalin-inactivated HIV have had some protection against infection. Rabbits infected with HIV also develop latent infection without progression to AIDS.

Several transgenic mouse models for AIDS studies have been established. One line contains complete copies of HIV genes. After the founder transgenic lineage was bred with nontransgenic animals, the F_1 progeny that contained the HIV transgene developed an AIDS-like syndrome. Another transgenic mouse line containing the HIV *tat* gene develops fibroblastic tumors similar to Kaposi's sarcomas.

A different mouse model has been produced by transfer of human fetal thymus, liver, and lymph node cells to SCID mice, which allows the proliferation of CD4+ and CD8+ human T cells, as well as production of human immunoglobulin. In situ hybridization has revealed the presence of HIV-infected cells in the thymus and lymph nodes of these mice. A similar model has been produced by injection of SCID mice with human blood lymphocytes. These mice develop wasting and severe lymphoid atrophy, and most die 6 to 8 weeks after infection with HIV. Finally, bg/nu/xid mice injected with human bone marrow serve as a host system for human cells of macrophage lineage. Each of these models has great promise in the study of certain aspects of AIDS infection, but considerable care will need to be taken in extrapolating any results on pathogenesis to the human situation. An additional model used to study pathogenesis, therapy, and vaccination is the related murine leukemia virus (MuLV) infection of mice, which has many features in common with human HIV infection.

Summary

AIDS is a secondary immunodeficiency caused by infection with HIV, a human retrovirus. The virus selectively infects and destroys CD4+ T-helper lymphocytes. This results in a loss of T-cell function and a severe immunodeficiency manifested by fatal opportunistic infections by infectious agents that are not pathogenic for individuals with normal immune systems. HIV infects selected cells in the macrophage lineage, such as glial cells, dendritic follicular cells, and Langerhans' cells in the skin. The virus is able to persist in these cells for long periods of time (inapparent infection) before the infection spreads to CD4+ T cells. The surface of the virus contains molecules that bind to CD4+ markers on CD4+ T cells. The virus then enters the cell by fusion or endocytosis. Once in the cell, the RNA core of the virus unravels, and complementary DNA is synthesized by reverse transcriptase. The DNA enters the nucleus where it integrates into the host DNA as a provirus. The virus may remain inapparent in this form for many years. A change from inapparent to latent infection is indicated by the production of circulating antibody to HIV core (p24 or p31) and surface (gp41 or gp120) antigens. Overt disease appears after a latent period of two to ten years. Activation of productive infection appears to result from immune stimulation, leading to activation of infected T cells by IL-1 and TNF produced by activated macrophages. This, in turn leads to synthesis of activation products of T cells, (NF-AT and NF-kB), which form a "transcription complex" that greatly increases HIV gene transcription.

The appearance of disease is heralded by the AIDS-related complex (ARC). The major features of ARC are presence of antibodies to HIV, lymphadenopathy, a decrease in the numbers of CD4+ lymphocytes in the blood, and symptoms of systemic disease, including fever, diarrhea, weight loss, and night sweats. The CDC has defined AIDS as evidence of HIV infection (seropositive) associated with CD4 cell counts less than $200/mm^3$. True AIDS occurs when an opportunistic infection is diagnosed on the ARC background. Among the most important of such agents are *Pneumocystic carinii*, cytomegalovirus, *Mycobacterium avium*, herpes simplex, and *Candida albicans*, although there are many others. In addition, other infectious agents such as *Mycobacterium tuberculosis* and *Treponema pallidum* are becoming increasingly important, as these may be transmitted to non-HIV–infected individuals. A number of immune abnormalities occur in AIDS patients, suggesting an immune-related pathogenesis that is much more complex than simply HIV destruction of T-helper cells. These include the production of anti-antibodies and autoreactive T-killer cells, leading to lymphopenia, thrombocytopenia, granulopenia, and anemia, and a stage of hyperplasia of lymphoid tissue followed by lymphoid organ depletion.

Since the spring of 1981, when a few unusual cases of *P. carinii* and Kaposi's sarcoma among young homosexual men in New York and California were reported by the Centers for Disease Control and Prevention in Atlanta, AIDS has grown to epidemic proportions and spread rapidly to the heterosexual community. Epidemiologic data indicate that the virus arose in central Africa and spread rapidly among sexually active populations, especially male homosexuals.

Transmission of the infection may occur by passage of the free virus or by infected cells. Natural infection of humans occurs most often by sexual activities in which blood, semen, or vaginal fluids carrying virus or infected cells comes into contact with breaks in the skin or mucous membranes, or through the use of contaminated needles or syringes by intravenous drug abusers. Transmission may also occur across the placenta from mother to fetus and actually occurs in about half of pregnancies in which the mother is infected with HIV.

Attempts to produce vaccines to prevent HIV have met with little success, as have attempts at therapy. The intracellular location of the virus, the marked variability that occurs in RNA sequences—particularly of the *env* region—during an infection, and the possibility of producing an immunopathologic effect by immunization are all contributing factors to difficulties in finding a vaccine. Clinical trials using synthetic HIV surface antigens (eg, gp160) demonstrate increased antibody and cellular immunity to HIV epitopes; trials are underway to determine if immunization with envelope proteins will delay the development of AIDS in HIV-infected individuals. Therapy directed to restoring immune reactivity by passive transfer of cells or serum, immunostimulating agents, or interleukins has not been successful. Drugs have also had little effect. Zidovudine, an inhibitor of reverse transcriptase, produces a temporary alleviation of some symptoms but is unsatisfactory in the long run. Animal models using macaques, chimpanzees, mice reconstituted with human cells, or transgenic mice that carry the HIV provirus, as well as rabbits infected with HIV, are being evaluated for use in vaccine and therapy trials, as well as for experimental studies of pathogenesis.

AIDS is the most threatening infectious disease to appear in the western world in this century. The rapid advances in immunology and molecular biology that have occurred in the last twenty years have provided an amazing variety of approaches to study the virus and learn how to modify its effects. Yet much more must be learned and accomplished before effective therapy or vaccination will be achieved. At present, infection can be prevented by appropriate behavior to avoid transmission of the virus.

Bibliography

GENERAL

Journal of Acquired Immune Deficiency Syndromes. New York, Raven Press.
AIDS: An International Bimonthly Journal. London, Gower Academic Journals.
AIDS Research and Human Retroviruses. New York, Mary Ann Liebert.
DeVita VT, Hillman S, Rosenberg SA (eds.): *AIDS: Etiology, Diagnosis, Treatment, and Prevention*, 2nd ed. Philadelphia, Lippincott, 1989.
Harawi SJ, O'Hara CJ (eds.): *Pathology and Pathophysiology of AIDS and HIV-related Diseases.* Boca Raton, FL, Mosby, CRC Press, 1989.
Ioachim HL: *Pathology of AIDS.* Philadelphia, Lippincott, 1989.

Neiburgs HE, Bekesi JG: *Immune Dysfunctions in Cancer and AIDS*. New York, Liss, 1988.

Relman AS (ed.): AIDS: Epidemiologic and clinical studies. *N Engl J Med* 1988.

Wormser GP (ed.): *AIDS and Other Manifestations of HIV Infection*, 2nd ed. New York, Raven Press, 1992.

AIDS VIRUSES/ MOLECULAR BIOLOGY/LIFE CYCLE

Clements JE, Gidovin SL, Montelaro RC, et al.: Antigenic variation in lentiviral diseases. *Annu Rev Immunol* 6:139–159, 1988.

Cullen BR: The HIV-1 tat protein: An RNA sequence-specific processing factor? *Cell* 63:655–657 1990.

Cullen BR: Regulation of HIV-1 expression. *FASEB J* 5:2361, 1991.

Haseltine WA: Molecular biology of the human immunodeficiency virus type I. *FASEB J* 5:2349, 1991.

Palker TJ: Human T-cell lymphotropic viruses: Review and prospects for antiviral therapy. *Antiviral Chem Chemother* 3:127, 1992.

Roberts JD, Bebnek K, Kunkel TA: The accuracy of reverse transcriptase from HIV. *Science* 242:1171.

Solomin L, Felber BK, Pavlakin GN: Different sites of interaction for rev, tev, and rex proteins within the rev-responsive element of human immunodeficiency virus type 1. *J Virol* 64:6010, 1990.

Strauss JH, Strauss EG: Evolution of RNA Viruses: *Annu Rev Microbiol* 42:657–683, 1988.

Truneh A, Buck D, Cassatt DR, et al.: A region in domain 1 of CD4 distinct from the primary gp120-binding site is involved in HIV infection and virus-mediated fusion. *J Biol Chem* 266:5942, 1991.

Wong-Staal F: Human immunodeficiency virus: Genetic structure and function. *Semin Hematol* 25:189, 1988.

EPIDEMIOLOGY/ TRANSMISSION

Blattner WA: HIV epidemiology: Past, present and future. *FASEB J* 5:2340, 1991.

Brookmeyer R: Reconstruction and future trends of the AIDS epidemic in the United States. *Science* 253:37, 1991.

Caussy D, Goedert JJ: The epidemiology of human immunodeficiency virus and acquired immunodeficiency syndrome. *Semin Oncol* 17:244–250, 1990.

Comstock GW: Tuberculosis: A bridge to chronic disease epidemiology. *Am J Epidemiol* 124:1–16, 1966.

Curran JW, Morgan WM, Hardy AM, et al.: The epidemiology of AIDS: Current status and future prospects. *Science* 279:1352–1357, 1985.

Garry RF, Witte MH, Gottleib A, et al.: Documentation of an AIDS virus infection in the United States in 1968. *JAMA* 260:2085–2087, 1988.

Jaffe HW, Bergman DJ, Selik RM: Acquired immune deficiency syndrome in the United States: The first 1,000 cases. *J Infect Dis* 148:339–345, 1983.

Lehner T, Bergmeier LA, Panagoitidi C, et al.: Induction of mucosal and systemic immunity to a recombinant simian immunodeficiency viral protein. *Science* 258:1365, 1992.

O'Brien TR, George JR, Holmberg SD: Human immunodeficiency virus type 2 infection in the United States. *JAMA* 267:2775, 1992.

Zolla-Pazner S, Gorny MK: Passive immunization for the prevention and treatment of HIV infection. *AIDS* 6:1235, 1992.

NATURAL HISTORY/ PATHOGENESIS

Armstrong D: Opportunistic infections in the acquired immune deficiency syndrome. *Semin Hematol* 14:40–47, 1987.

Ascher MA, Sheppard HW: AIDS as immune system activation. II. The panergic amnesia hypothesis. *J Acq Immun Def Syndr* 3:177–191, 1990.

Bednarik DP, Folks, TM: Mechanisms of HIV-1 latency. *AIDS* 6:3, 1992.

Cameron PU, Freudenthal PS, Barker JM, et al.: Dendritic cells exposed to human immunodeficiency virus type 1 transmit a vigorous cytopathic infection to CD4+ T cells. *Science:* 257:383, 1992.

Chang Y, Cesarman E, Pessin MS: Identification of herpes-like DNA sequences in AIDS-associated sarcoma. *Science* 266:1865–1869, 1994.

Edelman AS, Zolla-Pazner S: AIDS: A syndrome of immune dysregulation, dysfunction, and deficiency. *FASEB J* 3:22–30, 1989.

Farrar WF, Korner M, Clouse KA: Cytokine regulation of human immunodeficiency virus expression. *Cytokine* 3:531, 1991.

Fiala M, Mosca JD, Barry P, et al.: Multistep pathogenesis of AIDS: Role of cytomegalovirus. *Res Immunol* 142:87, 1991.

Germain RN: Antigen processing and CD4+ T-cell depletion in AIDS. *Cell* 54:441–444, 1988.

Ho DD, Neumann AU, Perelson AS, et al.: Rapid turnover of plasma virions and CD4 lymphocytes in HIV-1 infection. *Nature* 12:123–126, 1995.

Ho DD, Pomerantz RJ, Kaplan JC: Pathogenesis of infection with human immunodeficiency virus. *N Engl J Med* 317:278–286, 1987.

Johnson RT, McArthur JC, Narayan O.: The neurobiology of human immunodeficiency virus infections. *FASEB J* 2:2970–2981, 1988.

Lifson AR, Hessol NA, Rutherford GW: Progression and clinical outcome of infection due to human immunodeficiency virus. *Clin Infect Dis* 14:966, 1992.

McCune JM: HIV-1: The infective process in vivo. *Cell* 64:351, 1991.

Meltzer MS, Skillman DR, Gomatos PJ, et al.: Role of mononuclear phagocytes in the pathogenesis of human immunodeficiency virus infection: *Annu Rev Immunol* 8:169–194, 1990.

Merrill JE, Chen ISY: HIV-1, macrophages, glial cells, and cytokines in AIDS nervous system disease. *FASEB J* 5:2391, 1991.

Root-Bernstein RS: Multiple antigen-mediated autoimmunity (MAMA) in AIDS: A possible model for postinfectious antoimmune complications. *Res Immunol* 41:321–339, 1990.

Rosenberg ZF, Fauci AS: Immunopathogenesis of HIV infection. *FASEB J* 5:2382, 1991.

Rossi P, Moschese V: Mother-to-child transmission of human immunodeficiency virus. *FASEB J* 5:2419, 1991.

Shearer GM, Clerici M: Early T-helper cell defects in HIV infection. *AIDS* 5:245, 1991.

Sheppard HW, Lang W, Ascher MS, et al.: The characterization of nonprogressors: Long-term HIV-1 infection with stable CD4+ T-cell levels. *AIDS* 7:1159–1166, 1993.

Wei X, Ghosh SK, Taylor ME, et al.: Viral dynamics in human immunodeficiency virus type 1 infection. *Nature* 12:117–122, 1995.

Wormser GP (ed.): *AIDS and Other Manifestations of HIV Infection*, 2nd ed. New York, Raven Press, 1992.

DIAGNOSIS/
PATHOGENESIS/
IMMUNE
DYSFUNCTION/
STAGING

Armstrong JA: Ultrastructural and significance of the lymphoid tissue lesions in HIV infection. In Racz P, Dijkstra CD, Gluckman JC (eds.). Accessory cells in HIV and other retroviral infections. Basel, Karger, 1991, 69.

Bagasra O, Hauptman SP, Lischner HW, et al.: Detection of human immunodeficiency virus type 1 provirus in mononuclear cells by in situ polymerase chain reaction *N Engl J Med* 326:1385, 1992.

Bjork RL: HIV-1: Seven facets of functional molecular mimicry. *Immunol Lett* 28:91, 1991.

Blatt SP, Hendrix CW, Butzin CA, et al.: Delayed-type hypersensitivity skin testing predicts progression to AIDS in HIV-infected patients. *Ann Int Med* 119:177-184, 1993.

Buchbinder A, Josephs SF, Ablashi D, et al.: Polymerase chain reaction amplification and in situ hybridization for the detection of human T-lymphotrophic virus. *J Virol Meth* 21:191, 1988.

Centers for Disease Control: Interpretation and use of western blot assay for serodiagnosis of human immunodeficiency virus type 1 infections. *Morbid Mortal Weekly Rep* 38 (suppl. S-7):1, 1989.

Centers for Disease Control: Unexplained CD4+ T-lymphocyte depletion in persons without evident HIV infection—United States. *Morbid Mortal Weekly Rep* 41:541, 1992.

Consortium for Retrovirus Serology Standardization: Serologic diagnosis of human immunodeficiency virus infection by western blot testing. *JAMA* 260:674–679, 1988.

Constantine NT: Serologic tests for the retroviruses: Approaching a decade of evolution. *AIDS* 7:1, 1993.

Constantine NT, Callahan JD, Watts DM: Retroviral testing: Essentials for quality control and laboratory diagnosis: Boca Raton, FL, CRC Press, 1992.

Daar ES, Moudgil, T, Meyer RD, et al.: Transient high levels of viremia in patients with primary human immunodeficiency virus type 1 infection. *N Engl J Med* 324:961, 1991.

Defer C, Agut H, Garbatg-Chenon A, et al.: Multicenter quality control of polymerase chain reaction for detection of HIV DNA. *AIDS* 6:659, 1992.

Eble BE, Busch MP, Khayam-Bashi H, et al.: Resolution of infection status of HIV-seroindeterminate donors and high-risk seronegative individuals with polymerase chain reaction and virus culture: Absence of persistent silent HIV type 1 infection in a high-prevalence area. *Transfusion* 32:503, 1992.

Fox CH, Tenner-Racz K, Racz P, et al.: Lymphoid germinal centers are reservoirs of HIV-1 RNA. *J Infect Dis* 164:1051, 1991.

Grant MD, Smail FM, Rosenthal KL: Cytotoxic T-Lymphocytes that kill autologous CD4+ lymphocytes are associated with CD4+ lymphocyte depletion in HIV-1 infection. *J AIDS Synd* 7:571–579, 1994.

Imagawa DT, Lee MH, Wolinski SM, et al.: HIV-1 infection in homosexual men who remain seronegative for prolonged periods. *N Engl J Med* 320:1458–1462, 1989.

Jackson JB: HIV-indeterminate western blots and latent HIV infection. *Transfusion* 32:497, 1992.

Janossy G, Autran B, Miedema F: Immunodeficiency in HIV infection and AIDS. Farmington, CT, S Karger, 1992.

Krueger GRF, Ablashi DV, Lusso P, et al.: Immunologic dysregulation of lymph nodes in AIDS patients. *Curr Top Pathol* 84:157, 1991.

Lawrence J, Hodtsev AS, Posnett DN: Superantigen implicated in dependence of HIV-1 replication in T cells on TCR V_β expression. *Nature* 358:255, 1992.

Levine AM: Acquired immunodeficiency syndrome-related lymphoma. *Blood* 80:8, 1992.

Levy JA: Pathogenesis of human immunodeficiency virus infection. *Microbiol Rev* 57:183, 1993.

Littlefield JW: Possible supplemental mechanisms in the pathogenesis of AIDS. *Clin Immunol Immunopathol* 65:85, 1992.

Meyaard L, Otto SA, Jonker RR, et al.: Programmed death of T cells in HIV-1 infection. *Science* 257:217, 1992.

Miller CJ, McGhee Jr, Gardner MB: Mucosal immunity, HIV transmission, and AIDS. *Lab Invest* 68:129, 1992.

Milman G, D'Souza MP: HIV-mediated defects in immune regulations. *AIDS Res Hum Retrovir* 10:421–430, 1994.

Montagnier L, Gougeon ML, Oliver R, et al.: Factors and mechanisms of AIDS pathogenesis. In: *Science Challenging AIDS*. Rossi GB, Beth-Giraldo E., Chieco-Bianchi L, et al. (eds.). Basel, Karger, 1992, 51.

Morrow WJW, Isenberg DA, Sobol RE, et al.: AIDS virus infection and autoimmunity: A perspective of the clinical, immunologic, and molecular origins of the autoallergic pathologies associated with HIV disease. *Clin Immunol Immunopathol* 58:163, 1991.

Psallidopoulos MC, Schnittman SM, Thompson LM, et al.: Integrated proviral HIV-1 is present in CD4+ peripheral blood lymphocytes in healthy seropositive individuals. *J Virol* 63:4626–4631, 1989.

Richman DD, McCutchan JA, Spector SA: Detecting HIV RNA in peripheral blood mononuclear cells by nucleic acid hybridization. *J Infect Dis* 156:823–827, 1987.

Sharer LR: Pathology of HIV-1 infection of the central nervous system: A review. *J Neuropathol Exp Neurol* 51:3, 1992.

Stein DS, Korvick JA, Vermund SH: CD4+ lymphocyte cell enumeration for prediction of clinical course of HIV disease: A review. *J Infect Dis* 165:352, 1992.

Stellrecht KA, Sperber K, Pogo BGT: Activation of HIV-1 long-terminal repeat by vaccinia virus. *J Virol* 66:2051, 1992.

Stute R: Comparison in sensitivity of ten HIV antibody detection tests by serial dilutions of western blot confirmed samples. *J Virol Meth* 20:269–273, 1988.

Tsoukas CM, Bernard NF: Markers predicting progression of human immunodeficiency virus-related disease. *Clin Microbiol Rev* 7:14–28, 1994.

WHO Collaborating Group on Western Blotting: Proposed WHO criteria for interpreting results from western blot assays for HIV-1, HIV-2, and HTLV-1/HTLV-2. *WHO Weekly Epidemiol Rec* 37:281, 1990.

Wiley CA, Johnson RT, Reingold SC: Neurologic consequences of immune dysfunction: Lessons from HIV infection and multiple sclerosis. *J Neuroimmunol* 40:115, 1992.

THERAPY

Arnold E, Arnold GF: Human immunodeficiency virus structure: Implications for antiviral design. *Adv Virus Res* 39:1, 1991.

Cooper DA, Gatell JM, Kroon S, et al.: Zidovudine in persons with asymptomatic HIV infection and CD4+ cell counts greater than 400 per cubic millimeter. *N Engl J Med* 329:297–303, 1993.

Feinberg J, Hoth DF: Current status of HIV therapy. II. Opportunistic infections. *Hosp Pract* 27:107, 1992.

Graham NMH, Zeger SL, Lawrence LP, et al.: The effects on survival of early treatment of HIV infection. *N Engl J Med* 326:1037, 1992.

Hoth DF, Myers MW, Stein DS: Current status of HIV therapy. I. Retroviral agents. *Hosp Pract* 27:95, 1992.

Lane HC, Fauci AS: Immunologic reconstitution in the acquired immunodeficiency syndrome. *Ann Int Med* 103:714–718, 1985.

Mitsuya H, Yarchoan R, Kadeyama S, et al.: Targeted therapy of human immunodeficiency virus-related disease. *FASEB J* 5:2369, 1991.

Murphy PM, Lane HC, Gallin JI, et al.: Marked disparity in incidence of bacterial infections in patients with AIDS receiving interleukin-2 or interferon. *Ann Intern Med* 108:36–41, 1988.

Richman DD: Antiviral therapy of HIV infection. *Annu Rev Med* 42:69, 1991.

Sarver N, Rossi JJ: Gene therapy for HIV-1 infection: Progress and prospects. *J NIH Res* 5:63–67, 1993.

Schinazi RF, Mead JR, Feorino PM: Insights into HIV chemotherapy. *AIDS Res Human Retrovir* 8:963, 1992.

Tindall B, Cooper DA: Primary HIV infections: Host responses and intervention strategies. *AIDS* 5:1, 1991.

Yap PL, Williams PE: Immunoglobulin preparations for HIV-infected patients. *Vox Sang* 55:65–74, 1988.

Yeni P, Schooley R, Hammer S: Antiretroviral and immune-based therapies: Update. *Current Sci* 7 (Suppl. 1):S173–S184, 1993.

VACCINE DEVELOPMENT

Arthur LO, Bess JW, Sowder RC, et al.: Cellular proteins bound to immunodeficiency viruses: Implications for pathogenesis and vaccines. *Science* 258:1935, 1992.

Berman PW, Gregory TJ, Riddle L, et al.: Protection of chimpanzees from infection by HIV-1 after vaccination with recombinant glycoprotein gp120 but not gp160. *Nature* 345:622–625, 1990.

Berzofsky JA: Development of artificial vaccines against HIV using defined epitopes. *FASEB J* 5:2412–2418, 1991.

Bolognesi DP: Natural immunity to HIV and its possible relationship to vaccine strategies. *Microbiol Sci* 5:236–241, 1988.

Clerici M, Tacket CO, Via CS, et al.: Immunization with subunit HIV vaccine generates stronger T-helper cell immunity than natural infection. *Eur J. Immunol* 21:1345, 1991.

Cohen J: Pediatric AIDS vaccine trials set. *Science* 258:1568, 1992.

Cooney EL, McElrath MJ, Corey L, et al.: Enhanced immunity to HIV envelope elicited by a combined vaccine regimen consisting of priming with a vaccinia recombinant-expressing HIV envelope and boosting with gp160 protein. *Proc Natl Acad Sci USA* 90:1882–1886, 1993.

Daniel MD, Kirchhoff F, Czajak AC, et al.: Protective effects of a live, attenuated SIV vaccine with a deletion in the nef gene. *Science* 258:1938, 1992.

Dolin R, Graham BS, Greenberg SB, et al.: The safety and immunogenicity of an HIV-1 recombinant gp160 candidate vaccine in humans. *Ann Int Med* 114:119, 1991.

Gorny MK, Xu J-Y, Gianakakos V, et al.: Production of site-selected neutralizing human monoclonal antibodies against the third variable domain of the HIV-1 envelope glycoprotein. *Proc Natl Acad Sci USA* 88:3238, 1991.

Goudsmit J, Back NKT, Nara PF: Genomic diversity and antigenic variation of HIV-1: Links between pathogenesis, epidemiology, and vaccine development. *FASEB J* 5:2427, 1991.

Hinkuo J, Rosen J, Sundqvist V-A, et al.: Epitope mapping of the HIV-1 gag region with monoclonal antibodies. *Molec Immunol* 27:395–403, 1990.

Johnston MI, Noe JS Killen JY: Recent advances in AIDS vaccine research and development. *AIDS Res Human Retro* 10(Suppl 2):S317-S322, 1994.

Katzenstein DA, Sawyer LA, Quinnan GV: Issues in the evaluation of AIDS vaccines. *AIDS* 2:151,155, 1988.

Lasky LA: Current status of the development of an AIDS vaccine. *CRC Crit Rev Immunol* 9:153–168, 1989.

Nixon DF, Broliden K, Ogg G, et al.: Cellular and humoral antigenic epitopes in HIV and SIV. *Immunology* 76:515, 1992.

Nowak MA: Variability of HIV infections. *J Theor Biol* 155:1, 1992.

Prince AM, Horowita B, Baker L, et al.: Failure of an HIV immune globulin to protect chimpanzees against experimental challenge with HIV. *Proc Natl Acad Sci* 85:6944–6948, 1988.

Redfield RR, Birx DL: HIV-specific vaccine therapy: Concepts, status, and future directions. *AIDS Res Hum Retrovir* 8:1051, 1992.

Spear GT, Takefman DM, Sharpe S, et al.: Antibodies to HIV-1 V$_3$ loop in serum from infected persons constitute a major portion of immune effector functions including complement activation, antibody binding, and neutralization. *Virology* 204:609–615, 1994.

Takahashi H, Takeshita T, Merli S, et al.: Induction of CD8+ cytotoxic T cells by immunization with purified HIV-1 envelope protein in ISCOMs. *Nature* 344:873–875, 1990.

Wigzell H: Prospectus for an HIV vaccine. *FASEB J* 5:2406, 1991.

Zagury D, Gagne I, Reveil B, et al.: Repairing the T-cell defects in AIDS. *Lancet* 2:449, 1985.

ANIMAL MODELS

Brady HJM, Pennington DJ, Dzierak EA: Transgenic mice as models of human deficiency virus expression and related cellular effects. *J Gen Virol* 75:2549–2558, 1994.

Desrosiers RC: Simian immunodeficiency viruses. *Annu Rev Microbiol* 42:607–625, 1988.

Gardner MB, Luciw PA: Animal models of AIDS. *FASEB J* 3:2593–2606, 1989.

Hu S-L, Abrams K, Barber GN, et al.: Protection of macaques against SIV infection by subunit vaccines of SIV envelope glycoprotein gp160. *Science* 255:456, 1992.

Jolicoeur PJ: Murine-acquired immunodeficiency syndrome (MAIDS): An animal model to study AIDS pathogenesis. *FASEB J* 5:2398, 1991.

Kock JA: Ruprecht RM: Animal models for anti-AIDS therapy. *Antiviral Res* 19:81, 1992.

McCune JM, Namikawa R, Kaneshima H, et al.: The SCID-hu mouse: Murine model for the analysis of human hematolymphoid differentiation and function. *Science* 241:1632–1639, 1988.

Morse HC, Chattopadhyay SK, Makino M, et al.: Retrovirus-induced immunodeficiency in the mouse: MAIDS as a model for AIDS. *AIDS* 6:607, 1992.

Schellekens H, Horzinek M: *Animal Models in AIDS.* New York, Elsevier, 1990.

Simon MA, Chalifoux LV, Ringler DJ: Pathologic features of SIV-induced disease and the association of macrophage infection with disease evolution. *AIDS Res Hum Retrovir* 8:327, 1992.

30

Tumor Immunity

This chapter deals with the role of host immune mechanisms in the host–tumor relationship. The topics include the nature of tumor antigens, immune effector mechanisms against cancer, and prevention of growth of newly formed cancer (immunosurveillance), as well as immune approaches to the diagnosis, treatment, and prevention of human cancer. Cancer is the progressive replacement of normal tissue by an increase in the number of cells of one lineage. Instead of a steady-state relationship between the production and destruction of cells, cancer cells die at a slower rate than they are produced, leading to an increase in the number of cancer cells and the mass of cancerous tissue. In some cases, growth occurs at only one site, called the primary site. In others, the malignant cells seed to and grow at other "secondary" sites. This is called metastasis. The loss of the function of the normal tissue replaced by, or impinged upon by, the primary cancer and/or the metastases leads to the symptoms of the cancer and eventual death of the patient.

Host–Tumor Relationships

TUMOR AUTONOMY AND IMMUNITY

One of the key characteristics of a cancer is its autonomy, that is, its ability to grow independently of host mechanisms that limit the number of normal cells. On the other hand, some experimental tumors express antigens that can be recognized as foreign by the immune system. The immune system may be able to prevent the emergence of these tumors or eradicate small tumor masses (tumor immunity). A short history of observations supporting the concept of tumor immunity is given in Table 30–1.

TABLE 30–1. A SHORT HISTORY OF TUMOR IMMUNITY

1898	Halsted	Lymphocytic infiltration and lymph node hyperplasia seen in cancers with good prognoses
1900	Erlich	Proposed tumor-specific immunity
1904	Loeb	Tumor transplantation in inbred Japanese waltzing mice
1906	Schone	Tumor immunity induced by fetal tissues in outbred mice
1908	Wade	Tumor grafts rejected in outbred animals—associated with lymphocyte infiltration
1941	Gross	Tumor grafts rejected in partially inbred mice
1953	Foley	Tumor grafts rejected in fully inbred mice
1957	Prehn	Primary tumor used to immunize syngeneic mice
1960	Klein	Tumor-specific rejection in autochthonous hosts (mice)

EXPERIMENTAL TUMOR IMMUNITY

Studies on tumor immunity in animals have provided provocative insights into human disease. Normal animals make both cellular and humoral immune responses to tumor antigens. In some cases, strong cellular immune responses are able to effect destruction of well-established transplantable tumors. However, many spontaneously occurring tumors in animals do not have demonstrable tumor antigens. In addition, since immune products may affect tumor growth in a variety of ways, immunization may result in increased tumor growth, decreased tumor growth, or have no effect, depending on the nature of the tumor and the type of immune response stimulated.

From the animal models, one can predict that the immune response to tumors in humans will be enormously varied and difficult to control. Some tumors would be expected to be highly antigenic and responsive to immunotherapeutic and immunoprophylactic procedures. Unfortunately, most human tumors seem to be like spontaneously occurring tumors of animals. Thus, animal models of tumor-specific transplantation using highly antigenic tumors may have little relevance to human tumors. In addition, transplantation tumor immunity may not reflect what happens in the autochthonous host. What is true for one tumor may not be true for another. Even tumors of similar histologic type and growth pattern may provoke entirely different immune responses.

TUMOR IMMUNITY IN HUMANS

The evidence supporting the hypothesis that immune reactivity may control or limit the growth of human tumors is listed in Table 30–2. However, the evidence is circumstantial, and definitive proof of effective tumor immunity in humans has not been obtained.

Spontaneous remissions of different human tumors have been rec-

TABLE 30–2. EVIDENCE FOR TUMOR IMMUNITY IN HUMANS

Event	Comment
1. Spontaneous regression	Rare; usually tumors that could be controlled by developmental factors or contain foreign antigens (ie, paternal antigens in chorio-carcinomas)
2. Regression of metastases after removal of primary tumor	Rare, not necessarily immune-mediated
3. Reappearance of metastases after long latent periods	Not necessarily immune-mediated, determined by nature of the tumor
4. Failure of circulating cells to form metastases	Most likely not immune-mediated; circulating cells may not find supportive environment
5. Infiltration of tumors by mono-nuclear cells	Could be secondary effect; not always associated with tumor regression
6. High incidence of cancer in immunosuppressed, aged, or immunity deficient patients	Strong circumstantial evidence; usually lymphomas; may be due to loss of controlling T cells or virus infection
7. Depressed immune reactivity in cancer patients	Associated with debilitated state of patient; a secondary effect of cancer
8. Tumor antigens identified by in vitro assays on human cancers	In vitro assays not reliable indication of in vivo tumor rejection
9. Cancer patients may have delayed skin tests to cancer extracts	Significance of skin tests not clear
10. Immune complexes and glomerulo-nephritis are found in some cancer patients	Relationship of immune complexes to tumor resistance not documented, antigens in complexes may not be to tumor antigens; antibodies to tumor antigens may aid tumor growth

ognized. Although many claims of spontaneous remission of human cancer do not hold up to critical review, Emerson (after an extensive survey) accepted 130 cases of spontaneous regression of malignant tumors. Of these, 10% were choriocarcinomas, in which paternal antigens foreign to the maternal host are expressed. Spontaneous regressions have also been reported in about 15% of nodular lymphomas, a form of B-cell cancer subject to control by other cells in the lymphocyte series, and in malignant melanomas, the cancer most likely to elicit immune rejection.

Regression of metastases after removal of a primary tumor is a rare and complex phenomenon. One explanation is that removal of the primary tumor permits an immune response to tumor antigens to become directed to metastatic lesions. However, other complex phenomena involving the biology of the tumor and host factors, such as hormonal requirements for tumor growth being altered by removal of the primary tumor or dependence of the metastases on factors produced by the primary tumor, could be the explanation.

Reappearance of metastases after a long latent period is an example of tumor dormancy. It has been documented in experimental models that tumor cells may exist in a quiescent state for many years. Changes in blood supply, operative trauma, or other events are associated with tumor cells breaking out of the dormant state. This is sometimes related to an immunosuppressive event.

Failure of circulating tumor cells to form metastases has been well documented in both animal and human studies. During cancer surgery, large numbers of tumor cells may be released into the circulation, yet later, metastases are not found. This can be explained by a number of nonimmune mechanisms, such as the inability of the tumor cells to escape successfully from the circulation and proliferate away from the primary site, clearing of tumor cells from the circulation by the reticuloendothelial system, or distribution of tumor cells to nonsupportive environments.

Tumor tissue is often infiltrated by large numbers of lymphocytes, perhaps because of a cellular immunologic reaction to tumor antigens. In 1898, William Halsted described perivascular infiltration by lymphocytes and hyperplasia of draining lymph nodes in patients with large breast cancers that had a relatively prolonged course without metastases as compared to breast cancers without infiltrating lymphocytes. Lymphocytes infiltrating the base of a malignant melanoma are associated with a more favorable prognosis than melanomas in the vertical growth phase that lack a lymphocytic infiltrate. Lymphocytes that are found in tumors are known as "tumor infiltrating lymphocytes" (TILs). These cells can be isolated from tumors, expanded, and activated in vitro and used for passive immunotherapy of cancer (see below).

An increased incidence of cancer is found in patients with primary or secondary immune deficiency states. A tabulation of the occurrence of primary cancer in transplant patients during immunosuppressive therapy showed that the overall occurrence for all cancers was far greater (13:2000) than in the general population (8.2:100,000). However, immunosuppressed individuals have a preponderance of skin cancer and lymphomas, which may reflect abnormalities in control of lymphoid cell proliferation rather than suppression of immunity per se or susceptibility to cancer in general. A good case has been made that all cancers in immunosuppressed patients are viral or ultraviolet light-exposure associated.

Since the majority of cancers occur in patients over 65 years of age, it has been suggested that this is due to the age-associated decline in immune function. However, many important interactions of normal aging and carcinogenesis are incompletely understood. It is likely that other factors, such as the time required for the multistep process of carcinogenesis to become manifest and the effect of aging on DNA repair, are more important than the decline in immunity with aging.

Some cancer patients have decreased cell-mediated immune responses to a variety of antigens, and these patients appear to have more rapid tumor growth than cancer patients whose cell-mediated immunity is not decreased. In addition, cellular immune deficiency is more marked in patients with disseminated tumor growth or those who respond poorly to therapy. This may reflect more the debilitated state of a terminal cancer patient rather than a specific immune deficit, and some tumors may produce immunosuppressive products.

Some human tumors have tumor antigens detectable by in vitro assays. Several human tumor-specific antigens have been identified by these assays (see below). Although reasonable data have been obtained in various animal systems that correlate cellular immune reactivity to ability of an animal to resist tumor challenge, the specificity of cellular tests for human tumors has been questioned. One major problem has been the finding of lymphocytes that are cytotoxic for tumor cells in normal individuals. Thus, whereas lymphocytes from cancer patients may react with certain tumor target cells, similar cells from normal persons often react just as strongly. These are called natural killer (NK) cells. In addition, tumor cell lines have been used almost exclusively as target cells for human lymphocytic killer cells. These cell lines may not express the same antigenicity as the original tumor. Therefore, most of the data in which in vitro human tumor immunity was tested using cell lines is subject to different interpretations. In may be necessary to perform all such tests using primary cultures of freshly obtained tumor target cells.

A tumor-bearing patient may produce a delayed hypersensitivity skin reaction against a membrane extract of his own tumor cells, but the significance of such a reaction is difficult to evaluate. In addition, immediate (2-minute) skin reactions to tumor extracts preincubated with the patient's serum (Markari test) have been reported to be an indicator of the presence of tumors, but this has not been generally accepted.

Circulating immune complexes and glomerular immune complex disease, frequently subclinical, are found in about 10% of all cancer patients. In a few cases, the glomerular deposits of complexes have been demonstrated to contain tumor-associated antigen (carcinoembryonic antigen [CEA]) or antibody to CEA. The relationship of these complexes to tumor resistance is not known, but it suggests that an antibody to a tumor "antigen" is present. Such antibodies may actually aid tumor growth (see Immune Facilitation, below).

In summary, the evidence that an immune response does occur to some human tumors and that this response may, in rare cases, be responsible for regression of inoperable primary tumors remains circumstantial. Demonstrations of effective tumor resistance in humans due to an immune response to the tumor are exceptions to the general rule.

CARCINO-GENESIS AND TUMOR IMMUNITY

If the immune system is playing a prominent role in development of cancers, then agents that cause cancer (carcinogens), would be expected to be immunosuppressive and immunosuppressive agents would be expected to be carcinogenic. Two potent skin carcinogens, dimethylbenzeneanthracene and ultraviolet (UV) irradiation, cause convincing immune suppression, whereas most others do not. Thus, immunosuppression is not a common feature of carcinogens. UV exposure acts through alteration of DNA to induce mutations and transform epithelial cells (induce cancerous changes in growth behavior), as well as cause both local and systemic immune effects. Locally, there is a marked loss of Langerhans' cells in the skin, as well as T-suppressor cell activation that blocks an immune response to the developing tumors. UV-induced tumors are highly immunogenic in syngeneic nonirradiated mice, but UV irradiation suppresses the response in the original host. In addition, there is a transient depression of delayed hypersensitivity and contact dermatitis reactions to nontumor antigens, believed to be caused by release of suppressive cytokines from keratinocytes. UV irradiation thus produces both a tumor-specific and -nonspecific immunosuppression that allows strongly antigenic tumors to develop. UV-induced tumors to express not only tumor-specific antigens for T-effector cells but also shared antigens for T-suppressor cells. On the other hand, strong hepatocarcinogens, such as acetylaminofluorene and diethylnitrosamine, produce little, if any, immunosuppression. Phorbol esters, which are promoting agents, may produce up to a 50% reduction in NK activity, but they are also mitogenic for lymphocytes. With the high interest in this aspect of carcinogenesis, it is noteworthy that there are not more published results indicating that carcinogens are immunosuppressive. Thus, it appears that carcinogens, such as UV radiation, which induce tumors with relatively strong transplantation antigens, also cause immunosuppression, whereas carcinogens that do not induce transplantation antigens are not immunosuppressive.

IMMUNO-SUPPRESSION AND CARCINO-GENESIS

Although it is generally accepted that immunosuppressive drugs may act as carcinogens, based on the finding of high cancer rates in patients on immunosuppressive drugs, there are few data to support a direct relationship. In an extensive study in rats, the immunosuppressive drugs methotrexate, 5-fluorouracil, and azathioprine, were not carcinogenic, although a number of other nonimmunosuppressive anticancer drugs were carcinogenic. However, immunosuppressive drugs may act to enhance the carcinogenicity of other agents. Azathioprine appears to increase the carcinogenic effects of sunlight in renal transplant patients. In experimental models, immunosuppression may have different effects. A biphasic response was discovered when carcinogen-treated skin was grafted onto mice with different degrees of immuno-suppression. More tumors occurred in moderately immunosuppressed mice than in mice with high or low immunosuppressive doses of irra-diation, thus suggesting that immunity may either inhibit or stimulate tumor growth.

Tumor Antigens

A number of cell surface antigenic changes may occur in tissues that undergo malignant change. These include the loss of antigenic speci-ficities present in normal tissue, the addition of new antigenic specifici-ties not present in normal tissue, the appearance of markers present in fetal or embryonic tissue but not present in normal adult tissue (oncode-velopmental products), and combinations of the above (Fig. 30–1).

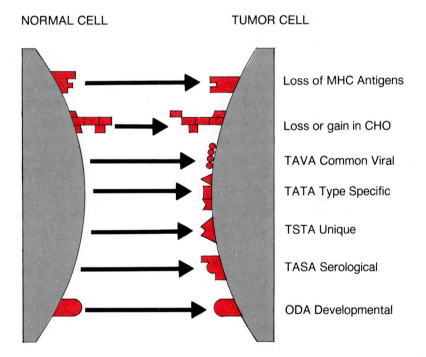

Figure 30–1. Some antigenic features of tumor cells. A number of changes in the cell surface of tumor cells has been noted, including loss or gain of histocompatibility antigen, loss or gain of cell surface carbo-hydrates, the appearance of viral-associated antigens (tumor-associated viral antigen [TAVA]), and tumor-associated transplantation antigens common for tumors of the same histologic type (TATA). Also seen are tumor-specific transplantation antigens present on only one tumor (TSTA), antigens detected by only serologic reactions that are unique for a given tumor (tumor-associated serologically defined antigens), and markers shared by embryonic or developing tumors and tumors (oncode-velopmental antigens [ODA]).

A fundamental problem in the study of tumor immunity is the identification of new tumor-specific antigens not present in normal tissues. At least three types of tumor antigens have been identified: Those found associated with chemically or physically induced tumors or with some spontaneous tumors of animals and humans, virus-induced tumor antigens, and oncodevelopmental antigens.

TUMOR-SPECIFIC TRANSPLANTATION ANTIGENS

The first type of tumor antigen includes those identified by transplantation in experimental animals (TSTAs) but not yet identified in human tumors. These antigens may be divided into two general classes—those that are specific for a given tumor and those that are shared by two or more tumors, generally of a particular histologic type. A given tumor may have both unique and shared antigens. For diagnostic and therapeutic purposes in humans, antigenic specificities shared by a large number of tumors of a given class are potentially much more valuable than unique antigens. Detection of a shared antigen could be used as a screening test for tumors in different persons or used for preventive immunization, whereas a unique antigen would not be detected by a common antigen screening test and would be effective as an immunogen only in the individual with that tumor. A skin tumor induced in a mouse by the carcinogen methylcholanthrene is usually antigenically different from every other skin tumor induced by methylcholanthrene. Indeed, two primary tumors induced in the same animal are antigenically distinct. This demonstration of tumor-specific antigens extends to other chemically induced tumors, including sarcomas induced by aromatic hydrocarbons, hepatomas induced by azo dyes, and mammary carcinomas induced by methylcholanthrene, as well as to tumors induced by physical agents, such as implantation of cellophane films or millipore filters.

Tumor-specific transplantation antigens may be related to, but are clearly different from, histocompatibility transplantation antigens. As early as 1910, it was observed that the serum of mice that had recovered from tumors inhibited tumor growth in other mice, sometimes causing regression and an apparent cure. Attempts were made to treat cancer with immunization methods similar to those that had proved successful with infectious diseases, and promising results were obtained in experimental animals. This raised hopes that tumor-specific immune reactions could cure cancer. However, it became apparent that the results obtained were not because of tumor-specific antigens but because of histocompatibility antigens. In other words, normal tissue and tumor tissue from the tumor donor were rejected in a similar manner by the same recipient. Terms used to identify host–tumor relationships are the same as those used for tissue graft donor–recipient relationships (Table 30–3). Both tissue and tumor

TABLE 30–3. TERMINOLOGY OF HOST–TUMOR GRAFT RELATIONSHIPS

Relationship	Terminology
Same individual	Autochthonous
Genetically identical (twin, inbred strain)	Syngeneic
Different individual, same species	Allogeneic
Different species	Xenogeneic

grafts will survive in autochthonous or syngeneic recipients, but not in allogeneic or xenogeneic recipients.

The inability to demonstrate TSTAs led to a general loss of interest in tumor immunity, until the development of inbred strains of mice. In 1943, Ludwig Gross transplanted tumors (sarcomas), induced by the chemical methylcholanthrene, in inbred mice. He found that tumor nodules appeared after tumor cells were injected into the skin, grew for a few days, and then regressed. After regression, reinjection of cells from the same tumor did not produce a tumor nodule, demonstrating that the syngeneic animals that had rejected the transplanted tumor were now resistant to it. Almost 20 years later, Prehn followed up Gross's observations. Prehn tested 3-methylcholanthrene–induced sarcomas of C_3H/He mouse origin. Immunization was accomplished by strangulation of the first or second transplant generation of tumor grafts. Following tumor regression, the animals were rechallenged with living cells, and the frequency of "takes" was then compared with that in untreated controls. Resistance to challenge was noted when the mice were reinjected with the same tumor. Appropriate controls involving skin grafts and immunization with normal tissue ruled out the possibility that rejection is caused by antigens present in normal tissue and not specific for the tumor. In 1957, Prehn extended these observations by showing that tumor-specific immunity could be produced by allowing a tumor to grow and then removing it by surgical excision. Animals that had been immunized in this way could then reject the same transplantable tumor, even if greater numbers of tumor cells were injected. He also found that chemically induced tumors possessed individually specific tumor antigens; immunization of an animal to one chemically induced tumor did not protect it from growth of a different chemically induced tumor.

IMMUNE RESPONSE OF THE PRIMARY TUMOR-BEARING HOST

The studies cited describe immunity to transplanted tumors in syngeneic animals, but can an individual make an immune response to his own "autochthonous" tumor? The term autochthonous is used to indicate the relationship between a tumor and the individual in which that tumor arose (primary host). To demonstrate autochthonous tumor immunity, primary methylcholanthrene-induced sarcomas were excised from the autochthonous animal and maintained by passage in syngeneic recipients. Transplantation of the passaged tumor back to the autochthonous host resulted in rejection of the tumor 3 to 4 weeks later (Fig. 30–2). Thus, an experimental animal may make an immune response to its own tumor, and this response may be effective in controlling the growth of the tumor (autochthonous tumor resistance). In some instances, the primary tumor-bearing animal (autochthonous host) may have an immune response that can be demonstrated by rejection upon transplantation of part of the tumor to another site or by in vitro tests, but in spite of this response, the primary tumor grows progressively in vivo. This is termed **"concomitant immunity."** Primary tumors in individuals with concomitant immunity are able to avoid immune attack that is effective if the same tumor cells are inoculated at another site.

ETIOLOGY AND IMMUNOGENICITY OF TUMORS

The immunogenicity of a given tumor-specific antigen is related to the etiology of the tumor. Virus-induced tumors have strong antigens that are shared by other tumors caused by the same virus. Skin cancers induced by ultraviolet light demonstrate both common and tumor-specific antigens and are much more immunogenic than tumors induced by chemicals. Tumors induced by large doses of carcinogens are generally more likely to express tumor-specific transplantation antigens than tumors induced by smaller doses of carcinogens. In addition, tumors induced by "strong" carcinogens are more likely to be immunogenic than tumors induced by "weak" carcinogens (Table 30–4).

Individual tumor-specific antigens are more easily demonstrated on chemically induced tumors than on virus-induced tumors because of the presence of common viral antigens on virus-induced tumors. Spontaneous tumors of mice may lack tumor antigens or express them very weakly. Some tumor antigens may be identified only serologically. Epitopes identified serologically do not necessarily induce a rejection reaction.

NATURE OF TUMOR-SPECIFIC ANTIGENS

The chemical nature of tumor-specific antigens remains unclear. Are these new molecules not present in normal tissues or rearrangements of normal structures? There is no conclusive evidence that TSTAs are caused by mutations of structural genes, despite the well-known mutagenic properties of carcinogens and the possibility that rearranged genes in tumors, such as leukemias, may code for new fusion proteins. It is likely that not all tumor antigens are specific for tumors but may be present in small amounts in normal tissue. These are called tumor-associated antigens. For instance, protection against some syngeneic tumors may be induced by inoculation of recipient animals with normal tissues prior to tumor challenge.

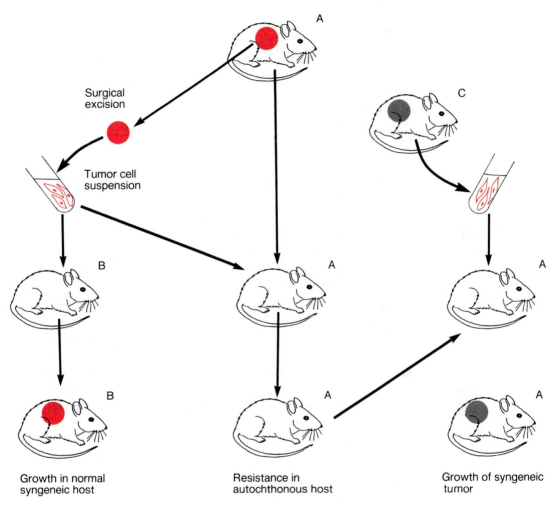

Figure 30–2. Demonstration of specific rejection of an autochthonous tumor. A chemically induced primary tumor is removed surgically and a suspension of the tumor cells made. A dose of tumor cells that will grow in a normal syngeneic mouse of the same strain (**B**) as that in which the tumor was induced is injected into the original primary tumor-bearing animal (autochthonous host). This tumor does not grow in the autochthonous host (**A**); the autochthonous host has developed immune resistance to growth of his own tumor. The tumor will grow when injected with a normal recipient of the same strain (**B**). However, a second tumor arising in another individual of the same strain (**C**) will grow when injected into the host of the first tumor (**A**). Thus, the tumor resistance is specific for the first tumor and does not extend to other tumors (tumor-specific transplantation immunity). This type of experiment demonstrates that an individual can develop immunity to his own tumor.

TABLE 30–4. IMMUNOGENICITY OF RAT TUMORS

Origin	Common Antigens	TSTA	ODA
Viral	++++	++	+
Ultraviolet radiation	++ (T_s)	++++	+
Methylcholanthrene	+	+++	+
Diaminoazobenzene	+	+	+
Acetylaminofluorene	0	+	+
Spontaneous	0	+/–	+

TSTA, tumor-specific transplantation antigens; ODA, oncodevelopmental (serologic); +, degree of immunogenicity; T_s, T-suppressor cells.

Some tumor-specific antigens may represent altered histocompatibility structures or peptides presented by MHC during induction of immunity. The selective loss of certain syngeneic class I MHC markers on tumors may significantly alter the immune response to antigens on the tumor. An inverse relationship was found between the expression of MHC class I products and TSTA in mouse sarcomas. Genetic analysis of hybrid cells has shown that MHC products and TSTA are controlled by different chromosomes. Different configurations or spatial arrangements of histocompatibility antigens may occur on tumor cells and be recognized as foreign by the immune system. New MHC antigens have been described on immune tumor cells after viral infections. In addition, infection of tumors with viruses leads to the appearance of virus-specific antigen as well as a marked increase in immunogenicity of nonviral tumor antigens (xenogenization). Thus, tumor antigens may be entirely new structures, modifications of existing structures, or realignments of existing cell surface structures.

Attempts have been made to solubilize cell surface TSTAs in order to isolate and characterize the tumor antigen. TSTAs are protein or glycoprotein components of the cell wall, but the exact biochemical nature of tumor antigens is still not well known. In addition, T cells recognize putative tumor antigens only as MHC-associated peptides, not the whole antigen. Extracting membrane antigens may yield only a peptide that is not immunogenic. Some soluble tumor-associated antigen extracts have been shown to possess antigenic activity, but the purity of such fractions is questionable. In other words, the tumor antigen extract may be contaminated with a variety of nonantigenic or non-tumor-specific molecules extracted from the tumor cell surface. Many "tumor antigens" identified serologically are carbohydrate structures formed by altered carbohydrate synthesis or processing by cancer cells (see below).

VIRUS-INDUCED TUMOR ANTIGENS

In contrast to chemically induced or spontaneous cancers, virus-induced tumors share common antigens. These shared antigens may be products encoded by the viral genome or cellular products not expressed in the virus itself.

DNA Viruses

Each DNA virus induces unique nuclear and cell surface antigens. A given virus induces the expression of the same antigens regardless of the tissue origin or animal species. Although these antigens are coded for by the virus, they are distinct from virion antigens and are referred to as tumor-associated antigens. Viral induced tumors may also express other antigens coded for by the host genome (such as TSTA or ODA) as a result of host gene deregulation by the transforming event.

The association of DNA viruses with cell transformation and cancer in animals is well established and is linked to certain human tumors. For example, Epstein-Barr virus (EBV), one of the herpesviruses, is the cause of human infectious mononucleosis, and is also associated with (but not proved to be the etiologic agent of) Burkitt's lymphoma and nasopharyngeal carcinoma. Similarly, papillomaviruses have been linked to human cervical carcinoma, and hepatitis B virus to hepatocellular carcinoma. In animals, herpesviruses have been shown to be oncogenic, as exemplified by Marek's lymphoma of chickens.

RNA Viruses

Tumors produced by RNA virus contain chromosomally integrated DNA that has been transcribed from the viral RNA by reverse transcriptase. When the oncogenic RNA viruses (oncornaviruses) infect the host cell, a double-stranded circular DNA copy of the RNA genome is synthesized and inserted into the host cell genome during cell transformation. Tumor cells induced by oncornaviruses express antigens coded for by both the viral and host genomes. These include: (1) The viral envelope antigens, mostly the envelope glycoprotein; (2) intrinsic viral proteins; and (3) virus-induced cell surface antigens. Whereas antibodies to viral envelope antigens will prevent infectivity, immunity against the neoplastic cell surface antigens is mainly responsible for the immunologic rejection of the malignant cell. These cell surface antigens are distinct from the viral antigens and also from the major histocompatibility antigens. The complexity of neoantigens expressed in virus-induced tumors is illustrated by the Rous sarcoma system of hamsters and HTLV-1 in humans: The antigens include virus envelope antigen (VEA), virus group-specific antigens (ggag), virus-coded non-viral proteins, cell-coded determinants activated by the virus, and oncodevelopmental antigens coded by cellular genes that are activated by virus-induced transformation.

A number of retroviruses have been identified as having oncogene sequences by their ability to transfect cultured cells and effect changes in growth of the transfected cells (transformation). Human T-cell leukemia/lymphoma virus (HTLV-1) is a prime example. In addition, the tumors of many human cancers have been found to contain cDNA sequences similar to transforming oncogenes. Normal human DNA has also been found to contain such DNA sequences (proto-oncogenes), and some oncogene products may be used to estimate the prognosis of patients with cancer (see below). These oncogenes code for cellular products, particularly kinases, growth factors, or growth factor receptors, which are produced normally during development but which are also believed to contribute to the altered growth characteristics of transformed adult cells. Monoclonal antibodies have been produced to oncogene products of human tumors and are being used to measure the altered or overexpressed product in neoplastic tissues.

ONCODEVELOP-MENTAL TUMOR ANTIGENS

Oncodevelopmental antigens (ODTAs) are found in embryonic or fetal tissues and in tumors of adults, but are not present or barely detectable in normal adult tissues. ODTAs were identified by transplantation as early as 1906, when Schone found that tumor transplants that would kill normal mice would be rejected by mice that had been previously immunized with fetal tissue; immunization with adult tissue was ineffective. In the 1930s, humoral antibodies that cross-reacted with fetal and tumor tissue were reported. These studies were complicated by histocompatibility differences and are difficult to duplicate. General interest in oncodevelopmental antigens received little attention until the late 1960s, when antigens common to embryonic tissue and tumors were demonstrated in inbred strains by serologic cross-reactivity. In 1970, it was reported that lymph node cells from pregnant mice incubated in vitro with chemically induced syngeneic sarcoma cells caused death of the tumor cells. Although extensive experimental investigation of ODTAs followed, the significance of such antigens in regard to tumor immunogenicity remains undefined. The following general conclusions seem valid. Tumors and fetal tissue may share antigens that are different from TSTAs. OD antigens are not specific for a given tumor but are shared by tumors of different histologic type and even of different species of origin. Immune products that react with tumors in vitro (antibody or sensitized cells) may be generated by immunization of adults with fetal tissue or by exposure to fetal antigen during pregnancy. However, no effect of this immunization on tumor incidence or growth has been consistently demonstrated. Animals that have in vitro immune reactivity to OD antigens may have resistance to tumor challenge, demonstrate no differences from nonimmune recipients, or have increased growth of transplanted tumors. In systems that have shown OD transplantation antigens, immunogenicity is much more difficult to demonstrate than in the case of TSTAs or viral tumor antigens. In humans, OD antigens have been tentatively identified by in vitro tests.

However, there is little or no evidence that immunization to fetal antigens protects against cancer in humans. Only one study has shown that the course of cancer differs in multiparous women from that in nulliparous women. Previously pregnant women, after treatment for malignant melanoma, had slightly better survival rates than women with no previous pregnancies. Multiparous women have a higher incidence of carcinoma of the cervix but a lower incidence of carcinoma of the breast, but these differences are believed to be due to hormonal rather than immunological differences. Oncodevelopmental antigens detected serologically are used as clinical "markers" of cancer (see below), but these epitopes are not involved in tumor rejection.

Autologous Antigens of Human Cancers

Evidence that humans do make immune responses against their own solid tumors is listed for breast cancer and melanoma in Table 30–5. Studies on human autologous antigens are at an early stage and as yet incomplete. Both antibody and T-cell responses have been found. Immune recognition of differentiation antigens of melanocytes is prominent and demonstrates that most human tumors "antigens" are developmental. One antigen, Melan-A or melanoma antigen recognized by T cells 1 (MART-1), is expressed by melanoma, melanocytes and pigmented retinal cells but not other normal tissues. When pre-

TABLE 30–5. ANTIGENS ON AUTOLOGOUS HUMAN CANCERS RECOGNIZED BY ANTIBODY OR T CELL RESPONSES

	Antigen	Tumor Type	Normal Tissue Expression	Comments
Antibody	gp75/brown	Melanoma	Melanocytes	Melanosomal protein
	Gangliosides (GM2, GD2)	Melanoma	Neuroectoderm-derived tissues	Carbohydrate antigens
	Melanotransferrin	Melanoma	Melanocytes, other tissues	Potential unique determinant
	HER2/neu	Breast	Epithelium	Overexpressed on a proportion of cancers
	p53, nonmutant	Breast	Most cells	No recognition of mutant p53
	T,Tn,sialylTn	Breast	Epithelium	Carbohydrate antigens
T cell	MAGE-1,3	Melanoma, lung, and other cancers	Testes	Not expressed by melanocytes
	Tyrosinase/albino	Melanoma	Melanocytes	Melanosomal protein
	MUC1	Pancreas, breast	Epithelium	Non-MHC restricted
	Melan-A/MART-1	Melanoma	Melanocytes	Melanocytes and retin
	pMel17/silver?	Melanoma	Melanocytes	Melanosomal protein

Antigens with known structures that are recognized on autologous tumor cells.

sented through class I MHC HLA-2.1 molecules expressed by melanoma cells, a MHC restricted T_{CTL} response can be demonstrated. Another melanoma peptide recognized by melanoma-specific cytotoxic T-cells from different patients has been shown to be a fragment of a protein called gp100 (pMel-17). This protein is produced by normal melanocytes and is involved in melanin synthesis. Normally these peptides appear to have a very low affinity for MHC molecules and are not expressed on the surface of normal cells. In melanoma cells upregulation of MHC expression may increase the cell-surface representation of such peptides, allowing them to be recogniezd by cytotoxic T-cells. The MAGE-1 and -3 antigen systems on melanoma appear to be restricted to testes in normal tissues. The melanoma antigens are clearly not tumor specific and there is no evidence yet that the auto-antibody or T-cell response has any effect on tumor incidence or growth. Attempts to produce melanoma vaccines using these "antigens" are now underway.

A partial listing of the methods used to demonstrate immune reactivity to tumors in vitro is given in Table 30–6. These include almost every conceivable method of measuring the reaction of antibody or sensitized cells with antigens. Tests for humoral (circulating) antibody to tumor antigens are hampered by the difficulty in obtaining soluble antigens from tumor cells and the lack of characterization of nonviral tumor-specific antigens. Both humoral and cellular reactions are usually measured by determining some effect of immune products on tumor target cells. The most frequently used assays measure target cell lysis (such as by ^{51}Cr release) as an endpoint.

Mechanisms of Tumor Cell Destruction by the Immune System

A. IN VITRO ASSAYS OF TUMOR IMMUNITY

TABLE 30–6. SOME IN VITRO ASSAYS FOR HUMAN ANTIGENS

Humoral	Cellular (CMI)
Immunodiffusion	Effect of immune cells on targets
Antibody binding	Reduction of cell number
Fluorescence	Cytotoxicity
Radiolabeled	Vital dye uptake
Immunoperoxidase	Visual cell death
Blocking of antibody binding	^{51}Cr release
Complement-dependent killing	Inhibition of metabolism
Complement fixation	Loss of cell adherence
Cl fixation and transfer	Cytostasis
Mixed hemadsorption	Colony inhibition
Cytostasis	In vitro incubation, in vivo growth (Winn assay)
Loss of cell adherence	Effect of targets on immune cells
Blocking of cellular reactions	Mixed lymphocyte-tumor reactions
Immune adherence	Lymphokine release (IL-2, IFN-γ, etc.)
ELISA	Leukocyte adherence inhibition
Cytofluorometry	Blastogenesis (T-cell proliferation)

Studies of these in vitro mechanisms have resulted in new insights into how immune mechanism might restrict the growth or kill tumor cells in vivo. Although humoral antibody/complement lysis of tumor cells in suspension in vitro may be demonstrated, this mechanism does not appear to act on solid tumors. Cellular-mediated tumor killing mechanisms are listed in Table 30–7. The major in vivo mechanism for tumor cell killing appears to be T-cell cytotoxicity or delayed hypersensitivity; the contribution of natural killer cells or antibody-dependent cell-mediated cytotoxicity as defined by in vitro assays to in vivo tumor killing is not clear, but there is evidence that NK cells may kill blood-borne tumor cells.

Humoral Antibody-mediated Tumor Cell Killing

This mechanism may operate directly to produce lesions in the cell membrane or indirectly by opsonization of target cells. It is usually effective only on cells that are in suspension and not on cells in solid tissue. This mechanism has been demonstrated to be active in certain animal models of leukemia.

T Cell–mediated Cytolysis (T_{CTL})

T_{CTL}s directly recognize cell surface peptides associated with class I MHC on the target cell via the T-cell receptor. One effector T cell can react with and lyse many target cells. The reaction of specific T cells with the target cell causes membrane alterations in the target cells and results in swelling of the target cell and eventual osmotic lysis (see

TABLE 30–7. PROPERTIES OF CELLS MEDIATING TUMOR IMMUNITY

Abbreviation	Name	Markers	Specificity	Mechanism	Function	MHC Restriction
T_{CTL}	Cytotoxic T cell	CD8+	Specific	Lysis	Tumor rejection	Class II
T_{DTH}	Delayed hypersensitivity T cell	CD4+	Specific	Macrophage activation	Tumor rejection	Class I
NK	Natural killer cell	CD16+	Nonspecific	Lysis	Tumor surveillance	NR
LAK	Lymphokine-activated killer cell	CD16+ IL-2R	Nonspecific	Lysis	Immunotherapy	NR
ADCC	Antibody dependent cell-mediated cytotoxic cell	FcR	Specific	Lysis	Uncertain	NR
TIL	Tumor-infiltrating lymphocyte	Mixed	Both	Lysis and activation	Uncertain	Both
AMØ	Activated macrophages	Monocyte	Nonspecific	Lysis and phagocytosis	Tumor rejection	None

Chapter 15). Lysis is frequently measured by the release of radiolabeled intracellular molecules (^{51}Cr release).

One of the first successful demonstrations of the effect of immune cells on tumor growth was accomplished by mixing effector lymphoid cells with tumor target cells in vitro, then injecting the mixture into a normal or irradiated syngeneic recipient. (Although first described by Klein, this has become known as the Winn assay.) (See Fig. 30–3.) If growth of the transplanted tumor cells is inhibited by the in vitro pretreatment, it may be concluded that the tumor cells were killed or damaged by the immune effector cells.

Delayed Hypersensitivity

T cells responsible for delayed hypersensitivity reactions (T_{DTH}) specifically recognize antigens in tissues and are activated to release

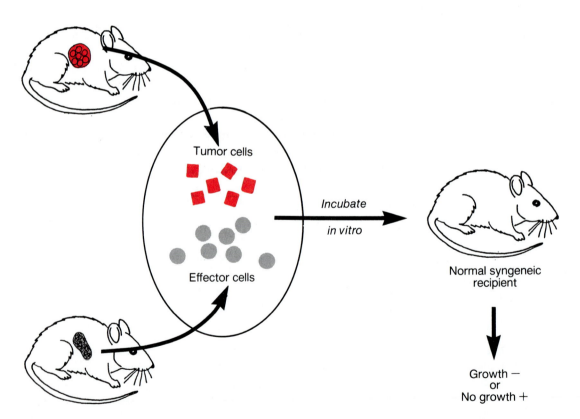

Figure 30–3. Winn assay. To determine the possible adverse or killing effect of lymphoid cells upon a given tumor, the effector lymphoid cells are admixed in vitro with the tumor target cells and the mixture transplanted into a normal syngeneic recipient. If growth of the tumor is inhibited in comparison to tumor cells alone or tumor cells treated with control (unsensitized) lymphoid cells, it may be concluded that tumor immunity exists in the tested lymphoid cells.

mediators that attract and activate macrophages. The activated macrophages are able to phagocytose cells and destroy them. In some animal models this mechanism is highly effective in killing tumors in vivo, but the mechanism cannot be duplicated in vitro.

Natural Killer Cells

Natural killer cells (NKs) are large granular lymphocytes of a particular lineage with defined markers (eg, CD16). They are operationally defined as cells present in normal individuals capable of cytotoxic activity against a variety of target cells. Lymphocytes from normal persons may be just as reactive against tumor cell lines as those from patients with tumors of the same or different histologic types. The role of NK cells in tumor surveillance in humans has recently been questioned on the basis of the finding that a patient with virtual lack of NK cells had problems with viral infections but did not have cancer.

Lymphokine-activated Killer Cells (LAKs)

In 1980, Elizabeth Grimm and others demonstrated that incubation of "normal" mouse spleen cells or human PBLs for 3 to 4 days in vitro with IL-2 resulted in the generation of "lymphokine-activated killer cells" that did not bear T-cell markers, were not MHC restricted, lysed cell lines resistant to NK killing, and were effective in reducing large tumor cell masses in mice. There has been some disagreement on the nature of the precursor cell for LAKs, but most evidence indicates that they arise from a common precursor of T and NK cells. LAK cells are being tested in clinical immunotherapy trials (see below). LAK cells are not immunologically specific and a given population of LAK cells will lyse a number of different tumor target cell lines, but not normal cells. Further stimulation of LAK cells with antibodies to the T-cell receptor (CD3, anti-TCR$\alpha\beta$) enhances release of IFN-γ from LAKs, but antibodies to other T-cell surface markers do not. This suggests that LAK cells may have receptors similar to conventional T-cells, but are not necessarily of the same lineage.

Antibody-dependent Cell-mediated Cytotoxicity (ADCC)

Effector cells that have surface receptors for the Fc of aggregated antibody (usually IgG) may react with antibody bound to target cells and cause lysis. The effector cell types are heterogeneous and include polymorphonuclear leukocytes, macrophages, and lymphocytes. The lymphocytes involved usually have no distinguishing T- or B-cell surface markers. They have been called null cells or killer cells. Presence of Fc receptor for IgG is a common feature of ADCC effector cells. Killing requires effector–target cell interaction accomplished by the antibody binding by its antigen recognition sites to the target cell and by its Fc to the effector cell. Lysis of the target cell by ADCC follows interaction with the killer cell. The mechanism of target cell destruction is not well understood, and in vivo significance remains unclear.

Tumor-infiltrating
Lymphocytes
(TILs)

The attempt to use specific autologous cells for treatment of cancers has met with limited success. Recently, the application of TILs or tumor-derived activated cells has been reported to have in vivo antitumor effects against both animal and human tumors. These cells are extracted from tumor tissue, treated with interleukin-2 in vitro, and injected back into the individual from which the tumor tissue was obtained. Cell lines with antitumor activity have been derived from TILs, and these are being used for passive immunotherapy (see below).

Activated
Macrophages

Macrophages are activated as a result of a delayed hypersensitivity reaction initiated by T_{DTH} cells or by nonspecific macrophage activators, such as polynucleotides. The role of macrophages as scavengers that "clean up" injured cells is well known. Macrophages may be activated and attracted to inflammatory sites by mediators released from T_{DTH} lymphocytes (delayed hypersensitivity) in vivo. Macrophages may also be activated by a variety of agents, including mycobacteria (BCG) and polynucleotides (see below). The mechanism of this type of killing involves the phagocytic activity of macrophages, through formation of oxygen radicals and activation of proteolytic enzymes.

IN VIVO TUMOR
KILLING/-
DELAYED
HYPER-
SENSITIVITY
VERSUS T-CELL
CYTOTOXICITY

The immune mechanism responsible for the rejection of solid tumors in experimental animals is essentially the same as that responsible for homograft rejection. The mechanism is either T_{CTL} lysis of tumor cells or T_{DTH}-mediated delayed hypersensitivity. However, through the use of diffusion chambers (permeable to antibody and complement, but not permeable to cells), it has been demonstrated that antibody and complement may cause the death of some kinds of tumor cells. Leukemias, which exist as single cells in suspension, are sensitive to antibody both in vivo and in vitro, whereas sarcoma and carcinoma cells that form solid tumor masses are usually resistant to the effect of antibody and complement. Thus, antibody-mediated cytotoxic reactions may be responsible for the death of tumor cells that grow primarily in suspension, whereas the T cell-mediated reactions are responsible for the rejection of solid tumors.

Studies of transplantable hepatomas in syngeneic guinea pigs have shown destruction of tumor cells in vivo by a two-step delayed hypersensitivity-like mechanism. Sensitized cells (T_{DTH}) are necessary to initiate the reaction with tumor cells, but macrophages accumulate at the site of the reaction with tumor cells and are responsible for the final tumor cell destruction. If macrophages are mixed with tumor cells, or if they are brought to the site of tumor cell inoculation by non-specific means, tumor cell destruction is still seen. The contribution of T_{CTL} in this model of tumor cell rejection is not clear but may be critical for effective destruction of tumor cells in other systems.

Immuno-surveillance

DOES THE IMMUNE SYSTEM PREVENT CANCER?

If tumors have specific antigens that are recognizable by the autochthonous host, then it is possible that such antigens may stimulate an "early warning" immune reaction that will eliminate small tumors or developing cancer cells. Sir MacFarland Burnet and Lewis Thomas separately developed the theory of immune surveillance and postulated that if it were not for the immune rejection mechanism, vertebrates would die at an early age from tumor growth. The immunosurveillance hypothesis states that potential malignant cells that develop new antigenic determinants are recognized as foreign by the immune system and are eliminated. Burnet went on to suggest that the allograft rejection mechanism prevents tumors from being contagious; if allogeneic tissue were not rejected, the tumors of one person could easily grow in another, such as occurs in nude mice.

IMMUNO-SURVEILLANCE IN NUDE MICE

The findings in nude mice illustrate the difficulty in using an experimental system to confirm or deny the hypothesis of immune surveillance. Nude mice do not have functional T cells, are unable to reject foreign tissue grafts, and will support the growth of allogeneic or even syngeneic tumors. In addition, the nude mouse is highly susceptible to virus-induced tumors. At first glance, these findings imply that the nude mouse proves the theory that the lack of an immune surveillance system leads to cancer. However, nude mice do not have an increased incidence of spontaneous tumors or increased susceptibility to chemical carcinogens. Therefore, at second glance, the lack of a T-cell surveillance system does not appear to result in an increase in tumor development. On the other hand, nude mice do have active NKs, even more than most normal mice. Thus, on third glance, it is possible that immune surveillance of tumors in nude mice may depend on the NK system. However, in mice deficient in NK activity, such as mice with the beige mutation, there is no increased susceptibility to chemically induced tumors. These findings and the lack of in vivo correlation between tumor development (either high or low) and NK activity in other models leave in doubt a role for NK as a general mechanism for immune surveillance.

NATURAL SELECTION AND TUMOR IMMUNITY

Immune surveillance may be weakened by natural selection mechanisms. There is a clear difference in the vigorous response to many virus-induced tumors in animals as compared to little or no response to spontaneously arising human tumors. There appears to be a host selection for an immune mechanism favoring prompt rejection of virus-transformed cells along the lines of the response to other infectious agents. On the other hand, there does not seem to be strong host selection for immune resistance to spontaneous tumors, presumably because most spontaneously occurring tumors arise after the host has passed the reproductive age. Thus, immune surveillance may be effective against "strongly antigenic" tumors, such as tumors caused by viruses, but not against spontaneously developing tumors. In support of the above hypothesis is the observation that strongly antigenic virus-induced tumors of humans are relatively rare compared to nonantigenic spontaneous tumors, except in immunosuppressed individuals. Alternatively, cancer may result from an adaptive mechanism of a cell line against toxic cell injury–an adaptation with advantages for the cell line, albeit at the expense of the whole organism.

FAILURE OF IMMUNO-SURVEILLANCE

If progressive growth of a tumor implies breakdown of an immune surveillance mechanism, then malignancy may represent a failure of the host's tumor immune defense. There are at least 14 explanations for the failure of the immune response in the tumor-bearing host (Table 30–8):

1. Nonantigenic tumors: Clearly, if a given tumor does not have an antigen that can be recognized by the autochthonous host, an immune response to the tumor will not take place. Spontaneous tumors in rodents frequently do not have demonstrable tumor antigens, and tumors induced with low doses of carcinogens are less immunogenic than those induced with higher doses. Antigenicity is not necessarily a constant feature of all tumors, and in some instances, tumor-specific antigens are undetectable even after extensive examination.

2. Tumor antigens may not be immunogenic in the primary (autochthonous) host: The tumor may contain an antigen that is recognized in another species, such as carcinoembryonic antigen, but is not immunogenic in the tumor-bearing animal. Most serologically defined tumor antigens are not able to induce an effective immune response in the autochthonous host.

3. Immune tolerance: Increasing evidence shows that the primary host responds immunologically even in the face of tumor growth (concomitant immunity); this suggests that tolerance to tumor antigens does not usually exist in the tumor-bearing animal. However, full tolerance was found to prevail in animal systems where an oncogenic virus was introduced into a fetal or newborn host capable of supporting virus proliferation and maturation. This included the RNA viruses such as mouse mammary tumor agent, murine leukemia agents of

TABLE 30–8. FACTORS RESPONSIBLE FOR FAILURE OF IMMUNE SURVEILLANCE OF CANCER

1. Lack of tumor antigen
2. Tumor antigen is not immunogenic
3. Immune tolerance to tumor antigen
4. Immune suppression
5. Immune enhancement
6. Antigenic modulation to tumor antigen
7. Immunoselection of nonantigenic clones
8. Imbalance of tumor growth and immune response
9. Suppressor cells for tumor immunity
10. Growth of tumor in privileged site
11. Lack of self MHC recognition
12. Immunostimulation
13. Alteration of T-cell receptor
14. Lack of expression of costimulatory molecules on tumor cells

Gross, and other mouse leukemia agents. A role for tolerance in human cancer victims cannot be ruled out.

4. Immunosuppression: Increased tumor incidence has been observed in patients who have been treated with immunosuppressive drugs or who have congenital immunologic deficiency diseases. As stated above, tumors in immunosuppressed individuals frequently arise in the lymphoreticular system and do not necessarily imply a loss of immune surveillance in general, but may indicate an abnormality in control of lymphoid cell proliferation. Surveys have generally concluded that whereas patients with solid tumors may have normal ability to form antibodies, they often have an impaired delayed cutaneous hypersensitivity. Even if impaired cellular immune mechanisms have no cause or effect relationship to the growth and/or development of the tumor, they have importance in respect to the problem of infectious diseases complicating cancer.

5. Immune enhancement: The tumor-bearing animal may not only make an ineffective immune response, but also the immune response to the tumor may allow the tumor to grow more readily. Immune enhancement was described by Kaliss in 1956 as the progressive growth of normally rejected strain-specific tumors in recipients who had been pretreated with either antiserum directed against the tumor (passive enhancement) or with repeated injections of antigenic material of the tumor (active enhancement). Although first seen in allogeneic systems, enhancement has been demonstrated to occur in syngeneic transplantation models with methylcholanthrene-induced sarcomas, mammary adenocarcinomas derived from mammary tumor virus-carrying mice, and possibly Moloney virus-induced lymphomas. Most of these later studies involved immunization of animals with tumor-

derived materials in such a way as to induce the formation of humoral antibody, but not delayed hypersensitivity. Transfer of tumors to such immunized recipients or to recipients injected with serum from immunized donors results in a more rapid growth than occurs in untreated tumor recipients. Growth of the tumor is enhanced in the presence of serum antibody, and such enhancement has been attributed to the presence of "blocking antibodies" (Fig. 30–4).

Mechanisms of enhancement in relation to the immune response may be afferent, efferent, or central. Afferent inhibition implies that the recipient did not become immunized by graft antigens because the simultaneous presence of antibody prevents antigen from becoming available to immune-responsive tissues. Central inhibition would occur if the host lymphoid cells failed to be stimulated, despite being presented with the antigen in a suitable immunogenic form. Efferent inhibition would apply if the recipient became immunized, but the response that resulted was ineffective against the tumor. It appears that enhancement is usually an efferent effect. In some instances, both cellular sensitivity and humoral factors are present in the autochthonous host, but the humoral factor blocks the colony-inhibiting effect of the sensitized cells (blocking factor). Although the term "blocking antibody" has been used to identify this factor, the antibody or immunoglobulin nature of the blocking factor has not been clearly established. It is possible that "blocking factor" is a complex of tumor antigen and antibody that inhibits the reaction of sensitized lymphocytes with antigen on the tumor cells or it may be free antigen. In addition, a serum factor that can decrease the effects of blocking factor has been described and is called "unblocking factor." Humoral factors may also cause enhanced tumor growth, either through physiologic changes in the tumor cells or through stimulation of a substance produced by tumor cells that produces unresponsiveness in lymphoid cells.

6. Antigenic modulation: Complete loss of antigenicity or a significant antigenic change with selective overgrowth of the changed variant has been demonstrated to be a mechanism of escape from immune rejection. Loss of the MHC antigens of one parental strain can be induced by passage of a tumor arising in an F_1 animal in the other parental strain; cell surface antigens of mouse leukemic cells (TL antigen) may disappear after treatment of the cells with antiserum to the TL antigen but reappear after removal of the antiserum. A stable subline of a Moloney tumor that is resistant to specific antiserum to the parent tumor has been produced by incubating tumor cells in cytotoxic antiserum in the presence of complement and then inoculating these samples into preimmunized mice. These observations support the concept that tumor cells under immunologic attack may be able to survive by not expressing the tumor-specific antigen to which the immune response is directed and thus thwarting immune surveillance.

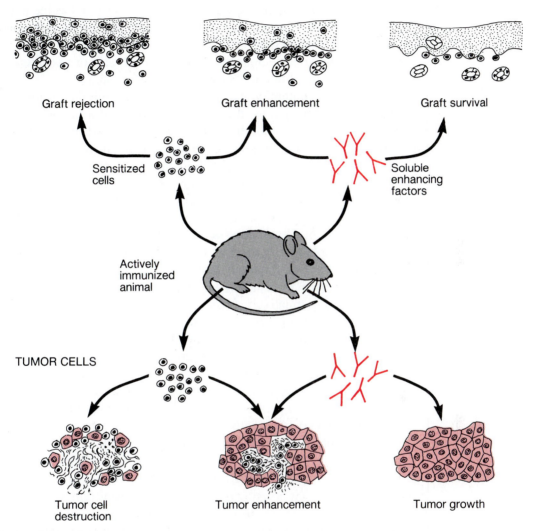

Figure 30–4. Tumor enhancement: Immune responses to tissue grafts and to tumors. An individual may produce two general types of immune reaction to tissue antigens—humoral antibody or cell-mediated immunity (CMI). The eventual outcome of a tissue graft (survival or rejection) or a tumor graft (growth or rejection) depends upon the relative response. If CMI is predominant, then sensitized cells will destroy the graft or kill the tumor cells. If humoral antibody is predominant, a foreign graft may survive, and tumor cells grow. If a mixture of sensitized cells and humoral antibody are produced, the eventual outcome will depend on their relative strength. When attempts are made to manipulate the immune response of an individual to prolong graft survival or to promote tumor rejection, the possibility of inducing an effect opposite than desired must be considered. Enhancing antibody is desirable for survival of a normal tissue graft but is undesirable for growth of a malignant tumor. The effects of humoral-enhancing antibody may be mediated by antibody-antigen complexes in some situations.

7. Immunoselection of nonantigenic clones: Spontaneous tumors may produce successive clonal variants that replace each other as the tumor progresses. Each successful variant has greater autonomy and is less affected by restricting host mechanisms. Thus, by natural selection, the tumor may evolve new clones with different antigens or nonantigenic clones that are not limited by host immune response.

8. Imbalance of immunity and tumor mass: The ability of an immune response to protect against the continued growth of a tumor depends upon the mass of the tumor that is being contained. Old and Boyse postulated that "sneaking through" of tumor cells might occur with a low number of tumor cells. In this situation, there may be insufficient antigenic stimulation to provide effective immunization until the tumor grows larger. At the higher cell number, antigenic stimulation is sufficient to provide effective immunization, which in turn prevents tumor growth. However, the presence of a large tumor mass may exhaust the supply of lymphocytes produced by the host (a form of desensitization). Most forms of immunotherapy effective in experimental animals may be overcome by a tumor of sufficient size. Immunotherapy is effective for only relatively small tumors or in preventing growth of small numbers of injected tumor cells. On the other hand, immune rejection can destroy huge tumor allografts.

9. Suppressor cells: Specific suppressor cells may depress the effect of an immune response to a tumor antigen. Thus, an immune response to a tumor might not result in the production of only killer cells to the tumor but also in suppressor cells that protect the tumor by inhibiting the production of T-killer cells.

10. Immune-privileged site: A tumor may arise in an immunologically sheltered site, where surveillance functions play no role in antagonizing tumor development. Such a site is known to occur in the hamster cheek pouch, which is frequently used to transplant tumors in a way that will avoid an immune reaction to the tumor. It is possible that such sites may serve as a locus for the development of primary tumors that avoid immune surveillance until growth of the tumor cannot be reversed by the immune mechanism. However, a high incidence of tumors in similar sites in humans is not observed.

11. Lack of self recognition: It is possible that progression, a change in the growth potential of a given tumor, may be related to selection for cellular variants of a tumor with altered class I gene expression. The expression of MHC antigens, especially class I antigens, have been demonstrated to play an important role in the behavior of tumors in experimental models. In mice, some tumors having a TSTA, but lacking the self class I antigen H2K, are resistant to T-cell killing and readily grow when transplanted into normal syngeneic hosts. However, if these same tumors are transfected with DNA coding for the H2K antigen and thereby induced to express the H2K antigen, the tumors are

then not transplantable. For these tumors, recognition of a TSTA in combination with self class I MHC antigen may be needed either for induction or expression of tumor rejection. In other systems, resistance to macrophage and/or natural killing may be correlated with a loss of class I antigen expression. In at least one instance of virus-transformed cell line, low class I MHC expression may be reversed by interferon treatment. In other instances, viral transfection or enhanced invasiveness of tumors is associated with increased class I antigen expression.

Skin cancers induced by UV irradiation express TSTAs and are rejected upon transplantation into syngeneic hosts. Yet UV-induced tumors grow progressively in the original UV-irradiated host. Margaret Kripke has shown that UV treatment induces suppressor components capable of specifically eliminating the T-cell response against the autochthonous tumor. This suppressor effect is not demonstrable against chemically induced tumors. Thus, alterations in self-recognition may be important in the host–tumor immune relationship for some cancers. Yet many metastatic tumors do not have demonstrable alterations in the level or nature of the class I products expressed as compared to normal tissue.

12. Immunostimulation: A major premise of tumor immunology is that a cell-mediated immune response to a given tumor is a beneficial reaction—that is, cell-mediated immunity, in contrast to humoral antibodies that may mediate enhancement, serves to limit or prevent tumor growth. However, Richmond Prehn has argued that, in some instances, the lymphocytic infiltrate seen in tumors is actually required for early stages of tumor growth. Under certain circumstances, immune reactions stimulate tumor target cells rather than inhibit or kill them. This result is dependent on dose. Immune cells that kill tumor target cells in vitro when added at high killer cell to target cell ratios in vitro (100:1 is commonly used) may actually increase tumor cell growth when present in smaller relative numbers in vivo. Although the specificity of immuno-stimulation has been questioned, it must be considered that tumors could escape immune surveillance by immunostimulation at a critical point in their development and later become resistant to the specific inhibitory effects of immune cells.

13. Alteration of T-cell receptors: T cells in tumor-bearing animals may have an altered T-cell receptor affecting the ability of T_{CTL} to become activated after reaction with tumor antigens. The expression of the CD3γ is low the T_{CTL} receptor may be unable to function. The role of this mechanism in humans has not been demonstrated.

14. Lack of expression of costimulatory molecules on tumor cells: Interaction of the B7 molecule on antigen-presenting cells with its receptors CD28 and CTLA-4 on T cells provides costimulatory signals for T-cell activation (Fig. 30–5). In experimental systems, trans-

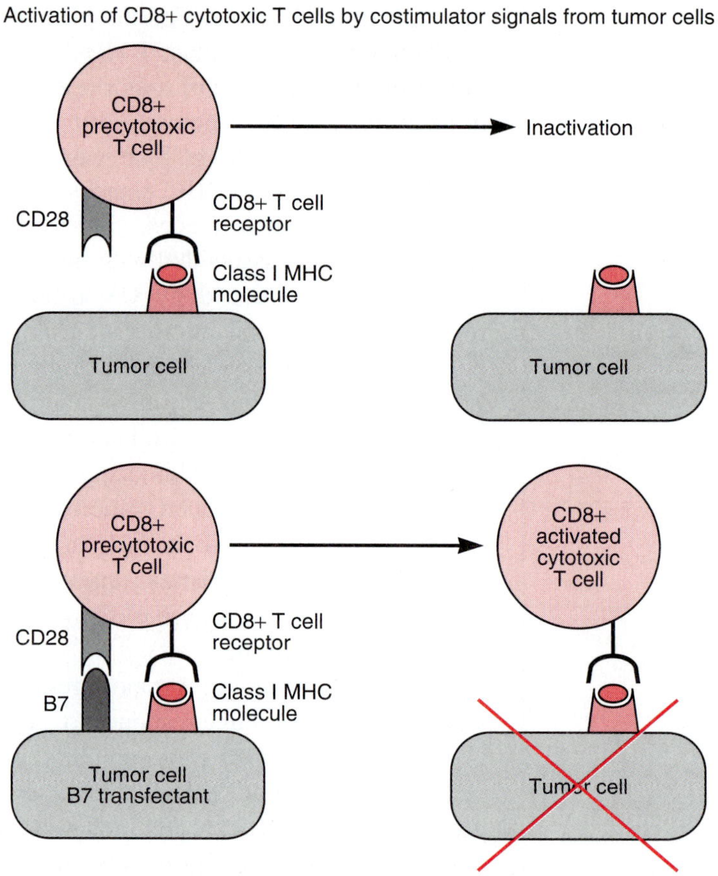

Figure 30–5. Activation of CD8+ cytotoxic T cells requires two signals: T-cell receptor with antigen presented by class I MHC molecule and interaction of CD28 with B7 on the tumor cell. Tumor cells that lack B7 will not activate CD8+ precytotoxic T cells. The same tumor cell transfected with B7 will activate T_{CTL} cells that will kill target cells that do not express B7. Interaction of TCR with antigen on class I MHC in the absence of costimulatory signals results in inactivation of the CD8+ precytotoxic cells.

plantable tumors which express B7 are rejected in syngeneic hosts, whereas tumors which lack B7 inactivate CD8+ T_{CTL} precursors, allowing the tumors to grow.

Immuno-diagnosis of Cancer

Pathologists recognize cancer tissue to be "less organized" and cancer cells to be "less differentiated" than normal tissue. Tumors are graded according to their degree of resemblance to normal tissue as being well differentiated; poorly differentiated; anaplastic (without form); or, if very close to normal, benign. Cancer markers are the biochemical or immunologic counterparts of the morphology of the tumors. During the last

TABLE 30–9. SOME CLINICAL APPLICATIONS OF CANCER MARKERS

Screen asymptomatic patients	Occult fecal blood
Screen high-risk patients	Complete blood count, AFP, PSA
Confirm a suspected clinical diagnosis	CEA, PSA, lymphocyte markers (CDs)
Monitor response to therapy	CEA, AFP, PSA, myeloma protein, carbohydrate and mucin epitopes (CAs)
Therapy (experimental)	
Antibody, monoclonal antibodies	CEA, AFP, anti-CDs
Antibody–drug/toxin conjugate	Ricin, diphtheria toxin, *Pseudomonas* exotoxin A, daunomycin
Radiolabeled antibody	Iodine 131, Yttrium 90

twenty years, there has been a growing appreciation that the morphologic resemblance of cancer cells to embryonic or fetal cells is also reflected in the production of cellular macromolecules by cancer cells that are more typical of embryonic or fetal cells than of adult tissue (Fig. 30–6).

Many of these macromolecules are not only present in the cell or on the cell surface, but are also secreted into the body fluids. Measurement of these "oncodevelopmental markers" by the clinical laboratory has become increasingly important in the diagnosis of cancer. In addition, antibodies to cancer markers are being used to localize tumor tissue in vivo and to treat certain selected cancers. Some clinical applications of cancer markers are listed in Table 30–9.

Examples of different types of cancer markers are listed in Table 30–10. These are only a few examples of an increasingly recognized number of markers associated with cancer. In most (if not all) instances, cancer markers are produced normally at some time during

TABLE 30–10. TYPES OF CANCER MARKERS

Type	Example
Deletions of blood group markers	ABH
Exposure of backbone or blood group markers	Monosialoganglioside
Cell surface glycoproteins	Carcinoembryonic antigen
Secreted proteins	Alpha-fetoprotein
Enzyme alterations	Glycosyltransferases, PSA
Isozymes	Alkaline phosphatase
Ectopic hormone	Human chorionic gonadotropin
Tumor antigens	Melanoma glycoproteins identified by monoclonal antibodies
Cytoskeletal elements	Epidermal tumors (cytokeratin)
Immunoglobulin gene rearrangements	B-cell tumors
Gene translocations	Lymphomas (Philadelphia chromosome)

TABLE 30–11. "LEVELS" OF EXPRESSION OF ONCODEVELOPMENTAL MARKER PRODUCTION BY TUMORS

Example	Normal Producing Tissue	Embryogenically Closely Related	Distantly Related	Different Germ Line
Carcinoembryonic antigen	Colon	Stomach, pancreas, liver	Lung, breast	Lymphoma
Alpha-fetoprotein	Liver, yolk sac	Colon, stomach, pancreas	Lung	Lymphoma
Serotonin	"Entero-endocrine"	Adrenal, carcinoid (GI)	Oat cell, lung	Epidermal, lung
Chorionic gonadotropin	Placenta	Germinal tumors	Liver	Epidermal, lung

development, but are present in low or undetectable amounts in the adult. The adult tumors that produce these oncodevelopmental markers usually originate from the tissue that normally produces the markers during development (Table 30–11). For instance, alpha-fetoprotein (AFP) is normally produced by the fetal liver and yolk sac. Tumors that arise from liver or germ cell tumors that contain yolk sac elements are the most frequent producers of AFP, and the order of frequency of other cancers correlates with embryonic lineage relationships—stomach > lung > lymphoma.

MYELOMA PROTEINS

The first cancer marker was recognized by Dr. H. Bence Jones in 1846. Bence Jones protein was identified as a urinary precipitate that occurred upon heating at pH 4 to 6 the urine of a patient with "mollities ossium," a bone disease now known as multiple myeloma. It is

Figure 30–6. Various oncodevelopmental markers are normally expressed at different stages of neonatal development and by proliferating tissues in the adult. The T-locus markers of the mouse and other differentiation antigens may be expressed on germinal cells and in the preimplantation embryo, as well as in primitive teratocarcinomas. Oncogene products are expressed during development, and their role in cancer is under active investigation. Placental hormones, isoenzymes, and proteins may be expressed in adult tumors of testes, ovary, liver, and breast. Other markers, such as AFP and CEA, are produced normally by developing liver or colonic mucosal cells, respectively, and are frequently expressed in tumors of these tissues, ie, hepatocellular carcinomas and adenocarcinomas of the colon, as well as other tumors of embryologically related tissues. Immunoglobulins and lymphocyte differentiation markers are found to be associated with lymphoproliferative tumors. Many surface glycoprotein and glycolipid carbohydrate differences are now being recognized using monoclonal antibodies. Gene rearrangements that occur normally during plasma cell development are used to identify clonality and B-cell origin of "null" lymphoid tumors.

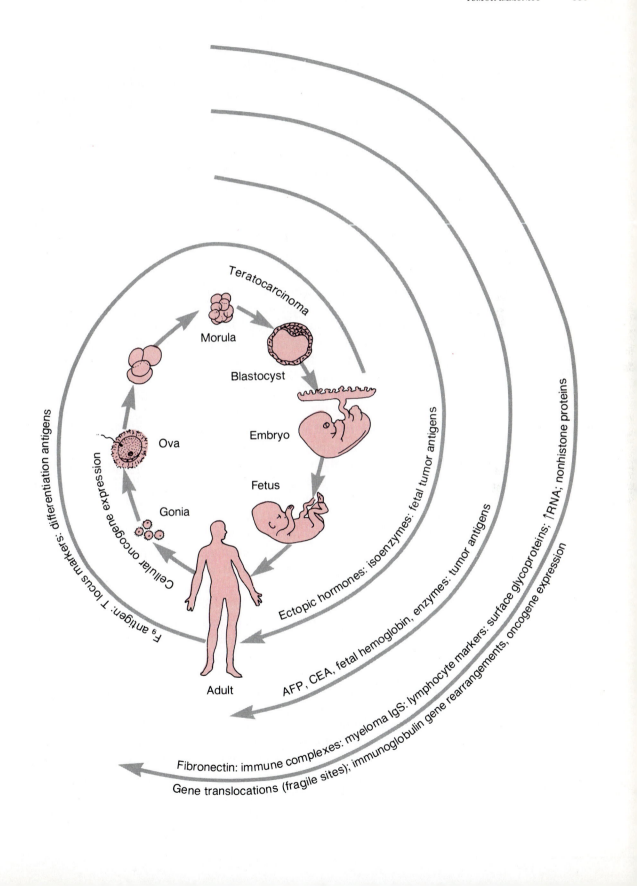

remarkable that it took over 100 years from the first recognition of Bence Jones protein to identify Bence Jones proteins as immunoglobulin light chains. Bence Jones proteins are produced in excess by about half of patients with plasmacytomas. The molecular weight of the light chain (about 22 kDa) is below that excluded by the basement membrane of glomerulus of the kidney, so that it appears in the urine as Bence Jones protein. It is associated with the presence of monoclonal immunoglobulins in the serum. The amount of Bence Jones protein found in urine or the amount of myeloma immunoglobulin in the serum may be used to follow the effects of therapy; the amount of these proteins in a given patient closely reflects the amount of myeloma tumor mass. This general principle also applies to other secreted tumor markers, including hormones and serum enzymes.

ALPHA-FETOPROTEIN (AFP)

The modern era of cancer markers began with the discovery of alpha-fetoprotein by Garri Abelev of the Soviet Union in 1963. He identified this protein in the sera of normal fetal mice and in the sera of adult mice with hepatocellular carcinoma, but not in normal adult mice. AFP is an antigenically distinct serum protein with properties similar to albumin. It is found in high concentrations (up to 10 mg/mL) in fetal serum and in the serum of patients with hepatocellular or teratocarcinomas, but in low concentrations (<10 ng/mL) in sera of adults. Elevations up to 500 ng/mL occur frequently in association with a variety of nonmalignant diseases, but elevations above this are essentially diagnostic of an AFP-producing tumor. Approximately half of the patients with hepatocellular carcinoma may be diagnosed by such an elevation. Serial determinations of AFP may be used clinically to determine the effectiveness of therapy (Fig. 30–7). Failure of elevated serum AFP to return to normal after surgery is an indication that the tumor has not been completely removed or that metastases are present. These patterns essentially hold true for other cancer markers found in the serum.

CARCINO-EMBRYONIC ANTIGEN (CEA)

Carcinoembryonic antigen is a cell surface glycoprotein that is normally produced by colonic epithelium and secreted in the intestine. In colonic and other CEA-producing cancers, alterations in the polarity of cells is associated with release of CEA in elevated levels into the blood. During development, CEA is produced by the fetal gastrointestinal tract; elevations of CEA associated with cancers in the adult reflect the developmental relationship to gastrointestinal tissue. CEA elevations also occur in association with nonmalignant diseases, so that elevated serum CEA can be used only as an adjunct to other diagnostic procedures (Table 30–12). In patients with colorectal cancer who have elevated serum CEA, the serum levels may be used to determine the effectiveness of therapy. Unfortunately, reelevation of CEA has not proven useful as an

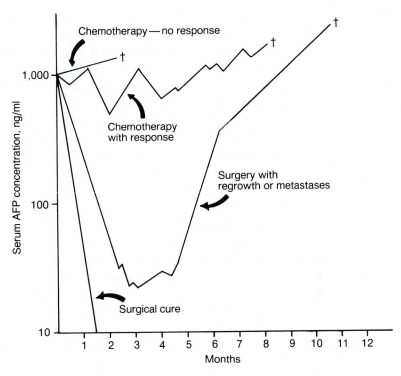

Figure 30–7. Representative responses of serum AFP to therapy. Changes in serum concentration of AFP correlate with growth of an AFP-producing tumor and reflect the response to therapy.

TABLE 30–12. CEA CONCENTRATIONS IN HUMAN SERA

Type of Patient	Number of Patients Tested	0–2.5 ng/mL (%)	2.6–5.0 ng/mL (%)	5.1–10 ng/mL (%)	10 ng/mL (%)
Healthy subjects					
Nonsmokers	892	97	3	0	0
Smokers	620	81	15	3	1
Colorectal carcinoma	544	28	23	14	35
Pulmonary carcinoma	181	24	25	25	26
Pancreatic carcinoma	55	9	31	25	35
Gastric carcinoma	79	39	32	10	19
Breast carcinoma	125	53	20	13	14
Other carcinoma	343	51	28	12	19
Benign breast disease	115	85	11	4	0
Severe alcoholic cirrhosis	120	29	44	25	2
Active ulcerative colitis	146	69	18	8	5
Pulmonary emphysema	49	43	37	16	4

Modified from Go V: Carcinoembryonic antigen. *Cancer* 37:562–566, 1976.

indication for "second-look" surgery. CEA levels in breast cancer become elevated when metastases occur, and serial CEA determination are useful for determining effectiveness of chemotherapy, for determining prognosis, and to measure progression of the disease.

Radiolabeled antibodies to AFP and CEA have been used to localize clandestine tumors by radioimmunescintigraphy. Labeled antibodies are injected into patients and localization of the label in tissues determined by scanning the body for radioactivity. Accuracy of diagnosis has been improved by application of computer analysis to the photoscans. Primary cancers have been localized in 83% of colorectal cancer, and in 22% of patients, cancer sites were located that no other detection method had found.

Antibodies to CEA and AFP have also been used to treat tumors producing these markers in animals. So far, the results, even when drugs such as daunomycin have been attached to the antibodies, have been equivocal. Trials in humans are not yet interpretable as being effective.

PROSTATE-SPECIFIC ANTIGEN (PSA)

The approval of PSA for clinical use in 1985 by the Food and Drug Administration represents the most important development in cancer markers since the early 1970s when CEA was approved. PSA is a single-chain 34-kDa protein (serine protease) containing 7% carbohydrate that is produced by normal prostate cells, but in increased amounts by prostatic cancer cells. An increase in serum PSA is now used clinically as a strong indication for prostate cancer. However, a rise in PSA may also occur with benign prostatic disease, such as prostatitis and benign prostatic hypertrophy, so that elevations of PSA should be followed by careful digital rectal exam (DRE) and transrectal ultrasound (TUS). The positive predictive values for positive findings are as follows:

+TUS alone	8%
+TUS+DRE	26%
+TUS+PSA	41%
+DRE+PSA	58%
+TUS+DRE+PSA	80%

PSA is now used to follow elderly men. Levels below 4 µg/L are considered normal. Although elevations above this level may occur with benign prostatic hypertrophy, any individual with a level above 4 µg/L or with increasing levels upon serial determinations should be examined by DRE and TUR. Many anecdotal cases where an elevated PSA has initiated further studies leading to identification of relatively small cancers curable by surgery have now been reported. However, the value of large-scale monitoring of PSA for men over 50 years of age has not yet been clearly established. Clinical trials now underway should resolve this question.

TABLE 30-13. COMPARISON OF CANCER MARKERS

Name	Nature	Normal Limit	Type of Cancer	USE			PERFORMANCE	
				Diagnosis	Prognosis	Monitoring	Sensitivity %	Specificity %
I. "Classic markers"								
AFP	70-Kda glycoprotein, 4% CHO	(≤) 15 µg/mL	Hepatocellular germ cell (yolk sac)	+++	+	+++	60–90	60–100
CEA	200-Kda glycoprotein up to 70% CHO	3–5 µg/mL	GI, pancreas, lung, breast, etc.	+	++	+++	42–96	10–90
βhCG	Glycopeptide hormone	3 IU/mL	Embryonal, choriocarcinoma	++	+++	+++	60–100	40–90
FER	450-Kda iron-binding protein	200 µg/UL	Liver, lung, breast, leukemia		++	++	5–56	76–97
PSA	33-Kda glycoprotein (7% CHO)	2.5 µg/mL	Prostate	+++	++	+++	33–89	89–97
II. Carbohydrates								
CA 19-9	Sialyated Lewis X^A	37 U/mL	GI pancreas, ovary	+	++	+++	33–89	82–97
CA-50	Sialyated Lewis X-1 afucosyl form	14 U/mL	GI, pancreas lung	+	++	+++	40–78	80–98
TAG-72	Sialyl Tn	4–7 U/mL	Breast, ovary GI	++	++		9–72	97
CA-242	Sialyated carbohydrate, co-expressed with CA-50	200 U/mL	GI, pancreas	+	++	++	44–83	75
III. Mucins								
CA 15-3	Transmembrane molecule-episialin 200 KDa, up to 50% CHO	30 U/mL	Breast, ovary lung (adeno)	+	++	+++	88–97	30–90
CA-125	High-molecular-weight glycoprotein	35 U/mL	Ovary (epidermal) endometrial	+	++	+++	40–86	86–99
DU-PAN-2	1,000-kDa mucin (peptide epitope)	400 U/mL	Pancreas, ovary GI, lung	+	+	+++	34	86
MCA	350-kDa glycoprotein	11 U/mL	Breast, ovary GI	+	++	+++	20–80	84–90
IV. Cytoplasmic Proteins								
SCC	48-kDa glycoprotein	1.5 ng/mL	Cervix, lung, head, neck (squamous)		+	+++	33–86	92–98
TPA	Cytokeratins 8, 18, and 19	85 U/L	Multiple, squamous		+	+++	67–80	75

Modified from Sell S: Cancer markers of the 1990s. *Clin Lab Med* 10:1–37, 1990.

MONOCLONAL ANTIBODIES TO CANCER MARKERS

The development of monoclonal antibodies to "cancer antigens" has produced a new generation of "cancer markers." These include carbohydrate and mucin epitopes, as well as cytoplasmic antigens and lymphocyte differentiation markers (CDs). A comparison of newly defined markers to "classic" cancer markers is given in Table 30–13. Use of a given marker for diagnosis requires a specificity of greater than 90%. Thus, most tumor markers are not sufficiently specific for diagnosis and must be used in conjunction with other diagnostic indicators. Lower specificities are acceptable for monitoring. A marker such as tissue polypeptide antigen (TPA) may not be at all useful for the diagnosis of cancer, but if a patient who is known to have cancer has an elevated TPA, serial determinations of TPA may be useful for follow-up. The markers that are the most useful for diagnosis include AFP, hCG, PSA, TAG-72, and terminal deoxytransferase (Tdt). On the other hand, many of the markers have proved useful for determining prognosis (high levels at the time of diagnosis indicate poor prognosis) or for monitoring the effects of therapy.

The application of monoclonal antibodies to lymphocyte differentiation antigens as applied to diagnosis and therapy of lymphomas is presented in Chapter 24. A summary of the CDs useful in human lymphomas is given in Table 30–14.

CELL SURFACE CARBOHYDRATES

As illustrated below, many of the "tumor markers" being detected by monoclonal antibodies are oligosaccharides. Oligosaccharides on the surface of mammalian cells are attached to lipid (glycosphingolipid [GSL]) or protein (glycoprotein [GP]). The lipid or protein is

TABLE 30–14. SOME IMPORTANT CLUSTER OF DIFFERENTIATION ANTIGENS FOR LYMPHOID TUMORS

CD	Normal Expression	Tumor Expression
3	Mature T and B cells	Good prognosis
4	T-helper/inducer cells	Not useful
5	Pan-T cell	Marker for CD5+ B-CLL
8	T-suppressor/cytotoxic	Not useful
10	Thymocytes, pre-B cells	Common leukemia antigen
15	Monocytes/myeloid cells (Leu-M1)	Hodgkin's, histiocytic lymphoma
16	Large granular lymphocytes (FcR)	LGL lymphomas
25	Tac (IL-2 receptor)	Prognosis related to serum level
38	Thymocytes, pre-B cells	Poor prognosis
Ki-1	Activated T cells	Some Hodgkin's cells
Ki-67	Cell cycle marker	Prognosis related to percentage of positive cells

hydrophobic and is located in the cell membrane, whereas the oligosaccharide is hydrophilic and extends from the cell surface, where it is readily accessible for reaction with antibody.

Of the more than 100 possible monosaccharides, only seven make up the oligosaccharides of the mammalian cell surface:

These oligosaccharides may be important in determining not only the biological behavior of cells but also the antigenicity of the cells. The composition and linkage of cell surface polysaccharides provide numerous epitopes that may be recognized by monoclonal antibodies. The appearance of "new" cell surface carbohydrates on cancer cells may be due to (1) the synthesis of different oligosaccharides by tumor cells, (2) the postsynthetic modification by glycolytic enzymes, or (3) the "unmasking" of cell surface carbohydrates by shedding or loss of masking cell surface material. Thus the changes found in cell surface carbohydrates in tumor cells as compared to normal cells are usually secondary to changes in activity or levels of glycosylating enzymes or glycosidases in cancer cells. The structural relationship of cell surface oligosaccharides is illustrated in Figure 30–8, and "cancer carbohydrates" identified by monoclonal antibodies in Figure 30–9. Cancer carbohydrates belong to four major structural classes—ganglio-, globo-, lacto-type 1, and lacto-type 2. The identification of monoclonal antibodies to cancer-associated carbohydrates may reflect the immunogenicity of the rigid restricted structure of the oligosaccharides or the relative stability of these structures to formalin fixation. This latter feature is important because many laboratories use formalin-fixed tissues to screen for monoclonal antibody activity.

A comparison of some carbohydrate epitopes in the diagnosis of colon and pancreatic cancer is given in Table 30–15.

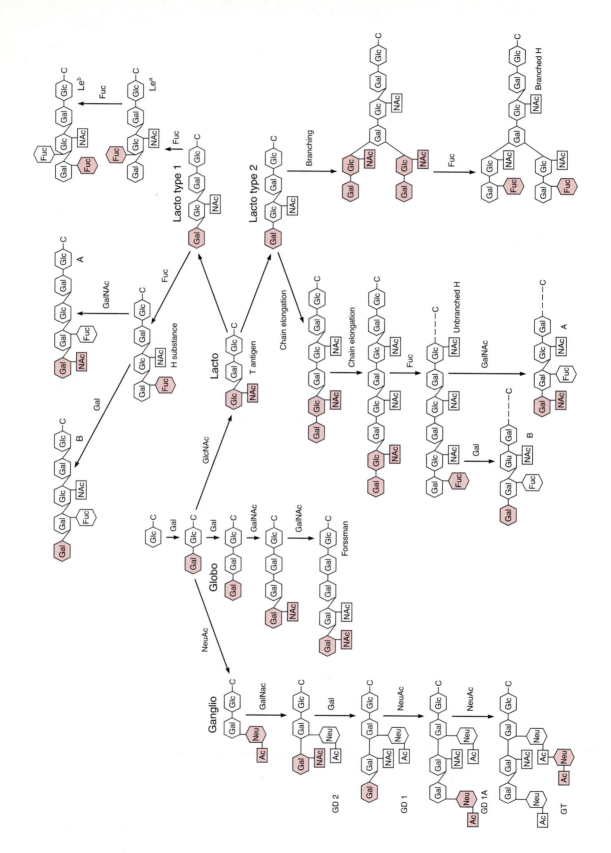

938

Figure 30–8. Cell surface carbohydrate structures. Cell surface carbohydrates are synthesized from a common gal-glu disaccharide by the addition of linear or branched monosaccharides. The four major classes are: Ganglio-, globo-, lacto-type 1, and lacto-type 2. The structures shown in this figure may be identified by monoclonal antibodies that recognize individual or shared carbohydrate epitopes. (From Sell S: Cancer-associated carbohydrates identified by monoclonal antibodies. *Hum Pathol* 21:1003, 1990.)

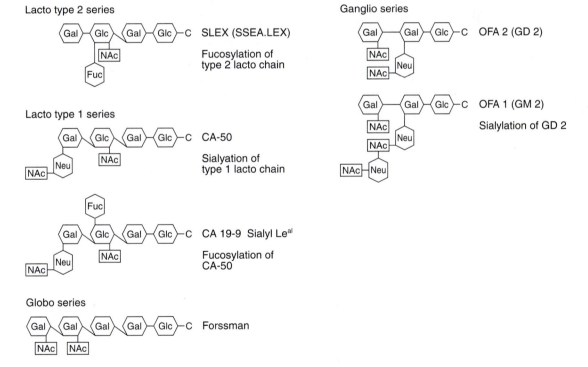

Figure 30–9. Carbohydrate structure of some major human cancer markers recognized by monoclonal antibodies. The epitope designated SLEX (SSEA, LEX) is formed by fucosylation of the type 2 lacto chain. CA-50 is formed by sialyation of the type 1 lacto chain, and CA-19.9 by fucosylation of CA-50. The Forssman antigen is not found normally on human cells, but may be identified on cancer cells because of an increase in expression of N-acetylgalactosamine transferase, producing the Forssman pentasaccharide in the globo series. OFA-2 (Oncofetal antigen 2) is produced by addition of the N-acetygalactosamine to the core trisaccharide of the globo series; OFA-1 is produced by sialyation of OFA-2. (From Sell S: Cancer-associated carbohydrates identified by monoclonal antibodies. *Hum Pathol* 21:1003, 1990.)

TABLE 30–15. COMPARISON OF CEA, CA-19.9, CA-50, AND CA-242 IN PATIENTS WITH COLORECTAL OR PANCREATIC–BILIARY CANCER (% POSITIVE)

	CEA	CA-19.9	CA-50	CA-242
Colorectal Cancer Sensitivity	>30 ng/mL*	>37 U/mL	>17 U/mL	>20 U/mL
Dukes A–B	32	16	26	47
Dukes C–D	71	44	47	59
Specificity	83	100	97	90
Pancreatic–Biliary				
Sensitivity	59	76	73	68
Specificity	79	74	67	95

*Recommended cutoff value.

MUCINS

Monoclonal antibodies have been made that react with epitopes of mucins produced by adenocarcinomas. These include: CA-15.3 (episialin), CA-125, DU-PAN-2 and mucinlike cancer-associated antigen (MCA). Mucins are high-molecular-weight glycoproteins with a high carbohydrate content (about 50%) that are secreted by glandular cells into glandular lumens and protect glands from self-digestion. With an increase in the number of cells in an adenocarcinoma producing these mucins and alterations in the polarity of the adenocarcinoma cells, the mucins are released into the circulation. For a given adenocarcinoma, the serum levels of a mucin epitope may be used to monitor the size of the adenocarcinoma and determine prognosis. Mucin antigens may also be detected by T-cell clones reactive with human breast and pancreatic cancers.

MIXED MARKERS

Since some tumors may produce more than one marker, the simultaneous measurement of more than one marker often provides information leading to a more precise diagnosis or prognosis than one marker alone. For instance, differentiation of germ cell tumor types can be accomplished on the basis of elevation of serum AFP or hCG (Table 30–16).

TABLE 30–16. PERCENTAGES OF PATIENTS WITH ELEVATION OF SERUM HCG OR AFP IN GERM CELL TUMORS

	hCG	AFP	Either
Seminoma	10	0	10
Seminoma, metastatic	38	0	0
Embryonal	60	70	87
Choriocarcinoma	100	0	100
Yolk sac	25	75	100
Teratoma	0	0	0

hCG, human chorionic gonadotropin.

The combined use of more than one cancer marker may greatly increase sensitivity, but also may greatly decrease the specificity of detection of cancer. For instance, using placental alkaline phosphatase and CA-125 as markers for ovarian cancer, the sensitivity was 59% for CA-125 and 31% for PL-ALP, but by using both CA-125 and PL-ALP, the sensitivity was increased to 67%. On the other hand, the specificity with PL-ALP 94% and with CA-125 was 87%, whereas using both, the specificity dropped to 82%. The application of multiple markers is fraught with many difficulties in interpretation. Setting the specificity of each cancer marker at the 95th percentile and using multiple markers greatly increases the likelihood of a false-positive diagnosis of cancer. A normal person who has thirteen separate cancer marker tests has, by chance alone, a probability of 50% of being diagnosed as having cancer. It is, in fact, the potential for the overdiagnosis of cancer that has contributed largely to the limited approval for cancer marker tests by the United States Food and Drug Administration panel. The application of multiple markers for screening is now being evaluated using higher cutoff values for each marker, thus decreasing the false positive rates.

CYTOSKELETAL ELEMENTS

Monoclonal antibodies to cytoskeletal elements have been used to identify the cellular origin of cancers by immunohistochemistry (Table 30–17). Glial fibrillary acidic protein (GFAP) is a major component of the intermediate filaments of astrocytes and appears to be useful for diagnosis of astrocytic neoplasms and mixed glial tumors, as it is not found in epidermal tumors, meningiomas or other nonastrocytic brain tumors. Prekeratin, in the form of intermediate-sized filaments, is found exclusively in cells of epidermal origin and may be used immunohistochemically to identify cancer cells of epithelial origin. Neurofilament antigens are found in neuroblastomas and pheochromocytomas; vimentin in sarcomas and lymphomas.

IMMUNO-GLOBULIN GENE REARRANGE-MENTS

The presence of immunoglobulin gene arrangements in lymphomas may give evidence of B-cell lineage even if the tumor cells do not produce cytoplasmic or surface monoclonal Ig. Immunoglobulin gene rearrangements that result in splicing out of an intervening DNA

TABLE 30–17. CYTOSKELETAL ELEMENTS IN CANCER

Element	Normal Distribution	In Cancers
Prekeratin	Epithelial cells	Epithelial cancers
GFAP	Astrocytes	Astrocytic tumors
Neurofilaments	Neural cells	Neuroblastomas, pheochromocytomas
Vimentin	Mesenchymal cells	Sarcomas, lymphomas
Desmin	Muscle	Myosarcomas

sequence has been associated with maturation of B cells and the ability to produce Ig. However, some gene rearrangements are not associated with the capacity to synthesize Ig, but are still believed to be characteristic of B cells. Some non-Ig producing null cell lymphomas will demonstrate gene rearrangements, whereas others will not. The finding of Ig gene rearrangements in a null cell tumor indicates (1) that the cell line is monoclonal and therefore probably neoplastic and (2) that the tumor is most likely of B-cell origin. (See Chapter 24 for further discussion of rearrangement of Ig genes and T-cell receptor genes in lymphomas.)

ONCOGENE PRODUCTS

Since oncogene activation is associated with cancer, products of oncogenes should be useful as cancer markers. The major oncogenes and their products under study as determinants of prognosis in human cancer are listed in Table 30–18. The expression of these genes in cancer tissue has also been measured by gene amplification and mRNA levels. In general, the higher the expression of the oncogene, the poorer the prognosis. The identification of *ras* oncogene mutations in the DNA of stool from patients with colorectal cancers has been reported to be an effective way to detect these tumors while still curable by surgery. Most patients with chronic myelogenous leukemia (CML) possess the Philadelphia chromosome, which is formed by a reciprocal translocation between chromosomes 9 and 22. This exchange joins the 5′ two-thirds of the BCR gene on chromosome 22 to a large portion of the *ABL* gene from chromosome 9. The detection of BCR-*ABL* fusion proteins in the blood cells of patients with CML by western blotting is now being used to follow patients with AML and CML.

TABLE 30–18. ONCOGENES BEING CONSIDERED AS CANDIDATES FOR EVALUATION OF PROGNOSIS OF HUMAN CANCER

Oncogene	Function and Product	Chromosomal Location	Change in Tumors	Detection Method	Types of Cancers
c-ras	Signal transduction (P21 tyrosinekinase)	IP (21 CEN)	Mutation/ Amplification	Immunohistology for P21	Breast, prostate, GI, neuroblastomas
n-myc	Transcription regulation (P62 DNA binding protein)	2P (23 TER)	Amplification	Immunohistology (p62), northern and southern blots	GI, SCLC, neuroblastomas, other
c-erbB-2	Growth factor receptor (p65 tyrosine kinase)	7P (G22 TER)	Amplification	Southern Blots	Ovary, breast
int-2/hst-1	Fibroblast growth factor	Hg 13	Amplification	Southern blots	Breast, head, neck

SUMMARY

Cancer markers include secreted proteins, cell surface molecules, hormones, enzymes and isozymes, and cytoplasmic constituents, as well as gene rearrangements and oncogene products. Many cancer markers are identified by heteroantisera or monoclonal antibodies. Cancer markers may be used for diagnosis, prognosis, or therapy. The most useful cancer markers are monoclonal immunoglobulins, alpha-fetoprotein, PSA, and CEA. Although the clinical applications of AFP and CEA have not fulfilled all the optimistic expectations that many predicted, these markers have achieved a place in cancer diagnosis and management. Many other cancer markers have not been nearly as useful and the verdict has not yet been returned on several now being studied. Claims of a universal cancer marker have been made repeatedly but have not been fulfilled. It is possible that molecular probes for human oncogenes or gene rearrangements might become a diagnostic approach in the future. A continued search for new tumor markers is more than justified by the tremendous potential for clinical applications.

Immunotherapy of Cancer

Immunotherapy of cancer is defined as any immune procedure that adversely affects the growth of an established tumor. Such immune procedures may be specific or nonspecific. Specific immunotherapy involves the use of tumor-specific antigens for targeting, whereas nonspecific therapy involves procedures that increase the activity of the effector arm of the rejection response in a manner that does not involve the recognition of a specific tumor antigen (Table 30–19). Specific immunotherapy may be accomplished by active or passive immunization. Active immunization with lysed melanoma cell culture lines or autologous cells mixed with BCG or conjugated to haptens has been under investigation for several years. Clinical trials of specific passive immunotherapy using monoclonal antibodies and nonspecific immunotherapy using interferon, interleukin-2, and LAKs have given promising, but mixed, results. The use of IL-12, which activates NK and T cells is also under study. Immunotherapy could be much improved if there was a way to predict which patients would respond favorably. There are data to indicate that cancer patients that are anergic to standard skin tests (tuberculin, *Candida,* etc.) will not respond to tumor immunotherapy, but many patients who do react to skin tests do not respond to immunotherapy, so that predictability of therapeutic outcome on this basis is limited.

ACTIVE
IMMUNIZATION

Active immunization of cancer patients against their own tumor has been an elusive goal of immunotherapy. Several requirements exist: The tumor must possess tumor-specific transplantation antigen(s) or tumor-associated antigen(s), the host must be able to recognize these

TABLE 30–19. IMMUNOTHERAPEUTIC APPROACHES TO HUMAN CANCER

Approaches	Status
SPECIFIC	
Active:	
Autologous tumor cells	Not effective
Autologous tumor extracts	Not effective
Autologous tumor lysates/BCG	Partial effect
Cell line lysates/BCG	Partial effect
Haptenated autologous cell lysates/BCG	Partial effect
Passive Cellular:	
Autologous lymphocytes	Not effective
Allogeneic lymphocytes	Some effect in bone marrow transplant recipients
Autologous stimulated lymphocytes (LAKs)	Clinical trials underway
Autologous gene modified lymphocytes	Clinical trials underway
Cytotoxic cell lines	Experimental
Transfer factor	Not effective
Immune RNA	Not effective
Passive Humoral:	
Xenogeneic antisera	Not effective
Monoclonal antibodies	Clinical trials underway
Antiidiotypic antibody	Experimental, clinical trials underway
Bispecific antibodies	Clinical trials underway
NONSPECIFIC	
BCG, *C. parvum*	Effective for bladder carcinoma
Mycobacterial extracts	Experimental
Levamisole, polynucleotides	Experimental
DNCB	Established for selected skin cancers
Lymphokines	Clinical trials underway

antigens, there must be an effective means of immunizing the host against the tumor to produce an immune response that results in tumor cell destruction, and a small tumor mass must be treated because immune reactions cannot be expected to affect a large tumor.

Tumor Vaccines

Autogenous human tumor vaccines using cells prepared from the tumor arising in the patient to be treated have generally been unsatisfactory. A variety of methods to accomplish immunization against the tumor have been attempted, including injection of living or killed tumor cells and coupling cell extracts with chemical haptens or foreign proteins, in the hope that some postulated cancer-specific antigen may be rendered more immunogenic. Attempts have also been made to immunize a patient with tumors from other patients. This therapy rests on the assumption that specific tumor antigens might be common to the cancers of other individuals. In humans, these approaches have given some encouraging anecdotal results but have generally been unsuccessful. In animal models, where experimental conditions and the time of immunization can be modified, better results have been observed. Caution must be exercised in attempts to immunize human patients actively, because the effects may be the opposite of those desired if blocking factors, tolerance, and/or suppressor cells are produced that might cause increased growth of the tumor. Active immunization has been attempted against melanoma using a variety of antigens (autologous cell lysates, lysates of mixtures of melanoma cell lines, oncolysates, allogeneic cells, etc.) with or without combination with nonspecific adjuvants (BCG, *Corynebacterium parvum,* lipopolysaccharides) with generally unimpressive results. Some patients developed antibodies or delayed hypersensitivity reactions with inflammation of cutaneous metastases, and some remissions were reported, but most patients had no clinical improvement. Two large-scale clinical trials are now testing vaccine-induced lysates of melanoma cells and two trials using ultrasonicated melanoma cells are now underway. More recently, three immunodominant melanoma antigens have been identified that hold promise for more effective active vaccination against melanoma. In addition, approaches such as the use of mouse monoclonal antiidiotope (anti-antimelanoma) immunization of humans, and haptenized autologous melanoma cells, have been reported to produce some beneficial effects in melanoma patients.

Direction of Vaccination to T-cell Epitopes

Although there are different immune mechanisms to affect tumor-specific immunity, there is general agreement that the most effective tumor immune mechanism in experimental models are T_{CTL} or T_{DTH} cells. Three developments in immunology have resulted in approaches to direct specific immunization to epitopes that will stimulate T_{CTL}. The first is molecular analysis of immunogens to identify epitopes that will be recognized by class I-restricted T cells. The second is the use of ISCOMs that direct antigens to class I-restricted (endogenous) processing. The third is the use of vaccinia vectors that infect epithelial cells and also lead to endogenous antigen processing. The classic or exogenous processing of immunogens is accomplished by class II MHC-positive antigen-presenting macrophages or activated B cells, which deliver the processed immunogen to CD4+ T-helper cells to induce delayed hypersensitivity and to B cells to induce antibody formation. The epitopes identified by the antibodies are to conformational or topographic surface epitopes formed by folding of the antigen. Because of this, parts of the epitope may be contributed by different amino acid sequences in the unfolded molecule. The endogenous pathway delivers peptide fragments associated with class I MHC molecules and can be accomplished by many nucleated cells. Immunogenic peptides that are presented by class I MHC molecules are directed to

CD8+ T cells that are the precursors of T-cytotoxic and T-suppressor cells. By analysis of the primary amino acid sequence of a potential immunogen, it is possible to predict peptides that will be recognized by CD8+ T cells. Such peptides are made up of seven to twelve amino acids that form amphipathic helixes. Amphipathicity refers to alternating hydrophobic and hydrophilic residues in an α-helix, so that hydrophobic and hydrophilic residues alternate about every three to four residues. Since there are about 3.6 residues per turn, this sequence aligns the hydrophobic residues on one side of the helix and hydrophilic residues on the other side of the helix. The hydrophobic side attaches to the cleft in the class I MHC molecule on the surface of the class I MHC-positive antigen-processing cell, whereas the hydrophilic side binds to the CD8+ T-cell receptor (see Fig. 29–2). Using this approach, a number of T-cell epitopes in antigens of infectious agents have been identified. Once the peptide having the putative T-cell epitope has been identified and synthesized, it is necessary to be able to deliver it to the endogenous processing system. This may be accomplished by the use of immunostimulating complexes (ISCOMs) (see Fig. 29–3). ISCOMs are glycosides that form micelles with the peptide that appear to be able to penetrate cell membranes, as liposomes do, and introduce the antigen into the endoplasmic reticulum, allowing endogenous processing and presentation by the class I pathway. This approach is now being applied to retroviruses such as feline leukemia virus and HIV. Such methods give promise of being able to direct vaccination to the type of cell-mediated immunity that is effective against tumor-specific antigens. However, T-suppressor cells also belong to the CD8+ population. In view of the effect of T-suppressor cells to inhibit induction of an immune effector mechanism against some experimental tumors, it may be that the use of peptides and ISCOMs that stimulate CD8+ cells may actually enhance carcinogenesis rather than inhibit it.

BCG/Macrophage Activation

The first attempt at active immunotherapy of cancer was immunization with "anticancer" vaccines made from microorganisms by William Coley (Coley's vaccines) in the late 1800s. This approach was replaced by the advent of radiotherapy in the early 1900s. It was not until the latter half of the next century that nonspecific immunity was first recognized as an acquired cellular resistance to microbial infections in animals whose mononuclear phagocytes have an apparently increased capacity to destroy unrelated microorganisms after inoculation of BCG, an attenuated tubercle bacillus. This capacity may be established by inoculation of a variety of agents, including BCG, *Listeria monocytogenes, Corynebacterium parvum* endotoxin, *Pseudomonas* vaccine, levamisole, mycobacterial extracts, and polynucleotides. For instance, an animal that has been inoculated with BCG develops an increased resistance to infection by unrelated organisms, which lasts for about one month. It has been postulated that such activation might also be operative against tumors.

In experimental studies, stimulation of guinea pigs bearing transplantable hepatomas with BCG may result in complete destruction of the tumor. This response is most effective when BCG is injected directly into the tumor. Intradermal inoculation of the transplantable tumor results in local growth, followed by metastases to the draining lymph node. After intralesional injection of BCG, there is not only total regression of the injected tumor but also regression of the growth in the lymph node. Both the tumor and the draining lymph node contain acid-fast bacilli and markedly increased numbers of macrophages. It is postulated that the tumor cells are destroyed because of the active host response to the injected BCG.

A number of studies in man suggest that under certain circumstances, inoculation of BCG may be effective in reducing tumor growth. BCG injected directly into melanoma nodules of patients with tuberculin sensitivity caused regression of some tumor nodules. Similar results have been obtained with metastatic breast tumors, basal cell tumors of the skin, and other solid tumor nodules. However, extensive clinical trials have not provided convincing evidence that BCG treatment is successful for noncutaneous tumors. There is no documented controlled study demonstrating that remission duration or survival in patients receiving BCG is longer than with other forms of therapy.

BCG has been found to be an effective treatment for prophylaxis and cure of superficial bladder cancers. For treatment of bladder cancer, BCG is repeatedly inoculated into the bladder lumen. This local application results in recruitment of activated lymphocytes into the bladder wall and increases of interleukins in the urine, as well as systemic immunity to BCG. Preliminary results indicate an improvement in survival from 68% to 86%, and a 20% decrease in treatment failures as compared to chemotherapy.

Other agents that may nonspecifically activate or potentiate a host response to a tumor include a variety of microorganisms, such as *C. parvum* and subcellular fractions of BCG, as well as polynucleotides and liposomes. More recently, attempts have been made to activate macrophages to a tumoricidal state by treatment with liposomes containing immunomodulators, such as muramyl dipeptide. In mouse models, such treatment may eradicate cancer metastases, and clinical trials in humans have resulted in significant improvement in patients with advanced osteosarcoma, with a doubling time of remission from four months to nine months.

Dinitro-chlorobenzene

Successful local therapy of tumors limited to the skin may be effected by elicitation of local contact dermatitis reactions to skin sensitizing haptens such as dinitrochlorobenzene (DNCB). Edmund Klein treated basal cell and squamous cell skin carcinomas by painting the skin lesions with contact sensitivity haptens such as DNCB, after the patients have been sensitized to DNCB. A delayed hypersensitivity reaction occurs to the sensitizing chemical, and the tumor tissue appears to be destroyed by the accumulation of macrophages that is stimulated by the reaction of sensitized lymphocytes to the DNCB. In persons sensitized systemically to this agent, skin painting of basal cell carcinomas with DNCB induces complete regression in approximately one-third of the treated lesions and partial regression in another third. Untreated lesions in patients with multiple basal cell carcinomas do not undergo regression at the time that other treated lesions are regressing. The mechanisms of the selective DNCB-induced regression of basal cell carcinoma is not well understood. Presumably, the tumor cells are more sensitive to delayed hypersensitivity reactions directed to DNCB than are normal epithelial cells. Such therapy is applicable to only cutaneous tumors.

Genetically Modified Tumor Cells

The apparent successful treatment of adenosine deaminase (ADA) deficiency by transplantation of lymphoid cells containing the inserted ADA gene has led to a blush of enthusiasm that genetically engineered tumor cells expressing interleukins or MHC antigens may be able to induce effective tumor immunity. In experimental models, tumor cells with inserted IL-4 or IL-6 genes have been used to induce immunity in mice with reduction of tumorigenicity and suppression of metastases. Clinical trials in humans include cancer cells with insertion of genes for tumor necrosis factor (TNF), IL-2, HLA-B7 (for melanoma), IL-4 and INF-8. In addition, transfer of a number of genes that inhibit oncogenes or growth factors have been proposed. At the time of this writing, there is no evidence in humans of a beneficial effect of such approaches for cancer prophylaxis or therapy. However, if the future can be predicted from the past, spectacular success will be reported with anecdotal cases; then limited positive effects will be found in larger controlled studies.

Growth Factors and Oncogene Products

Many tumors appear to be dependent on growth factors, some of which are products of oncogenes. Activation of expression of proto-oncogenes may result in increasing cell surface receptors for growth factors or production of factors with growth-stimulating activity. In some instances, the factor acts back on the tumor cell that produces it in an autocrine fashion. A short list of some oncogene-related growth factors, receptors, and cell transduction activators is given in Table 30–18. Lippman has recently reviewed eleven ways that intervention in growth factor-mediated pathways might be used to treat cancer. In an experimental system, immunization to K-*fgf/hst*–encoded fibroblast growth factor prevents growth of transplanted 3T3 cells. Of particular interest are antibodies that block epidermal growth factor (EGF) receptor, which may be cytostatic by itself, cytotoxic in the presence of monocytes for tumor cells with EGF receptors, or sensitize cells for TNF. In addition, it may be possible to direct T cells to react with and kill tumor cells that have EGF receptors.

PASSIVE IMMUNIZATION

Requirements for passive immunization include a donor of serum or cells that recognize tumor antigens but not the recipient's normal tissue, and a donor immune response that is effective in destroying tumor cells. Immune cells or cell products used for immunotherapy include monoclonal antibodies, as well as specific T_{CTL}, T_{DTH} (delayed hypersensitivity) cells; cell products, interferons and interleukin-2, as well as effector cells activated by IL-2 (LAKs). Tumor-bearing animals may be successfully treated with specifically sensitized lymphocytes or monoclonal antibodies against cancer tissue in selected model systems. These approaches are highly effective in "curing" nude mice bearing growing transplants of human tumors. However, the results of such procedures in humans have not been satisfactory. One major difficulty that is encountered in human passive immunotherapy is that of obtaining specific immunologically reactive cells to tumors in numbers sufficient to effect an antitumor response that do not also react with normal tissues. Passive immunotherapy using large numbers of autologous cultured lymphocytes has been attempted, but the immune potential of such cells has not been documented and the results are equivocal. However, since immune cells may have marked specificity for tumor cells and be active against a small tumor load while chemotherapy and radiotherapy can destroy a large tumor load but are limited because of nonspecificity, the combination of passive immunotherapy with radiation or chemotherapy might prove effective in some instances. The use of transfer factor and "immune RNA" as a means of converting nonimmune lymphocytes to specifically reactive cells has not yielded positive results, and such approaches have largely been abandoned in recent years.

Specific Cellular Transfer

Immune effector cell types used for passive immunotherapy include both tumor antigen-specific tumor infiltrating lymphocytes (TILs) and nonspecific LAK cells. In practice, it has been difficult to obtain specifically reactive T_{CTL} or T_{DTH} effector cells for specific adoptive immunotherapy. Lymphocytes extracted from tumors (TILs) as well as cultured cell lines with cytotoxic activity to cancer cells are now available. Cultured cells may respond to antigenic stimulation in vitro and produce long-lived clones in the presence of T-cell growth factors, such as IL-1 or IL-2. In addition, nonspecific cytotoxic activity and proliferation may be induced in vitro by treatment of cultured lymphocytes with IL-2, IL-12, or lectins. The ability to obtain "activated" T cells or cell lines from cultures of lymphocytes from a given patient permits passive specific immunotherapy using cells that will not be rejected or produce graft-versus-host disease. Particularly noteworthy would be the ability to produce a cell line from a given patient that could be passively transferred back to the patient and induce regression of cancer. Attempts to obtain lymphoid cells from tumor infiltrates (TILs), which presumably are reacting against the tumor, and expand them by in vitro cultivation with IL-2 have met with limited success due to the inability to obtain cells from some tumors and to induce sufficient proliferation of these cells in vitro. In addition, most TIL lines, when obtained, are not specifically reactive with their autochthonous tumor. However, in a large clinical trial, 60% of patients with metastatic malignant melanoma demonstrated some clinical response to TIL treatment. In experimental models, it has been possible to achieve eradication of disseminated cancer by infusion of tumor-specific cultured T-cell clones, but this approach has not been reproducible in humans.

Nonspecific Cellular Transfer–LAKs

The use of LAKs offers the opportunity to use lymphocytes from the same individual which had the tumor (autochthonous), avoiding problems with graft-versus-host reactions. The clinical use of LAKs was tested as a way of utilizing IL-2 for therapy, since IL-2 itself is very toxic and produces minimal antitumor effects. Although initially promising, the overall antitumor effects are similar to IL-2 alone. In many tumors, the majority of infiltrating mononuclear cells are macrophages. It is possible that some of the effects of IL-2–stimulated cells is the result of macrophage activation. LAKs release interferon-γ, TNF and macrophage colony-stimulating factor, each enhancing macrophage functions. In trials at NIH, there have been twelve CRs and seventeen PRs in 137 patients treated with LAKs. Again, most of these were in patients with renal cell carcinoma (17/54) or melanoma (6/34), tumors which occasionally have temporary remissions without treatment. Carefully controlled studies to determine if treatment produces a higher remission rate than occurs spontaneously have not been done. LAK therapy combined with IL-2 and chemotherapy, such as cyclophosphamide or dexorubicin, has been claimed to be beneficial in a small percentage of patients with metastatic disease. Thus, immunotherapy of cancer using LAKs remains experimental, and considerable improvements in results and cost effectiveness are needed before it can be considered for general use.

Biological Response Modifiers (BRMs)

BRMs are products of cells that may alter the individual's response to stress, infection, or neoplasia. The family of BRMs includes hematopoietic growth factors, lymphokines, TNF, and interleukins. Products of activated lymphocytes have been shown to have antitumor effects in experimental systems (see Tables 28–2 and 28–3). The most important of these are IFN and IL-2. The use of IFN, IL-2, and other

TABLE 30–20. BIOLOGICAL RESPONSE MODIFIERS IN CLINICAL TRIALS

Interferon-α	Used in combination with chemotherapy, preferred treatment for hairy cell leukemia
Interferon-γ	FDA approved for chronic granulomatous disease, used to modulate antigen expression with antibody immunotoxins
Interleukin-1α, β	In combination with growth factors as radio- or chemo-protectants
IL-2	FDA approval sought for treating renal cell carcinoma
IL-3	Alone and in combination with hematopoietic growth factors for stimulating bone marrow
IL-4	In phase 1 and 2 trials for B-cell tumors
IL-6	Phase 1 trials, also as platelet restoring factor
TNF	Toxicity limits use in humans
G-CSF	FDA-approved for chemotherapy myelosuppression, used with peripheral blood stem cell harvest and autologous bone marrow transplantation
GM-CSF	FDA approved for autologous bone marrow transplantation

lymphokines and interleukins as therapeutic agents is discussed in Chapter 28, and their present status is listed in Table 30–20. Theoretically, these agents have the potential to augment immune responses to tumor antigens, as well as having other effects detrimental to the tumor.

Interferon. Interferons may have a direct cytostatic effect on cancer cells, activate NK cells, or increase specific immune responses to tumors. Most experimental and clinical trials have employed interferon-α. In addition to its immunomodulating effects, IFN-α inhibits cell proliferation and has a cytostatic on tumors. For solid tumors, therapeutic responses are defined as follows. A complete response (CR) indicates disappearance of all clinically detectable tumor masses (by visual, palpation, or radiologic examination); a partial response (PR) means more than a 50% reduction in measurable disease. The responsiveness of different tumors to systemic IFN-α treatment is given in Table 30–21. The percent response includes both CR and PR. The most dramatic results have been obtained with hairy cell leukemia, with up to 20% CR and 60% PR, as well as with chronic myelogenous leukemia (45% CR, 20% PR) and cutaneous T-cell lymphoma (25% CR, 40% PR). However, to date, no patient has been cured of any cancer by IFN-α treatment. Eventually, the patient will develop progressive disease that is refractory to further treatment. The mechanism of effect in hairy cell leukemia is not clear, but it appears the IFN-α directly induces differentiation of the leukemia cells, so that they are less responsive to growth factors, and indirectly decreases the frequency of infectious complications.

TABLE 30–21. "MEDIAN" CLINICAL RESPONSE OF HUMAN TUMORS TO IFN-α

Type of Neoplasm	% of Response
Lymphoma	25
Hairy cell leukemia	73
Kaposi's sarcoma	34
Renal cell carcinoma	13
Melanoma	18
Multiple myeloma	21
Breast	0
Colon	0
Lung	0
Glioma	24
Ovary	14

The response of renal cell carcinomas to IFN-α may be used as a guide to further surgical treatment. Aggressive surgery for metastatic renal cell carcinoma is not generally recommended. However, in patients who have undergone clinical remission after initial IFN-α, surgery may result in increased disease-free survival in select patient who do not meet the traditional criteria for surgical resection of renal cell carcinoma.

Interleukin-2 (IL-2). IL-2 has undergone extensive trials, both as systemic therapy and as an activator of killer cells in vitro that are then inoculated into the tumor-bearing animal or patient (LAK cells, see below). Some beneficial effects of the systemic administration of IL-2 have been reported in phase 1 trials, but the dose is limited by toxic effects. These include hypotension (capillary leak syndrome), fever, nausea, chills, vomiting, diarrhea, cutaneous erythema, anemia, and moderate to severe renal or hepatic dysfunction, as well as thyroiditis. In addition, in trials conducted at NIH, the beneficial effect of IL-2 alone was limited to only 7 of 38 patients with renal cell carcinoma and 6 of 23 with melanoma, tumors that often show temporary spontaneous remissions. Controls of untreated patients with these tumors were not included. No beneficial effect was noted in 18 patients with other cancers. Because of the limited beneficial effect in the face of serious unwanted side effects, the clinical use of IL-2 has been shifted to regional inoculation, or to inducing LAK cells for passive immunotherapy. Phase 1 clinical trials with regional injection have produced fewer side effects, but in limited trials, so far, only marginal remissions have been noted.

Tumor Necrosis Factor (TNF). TNF has also been proposed for tumor therapy, but has not met with much success. TNF was originally found in the sera of mice infected with BCG and subsequently injected with bacterial lipopolysaccharide (endotoxin). Injection of sera from these mice into other mice sometimes caused necrosis of transplanted tumors. Human cell lines that produce TNF were used to clone the TNF gene and produce cloned TNF for human use. In phase 1 trials, considerable toxicity and little antitumor effect were found.

Monoclonal Antibodies

In 1906, Paul Ehrlich proposed antibodies ("bodies which possess a particular affinity for a certain organ") to serve as "magic bullets" to target cytotoxic agents to specific tissues. Over the next eighty years, attempts to effect this approach using conventional antibodies to cancers were not successful. With the development of hybridoma techniques, the possibility of the application of monoclonal antibodies as a new specific mode of cancer therapy for treatment of human cancers became possible. As described above, many monoclonal antibodies to human tumor-associated antigens are now available and theoretically could be used to treat human cancers. In an experimental model of leukemia, monoclonal antibodies have significantly prolonged survival of tumor-bearing mice, and anecdotal cases of prolonged remissions of some B- and T-cell tumors in humans have been reported. However, so far, the results of phase 1 and phase 2 clinical trials using monoclonal antibodies to human leukemia or lymphoma antigens, gastrointestinal antigen (CO17-1A), and melanoma antigens have been disappointing. Problems limiting the application of approaches to monoclonal antibodies and possible approaches to circumvent these problems are listed in Table 30–22. These approaches are not being used in both experimental animal models and in clinical trials. A recommended strategy for production, testing, and application of monoclonal antibody is given in Table 30–23. Presently, monoclonal antibodies are being tagged with radioisotopes, drugs, or toxins to increase their ability to kill target cells. A conjugate of ricin A chain with an antibody that is common to melanoma cells has been tested in clinical trials. In 58 patients, there were one CR and three PRs. Other trials are too small to allow satisfactory evaluation. Factors under evaluation in animal models include selection of radionucleotide or toxin, frequency of administration, regional administration, cocktails of antibodies, chimeric antibodies, use of a second antibody, and combined use with lymphokines. In addition to producing "immunoconjugates" of antibodies, strategies for directing recombinant toxins to cell surface receptors, such as the EGF receptor, IL-2 receptor, IL-6 receptor, and *erb*-B2 protein, are under investigation.

TABLE 30–22. PROBLEMS AND POSSIBLE SOLUTIONS TO MONOCLONAL ANTIBODY IMMUNOTHERAPY OF CANCER IN MAN

Problem	Possible Solution
Tumors not antigenic	Use of immune enhancing mechanisms (adjuvants, carriers, etc.)
Tumor antigens present in normal tissue	Selection of monoclonal antibodies that selectively react with tumor tissue
Presence of circulating free tumor antigen	Increasing doses of antibody to "clear" antigen
Modulation of tumor antigen	Use of mixtures (cocktails) or different antibodies sequentially
Selection of nonexpressing tumor cell clones	Use of mixtures (cocktails) or different antibodies sequentially
Immune response to foreign (mouse) monoclonal antibody	Use of human hybridomas to produce human monoclonal antibodies, construction of chimeric antibodies
Lack of cytotoxic effect of monoclonal antibody	Selection of cytotoxic monoclonal antibodies conjugation of cytotoxic drugs to monoclonal antibodies

In order to eliminate the human response to the foreign mouse antigens on monoclonal antibodies, efforts are directed to producing genetically engineered chimeric antibodies in which the mouse genes for the variable regions of the antibody are linked to the human genes for the immunoglobulin-constant regions. The construct is transfected into a mouse myeloma line for production of the chimeric antibody. Preliminary studies indicate that such antibodies have a longer half-life and are less immunogenic that mouse monoclonal antibodies. Production of human monoclonal antibodies has proven very difficult because of the lack of a suitable myeloma line for antibody formation. The difficulties in the use of monoclonal antibodies for tumor therapy have proven much more formidable than originally expected and at

TABLE 30–23. STRATEGY FOR DEVELOPMENT OF MONOCLONAL ANTIBODIES FOR USE IN HUMAN IMMUNOTHERAPY OF CANCER

1. Identification of "antigen" in cancer tissue, not detectable or present in low amounts in normal tissue
2. Production of hybridoma cell line producing monoclonal antibodies to tumor antigen
3. Selection of monoclonal antibody that binds and kills tumor cells in vitro, not toxic to normal cells
4. Isolation and characterization of monoclonal antibody
5. Demonstration of tumor binding and cytotoxic effect in vivo (nude mice bearing transplantable tumor)
6. Evaluation in clinical trials (Phases 1 and 2)

present the prognosis for developing effective immunotherapy with monoclonal antibody "magic bullets" must be guarded.

To develop a potential therapeutic monoclonal antibody, the antibody requires thorough testing in vitro and in animal model systems. The antibody should show relative specific binding to tumor cells and not normal cells and be able to kill tumor cells in vitro. It should localize and show some killing or growth retardation of tumor cells in animals. This latter effect is now tested by determining the effect of a monoclonal antibody on the growth of transplantable human cancers in nude mice. If a promising monoclonal antibody makes it through the steps in Table 30–23 and yet has no clearly demonstrable effect in clinical trials, further strategies to increase effectiveness include drug conjugation and use of mixtures of monoclonal antibodies. If a toxic drug is conjugated to a monoclonal antibody, it is necessary to repeat steps 3 to 6 in Table 30–23. Of particular importance is to test whether or not the drug antibody conjugate is more effective than drug alone, monoclonal antibody alone, or mixtures of drug and unconjugated monoclonal antibody. If mixtures of monoclonal antibodies are used, steps 3, 5, and 6 must be repeated. The expense of these approaches in time and money is enormous. Because of this, it will be some time before it can be determined if definitive monoclonal antibody treatment of human cancer will become generally available. At the time of this writing, no proven reproducible therapeutic reagent is available.

"Bispecific" antibodies, which contain two paratopes, one reacting with an immune cell, the other with a target cell, have been produced by chemically cross-linking a monoclonal antibody that reacts with a tumor-associated antigen to an antibody that reacts with the T-cell receptor complex (CD3) or other lymphocyte activation molecules, such as CD16. These bispecific antibodies then serve to bind the effector lymphocyte to the target cell and activate the release of lymphokines or lytic activity of the lymphocyte. Bispecific antibodies are now being evaluated in phase 1–2 clinical trials.

Antiidiotypic Antibodies

Antiidiotypic antibodies may also have a role in passive immunotherapy. Antiidiotypic antibodies have been used to treat human B-cell tumors that express an immunoglobulin idiotype. Antiidiotypic antibodies raised in rabbits to a mouse monoclonal antibody to human melanoma antigen p97 have been used to immunize mice to the idiotype. The immunized mice demonstrated delayed hypersensitivity when challenged with human melanoma cells. Similar antiidiotypic antibodies have been induced in humans to antigens of human gastrointestinal tumors by inoculation with mouse monoclonal antibodies. The presence of similar antiidiotypic antibodies in human sera are associated with long-term remissions in some patients. Thus, it is possible that induction of an antiidiotypic antibody with the internal image of the tumor antigen may be beneficial to the host. How this antibody could affect tumor growth remains unexplained.

Cell Adhesion Molecules

The interaction of tumor cells with other cells and with the extracellular matrix may be critical in determining invasiveness and metastatic behavior. Carcinoma cells have a reduced expression of adhesion receptors (integrins), and ICAM-1 can be upregulated on melanoma cells by interferon treatment. Monoclonal antibodies to integrins inhibit attachment of tumor cells to extracellular matrix. The ability to control tumor cell interactions by antibodies or biological treatment may lead to future therapeutic approaches.

EVALUATION OF IMMUNO-THERAPY

The variable course of cancer as a disease makes therapeutic assessment extremely difficult. One of the major problems in the past has been the inclusion of a valid control group. In addition, although the most desirable endpoint of any treatment is survival and quality of life, most clinical trials evaluate effectiveness in terms of complete or partial remission of tumor masses. In fact, remissions may be short-lived and have little long-term effect on survival. Regardless of the means of evaluation, the effect of immunotherapy on many solid nonlymphoid tumors has been limited to a few individual patients and is clinically unsatisfactory in most cases. The biologic problems involved in evaluating the effects of therapy are even more complicated for immunotherapy than for chemotherapy. For instance, there are a number of mechanisms whereby an otherwise immunologically adequate individual is unable to make an effective response to a tumor (see Table 30–9). It is possible that by attempting to immunize a person to his own tumor, the physician may actually cause the tumor to grow more rapidly by influencing the immune response in such a way as to inhibit or block the rejection mechanism.

The possibility of successful immunotherapy of cancer has raised great excitement. The introduction of a new approach usually generates great expectations. In the past, the enthusiasm of claims of success in the first clinical trials has been followed by the reality of limited or no beneficial effect. It is hoped that the clinical trials now underway will give more promising results.

Immuno-prophylaxis of Cancer

The goal of many immunologists, some of whom were eminently successful in producing vaccines for infectious diseases, has been to produce a "cancer vaccine" that could prevent tumors in humans. In theory, if human tumors are caused by viruses, a prophylactic tumor vaccine could be produced. Since virus-induced tumors share strong transplantation antigens, proper immunization might produce an immune response that would prevent development of primary tumors caused by oncogenic viruses. Less likely is a specific vaccine for chemically or spontaneously arising tumors. Nonspecific prophylaxis may also prove feasible, but the effect of this type of prophylaxis is also subject to doubt.

SPECIFIC IMMUNO-PREVENTION OF CANCER

Vaccination Against Virus-induced Tumors

Specific active vaccination to prevent virus-induced tumors of animals have been successful, but that application of this approach to human tumors is only beginning (Table 30–24). The most notable examples in animals are the use of turkey viruses to protect against Marek's disease in chickens and a 70,000-MW protein subunit vaccine used for immunization against feline leukemia virus in cats. Marek's disease vaccination has been extremely successful, whereas vaccination against FeLv needs to be improved. Recent approaches include the use of immunostimulating complexes (ISCOMs) to direct the immune response to produce cytotoxic T-cells (see Chapter 28).

Vaccination against human virus-induced tumors has not yet been accomplished. However, there are three candidates: Hepatitis B, papillomaviruses, and Epstein–Barr virus. Large-scale trials of hepatitis B vaccination in Africa have greatly reduced the incidence of overt hepatitis B infection in young children and may reduce the later high incidence of hepatocellular carcinoma in this population (see Chapter

TABLE 30–24. VACCINATION AGAINST VIRAL-INDUCED TUMORS

Animal:
SV40
Marek's disease
Feline leukemia virus
Simian immunodeficiency virus
Human candidates:
Hepatitis B
Papilloma
Epstein–Barr
Human possibilities:
HTLV-1
HIV
Herpes simplex
Cytomegalovirus

26). In addition, of course, is the extensive program to develop a vaccine for HTLV-1 and HIV infections of humans. Recent attempts to identify epitopes that select for cytotoxic T cells to HIV antigens has opened a new way to address immunization to tumor antigens.

Vaccination Against Chemically Induced Tumors

As noted above, there is considerable variation in the ability to demonstrate tumor transplantation antigens in chemically induced tumors. Even in the most highly quoted paper reporting the relatively high TSTA activity of methylcholanthrene-induced tumors by Prehn and Main, two of the fourteen tumors studied did not express TSTAs. Thus, the problem with specific immunointervention in the induction of cancers by chemicals is the question of identifying a specific antigen to which the immune cells could be directed. The problem may be even more in "spontaneously" arising tumors. Spontaneously arising mouse tumors may not express TSTAs. If this is the case, then immunoprevention of many human tumors may be impossible. On the other hand, others have found that tumor antigens may be demonstrated on spontaneously arising tumors after transplantation, metastasis, or mutagenesis, and that the resulting immune response may recognize the primary tumor cells. This indicates that spontaneously arising tumors may have antigens that can be seen by the immune system under other conditions.

Antibodies to Carcinogens

The possibility of using antibodies directed to carcinogens to prevent or block the carcinogenic effect has not received much attention. In 1986, Keren et al. proposed to induce "mucosal immunity" to the carcinogen acetylaminofluorene (2-AAF) to prevent intestinal absorption. In 1989, they reported that IgA antibodies induced in intestinal secretions by direct immunization with AAF conjugated to cholera toxin could reduce intestinal absorption by more than half after incubation in vitro. They propose that this approach could be used to develop oral vaccines against carcinogens. Another possible approach is to induce circulating anticarcinogen antibodies. Since circulating antigen–antibody complexes are usually picked up by the reticuloendothelial system (RES), the formation of such complexes could redirect a carcinogen from its target organ. Thus, hepatocarcinogens such as 2-AAF might be diverted from the hepatocyte to Kupffer cells. However, the carcinogens might still act on hepatocytes, and formation of soluble circulating complexes might cause serum sickness-like disease. In addition, RES clearance depends on formation of aggregated antibody. The fact that many carcinogens are simple chemicals that would not allow the binding of more than one antibody may make this approach not only untenable, but probably also hazardous.

T-suppressor
Cells

The ability of an individual to express tumor specific immunity depends upon the relatively greater activation of T-cytotoxic cells than T-suppressor cells. It is likely that for some tumors, such as highly immunogenic UV-induced skin cancers, the immune rejection system does not respond because of inhibition by T-suppressor (T_S) cells. It is possible that removal of the suppressor cells could result in immune rejection of the tumor. Therefore, presentation of antigens by mechanisms that direct immune stimulation to induction of T_{CTL} cells or to T_{DTH} cells that initiate killing or delayed hypersensitivity reactions rather than to suppressor T cells could allow the immune system to reject newly appearing cancer cells during the carcinogenic process.

Idiotype Vaccines

Theoretically, mouse antibodies to a human tumor antigen (Ab1) could be used to immunize other mice to produce an antiidiotypic antibody (Ab2) that would bear the mirror image of the idiotope of AB1 and therefore the tumor antigen epitope. The antiidiotype Ab2 would then be used to immunize humans to produce Ab3 that would react against the tumor epitope. This approach has worked in a few animal systems, resulting in protective immunity to some transplantable tumors in syngeneic mice and Ab3s have been produced in animals that react with human tumors. Clinical trials are now underway a mouse monoclonal antibody (Ab2) which mimics a unique tumor-associated cell surface glycoprotein 8P37 expressed on T-cell leukemia and lymphoma but not on normal T cells.

NONSPECIFIC
IMMUNO-
PREVENTION OF
CARCINOGEN-
ESIS

Antigen nonspecific prevention of carcinogenesis would employ effector mechanisms that may be activated in ways that bypass the requirement for specific recognition of antigen. For practical purposes, such approaches include activated macrophages and natural killer/lymphokine activated killer (NK/LAK) cells, as well as lymphokines and antibodies to oncogene products.

Activated
Macrophages

Several years ago, it was found that there was an up to 85% reduction in the risk of death from leukemia among children vaccinated neonatally with BCG to prevent tuberculosis. However, more extensive epidemiologic analysis has revealed that the difference between neonatally BCG vaccinated and nonvaccinated populations is very slight and there is no difference between vaccinated and nonvaccinated adults. At best, it is estimated that neonatal BCG vaccination may prevent cancer in 1 child per year for every 100,000 vaccinated. At this level, it is very difficult to demonstrate any statistically significant protective effect. In at least one experimental model immunization of rats with an extract of BCG inhibits DMBA-induced mammary neoplasias if given before DMBA but enhances tumor formation if given after the carcinogen. However, there are few data to justify the use of BCG to try to prevent cancer in humans.

NK/LAK

The use of LAKs to inhibit carcinogenesis appears to be worth trying in an experimental system. It is possible that LAKs might act on premalignant cells or newly appearing tumor cells and inhibit carcinogenesis. As noted above, NK activity in experimental animals is lowered by some carcinogens, but not by others. In one experimental model, it was found that inositol phosphate inhibited colon carcinogenesis in mice treated with dimethyhydrazine and that this inhibition was associated with an increase in NK activity.

Biological
Response
Modifiers
(BRMs)

There are few data on the possible role of BRMs in preventing cancer. On the one hand, interferon treatment may inhibit development of methylcholanthrene-induced sarcomas or development and progression of bladder cancers in mice treated with nitrofurylthiazolylformamide (FANFT). On the other hand, interferon may act a copromoter to increase the incidence of papillomas induced by DMBA and promoted with PMA. However, the mechanism of action of interferons is not clear because of their many biologic activities, including suppression of angiogenesis, inhibition of oncogene expression, modulation of cell differentiation, and inhibition of cell proliferation, as well as augmenting immune cell function. Since interleukins have many and varied growth and differentiation functions, it is likely that they may be involved in carcinogenic and/or promoting activities, particularly on lymphoid cells, as well as other cancers. For instance, IL-4 receptors are increased on a number of carcinomas; decreased availability of IL-4 could alter progression of such tumors.

Summary

There is documented evidence in experimental animals and circumstantial observations in humans that tumors contain specific antigens and that immune responses occur to these antigens. The identification of cancer-associated markers in the serum of affected patients has resulted in diagnostic tests for a few human tumors (hepatomas, teratocarcinomas, prostate cancer). Immune recognition of new tumor antigens may be important in preventing growth of newly mutated cancer cells (immune surveillance). Active or passive immunity to tumor antigens may restrict the growth of an established tumor under appropriate circumstances, but a number of coexisting phenomena may interfere with this effect. Specific passive immunotherapy using monoclonal antibodies and tumor-infiltrating lymphocytes (TILs), nonspecific immune stimulation using IFN, IL-2, and IL-2–activated killer cells (LAKs), as well as gene-modified cells and liposomes, are now being tested in clinical trials. Understanding and control of these phenomena may result in effective immunotherapy of cancer in humans.

Bibliography

TUMOR IMMUNITY

Berg JW: Morphologic evidence for immune response to breast cancer. *Cancer* 28:1453, 1971.

Brock N, Schnieder B, Stekar J, Pohl J: Experimental investigations into the carcinogenic effect of antitumor and immunosuppressive agents. *J Cancer Res Clin Oncol* 115:309, 1989.

Challis GB, Stam HJ: The spontaneous regression of cancer: A review of cases from 1900 to 1987. *Acta Oncologica* 29:545, 1990.

Chong ASF, Staren ED, Scuderi P: Monoclonal antibodies anti-CD3, anti-TCRαβ, and anti-CD2 act synergistically with tumor cells to stimulate lymphokine-activated killer cells and tumor-infiltrating lymphocytes to secrete interferon-γ. *Cancer Immunol Immunother* 35:335, 1992.

Emerson TC: Spontaneous regression of cancer. *Ann NY Acad Sci* 114:721, 1964.

Ershler WB: The influence of an aging immune system on cancer incidence and progression. *J Gerontol* 48:B3, 1993.

Foley EJ: Attempts to induce immunity against mammary adenocarcinoma in inbred mice. *Cancer Res* 13:578, 1953.

Foley EJ: Antigenic properties of methylcholanthrene-induced tumors in mice of strain of origin. *Cancer Res* 13:853, 1953.

Gatti RA, Good RA: Occurrence of malignancy in immunodeficiency diseases: A literature review. *Cancer* 28:89, 1971.

Gross L: Intradermal immunization of CSH mice against a sarcoma that originated in an animal of the same line. *Cancer Res* 3:326, 1943.

Hattler B, Amos B: The immunology of cancer: Tumor antigens and the responsiveness of the host. *Monogr Surg Sci* 3:1, 1966.

Hersy P, Stone DE, Morgan G, et al.: Previous pregnancy as a protective factor against death from melanoma. *Lancet* 1:451, 1977.

Hewitt HB, Blake ER, Walder AS: A critique of the evidence for active host defense against cancer, based on personal studies of 27 murine tumors of spontaneous origin. *Br J Cancer* 33:241, 1976.

Kaplan BS, Klassen J, Gault MH: Glomerular injury in patients with neoplasia. *Annu Rev Med* 27:117, 1976.

Klein G, Sjogren HO, Klein E, et al.: Demonstration of resistance against methylcholanthrene-induced sarcomas in the primary autochthonous host. *Cancer Res* 20:1561, 1960.

Klein G, Klein E: Immune surveillance against virus-reduced tumors and nonrejectability of spontaneous tumors: Contrasting consequences of host-versus-tumor evaluation. *Proc Nat Acad Med* 74:2121, 1977.

Korstein MJ, Guerry D: The immunopathology of the mononuclear cell infiltrate in malignant melanoma. *Pigment Cell* 8:147, 1987.

Kreider J, Bartlett WQ, Butkiewicz GL: Relationship of tumor leukocyte infiltration to host defense mechanisms and prognosis. *Cancer Metast Rev* 3:53, 1984.

Kripke ML: The immunology of skin cancer. In MD Anderson Symposium on Fundamental Cancer Research. Immunology and Cancer, Vol. 38. Kripke ML, Frost P (eds.). Austin, University Texas Press, 1986, 113–120.

Lewison EF: Conference on spontaneous regression of cancer. *Natl Cancer Inst Monogr* 44, 1976.

Loeb L: Further experimental evidence into the growth of tumors. Development of sarcoma and carcinoma after the inoculation of a carcinomatous tumor of the submaxillary gland in a Japanese mouse. *Univ Penn Med Bull* 19:113, 1906.

Mikulska ZB, Smith C, Alexander P: Evidence for an immunological reaction of the host directed against its own actively growing primary tumor. *J Natl Cancer Inst* 36:29, 1966.

Mueller BU, Pizzo PP: Cancer in children with primary or secondary immunodeficiencies. *J Pediat* 126:1-10, 1995.

Outzen HC: Development of carcinogen-induced skin tumors in mice with varied states of immune capacity. *Int J Cancer* 26:87, 1980.

Penn, I: Cancer in immunosuppressed patients. *Transplant Proc* 16:492, 1984.

Penn, I: Cancers after cyclosporine therapy. *Transplant Proc* 20:276, 1988.

Prehn RT: Relationship of tumor immunogenicity to concentration of the oncogen. *J Natl Cancer Inst* 55:189, 1975.

Prehn RT, Main JM: Immunity to methylcholanthrene induced sarcomas. *J Natl Cancer Inst* 18:769, 1957.

Prehn RT, Prehn LM: The autoimmune nature of cancer. *Cancer Res* 47:927, 1987.

Schone G: Untersuchungen uber Karzinomiummunitat bei Mausen. *Munch Med Wochenschr* 53:2517, 1906.

Scott OCA: Tumor transplantation and tumor immunity: A personal view. *Cancer Res* 51:757, 1991.

Sell S: Tumor immunity: Relevance of animal models to man. *Hum Pathol* 9:63, 1978.

Stutman O: Immunodepression and malignancy. *Adv Cancer Res* 22:261, 1975.

Svet-Moldavsky GS, Hamburg EA: Quantitative relationships in viral oncolysis and the possibility of artificial heterogenization of tumours. *Nature* 202:303, 1964.

Vose BM, Moore M: Human tumor-infiltrating lymphocytes: A marker of host response. *Semin Hematol* 22:27, 1985.

Waldmann TA, Strober W, Blaese RM: Immunodeficiency disease and malignancy: Various immunologic deficiencies of man and the role of immune processes in the control of malignant disease. *Ann Intern Med* 77:605, 1972.

TUMOR ANTIGENS

Alexander P: Fetal antigens in cancer. Nature 235:137, 1972.

Baldwin RW, Embleton MJ, Price MR, et al.: Embryonal antigen expression on experimental rat tumors. *Transplant Rev* 20:77, 1974.

Basombrio MA: Search for common antigenicities among twenty-five sarcomas induced by methylcholanthrene. *Cancer Res* 20:2458, 1970.

Chism SE, Wallis S, Burton RC, et al.: Analysis of murine oncofetal antigens as tumor associated transplantation antigens. *J Immunol* 117:1870, 1976.

Cox AJ, Skipper J, Chen Y, Henderson RA, Darrow TL, Shabanowitz J, Endelhard VH, Hunt DF, Slinguff CL: Identification of a peptide recognized by five melanoma-specific human cytotoxic T cell lines. *Science* 264:716–719, 1994.

Davidsohn I, Louisa YN: Loss of isoantigens A, B, and H in carcinoma of the lung. *J Pathol* 57:307, 1969.

Festenstein H: The biologic consequences of altered MHC expression on tumours. *Br Med Bull* 43:217, 1987.

Goodenow RS, Vogel JM, Linsk RL: Histocompatibility antigens on immune tumors. *Science* 230:777, 1985.

Klein G: Tumor specific transplantation antigens: GHA Clowes memorial lecture. *Cancer Res* 28:625, 1968.

Klein G, Klein E: Are methylcholanthrene-induced sarcoma-associated, rejection-inducing (TSTA) antigen modified forms of H-2 or linked determinants? *Int J Cancer* 15:879, 1975.

Kobayashi H, Kodama T, Gotohda E: *Xenogenization of Tumor Cells.* Sapporo, Japan, Hokkaido University Medical Library Series, 1977.

Old LJ, Boyse EA, Geering G, Oettgen HF: Serologic approaches to the study of cancer in animals and in man. *Cancer Res* 28:1288, 1968.

Pawelec G, Kalbacher H, Bruserud O: Tumor-specific antigens revisited: Presentation to the immune system of fusion peptides resulting solely from tumor-specific chromosomal translocations. *Oncol Res* 4:315–320, 1992.

Prehn RT: Tumor-specific antigens of nonviral tumors. Cancer Res 28:1326, 1968.

Schreiber H, Ward PL, Rowley DA, et al.: Unique tumor-specific antigens. *Ann Rev Immunol* 6:465, 1988.

Stonehill EH, Bendich A: Retrogenetic expression: The reappearance of embryonal antigens in cancer cells. *Nature* 228:370, 1970.

Witebsky E: Zur serologischen Spezifitat des Karzinomgewebes. *Klin Wochenschr* 9:58, 1930.

van Pel A, Vessiere F, Boon T: Protection against spontaneous mouse leukemias conferred by immunologic variants obtained by mutagenesis. *J Exp Med* 157:1992, 1983.

IN VITRO ASSAYS OF TUMOR IMMUNITY

Biron CA, Byron KS, Sullivan JL: Severe herpesvirus infections in an adolescent without natural killer cells. N Engl J Med 320:1731, 1989.

Bloom BR, Glade PR (eds.): *In Vitro Methods in Cell-mediated Immunity.* New York, Academic Press, 1971.

Cerittini J-C, Brunner KT: Cell-mediated cytotoxicity, allograft rejection, and tumor immunity. *Adv Immunol* 18:67, 1974.

Hellstrom KE, Hellstrom I: Lymphocyte-mediated cytotoxicity and blocking serum activity to tumor antigens. *Adv Immunol* 18:209, 1974.

Henkart PA: Mechanism of lymphocyte-mediated cytotoxicity. *Annu Rev Immunol* 3:31, 1985.

Herberman RB, Holden HT: Natural cell-mediated immunity. *Adv Cancer Res* 27:305, 1978.

Keller R: Cytostatic elimination of syngeneic rat tumor cells in vitro by nonspecifically activated macrophage. *J Exp Med* 138:625, 1973.

Moller E: Antagonistic effects of humoral isoantibodies on the in vitro cytotoxicity of immune lymphoid cells. *J Exp Med* 122:11, 1965.

Sjogren HO, Hellstrom I, Bansal SC, et al.: Elution of "blocking factors" from human tumors, capable of abrogating tumor cell destruction by specifically immune lymphocytes. *Int J Cancer* 9:274, 1972.

Takasugi M, Koide Y, Akira D, et al.: Specificities in natural cell-mediated cytotoxicity by the cross-competition assay. *Int J Cancer* 19:291, 1977.

Tshopp J, Nabholz M: Perforin-mediated target cell lysis by cytolytic T-lymphocytes. *Annu Rev Immunol* 8:279, 1990.

TUMOR ENHANCEMENT AND STIMULATION

Amos DB, Cohen I, Klein WS: Mechanisms of immunologic enhancement. Transplant Proc 2:68, 1970.

Hellstrom KE, Hellstrom I: Immunologic enhancement as studied by cell culture techniques. *Annu Rev Microbiol* 24:373, 1970.

Kaliss N: Immunological enhancement. *Int Rev Exp Pathol* 8:241, 1969.

Kaliss N: Dynamics of immunologic enhancement. *Transplant Proc* 2:59, 1970.

Lamon EW: Stimulation of tumor cell growth in vitro: A critical evaluation of immunologic specificity. *J Natl Cancer Inst* 59:769, 1977.

Prehn RT: Immunostimulation of the lymphodependent phase of neoplastic growth. *J Natl Cancer Inst* 59:1043, 1977.

IMMUNE SURVEILLANCE

Burnet FM: The concept of immunological surveillance. *Prog Exp Tumor Res* 13:1, 1970.

Chen L, Ashe S, Brady WA, et al.: Costimulation of antitumor immunity by the B7 counter-receptor for the T-lymphocyte molecules CD28 and CTLA-4. *Cell* 71:1093, 1992.

Fenyo EM, Klein E, Klein G, et al.: Selection of an immunoresistant Moloney lymphoma subline with decreased concentration of tumor-specific surface antigens. *J Natl Cancer Inst* 40:69, 1968.

Ioachim HL: The stromal reaction of tumors: An expression of immune surveillance. *J Natl Cancer Inst* 57:465, 1976.

Mizoguchi H, O'Shea JJ, Longo DL, et al.: Alterations in signal transduction molecules in T lymphocytes from tumor-bearing mice. *Science* 258:1795, 1992.

Moller G, Moller E: The concept of immunological surveillance against neoplasia. *Transplant Rev* 28:3, 1976.

Prehn RT: Immunosurveillance, regeneration, and oncogenesis. *Prog Exp Tumor Res* 14:1, 1970.

Prehn RT: Stimulatory effects of immune reactions upon the growths of untransplanted tumors. *Cancer Res.* 54:908-914, 1994.

Rygaard J, Poulsen CO: The nude mouse versus the hypothesis of immunologic surveillance. *Transplant Rev* 48:43, 1976.

Schwartz RH: Costimulation of T lymphocytes: The role of CD28, CTLA-4, and B7/BB1 in interleukin-2 production and immunotherapy. *Cell* 71:1065, 1992.

Stutman O: Tumor development after 3-methylcholanthrene in immunologically deficient athymic nude mice. *Science* 183:534, 1974.

Thomas L: Discussion. In *Cellular and Humoral Aspects of the Hypersensitive State.* Lawrence HS (ed.). New York, Harper & Row, 1959.

**IMMUNO-
DIAGNOSIS**

Abelev GI: Production of embryonal serum α-globulin by hepatomas: Review of experimental and clinical data. *Cancer Res* 28:1344, 1968.

Baylin JB: Ectopic production of hormones and other proteins by tumors. *Hosp Pract* 10:117, 1975.

Bence-Jones H: Papers on chemical pathology: Lecture III. *Lancet* 2:269–274, 1847.

Carter HB, Pearson JD, Metter EJ, et al.: Longitudinal evaluation of prostate-specific antigen levels in men with and without prostate disease. *JAMA* 267:2215, 1992.

Catalona WJ, Smith DS, Ratliff TL, et al.: Measurement of prostate-specific antigen in serum as a screening test for prostate cancer. *N Engl J Med* 324:1156, 1991.

Cooper GM: Cellular transforming genes. *Science* 217:801–806, 1982.

Gold P, Freedman SO: Specific carcinoembryonic antigens of the human digestive system. *J Exp Med* 122:467, 1965.

Guo JQ, Wang JYJ, Arlinghaus RB: Detection of BCR-ABL proteins in blood cells of benign phase chronic myelogenous leukemia patients. *Cancer Res* 51:3048, 1991.

Hakomori SI: Tumor-associated carbohydrate antigens. *Annu Rev Immunol* 2:103, 1984.

Hakomori S-I: Possible function of tumor-associated carbohydrate antigens. *Curr Opin Immunol* 3:646–653, 1991.

Klein G: Specific chromosomal translocations and genesis of B cell-derived tumors in mice and men. *Cell* 32:311–315, 1983.

McKenzie SJ: Diagnostic utility of oncogenes and their products in human cancer. *Biochim Biophysica Acta* 1072:193, 1991.

Mettlin C: The status of prostate cancer early detection. *Cancer* 72:1050–1055, 1993.

Sell S: Cancer markers of the 1990s: Comparison of the new generation of markers defined by monoclonal antibodies and oncogene probes to prototypic markers. *Clin Lab Med* 10:1, 1990.

Sell S: Cancer-associated carbohydrates identified by monoclonal antibodies. *Hum Pathol* 21:1003, 1990.

Sell S: *Serologic Cancer Markers.* Totowa, NJ, Humana Press, 1992.

Sell S, Becker FF; Guest editorial: Alpha-fetoprotein. *J Natl Cancer Inst* 60:19, 1978.

Sidransky D, Tokino T, Hamilton SR, et al.: Identification of *ras* oncogene mutations in the stool of patients with curable colorectal tumors. *Science* 256:102, 1992.

Tee DEH: Clinical evaluation of the Makari tumor skin test. *Brit J Cancer* 28:187, 1973.

Wolman SR, Henderson AS: Chromosomal aberrations as markers of oncogene amplification. *Hum Pathol* 20:309, 1989.

IMMUNO-THERAPY

Ascher MS, Gottlieb AA, Kirkpatrick CH (eds.): *Transfer Factor: Basic Properties and Clinical Application.* New York, Academic Press, 1976.

Bast RC Jr, Zbar B, Borsos T, Rapp HJ: BCG and cancer. *N Engl J Med* 290:1413, 1458, 1974.

Berd D, Macuire HC, Mastrangelo MJ: Treatment of human melanoma with a hapten-modified autologous vaccine. *Ann NY Acad Sci* 690:147–152, 1993.

Blakey DC: Drug targeting with monoclonal antibodies. *Rev Oncology* 1:91, 1992.

Bolhuis RLH, Sturm E, Braakman E: T-cell targeting in cancer therapy. *Cancer Immunol Immunother* 34:1, 1991.

Bonnem EM: Alpha-interferon: The potential drug of adjuvant therapy; past achievements and future challenges. *Eur J Cancer* 27(suppl. 4):52, 1991.

Britton KE: Overview of radioimmunotherapy: A European perspective. *Antibody Immunoconj Radiopharm* 4:133, 1991.

Buchsbaum DJ: Experimental radioimmunotherapy: Methods to increase therapeutic efficacy relevant to the study of human cancer. *Antibody Immunoconj Radiopharm* 4:693, 1991.

Bystryn J-C, Henn M, Li J, Shroba S: Identification of immunogenic human melanoma antigens in a polyvalent melanoma vaccine. *Cancer Res* 52:5948, 1992.

Carswell EA, Old LJ, Kassel RL, et al.: An endotoxin-induced serum factor that causes necrosis of tumors. *Proc Natl Acad Sci* 25:3660, 1975.

Chatterjee MB, Foon KA, Köhler H. Idiotypic antibody immunotherapy of cancer. *Cancer Immunol Immunother* 38:75-82, 1994.

Chiao JW: *Biological Response Modifiers and Cancer Therapy.* New York, Marcel Dekker, 1988.

Cornette JL, Margalit H, DeLisi C, et al.: Identification of T-cell epitopes and use in construction of synthetic vaccines. *Meth Enzymol* 178:611, 1989.

Culver KW: Clinical applications of gene therapy for cancer. *Clin Chem* 40:510–512, 1994.

Debruyne FMJ, Denis L, Van Der Meijden APM (eds.): EORTC genitourinary group monograph: BCG in superficial bladder cancer. *Prog Clin Biol Res* 6:310, 1989.

Esgro JJ, Whitworth P, Fidler IJ: Macrophages as effectors of tumor immunity. *Immunol Allergy Clin N Am* 10:705, 1990.

Fonn KA: Biological response modifiers: the new immunotherapy. *Cancer Res* 49:1621, 1989.

Gately MK: Interleukin-12: A recently discovered cytokine with potential for enhancing cell-mediated immune responses to tumors. *Cancer Invest* 11:500–506, 1993.

Goldstein D, Laszlo, J: Interferon therapy in cancer: From imagination to interferon. *Cancer Res* 46:4315, 1986.

Graham JB, Graham RM: Autogenous vaccine in cancer patients. *Surg Gynecol Obstet* 114:1, 1962.

Greenberg PD, Eiddell SR: Tumor-specific T-cell immunity: Ready for prime time? *J Natl Cancer Inst* 84:1059, 1992.

Grimm EA: Human lymphokine-activated killer (LAK) cells as a potential immunotherapeutic modality. *Biochim Biophys Acta* 865:267, 1986.

Hanna MG, Ransom JH, Pomato N, et al.: Active specific immunotherapy of human colorectal carcinoma with an autologous tumor cell/Bacillus Calmette–Guérin vaccine. *Ann NY Acad Sci* 690:135–146, 1993.

Harris DT, Mastrangelo MJ: Serotherapy of cancer. *Semin Oncol* 16:180, 1989.

Heaton KM, Grimm EA: Cytokine combinations in immunotherapy for solid tumors: A review. *Cancer Immunol Immunother* 37:213–219, 1993.

Heppner G, Fulton AM: *Macrophages and Cancer.* Boca Raton, FL, CRC Press, 1988.

Herlyn M, Koprowski H: Melanoma antigens: Immunologic and biologic characterization and clinical significance. *Annu Rev Immunol* 6:283, 1988.

Herlyn M, Menrad A, Koprowski H: Structure, function, and clinical significance of human tumor antigens. *J Natl Cancer Inst* 82:188, 1990.

Hersey P: Melanoma vaccines: Current status and future prospects. *Drugs* 47:373–382, 1994.

Klein E, Holterman OA, Helm F, et al.: Topical therapy for cutaneous tumors. *Transplant Proc* 16:507, 1984.

Kolitz JE, Mertelsmann R: The immunotherapy of human cancer with interleukin-2: Present status and future directions. *Cancer Invest* 9:529, 1991.

Lamm DL, Blumenstein BA, Crawford C, et al.: A randomized trial of intravesical doxorubicin and immunotherapy with Bacille Calmette–Guérin for transitional cell carcinoma of the bladder. *N Engl J Med* 325:1205, 1991.

Lamm DL, Thor DE, Stogdill VD, et al.: Bladder cancer immunotherapy. *J Urol* 128:931, 1982.

Lamoureaux G, Turcote R, Portelance V: *BCG in Cancer Immunotherapy.* New York, Grune & Stratton, 1976.

Levy R, Miller RA: Tumor therapy with monoclonal antibodies. *FASEB Proc* 42:2650, 1983.

Lotze MT, Kawakami Y, Rosenberg SA: Immunotherapy protocols at the National Cancer Institute: Current status and future prospects. *Colloque INSERM* 179:153, 1989.

Lotzova E, Herberman RB: Interleukin-2 and killer cells in cancer. Boca Raton, FL, CRC Press, 1989.

Lynch RG, Rohrer JW, Odermatt B, et al.: Immunoregulation of murine myeloma cell growth and differentiation: A monoclonal model of B-cell differentiation. *Immunol Rev* 48:81, 1979.

Maas RA, Dullens HFJ, Otter WD: Interleukin-2 in cancer treatment: Disappointing or (still) promising. *Cancer Immunol Immunother* 36:141–148, 1993.

Margalit H, Spouge JL, Cornette JL, et al.: Prediction of immunodominant helper T-cell antigenic sites from the primary sequence. *J Immunol* 138:2213, 1987.

Metzger RS, Mitchell MS (eds.): *Human Tumor Antigens and Specific Tumor Therapy.* New York, Liss, 1988.

Miller RA, Levy R: Response of cutaneous T-cell lymphoma to therapy with hybridoma monoclonal antibody. *Lancet* II:226, 1981.

Mitchell MS, Harel W, Kan-Mitchell J, et al.: Active specific immunotherapy of melanoma with allogeneic cell lysates. *Ann NY Acad Sci* 690:153–166, 1993.

Mittelman A, Chen ZJ, Yang J, et al.: Human high-molecular-weight melanoma-associated antigen (HMW-MAA) mimicry by mouse antiidiotypic monoclonal antibody MK2-23: Induction of humoral anti-HMW-MAA immunity and prolongation of survival in patients with stage IV melanoma. *Proc Natl Acad Sci USA* 89:466, 1992.

Moore GE, Moore MB: Auto-inoculation of cultured lymphocytes in malignant melanoma. *NY State J Med* 69:460, 1969.

Morein B, Sundquist B, Hoglund S, et al.: ISCOM, a novel structure for antigenic presentation on membrane proteins from enveloped viruses. *Nature* 308:457, 1984.

Murren JR, Buzaid AC: The role of interferons in the treatment of malignant neoplasms. *Yale J Biol Med* 62:271, 1989.

Nelson H: Targeted cellular immunotherapy with bifunctional antibodies. *Cancer* 3:163, 1991.

Nicola NA, Murphy MJ: The Beijing blood cell growth factors symposium. Blood cell growth factors: Their present and future use in hematology and oncology. *Cancer Res* 52:2012, 1992.

Old LJ, Stockert E, Boyse EA, et al.: Antigenic modulation. Loss of TL antigen from cells exposed to TL antibody: Study of the phenomenon in vitro. *J Exp Med* 127:523, 1968.

Pastan I, FitsGerald D: Recombinant toxins for cancer treatment. *Science* 254:1173, 1991.

Perussia B: Tumor-infiltrating cells. *Lab Invest* 67:155, 1992.

Quesada JR, Reuben JR, Manning JT, et al.: Alpha-interferon for induction of remission in hairy cell leukemia. *N Engl J Med* 30:15, 1984.

Reisfeld R, Sell S: Monoclonal antibodies and cancer therapy. New York, Liss, 1985.

Rosenberg SA: The immunotherapy and gene therapy of cancer. *J Clin Oncol* 10:180, 1992.

Rosenberg S, Lotze MT: Cancer immunotherapy using interleukin-2 and interleukin-2–activated lymphocytes. *Annu Rev Immunol* 4:681, 1986.

Roth AD, Kirkwood JM: New clinical trials with interleukin-2: Rationale for regional administration. *Nat Immun Cell Growth Regul* 8:153, 1989.

Schlom J: Basic principles and applications of monoclonal antibodies in the management of carcinomas: The Richard and Hinda Rosenthal Foundation award lecture. *Cancer Res* 46:3225, 1986.

Sell S, Reisfeld R (eds.): *Monoclonal Antibodies in Cancer Therapy.* Clifton, New Jersey, Humana, 1985.

Sella A, Swanson DA, Ro AY, et al.: Surgery following response to interferon-α–based therapy for residual renal cell carcinoma. *J Urol* 149:19, 1993.

Stevenson HC (ed.): Adoptive cellular immunotherapy of cancer. New York, Marcel Dekker, 1989.

Sznol M, Clark JW, Smith JW: Pilot study of interleukin-2 and lymphokine-activated killer cells combined with immunomodulatory doses of chemotherapy and sequenced with interferon-α-2a in patients with metastatic melanoma and renal cell carcinoma. *J Natl Cancer Inst* 84:929, 1992.

Talmadge JE: Development of immunotherapeutic strategies for the treatment of malignant neoplasms. *Biotherapy* 4:215, 1992.

Trinchieri G: Biology of natural killer cells. *Adv Immunol* 47:187, 1989.

Tukey JW: Some thoughts on clinical trials, especially problems of multiplicity. *Science* 198:679, 1977.

Vedantham S, Gamliel H, Golomb HM: Mechanism of interferon action in hairy cell leukemia: A model of effective cancer biotherapy. *Cancer Res* 52:1056, 1992.

Vitetta ES, Krolick KA, et al.: Immunotoxins: A new approach to cancer therapy. *Science* 219:644, 1983.

Waisbren BA: Observations on the combined systemic administration of mixed bacterial vaccine, bacillus Calmette–Guérin, transfer factor, and lymphoblastoid lymphocytes to patients with cancer, 1974–1985. *J Biol Resp Mod* 6:1, 1987.

Waldmann TA: Monoclonal antibodies in diagnosis and therapy. *Science* 252:1657, 1991.

IMMUNO-PREVENTION

Akerblom L, Stromstet K, Hoglund S, et al.: Formation and characterization of FeLv ISCOMs. *Vaccine* 7:142, 1989.

Biggs PM: Marek's disease: The disease and its prevention by vaccination. *Br J Cancer* 31:152, 1975.

Collumbek PR, Lazenby AJ, Levitsky HI, et al.: Treatment of established renal cancer by tumor cells engineered to secrete interleukin-4. *Science* 254:713, 1991.

Davignon L, Lemonde P, Robillard P, et al.: BCG vaccination and leukemia mortality. *Lancet* 2:638, 1970.

Epstein, M. A., Vaccine prevention of virus-induced human cancers. *Proc Royal Soc Lond (Biol)* 230:147, 1987.

Halliday GM, Wood RC, Muller HK: Presentation of antigen to suppressor cells by a dimethylbenz(a)anthracene resistant, Ia, Thy-1-negative, I-J restricted epidermal cell. *Immunology* 69:97, 1990.

Haubeck HD, Kolsh E: Tumor-specific T-suppressor cells induced at early stages of tumorigenesis act on the induction phase of cytotoxic T-cells. *Immunology* 47:503, 1982.

Miller AD: Human gene therapy comes of age. *Nature* 3357:455, 1992.

Miller RA, Levy R: Response of cutaneous T-cell lymphoma to therapy with hybridoma monoclonal antibody. *Lancet* II:226, 1981.

Hoover RN: Bacillus Calmette–Guérin vaccination and cancer prevention: A critical review of the human experience. *Cancer Res* 36:652, 1976.

Howie SM, McBride WH: Tumor-specific T-helper activity can be abrogated by two distinct suppressor cell mechanisms. *Eur J Immunol* 12:671, 1982.

Hurley DJ, Mastro AM: Induction of suppressor activity by tumor-promoting phorbol esters in primary cultures of lymph node cells. *Carcinogenesis* 8:357, 1987.

Keren DF, Silbart LK, Lincoln PM, et al.: Significance of immune responses to mucosal carcinogens: A hypothesis and a workable model system. *Pathol Immunopathol Res* 5:265, 1986.

Klinerman ES, et al.: Phase 2 study of liposomal muramyl tripeptide in osteosarcoma: The cytokine cascade and monocyte activation following administration. *J Clin Oncol* 10:1310, 1992.

Lippman ME: Growth factors, receptors, and breast cancer. *J NIH Res* 3:59, 1991.

Mastro JM, Lewis MG, Mathes LE, et al.: Feline leukemia vaccine: Efficiency, contents, and probable mechanism. *Vet Immunol Immunopathol* 11:205, 1986.

Maynard JE: Hepatitis B: Global importance and need for control. *Vaccine* 8 (suppl. p):18, 1990.

Okazaki W, Purchase HG, Burmester BR: Protection against Marek's disease by vaccination with a herpesvirus of turkey. *Avian Dis* 14:413, 1970.

Reiners JJ Jr, Pavone A, Rupp T, Cantu AR: Modulation of the copromoting activity of gamma interferon in SENCAR and C57BL/6 mouse skin by dinitromethylornithine and the scheduling and duration of interferon treatment. *Carcinogenesis* 11:129, 1990.

Rodeck U, Herlyn M, Herlyn D, et al.: Tumor growth modulation by a monoclonal antibody to the epidermal growth factor receptor: Immunologically mediated and effector cell-independent effects. *Cancer Res* 47:3692, 1987.

Salerno RA, Whitmire CE, Garcia IM, et al.: Chemical carcinogenesis in mice inhibited by interferon. *Nature* 239:31, 1972.

Silbart LK, Keren DF: Reduction of intestinal carcinogen absorption by carcinogen-specific secretory immunity. *Science* 243:1462, 1989.

Stevenson FK: Tumor vaccines. *FASEB J* 5:2250, 1991.

Talarico D, Ittmann M, Balsari A, et al.: Protection of mice against tumor growth by

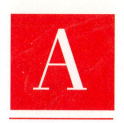

Appendix A:
Clinical Immunology Tests

Immunologically based tests are used for diagnosis and determination of prognosis for many human diseases. The tests may be classified as to which diseases they are used, as follows:

Serum proteins:	Immune deficiencies
	Inflammation
	Myeloma
Cell-mediated immunity:	Immune deficiencies
	Leukemia/lymphoma
	Cancer (prognosis)
Tissue-typing:	Blood transfusion
	Tissue grafting
Specific antibodies:	Infectious diseases
	Autoimmune diseases
	Allergic reactions (IgE)
Tumor-associated antigens:	Cancer

As techniques in molecular biology become more available and reagents better characterized, many assays (such as those for specific infectious agents or for determination of prognosis in cancer) are being replaced by assays using multiplication of DNA (polymerase chain reactions) and specific complementary DNA (cDNA) probes. Immune-labeling procedures for detection of organisms in tissues are being replaced by in situ hybridization using cDNA, a method that is also being applied to detect genetic changes in cancers. It is expected that molecular hybridization will soon replace serologic methods for determination of HLA phenotypes. Flow cytometry has been used increasingly for quantitation of expression of cell surface markers detected by antibodies. In addition, many colormetric-based assays have been automated, greatly decreasing cost and turnover time.

For more details on clinical immunologic testing see: Rose NR, de Macario EC, Fahey JL, Friedman H, Penn GM (Eds): Manual of Clinical Laboratory Immunology, 4th Ed, Washington, DC, 1992, 987 pp. or Rich RR, Fleisher TA, Schwartz BD, Shearer WT, Strober W (Eds): Clinical Immunology, St. Louis, Mosby, 1995, 2228 pp.

References

Osterlund CK: Laboratory diagnosis and monitoring in chronic systemic autoimmune diseases. Clin Chem 40:2146–2153, 1994.

Shearer WT, Adelman CD, Huston DP, Engler RJ, Gupta S, Ledford DK, Lopez M, Du Buske LM: Core content outline for clinical and laboratory immunology. J. Allergy Clin Immunol 94:933–941,1994.

TABLE A–1. SOME CLINICAL IMMUNOLOGY TESTS

Measurement	Assay Used	Diseases
SERUM PROTEINS; HUMORAL IMMUNITY		
Major globulins	Serum electrophoresis	Immune deficiencies, myeloma Other protein anomalies
Serum Ig classes	Nephelometry, RID	Immune deficiencies, myeloma
Serum proteins	Isoelectric focusing, immune fixation, isoelectric focusing, electrophoresis	Immune deficiencies, myeloma Immune globulin aberrations
Total complement	Hemolytic assay	Immune deficiencies, immune complex disorders
Serum complement components	Nephelometry, RID	Immune deficiencies, immune disorders
C1 esterase inhibitor	Nephlemetry, Inhibition of C1	Angioedema
C breakdown products	ELISA	Acute inflammation
Bence-Jones protein (urine)	Precipitation/nephelometry	Myeloma
Cryoglobulins	Cold precipitation	Raynauds phenomena, arthralgias
Immune complexes	RAJI cell binding, Ciq binding, Anti-Ig binding	Immune complex diseases
CELLULAR IMMUNITY (For cytokines see Appendix B; for CD markers see Appendix C)		
Total cells	Complete blood count, differential count	Infection, leukemia, immune deficiency
T-cells		
Total/subpopulations	Flow cytometry	Immune deficiency, leukemia/lymphoma, AIDS
Mitogen response	PHA, Concanavalin A	Immune deficiency, leukemia/lymphoma
Interleukins	ELISA	Immune deficiency, inflammation, etc.
Cytokine production	ELISA	Immune deficiency, inflammation, etc.
T-cell receptor	Flow cytometry	Immune deficiency
gene rearrangements	cDNA binding on gels	Leukemia/lymphoma
IL-2 receptors	Flow cytometry	Leukemia/lymphoma prognosis
Soluble IL-2R	ELISA	SLE, RA prognosis
ICAM-1	ELISA	Inflammation, RA, lymphoma
Neopterin (T-cell activation)	RIA	Infections, inflammation, lymphoma prognosis
B-cells		
sIg, subpopulations and Ig class clonality	Flow cytometry	Immune deficiency, leukemia/lymphoma
Ig gene rearrangements	cDNA binding on gels	Myeloma
Monocytes/macrophages		
Subpopulations	Flow cytometry	Leukemia/lymphoma
IL-1 production	Growth of T-cell lines	Immune deficiency

Continued

TABLE A–1. (CONTINUED)

Measurement	Assay Used	Diseases
Bacterial killing	Cytotoxicity in vitro	Immune deficiency
Activation (neutrophils)	Production of oxygen radicals	Immune deficiency
Subpopulations	Flow cytometry	Myeloid leukemia
Phagocytosis	Particle uptake	Immune deficiency
Digestion	Nitrobluetetrazolium prod.	Immune deficiency
Bacterial killing	Bactericidal test in vitro	Immune deficiency
Migration	Micropore filter in vitro	Immune deficiency
INFECTIOUS DISEASES (MICROBIOLOGY)		
Bacterial	Antibody titers, PCR	Specific diagnosis
Mycobacterial	Immunofluorescence (IF), PCR	Specific diagnosis
Parasites	Antibody, PCR	Specific diagnosis
Fungi	Antibody (ELISA), PCR, Immunofluor. western blot	Specific diagnosis
Viruses	Antibody, IF, PCR, ELISA, In situ hybrid, immunoblots, etc.	Specific diagnosis
Rickettsia	Antibody, PCR, immunoblots	Specific diagnosis
Chlamydia	IF, PCR, immunoblots	Specific diagnosis
TRANSFUSION		
Blood group antigens	Type and cross-match	Donor selection
Platelet antigens	Flow cytometry	Donor selection
Ig allotypes	Hemagglutination inhibition	Donor selection
HIV antibody	ELISA, western blot	Donor selection, diagnosis
HIV antigen	PCR	Donor selection, pediatric infection
Hepatitis antibody	ELISA	Donor selection. diagnosis
Hepatitis antigens	PCR (CDNA)	Donor selection, diagnosis
Fibrin split products	ELISA	Bleeding disorders
TRANSPLANTATION		
HLA (A–D) antigens	Serologic cytotoxicity, PCR	Donor selection
HLA D cellular antigens	Mixed lymph reaction, PCR	Donor selection
Lymphocyte killing	Cell-mediated cytotoxicity,	Rejection reaction
Antilymphocyte antibody	Serological cytotoxicity, flow cytometry	Donor activity
ALLERGIC REACTIONS		
Serum IgE	ELISA	Allergic predisposition
Allergen specific IgE	RAST, Immunoblot	Specific allergen
Basophil reactivity	Histamine release (fluorimetry)	Specific allergen
Skin test	Wheal and flare	Specific allergen
Schultz–Dale test	Constriction of smooth muscle in vitro	Specific allergen
ANTIBODY MEDIATED DISEASES		
Tissue Antibodies		
Acetylcholine receptor	ELISA, binding inhibition	Myasthenia gravis
Pancreatic islet cells	ELISA, IF	Type I diabetes mellitus
Basement membrane	ELISA, IF	Goodpasture's syndrome
Mitochondria	ELISA, IF	Primary biliary cirrhosis
TSH receptor	ELISA, IF	Graves' disease
Thyroglobulin	ELISA, IF, Passive Hemagglutination	Thyroiditis
Thryoid microsomes	IF, Passive Hemagglutination	Thyroid diseases
Adrenal antigens	IF	Idiopathic Addison's disease
Parathyroid antigens	IF	Idiopathis hypoparathyroidism
Striational	IF	Myasthenia gravis with thymoma
Smooth muscle antigens	IF	Chronic hepatitis, cirrhosis

Continued

Measurement	Assay Used	Diseases
Cardiac muscle	IF	Rheumatic myocarditis, bypass surgery
Gastric parietal cells	IF, ELISA to intrinsic fact.	Pernicious anemia
Gliadin, reticulin, endomysin	ELISA	Gluten sensitivity
Antineutrophil cytoplasmic abs	RIA, IF, Flow cytometry	Wegener's granulomatosis, vasculitis
Antiphospholipids	ELISA	SLE, fetal loss, PAPS
Antineurons	ELISA	SLE with CNS symptoms
Skin, basement membrane	IF	Pemphigus vulgaris
Skin, epidermal cells	IF	Bullous pemphigoid
Antinuclear Antibodies/Collagen Diseases		
Anti-ssDNA	ELISA	Scleroderma, SLE, etc.
Anti-dsDNA	ELISA	SLE
Anti-Sm	ELISA, immunoblot	SLE
Anti-RNP	ELISA, immunoblot	SLE, MCTD, Polymyositis, scleroderma
Anti-histones	Immunodiffusion, ELISA	SLE, drug-induced SLE
Anti-Scl 70	Immunodiffusion, ELISA	Scleroderma
Anti-centromere	IF	CREST syndrome
Anti-JO1	ELISA, immunodiffusion	Polymyositis, scleroderma
Anti-Pn-Acl (Pn-1)	ELISA, immunodiffusion	Polymyositis, scleroderma
Anti-Mi2	ELISA, immunodiffusion	Dermatomyositis
Anti-La (SS-B)	ELISA, immunodiffusion	SLE, Sjögren's syndrome
Anti-Ro (SS-A) (Cytoplasm)	ELISA, immunodiffusion	SLE, Sjögren's syndrome
Rheumatoid Factor	Nephelometry, Latex agg.	Rheumatoid arthritis
CANCER		
Tumor Immunity (see Chapter 33)		
Antitumor antibodies	ELISA, IF, cytotoxicity	Reactivity to specific tumor cell/antigen
Cell-mediated cytoxicity	Cell lysis (^{51}Cr release)	Specific and non specific killing
	Colony inhibition in vitro	
ADCC	Cell lysis	Antibody directed cell-mediated
Lymphocyte reactivity	Blast transformation, IL-2 and lymphokine production	Specific reactivity to tumors
Blocking factors	Inhibition of CMI	Blocking of tumor immunity
Tumor Markers, Serum (see Chapter 33 for other markers not listed)		
Alphafetoprotein	ELISA	Diagnosis, prognosis
Carcinoembryonic antigen	ELISA	Prognosis
Prostate specific antigen	ELISA	Screening, diagnosis, prognosis
Cancer carbohydrates	ELISA	Different cancers, prognosis
Cancer mucins	ELISA	Prognosis
Hormones[a]	ELISA	Differential diagnosis, prognosis
Myeloma proteins	Electrophoresis, immunofixation	Diagnosis, prognosis
Isoenzymes	Electrophoresis, immunofixation	Diagnosis
Melanoma antigen	ELISA	Diagnosis
Tumor Markers, Cellular		
Alpha-fetoprotein	IF or immunoperoxidase (IP)	Differential diagnosis
Carcinoembryronic antigen	IF or IP	Differential diagnosis
Prostate-specific antigen	IF, IP	Differential diagnosis
Pancreatic antigen	IF, IP	Differential diagnosis
Melanoma antigen	IF, IP	Differential diagnosis
Cancer carbohydrates	IF, IP	Differential diagnosis
Cancer mucins	IF, IP	Differential diagnosis
Lymphocyte markers	IF, IP	Differential diagnosis
Enzymes	Enzyme activity	Hematopoietic tumors
Molecular Biologic Markers		
Various oncogene products	IF, IP, Blots	Prognosis
Ig gene rearrangements	cDNA binding on gels	B-cell tumors
T-cell receptor rearrangements	cDNA binding on gels	T-cell tumors

[a]Insulin, gastrin, renin-angiotensis, growth hormone, placental hormones, thyroid hormones, cortisol, estradiol, testosterones, etc.

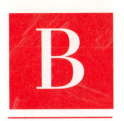

Appendix B:
Human Cytokines

The role of cytokines in human diseases, in particular those involving inflammation and immune reactions, is becoming better understood as more cytokines are identified and their biological activity determined. The following table lists most of the known cytokines, how they are assayed, and the human diseases in which they are found and may play a role in pathogenesis. Most of the assays involve effects on cell lines or cultures of normal cells *in vitro*. Thus most of the correlations listed in the table are derived from experimental work and the assays are not in general use in clinical immunology laboratories. There are ELISA assays using recombinant proteins for some of the human cytokines. These are listed in Appendix A. For more recent information on cytokines see: Thompson AW (Ed): Cytokine Handbook, 2nd Edition. Academic Press Ltd. London, 1994, 615 pp.

TABLE. HUMAN CYTOKINES

Cytokine	Bases of Assay	Cell/Assay System	Disease Association	Family	Size & Form
IL-1	IL-2 production Proliferation	IL-2 reactive cell line IL-1 reactive cell line	Inflammation, RA, CLL, etc.	Unassigned	153–159; monomer
IL-2	Proliferation	IL-2 reactive cell line	Inflammation, SLE, Autoimmune disease	Hematopoietin	133, monomer
IL-3	Proliferation	Bone marrow colony	Mastocytosis, malaria, asthma, allergy	Hematopoietin	133, monomer
IL-4	Proliferation CD23 expression	B-cell costimulation B-cell lines	Allergy, leukemia, immunosuppression	Hematopoietin	129, monomer
IL-5	Proliferation Eosinophil differentiation	Cell lines, lymphoma Bone marrow cells	Eosinophilia, rhinitis	Hematopoietin	115, homodimer
IL-6	Proliferation Acute phase proteins	Cell lines (B-cell) Hepatocyte lines	RA, psoriasis, myeloma, card. myxoma Castleman's disease	Hematopoietin	184, monomer
IL-7	Proliferation	pre-B-cell line Mitogen activated T-cells	Pre-B-cell tumors	Hematopoietin	152, monomer
IL-8	Neutrophil activation	Neutrophils	RA, inflammation, psoriasis, neutrophilia	Chemokine	69–79 dimers
IL-9	Proliferation	Cell lines, Bone marrow	Hodgkin's disease, large cell lymphomas	Hematopoietin	125, monomer
IL-10	Proliferation Decrease IFN-γ synthesis	Cell lines, mast cells Activated T-cells	Burkett's lymphoma	Unassigned	160, homodimer
IL-11	Proliferation Synergy with IL-3	Cell lines, plasmacytoma Bone marrow colony	Megakaryocytic leukemia	Hematopoietin	178, monomer
IL-12	Proliferation Increase IFN-γ	Mitogen activated T-cells T/NK cells	Leukemia	Unassigned	197 and 306 Heterodimer
IL-13	Proliferation	Cell lines (B-cell)	Leukemia Inflammation	Hematopoietin	132 monomer
IL-15	Proliferation	IL15 reactive cell lines	Leukemia	Hematopoietin	
Stem cell factor	Synergise with CSFs and cytokines	Progenitor bone marrow cells colony formation	Leukemia	Hematopoietin	
Erythropoiten	Red cell colony production	Bone marrow colonies	Polycythemia	Hematopoietin	monomer
G-CSF	Proliferation	BM colonies, cell lines	Chronic neutropenia, leukemia	Hematopoietin	174, monomer

(continued)

TABLE. HUMAN CYTOKINES (CONTINUED)

Cytokine	Bases of Assay	Cell/Assay System	Disease Association	Family	Size & Form
	Enhance superoxide	Neutrophils			
GM-CSF	Granulocyte colonies Neutrophil activation	BM colonies Neutrophils	Myelodysplasia, leukemia, osteosarcoma	Hematopoietin	127, monomer
M-CSF	Macrophage colonies IFN, TNF, G-CSF IL-1	BM colonies Macrophage synthesis	Leukemia	Hematopoietin	
TNFα/β	Increase MHCI, adhesion Cytotoxicity	Endothelial cells Fibroblast cell lines	Cachexia, RA, lymphomas, inflammation, infections, septic shock, multiple sclerosis	TNF Family	157–171, trimers
IFNα/β/γ	Increase MHCI/II Anti-viral effect Anti-proliferative	Different cell types Virus infected cell lines Tumor cell lines	SLE, Sjögren's, DTH, autoimmunity, etc.	Interferon	143–166, monomers
LIF	Proliferation Synergize with IL-3	Murine lymphoma lines BM colony assay	Cachexia, pancreatitis, osteoporosis	Hematopoietin	179, monomer
TGFβ	Inhibition of proliferation, Inhibition of CSF Chemotaxis	Fibroblast cell line BM colony assay Monocytes	RA, breast carcinoma, fibrosis	Unassigned	112, homo- & heteropolymers
MCP-1	Chemotaxis	Monocytes	Inflammation, atherosclerosis, cancer	Chemokine	76, monomer (?)
MIP-1α	Stem cell inhibition	BM colony assay	Immunosuppression, myleocytic leukemia	Chemokine	66, monomer (?)
MIP-1β	Chemotaxis	Neutrophils	Inflammation	Chemokine	
MIP-2	Neutrophil activation	Neutrophils	Inflammation	Chemokine	66, monomer (?)
MIF	Macrophage migration inhibition	Macrophages	Inflammation	Chemokine	115, monomer
RANTES	Chemotaxis	Monocytes	RA, inflammation, cancer	Chemokine	66, monomer

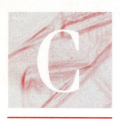

Appendix C:
Cluster of Differentation (CD) Molecules

Updated information on CD molecules is available through: Shaw, S. LEUKOCYTE DIFFERENTIATION ANTIGEN DATABASE. Available from Stephen Shaw, NIH, on disk: NIH ftp site (balrog.nci.nih.gov), Bethesda, 1995. See also: Shaw, S. Leukocyte Differentation Antigens: How to keep up with the litany of CD antigens. Human Immunol, 41:103-104, 1994.

CD Designation	Other Names	Molecular Structure	Cellular Expression	Family	Functions	Tumor Expressions
CD1 (a, b, c)	T6	43–49 kD; β_2 microglobulin-associated	Thymocytes, dendritic cells (incl. Langerhans cells)	Ig superfamily (IgSF)	? Ligand for some $\gamma\delta$ T cells	Langerhans cell histiocytosis
CD2	T11; LFA-2; sheep red blood cell receptor	50 kD	T cells, NK cells	Ig superfamily	Adhesion molecule (binds LFA-3); T cell activation	T-cell malignancies
CD3	T3; Leu-4	Composed of five chains	T cells	Ig superfamily	Signal transduction as a result of antigen recognition by T cells	T-cell malignancies
CD4	T4; Leu-3; L3T4 (mice)	55 kD	Class II MCH-restricted T cells	Ig superfamily	Adhesion molecule (binds to class II MHC); signal transduction	T-cell malignancies
CD5	T1; Lyt1	67 kD	T cells; B cell subset	Ig superfamily	?	T- and B-cell malignancies
CD6	T12	100 kD	Subset of T cells; some B cells	Scavenger receptor	?	T-cell malignancies
CD7	Leu-9	40 kD	Subset of T cells Hematopoietic precursors	Scavenger receptor	?	T-cell malignancies
CD8	T8; Leu-2; Lyt2	Composed of two 34 kD chains; expressed as $\alpha\alpha$ or $\alpha\beta$ dimer	Class I MHC-restricted T cells	Ig superfamily	Adhesion (binds to class I MHC); signal transduction	T-cell malignancies/LG L leukemia
CD9	BA-2, J-2	24 kD	Pre-B and immature B cells; monocytes, platelets	Ig superfamily	? Role in platelet activation	
CD10	CALLA	100 kD	Immature and some mature B cells; lymphoid progenitors, granulocytes	Tetraspanning membrane protein	Neural endopeptidase (enkephalinase)	ALLs, lymphomas
CD11a	LFA-1 α chain	180 kD; associates with CD18 to form LFA-1 integrin	Leukocytes		Adhesion (binds to ICAM-1)	
CD11b	Mac-1; CR3 (iCR3 (iC3B receptor) α chain Leu-15	165 kD; associates with CD18 to form Mac-1 integrin	Granulocytes, monocytes, NK cells		Adhesion; phagocytosis of iC3b-coated (opsonized) particles	NGL (NK) leukemia

CD Designation	Other Names	Molecular Structure	Cellular Expression	Family	Functions	Tumor Expressions
CD11c	p150, 95; CR4 α chain Leu M5	150 kD; associated with CD18 to form p150, 95 integrin	Monocytes, granulocytes, NK cells		Adhesion; ? phagocytosis of iC3b-coated (opsonized) particles	HCL, histiocytic tumors
CDw12§	—	? 90–120 kD			?	
CD13	My-7	150 kD	Monocytes, granulocytes Monocytes, granulocytes		Aminopeptidase; ? role in oxidative burst	AMLs
CD14	Leu M3, Mo2	55 kD; PI-linked	Monocytes		? Role in oxidative burst	AML (M4 and 5)
CD15	Leu M1	Carbohydrate epitope	Granulocytes		?	AMLs, Hodgkin's disease
CD16	FcRIII Leu II	50–70 kD; PI-linked and trans-membrane	NK cells, granulocytes, macrophages	Ig superfamily	Low-affinity Fcγ receptor; ADCC, activation of NK cells	LGL leukemia
CDw17	T5A7	Carbohydrate epitope (lactosyl-ceramide)	Granulocytes, macrophages, platelets		?	
CD18	β chain of LFA-1 family (β2 integrins	95 kD; noncovalently linked to CD11a, CD11b, or CD11c	Leukocytes		See CD11a, CD11b, CD11c	
CD19	Leu 12, B4	90 kD	Most B cells	Ig superfamily	? Role in B-cell activation or regulation	Lymphoid malignancies
CD20	Leu 16, B1	Heterodimer: 35- and 37-kD chains	Most of all B cells	Tetraspanning membrane protein	? Role in B-cell activation or regulation	Lymphoid malignancies
CD21	CR2; C3d receptor	145 kD	Mature B cells	Complement control protein (CCP) superfamily	Receptor for C3d, Epstein-Barr virus; ? role in B cell activation	Lymphoid malignancies
CD22	Leu 14	135 kD	B cells	Ig superfamily	?	Lymphoid malignancies
CD23	FcεRIIb	45–50 kD	Activated B cells, macrophages	C-type lectin	Low-affinity FcE receptor, induced by IL-4; function unknown	Lymphoid malignancies

CD	Common name	Molecular structure	Cellular expression	Family	Function	Disease association
CD24	BA-1	Heterodimer of 38 and 41 kD chains	B cells, granulocytes		?	
CD25	TAC; p55; low-affinity IL-2 receptor	55 kD	Activated T and B cells; activated macrophages	Complement control protein superfamily	complexes with p70 to form high-affinity IL-2 receptor; T cell growth	Lymphoid malignancies
CD26	—	120 kD	Activated T and B cells; macrophages		Serine peptidase, function unknown	T-cell tumors, HCL
CD27	—	Homodimer of 55 kD chains	Most T cells; ? some plasma cells	NGF receptor superfamily	? Role in B cell growth	
CD28	Tp44	Homodimer of 44 kD chains	T cells (most CD4+, some CD8+ cells)	Ig superfamily	? T cell receptor for costimulator molecule(s)	
CD29	β chain of VLA antigens (β1 integrins)	130 kD; noncovalently associated with VLA α chains (CD249)	Broad		Adhesion to extracellular matrix proteins, cell-cell adhesion (see CD249)	
CD30	Ki-1	105 kD	Activated T and B cells; Reed-Sternberg cells in Hodgkin's disease	NGF receptor superfamily	?	Lymphoma, Hodgkin's disease
CD31	Platelet gp11a	140 kD	Platelets; monocytes, granulocytes, B cells, endothelial cells	Ig superfamily	?	
CDw32	FcRII	~40 kD	Macrophages, granulocytes, B cells, eosinophils	Ig superfamily	?	
CD33	My 9	67 kD	Monocytes, myeloid progenitor cells	Ig superfamily	?	AMLs
CD34	MY 10	105–120 kD	Precursors of hematopoietic cells		?	Acute leukemias
CD35	CR1; C3b receptor	Polymorphic; four forms are 190–280 kD	Granulocytes, monocytes, erythrocytes, B cells	Complement control protein superfamily	Binding and phagocytosis of C3b-coated particles and immune complexes	
CD36	Platelet gpIIIb	90 kD	Monocytes, platelets		? Platelet adhesion	
CD37	—	Composed of 2 or 3 40–52 kD chains	B cells, some T cells	Tetraspanning membrane protein	?	

CD Designation	Other Names	Molecular Structure	Cellular Expression	Family	Functions	Tumor Expressions
CD38	T10, Leu 17	45 kD	Plasma cells, thymocytes, activated T cells		?	Multiple myeloma
CD39	—	70–100 kD	Mature B cells		?	
CD40	—	Heterodimer of 44 and 48 kD chains	B cells	NGF receptor superfamily	? Role in B cell growth, memory cell generation	
CD41	gpIIb/IIIa complex (gPIIIa is CD61)	Complex of gpIIb heterodimer (120 and 23 kD) and gpIIIa (CD61)	Platelets	TNF-like	Platelet aggregation and activation: receptor for fibrinogen, fibronectin (binds to R-G-D sequence)	AML (M7)
CD42a	Platelet gpIX	23 kD; forms complex with CD42b	Platelets, megakaryocytes		Platelet adhesion, binding to von Willeband factor	
CD42b	Platelet gpIb	Dimer of 135 and 25 kD chains, forms complex with CD42a	See CD42a		See CD42a	AML (M7)
CD43	Sialophorin	95 kD, highly sialylated	Leukocytes (except circulating B cells)		? Role in T cell activation	
CD44	Pgp-1: Hermes	88 → 100 kD, highly glycosylated	Leukocytes, erythrocytes		May function as homing receptor receptor for matrix components (e.g., hyaluronate)	
CD45	T200; leukocyte common antigen	Four isoforms, 180–220 kD	Leukocytes		? Role in signal transduction (tyrosine phosphatase)	Lymphomas
CD45R	Restricted forms of CD45 Leu 18 My 11	CD45RO: 180 kD CD45RA: 220 kD CD45RB: 190, 205 and 220 kD isoforms	CD45RO: memory T cells CD45RA: naive T cells CD45RB: B cells; subset of T cells		See CD45	
CD46	Membrane cofactor protein (MDP)	45–70 kD	Leukocytes; epithelial cells, fibroblasts	Complement control protein superfamily	Regulation of complement activation	

CD	Alternative name	Molecular characteristics	Cellular expression	Family	Function
CD47	—	47–52 kD	Broad	Ig superfamily	?
CD48	—	41 kD; PI-linked	Leukocytes		?
CDw49a	VLA α1 chain	210 kD; associates with CD29 to form VLA-1 (β1 integrin)	T cells, monocytes		Adhesion to collagen, laminin
CDw49b	VLA α2 chain; platelet gpla	170 kD; associates with CD29 to form VLA-2 (β1 integrin)	Platelets, activated T cells, monocytes, some B cells		Adhesion to extracellular matrix: receptor for collagen
CDw49c	VLA α3 chain	Dimer of 130 and 25 kD; associates with CD29 to form VLA-3 (β1 integrin)	T cells; some B cells, monocytes		Adhesion to fibronectin, laminin
CDw49d	VLA α4 chain	150 kD; associates with CD29 to form VLA-4 (β1 integrin)	T cells, monocytes, B cells		Peyer's patch homing receptor, binds to VCAM-1; adhesion to fibronectin
CDw49e	VLA α5 chain	Dimer of 135 and 25 kD; associates with CD29 to form VLA-5 (β1 integrin)	T cells; few B cells and monocytes		Adhesion to fibronectin
CDw49f	VLA α6 chain	150 kD; associates with CD29 to form VLA-6 (β1 antigrin)	Platelets, megakaryocytes; activated T cells		Adhesion to extracellular matrix: receptor for laminin
CDw50	—	108–140 kD; ?PI-linked	Leukocytes		?
CD51	α chain of vitronectin receptor	140 kD heterodimer, associates with CD61	Platelets		Adhesion: receptor for vitronectin, fibrinogen, von Willebrand factor (binds R-G-D sequence)
CDw52	—	? 21–28 kD	Leukocytes		?
CD53	—	32–40 kD	Leukocytes, plasma cells	Tetraspanning membrane protein	?
CD54	ICAM-1	80–114 kD	Broad; many activated cells (cytokine-inducible)	Ig superfamily	Adhesion: ligand for LFA-1

CD Designation	Other Names	Molecular Structure	Cellular Expression	Family	Functions	Tumor Expressions
CD55	Decay accelerating factor (DAF)	70 kD; PI-linked	Broad	Complement control protein superfamily	Regulation of complement activation	
CD56	Leu-19	Heterodimer of 135 and 220 kD chains	NK cells	Ig superfamily	Homotypic adhesion; isoform of neural cell adhesion molecule (N-CAM)	LGL leukemia
CD57	HNK-1, Leu-7	110 kD	NK cells, subset of T cells		?	LGL leukemia
CD58	LFA-3	55–70 kD; PI-linked	Broad	Ig superfamily	Adhesion: ligand for CD2	
CD59	Membrane inhibitor of reactive lysis (MIRL)	18–20 kD; PI-linked	Broad		Regulation of complement (MAC) action	
CDw60	—	Carbohydrate epitope	Subset of T cells, platelets		?	
CD61	β chain of vitronectin receptor (β3 integrin); gpIIIa	110 kD; associates with CD51 (α chain of vitronectin receptor)	Platelets, megakaryocytes		See CD51	
D62	GMP-140	140 kD; platelet granule protein that is translocated to cell surface upon activation	Platelets, endothelial cells		Neutrophil and monocyte adhesion to endothelium, platelets	
CD63	—	53 kD; present in platelet lysosomes, translocated to cell surface upon activation	Activated platelets; monocytes, macrophages		?	
CD64	FcRI	75 kD	Monocytes, macrophages		High-affinity Fcγ receptor: role in phagocytosis, ADCC, macrophage activation	
CDw65	—	Carbohydrate epitope	Granulocytes		? Role in neutrophil activation	

CD	Other names	Molecular structure	Cellular expression	Family	Function	Disease association
CD66	—	180–200 kD phosphorylated glycoprotein	Granulocytes		?	
CD67	—	100 kD; PI-linked	Granulocytes		?	
CD68	KP 1	100 kD intracellular protein, weak surface expression	Monocytes, macrophages		?	Histiocytic lesions
CD69	—	Homodimer of 28–34 kD chains, phosphorylated glycoprotein	Activated T and B cells, macrophages, NK cells		?	
CDw70	KI 24	?	Activated T and B cells		?	Lymphoid malignancies
CD71	T9; transferrin receptor	95-kD homodimer	Activated T and B cells, macrophages, proliferating cells		Receptor for transferrin: role in iron metabolism, cell growth	
CD72	Lyb-2	42 homodimer	B cells	C-type lectin	Unknown, ligand for CD5	Lymphoid malignancies
CD73		69	B-cell subsets, T-cell subsets		Ecto-5'-nucleotidase, dephosphorylates nucleotides to allow nucleoside uptake	
CD74	li, lγ	33, 35, 41, 43 (alternative initiation and splicing)	B cells, macrophages, monocytes, MHC class II positive cells		MHC class II-associated invariant chain	
CDw75	LN-1		Mature B cells, T-cell subsets		Unknown, possibly oligosaccharide, dependent on sialylation	Lymphoid malignancies
CDw76			Mature B cells, T-cell subsets		Unknown, possible oligosaccharide, dependent on sialylation	
CD77	Globotriaocyl-ceramide (Gb$_3$), p^k blood group		Germinal center B cells		Unkonwn	

CD Designation	Other Names	Molecular Structure	Cellular Expression	Family	Functions	Tumor Expressions
CDw78	Ba		B cells		Unknown	
CD79α, β	Igα, Igβ	α: 32–33 β: 37–39	B cells	Ig superfamily	Components of B-cell antigen receptor analogous to CD3, required for cell-surface expression and signal transduction	
CD80	B7 (now B7.1), BB1	60	B-cell subset	Ig superfamily	Co-stimulator, ligand for CD28 and CTLA-4	
CD81	Target of antiproliferative antibody (TAPA-1)	26	Lymphocytes	Tetraspanning membrane protein	Associates with CD19, CD21 to form B cell co-receptor	
CD82	R2	50–53	Leukocytes	Tetraspanning membrane protein	Unknown	
CD83	HB15	43	Activated B cells, activated T cells, circulating dendritic cells (veil cells)		Unknown	
CDw84	GR6	73	Monocytes, platelets, circulating B cells		Unknown	
CD85	GR4	120, 83	Monocytes, circulating B cells		Unknown	
CD86	FUN-1, GR65	80	Monocytes, activated B cells		Unknown	
CD87	UPA-R	50–65	Granulocytes, monocytes, macrophages, activated T cells		Urokinase plasminogen activator receptor	
CD88	C5aR	40	Polymorphonuclear leukocytes, macrophages, mast cells	Rhodopsin superfamily	Receptor for complement component C5a	
CD89	FcαR	50–70	Monocytes, macrophages, granulocytes, neutrophils, B-cell subsets, T-cell subsets	Ig superfamily	IgA receptor	

CD	Other names	MW (kDa)	Cellular expression	Family	Function/ligand
CDw90	Thy-1	18	CD34$^+$ prothymocytes (human) thymocytes, T cells (mouse)	Ig superfamily	Unknown
CD91		600	Monocytes		$\alpha_2$macroglobulin receptor
CDw92	GR9	70	Neutrophils, monocytes, platelets, endothelium		Unknown
CD93	GR11	120	Neutrophils, monocytes, endothelium		Unknown
CD94	KP43	43	T-cell subsets, natural killer cells		Unknown
CD95	Apo-1, Fas	43	Wide variety of cell lines, in vivo distribution uncertain	NGF receptor superfamily	Binds TNF-like Fas ligand, iduces apoptosis
CD96	T-cell activation increased late expression (TACTILE)	160	Activated T cells		Unknown
CD97	GR1	74, 80, 90	Activated cells		Unknown
CD98	4F2	80, 40 heterodimer	T cells, B cells, natural killer cells, granulocytes, all human cell lines		Unknown
CD99	MIC2, E2	32	Peripheral blood lymphocytes, thymocytes		Unknown
CD100	GR3	150	Broad expression on hematopoietic cells		Unknown
CDw101	BPC#4	140	Granulocytes, macrophages		Unknown
CD102	ICAM-2	55–65	Resting lymphocytes, monocytes, vascular endothelial cells (strongest)	Ig superfamily	Binds CD11a/CD18 (LFA-1) but not CD11b/CD18 (Mac-1)
CD103	HML-1, α_6, α_E integrin	150–25	Intraepithelial lymphocytes, 2–6%, peripheral blood lymphocytes		α_E integrin
CD104	β_4 integrin chain, β_4	220	Epithelia, Schwann cells, some tumor cells		β_4 integrin
CD105	Endoglin	95 homodimer	Endothelial cells, bone marrow cell subset, in vitro activated macrophages		Unknown, possibly ligand for an integrin

CD Designation	Other Names	Molecular Structure	Cellular Expression	Family	Functions	Tumor Expressions
CD106	VCAM-1	100, 110	Endothelial cells	Ig superfamily	Adhesion molecule, ligand for VLA-4	
CD107a	Lysosomal associated membrane protein-1 (LAMP-1)	110	Activated platelets		Unknown, is lysosomal membrane protein translocated to the cell surface after activation	
CD107b	LAMP-2	120	Activated platelets		Unknown, is lysosomal membrane protein translocated to the cell surface after activation	
CDw108	GR2	80	Activated T cells in spleen, some stromal cells		Unknown	
CDw109	Platelet activation factor, GR56		Not yet assigned			
CD110–CD114						
CD115	M-CSFR, c-fms	150	Monocytes, macrophages	Ig superfamily	Macrophage colony stimulating factor (M-CSF) receptor	
CDw116	GM-CSFRα	70–85	Monocytes, neutrophils, eosinophils, endothelium	Cytokine receptor superfamily	Granulocyte macrophage colony stimulating factor (GM-CSF) receptor α chain	
CD117	c-kit	145	Hematopoietic progenitors	Ig superfamily, tyrosine kinase	Stem cell factor (SCF) receptor	
CD118	IFN-α, βR		Broad cellular expression		Interferon-βR	
CD119	IFN-γR	90–100	Macrophages, monocytes, B cells, endothelium		Interferon-γ receptor	
CD120a	TNFR-I	50–60	Hematopoietic and non-hematopoietic cells, highest on epithelial cells	NFG receptor superfamily	TNF receptor, binds both TNF-α and TNF-β	

CD	Name	MW (kDa)	Cellular expression	Family	Function
CD120b	TNFR-II	75–85	Hematopoietic and non-hematopoietic cells, highest on myeloid cells	NFG receptor superfamily	TNF receptor, binds both TNF-α and TNF-β
CDw121a	IL-1R type I	80	Thymocytes, T cells	Ig superfamily	Type I interleukin-1 receptor, binds IL-1α and IL-1β
CDw121b	IL-1R type II	60–70	B cells, macrophages, monocytes	Ig superfamily	Type II interleukin-1 receptor, binds 1L-1α and IL-1β
CD122	IL-2Rβ	75	Natural killer cells, resting T-cell subpopulation, some B-cell lines		IL-2 receptor β chain
CD123	IL-3Rα	70	Bone marrow stem cells, granulocytes, monocytes, megakaryocytes	Cytokine receptor superfamily, fibronectin type III superfamily	IL-4 receptor
CD124	IL-4R	130–150	Mature B and T cells, hematopoietic precursor cells	Cytokine receptor superfamily, fibronectin type III superfamily	IL-4 receptor
CD125	IL-5Rα	55–60	Eosinophils, basophils	Cytokine receptor superfamily, fibronectin type III superfamily	IL-5 receptor α chain
CD126	IL-6Rα	80	Activated B cells and plasma cells (strong), most leukocytes (weak)	Ig superfamily, cytokine receptor superfamily, fibronectin type III superfamily	IL-6 receptor α subunit

CD Designation	Other Names	Molecular Structure	Cellular Expression	Family	Functions	Tumor Expressions
CDw127	IL-7R	68–79, possibly forms homodimers	Bone marrow lymphoid precursors, pro-B cells, mature T cells, monocytes	Fibronectin type III superfamily	IL-7 receptor	
CDw128	IL-8R	58–67	Neutrophils, basophils, T-cell subset	Rhodopsin superfamily	IL-8 receptor	
CD129			Not yet assigned			
CDw130	IL-6Rβ, IL-IIRβ, OSMRβ, LIFRβ	130	Activated B cells and plasma cells (strong), most leukocytes (weak), endothelial cells	Ig superfamily, Cytokine receptor superfamily, fibronectin type III superfamily		

Index

HIV infection (*cont.*)
  pathology and clinical staging,
      881–883
  stages, 871t
  therapy, 883–885, 884t
  transmission, 868–871, 869f
  vaccination, 885–892, 889f
HLA, 150–152
  class I antigens, 152f, 153t
  class II antigens, 152f, 154t
  inheritance within family, 155f
HLA-A2, peptide-binding groove, 157f
HLA-B8, Sjogren's syndrome and, 575
HLA-B27
  ankylosing spondylitis and, 539
  autoimmune disease and, 161
  binding groove, peptides eluted, 159f,
      160f
  inflammatory bowel disease and, 539
  spondylarthropathies associated,
      562–564, 563f
HLA-CW6, psoriasis and, 521
HLA-DR1, rheumatoid arthritis and, 562
HLA-DR3, Sjogren's syndrome and,
      575–576
HLA-DR4, rheumatoid arthritis and, 562
HLA testing, graft survival and, 593–594
HNP. *See* Human neutrophil protein
Hodgkin's disease, 654–657
  cell types, 656f
  cellular origin, 656–657
  histopathologic classification, 654–656,
      655t
  lymphocytopenia and, 806
  Reed-Sternberg cells, 655–656, 655f
  staging, 657, 658f
  treatment, 657
Holotoxoid, 747
Homing-associated cell adhesion
      molecule (H-CAM), 266
Homocytophilic, 392
Homograft rejection, 347
Homologous restriction factor (HRF),
      complement activation and, 237
Hormone receptors, structural/functional
      similarities with antibodies and
      enzymes, 319–320, 320f
Host-tumor relationship, 901–907
  terminology, 909t
HRF. *See* Homologous restriction factor
HSF. *See* Hepatocyte-stimulating factor
HSPG. *See* Heparan sulfate proteoglycan
HSV. *See* Herpes simplex virus
HTLV-1. *See* Human T-lymphotropic
      virus-1
Human antimouse antibody (HAMA), 134
Human chorionic gonadotropin (hCG)
  antibodies and, 308–309
  fertility and, 767
  germ cell tumors and, 940t
Human chromosome 6, MHC genes, 151f
Human growth hormone (hGH), epitopes,
      302–303
Human immunodeficiency virus (HIV),
      697–698, 861–867. *See also*
      HIV infection
  activation in stimulated lymphocytes,
      876f
  evasion of immune defenses, 712
  genome, 863–864, 863f
  life cycle, 865–867
  M cells and, 65

monoclonal antibodies and, 734
mutation and, 200–201
replication and gene expression,
      864–865, 866f
transmission, 868–871, 869f
Human neutrophil protein (HNP), 225
Human T-lymphotropic virus-1 (HTLV-1),
      861–862, 913
  adult T-cell leukemia/lymphoma and,
      653
  chronic fatigue syndrome and, 807
  encephalitis and, 699
  rheumatoid arthritis and, 560
Humoral antibody, 733–735
  bacterial infection and, 674
  graft facilitation and, 590
  tissue allograft rejection and, 439
  tumor cell killing and, 917
Humoral immunity, 6, 6t
  clinical tests, 970t
HUS. *See* Hemolytic-uremic syndrome
Hybridoma, 96
Hybrid resistance, bone marrow
      transplantation and, 612
Hydralazine
  autoimmune diseases induced, 504t
  systemic lupus erythematosus and, 573
Hydrocortisone, immune response and,
      840t
Hydroxychloroquine
  rheumatoid arthritis and, 561
  systemic lupus erythematosus and,
      573–574
Hydroxyurea
  allergic reactions, 502t
  immune response and, 840t
  mechanism of action, 803t
Hypercatabolic dysgammaglobulinemia,
      794–795
Hypercatabolic hypoproteinemia, familial,
      795
Hyperemia, inflammation and, 206
Hyperglobulinemia, adjuvant injection
      and, 826
Hyper-IgE syndrome, 794
Hyper-IgM syndrome, 192–194, 794
Hyperimmunoglobulin-IgE, 416
Hypersensitivity, 16, 290
  anaphylactic, chemical mediators, 214
  atopic, chemical mediators, 214
  basophil, cutaneous, 449–451
  delayed. *See* Delayed hypersensitivity
  granulomatous, infectious agents and,
      703
  granulomatous reactions, 464f, 466
  tuberculin-type, 446
Hypersensitivity pneumonitis, 477–478
Hypersensitivity vasculitis, vessels/sites
      involved, 377t
Hyperthyroidism
  antibodies to thyroid-stimulating
      hormone receptors and, 308
  long-acting thyroid stimulator and, 310
  pretibial myxedema and, 509–510
Hypocomplementemic
      glomerulonephritis, 369
Hypocomplementemic vasculitic urticarial
      syndrome, 375, 519
Hypogammaglobulinemia of infancy, 782
  phenotypic expression, 793t
Hypogammaglobulinemia with partial
      albinism, 789

Hypoproteinemia, hypercatabolic,
      familial, 795
Hyposensitization
  atopic allergy and, 413–415
  specific immunosuppression and, 838
Hypothyroidism
  antibodies and, 307–308
  autoimmune response and, 310
Hypoxanthine guanine
      phosphoribosyltransferase
      deficiency, 790t

IBD. *See* Inflammatory bowel disease
ICAM. *See* Intracellular adhesion
      molecule
ICL. *See* Idiopathic CD4+
      lymphocytopenia
IDDM. *See* Insulin-dependent diabetes
      mellitus
Idiopathic cardiomyopathy, 541
Idiopathic CD4+ lymphocytopenia (ICL),
      796–797
Idiopathic granulomatous hepatitis, 481
Idiopathic thrombocytopenic purpura
      (ITP), 345
  immunosuppressive drugs and, 855t
  intravenous immunogloblin and, 733
Idiotope, 106–107, 107f
Idiotype vaccine, 745–746
  cancer and, 959
IgA
  abundance in serum, 104
  celiac disease and, 513–514
  dermatitis herpetiformis and, 513
  properties, 103t
  secretion by intestinal epithelial cells,
      66f
IgA deficiency, phenotypic expression,
      793t
IgA nephritis, 369–370
IgA nephropathy, 374–375t
IgD
  abundance in serum, 103–1–4
  properties, 103t
IgE
  abundance in serum, 104
  allergic sensitization and, 388
  atopic allergy and, 416
  atopic/anaphylactic reactions and,
      420–422
  high-affinity receptors, 214
  properties, 103t
  radioimmunoabsorbent test and, 394
IgE antibody, 390–391
IGF. *See* Insulinlike growth factor
IgG, 97–99
  abundance in serum, 104–105
  cytotoxic/cytolytic reactions and,
      328–330
  malaria and, 685
  properties, 103t
  proteases cleaving, 98f
  rheumatoid factor and, 556–557
  structure, 100f
  subclasses, biologic properties, 97t
  warm antibody disease and, 338
IgM
  abundance in serum, 101–103
  cold antibody disease and, 339
  cytotoxic/cytolytic reactions and,
      328–330